Message from the Secretary

Healthy People 2010 provides our Nation with the wide range of public health opportunities that exist in the first decade of the 21st century. With 467 objectives in 28 focus areas, Healthy People 2010 will be a tremendously valuable asset to health planners, medical practitioners, educators, elected officials, and all of us who work to improve health. Healthy People 2010 reflects the very best in public health planning—it is comprehensive, it was created by a broad coalition of experts from many sectors, it has been designed to measure progress over time, and, most important, it clearly lays out a series of objectives to bring better health to all people in this country.

Achieving the vision of "Healthy People in Healthy Communities" represents an opportunity for individuals to make healthy lifestyle choices for themselves and their families. It challenges clinicians to put prevention into their practices. It requires communities and businesses to support health-promoting policies in schools, worksites, and other settings. It calls for scientists to pursue new research. Above all, it demands that all of us work together, using both traditional and innovative approaches, to help the American public achieve the 10-year targets defined by Healthy People 2010.

The 20th century brought remarkable and unprecedented improvements in the lives of the people of the United States. We saw the infant mortality rate plummet and life expectancy increase by 30 years. While we recognize that most of the advances came from prevention efforts, we also saw almost unimaginable improvements in medical technologies and health care. The challenge for the 21st century is twofold. First, we must ensure that this rate of advancement continues unabated. Second, we must make certain that all Americans benefit from advancements in quality of life, regardless of their age, race, ethnicity, gender, sexual orientation, disability status, income, educational level, or geographic location. These challenges are substantial, but with the objectives defined by Healthy People 2010, they are achievable.

I wholeheartedly commend Healthy People 2010, and I challenge all of us to work together to achieve its ambitious and important vision.

Donna E. Shalala
Secretary of Health and Human Services

Foreword

We have witnessed a great deal of progress in public health and medicine since our Nation first embarked on the national planning process for the Healthy People initiative. The process began in 1979 with *Healthy People: The Surgeon General's Report on Health Promotion and Disease Prevention*, which was followed in 1990 by *Healthy People 2000*. Healthy People 2010 represents the third time that the U.S. Department of Health and Human Services (HHS) has developed 10-year health objectives for the Nation.

Healthy People 2010 reflects the scientific advances that have taken place over the past 20 years in preventive medicine, disease surveillance, vaccine and therapeutic development, and information technology. It also mirrors the changing demographics of our country, the changes that have taken place in health care, and the growing impact of global forces on our national health status.

Healthy People 2010 incorporates input from a broad cross-section of people. Scientific experts from many Federal agencies took the lead in developing the focus areas and objectives. The Secretary's Council on National Health Promotion and Disease Prevention Objectives for 2010 and the Healthy People Steering Committee provided guidance to steer the process. The HHS Office of Public Health and Science, particularly the Office of Disease Prevention and Health Promotion, expertly managed the process. But perhaps most important to the success of this effort was the overwhelming and enthusiastic contribution made by the Healthy People Consortium and the public. We received more than 11,000 comments from people in every State by fax, Internet, letter, and in person through several public meetings.

The knowledge, commitment, and collaboration of these groups have combined to produce national health objectives that are even more comprehensive than their predecessors. There are 467 objectives in 28 focus areas, making Healthy People 2010 an encyclopedic compilation of health improvement opportunities for the next decade. Building on two decades of success in Healthy People initiatives, Healthy People 2010 is poised to address the concerns of the 21st century. Two major goals reflect the Nation's changing demographics. The first goal, which addresses the fact that we are growing older as a Nation, is to increase the quality and years of healthy life. The second goal, which addresses the diversity of our population, is to eliminate health disparities.

And, for the first time, a set of Leading Health Indicators will help individuals and communities target the actions to improve health. The Leading Health Indicators also will help communities track the success of these actions.

I sincerely appreciate the number of people, institutions, and organizations that have worked together to create this important document. But our journey has just begun. I encourage you to stay the course as we pursue the vision of Healthy People 2010 to create tomorrow's healthier people today.

David Satcher, M.D., Ph.D.
Assistant Secretary for Health and
Surgeon General

Contents

Healthy People 2010, Volume II

Healthy People 2010: Objectives for Improving Health (Part B)

Reader's Guide

This edition of Healthy People 2010 supersedes the January 2000 conference edition. Readers should review objectives of particular interest for editorial differences and the addition of new data. While most objectives are unchanged, some have been reworded. Updates to baselines and population group data tables may have resulted in revisions to the targets. In addition, a few developmental objectives are now measurable. Data included in this edition are as of June 1, 2000.

Healthy People 2010 will be updated on the Internet. Data for objectives are expected to be updated on an ongoing basis on the Centers for Disease Control and Prevention (CDC), National Center for Health Statistics (NCHS) Web site at http://www.cdc.gov/nchs/hphome.htm. Significant updates to the document will be posted on the Healthy People Web site at http://www.health.gov/healthypeople.

This document is in two sections:

- Understanding and Improving Health
- Objectives for Improving Health

Understanding and Improving Health

The first section explains the history of Healthy People 2010 and the overall Healthy People initiative, the model on which Healthy People is based, and how to use Healthy People as a systematic approach to health improvement, and the Leading Health Indicators (LHIs). It is also available as a separate publication (*Healthy People 2010: Understanding and Improving Health*).

Leading Health Indicators

To provide a snapshot of the health of the Nation, Healthy People 2010 identifies 10 Leading Health Indicators. The LHIs highlight major health priorities for the Nation and include the individual behaviors, physical and social environmental factors, and health system issues that affect the health of individuals and communities. Each of the 10 LHIs has one or more Healthy People measures associated with it. The selected objectives will be used to measure progress throughout the decade. (For a full discussion of the LHIs and the specific objectives, see Understanding and Improving Health.)

Leading Health Indicators	
Physical activity	Mental health
Overweight and obesity	Injury and violence
Tobacco use	Environmental quality
Substance abuse	Immunization
Responsible sexual behavior	Access to health care

Objectives for Improving Health

The second section provides detailed information on the 28 focus areas of Healthy People 2010. The focus area chapters were developed by work groups with experts in the subject area as well as through extensive public input. (See Appendices E and F for a list of work group coordinators and members, respectively.)

The focus area chapters are presented in alphabetical order. Each chapter contains the following sections:

Lead Agency

Each focus area is managed by a designated lead agency or co-lead agencies of the U.S. Department of Health and Human Services (HHS). These lead agencies have expertise in and responsibility for their respective focus areas. For two focus areas, the lead agency responsibilities are shared by other Federal Departments. The Disability and Secondary Conditions focus area is co-led by CDC and the U.S. Department of Education. The Food Safety focus area is co-led by the Food and Drug Administration and the Food Safety and Inspection Service of the U.S. Department of Agriculture. Lead agencies are responsible for undertaking activities to move the Nation toward achieving the year 2010 goals and for reporting progress on the focus area objectives over the course of the decade. (For contact information, see Appendix E. Healthy People 2010 Work Group Coordinators.)

Contents

This brief list details the specific organization of each chapter, including the descriptive headings for the types of objectives that are contained in the focus area.

Goal Statement

Each chapter contains a concise goal statement. This statement frames the overall purpose of the focus area.

Overview

The Overview provides the context and background for the objectives and identifies opportunities for prevention or interventions. The Overview addresses the following topics: nature of the issues; key trends or developments in the focus area; related costs and other pertinent information; relevant disparities among population groups (including race, ethnicity, gender, age, socioeconomic status, disability status, sexual orientation, and geographic location); and implications of such factors for prevention, other improvements, and promising research.

Interim Progress Toward Year 2000 Objectives

Because Healthy People 2010 builds on the experience of the preceding decade, this section provides a brief description of progress to date on year 2000 objectives pertaining to the focus area. A final report on the year 2000 objectives, *Healthy People 2000 Review*, will be published by NCHS, CDC.

Healthy People 2010 Objectives

This section begins with a restatement of the focus area goal and a list of short titles for all objectives in the focus area. In a majority of the focus areas, objectives are organized into sections with headings. These headings provide structure and appear in the list of short titles.

The objectives are designed to drive action. Therefore, each objective begins with a verb, followed by the subject.

Each objective is numbered for reference purposes (for example, 15-1, 15-2, etc.). Some objectives have multiple measures and are labeled sequentially with letters (for example, 15-1a, 15-1b, etc.). Numbering of objectives does not imply priority or importance. Explanatory text follows objectives as needed.

Types of Objectives

There are two types of objectives—measurable and developmental.

Measurable objectives. Measurable objectives provide direction for action. For measurable objectives, the current status is expressed with a national baseline. The baseline represents the starting point for moving the Nation toward the desired end. The baselines use valid and reliable data derived from currently established, nationally representative data systems. Some of these systems build on, or are comparable with, State and local data systems. However, State data are not a prerequisite to developing an objective. Non-national data may be used where national data are not available. These situations are noted in the baseline data for the objective. The data source for each measurable objective is identified. Baseline data provide the point from which a 2010 target is set. Where possible, objectives are measured with nationally representative data systems. (See *Tracking Healthy People 2010*, produced by NCHS, for an operational definition for each measurable objective.)

Developmental objectives. Developmental objectives provide a vision for a desired outcome or health status. Current national surveillance systems do not provide data on these subjects. The purpose of developmental objectives is to identify areas of emerging importance and to drive the development of data systems to measure them. Most developmental objectives have a potential data source with reasonable expectation of data points by the year 2004 to facilitate setting year 2010 targets in the mid-decade review. Developmental objectives with no baseline at the midcourse will be dropped.

Criteria for Developing Objectives

Criteria first published in *Developing Objectives for Healthy People 2010* in September 1997 call for objectives to be useful to national, State, and local agencies as well as to the private sector and the public. The objectives must have certain attributes, including the following:

- The result to be achieved should be **important and understandable** to a broad audience and relate to the two overarching Healthy People 2010 goals.

- Objectives should be **prevention oriented** and should address health improvements that can be achieved through population-based and health-service interventions.

- Objectives should **drive action** and suggest a set of interim steps that will achieve the proposed targets within the specified timeframe. Objectives should be **useful and relevant**. States, localities, and the private sector should be able to use the objectives to target efforts in schools, communities, worksites, health practices, and other settings.

- Objectives should be **measurable** and include a range of measures—health outcomes, behavioral and health-service interventions, and community capacity—directed toward improving health outcomes and quality of life. They should count assets and achievements and look to the positive.

- **Continuity** and **comparability** are important. Whenever possible, objectives should build on Healthy People 2000 and those goals and performance measures already established.

- Objectives must be supported by sound **scientific evidence.**

Population Group Data Table

Because eliminating health disparities is a goal of Healthy People 2010, a standard data table is used to display the baseline status of population groups for population-based objectives for which data are available. Generally, an objective is considered to be population based when its data source counts people. This table consists of a set of population variables that are to be considered a minimum breakout set for data collection. The minimum set includes race and ethnicity, gender, and measures of socioeconomic status. Within each category in the table, groups are alphabetized or shown by some gradient or level of achievement (such as educational or income levels). Depending on the parameters of the objective, some tables show more detailed or additional breakouts of population groups. In addition, some tables include population groups for which data are provided for informational purposes. In such cases, these population groups will not be tracked.

Sample Population-Based Table

NOTE: THE TABLE BELOW MAY CONTINUE TO THE FOLLOWING PAGE.

Population Group, year	Condition
	Measure
TOTAL	
Race and ethnicity	
American Indian or Alaska Native	
Asian or Pacific Islander	
Asian	
Native Hawaiian and other Pacific Islander	
Black or African American	
White	
Hispanic or Latino	
Not Hispanic or Latino	
Black or African American	
White	
Gender	
Female	
Male	
Family income level	
Poor	
Near poor	
Middle/high income	

Population Group, year	Condition
	Measure
Education level	
Less than high school	
High school graduate	
At least some college	
The following are additional categories included where appropriate.	
Geographic location	
Urban	
Rural	
Health insurance status	
Private health insurance	
Public health insurance	
Medicare	
Medicaid	
No health insurance	
Disability status	
Persons with disabilities or activity limitations	
Persons without disabilities or activity limitations	
Sexual orientation	
Select populations	
Age groups	
School grade levels	
Persons with select medical conditions	

DNA = Data have not been analyzed. DNC = Data are not collected. DSU = Data are statistically unreliable.
NA = Not applicable.

NOTE: THE TABLE ABOVE MAY HAVE CONTINUED FROM THE PREVIOUS PAGE.

Race and ethnicity. Following guidance issued by the Office of Management and Budget, Healthy People 2010 sets forth the current categories for reporting race and ethnicity. Federal data systems have until January 2003 to comply with these standards. "More than one race" will be displayed in this category when data are available. (See *Tracking Healthy People 2010* for further detail.)

Gender. In many instances, where the unique problem for each gender needs to be highlighted, data for all population groups in the table are presented for both genders.

Socioeconomic status (SES). SES is shown as income or education level breakouts or both. If income was selected, data are presented in three groups: poor, near poor, and middle/high income. In some objectives, programmatic data considerations may result in different income categories being displayed. If education was selected, data are presented in three groups: less than high school, high school graduate, and at least some college. (See *Tracking Healthy People 2010* for definitions of these categories.)

Age. Age is not included in the minimum table because showing inclusive age categories would add considerable complexity to the minimum set. Furthermore, age often is in the objective (for example, mammograms for women aged 40 years and over), and many objectives are relevant only for a subset of age groups. Age breakouts have been added to objectives where relevant and may not be inclusive of the total population. For example, data lines for elderly persons or children could be added to selected objectives without adding other groups. Age adjustment here is indicated for those objectives. (See *Tracking Healthy People 2010* for further explanation of age adjustment.)

Other Variables. Other population groups are shown in various objectives when scientific evidence shows that the group(s) may be at risk. Other population groups include urban/rural populations, health insurance status, persons with disabilities or activity limitations, and sexual orientation.

The following abbreviations are used in the data tables where data are not available:

DNA = Data have not been analyzed. Data in this category have been collected but not analyzed.

DNC = Data are not collected. The data source or sources listed for the objective do not collect data for the specific population group. A different or new data source may be required to measure progress for this population group.

DSU = Data are statistically unreliable. This category of analyzed data covers a number of situations, including the number of respondents is too small to produce a valid estimate, the proportion of respondents with missing information is too large, or the survey does not have representative data for certain population groups.

NA = Not applicable.

Targets for Measurable Objectives

Targets are based on national baseline data.

As a general rule, one target is set for all population groups to reach by the year 2010. This supports the overarching goal of eliminating health disparities. The guidelines used to develop targets are as follows:

■ One national target for the year 2010 is set for all measurable objectives and is applicable to most population groups. This target setting method supports the goal of eliminating health disparities and improving health for all segments of the total population.

■ For those measures contained in the HHS Initiative to Eliminate Racial and Ethnic Disparities in Health, the targets are set at "better than the best" of any racial or ethnic group. Data points for at least two population groups under the race and ethnicity category are needed to use "better than the best" as the target setting method.

■ For those objectives that in the short term can be influenced by lifestyle choices, behaviors, and health services (in other words, using existing and known interventions), the target also is set at "better than the best" currently achieved, at a minimum, by any racial and ethnic group.

■ For objectives for which achievement of an equal health outcome is unlikely within 10 years by applying known health interventions, the target is set at levels that represent improvements for a substantial proportion of the population. These targets are regarded as minimally acceptable improvements. Population groups already better than the identified target should continue to improve.

The following target setting methods have been used:

■ Better than the best.

■ __ percent improvement.

■ "Total coverage" or "Total elimination" (for targets like 100 percent, 0 percent, all States, etc.).

■ Consistent with _____ (another national program, for example, national education goals).

■ Retain year 2000 target (the Healthy People 2000 target has been retained).

Data Source/Potential Data Source

Data source is defined as the instrument that collects the measure indicated. Measurable objectives cite the data source for the baseline.

- For HHS data sets, surveys, and reports, the citation includes the name of the data set, the HHS agency, and the institute or center that serves as the source—for example, National Health Interview Survey, CDC, NCHS.

- For non-HHS or non-Federal data sets, surveys, and reports, the citation includes the name of the data set, cabinet-level agency, and bureau/agency/organization—for example, Fatality Analysis Reporting System, DOT, NHTSA.

Related Objectives

Each objective is placed in only one focus area, meaning there are no duplicate objectives in Healthy People 2010. There are, however, numerous linkages among focus areas, and these are represented in the list of related objectives from other focus areas.

Terminology

Terms are set up as dictionary definitions in alphabetical order. These definitions enable the reader to understand the concepts used in the chapter. A master list of abbreviations and acronyms used throughout the book appears in Appendix H.

References

The references cited throughout both the overview text and the objectives are listed at the end of each chapter.

Tracking Healthy People 2010

For more information on measuring the objectives, technical notes, or operational definitions, refer to the statistical compendium, *Tracking Healthy People 2010*. This volume is available on the CDC Web site at http://www.cdc.gov/nchs/hphome.htm.

For Further Information

Please visit the Healthy People Web site at http://www.health.gov/healthypeople or call 1-800-367-4725.

To obtain copies of Healthy People 2010 documents in print, see the order form at the end of this document or visit the U.S. Government Printing Office Web site at http://www.bookstore.gpo.gov/. For information about a Healthy People 2010 CD-ROM, visit the Healthy People 2010 Web site at http://www.health.gov/healthypeople.

Volume I

- **Understanding and Improving Health**
- **Objectives for Improving Health Part A: Focus Areas 1-14**

U.S. Department of Health and Human Services
November 2000

Introduction

Healthy People 2010 presents a comprehensive, nationwide health promotion and disease prevention agenda. It is designed to serve as a roadmap for improving the health of all people in the United States during the first decade of the 21st century.

Like the preceding Healthy People 2000 initiative—which was driven by an ambitious, yet achievable, 10-year strategy for improving the Nation's health by the end of the 20th century—Healthy People 2010 is committed to a single, overarching purpose: promoting health and preventing illness, disability, and premature death.

The History Behind the Healthy People 2010 Initiative

Healthy People 2010 builds on initiatives pursued over the past two decades. In 1979, *Healthy People: The Surgeon General's Report on Health Promotion and Disease Prevention* provided national goals for reducing premature deaths and preserving independence for older adults. In 1980, another report, *Promoting Health/Preventing Disease: Objectives for the Nation*, set forth 226 targeted health objectives for the Nation to achieve over the next 10 years.

Healthy People 2000: National Health Promotion and Disease Prevention Objectives, released in 1990, identified health improvement goals and objectives to be reached by the year 2000. The Healthy People 2010 initiative continues in this tradition as an instrument to improve health for the first decade of the 21st century.

Healthy People 2010 is grounded in science, built through public consensus, and designed to measure progress.

The Development of Healthy People 2010 Goals and Objectives

Healthy People 2010 represents the ideas and expertise of a diverse range of individuals and organizations concerned about the Nation's health. The Healthy People Consortium—an alliance of more than 350 national organizations and 250 State public health, mental health, substance abuse, and environmental agencies—conducted three national meetings on the development of Healthy People 2010. In addition, many individuals and organizations gave testimony about health priorities at five Healthy People 2010 regional meetings held in late 1998.

On two occasions—in 1997 and in 1998—the American public was given the opportunity to share its thoughts and ideas. More than 11,000 comments on draft materials were received by mail or via the Internet from individuals in every State, the District of Columbia, and Puerto Rico. All the comments received during the development of Healthy People 2010 can be viewed on the Healthy People Web site: http://www.health.gov/healthypeople/.

The final Healthy People 2010 objectives were developed by teams of experts from a variety of Federal agencies under the direction of Health and Human Services Secretary Donna Shalala, Assistant Secretary for Health and Surgeon General David Satcher, and former Assistant Secretaries for Health. The process was coordinated by the Office of Disease Prevention and Health Promotion, U.S. Department of Health and Human Services.

The Goals of Healthy People 2010

Healthy People 2010 is designed to achieve two overarching goals:

- Increase quality and years of healthy life.
- Eliminate health disparities.

These two goals are supported by specific objectives in 28 focus areas (see page 17). Each objective was developed with a target to be achieved by the year 2010. A full explanation of the two goals can be found in the next section of this document: "A Systematic Approach to Health Improvement."

Healthy People 2010: Understanding and Improving Health

The Relationship Between Individual and Community Health

Over the years, it has become clear that individual health is closely linked to community health—the health of the community and environment in which individuals live, work, and play. Likewise, community health is profoundly affected by the collective beliefs, attitudes, and behaviors of everyone who lives in the community.

Indeed, the underlying premise of Healthy People 2010 is that the health of the individual is almost inseparable from the health of the larger community and that the health of every community in every State and territory determines the overall health status of the Nation. That is why the vision for Healthy People 2010 is "Healthy People in Healthy Communities."

> Community health is profoundly affected by the collective beliefs, attitudes, and behaviors of everyone who lives in the community.

How Healthy People 2010 Will Improve the Nation's Health

One of the most compelling and encouraging lessons learned from the Healthy People 2000 initiative is that we, as a Nation, can make dramatic progress in improving the Nation's health in a relatively short period of time. For example, during the past decade, we achieved significant reductions in infant mortality. Childhood vaccinations are at the highest levels ever recorded in the United States. Fewer teenagers are becoming parents. Overall, alcohol, tobacco, and illicit drug use is leveling off. Death rates for coronary heart disease and stroke have declined. Significant advances have been made in the diagnosis and treatment of cancer and in reducing unintentional injuries.

But we still have a long way to go. Diabetes and other chronic conditions continue to present a serious obstacle to public health. Violence and abusive behavior continue to ravage homes and communities across the country. Mental disorders continue to go undiagnosed and untreated. Obesity in adults has increased 50 percent over the past two decades. Nearly 40 percent of adults engage in no leisure time physical activity. Smoking among adolescents has increased in the past decade. And HIV/AIDS remains a serious health problem, now disproportionately affecting women and communities of color.

Healthy People 2010 will be the guiding instrument for addressing these and emerging health issues, reversing unfavorable trends, and expanding past achievements in health.

The Key Role of Community Partnerships

Community partnerships, particularly when they reach out to nontraditional partners, can be among the most effective tools for improving health in communities.

For the past two decades, Healthy People has been used as a strategic management tool for the Federal Government, States, communities, and many other public- and private-sector partners. Virtually all States, the District of Columbia, and Guam have developed their own Healthy People plans modeled after the national plan. Most States have tailored the national objectives to their specific needs.

> **Partnerships are effective tools for improving health in communities.**

Businesses; local governments; and civic, professional, and religious organizations also have been inspired by Healthy People to print immunization reminders, set up hotlines, change cafeteria menus, begin community recycling, establish worksite fitness programs, assess school health education curriculums, sponsor health fairs, and engage in myriad other activities.

Everyone Can Help Achieve the Healthy People 2010 Objectives

Addressing the challenge of health improvement is a shared responsibility that requires the active participation and leadership of the Federal Government, States, local governments, policymakers, health care providers, professionals, business executives, educators, community leaders, and the American public itself. Although administrative responsibility for the Healthy People 2010 initiative rests in the U.S. Department of Health and Human Services, representatives of all these diverse groups shared their experience, expertise, and ideas in developing the Healthy People 2010 goals and objectives.

Healthy People 2010, however, is just the beginning. The biggest challenges still stand before us, and we all share a role in building a healthier Nation.

Regardless of your age, gender, education level, income, race, ethnicity, cultural customs, language, religious beliefs, disability, sexual orientation, geographic location, or occupation, Healthy People 2010 is designed to be a valuable resource in determining how you can participate most effectively in improving the Nation's health. Perhaps you will recognize the need to be a more active participant in decisions affecting your own health or the health of your children or loved ones. Perhaps you will assume a leadership role in promoting healthier behaviors in your neighborhood or community. Or perhaps you will use your influence and social stature to advocate for and implement policies and programs that can improve dramatically the health of dozens, hundreds, thousands, or even millions of people.

Whatever your role, this document is designed to help you determine what *you* can do—in your home, community, business, or State—to help improve the Nation's health.

Other Information Is Available About Healthy People 2010

Healthy People 2010: Understanding and Improving Health is the first of three parts in the Healthy People 2010 series. The second part, *Healthy People 2010*, contains detailed descriptions of 467 objectives to improve health. These objectives are organized into 28 specific focus areas. The third part, *Tracking Healthy People 2010*, provides a comprehensive review of the statistical measures that will be used to evaluate progress.

To receive more information about the Healthy People 2010 initiative, visit the Web site at http://www.health.gov/healthypeople/ or call 1-800-367-4725. To obtain copies of Healthy People 2010 documents in print or on a CD-ROM, see the order form at the end of this document or visit the U.S. Government Printing Office Web site at http://www.bookstore.gpo.gov/.

Healthy People 2010 contains 467 objectives to improve health, organized into 28 focus areas.

Healthy People in Healthy Communities

A Systematic Approach to Health Improvement

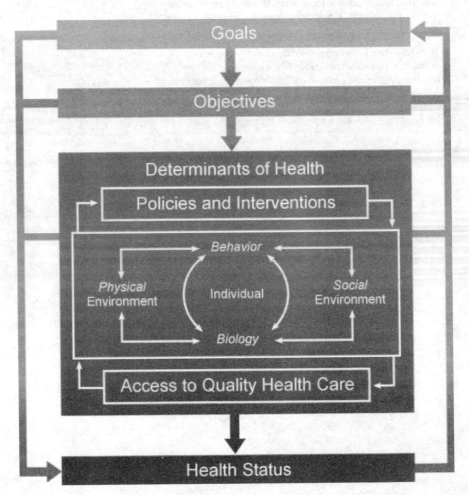

Healthy People 2010: Understanding and Improving Health

A Systematic Approach to Health Improvement

Healthy People 2010 is about improving health—the health of each individual, the health of communities, and the health of the Nation. However, the Healthy People 2010 goals and objectives cannot by themselves improve the health status of the Nation. Instead, they need to be recognized as part of a larger, systematic approach to health improvement.

This systematic approach to health improvement is composed of four key elements:

- Goals
- Objectives
- Determinants of health
- Health status

Whether this systematic approach is used to improve health on a national level, as in Healthy People 2010, or to organize community action on a particular health issue, such as promoting smoking cessation, the components remain the same. The goals provide a general focus and direction. The goals, in turn, serve as a guide for developing a set of objectives that will measure actual progress within a specified amount of time. The objectives focus on the determinants of health, which encompass the combined effects of individual and community physical and social environments and the policies and interventions used to promote health, prevent disease, and ensure access to quality health care. The ultimate measure of success in any health improvement effort is the health status of the target population.

> **Successful community partnerships use a systematic approach to health improvement.**

Healthy People 2010 is built on this systematic approach to health improvement.

Healthy People 2010 Goals

Goal 1: Increase Quality and Years of Healthy Life

The first goal of Healthy People 2010 is to help individuals of all ages increase life expectancy *and* improve their quality of life.

Life Expectancy

Life expectancy is the average number of years people born in a given year are expected to live based on a set of age-specific death rates. At the beginning of the 20th century, life expectancy at birth was 47.3 years. Fortunately, life expectancy has increased dramatically over the past 100 years (see figure 1). Today, the average life expectancy at birth is nearly 77 years.

Life expectancy for persons at every age group also has increased during the past century. Based on today's age-specific death rates, individuals aged 65 years can be expected to live an average of 18 more years, for a total of 83 years. Those aged 75 years can be expected to live an average of 11 more years, for a total of 86 years.

Differences in life expectancy between populations, however, suggest a substantial need and opportunity for improvement. At least 18 countries with populations of 1 million or more have life expectancies greater than the United States for both men and women (see figure 2).

Figure 1. Past and projected female and male life expectancy at birth, United States, 1900–2050.

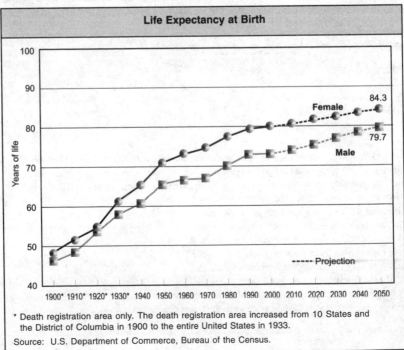

* Death registration area only. The death registration area increased from 10 States and the District of Columbia in 1900 to the entire United States in 1933.

Source: U.S. Department of Commerce, Bureau of the Census.

Healthy People 2010: Understanding and Improving Health

Figure 2. Life expectancy at birth by gender and ranked by selected countries, 1995.

Life Expectancy by Country

Female			Male		
	Country	Years of Life Expectancy		Country	Years of Life Expectancy
●	Japan	82.9	●	Japan	76.4
	France	82.6		Sweden	76.2
	Switzerland	81.9	☆	Israel	75.3
	Sweden	81.6		Canada	75.2
	Spain	81.5		Switzerland	75.1
	Canada	81.2		Greece	75.1
	Australia	80.9		Australia	75.0
	Italy	80.8		Norway	74.9
	Norway	80.7		Netherlands	74.6
	Netherlands	80.4		Italy	74.4
	Greece	80.3		England and Wales	74.3
	Finland	80.3		France	74.2
	Austria	80.1		Spain	74.2
	Germany	79.8		Austria	73.5
	Belgium	79.8		Singapore	73.4
	England and Wales	79.6		Germany	73.3
☆	Israel	79.3		New Zealand	73.3
	Singapore	79.0		Northern Ireland	73.1
	United States	**78.9**		Belgium	73.0
				Cuba	73.0
				Costa Rica	73.0
				Finland	72.8
				Denmark	72.8
				Ireland	72.5
				United States	**72.5**

Sources: World Health Organization; United
Nations; Centers for Disease
Control and Prevention; National
Center for Health Statistics;
National Vital Statistics System
1990–95 and unpublished data.

Healthy People 2010 Goals

There are substantial differences in life expectancy among different population groups within the United States. For example, women outlive men by an average of 6 years. White women currently have the greatest life expectancy in the United States. The life expectancy for African American women has risen to be higher today than that for white men. People from households with an annual income of at least $25,000 live an average of 3 to 7 years longer, depending on gender and race, than do people from households with annual incomes of less than $10,000.

Quality of Life

Quality of life reflects a general sense of happiness and satisfaction with our lives and environment. General quality of life encompasses all aspects of life, including health, recreation, culture, rights, values, beliefs, aspirations, and the conditions that support a life containing these elements. *Health-related quality of life* reflects a personal sense of physical and mental health and the ability to react to factors in the physical and social environments. Health-related quality of life is more subjective than life expectancy and therefore can be more difficult to measure. Some tools have been developed to measure health-related quality of life.

Global assessments, in which a person rates his or her health as "poor," "fair," "good," "very good," or "excellent," can be reliable indicators of one's perceived health. In 1996, 90 percent of people in the United States reported their health as good, very good, or excellent.

Healthy days is another measure of health-related quality of life that estimates the number of days of poor or impaired physical and mental health in the past 30 days. In 1998, adults averaged 5.5 days during the past month when their physical or mental health was not good—including 1.8 days when they were not able to do their usual activities. However, 52 percent of adults reported having good physical and mental health for the entire month in contrast with 10 percent of adults who were unhealthy for all 30 days. Typically, younger adults report more mentally unhealthy days while older adults report more physically unhealthy days.

Years of healthy life is a combined measure developed for the Healthy People initiative. The difference between life expectancy and years of healthy life reflects the average amount of time spent in less than optimal health because of chronic or acute limitations. Years of healthy life increased in 1996 to 64.2 years, a level that was only slightly above the 64.0 years at the beginning of the decade. During the same period, life expectancy increased a full year.

As with life expectancy, various population groups can show dramatic differences in quality of life. For example, people in the lowest income households are five times more likely to report their health as fair or poor than people in the highest income households (see figure 3). A higher percentage of women report their health as fair or poor compared to men. Adults in rural areas are 36 percent more likely to report their health status as fair or poor than are adults in urban areas.

Achieving a Longer and Healthier Life—the Healthy People Perspective

Healthy People 2010 seeks to increase life expectancy and quality of life over the next 10 years by helping individuals gain the knowledge, motivation, and opportunities they need to make informed decisions about their health. At the same time, Healthy People 2010 encourages local and State leaders to develop communitywide and statewide efforts that promote healthy behaviors, create healthy environments, and increase access to high-quality health care. Because individual and community health are virtually inseparable, both the individual and the community need to do their parts to increase life expectancy and improve quality of life.

Figure 3. Percentage of persons with perceived fair or poor health status by household income, United States, 1995.

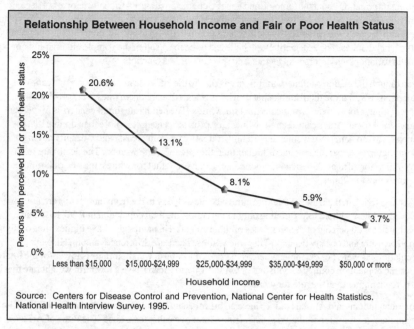

Relationship Between Household Income and Fair or Poor Health Status

Persons with perceived fair or poor health status

- 20.6% — Less than $15,000
- 13.1% — $15,000-$24,999
- 8.1% — $25,000-$34,999
- 5.9% — $35,000-$49,999
- 3.7% — $50,000 or more

Household income

Source: Centers for Disease Control and Prevention, National Center for Health Statistics. National Health Interview Survey. 1995.

Goal 2: Eliminate Health Disparities

The second goal of Healthy People 2010 is to eliminate health disparities among segments of the population, including differences that occur by gender, race or ethnicity, education or income, disability, geographic location, or sexual orientation. This section highlights ways in which health disparities can occur among various demographic groups in the United States.

Gender

Whereas some differences in health between men and women are the result of biological differences, others are more complicated and require greater attention and scientific exploration. Some health differences are obviously gender specific, such as cervical and prostate cancers.

Overall, men have a life expectancy that is 6 years less than that of women and have higher death rates for each of the 10 leading causes of death. For example, men are two times more likely than women to die from unintentional injuries and four times more likely than women to die from firearm-related injuries. Although overall death rates for women currently may be lower than for men, women have shown increased death rates over the past decade in areas where men have experienced improvements, such as lung cancer. Women also are at greater risk for Alzheimer's disease than men are and twice as likely as men to be affected by major depression.

Healthy People 2010 Goals

Race and Ethnicity

Current information about the biologic and genetic characteristics of African Americans, Hispanics, American Indians, Alaska Natives, Asians, Native Hawaiians, and Pacific Islanders does not explain the health disparities experienced by these groups compared with the white, non-Hispanic population in the United States. These disparities are believed to be the result of the complex interaction among genetic variations, environmental factors, and specific health behaviors.

Even though the Nation's infant mortality rate is down, the infant death rate among African Americans is still more than double that of whites. Heart disease death rates are more than 40 percent higher for African Americans than for whites. The death rate for all cancers is 30 percent higher for African Americans than for whites; for prostate cancer, it is more than double that for whites. African American women have a higher death rate from breast cancer despite having a mammography screening rate that is higher than the rate for white women. The death rate from HIV/AIDS for African Americans is more than seven times that for whites; the rate of homicide is six times that for whites.

Hispanics living in the United States are almost twice as likely to die from diabetes as are non-Hispanic whites. Although constituting only 11 percent of the total population in 1996, Hispanics accounted for 20 percent of the new cases of tuberculosis. Hispanics also have higher rates of high blood pressure and obesity than non-Hispanic whites. There are differences among Hispanic populations as well. For example, whereas the rate of low birth weight infants is lower for the total Hispanic population compared with that of whites, Puerto Ricans have a low birth weight rate that is 50 percent higher than the rate for whites.

American Indians and Alaska Natives have an infant death rate almost double that for whites. The rate of diabetes for this population group is more than twice that for whites. The Pima of Arizona have one of the highest rates of diabetes in the world. American Indians and Alaska Natives also have disproportionately high death rates from unintentional injuries and suicide.

Asians and Pacific Islanders, on average, have indicators of being one of the healthiest population groups in the United States. However, there is great diversity within this population group, and health disparities for some specific segments are quite marked. Women of Vietnamese origin, for example, suffer from cervical cancer at nearly five times the rate for white women. New cases of hepatitis and tuberculosis also are higher in Asians and Pacific Islanders living in the United States than in whites.

Income and Education

Inequalities in income and education underlie many health disparities in the United States. Income and education are intrinsically related and often serve as proxy measures for each other (see figure 4). In general, population groups that suffer the worst health status also are those that have the highest poverty rates and the least education. Disparities in income and education levels are associated with differences in the occurrence of illness and death, including heart disease, diabetes, obesity, elevated blood lead level, and low birth weight. Higher incomes permit increased access to medical care, enable people to afford better housing and live in safer neighborhoods, and increase the opportunity to engage in health-promoting behaviors.

Figure 4. Relationship between education and median household income among adults aged 25 years and older, by gender, United States, 1996.

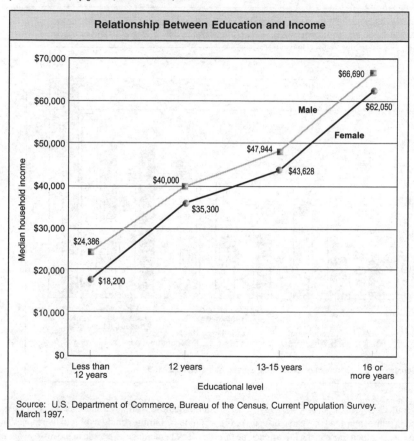

Source: U.S. Department of Commerce, Bureau of the Census. Current Population Survey. March 1997.

Income inequality in the United States has increased over the past three decades. There are distinct demographic differences in poverty by race, ethnicity, and household composition (see figure 5) as well as geographical variations in poverty across the United States. Recent health gains for the U.S. population as a whole appear to reflect achievements among the higher socioeconomic groups; lower socioeconomic groups continue to lag behind.

Figure 5. Percentage of persons below the poverty level by race and ethnicity and type of household, United States, 1996.

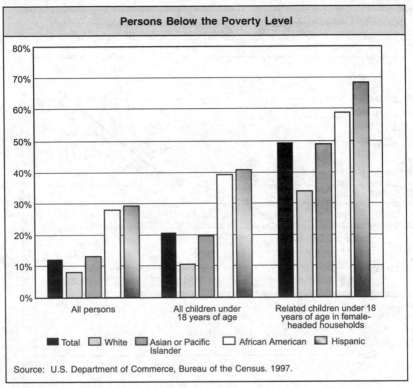

Persons Below the Poverty Level

Legend: ■ Total   □ White   ▨ Asian or Pacific Islander   □ African American   ▨ Hispanic

Source: U.S. Department of Commerce, Bureau of the Census. 1997.

Overall, those with higher incomes tend to fare better than those with lower incomes. For example, among white men aged 65 years, those in the highest income families could expect to live more than 3 years longer than those in the lowest income families. The percentage of people in the lowest income families reporting limitation in activity caused by chronic disease is three times that of people in the highest income families.

The average level of education in the U.S. population has increased steadily over the past several decades—an important achievement given that more years of education usually translate into more years of life. For women, the amount of education achieved is a key determinant of the welfare and survival of their children. Higher levels of education also may increase the likelihood of obtaining or understanding health-related information needed to develop health-promoting behaviors and beliefs in prevention. But again, educational attainment differs by race and ethnicity (see figure 6). Among people aged 25 to 64 years in the United States, the overall death rate for those with less than 12 years of education is more than twice that for people with 13 or more years of education. The infant mortality rate is almost double for infants of mothers with less than 12 years of education compared with those with an educational level of 13 or more years.

Figure 6. Percentage of adults aged 25 to 64 years by educational level, race and ethnicity, United States, 1996.

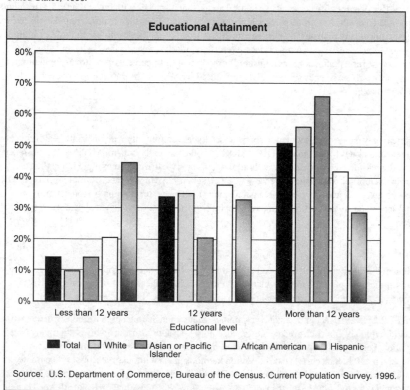

Source: U.S. Department of Commerce, Bureau of the Census. Current Population Survey. 1996.

Disability

People with disabilities are identified as persons having an activity limitation, who use assistance, or who perceive themselves as having a disability. In 1994, 54 million people in the United States, or roughly 21 percent of the population, had some level of disability. Although rates of disability are relatively stable or falling slightly for people aged 45 years and older, rates are on the rise among the younger population. People with disabilities tend to report more anxiety, pain, sleeplessness, and days of depression and fewer days of vitality than do people without activity limitations. People with disabilities also have other disparities, including lower rates of physical activity and higher rates of obesity. Many people with disabilities lack access to health services and medical care.

Healthy People 2010 Goals

Geographic Location

Twenty-five percent of Americans live in rural areas, that is, places with fewer than 2,500 residents. Injury-related death rates are 40 percent higher in rural populations than in urban populations. Heart disease, cancer, and diabetes rates exceed those for urban areas. People living in rural areas are less likely to use preventive screening services, exercise regularly, or wear safety belts. In 1996, 20 percent of the rural population was uninsured compared with 16 percent of the urban population. Timely access to emergency services and the availability of specialty care are other issues for this population group.

Sexual Orientation

America's gay and lesbian population comprises a diverse community with disparate health concerns. Major health issues for gay men are HIV/AIDS and other sexually transmitted diseases, substance abuse, depression, and suicide. Gay male adolescents are two to three times more likely than their peers to attempt suicide. Some evidence suggests lesbians have higher rates of smoking, overweight, alcohol abuse, and stress than heterosexual women. The issues surrounding personal, family, and social acceptance of sexual orientation can place a significant burden on mental health and personal safety.

Achieving Equity—The Healthy People Perspective

Although the diversity of the American population may be one of the Nation's greatest assets, it also represents a range of health improvement challenges—challenges that must be addressed by individuals, the community and State in which they live, and the Nation as a whole.

Healthy People 2010 recognizes that communities, States, and national organizations will need to take a multidisciplinary approach to achieving health equity—an approach that involves improving health, education, housing, labor, justice, transportation, agriculture, and the environment, as well as data collection itself. In fact, current data collection methods make it impossible to assess accurately the health status for some populations, particularly relatively small ones. However, the greatest opportunities for reducing health disparities are in empowering individuals to make informed health care decisions and in promoting communitywide safety, education, and access to health care.

Healthy People 2010 is firmly dedicated to the principle that—regardless of age, gender, race or ethnicity, income, education, geographic location, disability, and sexual orientation—every person in every community across the Nation deserves equal access to comprehensive, culturally competent, community-based health care systems that are committed to serving the needs of the individual and promoting community health.

Objectives

The Nation's progress in achieving the two goals of Healthy People 2010 will be monitored through 467 objectives in 28 focus areas. Many objectives focus on interventions designed to reduce or eliminate illness, disability, and premature death among individuals and communities. Others focus on broader issues, such as improving access to quality health care, strengthening public health services, and improving the availability and dissemination of health-related information. Each objective has a target for specific improvements to be achieved by the year 2010.

Together, these objectives reflect the depth of scientific knowledge as well as the breadth of diversity in the Nation's communities. More importantly, they are designed to help the Nation achieve Healthy People 2010's two overarching goals and realize the vision of healthy people living in healthy communities.

A list of the short titles of all Healthy People 2010 objectives by focus area can be found in the Appendix. In addition, *Healthy People 2010* provides an overview of the issues, trends, and opportunities for action in each of the 28 focus areas. It also contains detailed language of each objective, underlying rationale, target for the year 2010, and national data tables of its measures.

Healthy People 2010 Focus Areas

1. Access to Quality Health Services
2. Arthritis, Osteoporosis, and Chronic Back Conditions
3. Cancer
4. Chronic Kidney Disease
5. Diabetes
6. Disability and Secondary Conditions
7. Educational and Community-Based Programs
8. Environmental Health
9. Family Planning
10. Food Safety
11. Health Communication
12. Heart Disease and Stroke
13. HIV
14. Immunization and Infectious Diseases
15. Injury and Violence Prevention
16. Maternal, Infant, and Child Health
17. Medical Product Safety
18. Mental Health and Mental Disorders
19. Nutrition and Overweight
20. Occupational Safety and Health
21. Oral Health
22. Physical Activity and Fitness
23. Public Health Infrastructure
24. Respiratory Diseases
25. Sexually Transmitted Diseases
26. Substance Abuse
27. Tobacco Use
28. Vision and Hearing

Determinants of Health

Topics covered by the objectives in Healthy People 2010 reflect the array of critical influences that determine the health of individuals and communities.

For example, individual behaviors and environmental factors are responsible for about 70 percent of all premature deaths in the United States. Developing and implementing policies and preventive interventions that effectively address these determinants of health can reduce the burden of illness, enhance quality of life, and increase longevity.

Individual *biology* and *behaviors* influence health through their interaction with each other and with the individual's *social* and *physical environments*. In addition, *policies and interventions* can improve health by targeting factors related to individuals and their environments, including *access to quality health care* (see figure 7).

Figure 7. Determinants of health.

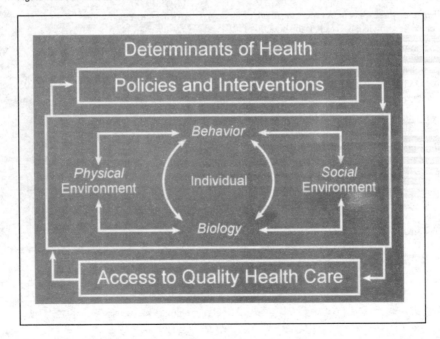

Healthy People 2010: Understanding and Improving Health

Biology refers to the individual's genetic makeup (those factors with which he or she is born), family history (which may suggest risk for disease), and the physical and mental health problems acquired during life. Aging, diet, physical activity, smoking, stress, alcohol or illicit drug abuse, injury or violence, or an infectious or toxic agent may result in illness or disability and can produce a "new" biology for the individual.

Behaviors are individual responses or reactions to internal stimuli and external conditions. Behaviors can have a reciprocal relationship to biology; in other words, each can react to the other. For example, smoking (behavior) can alter the cells in the lung and result in shortness of breath, emphysema, or cancer (biology) that then may lead an individual to stop smoking (behavior). Similarly, a family history that includes heart disease (biology) may motivate an individual to develop good eating habits, avoid tobacco, and maintain an active lifestyle (behaviors), which may prevent his or her own development of heart disease (biology).

Personal choices and the social and physical environments surrounding individuals can shape behaviors. The social and physical environments include all factors that affect the life of individuals, positively or negatively, many of which may not be under their immediate or direct control.

Social environment includes interactions with family, friends, coworkers, and others in the community. It also encompasses social institutions, such as law enforcement, the workplace, places of worship, and schools. Housing, public transportation, and the presence or absence of violence in the community are among other components of the social environment. The social environment has a profound effect on individual health, as well as on the health of the larger community, and is unique because of cultural customs; language; and personal, religious, or spiritual beliefs. At the same time, individuals and their behaviors contribute to the quality of the social environment.

Physical environment can be thought of as that which can be seen, touched, heard, smelled, and tasted. However, the physical environment also contains less tangible elements, such as radiation and ozone. The physical environment can harm individual and community health, especially when individuals and communities are exposed to toxic substances; irritants; infectious agents; and physical hazards in homes, schools, and worksites. The physical environment also can promote good health, for example, by providing clean and safe places for people to work, exercise, and play.

Policies and interventions can have a powerful and positive effect on the health of individuals and the community. Examples include health promotion campaigns to prevent smoking; policies mandating child restraints and safety belt use in automobiles; disease prevention services, such as immunization of children, adolescents, and adults; and clinical services, such as enhanced mental health care. Policies and interventions that promote individual and community health may be implemented by a variety of agencies, such as transportation, education, energy, housing, labor, justice, and other venues, or through places of worship, community-based organizations, civic groups, and businesses.

Determinants of Health

The health of individuals and communities also depends greatly on **access to quality health care**. Expanding access to quality health care is important to eliminate health disparities and to increase the quality and years of healthy life for all people living in the United States. Health care in the broadest sense not only includes services received through health care providers but also health information and services received through other venues in the community.

The determinants of health—individual biology and behavior, physical and social environments, policies and interventions, and access to quality health care—have a profound effect on the health of individuals, communities, and the Nation. An evaluation of these determinants is an important part of developing any strategy to improve health.

Our understanding of these determinants and how they relate to one another, coupled with our understanding of how individual and community health affects the health of the Nation, is perhaps the most important key to achieving our Healthy People 2010 goals of increasing the quality and years of life and of eliminating the Nation's health disparities.

Health Status

To understand the health status of a population, it is essential to monitor and evaluate the consequences of the determinants of health.

The health status of the United States is a description of the health of the total population, using information representative of most people living in this country. For relatively small population groups, however, it may not be possible to draw accurate conclusions about their health using current data collection methods. The goal of eliminating health disparities will necessitate improved collection and use of standardized data to identify correctly disparities among select population groups.

Health status can be measured by birth and death rates, life expectancy, quality of life, morbidity from specific diseases, risk factors, use of ambulatory care and inpatient care, accessibility of health personnel and facilities, financing of health care, health insurance coverage, and many other factors. The information used to report health status comes from a variety of sources, including birth and death records; hospital discharge data; and health information collected from health care records, personal interviews, physical examinations, and telephone surveys. These measures are monitored on an annual basis in the United States and are reported in a variety of publications, including *Health, United States* and *Healthy People Reviews*.

The leading causes of death are used frequently to describe the health status of the Nation. Over the past 100 years, the Nation has seen a great deal of change in the leading causes of death (see figure 8). At the beginning of the 1900s, infectious diseases ran rampant in the United States and worldwide and topped the leading causes of death. A century later, with the control of many infectious agents and the increasing age of the population, chronic diseases top the list.

A very different picture emerges when the leading causes of death are viewed for various population groups. Unintentional injuries, mainly motor vehicle crashes, are the fifth leading cause of death for the total population, but they are the leading cause of death for people aged 1 to 44 years. Similarly, HIV/AIDS is the 14th leading cause of death for the total population but the leading cause of death for African American men aged 25 to 44 years (see figure 9).

The leading causes of death in the United States generally result from a mix of behaviors; injury, violence, and other factors in the environment; and the unavailability or inaccessibility of quality health services. Understanding and monitoring behaviors, environmental factors, and community health systems may prove more useful to monitoring the Nation's *true* health, and in driving health improvement activities, than the death rates that reflect the cumulative impact of these factors. This more complex approach has served as the basis for developing the Leading Health Indicators.

Health Status

Figure 8. The leading causes of death as a percentage of all deaths in the United States, 1900 and 1997.

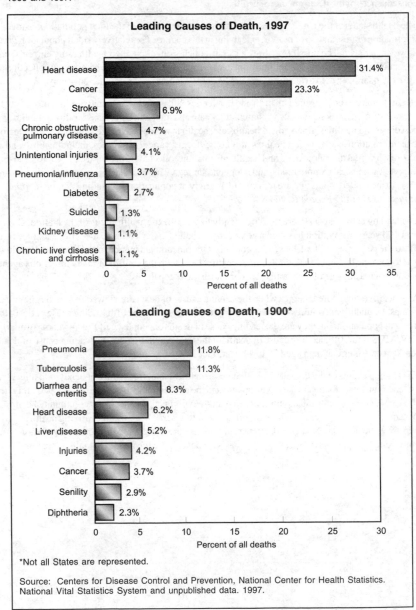

Leading Causes of Death, 1997

Cause	Percent
Heart disease	31.4%
Cancer	23.3%
Stroke	6.9%
Chronic obstructive pulmonary disease	4.7%
Unintentional injuries	4.1%
Pneumonia/influenza	3.7%
Diabetes	2.7%
Suicide	1.3%
Kidney disease	1.1%
Chronic liver disease and cirrhosis	1.1%

Percent of all deaths

Leading Causes of Death, 1900*

Cause	Percent
Pneumonia	11.8%
Tuberculosis	11.3%
Diarrhea and enteritis	8.3%
Heart disease	6.2%
Liver disease	5.2%
Injuries	4.2%
Cancer	3.7%
Senility	2.9%
Diphtheria	2.3%

Percent of all deaths

*Not all States are represented.

Source: Centers for Disease Control and Prevention, National Center for Health Statistics. National Vital Statistics System and unpublished data. 1997.

Healthy People 2010: Understanding and Improving Health

Figure 9. The three leading causes of death by age group, United States, 1997.

Leading Causes of Death by Age Group

Under 1 Year	Number of Deaths
Birth defects	6,178
Disorders related to premature birth	3,925
Sudden infant death syndrome	2,991
1-4 Years	
Unintentional Injuries	2,005
Birth defects	589
Cancer	438
5-14 Years	
Unintentional Injuries	3,371
Cancer	1,030
Homicide	457
15-24 Years	
Unintentional Injuries	13,367
Homicide	6,146
Suicide	4,186
25-44 Years	
Unintentional Injuries	27,129
Cancer	21,706
Heart disease	16,513
45-64 Years	
Cancer	131,743
Heart disease	101,235
Unintentional Injuries	17,521
65 Years and Older	
Heart disease	606,913
Cancer	382,913
Stroke	140,366

Source: Centers for Disease Control and Prevention, National Center for Health Statistics. National Vital Statistics System. 1999.

Leading Health Indicators

The Leading Health Indicators reflect the major public health concerns in the United States and were chosen based on their ability to motivate action, the availability of data to measure their progress, and their relevance as broad public health issues.

The Leading Health Indicators illuminate individual behaviors, physical and social environmental factors, and important health system issues that greatly affect the health of individuals and communities. Underlying each of these indicators is the significant influence of income and education (see Income and Education, page 12).

The process of selecting the Leading Health Indicators mirrored the collaborative and extensive efforts undertaken to develop Healthy People 2010. The process was led by an interagency work group within the U.S. Department of Health and Human Services. Individuals and organizations provided comments at national and regional meetings or via mail and the Internet. A report by the Institute of Medicine, National Academy of Sciences, provided several scientific models on which to support a set of indicators. Focus groups were used to ensure that the indicators are meaningful and motivating to the public.

Leading Health Indicators

- Physical activity
- Overweight and obesity
- Tobacco use
- Substance abuse
- Responsible sexual behavior
- Mental health
- Injury and violence
- Environmental quality
- Immunization
- Access to health care

For each of the Leading Health Indicators, specific objectives derived from Healthy People 2010 will be used to track progress. This small set of measures will provide a snapshot of the health of the Nation. Tracking and communicating progress on the Leading Health Indicators through national- and State-level report cards will spotlight achievements and challenges in the next decade. The Leading Health Indicators serve as a link to the 467 objectives in *Healthy People 2010* and can become the basic building blocks for community health initiatives.

A major challenge throughout the history of Healthy People has been to balance a comprehensive set of health objectives with a smaller set of health priorities.

The Leading Health Indicators are intended to help everyone more easily understand the importance of health promotion and disease prevention and to encourage wide participation in improving health in the next decade. Developing strategies and action plans to address one or more of these indicators can have a profound effect on increasing the quality of life and the years of healthy life and on eliminating health disparities—creating *healthy people in healthy communities*.

Physical Activity

Leading Health Indicator

Regular physical activity throughout life is important for maintaining a healthy body, enhancing psychological well-being, and preventing premature death.

In 1999, 65 percent of adolescents engaged in the recommended amount of physical activity. In 1997, only 15 percent of adults performed the recommended amount of physical activity, and 40 percent of adults engaged in no leisure-time physical activity.

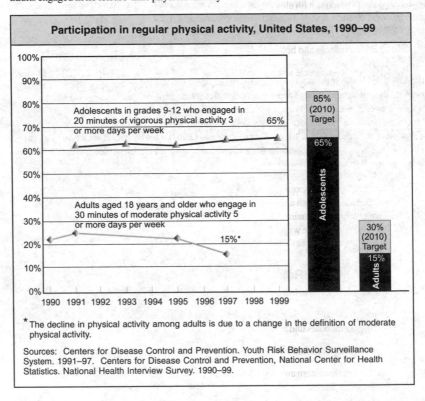

Participation in regular physical activity, United States, 1990–99

Adolescents in grades 9-12 who engaged in 20 minutes of vigorous physical activity 3 or more days per week — 65%

85% (2010) Target — 65% Adolescents

Adults aged 18 years and older who engage in 30 minutes of moderate physical activity 5 or more days per week — 15%*

30% (2010) Target — 15% Adults

*The decline in physical activity among adults is due to a change in the definition of moderate physical activity.

Sources: Centers for Disease Control and Prevention. Youth Risk Behavior Surveillance System. 1991–97. Centers for Disease Control and Prevention, National Center for Health Statistics. National Health Interview Survey. 1990–99.

The objectives selected to measure progress among adolescents and adults for this Leading Health Indicator are presented below. These are only indicators and do not represent all the physical activity and fitness objectives included in Healthy People 2010.

22-7. **Increase the proportion of adolescents who engage in vigorous physical activity that promotes cardiorespiratory fitness 3 or more days per week for 20 or more minutes per occasion.**

22-2. **Increase the proportion of adults who engage regularly, preferably daily, in moderate physical activity for at least 30 minutes per day.**

Health Impact of Physical Activity

Regular physical activity is associated with lower death rates for adults of any age, even when only moderate levels of physical activity are performed. Regular physical activity decreases the risk of death from heart disease, lowers the risk of developing diabetes, and is associated with a decreased risk of colon cancer. Regular physical activity helps prevent high blood pressure and helps reduce blood pressure in persons with elevated levels.

Regular physical activity also:

- Increases muscle and bone strength.

- Increases lean muscle and helps decrease body fat.

- Aids in weight control and is a key part of any weight loss effort.

- Enhances psychological well-being and may even reduce the risk of developing depression.

- Appears to reduce symptoms of depression and anxiety and to improve mood.

In addition, children and adolescents need weight-bearing exercise for normal skeletal development, and young adults need such exercise to achieve and maintain peak bone mass. Older adults can improve and maintain strength and agility with regular physical activity. This can reduce the risk of falling, helping older adults maintain an independent living status. Regular physical activity also increases the ability of people with certain chronic, disabling conditions to perform activities of daily living.

Populations With Low Rates of Physical Activity

- Women generally are less active than men at all ages.

- People with lower incomes and less education are typically not as physically active as those with higher incomes and education.

- African Americans and Hispanics are generally less physically active than whites.

- Adults in northeastern and southern States tend to be less active than adults in North-Central and Western States.

- People with disabilities are less physically active than people without disabilities.

- By age 75, one in three men and one in two women engage in *no* regular physical activity.

Other Issues

The major barriers most people face when trying to increase physical activity are lack of time, lack of access to convenient facilities, and lack of safe environments in which to be active.

For more information on Healthy People 2010 objectives or on physical activity and fitness, visit http://www.health.gov/healthypeople/ or call 1-800-336-4797.

HEALTHY
PEOPLE
2010

Overweight and Obesity

Leading Health Indicator

Overweight and obesity are major contributors to many preventable causes of death. On average, higher body weights are associated with higher death rates. The number of overweight children, adolescents, and adults has risen over the past four decades. Total costs (medical cost and lost productivity) attributable to obesity alone amounted to an estimated $99 billion in 1995.

During 1988–94, 11 percent of children and adolescents aged 6 to 19 years were overweight or obese. During the same years, 23 percent of adults aged 20 years and older were considered obese.

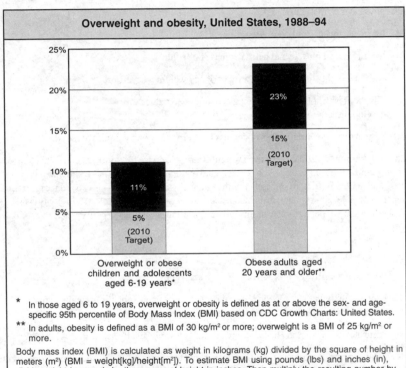

Overweight and obesity, United States, 1988–94

* In those aged 6 to 19 years, overweight or obesity is defined as at or above the sex- and age-specific 95th percentile of Body Mass Index (BMI) based on CDC Growth Charts: United States.

** In adults, obesity is defined as a BMI of 30 kg/m² or more; overweight is a BMI of 25 kg/m² or more.

Body mass index (BMI) is calculated as weight in kilograms (kg) divided by the square of height in meters (m²) (BMI = weight[kg]/height[m²]). To estimate BMI using pounds (lbs) and inches (in), divide weight in pounds by the square of height in inches. Then multiply the resulting number by 704.5 (BMI = weight[lbs]/height[in²] X 704.5).

Source: Centers for Disease Control and Prevention, National Center for Health Statistics. National Health and Nutrition Examination Survey. 1988–94.

The objectives selected to measure progress among children, adolescents, and adults for this Leading Health Indicator are presented below. These are only indicators and do not represent all the nutrition and overweight objectives included in Healthy People 2010.

19-3c. Reduce the proportion of children and adolescents who are overweight or obese.

19-2. Reduce the proportion of adults who are obese.

Health Impact of Overweight and Obesity

Overweight and obesity substantially raise the risk of illness from high blood pressure, high cholesterol, type 2 diabetes, heart disease and stroke, gallbladder disease, arthritis, sleep disturbances and problems breathing, and certain types of cancers. Obese individuals also may suffer from social stigmatization, discrimination, and lowered self-esteem.

Populations With High Rates of Overweight and Obesity

More than half of adults in the United States are estimated to be overweight or obese. The proportion of adolescents from poor households who are overweight or obese is twice that of adolescents from middle- and high-income households. Obesity is especially prevalent among women with lower incomes and is more common among African American and Mexican American women than among white women. Among African Americans, the proportion of women who are obese is 80 percent higher than the proportion of men who are obese. This gender difference also is seen among Mexican American women and men, but the percentage of white, non-Hispanic women and men who are obese is about the same.

Reducing Overweight and Obesity

Obesity is a result of a complex variety of social, behavioral, cultural, environmental, physiological, and genetic factors. Efforts to maintain a healthy weight should start early in childhood and continue throughout adulthood, as this is likely to be more successful than efforts to lose substantial amounts of weight and maintain weight loss once obesity is established.

A healthy diet and regular physical activity are both important for maintaining a healthy weight. Over time, even a small decrease in calories eaten and a small increase in physical activity can help prevent weight gain or facilitate weight loss. It is recommended that obese individuals who are trying to lose substantial amounts of weight seek the guidance of a health care provider.

Dietary and Physical Activity Recommendations

The *Dietary Guidelines for Americans* recommend that to build a healthy base, persons aged 2 years and older choose a healthful assortment of foods that includes vegetables; fruits; grains (especially whole grains); fat-free or low-fat milk products; and fish, lean meat, poultry, or beans. The guidelines further emphasize the importance of choosing foods that are low in saturated fat and added sugars most of the time and, whatever the food, eating a sensible portion size. It is recognized, however, that this guidance may be particularly challenging when eating out because the consumer may be offered large portion sizes with unknown amounts of saturated fat and added sugars.

The *Dietary Guidelines for Americans* recommend that all adults be more active throughout the day and get at least 30 minutes of moderate physical activity most, or preferably all, days of the week. Adults who are trying to maintain healthy weight after weight loss are advised to get even more physical activity. The guidelines also recommend that children get at least 60 minutes of physical activity daily and limit inactive forms of play such as television watching and computer games.

For more information on Healthy People 2010 objectives or on overweight and obesity, visit http://www.health.gov/healthypeople/ or call 1-800-336-4797.

Tobacco Use

Leading Health Indicator

Cigarette smoking is the single most preventable cause of disease and death in the United States. Smoking results in more deaths each year in the United States than AIDS, alcohol, cocaine, heroin, homicide, suicide, motor vehicle crashes, and fires—combined.

Tobacco-related deaths number more than 430,000 per year among U.S. adults, representing more than 5 million years of potential life lost. Direct medical costs attributable to smoking total at least $50 billion per year.

In 1999, 35 percent of adolescents were current cigarette smokers. In 1998, 24 percent of adults were current cigarette smokers.

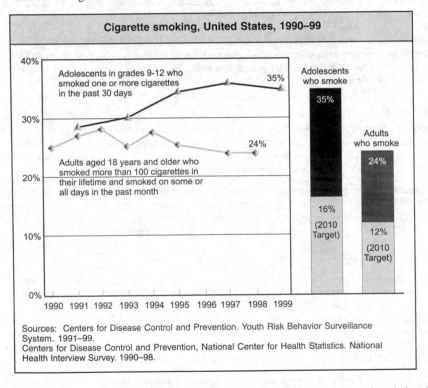

Cigarette smoking, United States, 1990–99

Adolescents in grades 9-12 who smoked one or more cigarettes in the past 30 days — 35%

Adults aged 18 years and older who smoked more than 100 cigarettes in their lifetime and smoked on some or all days in the past month — 24%

Adolescents who smoke 35% — 16% (2010 Target)

Adults who smoke 24% — 12% (2010 Target)

Sources: Centers for Disease Control and Prevention. Youth Risk Behavior Surveillance System. 1991–99.
Centers for Disease Control and Prevention, National Center for Health Statistics. National Health Interview Survey. 1990–98.

The objectives selected to measure progress among adolescents and adults for this Leading Health Indicator are presented below. These are only indicators and do not represent all the tobacco use objectives included in Healthy People 2010.

27-2b. Reduce cigarette smoking by adolescents.
27-1a. Reduce cigarette smoking by adults.

Health Impact of Cigarette Smoking

Smoking is a major risk factor for heart disease, stroke, lung cancer, and chronic lung diseases—all leading causes of death. Smoking during pregnancy can result in miscarriages, premature delivery, and sudden infant death syndrome. Other health effects of smoking result from injuries and environmental damage caused by fires.

Environmental tobacco smoke (ETS) increases the risk of heart disease and significant lung conditions, especially asthma and bronchitis in children. ETS is responsible for an estimated 3,000 lung cancer deaths each year among adult nonsmokers.

Trends in Cigarette Smoking

Adolescents. Overall, the percentage of adolescents in grades 9 through 12 who smoked in the past month increased in the 1990s. Every day, an estimated 3,000 young persons start smoking. These trends are disturbing because the vast majority of adult smokers tried their first cigarette before age 18 years; more than half of adult smokers became daily smokers before this same age. Almost half of adolescents who continue smoking regularly will die eventually from a smoking-related illness.

Adults. Following years of steady decline, rates of smoking among adults appear to have leveled off in the 1990s.

Populations With High Rates of Smoking

Adolescents. Adolescent rates of cigarette smoking have increased in the 1990s among white, African American, and Hispanic high school students after years of declining rates during the 1970s and 1980s. In 1999, 39 percent of white high school students currently smoked cigarettes compared with 33 percent for Hispanics and 20 percent for African Americans. Among African Americans in 1999, only 19 percent of high school girls, compared with 22 percent of boys, currently smoked cigarettes.

Adults. Overall, American Indians and Alaska Natives, blue-collar workers, and military personnel have the highest rates of smoking in adults. Rates of smoking in Asian and Pacific Islander men are more than four times higher than for women of the same race. Men have only somewhat higher rates of smoking than women within the total U.S. population. Low-income adults are more likely to smoke than are high-income adults. The percentage of people aged 25 years and older with less than 12 years of education who are current smokers is nearly three times that for persons with 16 or more years of education.

Other Important Tobacco Issues

There is no safe tobacco alternative to cigarettes. Spit tobacco (chew) causes cancer of the mouth, inflammation of the gums, and tooth loss. Cigar smoking causes cancer of the mouth, throat, and lungs and can increase the risk of heart disease and chronic lung problems.

For more information on Healthy People 2010 objectives or on tobacco use, visit http://www.health.gov/healthypeople/ or call 1-800-336-4797.

Substance Abuse

Leading Health Indicator

Alcohol and illicit drug use are associated with many of this country's most serious problems, including violence, injury, and HIV infection. The annual economic costs to the United States from alcohol abuse were estimated to be $167 billion in 1995, and the costs from drug abuse were estimated to be $110 billion.

In 1998, 79 percent of adolescents aged 12 to 17 years reported that they did *not* use alcohol or illicit drugs in the past month. In the same year, 6 percent of adults aged 18 years and older reported using illicit drugs in the past month; 17 percent reported binge drinking in the past month, which is defined as consuming five or more drinks on one occasion.

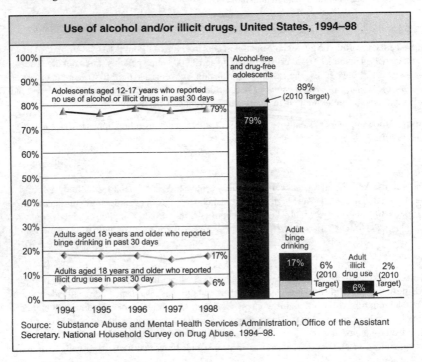

Use of alcohol and/or illicit drugs, United States, 1994–98

Source: Substance Abuse and Mental Health Services Administration, Office of the Assistant Secretary. National Household Survey on Drug Abuse. 1994–98.

The objectives selected to measure progress among adolescents and adults for this Leading Health Indicator are presented below. These are only indicators and do not represent all the substance abuse objectives in Healthy People 2010.

26-10a. **Increase the proportion of adolescents not using alcohol or any illicit drugs during the past 30 days.**

26-10c. **Reduce the proportion of adults using any illicit drug during the past 30 days.**

26-11c. **Reduce the proportion of adults engaging in binge drinking of alcoholic beverages during the past month.**

Healthy People 2010: Understanding and Improving Health

Health Impact of Substance Abuse

Alcohol and illicit drug use are associated with child and spousal abuse; sexually transmitted diseases, including HIV infection; teen pregnancy; school failure; motor vehicle crashes; escalation of health care costs; low worker productivity; and homelessness. Alcohol and illicit drug use also can result in substantial disruptions in family, work, and personal life.

Alcohol abuse alone is associated with motor vehicle crashes, homicides, suicides, and drowning—leading causes of death among youth. Long-term heavy drinking can lead to heart disease, cancer, alcohol-related liver disease, and pancreatitis. Alcohol use during pregnancy is known to cause fetal alcohol syndrome, a leading cause of preventable mental retardation.

Trends in Substance Abuse

Adolescents. Although the trend from 1994 to 1998 has shown some fluctuations, about 77 percent of adolescents aged 12 to 17 years report being both alcohol free and drug free in the past month.

Alcohol is the drug most frequently used by adolescents aged 12 to 17 years. In 1998, 19 percent of adolescents aged 12 to 17 years reported drinking alcohol in the past month. Alcohol use in the past month for this age group has remained at about 20 percent since 1992. Eight percent of this age group reported binge drinking, and 3 percent were heavy drinkers (five or more drinks on the same occasion on each of 5 or more days in the past 30 days).

Data from 1998 show that 10 percent of adolescents aged 12 to 17 years reported using illicit drugs in the past 30 days. This rate remains well below the all-time high of 16 percent in 1979. Current illicit drug use had nearly doubled for those aged 12 to 13 years between 1996 and 1997 but then decreased between 1997 and 1998. Youth are experimenting with a variety of illicit drugs, including marijuana, cocaine, crack, heroin, acid, inhalants, and methamphetamines, as well as misuse of prescription drugs and other "street" drugs. The younger a person becomes a habitual user of illicit drugs, the stronger the addiction becomes and the more difficult it is to stop use.

Adults. Binge drinking has remained at the same approximate level of 17 percent for all adults since 1988, with the highest current rate of 32 percent among adults aged 18 to 25 years. Illicit drug use has been near the present rate of 6 percent since 1980. Men continue to have higher rates of illicit drug use than women have, and rates of illicit drug use in urban areas are higher than in rural areas.

For more information on Healthy People 2010 objectives or on substance abuse, visit http://www.health.gov/healthypeople/ or call 1-800-336-4797.

Responsible Sexual Behavior

Leading Health Indicator

Unintended pregnancies and sexually transmitted diseases (STDs), including infection with the human immunodeficiency virus that causes AIDS, can result from unprotected sexual behaviors. Abstinence is the only method of complete protection. Condoms, if used correctly and consistently, can help prevent both unintended pregnancy and STDs.

In 1999, 85 percent of adolescents abstained from sexual intercourse or used condoms if they were sexually active. In 1995, 23 percent of sexually active women reported that their partners used condoms.

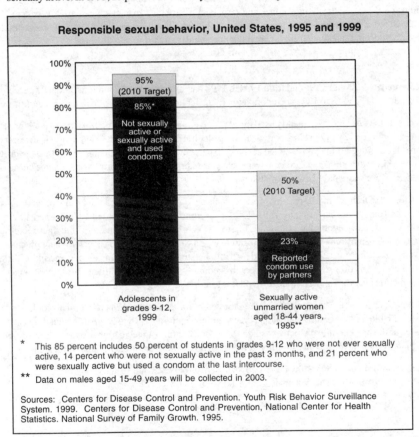

Responsible sexual behavior, United States, 1995 and 1999

*   This 85 percent includes 50 percent of students in grades 9-12 who were not ever sexually active, 14 percent who were not sexually active in the past 3 months, and 21 percent who were sexually active but used a condom at the last intercourse.

** Data on males aged 15-49 years will be collected in 2003.

Sources: Centers for Disease Control and Prevention. Youth Risk Behavior Surveillance System. 1999. Centers for Disease Control and Prevention, National Center for Health Statistics. National Survey of Family Growth. 1995.

The objectives selected to measure progress among adolescents and adults for this Leading Health Indicator are presented below. These are only indicators and do not represent all the responsible sexual behavior objectives in Healthy People 2010.

25-11. Increase the proportion of adolescents who abstain from sexual intercourse or use condoms if currently sexually active.

13-6a. Increase the proportion of sexually active persons who use condoms.

Healthy People 2010: Understanding and Improving Health

Trends in Sexual Behavior

In the past 6 years there has been both an increase in abstinence among all youth and an increase in condom use among those young people who are sexually active. Research has shown clearly that the most effective school-based programs are comprehensive ones that include a focus on abstinence *and* condom use. Condom use in sexually active adults has remained steady at about 25 percent.

Unintended Pregnancies

Half of all pregnancies in the United States are unintended; that is, at the time of conception the pregnancy was not planned or not wanted. Unintended pregnancy rates in the United States have been declining. The rates remain highest among teenagers, women aged 40 years or older, and low-income African American women. Approximately 1 million teenage girls each year in the United States have unintended pregnancies. Nearly half of all unintended pregnancies end in abortion.

The cost to U.S. taxpayers for adolescent pregnancy is estimated at between $7 billion and $15 billion a year.

Sexually Transmitted Diseases

Sexually transmitted diseases are common in the United States, with an estimated 15 million new cases of STDs reported each year. Almost 4 million of the new cases of STDs each year occur in adolescents. Women generally suffer more serious STD complications than men, including pelvic inflammatory disease, ectopic pregnancy, infertility, chronic pelvic pain, and cervical cancer from the human papilloma virus. African Americans and Hispanics have higher rates of STDs than whites.

The total cost of the most common STDs and their complications is conservatively estimated at $17 billion annually.

HIV/AIDS

Nearly 700,000 cases of AIDS have been reported in the United States since the HIV/AIDS epidemic began in the 1980s. The latest estimates indicate that 800,000 to 900,000 people in the United States currently are infected with HIV. The lifetime cost of health care associated with HIV infection, in light of recent advances in HIV diagnostics and therapies, is $155,000 or more per person.

About one-half of all new HIV infections in the United States are among people under age 25 years, and the majority are infected through sexual behavior. HIV infection is the leading cause of death for African American men aged 25 to 44 years. Compelling worldwide evidence indicates that the presence of other STDs increases the likelihood of both transmitting and acquiring HIV infection.

For more information on Healthy People 2010 objectives or on responsible sexual behavior, visit http://www.health.gov/healthypeople/ or call 1-800-336-4797.

Mental Health

Leading Health Indicator

Approximately 20 percent of the U.S. population is affected by mental illness during a given year; no one is immune. Of all mental illnesses, depression is the most common disorder. More than 19 million adults in the United States suffer from depression. Major depression is the leading cause of disability and is the cause of more than two-thirds of suicides each year.

In 1997, only 23 percent of adults diagnosed with depression received treatment.

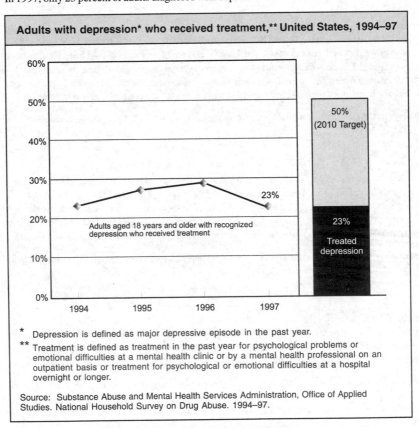

Adults with depression* who received treatment,** United States, 1994–97

* Depression is defined as major depressive episode in the past year.

** Treatment is defined as treatment in the past year for psychological problems or emotional difficulties at a mental health clinic or by a mental health professional on an outpatient basis or treatment for psychological or emotional difficulties at a hospital overnight or longer.

Source: Substance Abuse and Mental Health Services Administration, Office of Applied Studies. National Household Survey on Drug Abuse. 1994–97.

The objective selected to measure progress among adults for this Leading Health Indicator is presented below. This is only an indicator and does not represent all the mental health objectives in Healthy People 2010.

18-9b. Increase the proportion of adults with recognized depression who receive treatment.

Healthy People 2010: Understanding and Improving Health

Definition of Mental Health

Mental health is sometimes thought of as simply the absence of a mental illness but is actually much broader. Mental health is a state of successful mental functioning, resulting in productive activities, fulfilling relationships, and the ability to adapt to change and cope with adversity. Mental health is indispensable to personal well-being, family and interpersonal relationships, and one's contribution to society.

Impact of Depression

A person with a depressive disorder often is unable to fulfill the daily responsibilities of being a spouse, partner, or parent. The misunderstanding of mental illness and the associated stigmatization prevent many persons with depression from seeking professional help. Many people will be incapacitated for weeks or months because their depression goes untreated.

Depression is associated with other medical conditions, such as heart disease, cancer, and diabetes as well as anxiety and eating disorders. Depression also has been associated with alcohol and illicit drug abuse. An estimated 8 million persons aged 15 to 54 years had coexisting mental and substance abuse disorders within the past year.

The total estimated direct and indirect cost of mental illness in the United States in 1996 was $150 billion.

Treatment of Depression

Depression is treatable. Available medications and psychological treatments, alone or in combination, can help 80 percent of those with depression. With adequate treatment, future episodes of depression can be prevented or reduced in severity. Treatment for depression can enable people to return to satisfactory, functioning lives.

Populations With High Rates of Depression

Serious mental illness clearly affects mental health and can affect children, adolescents, adults, and older adults of all ethnic and racial groups, both genders, and people at all educational and income levels.

Adults and older adults have the highest rates of depression. Major depression affects approximately twice as many women as men. Women who are poor, on welfare, less educated, unemployed, and from certain racial or ethnic populations are more likely to experience depression. In addition, depression rates are higher among older adults with coexisting medical conditions. For example, 12 percent of older persons hospitalized for problems such as hip fracture or heart disease are diagnosed with depression. Rates of depression for older persons in nursing homes range from 15 to 25 percent.

For more information on Healthy People 2010 objectives or on mental health, visit http://www.health.gov/healthypeople/ or call 1-800-336-4797.

Injury and Violence

Leading Health Indicator

More than 400 Americans die each day from injuries due primarily to motor vehicle crashes, firearms, poisonings, suffocation, falls, fires, and drowning. The risk of injury is so great that most persons sustain a significant injury at some time during their lives.

Motor vehicle crashes are the most common cause of serious injury. In 1998, there were 15.6 deaths from motor vehicle crashes per 100,000 persons.

Because no other crime is measured as accurately and precisely, homicide is a reliable indicator of all violent crime. In 1998, the murder rate in the United States fell to its lowest level in three decades— 6.5 homicides per 100,000 persons.

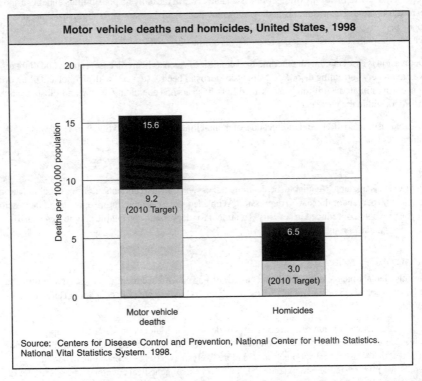

Motor vehicle deaths and homicides, United States, 1998

Deaths per 100,000 population

Motor vehicle deaths: 15.6 / 9.2 (2010 Target)
Homicides: 6.5 / 3.0 (2010 Target)

Source: Centers for Disease Control and Prevention, National Center for Health Statistics. National Vital Statistics System. 1998.

The objectives selected to measure progress for this Leading Health Indicator are presented below. These are only indicators and do not represent all the injury and violence prevention objectives in Healthy People 2010.

15-15a. Reduce deaths caused by motor vehicle crashes.
15-32.   Reduce homicides.

Impact of Injury and Violence

In 1995, the cost of injury and violence in the United States was estimated at more than $224 billion per year. These costs include direct medical care and rehabilitation as well as productivity losses to the Nation's workforce. The total societal cost of motor vehicle crashes alone exceeds $150 billion annually.

Motor Vehicle Crashes

Motor vehicle crashes are often predictable and preventable. Increased use of safety belts and reductions in driving while impaired are two of the most effective means to reduce the risk of death and serious injury of occupants in motor vehicle crashes.

Death rates associated with motor vehicle-traffic injuries are highest in the age group 15 to 24 years. In 1996, teenagers accounted for only 10 percent of the U.S. population but 15 percent of the deaths from motor vehicle crashes. Those aged 75 years and older had the second highest rate of motor vehicle-related deaths.

Nearly 40 percent of traffic fatalities in 1997 were alcohol related. Each year in the United States it is estimated that more than 120 million episodes of impaired driving occur among adults. In 1996, 21 percent of traffic fatalities of children aged 14 years and under involved alcohol; 60 percent of the time the driver of the car in which the child was a passenger was impaired.

The highest intoxication rates in fatal crashes in 1995 were recorded for drivers aged 21 to 24 years. Young drivers who have been arrested for driving while impaired are more than four times as likely to die in future alcohol-related crashes.

Homicides

In 1997, 32,436 individuals died from firearm injuries; of this number, 42 percent were victims of homicide. In 1997, homicide was the third leading cause of death for children aged 5 to 14 years, an increasing trend in childhood violent deaths. In 1996, more than 80 percent of infant homicides were considered to be fatal child abuse.

Many factors that contribute to injuries also are closely associated with violent and abusive behavior, such as low income, discrimination, lack of education, and lack of employment opportunities.

Males are most often the victims and the perpetrators of homicides. African Americans are more than five times as likely as whites to be murdered. There has been a decline in the homicide of intimates, including spouses, partners, boyfriends, and girlfriends, over the past decade, but this problem remains significant.

For more information on Healthy People 2010 objectives or on injury and violence, visit http://www.health.gov/healthypeople/ or call 1-800-336-4797.

Environmental Quality

Leading Health Indicator

An estimated 25 percent of preventable illnesses worldwide can be attributed to poor environmental quality. In the United States, air pollution alone is estimated to be associated with 50,000 premature deaths and an estimated $40 billion to $50 billion in health-related costs annually. Two indicators of air quality are ozone (outdoor) and environmental tobacco smoke (indoor).

In 1997, approximately 43 percent of the U.S. population lived in areas designated as nonattainment areas for established health-based standards for ozone. During the years 1988 to 1994, 65 percent of nonsmokers were exposed to environmental tobacco smoke (ETS).

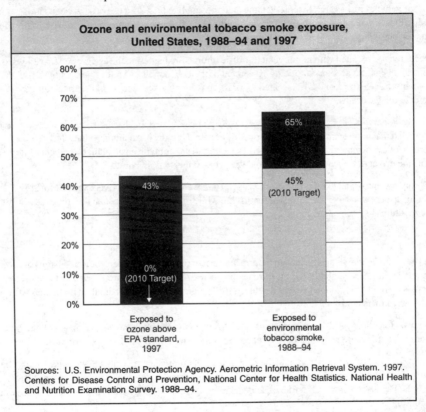

Ozone and environmental tobacco smoke exposure, United States, 1988–94 and 1997

Sources: U.S. Environmental Protection Agency. Aerometric Information Retrieval System. 1997. Centers for Disease Control and Prevention, National Center for Health Statistics. National Health and Nutrition Examination Survey. 1988–94.

The objectives selected to measure progress among children, adolescents, and adults for this Leading Health Indicator are presented below. These are only indicators and do not represent all the environmental quality objectives in Healthy People 2010.

8-1a. Reduce the proportion of persons exposed to air that does not meet the U.S. Environmental Protection Agency's health-based standards for ozone.

27-10. Reduce the proportion of nonsmokers exposed to environmental tobacco smoke.

Healthy People 2010: Understanding and Improving Health

Defining the Environment

Physical and social environments play major roles in the health of individuals and communities. The physical environment includes the air, water, and soil through which exposure to chemical, biological, and physical agents may occur. The social environment includes housing, transportation, urban development, land use, industry, and agriculture and results in exposures such as work-related stress, injury, and violence.

Global Concern

Environmental quality is a global concern. Ever-increasing numbers of people and products cross national borders and may transfer health risks such as infectious diseases and chemical hazards. For example, pesticides that are not registered or are restricted for use in the United States potentially could be imported in the fruits, vegetables, and seafood produced abroad.

Health Impact of Poor Air Quality

Poor air quality contributes to respiratory illness, cardiovascular disease, and cancer. For example, asthma can be triggered or worsened by exposure to ozone and ETS. The overall death rate from asthma increased 57 percent between 1980 and 1993, and for children it increased 67 percent.

Air Pollution. Dramatic improvements in air quality in the United States have occurred over the past three decades. Between 1970 and 1997, total emissions of the six principal air pollutants decreased 31 percent. Still, million of tons of toxic pollutants are released into the air each year from automobiles, industry, and other sources. In 1997, despite continued improvements in air quality, approximately 120 million people lived in areas with unhealthy air based on established standards for one or more commonly found air pollutants, including ozone. In 1996, a disproportionate number of Hispanics and Asian and Pacific Islanders lived in areas that failed to meet these standards compared with whites, African Americans, and American Indians or Alaska Natives.

Tobacco Smoke. Exposure to ETS, or secondhand smoke, among nonsmokers is widespread. Home and workplace environments are major sources of exposure. A total of 15 million children are estimated to have been exposed to secondhand smoke in their homes in 1996. ETS increases the risk of heart disease and respiratory infections in children and is responsible for an estimated 3,000 cancer deaths of adult nonsmokers.

Improvement in Environmental Quality

In the United States, ensuring clean water, safe food, and effective waste management has contributed greatly to a declining threat from many infectious diseases; however, there is still more that can be done. Work to improve the air quality and to understand better threats such as chronic, low-level exposures to hazardous substances also must continue.

For more information on Healthy People 2010 objectives or on environmental quality, visit http://www.health.gov/healthypeople/ or call 1-800-336-4797.

Immunization

Leading Health Indicator

Vaccines are among the greatest public health achievements of the 20th century. Immunizations can prevent disability and death from infectious diseases for individuals and can help control the spread of infections within communities.

In 1998, 73 percent of children received all vaccines recommended for universal administration.

In 1998, influenza immunization rates were 64 percent in adults aged 65 years and older—almost double the 1989 immunization rate of 33 percent. In 1998, only 46 percent of persons aged 65 years and older ever had received a pneumococcal vaccine.

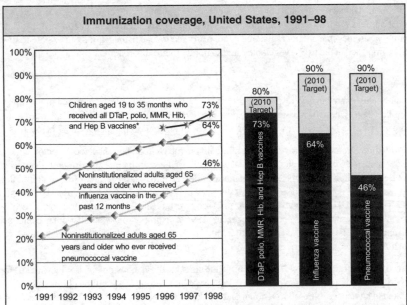

Immunization coverage, United States, 1991–98

Children aged 19 to 35 months who received all DTaP, polio, MMR, Hib, and Hep B vaccines* — 73%, 64%

Noninstitutionalized adults aged 65 years and older who received influenza vaccine in the past 12 months — 46%

Noninstitutionalized adults aged 65 years and older who ever received pneumococcal vaccine

Bars: DTaP, polio, MMR, Hib, and Hep B vaccines — 80% (2010 Target), 73%; Influenza vaccine — 90% (2010 Target), 64%; Pneumococcal vaccine — 90% (2010 Target), 46%

*Four or more doses of diphtheria/tetanus/acellular pertussis (DTaP) vaccine, three or more doses of polio vaccine, one or more dose of measles/mumps/rubella (MMR) vaccine, three or more doses of *Haemophilus influenzae* type b (Hib) vaccine, and three or more doses of hepatitis B (Hep B) vaccine.

Sources: Centers for Disease Control and Prevention, National Center for Health Statistics and National Immunization Program. National Immunization Survey. 1996–98. Centers for Disease Control and Prevention, National Center for Health Statistics. National Health Interview Survey. 1991–98.

The objectives selected to measure progress among children and adults for this Leading Health Indicator are presented below. These are only indicators and do not represent all the immunization and infectious diseases objectives in Healthy People 2010.

14-24a. Increase the proportion of young children who receive all vaccines that have been recommended for universal administration for at least 5 years.

14-29a, b. Increase the proportion of noninstitutionalized adults who are vaccinated annually against influenza and ever vaccinated against pneumococcal disease.

Healthy People 2010: Understanding and Improving Health

Impact of Immunization

Many once-common vaccine-preventable diseases now are controlled. Smallpox has been eradicated, poliomyelitis has been eliminated from the Western Hemisphere, and measles cases in the United States are at a record low.

Immunizations against influenza and pneumococcal disease can prevent serious illness and death. Pneumonia and influenza deaths together constitute the sixth leading cause of death in the United States. Influenza causes an average of 110,000 hospitalizations and 20,000 deaths annually; pneumococcal disease causes 10,000 to 14,000 deaths annually.

Recommended Immunizations

As of November 1, 1999, all children born in the United States (11,000 per day) should be receiving 12 to 16 doses of vaccine by age 2 years to be protected against 10 vaccine-preventable childhood diseases. This recommendation will change in the years ahead as new vaccines are developed, including combinations of current vaccines that may even reduce the number of necessary shots.

Recommended immunizations for adults aged 65 years and older include a yearly immunization against influenza (the "flu shot") and a one-time immunization against pneumococcal disease. Most of the deaths and serious illnesses caused by influenza and pneumococcal disease occur in older adults and others at increased risk for complications of these diseases because of other risk factors or medical conditions.

Trends in Immunization

National coverage levels in children now are greater than 90 percent for each immunization recommended during the first 2 years of life, except for hepatitis B and varicella vaccines. The hepatitis B immunization rate in children was 87 percent in 1998—the highest level ever reported. In 1998, 70 percent of children aged 19 to 35 months from the lowest income households received the combined series of recommended immunizations, compared with 77 percent of children from higher income households.

Both influenza and pneumococcal immunization rates are significantly lower for African American and Hispanic adults than for white adults.

Other Immunization Issues

Coverage levels for immunizations in adults are not as high as those achieved in children, yet the health effects may be just as great. Barriers to adult immunization include not knowing immunizations are needed, misconceptions about vaccines, and lack of recommendations from health care providers.

For more information on Healthy People 2010 objectives or on immunization and infectious diseases, visit http://www.health.gov/healthypeople/ or call 1-800-336-4797.

Access to Health Care

Leading Health Indicator

Strong predictors of access to quality health care include having health insurance, a higher income level, and a regular primary care provider or other source of ongoing health care. Use of clinical preventive services, such as early prenatal care, can serve as indicators of access to quality health care services.

In 1997, 83 percent of all persons under age 65 years had health insurance. In 1998, 87 percent of persons of all ages had a usual source of health care. Also in that year, 83 percent of pregnant women received prenatal care in the first trimester of pregnancy.

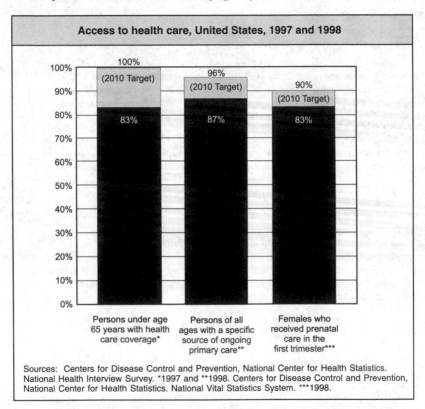

The objectives selected to measure progress for this Leading Health Indicator are presented below. These are only indicators and do not represent all the access to quality health services objectives in Healthy People 2010.

1-1. Increase the proportion of persons with health insurance.
1-4a. Increase the proportion of persons who have a specific source of ongoing care.
16-6a. Increase the proportion of pregnant women who begin prenatal care in the first trimester of pregnancy.

Health Insurance

Health insurance provides access to health care. Persons with health insurance are more likely to have a primary care provider and to have received appropriate preventive care such as a recent Pap test, immunization, or early prenatal care. Adults with health insurance are twice as likely to receive a routine checkup as are adults without health insurance.

More than 44 million persons in the United States do not have health insurance, including 11 million uninsured children. Over the past decade, the proportion of persons under age 65 years with health insurance remained steady at about 85 percent. About one-third of adults under age 65 years below the poverty level were uninsured. For persons of Hispanic origin, approximately one in three was without health insurance coverage in 1997. Mexican Americans had one of the highest uninsured rates at 40 percent.

Ongoing Sources of Primary Care

More than 40 million Americans do not have a particular doctor's office, clinic, health center, or other place where they usually go to seek health care or health-related advice. Even among privately insured persons, a significant number lacked a usual source of care or reported difficulty in accessing needed care due to financial constraints or insurance problems.

People aged 18 to 24 years were the most likely to lack a usual source of ongoing primary care. Only 80 percent of individuals below the poverty level and 79 percent of Hispanics had a usual source of ongoing primary care.

Barriers to Access

Financial, structural, and personal barriers can limit access to health care. Financial barriers include not having health insurance, not having enough health insurance to cover needed services, or not having the financial capacity to cover services outside a health plan or insurance program. Structural barriers include the lack of primary care providers, medical specialists, or other health care professionals to meet special needs or the lack of health care facilities. Personal barriers include cultural or spiritual differences, language barriers, not knowing what to do or when to seek care, or concerns about confidentiality or discrimination.

For more information on Healthy People 2010 objectives or on access to health care, visit http://www.health.gov/healthypeople/ or call 1-800-336-4797.

Bibliography

Introduction

McGinnis, J.M., and Maiese, D.R. Defining mission, goals, and objectives. In: Scutchfield, F.D., and Keck, C.W., eds. *Principles of Public Health Practice*. Albany, NY: Delmar Publishers, 1997, 140-141.

A Systematic Approach to Health Improvement

Goals

American College of Physicians. Rural primary care. *Annals of Internal Medicine* 122(5):380-390, 1995.

American Medical Association Council Report. Health care needs of gay men and lesbians in the United States. *Journal of the American Medical Association* 247:1354-1359, 1996.

Centers for Disease Control and Prevention (CDC). Behavioral Risk Factor Surveillance System Prevalence Data, 1998. <http://ww2.cdc.gov/nccdphp/brfss/index.asp>.

CDC. Health-related quality of life and activity limitation—eight states, 1995. *Morbidity and Mortality Weekly Report* 47(7):134-140, 1998.

CDC. Health-related quality-of-life measures—United States, 1993. *Morbidity and Mortality Weekly Report* 44:195-200, 1995.

U.S. Department of Health and Human Services (HHS). Terminology, Focus Area 6. Disability and Secondary Conditions. *Healthy People 2010*. 2nd ed. Vol. I. Washington, DC: U.S. Government Printing Office (GPO), November 2000, 24-25.

Institute of Medicine (IOM). *Improving Health in the Community*. Washington, DC: National Academy Press, 1997, 48-56.

National Center for Health Statistics (NCHS). *Health, United States, 1999*. With health and aging chartbook. Hyattsville, MD: HHS, 1999.

NCHS. *Healthy People 2000 Review, 1998-99*. Hyattsville, MD: HHS, 1999.

Barker, W.H. Prevention of disability in older persons. In: Wallace, R.B., ed. *Public Health and Preventive Medicine*. 14th ed. Stamford, CT: Appleton & Lange, 1998, 1063.

Braden, J., and Beauregard, K. *Health Status and Access to Care of Rural and Urban Populations*. AHCPR Pub. No. 94-0031. Rockville, MD: Public Health Service (PHS), Agency for Health Care Policy and Research (AHCPR), 1994.

Catalan, J., and Pugh, K. Suicidal behaviour and HIV infection—is there a link? *AIDS Care* 7(Suppl. 2):S117-S121, 1995.

Cochran, S.D., and Mays, V.M. Depressive distress among homosexually active African American men and women. *American Journal of Psychiatry* 151:524-529, 1994.

Davidson, L., and Linnoila, M., eds. *Report of the Secretary's Task Force on Youth Suicide, 2: Risk Factors for Youth Suicide*. Washington, DC: HHS, PHS, 1989.

Frumkin, H., and Walker, E.D. Minority workers and communities. In: Wallace, R.B., ed. *Public Health and Preventive Medicine*. 14th ed. Stamford, CT: Appleton & Lange, 1998, 685.

Hoyert, D.L.; Kochanek, K.D.; and Murphy, S.L. Deaths: Final data for 1997. *National Vital Statistics Reports* 47(19):1999.

Idler, E.L., and Benyamini, Y. Self-rated health and mortality: A review of twenty-seven community studies. *Journal of Health and Social Behavior* 38:21-37, 1997.

LaPlante, M.P.; Rice, D.P.; and Cyril, J. Health insurance coverage of people with disabilities in the U.S. *Disability Statistics Abstract.* Disability Statistics Rehabilitation. San Francisco, CA: Research and Training Center, 1994.

Last, J.M. The determinants of health. In: Scutchfield, F.D., and Keck, C.W., eds. *Principles of Public Health Practice.* Albany, NY: Delmar Publishers, 1997, 33-34.

Luepker, R.V. Heart disease. In: Wallace, R.B., ed. *Public Health and Preventive Medicine.* 14th ed. Stamford, CT: Appleton & Lange, 1998, 939-940.

McNeil, J.M. Americans with disabilities: 1994–95. *Current Population Reports.* Bureau of the Census (P70-61). Washington, DC: U.S. Department of Commerce, 1997.

Pamuk, E.; Makuc, D.; Heck, K.; et al. *Socioeconomic Status and Health Chartbook. Health, United States, 1998.* Hyattsville, MD: NCHS, 1998.

Pearson, T.A., and Lewis, C. Rural epidemiology: Insights from a rural population laboratory. *American Journal of Epidemiology* 148(10):949-957, 1998.

Solarz, A., ed. *Lesbian Health: Current Assessment and Directions for the Future.* Washington, DC: IOM, 1997.

Syme, S.L., and Balfour, J.L. Social determinants of disease. In: Wallace, R.B., ed. *Public Health and Preventive Medicine.* 14th ed. Stamford, CT: Appleton & Lange, 1998, 800-801.

Tissue, T. Another look at self-rated health among the elderly. *Journal of Gerontology* 27:91-94, 1972.

Vistnes, J.P., and Monheit, A.C. *Health Insurance Status of the Civilian Noninstitutionalized Population.* AHCPR Pub. No. 97-0030. Rockville, MD: AHCPR, 1997.

Determinants of Health

IOM. *Improving Health in the Community.* Washington, DC: National Academy Press, 1997, 48-56.

McGinnis, J.M., and Maiese, D.R. Defining mission, goals, and objectives. In: Scutchfield, F.D., and Keck, C.W., eds. *Principles of Public Health Practice.* Albany, NY: Delmar Publishers, 1997, 136-145.

Syme, S.L., and Balfour, J.L. Social determinants of disease. In: Wallace, R.B., ed. *Public Health and Preventive Medicine.* 14th ed. Stamford, CT: Appleton & Lange, 1998, 795.

Health Status

NCHS. *Health, United States, 1999.* With health and aging chartbook. Hyattsville, MD: HHS, 1999.

McGinnis, J.M., and Foege, W.H. Actual causes of death in the United States. *Journal of the American Medical Association* 270:2207-2212, 1993.

Physical Activity

CDC. Physical activity and the prevention of coronary heart disease. *Morbidity and Mortality Weekly Review* 42:669-672, 1993.

CDC. Prevalence of sedentary leisure-time behavior among adults in the United States. *Health E-Stats.* Atlanta, GA: CDC, NCHS, 1999.

NCHS. *Health, United States, 1999.* With health and aging chartbook. Hyattsville, MD: HHS, 1999.

NCHS. *Healthy People 2000 Review, 1998–99.* Hyattsville, MD: HHS, 1999.

HHS. *Physical Activity and Health: A Report of the Surgeon General.* Atlanta, GA: CDC, National Center for Chronic Disease Prevention and Health Promotion (NCCDPHP), 1996.

Pamuk, E.; Makuc, D.; Heck, K.; et al. *Socioeconomic Status and Health Chartbook. Health, United States, 1998.* Hyattsville, MD: NCHS, 1998.

Overweight and Obesity

Agricultural Research Service. Research News. Press release, U.S. Department of Agriculture (USDA), Washington, DC, November 20, 1996.

NCHS. *Health, United States, 1999.* With health and aging chartbook. Hyattsville, MD: HHS, 1999.

NCHS. *Healthy People 2000 Review, 1998–99.* Hyattsville, MD: HHS, 1999.

National Institutes of Health (NIH). *Statistics Related to Overweight and Obesity.* NIH Publication No. 96-4158. Bethesda, MD: HHS, National Institute of Diabetes and Digestive and Kidney Diseases, 1996.

USDA and HHS. *Dietary Guidelines for Americans.* 4th ed. USDA Home and Garden Bulletin No. 232. December 1995.

Lin, B.H., and Frazao, E. Nutritional quality of foods at and away from home. *Food Review* 20(2):33-40, 1997.

Pamuk, E.; Makuc, D.; Heck, K.; et al. *Socioeconomic Status and Health Chartbook. Health, United States, 1998.* Hyattsville, MD: NCHS, 1998.

Wolf, A.M., and Colditz, G.A. Current estimates of the economic cost of obesity in the United States. *Obesity Research* 6(2):97-106, 1998.

Tobacco Use

CDC. Guidelines for school health programs to prevent tobacco use and addiction. *Morbidity and Mortality Weekly Report* 43(RR-2), 1994.

CDC. Smoking-attributable mortality and years of potential life lost—United States, 1984. *Morbidity and Mortality Weekly Report* 46(20):441-451, 1997.

CDC. *Targeting Tobacco Use: The Nation's Leading Cause of Death.* Atlanta, GA: HHS, CDC, 1999.

CDC. Youth Risk Behavior Surveillance—United States, 1997. *Morbidity and Mortality Weekly Report* 47(SS-3):1998.

NCHS. *Health, United States, 1999.* With health and aging chartbook. Hyattsville, MD: HHS, 1999.

National Cancer Institute. *Cigars: Health Effects and Trends.* Bethesda, MD: HHS, NIH, 1998.

U.S. Environmental Protection Agency (EPA). *Respiratory Health Effects of Passive Smoking: Fact Sheet.* EPA Pub. No. EPA-43-F-93-003. Washington, DC: EPA, 1993.

HHS. *Tobacco Use Among U.S. Racial/Ethnic Minority Groups—African Americans, American Indians and Alaska Natives, Asian Americans and Pacific Islanders, and Hispanics: A Report of the Surgeon General.* Atlanta, GA: HHS, CDC, NCCDPHP, Office on Smoking and Health, 1998.

Substance Abuse

Center for Substance Abuse Prevention (CSAP), Substance Abuse and Mental Health Services Administration (SAMHSA). *Making the Link: Health Care Costs, the Deficit, & Alcohol, Tobacco, and Other Drugs.* NCADI Inventory No. ML007. Rockville, MD: CSAP, 1995.

SAMHSA. *Summary of Findings From the 1998 National Household Survey on Drug Abuse.* Rockville, MD: HHS, SAMHSA, Office of Applied Studies, 1999.

Harwood, H.; Fountain, D.; and Livermore, G. *The Economic Costs of Alcohol and Drug Abuse in the United States, 1992.* NIH Pub. No. 98-4327. Rockville, MD: HHS, NIH, 1998.

Responsible Sexual Behavior

American Social Health Association. *Sexually Transmitted Diseases in America: How Many Cases and At What Cost?* Menlo Park, CA: Kaiser Family Foundation, 1998.

CDC. CDC guidelines for national human immunodeficiency virus case surveillance, including monitoring for human immunodeficiency virus infection and acquired immunodeficiency syndrome. *Morbidity and Mortality Weekly Report* 48(RR013), 1999.

CDC. Fact sheet. *Youth Risk Behavior Trends.* Atlanta, GA: HHS, CDC, NCCDPHP, 1999.

CDC. *From Data to Action: CDC's Public Health Surveillance for Women, Infants, and Children.* Atlanta, GA: HHS, CDC, NCCDPHP, 1994.

CDC. *HIV/AIDS Surveillance Report.* Midyear ed. Atlanta, GA: HHS, CDC, 1999.

CDC. *PRAMS 1996 Surveillance Report.* Atlanta, GA: CDC, NCCDPHP, Division of Reproductive Health, 1999.

CDC. Trends in sexual risk behaviors among high school students—United States, 1991–1997. *Morbidity and Mortality Weekly Report* 47(36):749-752, 1998.

CDC. Young people at risk—epidemic shifts further toward young women and minorities. In: *CDC Update.* Atlanta, GA: HHS, CDC, National Center for HIV, STD, and TB Prevention, 1999.

CDC, Division of STD Prevention. *Sexually Transmitted Disease Surveillance, 1998.* Atlanta, GA: HHS, CDC, 1999.

NCHS. *Healthy People 2000 Review, 1998–99.* Hyattsville, MD: HHS, 1999.

Holtgrave, D.R., and Pinkerton, S.D. Updates of cost of illness and quality of life estimates for use in economic evaluations of HIV prevention programs. *Journal of Acquired Immune Deficiency Syndromes and Human Retrovirology* 16(1):54-62, 1997.

Hoyert, D.L.; Kochanek, K.D.; and Murphy, S.L. Deaths: Final data for 1997. *National Vital Statistics Reports* 47(19), 1999.

Maynard, R.A., ed. *Kids Having Kids; Economic Costs and Social Consequences of Teen Pregnancy.* Washington, DC: Urban Institute Press, 1997.

St. Louis, M.E.; Wasserheit, J.N.; and Gayle, H.D. Janus considers the HIV pandemic—harnessing recent advances to enhance AIDS prevention. *American Journal of Public Health* 87(1):10-12, 1997.

Mental Health

NCHS. *Healthy People 2000 Review, 1998–99.* Hyattsville, MD: HHS, 1999.

NIH, Consensus Development Panel on Depression in Late Life. Diagnosis and treatment of depression in late life. *Journal of the American Medical Association* 268:1018-1024, 1992.

National Institute of Mental Health (NIMH). *Depression.* Bethesda, MD: HHS, NIH, 1999. <http://www.nimh.nih.gov/depression/index.htm>.

NIMH. *The Invisible Disease—Depression.* Bethesda, MD: HHS, NIH, 1999. <http://www.nimh.nih.gov/publicat/invisible.cfm>.

SAMHSA, Office of Applied Studies. In: Rouse, B.A., ed. *SAMHSA Statistics Source Book, 1998.* Rockville, MD: HHS, 1998.

SAMHSA. *Mental Health: A Report of the Surgeon General.* Rockville, MD: HHS, NIH, 1999.

Bromet, E.J. Psychiatric disorders. In: Wallace, R.B., ed. *Public Health and Preventive Medicine.* 14th ed. Stamford, CT: Appleton & Lange, 1998, 1037.

Greenberg, P.E.; Stiglin, L.E.; Finkelstein, S.N.; et al. The economic burden of depression in 1990. *Journal of Clinical Psychiatry* 54:405-418, 1993.

Koenig, H.G., and Blazer, D.G. Mood disorders and suicide. In: Birren, J.E.; Sloane, R.B.; and Cohen, G.D.; eds. *Handbook of Mental Health and Aging.* 2nd ed. San Diego, CA: Academic Press, 1992, 379-407.

Weissman, M.M., and Klerman, J.K. Depression: Current understanding and changing trends. *Annual Review of Public Health* 13:319-339, 1992.

Injury and Violence

NCHS. *Healthy People 2000 Review, 1998–99.* Hyattsville, MD: HHS, 1999.

National Center for Injury Prevention and Control. *Impaired Driving Fact Sheet.* Atlanta, GA: HHS, CDC, 1999.

National Highway Traffic Safety Administration. *Traffic Safety Facts, 1998.* Washington, DC: U.S. Department of Transportation, 1998.

National Safety Council. *Accident Facts.* Washington, DC: the Council, 1995.

Baker, S.P.; O'Neill, B.; Ginsburg, M.J.; et al. *The Injury Fact Book.* 2nd ed. New York, NY: Oxford University Press, 1992.

Fox, J.A., and Zawitz, M.W. *Homicide Trends in the United States.* U.S. Department of Justice, Bureau of Justice Statistics, 1999.

Hoyert, D.L.; Kochanek, K.D.; and Murphy, S.L. Deaths: Final data for 1997. *National Vital Statistics Reports* 47(19), 1999.

Environmental Quality

American Lung Association. *Health Costs of Air Pollution.* Washington, DC: the Association, 1990.

California Environmental Protection Agency. *Health Effects of Exposure to Environmental Tobacco Smoke.* Final report. Sacramento, CA: the Agency, Office of Environmental Health Hazard Assessment, 1997.

CDC. Progress toward the elimination of tuberculosis—United States, 1998. *Morbidity and Mortality Weekly Report* 48:732-736, 1999.

CDC. State-specific prevalence of cigarette smoking among adults, and children's and adolescents' exposure to environmental tobacco smoke—United States. *Morbidity and Mortality Weekly Report* 46:1038-1043, 1997.

NCHS. *Health, United States, 1999.* With health and aging chartbook. Hyattsville, MD: HHS, 1999.

EPA. *National Air Quality and Trends Report.* Washington, DC: EPA, Office of Air and Radiation, 1997.

EPA. *Respiratory Health Effects of Passive Smoking: Lung Cancer and Other Disorders.* EPA Pub. No. EPA/600/6-90/006F. Washington, DC: EPA, 1992.

World Health Organization (WHO). Fact Sheet 170. Geneva, Switzerland: WHO, 1997.

Mannino, D.M.; Homa, D.M.; Pertowski, C.A.; et al. Surveillance for asthma—United States 1960–1995. In: CDC Surveillance Summaries, April 24, 1998. *Morbidity and Mortality Weekly Report* 47(SS-1):1-27, 1998.

Weiss, K.B.; Gergen, P.J; and Hodgson, T.A. An economic evaluation of asthma in the United States. *New England Journal of Medicine* 326:862-866, 1992.

Immunization

CDC, National Immunization Program, Immunization Services Division, Health Services Research and Evaluation Branch. Unpublished data, 1999.

CDC. National vaccination coverage levels among children aged 19-35 months—United States, 1998. *Morbidity and Mortality Weekly Report* 48:829-830, 1999.

CDC. Prevention and control of influenza: Recommendations of the Advisory Committee on Immunization Practices (ACIP). *Morbidity and Mortality Weekly Report* 48(RR-4), 1999.

CDC. Prevention of pneumococcal disease: Recommendations of the Advisory Committee on Immunization Practices (ACIP). *Morbidity and Mortality Weekly Report* 46(RR-8), 1997.

CDC. Reasons reported by Medicare beneficiaries for not receiving influcnza and pneumococcal vaccinations—United States, 1996. *Morbidity and Mortality Weekly Report* 48:886-890, 1999.

CDC. Recommended childhood immunization schedule—United States, 1999. *Morbidity and Mortality Weekly Report* 48:12-16, 1999.

CDC. Ten great public health achievements—United States, 1900–1999. *Morbidity and Mortality Weekly Report* 48:241-248, 1999.

NCHS. *Health, United States, 1999.* With health and aging chartbook. Hyattsville, MD: HHS, 1999.

Feiken, D.R.; Schuchat, A.; Kolczak, M.; et al. Mortality from invasive pneumococcal pneumonia in the era of antibiotic resistance, 1995–1997. *American Journal of Public Health,* in press.

Pamuk, E.; Makuc, D.; Heck, K.; et al. *Socioeconomic Status and Health Chartbook. Health, United States, 1998.* Hyattsville, MD: NCHS, 1998.

Access to Health Care

CDC. Health insurance coverage and receipt of preventive health services—United States, 1993. *Morbidity and Mortality Weekly Report* 44(11):219-225, 1995.

NCHS. *Health, United States, 1999.* With health and aging chartbook.Hyattsville, MD: HHS, 1999.

U.S. General Accounting Office (GAO). *Health Insurance: Coverage Leads to Increased Health Care Access for Children.* GAO/HEHS-98-14. Washington, DC: GAO, 1998, 4-20.

The Kaiser Commission on Medicaid and the Uninsured. *Uninsured in America: A Chart Book.* 2nd ed. Menlo Park, CA: the Commission, 2000.

Appendix: Short Titles for Healthy People 2010 Objectives

1. Access to Quality Health Services

Goal: Improve access to comprehensive, high-quality health care services.

Objective Number and Short Title

Clinical Preventive Care
1-1   Persons with health insurance
1-2   Health insurance coverage for clinical preventive services
1-3   Counseling about health behaviors

Primary Care
1-4   Source of ongoing care
1-5   Usual primary care provider
1-6   Difficulties or delays in obtaining needed health care
1-7   Core competencies in health provider training
1-8   Racial and ethnic representation in health professions
1-9   Hospitalization for ambulatory-care-sensitive conditions

Emergency Services
1-10   Delay or difficulty in getting emergency care
1-11   Rapid prehospital emergency care
1-12   Single toll-free number for poison control centers
1-13   Trauma care systems
1-14   Special needs of children

Long-Term Care and Rehabilitative Services
1-15   Long-term care services
1-16   Pressure ulcers among nursing home residents

2. Arthritis, Osteoporosis, and Chronic Back Conditions

Goal: Prevent illness and disability related to arthritis and other rheumatic conditions, osteoporosis, and chronic back conditions.

Objective Number and Short Title

Arthritis and Other Rheumatic Conditions
2-1   Mean number of days without severe pain
2-2   Activity limitations due to arthritis
2-3   Personal care limitations
2-4   Help in coping
2-5   Employment rate
2-6   Racial differences in total knee replacement
2-7   Seeing a health care provider
2-8   Arthritis education

Osteoporosis
2-9   Cases of osteoporosis
2-10   Hospitalization for vertebral fractures

Chronic Back Conditions
2-11   Activity limitations due to chronic back conditions

3. Cancer

Goal: Reduce the number of new cancer cases as well as the illness, disability, and death caused by cancer.

Objective Number and Short Title
3-1   Overall cancer deaths
3-2   Lung cancer deaths
3-3   Breast cancer deaths
3-4   Cervical cancer deaths
3-5   Colorectal cancer deaths
3-6   Oropharyngeal cancer deaths
3-7   Prostate cancer deaths
3-8   Melanoma deaths
3-9   Sun exposure and skin cancer
3-10   Provider counseling about cancer prevention

3-11	Pap tests
3-12	Colorectal cancer screening
3-13	Mammograms
3-14	Statewide cancer registries
3-15	Cancer survival

4. Chronic Kidney Disease

Goal: Reduce new cases of chronic kidney disease and its complications, disability, death, and economic costs.

Objective Number and Short Title

4-1	End-stage renal disease
4-2	Cardiovascular disease deaths in persons with chronic kidney failure
4-3	Counseling for chronic kidney failure care
4-4	Use of arteriovenous fistulas
4-5	Registration for kidney transplantation
4-6	Waiting time for kidney transplantation
4-7	Kidney failure due to diabetes
4-8	Medical therapy for persons with diabetes and proteinuria

5. Diabetes

Goal: Through prevention programs, reduce the disease and economic burden of diabetes, and improve the quality of life for all persons who have or are at risk for diabetes.

Objective Number and Short Title

5-1	Diabetes education
5-2	New cases of diabetes
5-3	Overall cases of diagnosed diabetes
5-4	Diagnosis of diabetes
5-5	Diabetes deaths
5-6	Diabetes-related deaths
5-7	Cardiovascular disease deaths in persons with diabetes
5-8	Gestational diabetes
5-9	Foot ulcers
5-10	Lower extremity amputations
5-11	Annual urinary microalbumin measurement
5-12	Annual glycosylated hemoglobin measurement
5-13	Annual dilated eye examinations
5-14	Annual foot examinations
5-15	Annual dental examinations
5-16	Aspirin therapy
5-17	Self-blood-glucose-monitoring

6. Disability and Secondary Conditions

Goal: Promote the health of people with disabilities, prevent secondary conditions, and eliminate disparities between people with and without disabilities in the U.S. population.

Objective Number and Short Title

6-1	Standard definition of people with disabilities in data sets
6-2	Feelings and depression among children with disabilities
6-3	Feelings and depression interfering with activities among adults with disabilities
6-4	Social participation among adults with disabilities
6-5	Sufficient emotional support among adults with disabilities
6-6	Satisfaction with life among adults with disabilities
6-7	Congregate care of children and adults with disabilities
6-8	Employment parity
6-9	Inclusion of children and youth with disabilities in regular education programs
6-10	Accessibility of health and wellness programs
6-11	Assistive devices and technology
6-12	Environmental barriers affecting participation in activities
6-13	Surveillance and health promotion programs

7. Educational and Community-Based Programs

Goal: Increase the quality, availability, and effectiveness of educational and community-based programs designed to prevent disease and improve health and quality of life.

Objective Number and Short Title

School Setting

7-1	High school completion
7-2	School health education
7-3	Health-risk behavior information for college and university students
7-4	School nurse-to-student ratio

Worksite Setting

7-5	Worksite health promotion programs
7-6	Participation in employer-sponsored health promotion activities

Health Care Setting

7-7   Patient and family education

7-8   Satisfaction with patient education

7-9   Health care organization sponsorship of community health promotion activities

Community Setting and Select Populations

7-10   Community health promotion programs

7-11   Culturally appropriate and linguistically competent community health promotion programs

7-12   Older adult participation in community health promotion activities

8. Environmental Health

Goal: Promote health for all through a healthy environment.

Objective Number and Short Title

Outdoor Air Quality

8-1   Harmful air pollutants

8-2   Alternative modes of transportation

8-3   Cleaner alternative fuels

8-4   Airborne toxins

Water Quality

8-5   Safe drinking water

8-6   Waterborne disease outbreaks

8-7   Water conservation

8-8   Surface water health risks

8-9   Beach closings

8-10   Fish contamination

Toxics and Waste

8-11   Elevated blood lead levels in children

8-12   Risks posed by hazardous sites

8-13   Pesticide exposures

8-14   Toxic pollutants

8-15   Recycled municipal solid waste

Healthy Homes and Healthy Communities

8-16   Indoor allergens

8-17   Office building air quality

8-18   Homes tested for radon

8-19   Radon-resistant new home construction

8-20   School policies to protect against environmental hazards

8-21   Disaster preparedness plans and protocols

8-22   Lead-based paint testing

8-23   Substandard housing

Infrastructure and Surveillance

8-24   Exposure to pesticides

8-25   Exposure to heavy metals and other toxic chemicals

8-26   Information systems used for environmental health

8-27   Monitoring environmentally related diseases

8-28   Local agencies using surveillance data for vector control

Global Environmental Health

8-29   Global burden of disease

8-30   Water quality in the U.S.-Mexico border region

9. Family Planning

Goal: Improve pregnancy planning and spacing and prevent unintended pregnancy.

Objective Number and Short Title

9-1   Intended pregnancy

9-2   Birth spacing

9-3   Contraceptive use

9-4   Contraceptive failure

9-5   Emergency contraception

9-6   Male involvement in pregnancy prevention

9-7   Adolescent pregnancy

9-8   Abstinence before age 15 years

9-9   Abstinence among adolescents aged 15 to 17 years

9-10   Pregnancy prevention and sexually transmitted disease (STD) protection

9-11   Pregnancy prevention education

9-12   Problems in becoming pregnant and maintaining a pregnancy

9-13   Insurance coverage for contraceptive supplies and services

10. Food Safety

Goal: Reduce foodborne illnesses.

Objective Number and Short Title

10-1   Foodborne infections

10-2   Outbreaks of foodborne infections

10-3   Antimicrobial resistance of *Salmonella* species

10-4   Food allergy deaths

10-5   Consumer food safety practices

10-6   Safe food preparation practices in retail establishments

10-7   Organophosphate pesticide exposure

11. Health Communication

Goal: Use communication strategically to improve health.

Objective Number and Short Title

11-1 Households with Internet access
11-2 Health literacy
11-3 Research and evaluation of communication programs
11-4 Quality of Internet health information sources
11-5 Centers for excellence
11-6 Satisfaction with health care providers' communication skills

12. Heart Disease and Stroke

Goal: Improve cardiovascular health and quality of life through the prevention, detection, and treatment of risk factors; early identification and treatment of heart attacks and strokes; and prevention of recurrent cardiovascular events.

Objective Number and Short Title

Heart Disease

12-1 Coronary heart disease (CHD) deaths
12-2 Knowledge of symptoms of heart attack and importance of calling 911
12-3 Artery-opening therapy
12-4 Bystander response to cardiac arrest
12-5 Out-of-hospital emergency care
12-6 Heart failure hospitalizations

Stroke

12-7 Stroke deaths
12-8 Knowledge of early warning symptoms of stroke

Blood Pressure

12-9 High blood pressure
12-10 High blood pressure control
12-11 Action to help control blood pressure
12-12 Blood pressure monitoring

Cholesterol

12-13 Mean total blood cholesterol levels
12-14 High blood cholesterol levels
12-15 Blood cholesterol screening
12-16 LDL-cholesterol level in CHD patients

13. HIV

Goal: Prevent HIV infection and its related illness and death.

Objective Number and Short Title

13-1 New AIDS cases
13-2 AIDS among men who have sex with men
13-3 AIDS among persons who inject drugs
13-4 AIDS among men who have sex with men and who inject drugs
13-5 New HIV cases
13-6 Condom use
13-7 Knowledge of serostatus
13-8 HIV counseling and education for persons in substance abuse treatment
13-9 HIV/AIDS, STD, and TB education in State prisons
13-10 HIV counseling and testing in State prisons
13-11 HIV testing in TB patients
13-12 Screening for STDs and immunization for hepatitis B
13-13 Treatment according to guidelines
13-14 HIV-infection deaths
13-15 Interval between HIV infection and AIDS diagnosis
13-16 Interval between AIDS diagnosis and death from AIDS
13-17 Perinatally acquired HIV infection

14. Immunization and Infectious Diseases

Goal: Prevent disease, disability, and death from infectious diseases, including vaccine-preventable diseases.

Objective Number and Short Title

Diseases Preventable Through Universal Vaccination

14-1 Vaccine-preventable diseases
14-2 Hepatitis B in infants and young children
14-3 Hepatitis B in adults and high-risk groups
14-4 Bacterial meningitis in young children
14-5 Invasive pneumococcal infections

Diseases Preventable Through Targeted Vaccination

14-6 Hepatitis A
14-7 Meningococcal disease
14-8 Lyme disease

Infectious Diseases and Emerging Antimicrobial Resistance

14-9 Hepatitis C
14-10 Identification of persons with chronic hepatitis C
14-11 Tuberculosis
14-12 Curative therapy for tuberculosis
14-13 Treatment for high-risk persons with latent tuberculosis infection

14-14 Timely laboratory confirmation of tuberculosis cases
14-15 Prevention services for international travelers
14-16 Invasive early onset group B streptococcal disease
14-17 Peptic ulcer hospitalizations
14-18 Antibiotics prescribed for ear infections
14-19 Antibiotics prescribed for common cold
14-20 Hospital-acquired infections
14-21 Antimicrobial use in intensive care units

Vaccination Coverage and Strategies

14-22 Universally recommended vaccination of children aged 19 to 35 months
14-23 Vaccination coverage for children in day care, kindergarten, and first grade
14-24 Fully immunized young children and adolescents
14-25 Providers who measure childhood vaccination coverage levels
14-26 Children participating in population-based immunization registries
14-27 Vaccination coverage among adolescents
14-28 Hepatitis B vaccination among high-risk groups
14-29 Influenza and pneumococcal vaccination of high-risk adults

Vaccine Safety

14-30 Adverse events from vaccinations
14-31 Active surveillance for vaccine safety

15. Injury and Violence Prevention

Goal: Reduce injuries, disabilities, and deaths due to unintentional injuries and violence.

Objective Number and Short Title

Injury Prevention

15-1 Nonfatal head injuries
15-2 Nonfatal spinal cord injuries
15-3 Firearm-related deaths
15-4 Proper firearm storage in homes
15-5 Nonfatal firearm-related injuries
15-6 Child fatality review
15-7 Nonfatal poisonings
15-8 Deaths from poisoning
15-9 Deaths from suffocation
15-10 Emergency department surveillance systems
15-11 Hospital discharge surveillance systems
15-12 Emergency department visits

Unintentional Injury Prevention

15-13 Deaths from unintentional injuries
15-14 Nonfatal unintentional injuries
15-15 Deaths from motor vehicle crashes
15-16 Pedestrian deaths
15-17 Nonfatal motor vehicle injuries
15-18 Nonfatal pedestrian injuries
15-19 Safety belts
15-20 Child restraints
15-21 Motorcycle helmet use
15-22 Graduated driver licensing
15-23 Bicycle helmet use
15-24 Bicycle helmet laws
15-25 Residential fire deaths
15-26 Functioning smoke alarms in residences
15-27 Deaths from falls
15-28 Hip fractures
15-29 Drownings
15-30 Dog bite injuries
15-31 Injury protection in school sports

Violence and Abuse Prevention

15-32 Homicides
15-33 Maltreatment and maltreatment fatalities of children
15-34 Physical assault by intimate partners
15-35 Rape or attempted rape
15-36 Sexual assault other than rape
15-37 Physical assaults
15-38 Physical fighting among adolescents
15-39 Weapon carrying by adolescents on school property

16. Maternal, Infant, and Child Health

Goal: Improve the health and well-being of women, infants, children, and families.

Objective Number and Short Title

Fetal, Infant, Child, and Adolescent Deaths

16-1 Fetal and infant deaths
16-2 Child deaths
16-3 Adolescent and young adult deaths

Maternal Deaths and Illnesses

16-4 Maternal deaths
16-5 Maternal illness and complications due to pregnancy

Prenatal Care

16-6 Prenatal care
16-7 Childbirth classes

Obstetrical Care

16-8   Very low birth weight infants born at level III hospitals
16-9   Cesarean births

Risk Factors

16-10 Low birth weight and very low birth weight
16-11 Preterm births
16-12 Weight gain during pregnancy
16-13 Infants put to sleep on their backs

Developmental Disabilities and Neural Tube Defects

16-14 Developmental disabilities
16-15 Spina bifida and other neural tube defects
16-16 Optimum folic acid levels

Prenatal Substance Exposure

16-17 Prenatal substance exposure
16-18 Fetal alcohol syndrome

Breastfeeding, Newborn Screening, and Service Systems

16-19 Breastfeeding
16-20 Newborn bloodspot screening
16-21 Sepsis among children with sickle cell disease
16-22 Medical homes for children with special health care needs
16-23 Service systems for children with special health care needs

17. Medical Product Safety

Goal: Ensure the safe and effective use of medical products.

Objective Number and Short Title

17-1   Monitoring of adverse medical events
17-2   Linked, automated information systems
17-3   Provider review of medications taken by patients
17-4   Receipt of useful information about prescriptions from pharmacies
17-5   Receipt of oral counseling about medications from prescribers and dispensers
17-6   Blood donations

18. Mental Health and Mental Illness

Goal: Improve mental health and ensure access to appropriate, quality mental health services.

Objective Number and Short Title

Mental Health Status Improvement

18-1   Suicide
18-2   Adolescent suicide attempts
18-3   Serious mental illness (SMI) among homeless adults
18-4   Employment of persons with SMI
18-5   Eating disorder relapses

Treatment Expansion

18-6   Primary care screening and assessment
18-7   Treatment for children with mental health problems
18-8   Juvenile justice facility screening
18-9   Treatment for adults with mental disorders
18-10 Treatment for co-occurring disorders
18-11 Adult jail diversion programs

State Activities

18-12 State tracking of consumer satisfaction
18-13 State plans addressing cultural competence
18-14 State plans addressing elderly persons

19. Nutrition and Overweight

Goal: Promote health and reduce chronic disease associated with diet and weight.

Objective Number and Short Title

Weight Status and Growth

19-1   Healthy weight in adults
19-2   Obesity in adults
19-3   Overweight or obesity in children and adolescents
19-4   Growth retardation in children

Food and Nutrient Consumption

19-5   Fruit intake
19-6   Vegetable intake
19-7   Grain product intake
19-8   Saturated fat intake
19-9   Total fat intake
19-10 Sodium intake
19-11 Calcium intake

Iron Deficiency and Anemia

19-12 Iron deficiency in young children and in females of childbearing age
19-13 Anemia in low-income pregnant females
19-14 Iron deficiency in pregnant females

Schools, Worksites, and Nutrition Counseling

19-15 Meals and snacks at school
19-16 Worksite promotion of nutrition education and weight management
19-17 Nutrition counseling for medical conditions

Food Security

19-18 Food security

20. Occupational Safety and Health

Goal: Promote the health and safety of people at work through prevention and early intervention.

Objective Number and Short Title

20-1 Work-related injury deaths
20-2 Work-related injuries
20-3 Overexertion or repetitive motion
20-4 Pneumoconiosis deaths
20-5 Work-related homicides
20-6 Work-related assaults
20-7 Elevated blood lead levels from work exposure
20-8 Occupational skin diseases or disorders
20-9 Worksite stress reduction programs
20-10 Needlestick injuries
20-11 Work-related, noise-induced hearing loss

21. Oral Health

Goal: Prevent and control oral and craniofacial diseases, conditions, and injuries and improve access to related services.

Objective Number and Short Title

21-1 Dental caries experience
21-2 Untreated dental decay
21-3 No permanent tooth loss
21-4 Complete tooth loss
21-5 Periodontal diseases
21-6 Early detection of oral and pharyngeal cancers
21-7 Annual examinations for oral and pharyngeal cancers
21-8 Dental sealants
21-9 Community water fluoridation
21-10 Use of oral health care system
21-11 Use of oral health care system by residents in long-term care facilities

21-12 Dental services for low-income children
21-13 School-based health centers with oral health component
21-14 Health centers with oral health service components
21-15 Referral for cleft lip or palate
21-16 Oral and craniofacial State-based surveillance system
21-17 Tribal, State, and local dental programs

22. Physical Fitness and Activity

Goal: Improve health, fitness, and quality of life through daily physical activity.

Objective Number and Short Title

Physical Activity in Adults

22-1 No leisure-time physical activity
22-2 Moderate physical activity
22-3 Vigorous physical activity

Muscular Strength/Endurance and Flexibility

22-4 Muscular strength and endurance
22-5 Flexibility

Physical Activity in Children and Adolescents

22-6 Moderate physical activity in adolescents
22-7 Vigorous physical activity in adolescents
22-8 Physical education requirement in schools
22-9 Daily physical education in schools
22-10 Physical activity in physical education class
22-11 Television viewing

Access

22-12 School physical activity facilities
22-13 Worksite physical activity and fitness
22-14 Community walking
22-15 Community bicycling

23. Public Health Infrastructure

Goal: Ensure that Federal, Tribal, State, and local health agencies have the infrastructure to provide essential public health services effectively.

Objective Number and Short Title

Data and Information Systems

23-1 Public health employee access to the Internet
23-2 Public access to information and surveillance data
23-3 Use of geocoding in health data systems
23-4 Data for all population groups
23-5 Data for Leading Health Indicators, Health Status Indicators, and Priority Data Needs at Tribal, State, and local levels

23-6 National tracking of Healthy People 2010 objectives
23-7 Timely release of data on objectives

Workforce
23-8 Competencies for public health workers
23-9 Training in essential public health services
23-10 Continuing education and training by public health agencies

Public Health Organizations
23-11 Performance standards for essential public health services
23-12 Health improvement plans
23-13 Access to public health laboratory services
23-14 Access to epidemiology services
23-15 Model statutes related to essential public health services

Resources
23-16 Data on public health expenditures

Prevention Research
23-17 Population-based prevention research

24. Respiratory Diseases

Goal: Promote respiratory health through better prevention, detection, treatment, and education efforts.

Objective Number and Short Title

Asthma
24-1 Deaths from asthma
24-2 Hospitalizations for asthma
24-3 Hospital emergency department visits for asthma
24-4 Activity limitations
24-5 School or work days lost
24-6 Patient education
24-7 Appropriate asthma care
24-8 Surveillance systems

Chronic Obstructive Pulmonary Disease (COPD)
24-9 Activity limitations due to chronic lung and breathing problems
24-10 Deaths from COPD

Obstructive Sleep Apnea (OSA)
24-11 Medical evaluation and followup
24-12 Vehicular crashes related to excessive sleepiness

25. Sexually Transmitted Diseases

Goal: Promote responsible sexual behaviors, strengthen community capacity, and increase access to quality services to prevent sexually transmitted diseases (STDs) and their complications.

Objective Number and Short Title

Bacterial STD Illness and Disability
25-1 Chlamydia
25-2 Gonorrhea
25-3 Primary and secondary syphilis

Viral STD Illness and Disability
25-4 Genital herpes
25-5 Human papillomavirus infection

STD Complications Affecting Females
25-6 Pelvic inflammatory disease (PID)
25-7 Fertility problems
25-8 Heterosexually transmitted HIV infection in women

STD Complications Affecting the Fetus and Newborn
25-9 Congenital syphilis
25-10 Neonatal STDs

Personal Behaviors
25-11 Responsible adolescent sexual behavior
25-12 Responsible sexual behavior messages on television

Community Protection Infrastructure
25-13 Hepatitis B vaccine services in STD clinics
25-14 Screening in youth detention facilities and jails
25-15 Contracts to treat nonplan partners of STD patients

Personal Health Services
25-16 Annual screening for genital chlamydia
25-17 Screening of pregnant women
25-18 Compliance with recognized STD treatment standards
25-19 Provider referral services for sex partners

26. Substance Abuse

Goal: Reduce substance abuse to protect the health, safety, and quality of life for all, especially children.

Objective Number and Short Title

Adverse Consequences of Substance Use and Abuse

26-1 Motor vehicle crash deaths and injuries
26-2 Cirrhosis deaths
26-3 Drug-induced deaths
26-4 Drug-related hospital emergency department visits
26-5 Alcohol-related hospital emergency department visits
26-6 Adolescents riding with a driver who has been drinking
26-7 Alcohol- and drug-related violence
26-8 Lost productivity

Substance Use and Abuse

26-9 Substance-free youth
26-10 Adolescent and adult use of illicit substances
26-11 Binge drinking
26-12 Average annual alcohol consumption
26-13 Low-risk drinking among adults
26-14 Steroid use among adolescents
26-15 Inhalant use among adolescents

Risk of Substance Use and Abuse

26-16 Peer disapproval of substance abuse
26-17 Perception of risk associated with substance abuse

Treatment for Substance Abuse

26-18 Treatment gap for illicit drugs
26-19 Treatment in correctional institutions
26-20 Treatment for injection drug use
26-21 Treatment gap for problem alcohol use

State and Local Efforts

26-22 Hospital emergency department referrals
26-23 Community partnerships and coalitions
26-24 Administrative license revocation laws
26-25 Blood alcohol concentration (BAC) levels for motor vehicle drivers

27. Tobacco Use

Goal: Reduce illness, disability, and death related to tobacco use and exposure to secondhand smoke.

Objective Number and Short Title

Tobacco Use in Population Groups

27-1 Adult tobacco use
27-2 Adolescent tobacco use
27-3 Initiation of tobacco use
27-4 Age at first tobacco use

Cessation and Treatment

27-5 Smoking cessation by adults
27-6 Smoking cessation during pregnancy
27-7 Smoking cessation by adolescents
27-8 Insurance coverage of cessation treatment

Exposure to Secondhand Smoke

27-9 Exposure to tobacco smoke at home among children
27-10 Exposure to environmental tobacco smoke
27-11 Smoke-free and tobacco-free schools
27-12 Worksite smoking policies
27-13 Smoke-free indoor air laws

Social and Environmental Changes

27-14 Enforcement of illegal tobacco sales to minors laws
27-15 Retail license suspension for sales to minors
27-16 Tobacco advertising and promotion targeting adolescents and young adults
27-17 Adolescent disapproval of smoking
27-18 Tobacco control programs
27-19 Preemptive tobacco control laws
27-20 Tobacco product regulation
27-21 Tobacco tax

28. Vision and Hearing

Goal: Improve the visual and hearing health of the Nation through prevention, early detection, treatment, and rehabilitation.

Objective Number and Short Title

Vision

28-1   Dilated eye examinations
28-2   Vision screening for children
28-3   Impairment due to refractive errors
28-4   Impairment in children and adolescents
28-5   Impairment due to diabetic retinopathy
28-6   Impairment due to glaucoma
28-7   Impairment due to cataract
28-8   Occupational eye injury
28-9   Protective eyewear
28-10 Vision rehabilitation services and devices

Hearing

28-11 Newborn hearing screening, evaluation, and intervention
28-12 Otitis media
28-13 Rehabilitation for hearing impairment
28-14 Hearing examination
28-15 Evaluation and treatment referrals
28-16 Hearing protection
28-17 Noise-induced hearing loss in children
28-18 Noise-induced hearing loss in adults

1

Access to Quality Health Services

Co-Lead Agencies: Agency for Healthcare Research and Quality
Health Resources and Services Administration

Contents

Goal

Improve access to comprehensive, high-quality health care services.

Overview

Access to quality care is important to eliminate health disparities and increase the quality and years of healthy life for all persons in the United States. This chapter focuses on four components of the health care system: clinical preventive care, primary care, emergency services, and long-term and rehabilitative care. Together with health care delivered by specialists and care received in hospital settings, these elements represent major components of the continuum of care. The public health system is important in each of these areas because it educates people about prevention and addresses the need to eliminate disparities by easing access to preventive services for people less able to use existing health services. It ensures the availability of primary care through direct funding of clinics and providers or by providing public insurance. It coordinates emergency services systems and oversees long-term and rehabilitative care. Tertiary services (for example, hospital and specialty care) currently are not included among the Healthy People 2010 objectives. The Agency for Healthcare Research and Quality (AHRQ), formerly the Agency for Health Care Policy and Research, is working in conjunction with the Centers for Disease Control and Prevention (CDC) and other agencies of the U.S. Department of Health and Human Services to develop a *National Report on Healthcare Quality*, which will report annually on a broader array of quality measures that will complement Healthy People 2010.

Issues

Access to high-quality health care across each of the components in the continuum of care must be improved to realize the full potential of prevention. For example, success in reducing the burden of heart disease and narrowing the gap in heart disease outcomes between different racial groups will depend on several factors. These factors include ensuring access to clinical preventive services, such as blood pressure and cholesterol screening; effective primary care to educate people about modifiable risk factors, such as smoking, and to manage effectively chronic conditions like hypertension; high-quality emergency services to improve outcomes of acute cardiac events; and access to rehabilitative and long-term care for heart disease patients.

Major changes in the structure of the U.S. health care system, including the increasing influence of market forces, changes in payment and delivery systems, and welfare reform, have significant implications for vulnerable and at-risk populations. In light of these systems changes, Federal, State, and local public health agencies must redouble their efforts to address access barriers and reduce disparities for these populations. It is increasingly important that health care communication and services be provided in a culturally and linguistically sensitive manner. Adequate access to health care and related services can increase appropriate patient use of the health care system and, ultimately, improve health outcomes. Consequently, measures of access across a continuum of care are an important way to evaluate the quality of the Nation's health care system.

Clinical preventive care. Clinical preventive services have a substantial impact on many of the leading causes of disease and death. People must have access to clinical preventive services that are effective in preventing disease (primary prevention) or in detecting asymptomatic disease or risk factors at early, treatable stages (secondary prevention). As in Healthy People 2000, the recommendations of the U.S. Preventive Services Task Force[1] serve as a guide to quality preventive health care. The task force was reconvened in 1998 and, in conjunction with AHRQ's Evidence-Based Practice Centers (EPCs), will provide additional information regarding the effectiveness and cost-effectiveness of individual clinical preventive services.

Improving access to appropriate preventive care requires addressing many barriers, including those that involve the patient, provider, and system of care.[2,3] Patient barriers include lack of knowledge, skepticism about the effectiveness of prevention, lack of a usual source of primary care, and lack of money to pay for preventive care. Although patient awareness and acceptance of some interventions are high (such as screening for breast cancer) other interventions (for example, colorectal cancer screening and sexually transmitted disease [STD] screening) are less uniformly accepted. A small but significant number of patients remain skeptical of even widely accepted preventive measures, such as immunizations. Having health insurance, a high income, and a primary care provider are strong predictors that a person will receive appropriate preventive care. Although reimbursement for common screening tests, such as mammograms and Pap tests, is provided by most health insurance plans (and is required by law in some States), reimbursement for effective counseling interventions, such as smoking cessation, is less common.[4]

Health provider barriers include limited time, lack of training in prevention, lack of perceived effectiveness of selected preventive services, and practice environments that fail to facilitate prevention. Although consensus is growing regarding the value of a range of preventive services, providers identify lack of time and reimbursement as specific barriers to more consistent delivery of counseling about behavioral risk factors such as diet and exercise.[5] Computerized or manual tracking systems, patient and clinician reminders, guidelines, and patient information materials can help providers improve delivery of necessary preventive care.[6]

System barriers can include lack of resources or attention devoted to prevention, lack of coverage or inadequate reimbursement for services, and lack of systems to track the quality of care.[3] Systems interventions that can increase delivery of health care include offering clinical preventive services among standard covered benefits, providing feedback on performance to providers and practices, offering incentives for improved performance, and developing and implementing systems to identify and provide outreach to patients in need of services.[2]

Measuring and reporting how well preventive care is provided under different systems are essential first steps in motivating those systems that are not performing well to develop the information, tools, and incentives to improve care.[7] Significant progress in the delivery of clinical preventive services (CPS) is unlikely without appropriate data systems to allow providers and administrators to identify those services and populations most in need of better delivery. To be effective, preventive care also must be linked to systems to ensure appropriate followup services or counseling for patients identified through risk assessment or screening. Comprehensive national data to track what systems of care are doing to monitor and improve the delivery of CPS will not be available in the first half of the decade. Thus, this issue is not addressed in this focus area's objectives but represents an important agenda for research and data collection for the coming decade.

Primary care. Improving primary care across the Nation depends in part on ensuring that people have a usual source of care. Having a primary care provider as the usual source of care is especially important because of the beneficial attributes of primary care. These benefits include the provision of integrated, accessible health care services by clinicians who are accountable for addressing a large majority of personal health care needs, developing a sustained partnership with patients, and practicing in the context of family and community.[8] Increasing the number and proportion of members of underrepresented racial and ethnic groups who are primary care providers also is important because they are more likely to practice in areas where health services are in short supply and in areas with high percentages of underrepresented racial and ethnic populations.

Emergency services. Prehospital emergency medical services (EMS), poison control centers (PCCs), and hospital-based emergency departments (EDs) are the most commonly sought sources of emergency care. Each year, they provide prompt first-contact care for millions of people regardless of their socioeconomic status, age, or special need. For many severely ill and injured persons, these settings are a crucial link in the chain of survival between the onset of symptoms and treatment in a hospital. For persons whose health problems are less pressing but who believe they need urgent medical attention, emergency services are a gateway to additional health care.

In addition to their central role in secondary and tertiary prevention, emergency services are increasingly contributing to primary prevention by providing immunizations and other preventive care in association with treatment for acute health problems.

Within the current health care delivery system, EDs are the only institutional providers required by Federal law to evaluate anyone seeking care.[9] They are expected at least to stabilize the most severely ill and injured patients, and they provide walk-in care for vast numbers of persons who face financial or other barriers to receiving care elsewhere.

Long-term care and rehabilitative services. People with physical or mental conditions that limit their capacity for self-care need long-term care and rehabilitative services. This population covers persons of all ages, from those who were born with physical or mental limitations or who developed such limitations later on in life, including those injured at any age, to those with diminishing functioning at older ages.[10] About 40 percent of the people in this population are under age 65 years.[11] The long-term care population includes individuals who need help or supervision to perform activities of daily living or instrumental activities of daily living.

The goals of long-term care services are to improve functioning, maintain existing functioning, or slow deterioration in functioning while delivering care in the least restrictive environment. Rehabilitative services, a critical component of long-term care, strive to return individuals to their optimal level of functioning. People in the long-term care population need access to a range of services, including nursing home care, home health care, adult day care, assisted living, and hospice care.

Trends

A significant measure of the access problem is the proportion of people who have health insurance. Following declines in the proportion of people with health insurance during the 1980s, the proportion has remained essentially level, at about 85 percent from 1989 to 1997 for persons under age 65 years.[12] Approximately 44.3 million persons lacked health insurance in 1998,[13] continuing an increase in the number of uninsured persons. At the same time, the proportion of adults with a usual source of care—an important predictor of access to needed services—fell from 83 percent to 78 percent between 1987 and 1992 before rising to 85 percent in 1998.[14] Although the lack of health insurance is clearly a major factor impeding access to care, having health insurance does not guarantee that health care will be accessible or affordable. Significant numbers of privately insured persons lack a usual source of care or report delays or difficulties in accessing needed care due to affordability or insurance problems.[15]

As a result of growing scientific evidence on the effectiveness of certain preventive services, 82 percent of employer-sponsored insurance plans include childhood immunizations, and 90 percent include Pap tests and mammograms. Nonetheless, gaps persist in coverage for effective preventive services, especially counseling.[4]

Concerns increasingly are focused on access to quality emergency services, long-term care, and rehabilitative services. Although emergency services are widely available in the United States, the range of services varies in accessibility and quality from region to region and, often, from neighborhood to neighborhood, raising additional concerns about care for vulnerable underserved populations. As the proportion of older people in the total U.S. population increases, the demand for quality long-term care services and facilities also will increase. Quality rehabilitative care needs are evident across all populations, and access to rehabilitative care is a significant problem for people who lack health insurance or who are underinsured and are unable to pay for the type and quality of health care they need.

During the 1990s and into the 21st century, increased attention has been paid at all levels of government as well as by the private sector to improving health care quality. The National Committee for Quality Assurance (NCQA), a managed care accreditation group, led a collaborative effort to develop the Health Plan Employer Data and Information Set (HEDIS), a widely used tool for evaluating health plan performance.[16] The Joint Commission for the Accreditation of Healthcare Organizations (JCAHO) also has developed performance measures. AHRQ has developed the Consumer Assessment of Health Plans Survey (CAHPS), an instrument to assess consumer experiences with health plans. AHRQ also has developed the Healthcare Cost and Utilization Project (HCUP), which makes available State and nationwide estimates of hospital use. These data can be used with the HCUP Quality Indicators to provide measures of ambulatory-care sensitive conditions, which can uncover potential problems in access to primary care services. Quality monitoring systems tend to emphasize measures that focus on delivery rates for clinical preventive services because access to and use of these services are an important indicator of the quality of health care providers and of delivery systems. The complementary *National Report on Healthcare Quality* will explore methods for integrating the data from these quality-monitoring systems with population-based data collected by the public sector.

The Federal Advisory Commission on Consumer Protection and Quality in the Health Care Industry was established in 1997 to study changes occurring in the health care system and recommend ways to ensure consumer protection and quality health care. The Commission's report[17] provides a foundation for the emerging issues of the next decade in monitoring and reporting on quality of health care. It also includes a "Consumer Bill of Rights and Responsibilities,"[18] which is designed to strengthen consumer confidence in the health care system while holding participants in the system accountable for improving quality.

One essential step to improving quality is to reduce errors. The Institute of Medicine issued a report in December 1999 documenting the magnitude of medical errors in U.S. hospitals. The report recommended strategies to reduce such errors, including better reporting of errors.[19]

Disparities

Limitations in access to care extend beyond basic causes, such as a shortage of health care providers or a lack of facilities. Individuals also may lack a usual source of care or may face other barriers to receiving services, such as financial barriers (having no health insurance or being underinsured), structural barriers (no facilities or health care professionals nearby), and personal barriers (sexual orientation, cultural differences, language differences, not knowing what to do, or environmental challenges for people with disabilities). Patients with disabilities may face additional barriers arising from facilities that are not physically accessible or from the attitudes of clinicians. Hispanics, young adults, and uninsured persons are least likely to have a usual source of care.[12] Hispanic persons and those with less than 12 years of education are least likely to have a usual primary care provider.[20] Certain people, such as those who are disabled, elderly, chronically ill, or HIV-infected, require access to health care providers who have the knowledge and skills to address their special needs.[21]

Substantial disparities remain in health insurance coverage for certain populations. Among the nonelderly population, approximately 33 percent of Hispanic persons lacked coverage in 1998, a rate that is more than double the national average.

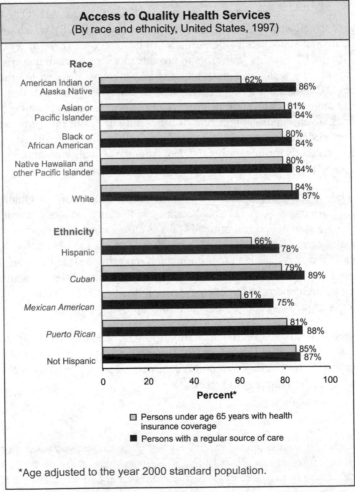

Source: CDC, NCHS. National Health Interview Survey (NHIS), 1997.

Healthy People 2010: Objectives for Improving Health

Mexican Americans had one of the highest uninsured rates at 40 percent. For adults under age 65 years, 34 percent of those below the poverty level were uninsured. Similar disparities exist in access to a specific source of ongoing care. An average of 85 percent of adults identified a specific source of ongoing care in 1998, but the proportions dropped to 76 percent for Hispanics and 77 percent for those below the poverty level.[12]

Opportunities

Increasing recognition of the critical role of preventive services across the continuum of care and the need for providers to incorporate preventive services into patient visits has led to the development of tools and projects designed to help providers and patients shift to a prevention-oriented health care system. HEDIS reports on the delivery of many clinical preventive services provided by participating health maintenance organizations (HMOs). The 1999 reporting set for HEDIS contained several measures of clinical preventive services, including childhood immunizations, adolescent immunizations, smoking cessation advice, influenza vaccinations for older adults, breast cancer screening, cervical cancer screening, and prenatal care in the first trimester. A CDC grant to the State of Massachusetts for a health assessment partnership has resulted in a collaborative effort in New England to increase HMO participation in HEDIS. The specific tools developed include the increased use of electronic birth certificates, which have assisted outreach programs to teach new mothers the value of periodic checkups for their infants.

One of the earliest and most recognized tool kits is the *Clinician's Handbook of Preventive Services,*[6] developed as part of the *Put Prevention Into Practice* initiative by the Office of Disease Prevention and Health Promotion and now the responsibility of AHRQ. It was produced as a companion to *Healthy People 2000* and the U.S. Preventive Services Task Force *Guide to Clinical Preventive Services.*[1] Under development is the CDC *Guide to Community Preventive Services*, due to be released in 2001.[22] The guide will assess the effectiveness of preventive services and interventions in community settings and at the clinical systems level. It will cover 15 topics in three areas: changing risk behaviors, such as eliminating tobacco use and increasing physical activity; reducing specific diseases and injuries, such as cancer and injuries from motor vehicle crashes; and addressing environmental challenges, such as changing the sociocultural environment.

Continued progress in the delivery of clinical preventive services will require better collection and reporting of data on the delivery of recommended services by providers and health plans. This information will allow providers and administrators to identify the services and groups of people where the biggest gaps exist in receiving needed health care services. The best information systems allow both cross-sectional comparisons of performance by providers, plans, systems, and localities as well as long-term analyses of the health and health care of individuals. These systems can facilitate interventions such as reminders for patients and providers, audit, and feedback, which have been shown to improve rates of immunization and screening.[23, 24]

In centralized health systems with stable populations (people who stay with one provider or health plan, for example), tracking of individuals has been used effectively for a limited number of services, primarily immunizations and cancer screenings. Expanding effective data collection efforts to cover additional services and to include more providers and health care systems is the current challenge. Measuring how well preventive care is provided under different systems is an essential first step in motivating those systems that are not performing well to develop the information, tools, and incentives to improve care.

Into the next decade, Healthy People and its partners will continue to promote communitywide efforts to provide clinical preventive services, using local leadership and insights to tailor and increase the accessibility of these services. Efforts will continue to promote the development of local prevention coalitions that include health departments, businesses, community institutions, and individuals from each community. Healthy People also will work to strengthen the capacity of States and localities to collect health data and conduct community health assessments for small geographic areas.

Advances in the use of genetic information may improve both clinical and preventive care by helping to identify high-risk individuals and populations who will benefit most from preventive services and other clinical interventions. It will be essential to develop policies that will ensure appropriate evaluation of new genetic services, quality assurance of available genetic technology, and access to genetic services of proven benefit.

Overcoming technological, financial, or organizational barriers that can slow or block access to emergency services and improving emergency care accessibility and quality will require the combined effort of health care providers, health plans, and health care consumers as well as government agencies at the Federal, Tribal, State, and local levels.

Interim Progress Toward Year 2000 Objectives

The proportion of adults under age 65 years without health care coverage has remained essentially the same, while the total number of uninsured persons has continued to increase. The proportion of the adult population with a specific source of primary care has increased, although Hispanic and African American adults and other subgroups continue to be less likely to have a specific source of primary care. Compared to 1991 and 1992 baseline data, the proportion of adults in 1995 who received selected recommended clinical preventive services (including tetanus boosters and routine mammograms) has increased. Progress also has been made in improving racial and ethnic representation in the health professions.

Note: Unless otherwise noted, data are from the Centers for Disease Control and Prevention, National Center for Health Statistics, *Healthy People 2000 Review, 1998–99*.

Access to Quality Health Services

Goal: Improve access to comprehensive, high-quality health care services.

Number	Objective Short Title

Clinical Preventive Care

1-1   Persons with health insurance

1-2   Health insurance coverage for clinical preventive services

1-3   Counseling about health behaviors

Primary Care

1-4   Source of ongoing care

1-5   Usual primary care provider

1-6   Difficulties or delays in obtaining needed health care

1-7   Core competencies in health provider training

1-8   Racial and ethnic representation in health professions

1-9   Hospitalization for ambulatory-care-sensitive conditions

Emergency Services

1-10   Delay or difficulty in getting emergency care

1-11   Rapid prehospital emergency care

1-12   Single toll-free number for poison control centers

1-13   Trauma care systems

1-14   Special needs of children

Long-Term Care and Rehabilitative Services

1-15   Long-term care services

1-16   Pressure ulcers among nursing home residents

Clinical Preventive Care

1-1. Increase the proportion of persons with health insurance.

Target: 100 percent.

Baseline: 83 percent of persons under age 65 years were covered by health insurance in 1997 (age adjusted to the year 2000 standard population).

Target setting method: Total coverage.

Data source: National Health Interview Survey (NHIS), CDC, NCHS.

NOTE: THE TABLE BELOW MAY CONTINUE TO THE FOLLOWING PAGE.

Persons Under Age 65 Years, 1997	Health Insurance
	Percent
TOTAL	83
Race and ethnicity	
American Indian or Alaska Native	62
Asian or Pacific Islander	81
Asian	81
Native Hawaiian and other Pacific Islander	80
Black or African American	80
White	84
Hispanic or Latino	66
Cuban	79
Mexican American	61
Puerto Rican	81
Not Hispanic or Latino	85
Black or African American	80
White	86
Gender	
Female	84
Male	81

Persons Under Age 65 Years, 1997	Health Insurance
	Percent
Family income level	
Poor	66
Near poor	69
Middle/high income	91
Geographic location	
Within MSA	83
Outside MSA	80
Disability status	
Persons with disabilities	83
Persons without disabilities	83
Sexual orientation	DNC
Select populations	
Age groups	
10 to 24 years	DNA
10 to 14 years	DNA
15 to 19 years	DNA
20 to 24 years	DNA

DNA = Data have not been analyzed. DNC = Data are not collected. DSU = Data are statistically unreliable.
MSA = Metropolitan statistical area.
Note: Age adjusted to the year 2000 standard population.
NOTE: THE TABLE ABOVE MAY HAVE CONTINUED FROM THE PREVIOUS PAGE.

Access to health services—including preventive care, primary care, and tertiary care—often depends on whether a person has health insurance.[25, 26, 27] Uninsured people are less than half as likely as people with health insurance to have a primary care provider; to have received appropriate preventive care, such as recent mammograms or Pap tests; or to have had any recent medical visits. Lack of insurance also affects access to care for relatively serious medical conditions. Evidence suggests that lack of insurance over an extended period significantly increases the risk of premature death and that death rates among hospitalized patients without health insurance are significantly higher than among patients with insurance.[28] As demonstrated by a study of data from the National Health Interview Survey (NHIS), Medicaid expansions that increase the proportion of a State's population eligible for Medicaid lead to increases in enrollment, enhanced utilization of medical services, and lower child death rates.[29] Another study showed that, among those without insurance, chronically ill persons are even less likely than those with acute conditions to get health care services they need.[30]

1-2. (Developmental) Increase the proportion of insured persons with coverage for clinical preventive services.

Potential data source: Medical Expenditure Panel Survey (MEPS), AHRQ.

Insurance coverage for clinical preventive services improved substantially during the 1990s, but significant variations remain in the services covered, depending on the plan and type of insurance. In 1988, among employers who offer health insurance, only 26 percent of their employees were covered for adult physical examinations, 35 percent for well-child care (including immunizations), and 43 percent for preventive screening tests.[31] In contrast, a 1997 national survey of over 3,000 employers found that 88 percent of employer-sponsored plans covered well-baby care, 89 percent covered adult physical examinations, 92 percent covered gynecologic examinations, and 89 and 91 percent covered Pap tests and mammograms, respectively. Coverage was highest in HMO plans and lowest in indemnity insurance plans.[4]

Including effective clinical preventive services among the services routinely covered by insurance is an effective way to emphasize the importance of clinical preventive services as an integral part of health care.[32] The Balanced Budget Act of 1997 (Public Law 105-33) added colorectal cancer screening among other new preventive benefits under the Medicare program and expanded Medicare coverage of mammography and cervical cancer screening. Although health insurance coverage by itself is not sufficient to eliminate existing gaps in the delivery of preventive services, it is an important factor influencing who gets recommended services.[33, 34]

Selected clinical preventive services have a positive influence on personal health, and many are cost-effective in comparison with the treatment of disease.[1, 35] Insurance coverage is especially problematic for counseling services, in part, because of the difficulty in proving the benefits of some counseling interventions. For example, only 22 percent of employer-sponsored plans cover medications or counseling for smoking cessation.[4] The effectiveness of smoking cessation counseling, however, is supported by strong evidence, with more intensive interventions having the greatest impact and most favorable cost-effectiveness ratios.[36]

1-3. Increase the proportion of persons appropriately counseled about health behaviors.

Target and baseline:

Objective	Increase in Counseling on Health Behaviors Among Persons at Risk With a Physician Visit in the Past Year	1995 Baseline	2010 Target
		Percent	
1-3a.	Physical activity or exercise (adults aged 18 years and older)	Developmental	
1-3b.	Diet and nutrition (adults aged 18 years and older)	Developmental	

1-3c.	Smoking cessation (adult smokers aged 18 years and older)	Developmental	
1-3d.	Reduced alcohol consumption (adults aged 18 years and older with excessive alcohol consumption)	Developmental	
1-3e.	Childhood injury prevention: vehicle restraints and bicycle helmets (children aged 17 years and under)	Developmental	
1-3f.	Unintended pregnancy (females aged 15 to 44 years)	19	50
1-3g.	Prevention of sexually transmitted diseases (males aged 15 to 49 years; females aged 15 to 44 years)	Developmental	
1-3h.	Management of menopause (females aged 46 to 56 years)	Developmental	

Target setting method: Better than the best.

Data sources: National Survey on Family Growth (NSFG), CDC, NCHS; National Health Interview Survey (NHIS), CDC, NCHS.

NOTE: THE TABLE BELOW MAY CONTINUE TO THE FOLLOWING PAGE.

Females Aged 15 to 44 Years With a Physician Visit in the Past Year, 1995	1-3f. Counseled About Unintended Pregnancy
	Percent
TOTAL	19
Race and ethnicity	
American Indian or Alaska Native	DSU
Asian or Pacific Islander	DSU
Asian	DNC
Native Hawaiian and other Pacific Islander	DNC
Black or African American	24
White	19
Hispanic or Latino	20
Not Hispanic or Latino	DNA
Black or African American	24
White	19

Females Aged 15 to 44 Years With a Physician Visit in the Past Year, 1995	1-3f. Counseled About Unintended Pregnancy
	Percent
Education level (females aged 22 to 44 years)	
Less than high school	15
High school graduate	20
At least some college	19
Sexual orientation	DNC
Select populations	
Age groups	
15 to 24 years	22
25 to 34 years	23
35 to 44 years	10

DNA = Data have not been analyzed. DNC = Data are not collected. DSU = Data are statistically unreliable.

NOTE: THE TABLE ABOVE MAY HAVE CONTINUED FROM THE PREVIOUS PAGE.

Substantial gaps remain in the delivery of appropriate screening and counseling services related to health behaviors. Unhealthy diets, smoking, physical inactivity, and alcohol use account for a majority of preventable deaths in the United States.[37] Data indicate that risk assessment and counseling interventions are delivered less frequently than other preventive interventions (for example, cancer screenings).[12] In addition, the attention physicians give to specific health-risk behaviors appears to be influenced by the socioeconomic status of their patients.[38] Although time is an important constraint in the primary care setting, evidence demonstrates that brief clinician counseling is effective in getting patients to stop smoking and reduce problem drinking.[1, 39] In addition, more intensive dietary counseling can lead to reduced dietary fat and cholesterol intake and increased fruit and vegetable consumption.[1] Effective primary care-based interventions to increase physical activity among patients have been more difficult to identify.[1, 40]

Some evidence shows that provider counseling can increase the use of seat belts, child safety seats, and bicycle helmets, especially when directed to parents of infants and young children.[1] Brief counseling interventions aimed at high-risk individuals can increase condom use and prevent the spread of sexually transmitted diseases.[41]

Clinician counseling should be tailored to the individual risk factors, needs, preferences, and abilities of each patient.[1] For some preventive interventions, such as hormone therapy in postmenopausal women, the optimal strategy depends on how individual women value potential benefits and risks. Counseling of perimenopausal and postmenopausal women should encourage shared decisionmaking based on individual risk factors and patient preferences.[1]

Primary Care

1-4. Increase the proportion of persons who have a specific source of ongoing care.

Target and baseline:

Objective	Increase in Persons With Specific Source of Ongoing Care	1998 Baseline*	2010 Target
		Percent	
1-4a.	All ages	87	96
1-4b.	Children and youth aged 17 years and under	93	97
1-4c.	Adults aged 18 years and older	85	96

*Age adjusted to the year 2000 standard population.

Target setting method: Better than the best.

Data source: National Health Interview Survey (NHIS), CDC, NCHS.

NOTE: THE TABLE BELOW MAY CONTINUE TO THE FOLLOWING PAGE.

Population by Age Group, 1998 (unless noted)	Specific Source of Ongoing Care		
	1-4a. All Ages	**1-4b. Aged 17 Years and Under**	**1-4c. Aged 18 Years and Older**
	Percent		
TOTAL	87	93	85
Race and ethnicity			
American Indian or Alaska Native	82	89	79
Asian or Pacific Islander	84	89	81
Asian	84	89	82
Native Hawaiian and other Pacific Islander	83	90	82
Black or African American	86	91	84
White	88	95	86

Healthy People 2010: Objectives for Improving Health

Population by Age Group, 1998 (unless noted)	Specific Source of Ongoing Care		
	1-4a. All Ages	1-4b. Aged 17 Years and Under	1-4c. Aged 18 Years and Older
	Percent		
Hispanic or Latino	79	86	76
Cuban	86	95	82
Mexican American	75	83	72
Puerto Rican	86	90	85
Not Hispanic or Latino	89	95	87
Black or African American	86	91	85
White	89	96	87
Gender			
Female	91	93	90
Male	84	94	81
Family income level			
Poor	80	88	77
Near poor	82	90	79
Middle/high income	91	97	88
Geographic location			
Urban	87	93	85
Rural	89	95	87
Disability status			
Persons with disabilities	89 (1997)	95 (1997)	86 (1997)
Persons without disabilities	86 (1997)	93 (1997)	84 (1997)
Sexual orientation	DNC	DNC	DNC
Select populations			
Age groups			
10 to 24 years	DNA	NA	NA
10 to 17 years	91 (1997)	NA	NA
18 to 24 years	72 (1997)	NA	NA

DNA = Data have not been analyzed. DNC = Data are not collected. DSU = Data are statistically unreliable. NA = Not applicable.

Note: Age adjusted to the year 2000 standard population.

NOTE: THE TABLE ABOVE MAY HAVE CONTINUED FROM THE PREVIOUS PAGE.

Access to care depends in part on access to an ongoing source of care. People with a usual source of health care are more likely than those without a usual source of care to receive a variety of preventive health care services.[42, 43] An estimated 15 percent of adults in the United States lack a usual source of care. Thus, more than 40 million persons have no particular doctor's office, clinic, health center, or other place where they go for health care advice. The National Health Interview Survey (NHIS) does not count emergency departments as a usual source of care.[12]

An estimated 93 percent of children aged 17 years and under have a specific source of ongoing care. The implementation of the Children's Health Insurance Program in 1999 provides a mechanism for increasing the proportion of children with an ongoing source of care.[12]

The usual source of care can vary among groups according to their age, race and ethnicity, and health insurance coverage. Young children and elderly adults aged 65 years and older are most likely to have a usual source of care, and adults aged 18 to 64 years are least likely. Young adults aged 18 to 24 years are the least likely of any age group to have a usual source of care. Among racial and ethnic groups, Hispanic persons are the least likely to have a usual source of care. Some 24 percent of the adult Hispanic population (and 28 percent of the Mexican American population) lack a usual source of care, compared to 15 percent of African Americans and 15 percent of the total adult population.[12]

Some 88 percent of persons with a usual source use an office-based provider, and 11 percent use a hospital outpatient department or clinic. African Americans and Hispanics are more likely to use hospital-based providers (including hospital clinics and outpatient departments) as their usual source of care.[15]

Uninsured persons under age 65 years are more likely to lack a usual source of care (38 percent) than those who have either public or private insurance. When compared with their counterparts who have private health insurance, uninsured people under age 65 years are 2.6 times more likely to lack a usual source of care.[15]

1-5. Increase the proportion of persons with a usual primary care provider.

Target: 85 percent.

Baseline: 77 percent of the population had a usual primary care provider in 1996.

Target setting method: Better than the best.

Data source: Medical Expenditure Panel Survey (MEPS), AHRQ.

Total Population, 1996	1-5. Have a Usual Primary Care Provider	Provider Has Office Hours at Night or on Weekends*	Provider Usually Asks About Prescription Medications and Treatments by Other Doctors*
	Percent		
TOTAL	77	37	59
Race and ethnicity			
American Indian or Alaska Native	79	37	64
Asian or Pacific Islander	72	36	57
Asian	DNC	DNC	DNC
Native Hawaiian and other Pacific Islander	DNC	DNC	DNC
Black or African American	74	34	60
White	77	37	59
Hispanic or Latino	64	32	52
Not Hispanic or Latino	78	37	60
Black or African American	74	34	60
White	79	38	60
Gender			
Female	80	37	61
Male	73	36	57
Education level (aged 18 years and older)			
Less than high school	69	24	53
High school graduate	74	32	58
At least some college	74	34	59
Geographic location			
Within MSA	76	39	59
Outside MSA	78	29	60
Disability status			
Persons with activity limitations	DNA	DNA	DNA
Persons without activity limitations	DNA	DNA	DNA

DNA = Data have not been analyzed. DNC = Data are not collected. DSU = Data are statistically unreliable. MSA = Metropolitan statistical area.

*Data for office hours, prescription medications, and treatments are displayed to further characterize the practices of primary care providers.

A usual source of primary care helps people clarify the nature of their health problems and can direct them to appropriate health services, including specialty care.[44] Primary care also emphasizes continuity, which implies that individuals use their primary source of care over time for most of their health care needs. More after-hours care, shorter travel time to a practice site, and shorter office waits have been associated with patients' beginning an acute episode of care with primary care physicians. Greater continuity has been observed for individuals with shorter appointment waits, insurance, and access to more after-hours care.[45] Other advantages of primary care are that a primary care provider deals with all common health needs (comprehensiveness) and coordinates health care services, such as referrals to specialists. Evidence suggests that first contact care provided by an individual's primary care provider leads to less costly medical care.[46]

1-6. Reduce the proportion of families that experience difficulties or delays in obtaining health care or do not receive needed care for one or more family members.

Target: 7 percent.

Baseline: 12 percent of families experienced difficulties or delays in obtaining health care or did not receive needed care in 1996.

Target setting method: Better than the best.

Data source: Medical Expenditure Panel Survey (MEPS), AHRQ.

NOTE: THE TABLE BELOW MAY CONTINUE TO THE FOLLOWING PAGE.

Families, 1996	Experienced Difficulty or Delay in Receiving Health Care or Received No Health Care
	Percent
TOTAL	12
Race and ethnicity (head of household)	
American Indian or Alaska Native	15
Asian or Pacific Islander	14
Asian	DNC
Native Hawaiian and other Pacific Islander	DNC
Black or African American	10
White	12
Hispanic or Latino	15
Not Hispanic or Latino	11
Black or African American	10

Families, 1996	Experienced Difficulty or Delay in Receiving Health Care or Received No Health Care
	Percent
White	11
Gender (head of household)	
Female	DNA
Male	DNA
Family income level	
Below poverty	17
Near poverty	17
Middle/high income	9
Geographic location	
Within MSA	12
Outside MSA	12
Health insurance status of family	
All members private insurance	7
All members public insurance	12
All members uninsured	27
Disability status	
Persons with activity limitations	DNA
Persons without activity limitations	DNA

DNA = Data have not been analyzed. DNC = Data are not collected. DSU = Data are statistically unreliable.
MSA = Metropolitan statistical area.

NOTE: THE TABLE ABOVE MAY HAVE CONTINUED FROM THE PREVIOUS PAGE.

In 1996, according to the Medical Expenditure Panel Survey (MEPS), 12.8 million families (11.6 percent) for a variety of reasons experienced difficulty or delay in obtaining care or did not receive health care services they thought they needed. In addition to a lack of insurance or underinsurance, barriers include a lack of appropriate referrals, travel distance to the provider, lack of transportation, and unavailability of specialists. Families experience barriers to care for a variety of reasons: inability to afford health care (60 percent); insurance-related causes (20 percent), including (1) the insurance company not approving, covering, or paying for care, (2) preexisting conditions for which insurance coverage often is restricted, (3) lack of access to required referrals, and (4) clinicians refusing to accept the family's insurance plan; and other problems (21 percent), such as transportation, physical barriers, communication problems, child care limitations, lack of time or information, or refusal of services.[15]

An additional source of information on obtaining services is the Robert Wood Johnson National Access to Care Survey. Results of the 1994 National Access to Care Survey suggest that some studies have missed substantial components of unmet needs by failing to include specific questions about supplementary health care services, such as prescription drugs, eyeglasses, dental care, and mental health care or counseling.[47] When specific questions were added about these services, the findings showed that 16.1 percent of respondents (approximately 41 million) were unable to obtain at least one service they believed they needed. The highest reported unmet need was for dental care. This problem can be attributed partly to insufficient provider reimbursement, which discourages participation in plans even when the service is covered.

1-7. (Developmental) Increase the proportion of schools of medicine, schools of nursing, and other health professional training schools whose basic curriculum for health care providers includes the core competencies in health promotion and disease prevention.

Potential data source: Adaptation of the Prevention Self-Assessment Analysis, Association of Teachers of Preventive Medicine (ATPM).

Significant changes in the health care system and in the expectations of consumers are influencing the education of health care providers in the United States. For example, many medical schools are assessing the content of their predoctoral and postgraduate curricula.[48] Medical educators and medical schools are recognizing that physicians will need to be prepared to provide population-based preventive health care as well as high-quality medical care to their patients.[49] This challenge exists for other health professionals, including nurses, nurse practitioners, physician assistants, and allied health personnel. This link between medicine and public health is essential to provide the highest quality health care possible to the U.S. population.

A core set of competencies for medical students in health promotion and disease prevention was developed by a task force established by the Association of Teachers of Preventive Medicine (ATPM) and the U.S. Department of Health and Human Services' Health Resources and Services Administration. The competencies, derived from the ATPM *Inventory of Knowledge and Skills Relating to Health Promotion and Disease Prevention,*[50] cover four categories: clinical prevention, quantitative skills, health services organization and delivery, and community dimensions of medical practice. Together, they address a wide spectrum of topics, including environmental health hazards and asthma management. This set of competencies will provide medical educators with measurable education outcomes in prevention education. The core competencies will be evaluated for potential adaptability to health provider education curricula in schools of nursing and health professional schools. The core competencies also will be reviewed for potential expansion to cover emerging issues and competencies in evaluating and responding to environmental health concerns and natural and man-made disasters.

Because health care providers will have to address new health issues, policies, technologies, and practice guidelines over their careers, continuing education programs also need to be updated periodically.

1-8. **In the health professions, allied and associated health profession fields, and the nursing field, increase the proportion of all degrees awarded to members of underrepresented racial and ethnic groups.**

Target and baseline:

Objective	Increase in Degrees Awarded to Underrepresented Populations	1996-97 Baseline (unless noted)	2010 Target
		Percent	
	Health professions, allied and associated health professions fields (For the baselines, health professions include medicine, dentistry, pharmacy, and public health.)		
1-8a.	American Indian or Alaska Native	0.6	1.0
1-8b.	Asian or Pacific Islander	16.2	4.0*
1-8c.	Black or African American	6.7	13.0
1-8d.	Hispanic or Latino	4.0	12.0
	Nursing		
1-8e.	American Indian or Alaska Native	0.7 (1995–96)	1.0
1-8f.	Asian or Pacific Islander	3.2 (1995–96)	4.0
1-8g.	Black or African American	6.9 (1995–96)	13.0
1-8h.	Hispanic or Latino	3.4 (1995–96)	12.0
	Medicine		
1-8i.	American Indian or Alaska Native	0.6	1.0
1-8j.	Asian or Pacific Islander	15.9	4.0*
1-8k.	Black or African American	7.3	13.0
1-8l.	Hispanic or Latino	4.6	12.0
	Dentistry		
1-8m.	American Indian or Alaska Native	0.5	1.0
1-8n.	Asian or Pacific Islander	19.5	4.0*
1-8o.	Black or African American	5.1	13.0
1-8p.	Hispanic or Latino	4.7	12.0
	Pharmacy		
1-8q.	American Indian or Alaska Native	0.4	1.0
1-8r.	Asian or Pacific Islander	17.5	4.0*

| 1-8s. | Black or African American | 5.7 | 13.0 |
| 1-8t. | Hispanic or Latino | 2.8 | 12.0 |

*The Asian or Pacific Islander population group has exceeded its target, which represents the minimum target based on this group's estimated proportion of the population.

Target setting method: Targets based on U.S. Bureau of the Census projections of the proportions of racial and ethnic groups in the population for the year 2000.

Data sources: Survey of Predoctoral Dental Educational Institutions, American Dental Association; Profile of Pharmacy Students, American Association of Colleges of Pharmacy; AAMC Data Book: Statistical Information Related to Medical Schools and Teaching Hospitals, Association of American Medical Colleges; Annual Data Report, American Association of Schools of Public Health; Annual Survey of RN (Registered Nurse) Programs, National League for Nursing, Center for Research in Nursing Education and Community Health.

Certain racial and ethnic groups and low-income communities lag behind the overall U.S. population on virtually all health status indicators, including life expectancy and infant death. Furthermore, access to health care is a problem, and these groups often lack a specific source of care. Increasing the number of health professionals from certain racial and ethnic groups is viewed as an integral part of the solution to improving access to care.

Members of underrepresented racial or ethnic groups make up about 25 percent of the U.S. population. Their representation among health professionals, however, is in the range of 10 percent. Several studies have shown that minority health professionals are more likely to serve areas with high proportions of underrepresented racial and ethnic groups and to practice in or near designated health care shortage areas.[51, 52]

Despite considerable efforts to increase the number of representatives of racial or ethnic groups in health profession schools (medicine, dentistry, nursing, pharmacy, and allied and associated health professions), the percentage of such entrants, enrollees, and graduates has not advanced significantly and in some cases has not advanced at all since 1990. The targets set for Healthy People 2000 for such enrollment and graduation were not achieved, and achieving the revised targets by 2010 presents a significant challenge. Additional attention will need to be given to such efforts as providing financial assistance for underrepresented racial and ethnic group students to pursue health care degrees, encouraging mentor relationships, promoting the early recruiting of students from racial and ethnic groups before they graduate from high school, and increasing the number of racial and ethnic group faculty and administrative staff members in schools that train health care professionals. Other suggested approaches to improving culturally appropriate care for ethnic and minority populations include increasing cultural competency among all health workers and increasing the number of lay health workers from underrepresented racial and ethnic groups.

1-9. Reduce hospitalization rates for three ambulatory-care-sensitive conditions—pediatric asthma, uncontrolled diabetes, and immunization-preventable pneumonia and influenza.

Target and baseline:

Objective	Reduction in Hospitalizations for Ambulatory-Care-Sensitive Conditions	1996 Baseline	2010 Target
		Admissions per 10,000 Population	
1-9a.	Pediatric asthma—persons under age 18 years	23.0	17.3
1-9b.	Uncontrolled diabetes—persons aged 18 to 64 years	7.2	5.4
1-9c.	Immunization-preventable pneumonia or influenza—persons aged 65 years and older	10.6	8.0

Target setting method: 25 percent improvement.

Data source: Healthcare Cost and Utilization Project (HCUP), AHRQ.

NOTE: THE TABLE BELOW MAY CONTINUE TO THE FOLLOWING PAGE.

Persons With Ambulatory-Care-Sensitive Conditions by Age Group, 1996	Hospitalizations		
	1-9a. Persons Under Age 18 Years With Asthma	1-9b. Persons Aged 18 to 64 Years With Diabetes	1-9c. Persons Aged 65 Years and Older With Preventable Pneumonia or Influenza
	Admissions per 10,000		
TOTAL	23.0	7.2	10.6
Race and ethnicity			
American Indian or Alaska Native	DNC	DNC	DNC
Asian or Pacific Islander	DNC	DNC	DNC
Asian	DNC	DNC	DNC
Native Hawaiian and other Pacific Islander	DNC	DNC	DNC
Black or African American	DNC	DNC	DNC
White	DNC	DNC	DNC

Persons With Ambulatory-Care-Sensitive Conditions by Age Group, 1996	Hospitalizations		
	1-9a. Persons Under Age 18 Years With Asthma	1-9b. Persons Aged 18 to 64 Years With Diabetes	1-9c. Persons Aged 65 Years and Older With Preventable Pneumonia or Influenza
	Admissions per 10,000		
Hispanic or Latino	DNC	DNC	DNC
Not Hispanic or Latino	DNC	DNC	DNC
Black or African American	DNC	DNC	DNC
White	DNC	DNC	DNC
Gender			
Female	18.2	7.0	9.1
Male	27.6	7.4	12.6
ZIP Code income level *			
$25,000 or less	52.0	18.8	21.1
$25,001 to $35,000	22.3	6.7	9.2
More than $35,000	10.6	2.9	6.0
Health insurance status			
Private	15.7	3.7	DNA
Medicaid	45.9	23.5	DNA
Uninsured	8.3	6.3	NA

DNA = Data have not been analyzed. DNC = Data are not collected. DSU = Data are statistically unreliable. NA = Not applicable.

*Income of patient is the median income for the postal ZIP Code of residence.

NOTE: THE TABLE ABOVE MAY HAVE CONTINUED FROM THE PREVIOUS PAGE.

Comprehensive primary care services can reduce the severity of certain illnesses. Hospital admission rates for "ambulatory-care-sensitive conditions" serve as an indicator for both limited access to primary care and evidence of low-quality primary care. Disparities in hospital admission rates for racial and ethnic groups and low-income populations have been well documented.[53, 54]

The three indicators selected here represent common problems encountered in primary care and allow monitoring of hospitalization rates for children (asthma), working-age adults (diabetes), and elderly persons (pneumonia and influenza). For each of these conditions, interventions can reduce hospitalization rates. Advances in the management of asthma have reduced its adverse health effects. Primary care can prevent both acute problems and long-term consequences of diabetes. Illness and death from preventable pneumonia and influenza among elderly persons can be avoided through the use of pneumococcal and influenza vaccines. These three conditions have been chosen because coordination of community preventive services, public health interventions, clinical preventive services, and primary care can reduce levels of these illnesses. To be effective, these services must be culturally competent and linguistically appropriate.[55]

This objective can be achieved by targeting high-risk populations. Because multiple factors besides access and quality contribute to the admission rates for ambulatory-care-sensitive conditions, each State will need to examine its rates and interpret them in the context of its population, health system, and community characteristics and will need to implement corresponding strategies. The objective is to improve primary care and preventive services and thereby reduce the need for hospital admission and the extended illness and costs associated with hospitalization.[56, 57, 58, 59]

It should be noted that persons who are privately insured have admission rates that are half those of the national average, indicating what is potentially achievable. Because of data limitations and potential access barriers to hospital admission among the uninsured, the Medicaid rate is artificially high and the uninsured rate is artificially low. (See *Tracking Healthy People 2010* for more information.) Data by race are not included because these data are reported at the State level. State-level hospital discharge databases can provide accurate estimates of racial and ethnic disparities in hospital admission rates at the State level. There are substantial disparities in hospital admission rates for pediatric asthma and uncontrolled diabetes by race and ethnicity. The magnitude of this disparity also fluctuates by State, suggesting that access to care and quality may play a role. Specifically, among seven States for which rates were determined, the age- and gender-adjusted relative risk of hospitalization for pediatric asthma ranged from 2.3 to 5.8 for African Americans and 1.3 to 2.6 for Hispanics compared to non-Hispanic whites. For uncontrolled diabetes, the relative risk of hospitalization ranged from 3.0 to 4.4 for African Americans and 1.2 to 2.0 for Latinos compared to non-Hispanic whites.[60] AHRQ is developing a "minority national inpatient sample" as part of HCUP that will provide national estimates of disparities in avoidable hospitalization rates by race and ethnicity.

Emergency Services

1-10. (Developmental) Reduce the proportion of persons who delay or have difficulty in getting emergency medical care.

Potential data source: National Health Interview Survey (NHIS), CDC, NCHS.

Emergency services are a vital part of access to health care in the United States. All population groups, regardless of their socioeconomic, health, or insurance status, want to know that emergency services will be available and will function quickly and effectively when needed.[61] This broadly shared social expectation was reinforced by landmark Federal legislation, the Emergency Medical Treatment and

Active Labor Act (EMTALA) of 1986. EMTALA stipulates that anyone seeking care at a hospital emergency department (ED) must receive a medical screening examination for an emergency medical condition and appropriate stabilizing measures.[62]

For many people, however, a variety of barriers continue to block access to emergency departments when the need for emergency medical care arises.[9] Among these barriers are psychological and cultural factors that may keep some people, even if insured, from seeking care promptly; financial constraints that may inhibit some people, even if insured, from seeking care promptly; and shortcomings in the number, location, or capability of EDs in a specified geographic area.

A significant component of this objective is to reduce the proportion of people whose access to emergency services is blocked by their health insurance coverage or payment policies. These policies affect access to hospital emergency departments and, in some instances, use of prehospital emergency services.[63] Typically, these policies stipulate that unless an enrollee's condition is life threatening, the enrollee or the ED must obtain authorization before an ED visit or risk that a claim for services will be denied. In some cases, claims for ED visits can be denied retroactively if they are deemed medically unnecessary. The rationale for these coverage and payment policies is clear: to manage care and contain costs. These policies, however, discourage some enrollees from receiving emergency treatment when and where it is warranted.[64]

Concerns about access barriers have prompted Federal, State, and organizational groups to seek assurances that health coverage or payment policies will provide payment when people go to an ED with acute symptoms of sufficient severity—including severe pain—such that a prudent layperson could reasonably expect that the lack of medical attention could result in serious jeopardy, serious impairment to bodily functions, or serious dysfunction of any bodily organ or part.

1-11. (Developmental) Increase the proportion of persons who have access to rapidly responding prehospital emergency medical services.

Potential data source: Annual Survey of EMS Operations, International Association of Fire Fighters.

The outcome of many medical emergencies depends on the prompt availability of appropriately trained and properly equipped prehospital emergency medical care providers. In urban areas, this capability is defined by an interval of less than 5 minutes from the time an emergency call is placed to arrival on the scene for at least 90 percent of first-responder emergency medical services and less than 8 minutes for at least 90 percent of transporting EMS. In rural areas, this capability is defined as an interval of less than 10 minutes from the time an emergency call is placed to arrival on the scene for at least 80 percent of EMS responses.

Assuring a prompt response requires a well-coordinated system of care involving a variety of organizations and agencies, some of which are outside the traditional health care arena. The components include public awareness of how and whom to call for emergency assistance and public education concerning initial lifesaving emergency care procedures to be followed until the arrival of EMS providers. They also include access via a 911 or enhanced 911 system or, in rural areas, a uniform addressing system that allows emergency responders to locate the person requesting emergency assistance quickly; the availability of well-trained and appropriately certified response personnel, who are frequently from law enforcement or fire services; transportation (ground, air, or water ambulance); medical direction and oversight; and destination hospitals that are well-equipped and appropriately staffed.

1-12. Establish a single toll-free telephone number for access to poison control centers on a 24-hour basis throughout the United States.

Target: 100 percent.

Baseline: 15 percent of poison control centers shared a single toll-free number in 1999.

Target setting method: Total coverage.

Data source: American Association of Poison Control Centers Survey, U.S. Poison Control Centers.

Poison control centers (PCCs) are staffed on a 24-hour basis by toxicologists and specialists in poison information who respond to requests from the general public and health care professionals for immediate information and treatment advice about poisonings and toxic exposures. Local or toll-free telephone calls to PCC hotline numbers provide primary access to these services. Each year more than 2 million callers seek telephone assistance from PCCs throughout the United States.[65] When a caller reports a poisoning or toxic exposure, a PCC toxicologist or specialist in poison information assesses the severity of the incident, advises the caller about treatment, and makes referrals for further medical attention when necessary. PCCs respond to inquiries in languages other than English by using language-translation services, interpreters, or bilingual staff members. PCCs manage most incidents by providing telephone advice to a caregiver at home, avoiding the need for more costly care at a hospital emergency department or another health care facility.

Linking all PCCs in the United States through a single toll-free telephone number and consolidating several key PCC functions can make contacting PCCs easier and more cost-effective.[66, 67] When PCCs are linked through a common telephone number, callers can be routed automatically to the nearest PCC based on their area code, telephone exchange number, and ZIP Code. Educational efforts could focus on a single easy-to-remember emergency number that permits callers to access PCCs quickly. Incorporating all PCCs under the umbrella of a toll-free nationwide telephone number will help ensure access to poison control services when and where they are needed.

1-13. Increase the number of Tribes, States, and the District of Columbia with trauma care systems that maximize survival and functional outcomes of trauma patients and help prevent injuries from occurring.

Target: All Tribes, States, and the District of Columbia.

Baseline: 5 States had trauma care systems in 1998.

Target setting method: Total coverage. (Tribal trauma systems are measured differently because they frequently are regional and often are linked to a State EMS.)

Data sources: State EMS Directors Survey, National Association of State EMS Directors; IHS (Tribal data are developmental).

A trauma care system is an organized and coordinated effort in a defined geographic area to deliver the full spectrum of care to injured patients. The main goals of the system are to match the available trauma care resources in a community, region, or State with the needs of individual patients and to ensure that patients have rapid access to the acute care facility and rehabilitation services they need. In a trauma care system, prehospital, acute care, and rehabilitation services are integrated and administered by a public agency that provides leadership, coordinates service delivery, establishes minimum standards of care, designates trauma centers (which offer 24-hour specialized treatment for the most severely injured patients), and fosters ongoing system evaluation and quality improvement.

Trauma care systems traditionally have focused on preventing adverse outcomes in the event of injury. Many trauma care professionals and people in the public health field believe that trauma care systems also should contribute to the prevention of injuries.[68] Trauma care professionals are in a good position to provide leadership in injury surveillance, clinical preventive services, and communitywide injury prevention programs. Recent Federal initiatives in trauma care have resulted in the design of a model system that incorporates public information, education, and prevention of injuries as key features.[69]

Results of a national survey conducted in 1993 indicated that only 5 States had complete trauma systems, but 19 other States and the District of Columbia had at least some trauma system components in place.[70] A survey of all 50 States and the District of Columbia in 1998 again indicated that only 5 States satisfied all trauma care system criteria.[71] However, results from this survey also showed that 37 other States and the District of Columbia had at least some trauma system components in place.

1-14. Increase the number of States and the District of Columbia that have implemented guidelines for prehospital and hospital pediatric care.

1-14a. Increase the number of States and the District of Columbia that have implemented statewide pediatric protocols for online medical direction.

Target: All States and the District of Columbia.

Baseline: 18 States had implemented statewide pediatric protocols for online medical direction in 1997.

Target setting method: Total coverage.

Data source: Emergency Medical Services for Children Annual Grantees Survey, HRSA.

Emergency medical service systems try to bring essential prehospital medical treatment to patients as quickly as possible. Emergency care of children presents a particular challenge because prehospital providers often treat fewer children and have limited pediatric experience and assessment skills. It can be more difficult to assess the severity of illness or injury because characteristic changes in vital signs that signal deterioration in adults may not occur in children. Important anatomic, physiologic, and developmental differences exist between children and adults that affect their responses to medical care and their risk of injury and illness.[72] Most EMS systems operate independently of hospitals or other facilities and typically have few physicians to ensure appropriateness of care.

Experienced providers can offer medical direction in two ways, either online or offline. Online direction involves direct communication (for example, voice) between EMS medical directors (for example, at hospitals) and emergency medical technicians (EMTs) and paramedics to authorize and guide the care of patients at the scene and during transport. Offline medical direction includes the development of guidelines, protocols, procedures, and policies, as well as planning for, training in, and evaluation of their use.

1-14b. Increase the number of States and the District of Columbia that have adopted and disseminated pediatric guidelines that categorize acute care facilities with the equipment, drugs, trained personnel, and other resources necessary to provide varying levels of pediatric emergency and critical care.

Target: All States and the District of Columbia.

Baseline: 11 States had adopted and disseminated pediatric guidelines that categorize acute care facilities with the equipment, drugs, trained personnel, and other resources necessary to provide varying levels of pediatric emergency and critical care in 1997.

Target setting method: Total coverage.

Data source: Emergency Medical Services for Children Annual Grantees Survey, HRSA.

Emergency care for life-threatening pediatric illness and injury requires specialized resources, medical direction, equipment, drugs, trained personnel, and properly staffed and equipped hospitals.[72] Children, however, receive emergency care in a variety of settings—from rural community hospitals to large urban medical centers. Hospitals vary in terms of their readiness to treat children's emergencies. If the hospitals are properly equipped and staffed, children frequently can receive the care that they need at local hospitals, but some children require the advanced care available only at regional specialty centers. Categorization is essentially an effort to identify the readiness and capability of a hospital and its staff to provide optimal emergency care.[73] Compliance can be voluntary or assigned by official agencies.

Long-Term Care and Rehabilitative Services

1-15. (Developmental) Increase the proportion of persons with long-term care needs who have access to the continuum of long-term care services.

Potential data sources: National Long-Term Care Survey, Medicare Current Beneficiary Survey, HCFA; National Health Interview Survey (NHIS), CDC, NCHS; Medical Expenditure Panel Survey (MEPS), AHRQ.

The long-term care population needs access to a range of services, including nursing home care, home health care, adult day care, assisted living, and hospice care.[74] Persons with long-term care needs require the help of other persons to perform activities of daily living (personal care activities) and instrumental activities of daily living (routine needs). Access problems are viewed as a need for specified long-term care services that were not received in the past 12 months.

Long-term care crosses the boundaries of different types of care—from health to social—and intensity of services—from periodic home health and homemaker visits to round-the-clock subacute care. Access to the full range of long-term care services continues to be a problem because of financial barriers and the limited availability of specific services.[11, 75] Although people in the long-term care population and their caregivers prefer long-term care to be delivered in the least restrictive environment, limited access and limited knowledge about care options can result in a long-term care population that is more dependent than necessary. The long-term care services selected cover key services in institutions, in the home, and in the community. Access to this range of services in rural areas is often difficult.

Healthy People 2010: Objectives for Improving Health

1-16. Reduce the proportion of nursing home residents with a current diagnosis of pressure ulcers.

Target: 8 diagnoses per 1,000 residents.

Baseline: 16 diagnoses of pressure ulcers per 1,000 nursing home residents were made in 1997.

Target setting method: Better than the best.

Data source: National Nursing Home Survey (NNHS), CDC, NCHS.

NOTE: THE TABLE BELOW MAY CONTINUE TO THE FOLLOWING PAGE.

Nursing Home Residents, 1997	Pressure Ulcers
	Diagnoses per 1,000
TOTAL	16
Race and ethnicity	
American Indian or Alaska Native	DSU
Asian or Pacific Islander	DSU
Asian	DSU
Native Hawaiian and other Pacific Islander	DSU
Black or African American	DSU
White	14
Hispanic or Latino	DSU
Not Hispanic or Latino	15
Black or African American	DSU
White	13
Gender	
Female	14
Male	20
Education level	
Less than high school	DNC
High school graduate	DNC
At least some college	DNC

Nursing Home Residents, 1997	Pressure Ulcers
	Diagnoses per 1,000
Geographic location	
Within MSA	17
Outside MSA	12
Disability status	
Persons with disabilities	16
Persons without disabilities	DSU

DNA = Data have not been analyzed. DNC = Data are not collected. DSU = Data are statistically unreliable.
MSA = Metropolitan statistical area.

NOTE: THE TABLE ABOVE MAY HAVE CONTINUED FROM THE PREVIOUS PAGE.

Pressure ulcers in all settings are sufficiently common to warrant concern, particularly as a quality-of-care issue. A significant number of people are at risk for pressure ulcers in nursing homes. Older adults are particularly prone to pressure ulcers as a result of decreased mobility, multiple contributing diagnoses, loss of muscle mass, and poor nutrition. About 24 percent of the Nation's 1.4 million nursing home residents require the assistance of another person to transfer from bed to chair.

According to studies of the treatment of pressure ulcers, it is difficult to determine the exact extent of the problem, including the number of new cases and the number of people who have pressure ulcers. Pressure ulcers have long been recognized as a serious quality-of-care problem in both acute care facilities and nursing homes.[76, 77] The prevention of pressure ulcers depends on close observation, appropriate nutrition, and effective nursing care. The number of new cases of pressure ulcers could indicate the overall quality of care provided to nursing home residents. Evidence-based guidelines have been issued on the prevention and treatment of pressure ulcers.[78]

Related Objectives From Other Focus Areas

2. **Arthritis, Osteoporosis, and Chronic Back Conditions**
   2-2. Activity limitations due to arthritis
   2-3. Personal care limitations
   2-6. Racial differences in total knee replacement
   2-7. Seeing a health care provider
   2-11. Activity limitations due to chronic back conditions
3. **Cancer**
   3-10. Provider counseling about cancer prevention
   3-11. Pap tests
   3-12. Colorectal cancer screening
   3-13. Mammograms

5. **Diabetes**
   5-1. Diabetes education
   5-4. Diagnosis of diabetes
   5-11. Annual urinary microalbumin measurement
   5-12. Annual glycosylated hemoglobin measurement
   5-13. Annual dilated eye examinations
   5-14. Annual foot examinations
   5-16. Aspirin therapy

6. **Disability and Secondary Conditions**
   6-7. Congregate care of children and adults with disabilities
   6-10. Accessibility of health and wellness programs

7. **Educational and Community-Based Programs**
   7-2. School health education
   7-3. Health-risk behavior information for college and university students
   7-5. Worksite health promotion programs
   7-7. Patient and family education
   7-8. Satisfaction with patient education
   7-12. Older adult participation in community health promotion activities

9. **Family Planning**
   9-1. Intended pregnancy
   9-2. Birth spacing
   9-3. Contraceptive use
   9-5. Emergency contraception
   9-6. Male involvement in pregnancy prevention
   9-10. Pregnancy prevention and sexually transmitted disease (STD) protection
   9-11. Pregnancy prevention education
   9-13. Insurance coverage for contraceptive supplies and services

11. **Health Communication**
    11-2. Health literacy
    11-6. Satisfaction with health care providers' communication skills

12. **Heart Disease and Stroke**
    12-1. Coronary heart disease (CHD) deaths
    12-15. Blood cholesterol screening

13. **HIV**
    13-6. Condom use
    13-8. HIV counseling and education for persons in substance abuse treatment
    13-9. HIV/AIDS, STD, and TB education in State prisons
    13-10. HIV counseling and testing in State prisons

14. **Immunization and Infectious Diseases**
    14-5. Invasive pneumococcal infections
    14-22. Universally recommended vaccination of children aged 19 to 35 months
    14-23. Vaccination coverage for children in day care, kindergarten, and first grade
    14-24. Fully immunized young children and adolescents
    14-25. Providers who measure childhood vaccination coverage levels
    14-26. Children participating in population-based immunization registries
    14-27. Vaccination coverage among adolescents
    14-28. Hepatitis B vaccination among high-risk groups
    14-29. Influenza and pneumococcal vaccination of high-risk adults

22. **Physical Activity and Fitness**
    22-12. School physical activity facilities
    22-13. Worksite physical activity and fitness
    22-14. Community walking
    22-15. Community bicycling

23. **Public Health Infrastructure**
    23-1. Public health employee access to the Internet
    23-2. Public access to information and surveillance data
    23-3. Use of geocoding in health data systems
    23-8. Competencies for public health workers
    23-9. Training in essential public health services
    23-10. Continuing education and training by public health agencies
    23-12. Health improvement plans
    23-13. Access to public health laboratory services
    23-14. Access to epidemiology services

24. **Respiratory Diseases**
    24-6. Patient education
    24-7. Appropriate asthma care
    24-11. Medical evaluation and followup

25. **Sexually Transmitted Diseases**
    25-11. Responsible adolescent sexual behavior
    25-13. Hepatitis B vaccine services in STD clinics
    25-14. Screening in youth detention facilities and jails
    25-15. Contracts to treat nonplan partners of STD patients
    25-16. Annual screening for genital chlamydia
    25-17. Screening of pregnant women
    25-18. Compliance with recognized STD treatment standards
    25-19. Provider referral services for sex partners

26. **Substance Abuse**
    26-18. Treatment gap for illicit drugs
    26-20. Treatment of injection drug use
    26-21. Treatment gap for problem alcohol use
    26-22. Hospital emergency department referrals

27. **Tobacco Use**
    27-5. Smoking cessation by adults
    27-7. Smoking cessation by adolescents
    27-8. Insurance coverage of cessation treatment

28. **Vision and Hearing**
    28-1. Dilated eye examinations
    28-2. Vision screening for children
    28-10. Vision rehabilitation services and devices
    28-11. Newborn hearing screening, evaluation, and intervention
    28-13. Rehabilitation for hearing impairment
    28-14. Hearing examination
    28-15. Evaluation and treatment referrals

Terminology

(A listing of abbreviations and acronyms used in this publication appears in Appendix H.)

Access: According to the Institute of Medicine, "The timely use of personal health services to achieve the best possible health outcomes."[79] This definition includes both the use and effectiveness of health services. The concept of access also encompasses physical accessibility of facilities.

Activities of daily living (ADL): Personal care activities, such as bathing, dressing, eating, and getting around (with special equipment, if needed) inside the home.

Acute care facility: A health facility that provides care on a short-term basis. Included are community hospitals with an average length of stay of less than 30 days for all patients.

Ambulatory care: Health care that does not require the patient to stay in a hospital or other facility, such as care provided on an outpatient basis.

Ambulatory-care-sensitive conditions: Conditions resulting in hospitalization that could potentially have been prevented if the person had improved access to high-quality primary care services outside the hospital setting.

Asymptomatic: Without symptoms. This term may apply either to healthy persons or to persons with preclinical (prior to clinical diagnosis) disease in whom symptoms are not yet apparent.

Clinical care: The provision of health care services to individual patients by trained health care professionals.

Clinical preventive services (CPS): Common screening tests, immunizations, risk assessment, counseling about health risk behaviors, and other preventive services routinely delivered in the clinical setting for the primary prevention of disease or for the early detection of disease in persons with no symptoms of illness.

Continuum of care: The array of health services and care settings that address health promotion, disease prevention, and the diagnosis, treatment, management, and rehabilitation of disease, injury, and disability. Included are primary care and specialized clinical services provided in community and primary care settings, hospitals, trauma centers, and rehabilitation and long-term care facilities.

Core competencies: A defined set of skills and knowledge considered necessary in the educational curricula for training health care providers. Examples of core competencies include skills in prevention education; skills in using sources of health data to identify what clinical preventive services should be delivered to the individual patient based on that person's age, gender, and risk factor status; an understanding of the U.S. public health system (local and State health departments) and its role in monitoring and maintaining the health of the community; and skills to evaluate and translate medical and scientific research reports into clinical practice.

Emergency services: Health care services that are or appear to be needed immediately because of injury or sudden illness that threatens serious impairment of any bodily function or serious dysfunction of any bodily part or organ.[18]

Functional assessment: A health care provider's review of a patient for the ability to perform activities of daily living (personal care activities) and instrumental activities (routine needs) of daily living. (See also *Persons with long-term care needs*.)

Health insurance: Any type of third party payment, reimbursement, or financial coverage for an agreed-upon set of health care services. Includes private insurance obtained through employment or purchased directly by the consumer, or health insurance provided through publicly funded programs, including Medicare, Medicaid, CHAMPUS/CHAMPVA, or other public hospital or physician programs.

Health intervention: Any measure taken to improve or promote health or to prevent, diagnose, treat, or manage disease, injury, or disability.

Health outcomes: The results or consequences of a process of care. Health outcomes may include satisfaction with care as well as the use of health care resources. Included are clinical outcomes, such as changes in health status and changes in the length and quality of life as a result of detecting or treating disease.

Instrumental activities for daily living: Routine activities, such as everyday household chores, shopping, or getting around for other purposes, that enable a person to live independently in the community.

Long-term care (LTC): A broad range of health and social services delivered in institutions, in the community, and at home. Long-term care services include institutional services, such as those delivered in nursing homes, rehabilitation hospitals, subacute care facilities, hospice facilities, and assisted living facilities; services delivered in the home, such as home health and personal care, hospice, homemaker, and meals; and community-based services, such as adult day care, social services, congregate meals, transportation and escort services, legal protective services, and counseling for clients as well as their caregivers.[10]

Managed care: According to the Institute of Medicine, "a set of techniques used by or on behalf of purchasers of health care benefits to manage health care costs by influencing patient care decisionmaking through case-by-case assessments of the appropriateness of care prior to its provision."[80]

Patient barriers: Any mental, physical, or psychosocial condition that prevents an individual from accessing needed health care. Examples include attitudes or biases, mental disorders or illnesses, behavioral disorders, physical limitations, cultural or linguistic factors, sexual orientation, and financial constraints.

Persons with long-term care needs: Persons who need the help of other persons to perform activities of daily living (personal care activities) and instrumental activities of daily living (routine needs).

Primary care: According to the Institute of Medicine, "The provision of integrated, accessible health care services by clinicians who are accountable for addressing a large majority of personal health care needs, developing a sustained partnership with patients, and practicing in the context of family and community."[8]

Primary care provider: A physician who specializes in general and family practice, general internal medicine, or general pediatrics, or a nonphysician health care provider, such as a nurse practitioner, physician assistant, or certified nurse midwife.

Primary prevention: Health care services, medical tests, counseling, and health education and other actions designed to prevent the onset of a targeted condition. Routine immunization of healthy individuals is an example of primary prevention.[1]

Provider barriers: Any mental, physical, psychosocial, or environmental condition that prevents or discourages health care providers from offering preventive services. Examples of provider barriers include a poor practice environment, lack of knowledge, and lack of efficacy studies.

Quality: According to the Institute of Medicine, "The degree to which health services for individuals and populations increase the likelihood of desired health outcomes and are consistent with current professional knowledge."[79] Simply stated, it is doing the right thing, for the right patient, at the right time, with the right outcome.

Rehabilitative services: Services to restore specific skills, including overall physical mobility and functional abilities.

Secondary prevention: Measures such as health care services designed to identify or treat individuals who have a disease or risk factors for a disease but who are not yet experiencing symptoms of the disease. Pap tests and high blood pressure screening are examples of secondary prevention.[1]

System barriers: Conditions within a health care system that prevent people from accessing needed services or prevent health care providers from delivering those services. System barriers include physical, cultural, linguistic, and financial barriers as well as the availability of health care facilities or providers with special skills, such as eye, ear, nose, and throat specialists.

Tertiary prevention: Preventive health care measures or services that are part of the treatment and management of persons with clinical illnesses. Examples of tertiary prevention include cholesterol reduction in patients with coronary heart disease and insulin therapy to prevent complications of diabetes.[1]

Usual source of care: A particular doctor's office, clinic, health center, or other health care facility to which an individual usually would go to obtain health care services. Having a usual source of care is associated with improved access to preventive services and followup care.

Vulnerable and at-risk populations: High-risk groups of people who have multiple health and social needs. Examples include pregnant women, people with human immunodeficiency virus infection, substance abusers, migrant farm workers, homeless people, poor people, infants and children, elderly people, people with disabilities, people with mental illness or mental health problems or disorders, and people from certain ethnic or racial groups who do not have the same access to quality health care services as other populations.

References

[1] U.S. Preventive Services Task Force. *Guide to Clinical Preventive Services.* 2nd ed. Washington, DC: U.S. Department of Health and Human Services (HHS), 1995.

[2] Thompson, R.S.; Taplin, S.H.; McAfee, T.A.; et al. Primary and secondary prevention services in clinical practice. Twenty years' experience in development, implementation, and evaluation. *Journal of the American Medical Association* 273:1130-1135, 1995.

[3] Solberg, L.I.; Kottke, T.E.; Brake, M.L.; et al. The case of the missing clinical preventive services systems. *Effective Clinical Practice* 1(1):33-38, 1998.

[4] Partnership for Prevention. *Results From the William M. Mercer Survey of Employer Sponsored Health Plans.* Washington, DC: the Partnership, 1999.

[5] American College of Preventive Medicine. *1998 National Prevention in Primary Care Study.* Washington, DC: the College, 1998.

[6] HHS. *Clinician's Handbook of Preventive Services.* 2nd ed. Washington, DC: HHS, 1998.

[7] National Committee for Quality Assurance (NCQA). *The State of Managed Care Quality.* Washington, DC: NCQA, 1999.

[8] Institute of Medicine (IOM). Donaldson, M.S.; Yordy, K.D.; Lohr, K.N., eds. *Primary Care In: America's Health in a New Era.* Washington, DC: National Academy Press, 1996.

[9] Josiah Macy, Jr. Foundation. The role of emergency medicine in the future of American medical care: Summary of the conference. *Annals of Emergency Medicine* 25:230-233, 1995.

[10] Kane, R.A., and Kane, R.L. *Long Term Care: Principles, Programs, and Policies.* New York, NY: Springer, 1987.

[11] Wiener, J.M.; Illston, L.H.; and Hanley, R.J. *Sharing the Burden: Strategies for Public and Private Long Term Care Insurance.* Washington, DC: The Brookings Institution, 1994.

[12] National Center for Health Statistics (NCHS). *National Health Interview Survey.* Hyattsville, MD: NCHS, unpublished data.

[13] U.S. Bureau of the Census. *Current Population Survey.* Washington, DC: the Bureau, 1999.

[14] Benson, V., and Marano, M.A. Current estimates from the National Health Interview Survey, 1995. *Vital and Health Statistics* 10(199), 1998.

[15] Weinick, R.M.; Zuvekas, S.H.; and Drilea, S.K. *Access to Health Care—Sources and Barriers, 1996.* MEPS Research Findings No. 3. AHCPR Pub. No. 98-0001. Rockville, MD: Agency for Health Care Policy and Research (AHCPR), 1997.

[16] NCQA. *Health Plan Employer Data and Information Set (HEDIS 3.0).* Washington, DC: NCQA, 1997.

[17] President's Advisory Commission on Consumer Protection and Quality in the Health Care Industry. *Quality First: Better Health Care for All Americans: Final Report to the President of the United States.* Washington, DC: U.S. Government Printing Office, 1998.

[18] President's Advisory Commission on Consumer Protection and Quality in the Health Care Industry. *Consumer Bill of Rights and Responsibilities—Report to the President.* Washington, DC: the Commission, 1997.

[19] Kohn, L.; Corrigan, J.; and Donaldson, M., eds. Committee on Quality of Health Care in America. *To Err Is Human: Building a Safer Health System.* Washington, DC: IOM, 1999.

[20] Agency for Healthcare Research and Quality (AHRQ). Unpublished tabulations of Medical Expenditure Panel Survey (MEPS) data, 1996.

[21] Bierman, A.S.; Magari, E.S.; Splaine, M.; et al. *Journal of Ambulatory Care Management* 21(3):17-26, 1998.

[22] Truman, B.I.; Smith-Akin, C.K.; Hinman, A.R.; et al. Developing the *Guide to Community Preventive Services*—Overview and rationale. *American Journal of Preventive Medicine* 18(2):18-26, 2000.

[23] Centers for Disease Control and Prevention (CDC). Vaccine-preventable diseases: Improving vaccination coverage in children, adolescents, and adults. A report on recommendations of the Task Force on Community Preventive Services. *Morbidity and Mortality Weekly Report* 48(No. RR-8):1-16, 1999.

[24] National Health Service, Center for Reviews and Dissemination. Getting evidence into practice. *Effective Health Care.* 5(1), 1999.

[25] CDC. Health insurance coverage and receipt of preventive health services—United States, 1993. *Morbidity and Mortality Weekly Report* 44:219-225, 1995.

[26] Weissman, J.S., and Epstein, A.M. The insurance gap: Does it make a difference? *Annual Review of Public Health* 14:243-270, 1993.

[27] U.S. General Accounting Office (GAO). *Health Insurance: Coverage Leads to Increased Health Care Access for Children.* GAO/HEHS-98-14. Washington, DC: GAO, 1998.

[28] Reinhardt, U.E. Coverage and access in health care reform. *New England Journal of Medicine* 330:1452-1453, 1994.

[29] Currie, J., and Gruber, J. Health insurance eligibility, utilization of medical care, and child health. *Quarterly Journal of Economics* 111(2):431-466, 1996.

[30] Hafner-Eaton, C. Physician utilization disparities between the uninsured and insured: Comparisons of the chronically ill, acutely ill, and well nonelderly populations. *Journal of the American Medical Association* 269:787-792, 1993.

[31] Health Insurance Association of America. *Research Bulletin: A Profile of Employer-Sponsored Group Health Insurance.* Washington, DC: the Association, 1989.

[32] Davis, K.; Bialek, R.; Parkinson, M.; et al. Paying for preventive care: Moving the debate forward. *American Journal of Preventive Medicine* 64(Suppl.):7-30, 1990.

[33] Faust, H.S. Strategies for obtaining preventive services reimbursement. *American Journal of Preventive Medicine* 64(Suppl.):1-5, 1990.

[34] Faulkner, L.A., and Schauffler, H.H. The effect of health insurance coverage on the appropriate use of recommended clinical preventive services. *American Journal of Preventive Medicine* 13(6):453-458, 1997.

[35] Tengs, T.O.; Adams, M.E.; Pliskin, J.S.; et al. Five-hundred life-saving interventions and their cost-effectiveness. *Risk Analysis* 15:369-390, 1995.

[36] Cromwell, J.; Bartosch, W.J.; Fiore, M.C.; et al. Cost-effectiveness of the clinical practice recommendations in the AHCPR guideline for smoking cessation. *Journal of the American Medical Association* 278:1759-1766, 1997.

[37] McGinnis, J.M., and Foege, W.H. Actual causes of death in the United States. *Journal of the American Medical Association* 270:2207-2212, 1993.

[38] Taira, D.A.; Safran, D.G.; Seto, T.B.; et al. The relationship between patient income and physician discussion of health risk behaviors. *Journal of the American Medical Association* 278:1412-1417, 1997.

[39] Fiore, M.C.; Bailey, W.C.; Cohen, S.J.; et al. *Smoking Cessation. Clinical Practice Guideline No. 18.* AHCPR Pub. No. 96-0692. Rockville, MD: HHS, AHCPR, 1996.

[40] HHS. *Physical Activity and Health: A Report of the Surgeon General.* Atlanta, GA: HHS, CDC, National Center for Chronic Disease Prevention and Health Promotion, 1996.

[41] Kamb, M.L.; Fishbein, M.; Douglas, J.M.; et al. Efficiency of risk reduction counseling to prevent human immunodeficiency virus and sexually transmitted diseases. *Journal of the American Medical Association* 280:1161-1167, 1998.

[42] Moy, E.; Bartman, B.A.; and Weir, M.R. Access to hypertensive care: Effects of income, insurance, and source of care. *Archives of Internal Medicine* 155(14):1497-1502, 1995.

[43] Ettner, S.L. The timing of preventive services for women and children: The effect of having a usual source of care. *American Journal of Public Health* 86:1748-1754, 1996.

[44] Starfield, B. *Primary Care: Balancing Health Needs, Services and Technology.* New York, NY: Oxford University Press, 1998.

[45] Forrest, C.B., and Starfield, B. Entry into primary care and continuity: The affects of access. *American Journal of Public Health* 88:1334, 1998.

[46] Forrest, C.B., and Starfield, B. The effect of first-contact care with primary care clinicians on ambulatory health care expenditures. *Journal of Family Practice* 43:40-48, 1996.

[47] Berk, M.L.; Schur, C.L.; and Cantor, J.C. Ability to obtain health care: Recent estimates from the Robert Wood Johnson Foundation National Access to Care Survey. *Health Affairs* 14(3):139-146, 1995.

[48] Wallace, R.B.; Wiese, W.H.; Lawrence, R.S.; et al. Inventory of knowledge and skills relating to disease prevention and health promotion. *American Journal of Preventive Medicine* 6:51-56, 1990.

[49] Report on the population health perspective panel. *Academic Medicine* 74:138-141, 1999.

[50] Wallace, R.B.; Wiese, W.H.; Lawrence, R.S.; et al. Inventory of knowledge and skills relating to disease prevention and health promotion. *American Journal of Preventive Medicine* 6:51-56, 1990.

[51] Komaromy, M.; Grumbach, K.; Drake, M.; et al. The role of black and Hispanic physicians in providing health care for underserved populations. *New England Journal of Medicine* 334:1305-1310, 1996.

[52] Cooper-Patrick, L.; Gallo, J.; Gonzales, J.; et al. Race, gender, and partnership in the patient-physician relationship. *Journal of the American Medical Association* 282:583-589, 1999.

[53] Goodman, D.C.; Stukel, T.A.; and Chang, C.H. Trends in pediatric asthma hospitalization rates: Regional and socioeconomic differences. *Pediatrics* 101:208-213, 1998.

[54] Pappas, G.; Hadden, W.C.; Kozak, L.J.; et al. Potentially avoidable hospitalizations: Inequalities in rates between U.S. socioeconomic groups. *American Journal of Public Health* 87:811-816, 1997.

[55] Carillo, J.E.; Green, A.R.; and Betancourt, J.R. Crosscultural primary care: A patient-based approach. *Annals of Internal Medicine* 130(1):829-834, 1999.

[56] Billings, J.; Anderson, G.M.; and Newman, L.S. Recent findings on preventable hospitalizations. *Health Affairs* 15(3):239-249, 1996.

[57] Billings, J.; Zeitel, L.; Lukomnik, J.; et al. Impact of socioeconomic status on hospital use in New York City. *Health Affairs* 12(1):162-173, 1993.

[58] Bindman, A.B.; Grumbach, K.; Osmond, D.; et al. Preventable hospitalizations and access to health care. *Journal of the American Medical Association* 274(4):305-311, 1995.

[59] Weissman, J.S.; Gatsonis, C.; and Epstein, A.M. Rates of avoidable hospitalization by insurance status in Massachusetts and Maryland. *Journal of the American Medical Association* 268(17):2388-2394, 1992.

[60] AHRQ. Hospital Cost and Utilization Project (HCUP), State Inpatient Database (SID). Unpublished data, 1996.

[61] Institute of Medicine (IOM). In: Millman, M., ed. *Access to Health Care in America.* Washington, DC: National Academy Press, 1993.

[62] Dane, L.A. The Emergency Medical Treatment and Active Labor Act: The anomalous right to health care. *Health Matrix* 8:3-28, 1998.

[63] Young, C.J. Emergency! Says who?: Analysis of the legal issues concerning managed care and emergency medical services. *Journal of Contemporary Health Law and Policy* 13:553-579, 1997.

[64] Young, G.P., and Lowe, R.A. Adverse outcomes of managed care gatekeeping. *Academic Emergency Medicine* 4:1129-1136, 1997.

[65] Litovitz, T.L.; Klein-Schwartz, W.; Caravati, E.M.; et al. Annual report of the American Association of Poison Control Centers: Toxic Exposure Surveillance System. *American Journal of Emergency Medicine* 17:435-487, 1999.

[66] Zuvekas, A.; Nolan, L.S.; Azzouzi, A.; et al. *An Analysis of Potential Economies of Scale in Poison Control Centers: Final Report.* Washington, DC: Center for Health Policy Research, Georgetown University Medical Center, 1997.

[67] Poison Control Center Advisory Work Group. *Final Report.* Atlanta, GA, and Rockville, MD: National Center for Injury Prevention and Control, CDC, and Maternal and Child Health Bureau, Health Resources and Services Administration (HRSA), 1997.

[68] IOM, Committee on Injury Prevention and Control. In: Bonnie, R.J.; Fulco, C.E.; and Liverman, C.T., eds. *Reducing the Burden of Injury: Advancing Treatment and Prevention.* Washington, DC: National Academy Press, 1999.

[69] HRSA. *Model Trauma Care System Plan.* Rockville, MD: HRSA, Division of Trauma and Emergency Medical Systems, 1992.

[70] Bazzoli, G.J.; Madura, K.J.; Cooper, G.F.; et al. Progress in the development of trauma systems in the United States: Results of a national survey. *Journal of the American Medical Association* 273:395-401, 1995.

[71] Bass, R.R.; Gainer, P.S.; and Carlini, A.R. Update on trauma system development in the United States. *Journal of Trauma* 47(Suppl. 3):515-521, 1999.

[72] IOM, Committee on Pediatric Emergency Medical Services. In: Durch, J.S., and Lohr, K.N., eds. *Emergency Medical Services for Children.* Washington, DC: National Academy Press, 1993.

[73] American Academy of Pediatrics. Guidelines for pediatric emergency care facilities. *Pediatrics* 96:526-537, 1995.

[74] Havens, B., and Beland, F., eds. Long-term care in five countries. *Canadian Journal on Aging* 15(Suppl. 1):1-102, 1996.

[75] Estes, C.L., and Swann, J.H. *The Long Term Care Crisis.* Newbury Park, CA: Sage Publications, 1993.

[76] Spector, W., and Fortinsky, W. Pressure ulcer prevalence in Ohio nursing homes. *Journal of Aging and Health* 10(1):62-80, 1998.

[77] Spector, W. Correlates of pressure sores in nursing homes: Evidence from the National Medical Expenditure Survey. *Journal of Investigative Dermatology* 102(6):425-455, 1994.

[78] The Pressure Ulcer Guideline Panel. *Treating Pressure Ulcers: Guideline Technical Report*. No. 15, Vols. 1 and 2. AHCPR Pub. No. 96-N014. Rockville, MD: AHCPR, 1996.

[79] IOM. *Medicare: A Strategy for Quality Assurance*. Vol. 1. Lohr, K.N., ed. Washington, DC: National Academy Press, 1998.

[80] Halverson, P.K.; Kaluzny, A.D.; McLaughln, C.P.; et al., eds. *Managed Care and Public Health*. Gaithersburg, MD: Aspen Publishers, Inc., 1998.

2

Arthritis, Osteoporosis, and Chronic Back Conditions

Co-Lead Agencies: Centers for Disease Control and Prevention
National Institutes of Health

Contents

Goal

Prevent illness and disability related to arthritis and other rheumatic conditions, osteoporosis, and chronic back conditions.

Overview

The current and projected growth in the number of people aged 65 years and older in the United States has focused attention on preserving quality of life as well as length of life. Chief among the factors involving preserving quality of life are the prevention and treatment of musculoskeletal conditions—the major causes of disability in the United States. Among musculoskeletal conditions, arthritis and other rheumatic conditions, osteoporosis, and chronic back conditions have the greatest impact on public health and quality of life.

Demographic trends suggest that people will need to continue working at older ages (for example, beyond age 65 years), increasing the adverse social and economic consequences of the high rates of activity limitation and disability of older persons with these conditions. At the same time, effective public health interventions exist to reduce the burden of all three conditions. (See Focus Area 6. Disability and Secondary Conditions.)

Issues and Trends

Arthritis

The various forms of arthritis affect more than 15 percent of the U.S. population—over 43 million persons—and more than 20 percent of the adult population, making arthritis one of the most common conditions in the United States.[1, 2, 3, 4]

The significant public health impact of arthritis is reflected in a variety of measures. First, arthritis is the leading cause of disability.[5] Arthritis limits the major activities (for example, working, housekeeping, school) of nearly 3 percent of the entire U.S. population (7 million persons), including nearly 1 out of every 5 persons with arthritis.[1, 2, 3] Arthritis trails only heart disease as a cause of work disability.[6] As a consequence, arthritis limits the independence of affected persons and disrupts the lives of family members and other caregivers.

Second, health-related quality-of-life measures are consistently worse for persons with arthritis, whether the measure is healthy days in the past 30 days, days without severe pain, "ability days" (that is, days without activity limitations), or difficulty in performing personal care activities.[7, 8]

Leading Causes of Disability
(Persons aged 15 years and older, United States, 1991–92)

	Percent
Arthritis or rheumatism	17.1%
Back or spine problem	13.5%
Heart trouble	11.1%
Lung or respiratory trouble	6.8%
High blood pressure	5.2%
Stiffness or deformity of the foot, leg, arm, or hand	4.8%
Diabetes	3.9%
Blindness or other visual impairment	3.5%
Deafness or serious trouble hearing	2.6%
Stroke	2.5%

Percent of all disabilities

Source: CDC. Prevalence of disabilities and associated health conditions—United States, 1991–92. *Morbidity and Mortality Weekly Report* 43(40):730-731, 737-739, 1994.

Third, arthritis has a sizable economic impact. Arthritis is the source of at least 44 million visits to health care providers, 744,000 hospitalizations, and 4 million days of hospital care per year.[4, 9] Estimated medical care costs for persons with arthritis were $15 billion, and total costs (medical care plus lost productivity) were $65 billion in 1992.[10] This latter amount is equal to 1.1 percent of the gross domestic product. Nearly 60 percent of persons with arthritis are in the working-aged population[1, 2, 3] and they have a low rate of labor force participation.[11]

Fourth, arthritis, like other chronic pain conditions, has an important negative effect on a person's mental health.[12, 13]

Fifth, although death is not a frequent outcome of arthritis, persons with certain forms of arthritis have higher death rates than the general population. For example, the 2 million persons in the United States with rheumatoid arthritis are at greater risk of premature death from respiratory and infectious diseases than the overall U.S. population.[14]

A variety of demographic trends indicate that the impact of arthritis will only increase.[15] Given current population projections, arthritis will affect over 18 percent of all persons in the United States (nearly 60 million persons) in the year

2020 and will limit the major activities of nearly 4 percent (11.6 million).[1, 2, 3] Direct and indirect costs are expected to rise proportionately.

Osteoporosis

About 13 to 18 percent of women aged 50 years and older and 3 to 6 percent of men aged 50 years and older have osteoporosis, a reduction in bone mass or density that leads to deteriorated and fragile bones. These rates correspond to 4 million to 6 million women and 1 million to 2 million men in the United States who have osteoporosis.[16] Another 37 to 50 percent of women aged 50 years and older and 28 to 47 percent of men of the same age group have some degree of osteopenia, reduction in bone mass that is not as severe as osteoporosis.

The major health consequence of osteoporosis is an increased risk of fractures. Approximately 1.5 million fractures per year are attributed to osteoporosis.[17] One in three women and one in eight men aged 50 years and older will experience an osteoporotic-related fracture in their lifetime.[17] Health care costs for these fractures are estimated at $13.8 billion per year in 1996 dollars.[18]

The risk of any fracture increases with the presence of osteoporosis, but hip fractures represent the most serious impact in terms of health care costs and consequences for the individual. In 1994, there were 281,000 hospital discharges for hip fracture among people aged 45 years and older. Of these, 74,000, or 26 percent, were among men.[16] In all, 1 out of 6 white women and 1 out of 17 white men will experience a hip fracture by the time they reach age 90 years.[19] Although the hip fracture rate among women seems relatively constant, the rate among men seems to be increasing over time.[20]

An average of 24 percent of hip fracture patients aged 50 years and older die in the year following fracture, with higher death rates among men than among women.[21] Also, hip fracture is more likely to lead to functional impairment than are other serious medical conditions, including heart attack, stroke, and cancer.[21] For example, half of all hip fracture patients will be unable to walk without assistance.[17]

Chronic Back Conditions

Chronic low back pain is described in different ways, such as the occurrence of back pain lasting for more than 7 to 12 weeks, back pain lasting beyond the expected period of healing, or frequently recurring back pain. Moreover, a wide range of outcome measures are used to describe chronic back problems, such as low back pain (LBP), activity limitation, impairment, and disability. Compounding the problem is the lack of a single data source to track chronic back problems. Sources that have been used include workers compensation data, Occupational Safety and Health Administration and Bureau of Labor Statistics records, and data from national health surveys.

Chronic back conditions are both common and debilitating. Back pain occurs in 15 to 45 percent of people each year,[22, 23, 24, 25, 26] and 70 to 85 percent of people have back pain some time in their lives. In the United States, back pain is the most frequent cause of activity limitation in people under age 45 years,[27, 28] the second most frequent reason for physician visits, the fifth-ranking reason for hospitalization, and the third most common reason for surgical procedures.[29]

Work-related risk factors, such as heavy physical work, lifting and forceful movements, awkward postures, and whole body vibration, are associated with low back disorders. Work-related risk factors account for 28 to 50 percent of the low back problems in an adult population.[30] A number of personal factors may be risk factors for low back pain. These include nonmodifiable factors, such as age and gender, some anthropometric characteristics (for example, height and body build), history of low back problems, and spinal abnormalities as well as modifiable factors, such as weight, physical fitness, smoking, some aspects of lumbar flexibility, trunk muscle strength, and hamstring elasticity. A history of low back problems is one of the most reliable predictors of subsequent back problems.[31]

Disparities

Arthritis is a leading health problem among all demographic groups, although significant and sometimes surprising disparities exist. Arthritis affects 50 percent of people aged 65 years and older. However, most people with arthritis are younger than age 65 years and of working age.[1, 2, 3] Arthritis also affects 285,000 children,[32] making it one of the more common chronic conditions of childhood. Arthritis is more common in women aged 18 years and older than in men and is the leading chronic condition and cause of activity limitation among women.[33, 34]

Whites and African Americans have similar rates of disease, but African Americans have greater rates of activity limitation.[1, 2, 3] For African Americans, arthritis is the third most common chronic condition and the leading cause of activity limitation.[35] For Hispanics and American Indians or Alaska Natives, arthritis is the second most common chronic condition and the second leading cause of activity limitation.[35] For Asians or Pacific Islanders, arthritis is the fourth most common chronic condition and the second leading cause of activity limitation.[35] For whites, arthritis is the most common chronic condition and the second leading cause of activity limitation.[35]

The rate of arthritis and its associated disabilities is higher among persons with low education and low income.[1, 2, 3] African Americans have lower rates of total joint replacement, a surgical procedure that is highly successful in reducing the impact of arthritis in persons with severe pain or disability, than do whites.[36] Certain types of jobs, such as shipyard work, farm work, and occupations that place high knee-bending demands on workers, increase the risks for osteoarthritis.[37, 38]

Osteoporosis is more common among women than men. The rates of disease increase markedly with increasing age. Rates are higher among non-Hispanic white Americans than among Mexican Americans or non-Hispanic African Americans.[16] White postmenopausal women are at highest risk of the disease.

The risk for chronic back pain increases with age. Although back pain appears to be equally common in men and women, impairment from back and spine conditions is more common in women.

Opportunities

The importance of physical activity for bone and joint health was highlighted in a 1996 report *Physical Activity and Health: A Report of the Surgeon General.*[39] Although behavioral interventions seem to have potential benefits, risk factors for the various types of arthritis need to be identified. Recreational or occupational joint injury has been identified as a risk factor for later osteoarthritis, and overweight is a risk factor for osteoarthritis of the knee and possibly the hip and hand.[40] Overweight appears to be a risk factor associated with the progression and severity of osteoarthritis.[40, 41]

Genetic research may soon identify persons at high risk for certain types of arthritis and thereby offer a better target for interventions. Current medical care offers considerable relief from pain and other symptoms for all types of arthritis. Available interventions often are not used, however, because of the popular belief that arthritis is part of normal aging, that a person can do nothing about it, and that it affects only old persons. However, early diagnosis and aggressive treatment of rheumatoid arthritis with disease-modifying drugs, for example, appear to reduce its symptoms and related disability.[42, 43, 44, 45, 46, 47]

Educational and behavioral interventions also can relieve symptoms and reduce disability. Telephone contacts with clinicians and several land-based and water exercise programs have had beneficial outcomes.[48, 49, 50, 51] The Arthritis Self-Help Course, a 6-week, 2-hour per week educational intervention, has been shown to reduce pain up to 20 percent beyond what was achieved through conventional medical care.[52] The course has the additional benefit of reducing medical care costs by reducing the number of physician visits for arthritis.[52, 53] These and other effective interventions currently are underused, with some reaching less than 1 percent of target populations.[54] Countering myths about arthritis and applying available interventions can help reduce the impact of this health problem. (See Focus Area 6. Disability and Secondary Conditions.)

Interventions for osteoporosis and fractures can be designed to prevent the development of the disease, reduce further bone loss after the occurrence of the disease, and lessen the risk of fractures. Opportunities for primary prevention occur throughout the lifespan and include programs to promote exercise, avoid smoking, reduce excessive alcohol consumption, and improve nutrition, particularly the amount of calcium and vitamin D in the diet. (See Focus Area 19.

Nutrition and Overweight.) These approaches may be important in achieving a high peak bone mass during adolescence to delay the onset of osteoporosis as bone mass declines with age. The approaches also may reduce the rate of bone loss later in life.

Women need to be particularly concerned about bone loss occurring at the time of menopause, when bone can be lost at the rate of 2 to 4 percent per year. Women should be counseled on methods to minimize their bone loss. Evidence indicates that older persons, even those who have had a fracture, can benefit from treatment to prevent further bone loss or restore some lost bone to decrease the risk of subsequent fractures.[55]

A wide range of interventions prevent or reduce low back problems. These interventions may include activities designed to reduce the physical demands of work activities by redesigning the task or to address the individual's specific needs, such as strength or endurance training or counseling for nutrition and lifestyle changes. Ergonomic interventions that are directed at changing the job or work environment have proved effective in reducing risk of occupational low back pain. (See Focus Area 20. Occupational Safety and Health.) Thus, it is reasonable to assume that ergonomic approaches would be effective in preventing chronic LBP as well. Even in a nonwork environment, the physical demands of an activity can be reduced by using ergonomic principles. Interventions involving training in proper lifting techniques, physical conditioning, and weight loss have been investigated in programmatically oriented studies. These have shown that workplace interventions may have an effect on low back disorders.[56] The overall benefits of exercise, nutrition, and lifestyle changes on an individual's health and well-being would certainly justify efforts in this area. Also, interventions directed at improving strength and endurance may have an important impact on reducing activity limitations due to chronic LBP.

Because national data systems will not be available in the first half of the decade for tracking progress, four subjects of interest concerning arthritis and osteoporosis are not covered in this focus area's objectives. Representing a research and data collection agenda for the coming decade, the topics involve appropriate management, patient education, provider counseling, and bone fracture prevention. The first addresses persons with systemic rheumatic disease who receive an early specific diagnosis and appropriate management plan. The second topic concerns hospitals, managed care organizations, and large group practices that provide effective, evidence-based arthritis education (including information about community and self-help resources) for patients to use as an integral part of the management of their condition. The third topic concerns health care provider counseling for persons at risk for or who have arthritis. Women aged 65 years and older who are eligible under Medicare criteria to have an initial bone density measurement are the focus of the fourth topic about bone fracture prevention.

The national health objectives for the year 2000 included two objectives for osteoporosis, one objective for chronic back conditions, and no objectives for arthritis. The objective of increasing the proportion of women of menopausal age who have been counseled about estrogen replacement therapy for the prevention of osteoporosis had no data subsequent to the 1994 baseline to chart progress. Annual hip fracture rates increased among people aged 65 years and older, and rates of activity limitation due to chronic back conditions increased from the 1986–88 baseline.

Note: Unless otherwise noted, data are from the Centers for Disease Control and Prevention, National Center for Health Statistics, *Healthy People 2000 Review, 1998–99.*

Arthritis, Osteoporosis, and Chronic Back Conditions

Goal: Prevent illness and disability related to arthritis and other rheumatic conditions, osteoporosis, and chronic back conditions.

Number Objective Short Title

Arthritis and Other Rheumatic Conditions

2-1	Mean number of days without severe pain
2-2	Activity limitations due to arthritis
2-3	Personal care limitations
2-4	Help in coping
2-5	Employment rate
2-6	Racial differences in total knee replacement
2-7	Seeing a health care provider
2-8	Arthritis education

Osteoporosis

2-9	Cases of osteoporosis
2-10	Hospitalization for vertebral fractures

Chronic Back Conditions

2-11	Activity limitations due to chronic back conditions

Arthritis and Other Rheumatic Conditions

2-1. (Developmental) Increase the mean number of days without severe pain among adults who have chronic joint symptoms.

Potential data sources: Behavioral Risk Factor Surveillance System (BRFSS), CDC, NCCDPHP; National Health Interview Survey (NHIS), CDC, NCHS.

Public health researchers measure days without severe pain by asking, "During the past 30 days, for about how many days did pain make it hard for you to do your usual activities, such as self-care, work, or recreation?" Pain is the most important symptom among persons with arthritis, resulting in the widespread use of conventional prescription and nonprescription medications, surgical interventions, and alternative medical treatments. A measure of pain-free days provides a pertinent and understandable performance-based approach for tracking this key health-related quality of life (HRQOL) determinant for persons with arthritis. Increasing days without severe pain is a feasible target, given more widespread use of available interventions (medical, educational, exercise, nutritional) that are likely to affect this measure. Health surveys variously ask about chronic joint symptoms or arthritis in addressing arthritis and other rheumatic conditions, which is why both terms are used for these objectives.

2-2. Reduce the proportion of adults with chronic joint symptoms who experience a limitation in activity due to arthritis.

Target: 21 percent.

Baseline: 27 percent of adults aged 18 years and older with chronic joint symptoms experienced a limitation in activity due to arthritis in 1997 (age adjusted to the year 2000 standard population).

Target setting method: Better than the best.

Data source: National Health Interview Survey (NHIS), CDC, NCHS.

Adults Aged 18 Years and Older With Chronic Joint Symptoms, 1997	Limitation in Activity Due to Arthritis
	Percent
TOTAL	27
Race and ethnicity	
American Indian or Alaska Native	27
Asian or Pacific Islander	18
Asian	16
Native Hawaiian and other Pacific Islander	DSU
Black or African American	32
White	27
Hispanic or Latino	28
Not Hispanic or Latino	27
Black or African American	32
White	27
Gender	
Female	31
Male	22
Family income level	
Poor	36
Near poor	30
Middle/high income	24
Education level (aged 25 years and older)	
Less than high school	34
High school graduate	32
At least some college	26

DNA = Data have not been analyzed. DNC = Data are not collected. DSU = Data are statistically unreliable.
Note: Age adjusted to the year 2000 standard population.

2-3. Reduce the proportion of all adults with chronic joint symptoms who have difficulty in performing two or more personal care activities, thereby preserving independence.

Target: 1.4 percent.

Baseline: 2.0 percent of adults aged 18 years and older with chronic joint symptoms experienced difficulty performing two or more personal care activities in 1997 (age adjusted to the year 2000 standard population).

Target setting method: Better than the best.

Data source: National Health Interview Survey (NHIS), CDC, NCHS.

Adults Aged 18 Years and Older With Chronic Joint Symptoms, 1997	Personal Care Limitations
	Percent
TOTAL	2.0
Race and ethnicity	
American Indian or Alaska Native	DSU
Asian or Pacific Islander	DSU
Asian	DSU
Native Hawaiian and other Pacific Islander	DSU
Black or African American	3.6
White	1.8
Hispanic or Latino	3.5
Not Hispanic or Latino	1.9
Black or African American	3.4
White	1.7
Gender	
Female	2.2
Male	1.6
Family income level	
Poor	5.4
Near poor	2.4
Middle/high income	0.9
Education level (aged 25 years and older)	
Less than high school	3.4
High school graduate	2.2
At least some college	1.4

DNA = Data have not been analyzed. DNC = Data are not collected. DSU = Data are statistically unreliable.
Note: Age adjusted to the year 2000 standard population.

Arthritis and other rheumatic conditions affect quality of life in many ways and are key items of personal interest to individuals with these conditions.[7, 8, 57, 58, 59, 60, 61] From a public health perspective, validated measures of HRQOL are essential for monitoring the impact of clinical and public health interventions.

Activity limitation occurs frequently among persons with arthritis and is an important functional element that can compromise independence. Activity limitation affects 27 percent of all persons who have arthritis,[1] making it the number one cause of activity limitations in the United States.[5] The activity limitations of arthritis also indirectly affect health and independence by decreasing physical activity, increasing weight, and placing persons at higher risk for all the adverse outcomes of those risk factors.

As the leading cause of disability, arthritis is a leading cause of difficulty in performing personal care activities and thereby a leading cause of loss of independence. Therefore, maintaining independence, especially in personal care, is important for persons with arthritis.

2-4.   (Developmental) Increase the proportion of adults aged 18 years and older with arthritis who seek help in coping if they experience personal and emotional problems.

Potential data sources: National Health Interview Survey (NHIS), CDC, NCHS; Behavioral Risk Factor Surveillance System (BRFSS), CDC, NCCDPHP.

Coping difficulties, depression, anxiety, and low self-efficacy are recognized as major personal and emotional problems among persons with arthritis.[12] These problems are especially frequent among persons who experience physical pain. Because arthritis is a leading cause of chronic pain, monitoring these mental health outcomes can help assess the success of applied interventions.[13]

2-5.   Increase the employment rate among adults with arthritis in the working-aged population.

Target: 78 percent.

Baseline: 67 percent of adults aged 18 to 64 years with arthritis were employed in the past week in 1997 (age adjusted to the year 2000 standard population).

Target setting method: Better than the best.

Data source: National Health Interview Survey (NHIS), CDC, NCHS.

NOTE: THE TABLE BELOW MAY CONTINUE TO THE FOLLOWING PAGE.

Adults Aged 18 to 64 Years With Arthritis, 1997	Employed in Past Week
	Percent
TOTAL	67
Race and ethnicity	
American Indian or Alaska Native	46
Asian or Pacific Islander	56
Asian	54
Native Hawaiian and other Pacific Islander	DSU

Adults Aged 18 to 64 Years With Arthritis, 1997	Employed in Past Week
	Percent
Black or African American	52
White	69
Hispanic or Latino	60
Not Hispanic or Latino	67
Black or African American	53
White	70
Gender	
Female	60
Male	74
Family income level	
Poor	39
Near poor	54
Middle/high income	77
Education level (aged 25 to 64 years)	
Less than high school	47
High school graduate	65
At least some college	78

DNA = Data have not been analyzed. DNC = Data are not collected. DSU = Data are statistically unreliable.
Note: Age adjusted to the year 2000 standard population.
NOTE: THE TABLE ABOVE MAY HAVE CONTINUED FROM THE PREVIOUS PAGE.

Labor force participation rates (which parallel employment rates) for all persons of working age (18 to 64 years) in 1994 were 71 percent for females and 87 percent for males.[11] Rates for persons with arthritis, however, are far below these numbers.[11] A part of this low rate may be increased through early diagnosis and appropriate management, improved self-management, and improved job retention efforts. Raising this low rate will help foster independence for affected persons and reduce the demands on families and society. Reducing demands on families and society is particularly important as demographic changes lead to fewer workers for each nonworker.

2-6. (Developmental) Eliminate racial disparities in the rate of total knee replacements.

Potential data sources: Medicare data, HCFA; National Hospital Discharge Survey (NHDS), CDC, NCHS; Hospital Cost and Utilization Project (HCUP), AHRQ.

Studies have shown that African Americans have much lower rates of total knee replacement than whites, even when adjusted for age, gender, and insurance coverage.[36] The reasons for this difference are unclear, but the effect is that many persons are not getting needed interventions to reduce pain and disability. This is one component of a more widespread problem of racial differences in medical care that is difficult to explain by financial or access-to-care issues.

2-7. (Developmental) Increase the proportion of adults who have seen a health care provider for their chronic joint symptoms.

Potential data source: National Health Interview Survey (NHIS) CDC, NCHS.

Studies using the 1989 National Health Interview Survey have shown that 16 percent of adults aged 18 years and older have not seen a doctor for their arthritis.[62] Appropriate medical management, patient and provider education, improved self-management, and physical activity—all encouraged by providers—can reduce arthritis pain and disability. Increasing the percentage of persons who seek a diagnosis and treatment from a health care provider for their chronic joint symptoms is an objective amenable to public awareness campaigns to counter the myths that arthritis is part of normal aging and nothing can be done for it. This objective is especially important for the working-aged population, the upper age limit of which is likely to rise as the overall population ages through the 2030s.

2-8. (Developmental) Increase the proportion of persons with arthritis who have had effective, evidence-based arthritis education as an integral part of the management of their condition.

Potential data sources: National Health Interview Survey (NHIS), CDC, NCHS; Behavioral Risk Factor Surveillance System (BRFSS), CDC, NCCDPHP.

Existing evidence-based education interventions, such as the Arthritis Self-Help Course, are effective in reducing arthritis pain and reducing physician visits for arthritis.[52] These beneficial interventions, which include information about community and self-help resources, are estimated to reach less than 1 percent of the population with arthritis.[54] Expanding the dissemination of the benefits of interventions currently available offers the opportunity of quickly improving the health of all persons with arthritis and reducing the impact of arthritis nationally. Education efforts should be provided in a culturally and linguistically competent manner.

2-9. Reduce the proportion of adults with osteoporosis.

Target: 8 percent.

Baseline: 10 percent of adults aged 50 years and older had osteoporosis as measured by low total femur bone mineral density (BMD) in 1988–94 (age adjusted to the year 2000 standard population).

Target setting method: 20 percent improvement.

Data source: National Health and Nutrition Examination Survey (NHANES), CDC, NCHS.

Adults Aged 50 Years and Older, 1988–94	Osteoporosis as Measured by Low Bone Mineral Density
	Percent
TOTAL	10
Race and ethnicity	
American Indian or Alaska Native	DSU
Asian or Pacific Islander	DSU
Asian	DNC
Native Hawaiian and other Pacific Islander	DNC
Black or African American	7
White	10
Hispanic or Latino	DSU
Mexican American	10
Not Hispanic or Latino	10
Black or African American	7
White	10
Gender	
Female	16
Male	3
Education level	
Less than high school	11
High school graduate	11
At least some college	9

DNA = Data have not been analyzed. DNC = Data are not collected. DSU = Data are statistically unreliable.
Note: Age adjusted to the year 2000 standard population.

BMD has been identified as one of the primary predictive factors for osteoporosis-related fractures.[63, 64, 65] Osteoporosis is defined as a BMD value that is more than 2.5 standard deviations below that of an average young adult.[66]

The proportion of adults aged 50 years and older with osteoporosis in the total femur region is 10 percent (16 percent in women and 3 percent in men). Osteoporosis occurs in nonwhite women and in men, although the rates of disease are not as high as the rates found among white women. These estimates are based on the total femur; estimates based on a different skeletal site (or combination of sites) may differ. For example, the proportion of white women with osteoporosis in Olmsted County, Minnesota, was established to be approximately 16 to 17 percent at the femur, lumbar spine, or wrist when each site was considered separately. However, 30 percent of women had osteoporosis in at least one of the three sites.[67]

Osteoporosis is a major risk factor for hip fracture. Virtually all persons with a hip fracture are hospitalized for treatment.[21] Two-thirds of persons who fracture a hip do not return to their prefracture level of functioning. Health care expenditures for hip fractures in 1995 have been estimated at $8.7 billion.[18] Interventions that reduce the rate of osteoporosis should have a marked impact on the rate of hip fractures. Estimates indicate that osteoporosis contributes to 90 percent of hip fractures in women and 80 percent of hip fractures in men.[65] Increasing BMD by 5 percent may decrease the risk of fractures by 25 percent.[68]

Although osteoporosis increases the risk of fractures, most hip fractures result from falls.[66] Some risk factors associated with falls may be amenable to interventions. These risk factors include impaired vision, use of long-acting psychotropic drugs, physical inactivity, muscle weakness, and poor health.[69] (See Focus Area 15. Injury and Violence Prevention.)

2-10. Reduce the proportion of adults who are hospitalized for vertebral fractures associated with osteoporosis.

Target: 14.0 hospitalizations per 10,000 adults aged 65 years and older.

Baseline: 17.5 hospitalizations per 10,000 adults aged 65 years and older were for vertebral fractures associated with osteoporosis in 1998 (age adjusted to the year 2000 standard population).

Target setting method: 20 percent improvement.

Data source: National Hospital Discharge Survey (NHDS), CDC, NCHS.

Adults Aged 65 Years and Older, 1998	Hospitalizations for Vertebral Fractures Associated With Osteoporosis
	Rate per 10,000
TOTAL	17.5
Race and ethnicity	
American Indian or Alaska Native	DSU
Asian or Pacific Islander	DSU
Asian	DNC
Native Hawaiian and other Pacific Islander	DNC
Black or African American	DSU
White	14.0
Hispanic or Latino	DSU
Not Hispanic or Latino	DSU
Black or African American	DSU
White	DSU
Gender	
Female	19.6
Male	13.9
Select populations	
Age groups (not age adjusted)	
65 to 74 years	6.7
75 to 84 years	26.0
85 years and older	39.0

DNA = Data have not been analyzed. DNC = Data are not collected. DSU = Data are statistically unreliable.
Note: Age adjusted to the year 2000 standard population.

Vertebral fractures are the most common fracture due to osteoporosis.[70] About 30 to 50 percent of women and 20 to 30 percent of men will experience vertebral fractures in their lifetime.[70] The overall number of cases of these fractures rises rapidly with increasing age. Among white women, the rate rises from 6 percent among those aged 50 to 59 years to about 75 percent among those aged 90 years and older.[71] Most of these fractures cause little difficulty and go unrecognized. However, 33 percent of the fractures will be diagnosed clinically, 8 percent will require hospitalization,[72] and about 2 percent will require long-term nursing care.[73]

The most common symptom of vertebral fractures is back pain, which is reported in about half of the cases. People with these fractures are more likely to have difficulty performing activities of daily living, such as bending, reaching above the head, and walking. Changes in the outward appearance of people experiencing these fractures is a loss of height and the development of a humped back.[70]

Interventions that reduce the number of persons with osteoporosis should reduce the rates of vertebral fractures. Falls associated with fractures at other sites do not play a prominent role in these fractures. Normal daily activities can place sufficient stress on the vertebra to cause fractures.[71]

For discussion of calcium and vitamin D, see Focus Area 19. Nutrition and Overweight.

Chronic Back Conditions

2-11. Reduce activity limitation due to chronic back conditions.

Target: 25 adults per 1,000 population aged 18 years and older.

Baseline: 32 adults per 1,000 population aged 18 years and older experienced activity limitation due to chronic back conditions in 1997 (age adjusted to the year 2000 standard population).

Target setting method: Better than the best.

Data source: National Health Interview Survey (NHIS), CDC, NCHS.

NOTE: THE TABLE BELOW MAY CONTINUE TO THE FOLLOWING PAGE.

Adults Aged 18 Years and Older, 1997	Activity Limitation Due to Chronic Back Conditions
	Rate per 1,000
TOTAL	32
Race and ethnicity	
American Indian or Alaska Native	68
Asian or Pacific Islander	18
Asian	15
Native Hawaiian and other Pacific Islander	DSU
Black or African American	36
White	31
Hispanic or Latino	28
Not Hispanic or Latino	32
Black or African American	36
White	32

Adults Aged 18 Years and Older, 1997	Activity Limitation Due to Chronic Back Conditions
	Rate per 1,000
Gender	
Female	32
Male	31
Family income level	
Poor	77
Near poor	53
Middle/high income	24
Education level (aged 25 years and older)	
Less than high school	54
High school graduate	35
Some college	28

DNA = Data have not been analyzed. DNC = Data are not collected. DSU = Data are statistically unreliable.
Note: Age adjusted to the year 2000 standard population.
NOTE: THE TABLE ABOVE MAY HAVE CONTINUED FROM THE PREVIOUS PAGE.

Persons who are overweight and persons who frequently bend over or lift heavy objects are at risk for low back injuries.[74] Occupations that require repetitive lifting, particularly in a forward bent and twisted position, place employees at especially high risk. Other risk factors for low back injury include exposure to vibration produced by vehicles or industrial machinery, prolonged vehicle driving, and certain sports activities.[24, 25, 26, 75, 76] Predictors of back problems may include diminished lumbar flexibility, trunk muscle strength, and hamstring elasticity.[77] Osteoporosis increases the risk of vertebral compression, which may account for the increase in reported low back pain in older females.[78, 79] Increased age also is associated with back pain.[80] In addition, persons who have experienced back problems in the past are at increased risk for future injury.[80, 81]

Related Objectives From Other Focus Areas

1. **Access to Quality Health Services**
   1-3. Counseling about health behaviors
3. **Cancer**
   3-10. Provider counseling about cancer prevention
6. **Disability and Secondary Conditions**
   6-4. Social participation among adults with disabilities
   6-5. Sufficient emotional support among adults with disabilities
   6-8. Employment parity

7. **Educational and Community-Based Programs**
   7-5.   Worksite health promotion programs
   7-6.   Participation in employer-sponsored health promotion activities
   7-10. Community health promotion programs
   7-12. Older adult participation in community health promotion activities

15. **Injury and Violence Prevention**
   15-28. Hip fractures

19. **Nutrition and Overweight**
   19-1.   Healthy weight in adults
   19-2.   Obesity in adults
   19-11. Calcium intake
   19-16. Worksite promotion of nutrition education and weight management
   19-17. Nutrition counseling for medical conditions

20. **Occupational Safety and Health**
   20-2.   Work-related injuries
   20-3.   Overexertion or repetitive motion

22. **Physical Activity and Fitness**
   22-1.   No leisure-time physical activity
   22-2.   Moderate physical activity
   22-3.   Vigorous physical activity
   22-4.   Muscular strength and endurance
   22-5.   Flexibility
   22-8.   Physical education requirement in schools
   22-10. Physical activity in physical education class

27. **Tobacco Use**
   27-1.   Adult tobacco use
   27-5.   Smoking cessation by adults
   27-7.   Smoking cessation by adolescents
   27-17. Adolescent disapproval of smoking

Terminology

(A listing of abbreviations and acronyms used in this publication appears in Appendix H.)

Activity limitations: Problems in a person's performance of everyday functions such as communication, self-care, mobility, learning, and behavior.

Arthritis: Shorthand for arthritis and other rheumatic conditions.

Arthritis and other rheumatic conditions: More than 100 conditions (or diseases or problems) that primarily affect the joints, muscles, fascia, tendons, bursa, ligaments, and other connective tissues of the body.

Bone mineral density (BMD): Measurement used to determine the presence of osteoporosis.

Chronic back conditions: Low back pain and other conditions affecting only the back.

Chronic joint symptoms: Pain, aching, stiffness, or swelling in or around a joint that was present on most days for at least 1 month in the past 12 months.

Disability: General term used to represent the interactions between individuals with a health condition and barriers in their environment. The term disability is operationalized as self-reported activity limitations or use of assistive devices or equipment related to an activity limitation.

Musculoskeletal conditions: Problems that affect the skeleton, joints, muscles, and connective tissues of the body.

Osteoarthritis: A slowly progressive, degenerative joint disease that results from the breakdown of cartilage and leads to pain and stiffness; usually affects the knees, hips, and hands; the most common form of arthritis.

Osteopenia: A condition similar to osteoporosis (see below) except the reduction in bone mass is not as severe.

Osteoporosis: Bone disease characterized by a reduction of bone mass and a deterioration of the microarchitecture of the bone leading to bone fragility.

Personal care activities: Eating, bathing, dressing, or getting around inside the home, including getting in or out of bed or chairs and using the toilet (including getting to the toilet).

Rheumatoid arthritis: A chronic, inflammatory disease of the body that produces its most prominent manifestations in joints, often leading to joint pain, stiffness, and deformity.

Work disability: Limited in the amount or kind of work; unable to work.

References

[1] Centers for Disease Control and Prevention (CDC). Arthritis prevalence and activity limitations—United States, 1990. *Morbidity and Mortality Weekly Report* 43(24):433-438, 1994.

[2] Lawrence, R.C.; Helmick, C.G.; Arnett, F.C.; et al. Estimates of the prevalence of arthritis and selected musculoskeletal disorders in the United States. *Arthritis & Rheumatism* 41(5):778-799, 1998.

[3] Helmick, C.G.; Lawrence, R.C.; Pollard, R.A.; et al. Arthritis and other rheumatic conditions: Who is affected now, who will be affected later? *National Arthritis Data Workgroup Arthritis Care and Research* 8:203-211, 1995.

[4] CDC. Impact of arthritis and other rheumatic conditions on the health-care system. *Morbidity and Mortality Weekly Report* 48(17):349-353, 1999.

[5] CDC. Current trends: Prevalence of disabilities and associated health conditions—United States, 1991–1992. *Morbidity and Mortality Weekly Report* 43(40):730-731, 737-739, 1994.

[6] LaPlante, M.P. *Data on Disability from the National Health Interview Survey, 1983–1985.* Washington, DC: National Institute on Disability and Rehabilitation Research (NIDRR), U.S. Department of Education (DOE), 1988.

[7] CDC. Health-related quality of life and activity limitation—8 states, 1995. *Morbidity and Mortality Weekly Report* 47(67):134-140, 1998.

[8] CDC. State differences in reported healthy days among adults—United States, 1993–1996. *Morbidity and Mortality Weekly Report* 47(12):239-243, 1998.

[9] CDC. *Targeting Arthritis: The Nation's Leading Cause of Disability. At-a-Glance, 1998.* Atlanta, GA: Technical Information and Editorial Services Branch, National Center for Chronic Disease Prevention and Health Promotion (NCCDPHP), CDC, 1998.

[10] Yelin, E., and Callahan, L.F. The economic cost and social and psychological impact of musculoskeletal conditions. *Arthritis & Rheumatism* 38(10):1351-1362, 1995.

[11] Trupin, L.; Sebesta, D.S.; Yelin, E.; et al. *Trends in Labor Force Participation Among Persons With Disability, 1983–1994. Disability Statistics Report 10.* Washington, DC: DOE, NIDRR, 1997.

[12] Frank, R.G., and Hagglund, K.J. Mood disorders. In: Wegener, S.T., ed. *Clinical Care in the Rheumatic Diseases.* Atlanta, GA: American College of Rheumatology, 1996, 125-130.

[13] Bradley, L.A.; Wegener, S.T.; Belza, B.L.; et al. Pain management interventions for patients with rheumatic diseases. In: Melvin, J., and Jensen, G., eds. *Rheumatologic Rehabilitation Series Volume I: Assessment and Management.* Rockville, MD: American Occupational Therapy Association, 1998, 259-278.

[14] Wolf, F. The natural history of rheumatoid arthritis. *Journal of Rheumathology* 23(Suppl. 44):13-22, 1996.

[15] Boult, C.; Altmann, M.; Gilbertson, D.; et al. Decreasing disability in the 21st century: The future effects of controlling six fatal and non-fatal conditions. *American Journal of Public Health* 86:1388-1393, 1996.

[16] Looker, A.C.; Orwoll, E.S.; Johnston, C.C.; et al. Prevalence of low femoral bone density in older U.S. adults from NHANES III. *Journal of Bone and Mineral Research* 12(11):1761-1768, 1997.

[17] Riggs, B.L., and Melton, III, L.J. The worldwide problem of osteoporosis: Insights afforded by epidemiology. *Bone* 17(Suppl. 5):505S-511S, 1995.

[18] Ray, N.F.; Chan, J.K.; Thamer, M.; et al. Medical expenditures for the treatment of osteoporotic fractures in the United States in 1995: Report from the National Osteoporosis Foundation. *Journal of Bone and Mineral Research* 12(1):24-35, 1997.

[19] Melton, III, L.J.; Chrischilles, E.A.; Cooper, C.; et al. How many women have osteoporosis? *Journal of Bone and Mineral Research* 7:1005-1010, 1992.

[20] Bacon, W.E. Secular trends in hip fracture occurrence and survival: Age and sex differences. *Journal of Aging Health* 8(4):538-553, 1996.

[21] U.S. Congress, Office of Technology Assessment. *Hip Fracture Outcomes in People Age 50 and Over—Background Paper.* OTA-BP-H-120. Washington, DC: U.S. Government Printing Office, July 1994.

[22] Anderson, G.B.J. The epidemology of spinal disorders. In: Frymoyer, J.W., ed. *The Adult Spine: Principles and Practice.* 2nd ed. Philadelphia, PA: Lippencott-Raven, 1997.

[23] Biering-Sorensen, F. Physical measurements as risk indicators for low-back trouble over a one year period. *Spine* 9:106-119, 1984.

[24] Frymoyer, J.W.; Pope, M.H.; Clements, J.H.; et al. Risk factors in low-back pain: An epidemiological survey. *Journal of Bone and Joint Surgery* 65(2):213-218, 1983.

[25] Frymoyer, J.W. Back pain and sciatica. *New England Journal of Medicine* 318(5):291-300, 1988.

[26] Svensson, H.O., and Anderson, G.B.J. Low-back pain in 40- to 47-year-old men: Work history and work environment factors. *Spine* 8(3):272-276, 1983.

[27] Anderson, G.B. Epidemiological aspects on low back pain in industry. *Spine* 6(1):53-60, 1981.

[28] Kelsey, J.L.; White, A.A.; Pastides, H.; et al. The impact of musculoskeletal disorders on the population of the United States. *Journal of Bone and Joint Surgery* 61(7):959-964, 1979.

[29] Praemer, A.; Furner, S.; and Rice, D.P. Musculoskeletal conditions in the United States. Park Ridge, IL: American Academy of Orthoscopic Surgery, 1992.

[30] Wegman, D.H., and Fine, L.J. Occupational and Environmental Medicine. *Journal of the American Medical Association* 275(23):1831-1832, 1996.

[31] Shelerud, R. Epidemiology of Occupational Low Back Pain. In: *Occupational Medicine: State of the Art Reviews.* Philadelphia, PA: Hanley and Belfus, 1998, 1-22.

[32] CDC. NCCDPHP, Division of Adult and Community Health, Health Care and Aging Studies Branch, Atlanta, GA, unpublished data, 1990.

[33] CDC. Prevalence and impact of arthritis among women. United States, 1989–1991. *Morbidity and Mortality Weekly Report* 44(17):329-334, 517-518, 1995.

[34] Callahan, L.F.; Rao, J.; and Boutaugh, M. Arthritis and women's health: Prevalence, impact, and prevention. *American Journal of Preventive Medicine* 12(5):401-409, 1996.

[35] CDC. Prevalence and impact of arthritis by race and ethnicity—United States, 1989–1991. *Morbidity and Mortality Weekly Report* 45(18):373-378, 1996.

[36] Wilson, M.G.; May, D.S.; and Kelly, J.J. Racial differences in the use of total knee arthroplasty for osteoarthritis among older Americans. *Ethnicity & Disease* 4(1):57-67, 1994.

[37] Hochberg, J.C. Osteoarthritis. In: Silman, A.J., and Hochberg, J.C., eds. *Epidemiology of the Rheumatic Diseases.* Oxford: Oxford University Press, 1993, 257-288.

[38] Felson, D.T. Epidemiology of hip and knee osteoarthritis. *Epidemiologic Reviews* 10:1-28, 1988.

[39] U.S. Department of Health and Human Services (HHS). *Physical Activity and Health: A Report of the Surgeon General.* Atlanta, GA: HHS, CDC, 1996.

[40] Felson, D.T., and Zhang, Y. Personal communication. An update on the epidemiology of knee and hip osteoarthritis with a view to prevention. August 1998.

[41] Felson, D.T.; Zhang, Y.; Anthony, J.M.; et al. Weight loss reduces the risk for symptomatic knee osteoarthritis in women. The Framingham Study. *Annals of Internal Medicine* 116(7):535-539, 1992.

[42] Weinblatt, M.E. Rheumatoid arthritis: Treat now, not later! (Editorial). *Annals of Internal Medicine* 124:773-774, 1996.

[43] Van der Heide, A.; Jacobs, J.W.; Bijlsma, J.W.; et al. The effectiveness of early treatment with "second-line" antirheumatic drugs. A randomized, controlled trial. *Annals of Internal Medicine* 124(8):699-707, 1996.

[44] Fries, J.F.; Williams, C.A.; Morrfeld, D.; et al. Reduction in long-term disability in patients with rheumatoid arthritis by disease-modifying antirheumatic drug-based treatment strategies. *Arthritis & Rheumatism* 39:616-622, 1996.

[45] Egsmose, C.; Lund, B.; Borg, G.; et al. Patients with rheumatoid arthritis benefit from early 2nd line therapy: 5-year follow up of a prospective double blind placebo controlled study. *Journal of Rheumatology* 22:2208-2213, 1995.

[46] Kirwan, J.R. The Arthritis and Rheumatism Council, Low-Dose Glucocorticoid Study Group. The effect of glucocorticoids on joint destruction in rheumatoid arthritis. *New England Journal of Medicine* 333(3):142-146, 1995.

[47] Emery, P., and Salmon, M. Early rheumatoid arthritis: Time to aim for remission? *Annals of Rheumatic Diseases* 54:944-947, 1995.

[48] Maisiak, R.; Austin, J.; and Heck, L. Health outcomes of two telephone interventions for patients with rheumatoid arthritis or osteoarthritis. *Arthritis & Rheumatism* 39:1391-1399, 1996.

[49] Minor, M.A. Arthritis and exercise: The times they are a-changin' (Editorial). *Arthritis Care and Research* 9:9-81, 1996.

[50] Minor, M.A., and Kay, D.R. Arthritis. In: *Exercise Management for Persons With Chronic Diseases and Disabilities.* Champaign, IL: Human Kinetics, 1997.

[51] Puett, D.W., and Griffin, M.R. Published trials of nonmedicinal and noninvasive therapies for hip and knee osteoarthritis. *Annals of Internal Medicine* 121(2):133-140, 1994.

[52] Lorig, K.R.; Mazonson, P.D.; and Holman, H.R. Evidence suggesting that health education for self-management in patients with chronic arthritis has sustained health benefits while reducing health care costs. *Arthritis & Rheumatism* 36(4):439-446, 1993.

[53] Kruger, J.M.S.; Helmick, C.G.; Callahan, L.F.; et al. Cost-effectiveness of the Arthritis Self-Help Course. *Archives of Internal Medicine,* 1998.

[54] Boutaugh, M., Group Vice President, Health Promotion, Arthritis Foundation. Personal communication. August 1999.

[55] Seeman, E. Introduction. *American Journal of Medicine* 103(Suppl. 2a):1S-2S, 1997.

[56] Violinn, E. Do workplace interventions prevent low-back disorders? If so: Why?: A methodological commentary. *Erognomics* 42(1):258-272, 1999.

[57] Hennessy, C.H.; Moriarty, D.G.; Zack, M.M.; et al. Measuring health-related quality of life for public health surveillance. *Public Health Reports* 109(5):665-672, 1994.

[58] CDC. Quality of life as a new public health measure—Behavioral Risk Factor Surveillance System, 1993. *Morbidity and Mortality Weekly Report* 43(20):375-380, 1994.

[59] CDC. Health-related quality-of-life measures—United States, 1993. *Morbidity and Mortality Weekly Report* 44(11):195-200, 1995.

[60] Newschaffer, C.J. *Validation of BRFSS HRQOL Measures in a Statewide Sample.* Atlanta, GA: HHS, Public Health Service, CDC, NCCDPHP, 1998.

[61] Verbrugge, L.M.; Merrill, S.S.; and Liu, X. Measuring disability with parsimony. *Disability Rehabilitation* 21(5-6):295-306, 1999.

Healthy People 2010: Objectives for Improving Health

[62] Rao, J.K.; Callahan, L.F.; and Helmick, C.G. Characteristics of persons with self-reported arthritis and other rheumatic conditions who do not see a doctor. *Journal of Rheumatology* 24:169-173, 1997.

[63] Cummings, S.R.; Black, D.M.; Nevitt, M.C.; et al. Bone density at various sites for prediction of hip fractures. *Lancet* 341(8837):72-75, 1993.

[64] Melton, III, L.J.; Atkinson, E.J.; O'Fallon, W.M.; et al. Long-term fracture prediction by bone mineral assessed at different skeletal sites. *Journal of Bone and Mineral Research* 8(10):1227-1233, 1993.

[65] Melton, III, L.J.; Thamer, M.; Ray, N.F.; et al. Fractures attributable to osteoporosis: Report from the National Osteoporosis Foundation. *Journal of Bone and Mineral Research* 12(1):16-23, 1997.

[66] World Health Organization (WHO). *Assessment of Fracture Risk and Its Application to Screening for Postmenopausal Osteoporosis.* Technical Report Series No. 843. Geneva, Switzerland: WHO, 1994.

[67] Melton, III, L.J. How many women have osteoporosis now? *Journal of Bone and Mineral Research* 10(2):175-177, 1995.

[68] Lips, P. Prevention of hip fractures: Drug therapy. *Bone* 18(Suppl. 3):159S-163S, 1996.

[69] Cummings, S.R. Treatable and untreatable risk factors for hip fracture. *Bone* 18 (Suppl. 3):165S-176S, 1996.

[70] Ross P.D. Clinical consequences of vertebral fractures. *American Journal of Medicine* 103:30S-43S, 1997.

[71] Melton, III, L.J.; Kan, S.H.; Frye, M.A.; et al. Epidemiology of vertebral fractures in women. *American Journal of Epidemiology* 129:1000-1011, 1989.

[72] Jacobsen, S.J.; Cooper, C.; Gottlieb, M.S.; et al. Hospitalization with vertebral fracture among the aged: A national population-based study 1986–1989. *Epidemiology* 3(6):515-518, 1992.

[73] Chrischilles, E.A.; Butler, C.D.; Davis, S.C.; et al. A model of lifetime osteoporosis impact. *Archives of Internal Medicine* 151(10):2026-2032, 1991.

[74] Schuchmann, J.A. Low back pain: A comprehensive approach. *Comprehensive Therapy* 14(1):14-18, 1988.

[75] Kelsey, J.L.; Githens, P.B.; White, III, A.A.; et al. An epidemiologic study of lifting and twisting on the job and risk for acute, prolapsed lumbar vertebral disc. *Journal of Orthopaedic Research* 2(1):61-66, 1984.

[76] Kelsey, J.L.; Githens, P.B.; O'Conner, T.; et al. Acute prolapsed lumbar intervertebral disc. An epidemiologic study with special reference to driving automobiles and cigarette smoking. *Spine* 9(6):608-613, 1984.

[77] Parnianpour, M.; Bejjani, F.J.; and Pavlidis, L. Worker training: The fallacy of single, correct lifting technique. *Ergonomics* 30(2):331-334, 1987.

[78] Porter, R.W.; Hibbert, C.; and Wellman, P. Backache and the lumbar spinal canal. *Spine* 5(2):99-105, 1980.

[79] Buchanan, J.R.; Myers, C.; Greer, III, R.B.; et al. Assessment of the risk of vertebral fracture in menopausal women. *Journal of Bone and Joint Surgery* 69(2):212-218, 1987.

[80] Chaffin, D.B., and Park, K.S. A longitudinal study of low back pain as associated with occupational weight lifting factors. *American Industrial Hygiene Association Journal* 34(12):513-525, 1973.

[81] Venning, P.J.; Walter, S.D.; and Stitt, L.W. Personal and job-related factors as determinants of incidence of back injuries among nursing personnel. *Journal of Occupational Medicine* 29(10):820-825, 1987.

3

Cancer

Co-Lead Agencies: Centers for Disease Control and Prevention
National Institutes of Health

Contents

Goal

Reduce the number of new cancer cases as well as the illness, disability, and death caused by cancer.

Overview

Cancer is the second leading cause of death in the United States. During 2000, an estimated 1,220,100 persons in the United States were expected to be diagnosed with cancer; 552,200 persons were expected to die from cancer.[1] These estimates did not include most skin cancers, and new cases of skin cancer are estimated to exceed 1 million per year. One-half of new cases of cancer occur in people aged 65 years and over.[2]

About 491,400 persons who get cancer in a given year, or 4 in 10 patients, are expected to be alive 5 years after diagnosis. When adjusted for normal life expectancy (accounting for factors such as dying of heart disease, injuries, and diseases of old age), a relative 5-year survival rate of 60 percent is seen for all cancers.[1] This rate means that the chance of a person recently diagnosed with cancer being alive in 5 years is 60 percent of the chance of someone not diagnosed with cancer. Five-year relative survival rates commonly are used to monitor progress in the early detection and treatment of cancer and include persons who are living 5 years after diagnosis, whether in remission, disease free, or under treatment.

Issues and Trends

Cancer death rates for all sites combined decreased an average of 0.6 percent per year from 1990 to 1996.[3] This decrease occurred after rates had increased by 0.4 percent per year from 1973 to 1990.[4] Death rates for male lung, female breast, prostate, and colorectal cancers decreased significantly during the 1990–96 period.[3] The lung and bronchus, prostate, female breast, and colon and rectum were the most common cancer sites for all racial and ethnic populations in the United States and together accounted for approximately 54 percent of all newly diagnosed cancers.[1]

In addition to the human toll of cancer, the financial costs of cancer are substantial.[5] The overall annual costs for cancer are estimated at $107 billion, with $37 billion for direct medical costs (the total of all health expenditures), $11 billion for costs of illness (the cost of low productivity due to illness), and $59 billion for costs of death (the cost of lost productivity due to death). Treatment for lung, breast, and prostate cancers alone accounts for more than half of the direct medical costs.

Disparities

Cancer death rates vary by gender, race, and ethnicity.[3] Male cancer death rates peaked in 1990 at 220.8 per 100,000, and female death rates peaked a year later at 142.2 per 100,000. After the peak year, through 1996, male cancer deaths for all sites decreased on average by 1 percent per year, and female deaths decreased on average by 0.4 percent per year. There were significant decreases in death for lung, prostate, brain, and other nervous system cancers in males and a significant decrease in breast cancer death for females.[3] Among males, lung cancer death

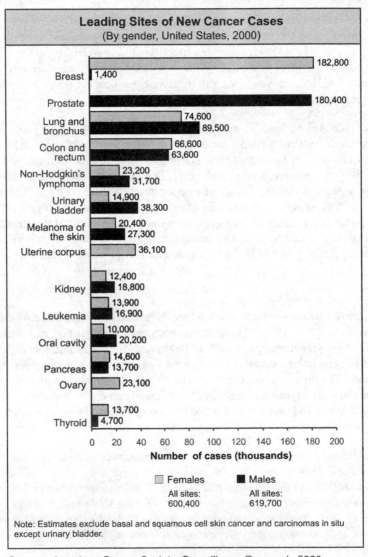

Leading Sites of New Cancer Cases
(By gender, United States, 2000)

Site	Females	Males
Breast	182,800	1,400
Prostate		180,400
Lung and bronchus	74,600	89,500
Colon and rectum	66,600	63,600
Non-Hodgkin's lymphoma	23,200	31,700
Urinary bladder	14,900	38,300
Melanoma of the skin	20,400	27,300
Uterine corpus	36,100	
Kidney	12,400	18,800
Leukemia	13,900	16,900
Oral cavity	10,000	20,200
Pancreas	14,600	13,700
Ovary	23,100	
Thyroid	13,700	4,700

Number of cases (thousands)

☐ Females   ■ Males

All sites: 600,400   All sites: 619,700

Note: Estimates exclude basal and squamous cell skin cancer and carcinomas in situ except urinary bladder.

Source: American Cancer Society. *Surveillance Research,* 2000.

Healthy People 2010: Objectives for Improving Health

rates have declined since 1990. In contrast, lung cancer death rates have continued to increase among females. Since 1987, more females have died from lung cancer than breast cancer.

African Americans are about 34 percent more likely to die of cancer than are whites and more than two times more likely to die of cancer than are Asian or Pacific Islanders, American Indians, and Hispanics.[1] African American women are more likely to die of breast and colon cancers than are women of any other racial and ethnic group, and they have approximately the same lung cancer death rates as white women. African American men have the highest death rates of colon and rectum, lung, and prostate cancers. Age-adjusted lung cancer death rates are approximately 40 percent higher among African American males than white males. Little difference in age-adjusted lung cancer death rates has been observed between African American females and white females. Hispanics have higher rates of cervical, esophageal, gallbladder, and stomach cancers. Similarly, some specific forms of cancer affect other ethnic groups at rates higher than the national average (for example, stomach and liver cancers among Asian American populations and colorectal [CRC] cancer among Alaska Natives). Certain racial and ethnic groups have lower survival rates than whites for most cancers.[1]

Differences among the races represent both a challenge to understand the reasons and an opportunity to reduce illness and death and to improve survival rates.

The Hispanic cancer experience also differs from that of the non-Hispanic white population, with Hispanics having higher rates of cervical, esophageal, gallbladder, and stomach cancers. New cases of female breast and lung cancers are increasing among Hispanics, who are diagnosed at later stages and have lower survival rates than whites.

The recent decrease in deaths from breast cancer in white females is attributed to greater use of breast cancer screening in regular medical care. However, deaths due to breast cancer in African American females continue to increase, in part, because breast cancer is diagnosed at later stages in African American females.[1]

Data on CRC show a decline in new cases and death rates in white males and females, stable new case rates in African Americans, and a continued rise in death rates in African American males. Five-year survival rates for the 1989–94 period are 64 percent in whites and 52 percent in African Americans.[3] Early detection and treatment play a key role in these survival rates.

New cases of prostate cancer peaked in 1992 at 190.8 per 100,000 people and declined on average by 8.5 percent each year from 1992 to 1996. Prostate cancer death rates peaked in 1991 at 26.7 per 100,000 people; rates decreased on average by 2.1 percent each year from 1991 to 1995.[3] Causes of the trends are unclear but may be attributed to a number of factors that are under investigation.

Possible disparities regarding the health status of lesbian women and possible barriers to access to health services by lesbians have been identified by the Institute of Medicine as a research priority.[6]

Opportunities

Evidence suggests that several types of cancer can be prevented and that the prospects for surviving cancer continue to improve. The ability to reduce cancer death rates depends, in part, on the existence and application of various types of resources. First, the means to provide culturally and linguistically appropriate information on prevention, early detection, and treatment to the public and to health care professionals are essential. Second, mechanisms or systems must exist for providing people with access to state-of-the-art preventive services and treatment. Where suitable, participation in clinical trials also should be encouraged. Third, a mechanism for maintaining continued research progress and for fostering new research is essential. Genetic information that can be used to improve disease prevention strategies is emerging for many cancers and may provide the foundation for improved effectiveness in clinical and preventive medicine services.

To provide new opportunities for cancer prevention and control in the future, there is a continuing and vital need to foster new, innovative research on both the causes of cancer (including genetic and environmental causes) and on methods to translate biologic and epidemiologic findings into effective prevention and control programs for use by government and community organizations to reduce further the Nation's cancer burden.

These needs can be met, in part, with the network of cancer control resources now in place. This network has the organizational and personnel capabilities for various cancer interventions. Despite the extent of these resources, they alone are insufficient to reduce deaths from cancer. Gaps exist in information transfer, optimal practice patterns, research capabilities, and other areas. These gaps must be recognized and filled to meet cancer prevention and control needs.

It is estimated that as much as 50 percent or more of cancer can be prevented through smoking cessation and improved dietary habits, such as reducing fat consumption and increasing fruit and vegetable consumption.[7, 8] Physical activity and weight control also can contribute to cancer prevention.[9, 10]

Scientific data from randomized trials of cancer screening together with expert opinions indicate that adherence to screening recommendations for cancers of the breast, cervix, and colon/rectum reduces deaths from these cancers.

To reduce breast cancer deaths in the United States, a high percentage of females aged 40 years and older need to comply with screening recommendations. A reduction in breast cancer deaths could be expected to occur after a delay of roughly 7 years.[11] To reduce cervical cancer deaths, a high percentage of females in the United States who are aged 18 years and older need to comply with screening recommendations. Evidence from randomized preventive trials is unavailable, but expert opinion suggests that a beneficial impact on cervical cancer death rates would be expected to occur after a delay of a few years.

Evidence shows that a reduction in CRC deaths can be achieved through detection and removal of precancerous polyps and treatment of CRC in its earliest stages. The findings from three randomized controlled trials indicate that biennial screening with fecal occult blood tests (FOBT) can reduce deaths from CRC by 15 to 21 percent in people aged 45 to 80 years.[12, 13, 14] One trial[15] reported a 33 percent reduction in deaths with annual screening in the same age groups, and a simulation model showed a 56 percent reduction.[16] The efficacy of sigmoidoscopy has been supported by three case-control studies[17, 18, 19] that showed 59 to 79 percent reductions in CRC deaths from cancers within reach of the sigmoidoscope in age groups 45 years and older.

Prostate cancer prevention strategies are not available at this time. Race and age are the only clearly identified risk factors for prostate cancer. African Americans and older men are at higher risk. There is no scientific agreement on the benefits of screening for prostate cancer, and screening is not recommended in the general population or in high-risk groups because it is unclear if screening and treatment do more good than harm.[20] Clinical trials currently are under way to assess the benefits and risks of screening and treatments, and additional research is needed to identify modifiable risk factors for prostate cancer.

Melanoma and other skin cancers were expected to claim the lives of almost 9,600 persons in 2000.[1] Insufficient evidence exists to determine whether routine skin examinations (self or physician) decrease deaths from melanoma or other skin cancers. However, many of the skin cancers diagnosed each year could be prevented by limiting exposure to the sun, by wearing protective clothing, and by using sunscreen.

For all cancers, treatments designed to increase survival are needed along with improved access to state-of-the-art care. In addition to measurements of survival, indices of quality of life for both the short term and long term are regarded as important considerations.

Interim Progress Toward Year 2000 Objectives

The Healthy People 2000 objective for total cancer deaths was achieved for the total population by 1995. Lung cancer deaths declined for the first time in 50 years in 1991, declined again in 1992, remained level in 1993, and then dropped again in 1994, 1995, and 1996. The decline in the age-adjusted death rate for CRC for the total population has gone beyond the year 2000 target, but declines in death rates have not been as substantial for the black population. Improvements were observed in cancer risk factors, such as tobacco use and dietary fat intake. Data also showed some improvement in the proportion of women receiving mammograms and Pap tests. In addition, for both mammograms and Pap tests, the disparity in use rates for most of the population subgroups and those for all women either has been reduced or eliminated.

Note: Unless otherwise noted, data are from the Centers for Disease Control and Prevention, National Center for Health Statistics, *Healthy People 2000 Review, 1998–99.*

Cancer

Goal: Reduce the number of new cancer cases as well as the illness, disability, and death caused by cancer.

Number	Objective Short Title
3-1	Overall cancer deaths
3-2	Lung cancer deaths
3-3	Breast cancer deaths
3-4	Cervical cancer deaths
3-5	Colorectal cancer deaths
3-6	Oropharyngeal cancer deaths
3-7	Prostate cancer deaths
3-8	Melanoma deaths
3-9	Sun exposure and skin cancer
3-10	Provider counseling about cancer prevention
3-11	Pap tests
3-12	Colorectal cancer screening
3-13	Mammograms
3-14	Statewide cancer registries
3-15	Cancer survival

3-1. Reduce the overall cancer death rate.

Target: 159.9 deaths per 100,000 population.

Baseline: 202.4 cancer deaths per 100,000 population occurred in 1998 (age adjusted to the year 2000 standard population).

Target setting method: 21 percent improvement.

Data source: National Vital Statistics System (NVSS), CDC, NCHS.

Total Population, 1998	Cancer Deaths
	Rate per 100,000
TOTAL	202.4
Race and ethnicity	
American Indian or Alaska Native	129.3
Asian or Pacific Islander	124.2
Asian	DNC
Native Hawaiian and other Pacific Islander	DNC
Black or African American	255.1
White	199.3
Hispanic or Latino	123.7
Not Hispanic or Latino	206.6
Black or African American	261.8
White	203.0
Gender	
Female	169.2
Male	252.4
Education level (aged 25 to 64 years)	
Less than high school	137.8
High school graduate	139.7
At least some college	79.6

DNA = Data have not been analyzed. DNC = Data are not collected. DSU = Data are statistically unreliable.
Note: Age adjusted to the year 2000 standard population.

3-2. Reduce the lung cancer death rate.

Target: 44.9 deaths per 100,000 population.

Baseline: 57.6 lung cancer deaths per 100,000 population occurred in 1998 (age adjusted to the year 2000 standard population).

Target setting method: 22 percent improvement.

Data source: National Vital Statistics System (NVSS), CDC, NCHS.

Total Population, 1998	Lung Cancer Deaths
	Rate per 100,000
TOTAL	57.6
Race and ethnicity	
American Indian or Alaska Native	38.2
Asian or Pacific Islander	29.3
Asian	DNC
Native Hawaiian and other Pacific Islander	DNC
Black or African American	66.7
White	57.5
Hispanic or Latino	22.7
Not Hispanic or Latino	59.6
Black or African American	68.6
White	59.6
Gender	
Female	41.5
Male	79.9
Education level (aged 25 to 64 years)	
Less than high school	49.0
High school graduate	41.8
At least some college	17.6

DNA = Data have not been analyzed. DNC = Data are not collected. DSU = Data are statistically unreliable.
Note: Age adjusted to the year 2000 standard population.

Lung cancer is the most common cause of cancer death among both females and males in the United States. Estimates indicated that 164,100 (74,600 females and 89,500 males) new cases of lung cancer would be diagnosed in 2000; 156,900 persons (67,600 females and 89,300 males) would die from lung cancer in 2000, accounting for 28 percent of all cancer deaths.[1]

Cigarette smoking is the most important risk factor for lung cancer, accounting for 68 to 78 percent of lung cancer deaths among females and 88 to 91 percent of lung cancer deaths among males.[21] Other risk factors include occupational exposures (radon, asbestos) and indoor and outdoor air pollution (radon, environmental tobacco smoke).[22] One to two percent of lung cancer deaths are attributable to air pollution.[23] After 10 years of abstinence, smoking cessation decreases the risk of lung cancer to 30 to 50 percent of that of continuing smokers.[7]

3-3.   Reduce the breast cancer death rate.

Target: 22.3 deaths per 100,000 females.

Baseline: 27.9 breast cancer deaths per 100,000 females occurred in 1998 (age adjusted to the year 2000 standard population).

Target setting method: 20 percent improvement.

Data source: National Vital Statistics System (NVSS), CDC, NCHS.

Females, 1998	Breast Cancer Deaths
	Rate per 100,000
TOTAL	27.9
Race and ethnicity	
American Indian or Alaska Native	14.2
Asian or Pacific Islander	13.1
Asian	DNC
Native Hawaiian and other Pacific Islander	DNC
Black or African American	35.7
White	27.3
Hispanic or Latino	16.8
Not Hispanic or Latino	28.5
Black or African American	36.7
White	27.9
Education level (aged 25 to 64 years)	
Less than high school	20.0
High school graduate	28.4
At least some college	22.0

DNA = Data have not been analyzed. DNC = Data are not collected. DSU = Data are statistically unreliable.
Note: Age adjusted to the year 2000 standard population.

Breast cancer is the most common cancer among women in the United States. An estimated 184,200 new cases were expected to be diagnosed in 2000. About 40,800 U.S. women were expected to die from breast cancer in 2000, accounting for about 15.2 percent of cancer deaths among women.[1] Death from breast cancer can be reduced substantially if the tumor is discovered at an early stage. Mammography is the most effective method for detecting these early malignancies. Clinical trials have demonstrated that mammography screening can reduce breast cancer deaths by 20 to 39 percent in women aged 50 to 74 years and about 17 percent in women aged 40 to 49 years.[24] Breast cancer deaths can be reduced through increased adherence with recommendations for regular mammography screening.

Many breast cancer risk factors, such as age, family history of breast cancer, reproductive history, mammographic densities, previous breast disease, and race and ethnicity, are not subject to intervention.[25, 26] However, being overweight is a well-established breast cancer risk for postmenopausal women that can be addressed.[25] Avoiding weight gain is one method by which older women may reduce their risk of developing breast cancer.

3-4. Reduce the death rate from cancer of the uterine cervix.

Target: 2.0 deaths per 100,000 females.

Baseline: 3.0 cervical cancer deaths per 100,000 females occurred in 1998 (age adjusted to the year 2000 standard population).

Target setting method: Better than the best.

Data source: National Vital Statistics System (NVSS), CDC, NCHS.

NOTE: THE TABLE BELOW MAY CONTINUE TO THE FOLLOWING PAGE.

Females, 1998	Cervical Cancer Deaths
	Rate per 100,000
TOTAL	3.0
Race and ethnicity	
American Indian or Alaska Native	2.5
Asian or Pacific Islander	3.3
Asian	DNC
Native Hawaiian and other Pacific Islander	DNC
Black or African American	6.0
White	2.7

Females, 1998	Cervical Cancer Deaths
	Rate per 100,000
Hispanic or Latino	3.3
Not Hispanic or Latino	3.0
Black or African American	6.2
White	2.6
Education level (aged 25 to 64 years)	
Less than high school	7.2
High school graduate	4.8
At least some college	2.1

DNA = Data have not been analyzed. DNC = Data are not collected. DSU = Data are statistically unreliable.
Note: Age adjusted to the year 2000 standard population.

NOTE: THE TABLE ABOVE MAY HAVE CONTINUED FROM THE PREVIOUS PAGE.

Cervical cancer is the 10th most common cancer among females in the United States, with an estimated 12,800 new cases in 2000. The number of new cases of cervical cancer is higher among females from racial and ethnic groups than among white females. An estimated 4,600 U.S. females were expected to die from cervical cancer in 2000.[1] Cervical cancer accounts for about 1.7 percent of cancer deaths among females. Infections of the cervix with certain types of sexually transmitted human papilloma virus increase risk of cervical cancer and may be responsible for most cervical cancer in the United States.[27]

Considerable evidence suggests that screening can reduce the number of deaths from cervical cancer. Invasive cervical cancer is preceded in a large proportion of cases by precancerous changes in cervical tissue that can be identified with a Pap test. If cervical cancer is detected early, the likelihood of survival is almost 100 percent with appropriate treatment and followup; that is, almost all cervical cancer deaths could be avoided if all females complied with screening and followup recommendations.[28] Risk is substantially decreased among former smokers in comparison to continuing smokers.[7]

3-5.   Reduce the colorectal cancer death rate.

Target: 13.9 deaths per 100,000 population.

Baseline: 21.2 colorectal cancer deaths per 100,000 population occurred in 1998 (age adjusted to the year 2000 standard population).

Target setting method: 34 percent improvement.

Data source: National Vital Statistics System (NVSS), CDC, NCHS.

Total Population, 1998	Colorectal Cancer Deaths
	Rate per 100,000
TOTAL	21.2
Race and ethnicity	
American Indian or Alaska Native	13.3
Asian or Pacific Islander	13.7
Asian	DNC
Native Hawaiian and other Pacific Islander	DNC
Black or African American	28.2
White	20.8
Hispanic or Latino	12.8
Not Hispanic or Latino	21.7
Black or African American	28.9
White	21.1
Gender	
Female	18.2
Male	25.4
Education level (aged 25 to 64 years)	
Less than high school	10.4
High school graduate	12.0
At least some college	7.5

DNA = Data have not been analyzed. DNC = Data are not collected. DSU = Data are statistically unreliable.
Note: Age adjusted to the year 2000 standard population.

Colorectal cancer is the second leading cause of cancer-related deaths in the United States. An estimated 130,200 cases (66,600 females and 63,600 males) of CRC and 56,300 deaths (28,500 females and 27,800 males) from CRC were expected to occur in 2000. When cancer-related deaths are estimated separately for males and females, however, CRC becomes the third leading cause of cancer death behind lung and breast cancers for females and behind lung and prostate cancers for males.[1]

Risk factors for CRC may include age, personal and family history of polyps or colorectal cancer, inflammatory bowel disease, inherited syndromes, physical inactivity (colon only), obesity, alcohol use, and a diet high in fat and low in fruits and vegetables.[29] Detecting and removing precancerous colorectal polyps and detecting and treating the disease in its earliest stages will reduce deaths from CRC. FOBT and sigmoidoscopy are widely used to screen for CRC, and barium enema and colonoscopy are used as diagnostic tests.

3-6.   Reduce the oropharyngeal cancer death rate.

Target: 2.7 deaths per 100,000 population.

Baseline: 3.0 oropharyngeal cancer deaths per 100,000 population occurred in 1998 (age adjusted to the year 2000 standard population).

Target setting method: 10 percent improvement.

Data source: National Vital Statistics System (NVSS), CDC, NCHS.

Total Population, 1998	Oropharyngeal Cancer Deaths
	Rate per 100,000
TOTAL	3.0
Race and ethnicity	
American Indian or Alaska Native	2.1
Asian or Pacific Islander	2.2
Asian	DNC
Native Hawaiian and other Pacific Islander	DNC
Black or African American	4.5
White	2.8
Hispanic or Latino	1.8
Not Hispanic or Latino	3.1
Black or African American	4.7
White	2.9
Gender	
Female	1.7
Male	4.5
Education level (aged 25 to 64 years)	
Less than high school	3.6
High school graduate	3.0
At least some college	1.2

DNA = Data have not been analyzed. DNC = Data are not collected. DSU = Data are statistically unreliable.
Note: Age adjusted to the year 2000 standard population.

Oral and pharyngeal (oropharyngeal) cancers comprise a diversity of malignant tumors that affect the oral cavity and pharynx; the overwhelming majority of these tumors are squamous cell carcinomas. In 2000, 30,200 new cases of oropharyngeal cancer were expected to be diagnosed, and approximately 7,800 deaths were expected to occur from the disease. Oropharyngeal cancer is the 10th most common cancer among U.S. men and the 14th most common among U.S. women.[1] Its

5-year survival rate is only 53 percent. The risk of oral cancer is increased in current smokers. Alcohol consumption is an independent risk factor, and when alcohol is combined with use of tobacco products, 90 percent of all oral cancers are explained.[30]

3-7.   Reduce the prostate cancer death rate.

Target: 28.8 deaths per 100,000 males.

Baseline: 32.0 prostate cancer deaths per 100,000 males occurred in 1998 (age adjusted to the year 2000 standard population).

Target setting method: 10 percent improvement.

Data source: National Vital Statistics System (NVSS), CDC, NCHS.

Males, 1998	Prostate Cancer Deaths
	Rate per 100,000
TOTAL	32.0
Race and ethnicity	
American Indian or Alaska Native	15.9
Asian or Pacific Islander	12.4
Asian	DNC
Native Hawaiian and other Pacific Islander	DNC
Black or African American	68.7
White	29.4
Hispanic or Latino	20.9
Not Hispanic or Latino	32.4
Black or African American	70.2
White	29.7
Education level (aged 25 to 64 years)	
Less than high school	4.4
High school graduate	5.0
At least some college	2.8

DNA = Data have not been analyzed. DNC = Data are not collected. DSU = Data are statistically unreliable.
Note: Age adjusted to the year 2000 standard population.

Prostate cancer is the most commonly diagnosed form of cancer (other than skin cancer) in males and the second leading cause of cancer death among males in the United States. Prostate cancer was expected to account for an estimated 180,400 cases and 31,900 deaths in 2000, or about 29 percent and 11 percent of the cases and deaths due to all cancers, respectively.[1] Prostate cancer is most common in men aged 65 years and older, who account for approximately 80 percent of all cases of prostate cancer.

Digital rectal examination (DRE) and the prostate-specific antigen (PSA) test are two commonly used methods for detecting prostate cancer. Clinical trials of the benefits of DRE and PSA screening are under way, with results expected in the early 21st century.

Although several treatment alternatives are available for prostate cancer, their impact on reducing death from prostate cancer when compared with no treatment in patients with operable cancer is uncertain.[31, 32, 33] Efforts aimed at reducing deaths through screening and early detection remain controversial because of the uncertain benefits and potential risks of screening, diagnosis, and treatment.

3-8. Reduce the rate of melanoma cancer deaths.

Target: 2.5 deaths per 100,000 population.

Baseline: 2.8 melanoma cancer deaths per 100,000 population occurred in 1998 (age adjusted to the year 2000 standard population).

Target setting method: 11 percent improvement.

Data source: National Vital Statistics System (NVSS), CDC, NCHS.

NOTE: THE TABLE BELOW MAY CONTINUE TO THE FOLLOWING PAGE.

Total Population, 1998	Melanoma Cancer Deaths
	Rate per 100,000
TOTAL	2.8
Race and ethnicity	
American Indian or Alaska Native	DSU
Asian or Pacific Islander	0.3
Asian	DNC
Native Hawaiian and other Pacific Islander	DNC
Black or African American	0.5
White	3.1
Hispanic or Latino	0.8
Not Hispanic or Latino	2.9
Black or African American	0.5
White	3.3

Healthy People 2010: Objectives for Improving Health

Total Population, 1998	Melanoma Cancer Deaths
	Rate per 100,000
Gender	
Female	1.8
Male	4.1
Education level (aged 25 to 64 years)	
Less than high school	1.8
High school graduate	2.7
At least some college	2.3

DNA = Data have not been analyzed. DNC = Data are not collected. DSU = Data are statistically unreliable.
Note: Age adjusted to the year 2000 standard population.
NOTE: THE TABLE ABOVE MAY HAVE CONTINUED FROM THE PREVIOUS PAGE.

Melanoma, the deadliest of all skin cancers, was expected to account for an estimated 47,700 new cancer cases and 7,700 deaths in 2000.[1] Trends show annual rises in the number of new cases of 4.3 percent (1973–90) and 2.5 percent (1990–95) and an annual rise in deaths of 1.7 percent (1973–90) followed by a decline of 0.4 percent in 1990–95. In whites, the population at highest risk, death rates are twice as high in males as in females.[3]

Although the cause of melanoma is unknown, risk factors include a personal or family history of melanoma, the presence of atypical moles, a large number of moles, intermittent sun exposure, a history of sunburns early in life, freckles, and sun-sensitive skin (as measured by poor tanning ability and light skin, eye, or hair color).[34] Evidence is insufficient to determine whether early detection through routine skin examination (self or physician) decreases the number of deaths from melanoma, but reduced ultraviolet exposure is likely to have a beneficial impact on the risk of melanoma and other skin cancers (basal and squamous cell skin cancers).[33]

3-9. **Increase the proportion of persons who use at least one of the following protective measures that may reduce the risk of skin cancer: avoid the sun between 10 a.m. and 4 p.m., wear sun-protective clothing when exposed to sunlight, use sunscreen with a sun-protective factor (SPF) of 15 or higher, and avoid artificial sources of ultraviolet light.**

3-9a. (Developmental) Increase the proportion of adolescents in grades 9 through 12 who follow protective measures that may reduce the risk of skin cancer.

Potential data source: Youth Risk Behavior Surveillance System (YRBSS), CDC, NCCDPHP.

3-9b. Increase the proportion of adults aged 18 years and older who follow protective measures that may reduce the risk of skin cancer.

Target: 75 percent of adults aged 18 years and older use at least one of the identified protective measures.

Baseline: 47 percent of adults aged 18 years and older regularly used at least one protective measure in 1998 (age adjusted to the year 2000 standard population).

Target setting method: Better than the best.

Data source: National Health Interview Survey (NHIS), CDC, NCHS. Data on artificial ultraviolet light source are developmental.

NOTE: THE TABLE BELOW MAY CONTINUE TO THE FOLLOWING PAGE.

Persons Aged 18 Years and Older, 1998 (unless noted)	Type of Protective Measure			
	3-9b. Regularly Used at Least One Protective Measure	Limited Sun Exposure*	Wore Protective Clothing*	Used Sunscreen*
	Percent			
TOTAL	47	28	24	31
Race and ethnicity				
American Indian or Alaska Native	48	28	26	31
Asian or Pacific Islander	44	34	25	22
Asian	44	34	25	23
Native Hawaiian and other Pacific Islander	50	39	31	17
Black or African American	44	37	23	12
White	49	26	24	34
Hispanic or Latino	41	30	24	22
Not Hispanic or Latino	48	27	24	32
Black or African American	44	37	24	12
White	49	26	24	35
Gender				
Female	54	33	25	39
Male	40	22	24	22

Healthy People 2010: Objectives for Improving Health

	Type of Protective Measure			
Persons Aged 18 Years and Older, 1998 (unless noted)	**3-9b. Regularly Used at Least One Protective Measure**	**Limited Sun Exposure***	**Wore Protective Clothing***	**Used Sunscreen***
	Percent			
Education level (aged 25 years and older)				
Less than high school	41	29	24	17
High school graduate	45	28	24	27
Some college	54	30	29	39
Family income level				
Poor	43	33	25	19
Near poor	46	32	25	24
Middle/high income	51	27	26	35
Geographic location				
Urban	49	29	25	32
Rural	44	25	24	28
Disability status				
Persons with activity limitations	57 (1992)	38 (1992)	33 (1992)	27 (1992)
Persons without activity limitations	53 (1992)	31 (1992)	28 (1992)	29 (1992)

DNA = Data have not been analyzed. DNC = Data are not collected. DSU = Data are statistically unreliable.

Note: Age adjusted to the year 2000 standard population.

*Data for limited sun exposure, used sunscreen, and wore protective clothing are displayed to further characterize the issue.

NOTE: THE TABLE ABOVE MAY HAVE CONTINUED FROM THE PREVIOUS PAGE.

3-10. Increase the proportion of physicians and dentists who counsel their at-risk patients about tobacco use cessation, physical activity, and cancer screening.

Target and baseline:

Objective	Increase in Counseling About Tobacco Use Cessation, Physical Activity, and Cancer Screening	1988 Baseline (unless noted)	2010 Target
		Percent	
3-10a.	Internists who counsel about smoking cessation	50	85
3-10b.	Family physicians who counsel about smoking cessation	43	85
3-10c.	Dentists who counsel about smoking cessation	59 (1997)	85
3-10d.	Primary care providers who counsel about blood stool tests	56	85
3-10e.	Primary care providers who counsel about proctoscopic examinations	23	85
3-10f.	Primary care providers who counsel about mammograms	37	85
3-10g.	Primary care providers who counsel about Pap tests	55	85
3-10h.	Primary care providers who counsel about physical activity	22 (1995)	85

Target setting method: Better than the best.

Data sources: Survey of Physicians' Attitudes and Practices in Early Cancer Detection, NIH, NCI; National Ambulatory Medical Care Survey (NAMCS), CDC, NCHS; Survey of Current Issues in Dentistry, American Dental Association.

Smoking cessation,[7, 21] adoption of healthy diets,[8] increased physical activity,[9, 10] and increased cancer screening[11, 12, 13, 14, 15, 16, 17, 18, 19] can all contribute to reduced numbers of cancer deaths. Experts recommend that providers screen patients for breast, cervical, and colorectal cancers and counsel patients to prevent or reduce tobacco use, promote physical activity, and promote a healthy diet.[32] Provider counseling should be conducted in a linguistically and culturally appropriate manner.

3-11. Increase the proportion of women who receive a Pap test.

Target and baseline:

Objective	Increase in Pap Testing	1998 Baseline*	2010 Target
		Percent	
3-11a.	Women aged 18 years and older who have ever received a Pap test	92	97
3-11b.	Women aged 18 years and older who received a Pap test within the preceding 3 years	79	90

*Age adjusted to the year 2000 standard population. Includes women without a uterine cervix.

Target setting method: Better than the best.

Data source: National Health Interview Survey (NHIS), CDC, NCHS.

NOTE: THE TABLE BELOW MAY CONTINUE TO THE FOLLOWING PAGE.

Women Aged 18 Years and Older, 1998 (unless noted)	Pap Test	
	3-11a. Ever	3-11b. In Preceding 3 Years
TOTAL	92	79
Race and ethnicity		
American Indian or Alaska Native	88	72
Asian or Pacific Islander	78	67
Asian	78	67
Native Hawaiian and other Pacific Islander	80	66
Black or African American	94	83
White	93	79
Hispanic or Latino	85	74
Not Hispanic or Latino	93	80
Black or African American	94	83
White	94	80
Education level (aged 25 years and older)		
Less than high school	89	69
High school graduate	95	78
At least some college	97	83

Women Aged 18 Years and Older, 1998 (unless noted)	Pap Test	
	3-11a. Ever	3-11b. In Preceding 3 Years
Family income level		
Poor	88	69
Near poor	92	73
Middle/high income	94	83
Geographic location		
Urban	92	80
Rural	93	78
Disability status		
With activity limitations	95 (1994)	74 (1994)
Without activity limitations	94 (1994)	78 (1994)

DNA = Data have not been analyzed. DNC = Data are not collected. DSU = Data are statistically unreliable.

Note: Age adjusted to the year 2000 standard population. Includes women without a uterine cervix.

NOTE: THE TABLE ABOVE MAY HAVE CONTINUED FROM THE PREVIOUS PAGE.

3-12. Increase the proportion of adults who receive a colorectal cancer screening examination.

Target and baseline:

Objective	Increase in Colorectal Cancer Screening	1998 Baseline*	2010 Target
		Percent	
3-12a.	Adults aged 50 years and older who have received a fecal occult blood test (FOBT) within the preceding 2 years	35	50
3-12b.	Adults aged 50 years and older who have ever received a sigmoidoscopy	37	50

*Age adjusted to the year 2000 standard population.

Target setting method: Better than the best.

Data source: National Health Interview Survey (NHIS), CDC, NCHS.

Adults Aged 50 Years and Older, 1998 (unless noted)	Colorectal Cancer Screening	
	3-12a. Fecal Occult Blood Test	3-12b. Sigmoidoscopy
	Percent	
TOTAL	35	37
Race and ethnicity		
American Indian or Alaska Native	24	29
Asian or Pacific Islander	31	34
Asian	33	35
Native Hawaiian and other Pacific Islander	DSU	DSU
Black or African American	30	32
White	35	38
Hispanic or Latino	23	27
Not Hispanic or Latino	35	38
Black or African American	30	32
White	36	39
Gender		
Female	34	33
Male	36	43
Education level		
Less than high school	26	29
High school graduate	34	35
At least some college	41	44
Family income level		
Poor	23	28
Near poor	31	31
Middle/high income	39	43
Geographic location		
Urban	36	38
Rural	31	36
Disability status		
Persons with activity limitations	32 (1992)	37 (1992)
Persons without activity limitations	28 (1992)	31 (1992)

DNA = Data have not been analyzed. DNC = Data are not collected. DSU = Data are statistically unreliable.
Note: Age adjusted to the year 2000 standard population.

3-13. Increase the proportion of women aged 40 years and older who have received a mammogram within the preceding 2 years.

Target: 70 percent.

Baseline: 67 percent of women aged 40 years and older received a mammogram within the preceding 2 years in 1998 (age adjusted to the year 2000 standard population).

Target setting method: Better than the best.

Data source: National Health Interview Survey (NHIS), CDC, NCHS.

NOTE: THE TABLE BELOW MAY CONTINUE TO THE FOLLOWING PAGE.

Women Aged 40 Years and Older, 1998 (unless noted)	Mammogram
	Percent
TOTAL	67
Race and ethnicity	
American Indian or Alaska Native	45
Asian or Pacific Islander	61
Asian	61
Native Hawaiian and other Pacific Islander	DSU
Black or African American	66
White	67
Hispanic or Latino	61
Not Hispanic or Latino	68
Black or African American	66
White	68
Education level	
Less than high school	53
High school graduate	66
At least some college	73
Family income level	
Poor	50
Near poor	54
Middle/high income	73
Geographic location	
Urban	68
Rural	65

Women Aged 40 Years and Older, 1998 (unless noted)	Mammogram
	Percent
Disability status	
Persons with activity limitations	55 (1994)
Persons without activity limitations	61 (1994)

DNA = Data have not been analyzed. DNC = Data are not collected. DSU = Data are statistically unreliable.
Note: Age adjusted to the year 2000 standard population.

NOTE: THE TABLE ABOVE MAY HAVE CONTINUED FROM THE PREVIOUS PAGE.

3-14. Increase the number of States that have a statewide population-based cancer registry that captures case information on at least 95 percent of the expected number of reportable cancers.

Target: 45 States.

Baseline: 21 States had a statewide population-based cancer registry that captured case information on at least 95 percent of the expected number of reportable cancers in 1999.

Target setting method: 114 percent improvement.

Data source: National Program of Cancer Registries, CDC.

Cancer surveillance serves as the foundation for a national comprehensive strategy to reduce illness and death from cancer. Such surveillance is the indispensable tool that enables public health professionals at the national, State, and community levels to better understand and tackle the cancer burden while advancing clinical, epidemiologic, and health services research. In addition, surveillance data from cancer registries, such as cancer incidence and deaths, stage at diagnosis, treatment, and demographics of cancer patients, are essential for planning and evaluating cancer control programs, allocating preventive and treatment resources, targeting and conducting research, and responding to concerns from citizens about the occurrence of cancer in their communities.

Population-based State cancer registries that provide accurate, complete, and timely data are a critical component of the public health infrastructure in the United States. The National Program of Cancer Registries (NPCR) provides funds to 45 States to assist in planning or enhancing cancer registries; develop model legislation and regulations for programs to increase the viability of registry operations; set standards for data quality, completeness, and timeliness; provide training for registry personnel; and help establish computerized reporting and data processing systems. The National Cancer Institute's SEER Program covers the remaining 5 States.

3-15. Increase the proportion of cancer survivors who are living 5 years or longer after diagnosis.

Target: 70 percent.

Baseline: 59 percent of persons with invasive cancer of any type were living 5 years or longer after diagnosis in 1989–95.

Target setting method: 19 percent improvement.

Data source: Surveillance, Epidemiology, and End Results (SEER) Program, NIH, NCI.

Persons With Invasive Cancer of Any Type, 1989–95	5 Years or Longer Survival
	Percent
TOTAL	59
Race and ethnicity	
American Indian or Alaska Native	DNA
Asian or Pacific Islander	DNA
Asian	DNA
Native Hawaiian and other Pacific Islander	DNA
Black or African American	48
White	61
Hispanic or Latino	DNA
Not Hispanic or Latino	DNA
Black or African American	DNA
White	DNA
Gender	
Female	61
Male	58
Education level (aged 25 to 64 years)	
Less than high school	DNA
High school graduate	DNA
At least some college	DNA

DNA = Data have not been analyzed. DNC = Data are not collected. DSU = Data are statistically unreliable.

19. **Nutrition and Overweight**
    19-5. Fruit intake
    19-6. Vegetable intake
    19-8. Saturated fat intake
    19-9. Total fat intake

21. **Oral Health**
    21-6. Early detection of oral and pharyngeal cancers
    21-7. Annual examinations for oral and pharyngeal cancers

27. **Tobacco Use**
    27-1. Adult tobacco use
    27-2. Adolescent tobacco use
    27-5. Smoking cessation by adults
    27-7. Smoking cessation by adolescents
    27-8. Insurance coverage of cessation treatment

Terminology

(A listing of abbreviations and acronyms used in this publication appears in Appendix H.)

Cancer: A term for diseases in which abnormal cells divide without control. Cancer cells can invade nearby tissue and can spread through the bloodstream and lymphatic system to other parts of the body.

Cancer screening: Checking for changes in tissue, cells, or fluids that may indicate the possibility of cancer when there are no symptoms.

Carcinoma: Cancer that begins in the epithelial tissue that lines or covers an organ.

Clinical trials: Research studies that evaluate the effectiveness of new treatment or disease prevention methods on patients.

Colonoscopy: An examination of the rectum and entire colon using a lighted instrument called a colonoscope. A colonoscope allows the physician to remove polyps or other abnormal tissue for examination under a microscope.

Digital rectal exam (DRE): A test in which the health care provider inserts a lubricated, gloved finger into the rectum to feel for abnormal areas.

Fecal occult blood test (FOBT): A test to check for small amounts of hidden blood in stool.

Grade: A system for classifying cancer cells in terms of how abnormal they appear under a microscope. The grading system provides information about the probable growth rate of the tumor and its tendency to spread. The systems used to grade tumors vary with each type of cancer. Grading plays a role in treatment decisions.

Invasive cervical cancer: Cancer that has spread from the surface of the cervix to tissue deeper in the cervix or to other parts of the body.

Malignant: Cancerous.

Mammogram: An x ray of the breast.

Melanoma: Cancer of the cells that produce pigment in the skin.

Pap (Papanicolaou) test: Microscopic examination of cells collected from the cervix. The Pap test is used to detect cancer, changes in the cervix that may lead to cancer, and non-cancerous conditions, such as infection or inflammation.

PSA (prostate-specific antigen) test: A test that measures the level of an enzyme (PSA) in the blood that increases due to diseases of the prostate gland, including prostate cancer.

Risk factor: Something that increases a person's chance of developing a disease.

Sigmoidoscopy: A procedure in which the physician or health care provider looks inside the rectum and the lower part of the colon (sigmoid colon) through a flexible lighted tube. During the procedure, the physician or health care provider may collect samples of tissues or cells for closer examination.

Squamous cells: Flat cells that look like fish scales. These cells are found in the tissue that forms the surface of the skin, the lining of the hollow organs of the body, and the passages of the respiratory and digestive tracts.

Stage: The size and extent of a cancer, including whether the disease has spread from the original site into surrounding tissue and other parts of the body.

References

[1] Landis, S.H.; Murray, T.; Bolden, S.; et al. Cancer statistics, 2000. *CA: A Cancer Journal for Clinicians* 50(1):2398-2424, 2000.

[2] Ries, L.A.G.; Kosary, C.L.; Hankey, B.F.; et al. *SEER Cancer Statistics Review, 1973–1996.* Bethesda, MD: National Cancer Institute, 1999.

[3] Wingo, P.A.; Ries, L.A.G.; Giovino, G.A.; et al. Annual report to the nation on the status of cancer, 1973–1996, with a special section on lung cancer and tobacco smoking. *Journal of the National Cancer Institute* 91(8):675-690, 1999.

[4] Wingo, P.A.; Ries, L.A.; Rosenberg, H.M.; et al. Cancer incidence and mortality 1973–1995: A report card for the U.S. *Cancer* 82(6):1197-1207, 1998.

[5] Brown, M.L.; Hodgson, T.A.; and Rice, D.P. Economic impact of cancer in the United States. In: Schottenfeld, D., and Fraumeni, Jr., J.F.; eds. *Cancer Epidemiology and Prevention.* 2nd ed. New York, NY: Oxford University Press, 1996.

[6] Solarz, A., ed. *Lesbian Health: Current Assessment and Directions for the Future 1999.* Washington, DC: National Academy Press, 1999.

[7] U.S. Department of Health and Human Services (HHS). *The Health Benefits of Smoking Cessation.* DHHS Publication No. CDC 90-8416. Atlanta, GA: Public Health Service, Centers for Disease Control, Center for Chronic Disease Prevention and Health Promotion, Office on Smoking and Health, 1990.

[8] Willet, W. Diet and nutrition. In: Schottenfeld, D., and Fraumeni, Jr., J.F.; eds. *Cancer Epidemiology and Prevention.* 2nd ed. New York, NY: Oxford University Press, 1996, 438-461.

[9] Greenwald, P.; Kramer, B.; and Weed, D.L.; eds. *Cancer Prevention and Control.* New York, NY: Marcel Dekker, 1995, 303-327.

[10] HHS. *Physical Activity and Health: A Report of the Surgeon General.* Atlanta, GA: Centers for Disease Control and Prevention (CDC), 1996.

[11] Fletcher, S.W.; Black, W.; Harris, R.; et al. Report of the International Workshop on Screening for Breast Cancer. *Journal of the National Cancer Institute* 85(20):1644-1656, 1993.

[12] Kronborg, O.; Fenger, C.; Olsen, J.; et al. Randomized study of screening for colorectal cancer with faecal-occult-blood test. *Lancet* 348(9640):1467-1471, 1996.

[13] Hardcastle, J.D.; Chamberlain, J.O.; Robinson, M.H.E.; et al. Randomized controlled trial of faecal-occult-blood screening for colorectal cancer. *Lancet* 348(9040):1472-1477, 1996.

[14] Mandel, J.S. Reducing mortality from colorectal cancer by screening for fecal occult blood. *Journal of the National Cancer Institute* 91(5): 434-437, 1999.

[15] Mandel, J.S.; Bond, J.H.; Church, T.R.; et al. Reducing mortality from colorectal cancer by screening for fecal occult blood. *New England Journal of Medicine* 328(19):1365-1371, 1993.

[16] Winawer, S.; Fletcher, R.; Miller, L.; et al. Colorectal cancer screening: Clinical guidelines and rationale. *Gerontology* 112:594-642, 1997.

[17] Selby, J.V.; Freidman, G.D.; Quesenberry, Jr., C.P.; et al. A case-control study of screening sigmoidoscopy and mortality from colorectal cancer. *New England Journal of Medicine* 326(10):653-657, 1992.

[18] Muller, A.D., and Sonnenberg, A. Protection by endoscopy against death from colorectal cancer—A case-control study among veterans. *Archives of Internal Medicine* 155:1741-1748, 1995.

[19] Newcomb, P.A.; Norfleet, R.G.; Storer, B.E.; et al. Screening sigmoidoscopy and colorectal cancer mortality. *Journal of the National Cancer Institute* 84(20):1572-1575, 1992.

[20] Alexander, F.E.; Edinburgh, G.L.; Andriole, G.L.; et al. Rationale for randomized trials of prostate cancer screening. *European Journal of Cancer* 35(2):262-271, 1999.

[21] CDC. Cigarette smoking-attributable mortality and years of potential life lost—United States, 1990. *Morbidity and Mortality Weekly Report* 42(33):645-649, 1993.

[22] Greenwald, P.; Kramer, B.S.; and Weed, D.L.; eds. *Cancer Prevention and Control.* New York, NY: Marcel Dekker, 1995, 568-569.

[23] Doll, R., and Peto, R. *The Causes of Cancer. Quantitative Estimates of Avoidable Risks of Cancer in the United States Today.* New York, NY: Oxford University Press, 1981.

[24] Kerlikowske, K.; Grady, D.; Rubin, S.M.; et al. Efficacy of screening mammography. A meta-analysis. *Journal of the American Medical Association* 273:149-154, 1995.

[25] Henderson, B.E.; Pike, M.C.; Bernstein, L.; et al. Breast cancer. In: Schottenfeld, D., and Fraumeni, Jr., J.F., eds. *Cancer Epidemiology and Prevention.* 2nd ed. New York, NY: Oxford University Press, 1996, 1022-1039.

[26] Harvard report on cancer prevention. Vol. 1. Causes of human cancer. *Cancer Causes & Control* 7(Suppl. 1):53-59, 1996.

[27] National Institutes of Health. Cervical cancer. *NIH Consensus Statement* 14(1):1-38, 1996.

[28] Schiffman, M.H.; Brinton, L.A.; Devesa, S.S.; et al. Cervical cancer. In: Schottenfeld, D., and Fraumeni, Jr., J.F., eds. *Cancer Epidemiology and Prevention.* 2nd ed. New York, NY: Oxford University Press, 1996, 1090-1116.

[29] Schottenfeld, D., and Winawer, S.J. Cancers of the large intestine. In: Schottenfeld, D., and Fraumeni, Jr., J.F., eds. *Cancer Epidemiology and Prevention.* 2nd ed. New York, NY: Oxford University Press, 1996, 813-840.

[30] Silverman, S. *Oral Cancer.* 4th ed. Hamilton, Ontario, Canada: American Cancer Society, B.C. Decker, Inc., 1998.

[31] Chodak, G.W.; Thisted, R.A.; Gerber, G.S.; et al. Results of conservative management of clinically localized prostate cancer. *New England Journal of Medicine* 330(4):242-248, 1994.

[32] Gerber, G.S.; Thisted, R.A.; Scardino, P.T.; et al. Results of radical prostatectomy in men with clinically localized prostate cancer: Multi-institutional pooled analysis. *Journal of the American Medical Association* 276(8):615-619, 1996.

[33] U.S. Preventive Services Task Force. *Guide to Clinical Preventive Services.* 2nd ed. Washington, DC: HHS, 1996.

[34] Armstrong, B.K., and English, D.R. Cutaneous malignant melanoma. In: Schottenfeld, D., and Fraumeni, Jr., J.F., eds. *Cancer Epidemiology and Prevention.* 2nd ed. New York, NY: Oxford University Press, 1996, 1282-1312.

4

Chronic Kidney Disease

Lead Agency: National Institutes of Health

Contents

Goal

Reduce new cases of chronic kidney disease and its complications, disability, death, and economic costs.

Overview

Issues and Trends

Chronic kidney failure is the most significant result of chronic kidney disease. When kidney function has deteriorated and is no longer adequate to sustain life and the process is considered irreversible, renal replacement therapy (RRT)—dialysis or transplantation—becomes necessary to maintain life. Treated chronic kidney failure, also called end-stage renal disease (ESRD), is the most feared consequence of kidney disease. Chronic renal insufficiency, however, is more common than treated chronic kidney failure and can also severely affect health and well-being. Therefore, ideally, programs should be directed at preventing the development of chronic renal insufficiency and its subsequent progression to ESRD.

Unfortunately, chronic renal insufficiency is usually asymptomatic, and the exact number of people affected is unknown. The best available estimates are based on national surveys. Current estimates indicate approximately 10 million persons aged 12 years and older have some form of chronic kidney disease.[1] People with end-stage kidney failure represent a small fraction of all individuals with chronic kidney disease. A significant proportion of people with chronic kidney failure

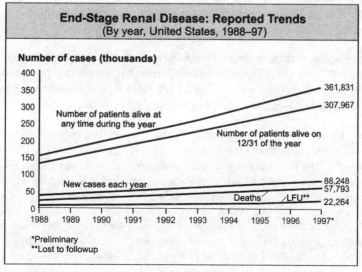

End-Stage Renal Disease: Reported Trends
(By year, United States, 1988–97)

Number of cases (thousands)

Number of patients alive at any time during the year — 361,831

Number of patients alive on 12/31 of the year — 307,967

New cases each year — 88,248 / 57,793

Deaths / LFU** — 22,264

*Preliminary
**Lost to followup

Source: NIH. U.S. Renal Data System, *1999 Annual Data Report.*

progress to end stage. The challenge is to initiate effective programs to prevent progression of established kidney disease and to institute methods to assess the progress of such initiatives.

In 1997, 80,248 new cases of end-stage kidney failure were reported.[2] Virtually all of these patients became permanently dependent on renal replacement therapy to stay alive.

Dialysis and kidney transplantation are the two methods of treatment available to people with kidney disease when they reach end stage. In 1997, 361,031 people in the United States depended on either dialysis or transplants to replace the function of their own failed kidneys.[3] Although these treatments are lifesaving, dialysis and transplants have substantial limitations. Neither treatment restores normal health, and both are expensive.[4] The rates of illness, disability, and death experienced by individuals with treated chronic kidney failure are substantially higher than those of the general population.[5]

In most instances, terminal kidney failure develops as the result of progressive damage to the kidneys over a decade or more. A number of underlying diseases can cause progressive kidney failure. The two most important of these are diabetes, which in 1997 accounted for 42 percent of the new cases of chronic kidney failure, and high blood pressure, which was responsible for 26 percent of the new cases.[6] Other conditions that contribute significantly include glomerulonephritis, vasculitis, interstitial nephritis, and genetic and congenital disorders, particularly polycystic kidney disease.[7]

Chronic kidney failure affects people of all ages. The number of new cases peaks in the sixth decade of life, but 25 percent of persons arriving at end stage in 1997 were under age 45 years, and 1.5 percent—nearly 1,100—were under age 20 years.[6] Kidney failure is particularly devastating in childhood, often resulting in impaired growth and development.

A worrisome increase in the number of new cases of kidney failure occurred between 1987 and 1997. The rate increased from 142 per million population in 1987 to 296 per million population in 1997,[8] representing an increase in the annual number of new cases from 34,797 to 80,248,[9] respectively.

This relentless growth in new cases of kidney failure has occurred in spite of the fact that death rates from other diseases, especially cardiovascular diseases, have declined.[10] The increase has not been confined to a single age group. Although the rates of new cases have grown slightly more rapidly for individuals aged 75 years and older, sizable increases have been noted in every age group.[11]

The causes of these increases are not completely understood, but one major factor appears to be an increase in the number of new cases of diabetes, particularly type 2 diabetes.[12, 13] In 1987, the rate of new cases of treated chronic kidney failure due to diabetes was 45 per million population. By 1997, the rate had increased to 124 per million population.[14]

Treatment for end-stage kidney failure has a substantial impact on Federal resources for health care. The 1972 Social Security Amendment (Public Law 92-603) instituted federally financed health care coverage for dialysis and renal transplantation, effective July 1, 1973. The cost of this program has far exceeded original expectations. Medicare spending in 1996 was estimated to be $10.96 billion, a 12.5 percent increase from the $9.74 billion spent in 1995. The total expenditure by all payers for treating these patients in 1996 was estimated at $14.55 billion, up from $13.05 billion in 1995.[15] Although this patient population made up only 0.6 percent of the total Medicare population in 1994, it consumed 5.1 percent of Medicare expenditures.[16] The increases in the cost per patient have been modest, but the driving force behind the growth in these expenditures has been the growing number of patients.

Kidney disease develops and progresses more rapidly to end stage in people with chronic health problems (such as type 1 or type 2 diabetes or high blood pressure) or with a family history of genetic kidney diseases. Therefore, people with these chronic health problems require counseling about the possibility of kidney disease and the steps they must take to avoid serious kidney complications. Also, people who have proteinuria and/or elevated serum creatinine have a greater likelihood of developing serious cardiovascular disease (CVD) complications. Therefore, cardiovascular risk assessment and management should include kidney function to prevent the consequences of kidney failure. Because national data systems will not be available in the first half of the decade to track progress, these issues are not addressed in the chapter.

Disparities

Kidney disease has a disproportionate impact on certain racial and ethnic groups, especially African Americans and American Indians or Alaska Natives. African Americans have the highest overall risk of chronic kidney disease. The reasons are not entirely explained by the higher number of persons in this population who have diabetes and high blood pressure.[17, 18] On average, African Americans develop end-stage kidney failure at an earlier age than whites (55.8 years compared to 62.2 years).[19] American Indians or Alaska Natives have a much higher risk of chronic kidney disease due to diabetes than whites. Overall, the rates of new cases are 4 times higher in African Americans and American Indians or Alaska Natives and 1.5 times higher in Asians or Pacific Islanders than in whites.

Annual increases in ESRD rates are greater in certain racial and ethnic populations than in white populations. Rates of new cases are increasing by 7 percent per year for African Americans, 10 percent per year for American Indians or Alaska Natives, and 11 percent for Asians or Pacific Islanders, compared to 6 percent per year for whites. Two communities of an American Indian Tribe, the Zuni Pueblo in New Mexico and in Sacaton, Arizona, may have the highest rates of chronic kidney failure in the world, at 12.6 and 14.0 times the overall average U.S. rate, respectively. Projections indicate that increases in the rates of new cases will continue in American Indians or Alaska Natives.

Although complete data are not yet available, some evidence indicates that persons of Mexican ancestry also may have a high risk of developing chronic kidney failure, particularly due to diabetes.[20, 21] In 1995, the Health Care Financing Administration changed the way in which data on race and ethnicity are collected on the Medical Evidence Form used to enroll patients into the Medicare End-Stage Renal Disease Program. Data from 1997 suggest that 7 percent of the ESRD patients are of Mexican ancestry and another 4 percent are of Hispanic ancestry from areas other than Mexico.[22]

The disproportionately high rates of chronic kidney failure among certain racial and ethnic groups have resulted in a greater burden of disease in these communities. In 1996, African Americans constituted 12.6 percent of the U.S. population but 29.8 percent of ESRD patients; American Indians or Alaska Natives constituted 0.9 percent of the U.S. population but 1.7 percent of those receiving renal replacement therapy.[23] On December 31, 1996, the point-prevalent rate per million population (adjusted for age and gender) was 3,404 in African Americans and 2,761 in American Indians or Alaska Natives, compared to 754 in whites, differences of 4.5- and 3.7-fold, respectively.[24] Data on persons of Asian or Pacific Islander ancestry indicate slightly higher incidence and prevalence rates than those for whites.[25]

There is a slight preponderance of kidney failure in men. In 1997, the incidence of treated chronic kidney failure was 322 per million population in men, compared with 271 per million in women.[8]

Renal transplantation is an important lifesaving renal replacement therapy and has been shown to offer many advantages when compared with dialysis.[26, 27] In 1997, 12,445 transplants were performed in the United States. There was significant gender discrepancy, with 7,352 transplants for men, compared with 4,948 for women.[28] Racial and ethnic disparities also exist. Between 1994 and 1997, the first cadaveric transplantation rates (per 100 patient years) in the pediatric age group were 31 for black males, 28 for white males, 19 for black females, and 26 for white females. For recipients between the ages of 20 and 44 years, the rates were 7 for black males, 17 for white males, 7 for black females, and 15 for white females. In the 45- to 65-year age group, the rates were 4 for black males, 8 for white males, 2 for black females, and 6 for white females.[29] The data from the U.S. Renal Data System (USRDS) database also confirm that the transplantation rate is lower for Native Americans. The transplantation rate in Asians is equivalent to the rate in whites.[30] Reasons for the racial and ethnic disparities in the rate of transplantation are varied and include differences in finding human leukocyte antigen matches, cultural attitudes and beliefs on the part of both patients and health care providers, socioeconomic status, rates of organ donation, and geographic location.

Major risk factors for the development and progression of chronic kidney disease include diabetes, high blood pressure, environmental exposures, proteinuria, family history of kidney disease, and increasing age. African Americans and American Indians or Alaska Natives who have these risk factors are especially susceptible to the development of chronic and progressive kidney disease.[31, 32] Strategies for preventing the development of chronic kidney disease, therefore, should use appropriate methods to target these populations.

Under certain circumstances, the progression of kidney disease to end stage can be slowed or halted. Three interventions are effective in certain defined populations: glycemic control (for patients with diabetes), blood pressure control (for patients with high blood pressure), and use of angiotensin-converting enzyme (ACE) inhibitors. Interventions to slow the progression of kidney disease and prevent chronic kidney failure are likely to have the greatest impact if applied early in the course of the disease. Unfortunately, because kidney disease in its early stages is generally asymptomatic, many people who would benefit from these interventions are not identified. Early identification of patients at risk for chronic kidney disease is essential in reducing the growth in the number of new cases of treated chronic kidney failure. For example, microalbuminuria screening and more intensive treatment of patients with microalbuminuria are an important part of a strategy to reduce nephropathy in persons with type 1 diabetes, both in terms of economic indices and clinical outcomes.[33, 34, 35] This strategy also may be useful in type 2 diabetes.

Patient care must continue to emphasize interventions to conserve residual renal function. At a certain stage, however, providing appropriate preparation for renal replacement therapy becomes advisable. Several studies show that many patients with chronic kidney failure do not receive optimum preparation for treated chronic kidney failure in the year prior to the commencement of RRT. This lack of optimal preparation has a substantial effect on the cost of care and on illness and disability at the time of RRT.[36]

Kidney transplantation has emerged as the preferred therapy for many patients with treated chronic kidney failure, particularly children. Kidney transplantation confers a survival advantage over dialysis.[37] Over the past decade, transplantation success rates, especially 1-year patient and graft survival, have improved steadily. This improvement has been observed in both cadaveric and living-related transplants.[38, 39] For young children, kidney transplantation results in improved rates of growth.[40] Because of accumulating evidence on the advantages of transplantation, equal access of all population groups to transplantation is a substantial concern. Certain racial and ethnic groups and women consistently have longer waiting times and lower rates of kidney transplantation than white males.[41, 42, 43, 44, 45, 46]

Attention to risk factors for kidney disease and interventions to slow its progression are urgently needed. This need is driven by the increasing number of cases of treated chronic kidney failure, its disproportionate effect on certain racial and ethnic groups, the high societal cost of the disease, and the impact on Federal health care resources.

Interim Progress Toward Year 2000 Objectives

Healthy People 2000 did not include a chapter on chronic kidney disease. However, objectives relating to chronic kidney disease were included in several chapters. Since the mid-1980s, the number of new cases of ESRD has grown steadily. One objective concerning diabetes addressed ESRD. Results show that ESRD among people with diabetes has more than doubled since 1987 and is moving away from the target. Subobjectives tracking ESRD due to diabetes among African Americans and American Indians or Alaska Natives also are moving away from their targets.

Note: Unless otherwise noted, data are from the Centers for Disease Control and Prevention, National Center for Health Statistics, *Healthy People 2000 Review, 1998–99*.

Chronic Kidney Disease

Goal: Reduce new cases of chronic kidney disease and its complications, disability, death, and economic costs.

Number **Objective Short Title**

4-1   End-stage renal disease

4-2   Cardiovascular disease deaths in persons with chronic kidney failure

4-3   Counseling for chronic kidney failure care

4-4   Use of arteriovenous fistulas

4-5   Registration for kidney transplantation

4-6   Waiting time for kidney transplantation

4-7   Kidney failure due to diabetes

4-8   Medical therapy for persons with diabetes and proteinuria

4-1. Reduce the rate of new cases of end-stage renal disease (ESRD).

Target: 217 new cases per million population.

Baseline: 289 new cases of end-stage renal disease per million population were reported in 1997.

Target setting method: Better than the best.

Data source: U.S. Renal Data System (USRDS), NIH, NIDDK.

NOTE: THE TABLE BELOW MAY CONTINUE TO THE FOLLOWING PAGE.

Total Population, 1997	New Cases of End-Stage Renal Disease
	Rate per Million
TOTAL	289
Race and ethnicity	
American Indian or Alaska Native	586
Asian or Pacific Islander	344
Asian	DNC
Native Hawaiian and other Pacific Islander	DNC
Black or African American	873
White	218
Hispanic or Latino	DNA
Not Hispanic or Latino	DNA
Black or African American	DNA
White	DNA
Gender	
Female	242
Male	348
Family income level	
Poor	DNC
Near poor	DNC
Middle/high income	DNC

Total Population, 1997	New Cases of End-Stage Renal Disease
	Rate per Million
Select populations	
Age groups	
Under 20 years	13
20 to 44 years	109
45 to 64 years	545
65 to 74 years	1,296
75 years and older	1,292

DNA = Data have not been analyzed. DNC = Data are not collected. DSU = Data are statistically unreliable.

NOTE: THE TABLE ABOVE MAY HAVE CONTINUED FROM THE PREVIOUS PAGE.

The current average annual increase in new cases of treated chronic kidney failure rates is 6 percent. Therefore, the expected rate in 2010 would be 612 new cases per million population. Without improvements in prevention and because of changes in demographics and increases in the number of cases of diabetes, rates of new cases of treated chronic kidney failure are expected to continue to rise 5 to 8 percent per year.

4-2. Reduce deaths from cardiovascular disease in persons with chronic kidney failure.

Target: 52 deaths per 1,000 patient years at risk.

Baseline: 70 deaths from cardiovascular disease per 1,000 patient years at risk (in persons with ESRD) occurred in 1997.

Target setting method: Better than the best.

Data source: U.S. Renal Data System (USRDS), NIH, NIDDK.

NOTE: THE TABLE BELOW MAY CONTINUE TO THE FOLLOWING PAGE.

Persons With Treated Chronic Kidney Failure, 1997	Deaths From Cardiovascular Disease
	Per 1,000 Patient Years at Risk
TOTAL	70
Race and ethnicity	
American Indian or Alaska Native	63
Asian or Pacific Islander	60
Asian	DNC

Persons With Treated Chronic Kidney Failure, 1997	Deaths From Cardiovascular Disease
	Per 1,000 Patient Years at Risk
Native Hawaiian and other Pacific Islander	DNC
Black or African American	62
White	75
Hispanic or Latino	DNA
Not Hispanic or Latino	DNA
Black or African American	DNA
White	DNA
Gender	
Female	73
Male	67
Family income level	
Poor	DNC
Near poor	DNC
Middle/high income	DNC

DNA = Data have not been analyzed. DNC = Data are not collected. DSU = Data are statistically unreliable.

NOTE: THE TABLE ABOVE MAY HAVE CONTINUED FROM THE PREVIOUS PAGE.

Cardiovascular disease is the major cause of death among patients with chronic renal failure and ESRD. Therefore, targeting reduction in CVD deaths will lead to a significant decrease in deaths for this population. The increased risk of CVD in kidney disease patients is evident before the onset of terminal kidney failure. Increases in the number of CVD deaths also are seen in individuals with proteinuria or elevated creatinine (both are markers of declining kidney function). CVD death rates in the treated chronic kidney failure population are estimated to be 30-fold higher than in the general population.[47] The known risk factors for CVD in the general population include age, male gender, diabetes, elevated cholesterol, high blood pressure, smoking, and family history. Elevated homocysteine levels in the blood also may be an important risk factor in treated chronic kidney failure patients and at earlier stages in the progression of kidney disease.[48, 49, 50] Strategies to reduce CVD deaths should target risk reduction before terminal kidney failure.[51] All responsible health care providers can initiate the strategies to reduce CVD deaths as suggested in published guidelines.[51]

4-3. Increase the proportion of treated chronic kidney failure patients who have received counseling on nutrition, treatment choices, and cardiovascular care 12 months before the start of renal replacement therapy.

Target: 60 percent.

Baseline: 45 percent of newly diagnosed patients with treated chronic kidney failure received counseling on nutrition, treatment choices, and cardiovascular care in 1996.

Target setting method: 33 percent improvement. (Better than the best will be used when data are available.)

Data source: U.S. Renal Data System (USRDS), NIH, NIDDK.

Newly Diagnosed Patients With Treated Chronic Kidney Failure, 1996	Received Counseling Prior to Renal Replacement Therapy
	Percent
TOTAL	45
Race and ethnicity	
American Indian or Alaska Native	DNA
Asian or Pacific Islander	DNA
Asian	DNC
Native Hawaiian and other Pacific Islander	DNC
Black or African American	DNA
White	DNA
Hispanic or Latino	DNA
Not Hispanic or Latino	DNA
Black or African American	DNA
White	DNA
Gender	
Female	DNA
Male	DNA
Family income level	
Poor	DNC
Near poor	DNC
Middle/high income	DNC

DNA = Data have not been analyzed. DNC = Data are not collected. DSU = Data are statistically unreliable.

Medically appropriate care of kidney disease patients within 12 months before the start of renal replacement therapy reduces the substantial illness, disability, and death associated with treated chronic kidney failure.[52] Appropriate preparation for RRT includes reduction in CVD risk factors, treatment of anemia, optimum therapy to preserve residual renal function, consultation about nutrition, and patient education about RRT methods. Patients should be seen by a specialist in RRT at least 12 months prior to initiation of RRT for general counseling. However, specific issues—such as vascular access and estimation of residual renal function—need to be addressed at least 6 months prior to RRT. Many patients with chronic renal failure are not seen by health care professionals who have RRT expertise until very near the time that RRT will be required. In a USRDS survey of 3,468 new dialysis patients, 55 percent had not been seen by a nephrologist 1 year prior to the start of RRT, and 33 percent had not been seen even 3 months before RRT.[53] Although control of diet is a major aspect of care for patients with chronic kidney failure and terminal kidney failure, by the start of RRT, 46 percent of the patients had not seen a dietitian.

4-4. Increase the proportion of new hemodialysis patients who use arteriovenous fistulas as the primary mode of vascular access.

Target: 50 percent.

Baseline: 29 percent of newly diagnosed patients with treated chronic kidney failure on hemodialysis used arteriovenous fistulas as the primary mode of vascular access in 1997.

Target setting method: 72 percent improvement (consistent with Dialysis Outcomes Quality Initiative [DOQI] guidelines). (Better than the best will be used when data are available.)

Data source: U.S. Renal Data System (USRDS), NIH, NIDDK.

NOTE: THE TABLE BELOW MAY CONTINUE TO THE FOLLOWING PAGE.

Newly Diagnosed Patients With Treated Chronic Kidney Failure on Hemodialysis, 1997	Arteriovenous Fistula Use
	Percent
TOTAL	29
Race and ethnicity	
American Indian or Alaska Native	DNA
Asian or Pacific Islander	DNA
Asian	DNC
Native Hawaiian and other Pacific Islander	DNC
Black or African American	DNA
White	DNA

Newly Diagnosed Patients With Treated Chronic Kidney Failure on Hemodialysis, 1997	Arteriovenous Fistula Use
	Percent
Hispanic or Latino	DNA
Not Hispanic or Latino	DNA
Black or African American	DNA
White	DNA
Gender	
Female	DNA
Male	DNA
Family income level	
Poor	DNC
Near poor	DNC
Middle/high income	DNC

DNA = Data have not been analyzed. DNC = Data are not collected. DSU = Data are statistically unreliable.

NOTE: THE TABLE ABOVE MAY HAVE CONTINUED FROM THE PREVIOUS PAGE.

Patients receiving renal replacement therapy as of December 31, 1997, were treated predominantly (72 percent) with dialysis. Of these, 88 percent were on hemodialysis. Vascular access is the major lifeline for hemodialysis patients. The presence of a functioning vascular access site represents a critical factor in the well-being of these patients. Unfortunately, however, it also is the largest single cause of illness and disability in patients receiving hemodialysis for renal replacement therapy, accounting for nearly 25 percent of all hospitalizations. Complications and problems related to vascular access have been estimated to account for as much as 17 percent of the health care costs associated with treated chronic kidney failure.[54]

Monitoring the type of vascular access for dialysis in new patients is an important method to assess the adequacy of preparation for RRT. Clinical evidence shows that patients with endogenous arteriovenous fistulas experience lower complication rates than patients with synthetic grafts. In the United States, the use rate for arteriovenous fistulas is under 30 percent.[55] Arteriovenous fistulas, ideally, should be placed at least 6 months before the start of dialysis. Early placement of arteriovenous fistulas is particularly important for elderly persons, because atherosclerotic vessels may take a much longer time to dilate to a usable diameter.

4-5. Increase the proportion of dialysis patients registered on the waiting list for transplantation.

Target: 66 percent of dialysis patients.

Baseline: 20 percent of newly diagnosed treated chronic kidney failure patients under age 70 years were registered on the waiting list in 1994–96.

Target setting method: Better than the best.

Data source: U.S. Renal Data System (USRDS), NIH, NIDDK.

Dialysis Patients Under Age 70 Years, 1994–96	Transplant Waiting List
	Percent
TOTAL	20
Race and ethnicity	
American Indian or Alaska Native	2
Asian or Pacific Islander	4
Asian	DNC
Native Hawaiian and other Pacific Islander	DNC
Black or African American	29
White	65
Hispanic or Latino	12
Not Hispanic or Latino	DNA
Black or African American	DNA
White	DNA
Gender	
Female	40
Male	60
Family income level	
Poor	DNC
Near poor	DNC
Middle/high income	DNC
Select populations	
Age groups	
Under 20 years	3
20 to 39 years	31
40 to 59 years	51
60 to 69 years	15

DNA = Data have not been analyzed. DNC = Data are not collected. DSU = Data are statistically unreliable.

Healthy People 2010: Objectives for Improving Health

Successful renal transplantation confers many advantages, including improvements in physical and psychological growth in children and improved survival and quality of life for recipients in general. The prospects of receiving a kidney transplant, however, are determined by a number of factors. These factors include age, primary cause of kidney failure, race and ethnic origin, gender, geographic location, and availability of suitable donors. Any combination of these factors may directly influence the first important step in the process of receiving a kidney transplant—namely, being registered on the waiting list. Significant disparities exist in the people who are registered on the waiting list. Women and people from certain racial and ethnic groups—particularly, African Americans—are less likely than other kidney transplant candidates to be registered on the waiting list.[40, 55, 56]

4-6. Increase the proportion of patients with treated chronic kidney failure who receive a transplant within 3 years of registration on the waiting list.

Target: 51 registrants per 1,000 patient years at risk.

Baseline: 41 registrants per 1,000 patient years at risk (since placed on dialysis) received a transplant within 3 years in 1995–97.

Target setting method: Better than the best.

Data source: U.S. Renal Data System (USRDS), NIH, NIDDK.

DATA NOTE: THE TABLE BELOW MAY CONTINUE TO THE FOLLOWING PAGE.

Renal Transplant Waiting List Registrants, 1995–97	Transplant Within 3 Years
	Rate per 1,000 Patient Years
TOTAL	41
Race and ethnicity	
American Indian or Alaska Native	30
Asian or Pacific Islander	DNA
Asian	50
Native Hawaiian and other Pacific Islander	DNA
Black or African American	30
White	49
Hispanic or Latino	DNA
Not Hispanic or Latino	DNA
Black or African American	DNA
White	DNA

Renal Transplant Waiting List Registrants, 1995–97	Transplant Within 3 Years
	Rate per 1,000 Patient Years
Gender	
Female	33
Male	49
Family income level	
Poor	DNC
Near poor	DNC
Middle/high income	DNC
Select populations	
Age groups	
Under 20 years	282
20 to 44 years	110
45 to 64 years	52
65 years and older	6

DNA = Data have not been analyzed. DNC = Data are not collected. DSU = Data are statistically unreliable.

NOTE: THE TABLE ABOVE MAY HAVE CONTINUED FROM THE PREVIOUS PAGE.

Individuals from certain racial and ethnic populations (specifically, African Americans) move up the waiting list to receive kidney transplants at a slower rate than whites.[57, 58] The exact causes are unclear. Racial and ethnic disparities in waiting times may be influenced by genetic and biological factors (such as HLA types),[59] the request and consent procedures of organ procurement organizations, patient registration practices for a center or region, organ acceptance practices at each transplant center, geographic location, socioeconomic status, cultural attitudes and beliefs about organ donation, rates of organ donation within each local area, and the donor pool.[42, 60]

Reports also have documented a lower rate of transplantation in women.[55] The U.S. Department of Health and Human Services (HHS) is working toward the goal of making sure that all persons in the United States have an equal opportunity to receive a transplant, regardless of who they are or where they live. To increase access to transplantation, HHS launched the National Organ and Tissue Donation Initiative to increase overall organ and tissue donation. One aspect of the initiative is to learn more about the factors that influence organ and tissue donation, with a special emphasis on certain racial and ethnic communities. Health care workers, particularly in the area of transplantation, need to understand the various obstacles to organ donation and transplantation, especially in the groups with which they work, and to initiate programs and policies that are culturally sensitive and meaningful.

4-7. Reduce kidney failure due to diabetes.

Target: 78 diabetic persons with new cases of ESRD per million population.

Baseline: 113 diabetic persons with new cases of ESRD per million population were reported in 1996.

Target setting method: Better than the best.

Data source: U.S. Renal Data System (USRDS), NIH, NIDDK.

NOTE: THE TABLE BELOW MAY CONTINUE TO THE FOLLOWING PAGE.

Persons With Diabetes, 1996	New Cases of ESRD
	Rate per Million
TOTAL	113
Race and ethnicity	
American Indian or Alaska Native	482
Asian or Pacific Islander	156
Asian	DNC
Native Hawaiian and other Pacific Islander	DNC
Black or African American	329
White	79
Hispanic or Latino	DNA
Not Hispanic or Latino	DNA
Black or African American	DNA
White	DNA
Gender	
Female	103
Male	112
Family income level	
Poor	DNC
Near poor	DNC
Middle/high income	DNC
Select populations	
Age groups	
Under 20 years	0
20 to 44 years	35
45 to 64 years	276

Persons With Diabetes, 1996	New Cases of ESRD
	Rate per Million
65 to 74 years	514
75 years and older	263

DNA = Data have not been analyzed. DNC = Data are not collected. DSU = Data are statistically unreliable.
NOTE: THE TABLE ABOVE MAY HAVE CONTINUED FROM THE PREVIOUS PAGE.

Convincing, consistent, and continuing scientific evidence shows that with secondary and tertiary prevention, microvascular complications of diabetes, especially diabetic kidney disease, can be reduced substantially. Enhanced quality of life, reductions in death rates, and reduced costs can result from improved clinical and public health diabetes prevention strategies directed at kidney disease and other microvascular and metabolic complications of diabetes. Monitoring the consequences of these strategies, including reductions in the magnitude of chronic renal insufficiency, terminal kidney failure, and other microvascular complications, should be an important component of an effective national public health program.

4-8. **(Developmental) Increase the proportion of persons with type 1 or type 2 diabetes and proteinuria who receive recommended medical therapy to reduce progression to chronic renal insufficiency.**

Potential data sources: National Ambulatory Medical Care Survey (NAMCS), CDC, NCHS; National Hospital Ambulatory Medical Care Survey (NHAMCS), CDC, NCHS.

Related Objectives From Other Focus Areas

1. **Access to Quality Health Services**
    1-2. Health insurance coverage for clinical preventive services
    1-3. Counseling about health behaviors
    1-7. Core competencies in health provider training
5. **Diabetes**
    5-2. New cases of diabetes
    5-3. Overall cases of diagnosed diabetes
    5-4. Diagnosis of diabetes
    5-7. Cardiovascular disease deaths in persons with diabetes
    5-11. Annual urinary microalbumin measurement
    5-12. Annual glycosylated hemoglobin measurement
6. **Disability and Secondary Conditions**
    6-1. Standard definition of people with disabilities in data sets
    6-2. Feelings and depression among children with disabilities

6-3. Feelings and depression interfering with activities among adults with disabilities

6-5. Sufficient emotional support among adults with disabilities

6-6. Satisfaction with life among adults with disabilities

6-8. Employment parity

7. Educational and Community-Based Programs

7-7. Patient and family education

7-8. Satisfaction with patient education

7-9. Health care organization sponsorship of community health promotion activities

7-10. Community health promotion programs

7-11. Culturally appropriate and linguistically competent community health promotion programs

8. Environmental Health

8-11. Elevated blood lead levels in children

8-14. Toxic pollutants

8-20. School policies to protect against environmental hazards

8-22. Lead-based paint testing

8-25. Exposure to heavy metals and other toxic chemicals

8-26. Information systems used for environmental health

8-27. Monitoring environmentally related diseases

8-29. Global burden of disease

10. Food Safety

10-1. Foodborne infections

10-2. Outbreaks of foodborne infections

10-5. Consumer food safety practices

10-6 Safe food preparation practices in retail establishments

11. Health Communication

11-2. Health literacy

11-4. Quality of Internet health information sources

11-6. Satisfaction with health care providers' communication skills

12. Heart Disease and Stroke

12-1. Coronary heart disease (CHD) deaths

12-2. Knowledge of symptoms of heart attack and importance of calling 911

12-6. Heart failure hospitalizations

12-8. Knowledge of early warning symptoms of stroke

12-9. High blood pressure

12-10. High blood pressure control

12-11. Action to help control blood pressure

12-12. Blood pressure monitoring

12-16. LDL-cholesterol level in CHD patients

13. HIV

13-1. New AIDS cases

13-3. AIDS among persons who inject drugs

13-5. New HIV cases

13-8. HIV counseling and education for persons in substance abuse treatment

13-12. Screening for STDs and immunization for hepatitis B

13-17. Perinatally acquired HIV infection

(A listing of abbreviations and acronyms used in this publication appears in Appendix H.)

Arteriovenous fistula: The type of vascular access created by joining a person's own (endogenous) artery to the nearby vein. The increase in blood flow in the vein leads to marked dilation of the vein and permits an easier insertion of needles for dialysis.

Chronic renal insufficiency, chronic renal failure, and end-stage renal disease (ESRD) (defined in this chapter as treated chronic kidney failure): Terms describing the continuum of increasing renal dysfunction and decreasing glomerular filtration rate (GFR). Because of the progressive nature of kidney disease, these terms represent successive stages of disease in most patients.

Chronic renal insufficiency: The stage in chronic kidney disease in which damage to the kidney already has resulted in significant impairment of renal function, but systemic manifestations are minimal. Most patients who have chronic renal insufficiency are asymptomatic. Chronic renal insufficiency usually is identified because the serum creatinine is slightly elevated (greater than 1.5 mg/dL in males or 1.2 mg/dL in females and greater than age-specific normative values in children). The serum creatinine test is insensitive and does not identify all persons who have chronic renal insufficiency. Although precise GFR limits cannot be assigned to this stage of disease, typically patients with chronic renal insufficiency have a GFR between 30 ml/min and 75 ml/min.

Chronic renal failure: The stage in chronic renal disease in which renal dysfunction has progressed to a level resulting in systemic manifestations. These manifestations include a rise in the blood concentration of urea, creatinine, and phosphate, which are removed by the kidneys, and other problems, such as anemia, bone disease, acidosis, and salt and fluid retention. Growth failure may be seen in children. Most patients with chronic renal failure progress to treated chronic kidney failure (end-stage renal disease).

End-stage renal disease (ESRD) (referred to in this focus area as treated chronic kidney failure): The stage in chronic renal disease in which renal replacement therapy, dialysis, or kidney transplantation is needed to sustain life. Treated chronic kidney failure is generally an irreversible state. The glomerular filtration rate is usually less than 10 ml/min.

Diabetes (diabetes mellitus): A chronic disease due to insulin deficiency or resistance to insulin action and associated with hyperglycemia (elevated blood glucose levels). Over time, without proper preventive treatment, organ complications related to diabetes develop, including heart, nerve, foot, eye, and kidney damage as well as problems with pregnancy. Diabetes is classified into two major categories.

Type 1 diabetes (previously called insulin-dependent diabetes mellitus [IDDM] or juvenile-onset diabetes [JODM]): Represents clinically about 5 percent of all persons with diagnosed diabetes. Its clinical onset typically occurs at ages under 30 years, with more gradual development after age 30. Most often type 1 diabetes represents an autoimmune destructive disease in the beta (insulin-producing) cells of the pancreas in genetically susceptible individuals. Insulin therapy always is required to sustain life and maintain diabetes control.

Type 2 diabetes (previously called noninsulin-dependent diabetes mellitus [NIDDM] or adult-onset diabetes [AODM]): Refers to the most common form of diabetes in the United States and the world, especially in certain racial and ethnic groups and in elderly persons. Women who develop diabetes during pregnancy also are at increased risk of developing this type of diabetes later in life. In the United States, approximately 95 percent of all persons with diagnosed diabetes (10.5 million) and 100 percent of all persons with undiagnosed (5.5 million) diabetes probably have type 2 diabetes.

Diabetic kidney disease: Kidney disease and resultant kidney functional impairment due to the longstanding effects of diabetes on the microvasculature of the kidney. Features include increased urine protein and decreased kidney function.

Dialysis: The process by which metabolic waste products are removed by cleansing of the blood directly through extracorporeal filtration membranes (hemodialysis) or indirectly by diffusion of waste products through the peritoneal membranes into instilled fluids (peritoneal dialysis).

End-stage renal disease: See above.

Glomerular filtration: The process by which the kidneys filter the blood, clearing it of toxins.

Glomerular filtration rate (GFR): The rate at which the blood is cleared by glomerular filtration and an important measure of kidney function. Normal GFR values in adults are between 100 and 150 ml/min. One of the most important hallmarks of chronic renal disease is a progressive decline in the rate of glomerular filtration. Generally, a GFR below 75 ml/min represents clinically significant renal insufficiency. A GFR of less than 10 ml/min represents kidney failure severe enough to require renal replacement therapy to maintain life.

Hemodialysis: The process by which biologic waste products are removed from the body through external blood circuit and external (artificial) membranes.

Glomerulonephritis: Inflammation in the primary filtration units (glomeruli) of the kidneys. Typically, this process leads to loss of blood, blood products, and protein into the urine. Unchecked or without effective treatment, this process could lead ultimately to permanent kidney damage and loss of kidney function and chronic kidney failure.

Incidence rate: A measure of the number of new cases of disease occurring in a specific population over a specific period of time, usually 1 year. For end-stage renal disease, the best information is based on the incidence of treated end-stage kidney disease reported through Medicare to the U.S. Renal Data System. Available data exclude those patients who die without receiving treatment.

Interstitial nephritis: Inflammation in the supporting matrix of the kidneys. This process could result from damage caused by microorganisms (such as bacteria and viruses) or from toxic reaction to drugs or other substances such as lead and mercury.

Microalbuminuria: Abnormally elevated levels of albumin in the urine—but at levels too low to be detectable by the dipstick method used to test for protein in the urine. Increased urinary excretion of albumin, even if the concentration is too low to be detectable as dipstick proteinuria, has been associated with increased risk of progressive kidney disease in people with diabetes[6, 7] and increased risk of subsequent death in persons with[8] and without diabetes[9, 10] and in elderly individuals.[11] Microalbuminuria can be measured in several ways. If a random urine sample is used, the albumin concentration in the first-voided morning urine or the ratio of urine albumin to urine creatinine can be used. If a timed urine collection is available, an albumin excretion rate can be determined. Urine albumin concentrations of 30 to 300 µg/ml, urinary albumin to creatinine ratios of less than 3.5 mg/mmol, and urine albumin excretion rates of less than 15 µg/min all have been used as cutoff values for detection of microalbuminuria.

Patient year (at risk): A measure of the duration (in years) a patient has been exposed to the effects of a particular biologic or physiologic condition, such as chronic renal insufficiency or the effects of dialysis.

Polycystic kidney disease: A disorder (usually inherited) of the kidneys in which the normal kidney structures (particularly, the tubules) are replaced by sacs (or cysts) that ultimately increase in size and lead to further destruction of the supporting matrix of the kidneys. The most common variety is the adult polycystic kidney disease (ADPKD), which is inherited as an autosomal dominant genetic disease. ADPKD is usually characterized by elevated blood pressure, pain from enlarged cysts, blood in the urine, and a relentless progression to terminal kidney failure.

Prevalence rate: A measure of the total number of cases of disease existing in a specific population at a certain point in time (point prevalence) or over a certain period of time (period prevalence). Point-prevalence rates reflect the number of individuals at the stated date.

Proteinuria: Abnormal levels of protein in the urine. Proteinuria is a marker for structural kidney damage or inflammation and also may be involved in the pathogenesis of progressive renal injury. Increased risks of developing progressive renal disease,[1,2] of death,[3,4] and of death due to cardiovascular disease[5] have been documented in persons with persistent proteinuria. Urine protein can be estimated by a dipstick method, which provides a semiquantitative estimate of concentration. More accurate measures include determining the ratio of urine protein to urine creatinine or the amount of protein excreted by a person in a 24-hour period.

Renal disease: A synonym for kidney disease.

Serum creatinine: A blood chemistry measurement used to estimate the level of kidney function. Serum creatinine is an important index for monitoring progression of disease in persons with chronic renal disease. Elevations in serum creatinine are an insensitive marker of early chronic renal insufficiency. In advanced renal failure, however, a change in serum creatinine is a more reliable indicator. This test remains the most widely available method used to estimate the glomerular filtration rate or to monitor changes in level of renal function.[12]

U.S. Renal Data System (USRDS): A national database of information on treated chronic kidney failure patients—new cases, illness, disability, and death outcomes. USRDS is based predominantly on data collected by the Health Care Financing Administration's Medicare treated chronic kidney failure program and is funded by a contract from the National Institutes of Health.[13] This database contains information on approximately 93 percent of all patients treated for treated chronic kidney failure in the United States. Most of the data cited in this focus area derive from USRDS reports. As noted, these numbers reflect reported cases of treated end-stage renal disease and, therefore, do not include patients who die without treatment or patients whose care is not reported to USRDS.

Vascular access: The means by which blood is removed from a person for cleansing during dialysis and safely and easily returned, when cleaned, into the body.

Vasculitis: Inflammation of the blood vessels. Typically, the cause of this process is unknown. Untreated, it leads to progression to relentless and specific organ failures, including chronic kidney failure, or death.

References

[1] Jones, C.A.; McQuillan, G.M.; Kusek, J.W.; et al. Serum creatinine levels in the U.S. population: Third National Health and Nutrition Examination Survey. *American Journal of Kidney Diseases* 32:992-999, 1998.

[2] U.S. Renal Data System (USRDS). *1999 Annual Data Report (ADR)*. Bethesda, MD: National Institutes of Health (NIH), National Institute of Diabetes and Digestive and Kidney Diseases (NIDDK), April 1999, Appendix, Table A-1.

[3] USRDS. *1999 ADR*. Bethesda, MD: NIH, NIDDK, April 1999, Appendix, Tables A-1 and B-3.

[4] USRDS. *1999 ADR*. Bethesda, MD: NIH, NIDDK, April 1999, Chapter X, 133-148.

[5] USRDS. *1999 ADR*. Bethesda, MD: NIH, NIDDK, April 1999, Chapter V, 63-78.

[6] USRDS. *1999 ADR.* Bethesda, MD: NIH, NIDDK, April 1999, Appendix, Table A-1.

[7] USRDS. *1999 ADR.* Bethesda, MD: NIH, NIDDK, April 1999, Appendix, Table A-15.

[8] USRDS. *1999 ADR.* Bethesda, MD: NIH, NIDDK, April 1999, Appendix, Table A-3.

[9] USRDS. *1999 ADR.* Bethesda, MD: NIH, NIDDK, April 1999, Appendix, Table A-1.

[10] National Heart, Lung, and Blood Institute. *Morbidity and Mortality Chartbook on Cardiovascular Disease, Lung and Blood Diseases.* Bethesda, MD: Public Health Service, 1998.

[11] USRDS. *1999 ADR.* Bethesda, MD: NIH, NIDDK, April 1999, Appendix, Tables A-1, A-2, and A-3.

[12] Clark, C. How should we respond to the worldwide diabetes epidemic? *Diabetes Care* 21:475-476, 1998.

[13] Centers for Disease Control and Prevention (CDC). *National Diabetes Fact Sheet: National Estimates and General Information on Diabetes in the United States.* Atlanta, GA: U.S. Department of Health and Human Services, 1997.

[14] USRDS. *1999 ADR.* Bethesda, MD: NIH, NIDDK, April 1999, Appendix, Table A-6.

[15] Eggers, P.W. Personal communication. Health Care Financing Administration. 1999.

[16] Perneger, T.V.; Klag, M.J.; Feldman, H.I.; et al. Projection of hypertension related renal disease in middle-aged residents of the United States. *Journal of the American Medical Association* 269(10):1272-1277, 1993.

[17] Whittle, J.C.; Whelton, P.K.; Seidler, A.J.; et al. Does racial variation in risk factors explain black-white differences in the incidence of hypertensive end-stage renal disease? *Archives of Internal Medicine* 151:1359-1364, 1991.

[18] Brancati, F.L.; Whittle, J.C.; Whelton, P.K.; et al. The excess incidence of diabetic end-stage renal disease among blacks. A population based study of potential explanatory factors. *Journal of the American Medical Association* 268:3079-3084, 1992.

[19] USRDS. *1999 ADR.* Bethesda, MD: NIH, NIDDK, April 1999, Appendix, Tables A-1 and A-14.

[20] Gonzales Villalpano, C.G.; Stern, M.P.; Arrendondo Perez, B.; et al. Nephropathy in low income diabetics: The Mexico City Diabetes Study. *Archives of Medical Research* 27:367-372, 1996.

[21] Pugh, J.A.; Stern, M.P.; Haffner, S.M.; et al. Excess incidence of treatment of end-stage renal disease in Mexican Americans. *American Journal of Epidemiology* 127:135-144, 1998.

[22] Agodoa, L.Y.C.; Roys, E.C.; Wolfe, R.A.; et al. ESRD among Hispanics in the U.S. *Journal of the American Society of Nephrology* 10:232A, 1999.

[23] USRDS. *1999 ADR.* Bethesda, MD: NIH, NIDDK, April 1999, Appendix, Table B-3.

[24] USRDS. *1999 ADR.* Bethesda, MD: NIH, NIDDK, April 1999, Appendix, Table ES-1.

[25] USRDS. *1999 ADR.* Bethesda, MD: NIH, NIDDK, April 1999, Appendix, Table A-6.

[26] Rettig, R., and Levinsky, N.G. *Kidney Failure and the Federal Government.* Washington, DC: National Academy Press, 1991.

[27] Port, F.K.; Wolfe, B.A.; Mauger, E.A.; et al. Comparison of survival probabilities for dialysis patients vs. cadaveric renal transplant recipients. *Journal of the American Medical Association* 270(11):1339-1343, 1993.

[28] USRDS. *1999 ADR*. Bethesda, MD: NIH, NIDDK, April 1999, Appendix, Table F-1.

[29] USRDS. *1999 ADR*. Bethesda, MD: NIH, NIDDK, April 1999, Chapter VII, 104-106.

[30] USRDS. *1999 ADR*. Bethesda, MD: NIH, NIDDK, April 1999, Appendix, Table F-2.

[31] Freedman, B.I.; Tuttle, A.B.; and Spray, B.J. Familial predisposition to nephropathy in African Americans with non-insulin-dependent diabetes mellitus. *Kidney Diseases* 25(5):710-713, 1995.

[32] Siegel, J.; Krolewski, A.; Warran, J.; et al. Cost-effectiveness of screening and early treatment of nephropathy in patients with insulin-dependent diabetes mellitus. *Journal of the American Society of Nephrology* 3:S111-S119, 1992.

[33] Kiberd, B., and Jindal, K. Screening to prevent renal failure in insulin dependent diabetic patients: An economic evaluation. *British Medical Journal* 311:1595-1599, 1995.

[34] Borch-Johnsen, K.; Wenzel, H.; Viberti, G.; et al. Is screening and intervention for microalbuminuria worthwhile in patients with insulin dependent diabetes? *British Medical Journal* 306:1722-1725, 1993.

[35] Ifudu, O.; Dawood, M.; Homel, P.; et al. Excess morbidity in patients starting uremia therapy without prior care by a nephrologist. *American Journal of Kidney Diseases* 28:841-845, 1996.

[36] USRDS. *1997 ADR*. Bethesda, MD: NIH, NIDDK, April 1997, 49-60.

[37] USRDS. *1998 ADR*. Bethesda, MD: NIH, NIDDK, April 1998, Table G-19.

[38] USRDS. *1998 ADR*. Bethesda, MD: NIH, NIDDK, April 1998, Appendix, Table G-43.

[39] Turenne, M.N.; Port, F.K.; Strawderman, R.L.; et al. Growth rates in pediatric dialysis patients and renal transplant recipients. *American Journal of Kidney Diseases* 30(2):193-203, 1997.

[40] United Network for Organ Sharing (UNOS). *1997 Report of the Organ Procurement and Transplantation Network: Waiting List Activity and Donor Procurement.* Executive Summary, Kidney Volume. Richmond, VA: UNOS, 1997.

[41] Alexander, G.C., and Sehgal, A.R. Barriers to cadaveric renal transplantation among blacks, women, and the poor. *Journal of the American Medical Association* 280(13):1148-1152, 1998.

[42] Bloembergen, W.E.; Mauger, E.A.; and Wolfe, R.A. Association of gender and access to cadaveric renal transplantation. *American Journal of Kidney Diseases* 30(6):733-738, 1997.

[43] Narva, A.; Stiles, S.; Karp, S.; et al. Access of Native Americans to renal transplantation in Arizona and New Mexico. *Blood Purification* 14:293-304, 1996.

[44] Ozminkowski, R.J.; White, A.J.; Hassol, A.; et al. Minimizing racial disparity regarding receipt of a cadaver kidney transplant. *American Journal of Kidney Diseases* 30:749-759, 1997.

[45] USRDS. *1997 ADR*. Bethesda, MD: NIH, NIDDK, April 1997, 107-112.

[46] Levey, A.S.; Beto, J.A.; Coronado, B.E.; et al. Controlling the epidemic of cardiovascular disease in chronic renal disease. What do we know? What do we need to learn? Where do we go from here? *Report of the National Kidney Foundation Task Force on Cardiovascular Disease.* New York, NY: National Kidney Foundation, July 1998.

[47] Bostom, A.G.; Shemin, D.; Verhoef, P.; et al. Elevated fasting total plasma homocysteine levels and cardiovascular disease outcomes in maintenance dialysis patients: A prospective study. *Arteriosclerosis, Thrombosis, and Vascular Biology* 17(11):2554-2558, 1997.

[48] Bostom, A.G., and Lathrop, L. Hyperhomocysteinemia in end-stage renal disease: Prevalence, etiology, and potential relationship to arteriosclerotic outcomes. *Kidney International* 52(1):10-20, 1997.

[49] Bostom, A.G.; Shemin, D.; Lapane, K.L.; et al. Hyperhomocysteinemia, hyperfibrinogenemia, and lipoprotein (a) excess in maintenance dialysis patients: A matched case-control study. *Arteriosclerosis* 125(1):91-101, 1996.

[50] Perneger, T.V.; Klag, M.J.; and Whelton, P.K. Cause of death in patients with end-stage renal disease: Death certificates vs. registry reports. *American Journal of Public Health* 83(12):1735-1738, 1993.

[51] USRDS. *1997 ADR.* Bethesda, MD: NIH, NIDDK, April 1997, Figure IV-3, 52.

[52] National Kidney Foundation. *Dialysis Outcomes, Quality Initiatives, Clinical Practice Guidelines.* Executive Summaries. New York, NY: the Foundation, 1997.

[53] USRDS. *1999 ADR.* Bethesda, MD: NIH, NIDDK, April 1999, 159.

[54] Hirth, R.A.; Turenne, M.N.; Woods, J.D.; et al. Vascular access in newly treated U.S. hemodialysis patients: Predictors and trends. *Journal of the American Medical Association* 276:1303-1308, 1996.

[55] Soucie, J.M.; Neylan, J.F.; and McClellan, W. Race and sex differences in the identification of candidates for renal transplantation. *American Journal of Kidney Diseases* 19:414-419, 1992.

[56] Kasiske, B.L.; London, W.; and Ellison, M.D. Race and socioeconomic factors influencing early placement on the kidney transplant waiting list. *Journal of the American Society of Nephrology* 9:2142-2147, 1998.

[57] Ellison, M.D.; Breen, T.J.; Guo, T.G.; et al. Blacks and whites on the UNOS renal waiting list: Waiting times and patient demographics compared. *Transplantation Proceedings* 25(4):2462-2466, 1993.

[58] Thompson, J.S. American Society of Histocompatibility and Immunogenetics Cross-Match Study. *Transplantation* 59(11):1636-1638, 1995.

[59] Sanfilippo, F.P.; Vaughn, W.K.; Peters, T.G.; et al. Factors affecting the waiting time of cadaveric kidney transplant candidates in the United States. *Journal of the American Medical Association* 267:247-252, 1992.

[60] McCauley, J.; Irish, W.; Thompson, L.; et al. Factors determining the rate of referral, transplantation, and survival on dialysis in women with ESRD. *American Journal of Kidney Diseases* 30:739-748, 1997.

5

Diabetes

Co-Lead Agencies: Centers for Disease Control and Prevention
                    National Institutes of Health

Contents

Goal

Through prevention programs, reduce the disease and economic burden of diabetes, and improve the quality of life for all persons who have or are at risk for diabetes.

Overview

Diabetes poses a significant public health challenge for the United States. Some 800,000 new cases are diagnosed each year, or 2,200 per day.[1,2] The changing demographic patterns in the United States are expected to increase the number of people who are at risk for diabetes and who eventually develop the disease. Diabetes is a chronic disease that usually manifests itself as one of two major types: type 1, mainly occurring in children and adolescents 18 years and younger, in which the body does not produce insulin and thus insulin administration is required to sustain life; or type 2, occurring usually in adults over 30 years of age, in which the body's tissues become unable to use its own limited amount of insulin effectively. While all persons with diabetes require self-management training, treatment for type 2 diabetes usually consists of a combination of physical activity, proper nutrition, oral tablets, and insulin. Previously, type 1 diabetes has been referred to as juvenile or insulin-dependent diabetes and type 2 diabetes as adult-onset or noninsulin dependent diabetes.

Issues

The occurrence of diabetes, especially type 2 diabetes, as well as associated diabetes complications, is increasing in the United States.[1,2,3] The number of persons with diabetes has increased steadily over the past decade; presently, 10.5 million persons have been diagnosed with diabetes, while 5.5 million persons are estimated to have the disease but are undiagnosed. This increase in the number of cases of diabetes has occurred particularly within certain racial and ethnic groups.[4] Over the past decade, diabetes has remained the seventh leading cause of death in the United States, primarily from diabetes-associated cardiovascular disease. While premenopausal nondiabetic women usually are at less risk of cardiovascular disease than men, the presence of diabetes in women is associated with a three- to four-fold increase in coronary heart disease compared to nondiabetic females.[5] In the United States, diabetes is the leading cause of nontraumatic amputations (approximately 57,000 per year or 150 per day); blindness among working-aged adults (approximately 20,000 per year or 60 per day); and end-stage renal disease (ESRD) (approximately 28,000 per year or 70 per day).[6] (See Focus Area 4. Chronic Kidney Disease and Focus Area 28. Vision and Hearing.)

These and other health problems associated with diabetes contribute to an impaired quality of life and substantial disability among people with diabetes.[7] Diabetes is a costly disease; estimates of the total attributable costs of diabetes are around $100 billion ($43 billion direct; $45 billion indirect).[8,9] Hospitalizations for diabetes-associated cardiovascular disease account for the largest component of the direct costs. However, diabetes management is occurring increasingly in the outpatient setting, and more people with diabetes are using nursing home facilities.[8, 9]

Diabetes is a major clinical and public health challenge within certain racial and ethnic groups where both new cases of diabetes and the risk of associated complications are great.[4, 10]

These realities are especially disturbing given the validated efficacy and economic benefits of secondary prevention (controlling glucose, lipid, and blood pressure levels) and tertiary prevention (screening for early diabetes complications [eye, foot, and kidney abnormalities], followed by appropriate treatment and prevention strategies).[11, 12, 13, 14, 15, 16, 17] For many reasons, however, these scientifically and economically justified prevention programs are not used routinely in daily clinical management of persons with diabetes.[18, 19, 20] Diabetes is thus a "wasteful" disease. Strategies that would lessen the burden of this disease are not used regularly, resulting in unnecessary illness, disability, death, and expense.

Trends

The toll of diabetes on the health status of people in the United States is expected to worsen before it improves, especially in vulnerable, high-risk populations—African Americans, Hispanics, American Indians or Alaska Natives, Asians or other Pacific Islanders, elderly persons, and economically disadvantaged persons. Several factors account for this chronic disease epidemic, including behavioral elements (improper nutrition, for example, increased fat consumption; decreased physical activity; obesity); demographic changes (aging, increased growth of at-risk populations); improved ascertainment and surveillance systems that more completely capture the actual burden of diabetes; and the relative weakness of interventions to change individual, community, or organizational behaviors.[1, 3, 7, 21] Several other interrelated factors influence the present and future burden of diabetes, including genetics, cultural and community traditions, and socioeconomic status (SES). In addition, unanticipated scientific breakthroughs, the characteristics of the health care system, and the level of patient knowledge and empowerment all have a great impact on the disease burden associated with diabetes.

Personal behaviors. "Westernization," which includes a diet high in fat and processed foods as well as total calories, has been associated with a greater number of overweight persons in the United States when compared to a decade ago, especially within certain racial and ethnic groups, for example, African American females.[22, 23] Obesity, improper nutrition (including increased ingestion of fats and processed foods), and lack of physical activity are occurring in persons under age 15 years. These behaviors and conditions may explain the increasing diagnosis of type 2 diabetes in teenagers.[24, 25] Increased television watching associated with diminished physical activity also may contribute to the emergence of type 2 diabetes in youth.[24, 25, 26, 27]

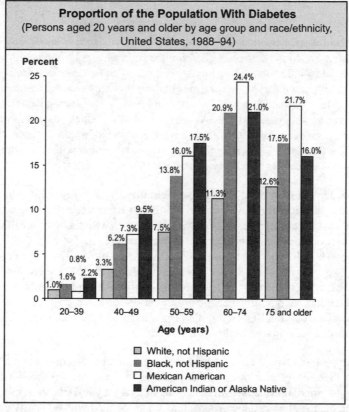

Proportion of the Population With Diabetes
(Persons aged 20 years and older by age group and race/ethnicity,
United States, 1988–94)

Percent

Age (years)

☐ White, not Hispanic
■ Black, not Hispanic
☐ Mexican American
■ American Indian or Alaska Native

Sources: Harris, M.; Flegal, K., Cowie, C.; et al. Prevalence of diabetes,
impaired fasting glucose, and impaired glucose tolerance in U.S. adults:
The Third National Health and Nutrition Examination Survey, 1998–1994.
Diabetes Care 21(4):518–524, 1998. Indian Health Service, national
outpatient database.

Demographics. Diabetes is most common in persons over age 60 years.[28] Increased insulin resistance and gradual deterioration in the function of insulin-
producing cells may account for this phenomenon. As the population in the
United States ages, especially as the number of persons aged 60 years and older
grows, an increase in the number of people with diabetes is expected. While studies indicate that aging itself may not be a major factor in the substantial increase
in the number of persons with diabetes,[21] present and future prevention strategies
for diabetes will be associated with a greater lifespan for persons with diabetes.[29]

Other changes in the U.S. population can be expected to affect the number of persons with diabetes. By 2050, almost half of the population will be other than
white (53 percent white, 24 percent Hispanic, 14 percent African American, and 8
percent Asian).[30] Because these racial and ethnic groups are at greater risk for
diabetes and associated complications, and because of rising levels of obesity and

physical inactivity in the general population, the number of persons with diabetes is expected to continue to increase into the first few decades of the 21st century.[31]

Ascertainment. Known as the "hidden" disease, diabetes is undiagnosed in an estimated 5 million persons.[32, 33] In addition, complications and health services associated with diabetes frequently are not recorded on death certificates,[34, 35] hospital discharge forms,[36] emergency department paperwork, and other documents. Much of this "missing" burden of diabetes is being captured due to improved surveillance and data systems,[37] including boxes on data forms to indicate the presence of diabetes and screening programs for undiagnosed diabetes in high-risk persons.[32] Thus, the real—but previously undocumented—burden of diabetes is becoming better recognized.

Limitations in programs to change behaviors. Scientific evidence indicates that secondary and tertiary prevention programs are effective in reducing the burden of diabetes. Yet changing the behaviors of persons with diabetes, health care providers, or other individuals or organizations involved in diabetes health care (for example, health maintenance organizations and employers) is difficult. Although many factors account for these challenges,[38] more effective interventions will need to be developed and implemented to improve the practice of diabetes care. Several other factors influence the present and future burden of diabetes, including genetics, culture, SES, scientific discoveries, and the characteristics of both chronic diseases and the health care system.

Both type 1 and type 2 diabetes have a significant genetic component.[39, 40] For type 1 diabetes, genetic markers that indicate a greater risk for this condition have been identified; they are sensitive but not specific. Type 2 diabetes, especially in vulnerable racial and ethnic groups, may be associated with a "thrifty gene."[40, 41] Family and twin studies demonstrate considerable influence of genetics for type 2 diabetes, but a specific genetic marker for the common variety of type 2 diabetes has not been identified. The degree to which such genetic indicators can be both validated and clinically available will determine the effectiveness of primary prevention trials.[42, 43]

Personal behaviors are influenced by beliefs and attitudes, and these are greatly affected by community and cultural traditions.[44, 45] In many racial and ethnic communities, fatalism, use of alternative medicine, desirability of rural living conditions, lack of economic resources, and other factors will influence significantly both availability of health care and the capabilities of persons with diabetes in handling their own care. Thirteen percent of the total U.S. population speak a language at home other than English. Cultural and linguistic factors affect interactions with health care providers and the system. The degree to which diabetes prevention strategies recognize and incorporate these traditions will largely determine program effectiveness.[46, 47]

The public health and medical communities increasingly are recognizing the influence of SES in the occurrence of new cases and progression of chronic diseases.[48, 49, 50] Chronic diseases, such as diabetes, reflect the social fabric of our society: the degree to which employment, financial security, feelings of safety, education, and the availability of health care are addressed and improved within the United States will influence the likelihood of developing type 2 diabetes as well as effectively managing both types of diabetes.[51] For example, unemployment without access to health insurance will substantially limit attention to and expenditures for preventive health practices.

Because acute infectious diseases were the dominant health threats during the first half of the 20th century, a dichotomous view of health developed: for example, people were either alive or dead, vaccinated or not vaccinated. Death and length of life were the most important markers of disease burden and program effectiveness during those years. Chronic diseases, such as diabetes, pose different challenges because qualitative terms such as "doing better" are valid indicators of health improvement, as are measures of quality of life and disability. Further, a variety of nonphysician health professionals (for example, nurses or pharmacists) and nonhealth care professionals (for example, faith or community leaders, employers) can be involved in critical decisions affecting chronic diseases. Diabetes, like other chronic conditions, is long term and is affected by the environment where people live, work, and play. For diseases like diabetes, the accurate measurement of quality of life as an indicator of program effectiveness and the incorporation of nonhealth professionals at work or worship on the health team will influence the successes of preventive treatment programs.[37, 45, 46]

The rapidity and utility of scientific discoveries also will influence the control of the diabetes burden. In all aspects of scientific investigation, important observations about diabetes will continue to occur. These scientific results will greatly influence diabetes prevention and management,[52, 53, 54] but any scientific study that is not translated and used in daily practice ultimately is "wasted."[10, 55]

The availability of a responsive and effective health care system will determine access to quality care, especially in secondary and tertiary prevention.[56, 57] With the emergence of managed care, a person with diabetes theoretically could receive effective, economical, and planned preventive care that would minimize the diabetes burden.[58] Several additional changes need to occur within the managed care setting, however, to maximize fully this theoretical opportunity for persons with diabetes, including managed care (1) not denying access to potentially expensive patients, (2) allowing adequate time for health professionals to interact with patients, and (3) ensuring patient protection rights.

In addition, the apparent movement toward primary care will affect diabetes management and outcomes. At present, about 90 percent of all persons with diabetes receive continuous care from the primary care community. This is highly unlikely to change. Thus, the degree that improved relationships can be established between diabetes specialists and primary care health providers will determine the quality of diabetes care.[59]

People with diabetes spend a small percentage of their time in contact with health professionals. In addition to family, friends, and work colleagues, individual patient knowledge, beliefs, and attitudes affect diabetes management and outcomes. The ability to understand and influence individual, community, and organizational behaviors will influence significantly the success of preventive programs in diabetes.[60, 61, 62]

Disparities

Gaps exist among racial and ethnic groups in the rate of diabetes and its associated complications in the United States. Certain racial and ethnic communities, including African Americans, Hispanics, American Indians, and certain Pacific Islander and Asian American populations as well as economically disadvantaged or older people, suffer disproportionately compared to white populations. For example, the relative number of persons with diabetes in African American, Hispanic, and American Indian communities is one to five times greater than in white communities.[4] Deaths from diabetes are 2 times higher in the African American population than they are in the white population, and diabetes-associated renal failure is 2.5 times higher in the African American population than it is in the Hispanic population.[1, 6, 7]

Particularly within certain racial and ethnic groups, there are four potential individual reasons for the greater burden of diabetes:

Greater number of cases of diabetes. If diabetes is more common, then more amputations, death, and other complications from diabetes would be expected.

Greater seriousness of diabetes. If hyperglycemia or other serious comorbid conditions, such as high blood pressure or elevated blood lipids, are present in certain racial and ethnic groups, a greater diabetes-related disease burden will occur. Many other factors could be involved, including genetics and excess weight. Greater seriousness of diabetes can be determined by comparing, for example, death or amputation rates for specific racial and ethnic diabetic groups with those rates in the general diabetic population.

Inadequate access to proper diabetes prevention and control programs. If proven diabetes services, such as self-management training programs or eye-retina examinations, are not a part of routine diabetes care, then effective programs to reduce the burden of diabetes will not be accessed and used. These essential diabetes services often are provided by specialists. Unfortunately, many diabetes at-risk groups reside in medically underserved areas or are without adequate insurance and thus do not receive these types of preventive services.

Improper quality of care. If diabetes management services are available, but the quality of that service is inadequate, prevention programs would not be effective in reducing the burden of diabetes.

Identifying the reasons for disparities in diabetes health outcomes is important in tailoring programs to those specific areas where deficiencies exist. Collection of racial and ethnic health services data for all health activities is critical to designate the reason for the greater disease burden.

Opportunities to meet the challenges of diabetes lie in four transition points in the natural history of this disease and the preventive interventions that target them: primary prevention, screening and early diagnosis, access, and quality of care (secondary and tertiary prevention).[63]

The transition points and associated public health interventions are as follows:

- Transition Point 1: From No Diabetes to Diabetes Present (although not recognized). Intervention, *Primary Prevention.*

- Transition Point 2: From Diabetes Not Recognized to Diabetes Recognized (but preventive diabetes care not provided). Intervention, *Screening/Early Diagnosis.*

- Transition Point 3: From No Care to Diabetes Care Applied. Intervention, *Access.*

- Transition Point 4: From Improper Care to Proper Care. Intervention, *Quality of Care.* (Secondary and Tertiary Prevention—for example, glucose control and decreasing diabetes complications.)

Each transition point represents a diabetes prevention and control opportunity that is contained in the diabetes objectives of Healthy People 2010. Objectives are categorized as: (1) diabetes education, (2) burden of disease (new cases, existing cases, undiagnosed diabetes, death, pregnancy complications), (3) macrovascular, microvascular, and metabolic complications, (4) laboratory services (lipids, glycosylated hemoglobin, microalbumin measurements), (5) health provider services (eye, foot, and dental examinations), and (6) patient protection behaviors (aspirin, self-blood-glucose-monitoring). These objectives measure both the processes and outcomes of preventive diabetes programs.

To improve the quality of diabetes care, the Diabetes Quality Improvement Project (DQIP)—a joint public/private effort—has identified a set of measures to track critical performance measures of diabetes management. Through the Quality Interagency Coordination (QuIC) task force, Federal agencies with health care responsibilities are collaborating to use DQIP to better focus efforts to improve diabetes care.

Interim Progress Toward Year 2000 Objectives

In Healthy People 2000, five diabetes-related objectives were included in a group of objectives addressing chronic conditions linked by their potential impact on quality of life and disability. Of these five objectives, eye examinations is moving toward the 2000 target. Death from diabetes, nonretinal diabetes complications, new cases of diabetes, and the number of existing cases all are moving away from the 2000 targets. Diabetes education is increasing in frequency among persons with diabetes.

These changes in direction need to be considered carefully with regard to significance, causes, and implications. The greater number of new cases of ESRD among persons with diabetes may in part be due to "ascertainment"; that is, persons with diabetes were not in the past but now are allowed access to ESRD treatment programs. Similarly, while new cases of type 2 diabetes truly may be increasing in association with obesity and inactivity, a higher number of cases of diabetes also may reflect increased efforts to screen for previously undiagnosed diabetes as well as decreased deaths from such conditions as diabetic acidosis or amputations. Thus, an increased number of existing cases of type 2 diabetes may in part reflect successes in other types of diabetes prevention programs.

Note: Unless otherwise noted, data are from the Centers for Disease Control and Prevention, National Center for Health Statistics, *Healthy People 2000 Review, 1998–99.*

Diabetes

Goal: Through prevention programs, reduce the disease and economic burden of diabetes, and improve the quality of life for all persons who have or are at risk for diabetes.

Number	Objective Short Title
5-1	Diabetes education
5-2	New cases of diabetes
5-3	Overall cases of diagnosed diabetes
5-4	Diagnosis of diabetes
5-5	Diabetes deaths
5-6	Diabetes-related deaths
5-7	Cardiovascular disease deaths in persons with diabetes
5-8	Gestational diabetes
5-9	Foot ulcers
5-10	Lower extremity amputations
5-11	Annual urinary microalbumin measurement
5-12	Annual glycosylated hemoglobin measurement
5-13	Annual dilated eye examinations
5-14	Annual foot examinations
5-15	Annual dental examinations
5-16	Aspirin therapy
5-17	Self-blood-glucose-monitoring

5-1. **Increase the proportion of persons with diabetes who receive formal diabetes education.**

Target: 60 percent.

Baseline: 45 percent of persons with diabetes received formal diabetes education in 1998 (age adjusted to the year 2000 standard population).

Target setting method: Better than the best.

Data source: National Health Interview Survey (NHIS), CDC, NCHS.

NOTE: THE TABLE BELOW MAY CONTINUE TO THE FOLLOWING PAGE.

Persons With Diabetes, 1998	Diabetes Education
	Percent
TOTAL	45
Race and ethnicity	
American Indian or Alaska Native	DSU
Asian or Pacific Islander	DSU
Asian	DSU
Native Hawaiian and other Pacific Islander	DSU
Black or African American	45
White	46
Hispanic or Latino	34
Not Hispanic or Latino	47
Black or African American	46
White	48
Gender	
Female	49
Male	42
Education level (aged 25 years and older)	
Less than high school	26
High school graduate	43
At least some college	56
Geographic location	
Urban	49
Rural	37

Persons With Diabetes, 1998	Diabetes Education
	Percent
Disability status	
Persons with activity limitation	DNA
Persons without activity limitations	DNA
Select populations	
Age groups (not age adjusted)	
Under 18 years	DNC
18 to 44 years	48
45 to 64 years	47
65 to 74 years	40
75 years and older	27

DNA = Data have not been analyzed. DNC = Data are not collected. DSU = Data are statistically unreliable.
Note: Age adjusted to the year 2000 standard population.

NOTE: THE TABLE ABOVE MAY HAVE CONTINUED FROM THE PREVIOUS PAGE.

Diabetes patient education is viewed uniformly as effective and economical in the ultimate prevention of long-term complications from diabetes. An individual with diabetes spends less than 1 percent of his or her time in contact with the health care system and on a daily basis must make a variety of critical decisions about diabetes. An informed and motivated patient is essential in managing the disease and reducing the risk of complications (for example, foot ulcers, hypoglycemia, and hypertension).[64, 65]

5-2.   Prevent diabetes.

Target: 2.5 new cases per 1,000 population per year.

Baseline: 3.5 new cases of diabetes per 1,000 population (3-year average) occurred in 1994–96 (age adjusted to the year 2000 standard population).

Target setting method: Better than the best (retain year 2000 target).

Data source: National Health Interview Survey (NHIS), CDC, NCHS.

NOTE: THE TABLE BELOW MAY CONTINUE TO THE FOLLOWING PAGE.

Total Population, 1994–96	New Cases of Diabetes
	Rate per 1,000
TOTAL	3.5
Race and ethnicity	
American Indian or Alaska Native	DSU
Asian or Pacific Islander	DSU

Total Population, 1994–96	New Cases of Diabetes
	Rate per 1,000
Asian	DSU
Native Hawaiian and other Pacific Islander	DSU
Black or African American	5.7
White	3.2
Hispanic or Latino	5.7
Not Hispanic or Latino	3.3
Black or African American	5.9
White	3.0
Gender	
Female	3.9
Male	3.1
Education level (aged 25 years and older)	
Less than high school	6.9
High school graduate	4.5
At least some college	4.3
Geographic location	
Urban	3.5
Rural	3.7
Disability status	
Persons with activity limitations	6.4
Persons without activity limitations	2.5
Select populations	
Age groups (not age adjusted)	
Under 18 years	DSU
18 to 44 years	2.0
45 to 64 years	6.9
65 to 74 years	9.3
75 years and older	9.4

DNA = Data have not been analyzed. DNC = Data are not collected. DSU = Data are statistically unreliable.
Note: Age adjusted to the year 2000 standard population.
NOTE: THE TABLE ABOVE MAY HAVE CONTINUED FROM THE PREVIOUS PAGE.

5-3.   Reduce the overall rate of diabetes that is clinically diagnosed.

Target: 25 overall cases per 1,000 population.

Baseline: 40 overall cases (including new and existing cases) of diabetes per 1,000 population occurred in 1997 (age adjusted to the year 2000 standard population).

Target setting method: Better than the best (retain year 2000 target).

Data source: National Health Interview Survey (NHIS), CDC, NCHS.

NOTE: THE TABLE BELOW MAY CONTINUE TO THE FOLLOWING PAGE.

Total Population, 1997	Overall Cases of Diagnosed Diabetes
	Rate per 1,000
TOTAL	40
Race and ethnicity	
American Indian or Alaska Native	DSU
Asian or Pacific Islander	DSU
Asian	DSU
Native Hawaiian and other Pacific Islander	DSU
Black or African American	74
White	36
Hispanic or Latino	61
Not Hispanic or Latino	38
Black or African American	74
White	34
Gender	
Female	40
Male	39
Education level (aged 25 years and older)	
Less than high school	95
High school graduate	58
At least some college	44
Geographic location	
Urban	40
Rural	38
Disability status	
Persons with disabilities	87
Persons without disabilities	28

Total Population, 1997	Overall Cases of Diagnosed Diabetes
	Rate per 1,000
Select populations	
Age groups (not age adjusted)	
Under 18 years	DSU
18 to 44 years	15
45 to 64 years	76
65 to 74 years	143
75 years and older	117

DNA = Data have not been analyzed. DNC = Data are not collected. DSU = Data are statistically unreliable.
Note: Age adjusted to the year 2000 standard population.

NOTE: THE TABLE ABOVE MAY HAVE CONTINUED FROM THE PREVIOUS PAGE.

5-4. Increase the proportion of adults with diabetes whose condition has been diagnosed.

Target: 80 percent.

Baseline: 68 percent of adults aged 20 years and older with diabetes had been diagnosed in 1988–94 (age adjusted to the year 2000 standard population).

Target setting method: Better than the best.

Data source: National Health and Nutrition Examination Survey (NHANES), CDC, NCHS.

NOTE: THE TABLE BELOW MAY CONTINUE TO THE FOLLOWING PAGE.

Adults Aged 20 Years and Older With Diabetes, 1988–94 (unless noted)	Persons Whose Diabetes Has Been Diagnosed
	Percent
TOTAL	68
Race and ethnicity	
American Indian or Alaska Native	DSU
Asian or Pacific Islander	DSU
Asian	DNC
Native Hawaiian and other Pacific Islander	DNC
Black or African American	68
White	68
Hispanic or Latino	DSU
Mexican American	55
Not Hispanic or Latino	71

Healthy People 2010: Objectives for Improving Health

Adults Aged 20 Years and Older With Diabetes, 1988–94 (unless noted)	Persons Whose Diabetes Has Been Diagnosed
	Percent
Black or African American	67
White	73
Gender	
Female	68
Male	66
Education level (aged 25 years and older)	
Less than high school	64
High school graduate	66
At least some college	56
Geographic location	
Urban	64
Rural	71
Disability status	
Persons with disabilities	66 (1991–94)
Persons without disabilities	69 (1991–94)
Select populations	
Age groups (not age adjusted)	
20 to 44 years	67
45 to 64 years	62
65 to 74 years	70
75 years and older	70

DNA = Data have not been analyzed. DNC = Data are not collected. DSU = Data are statistically unreliable.
Note: Age adjusted to the year 2000 standard population.
NOTE: THE TABLE ABOVE MAY HAVE CONTINUED FROM THE PREVIOUS PAGE.

Diabetes is increasingly common in the United States and the world. Many factors could be contributing to this "chronic disease epidemic," including an increase in new cases, a decrease in deaths, and improvements in detection.[1, 2, 3, 21, 63] Given the seriousness and costs associated with diabetes and the complexities of the disease, factors that account for the increasing frequency of diabetes should be identified.[66, 67, 68, 69]

5-5. Reduce the diabetes death rate.

Target: 45 deaths per 100,000 population.

Baseline: 75 deaths per 100,000 population were related to diabetes in 1997 (age adjusted to the year 2000 standard population).

Target setting method: 43 percent improvement.

Data source: National Vital Statistics System (NVSS), CDC, NCHS.

Total Population, 1997	Diabetes Deaths
	Rate per 100,000
TOTAL	75
Race and ethnicity	
American Indian or Alaska Native	107
Asian or Pacific Islander	62
Asian	DNC
Native Hawaiian and other Pacific Islander	DNC
Black or African American	130
White	70
Hispanic or Latino	86
Mexican American	115
Puerto Rican	87
Cuban	39
Not Hispanic or Latino	74
Black or African American	133
White	68
Gender	
Female	67
Male	87
Education level (aged 25 years and older)	
Less than high school	48
High school graduate	38
At least some college	17
Select populations	
Age groups	
Under 45 years	3
45 to 64 years	64
65 to 74 years	281
75 years and older	673

DNA = Data have not been analyzed. DNC = Data are not collected. DSU = Data are statistically unreliable.
Note: Age adjusted to the year 2000 standard population.

5-6. Reduce diabetes-related deaths among persons with diabetes.

Target: 7.8 deaths per 1,000 persons with diabetes.

Baseline: 8.8 deaths per 1,000 persons with diabetes listed anywhere on the death certificate occurred in 1997 (age adjusted to the year 2000 standard population).

Target setting method: 11 percent improvement.

Data sources: National Vital Statistics System (NVSS), CDC, NCHS; National Health Interview Survey (NHIS), CDC, NCHS.

NOTE: THE TABLE BELOW MAY CONTINUE TO THE FOLLOWING PAGE.

Persons With Diabetes, 1997	Diabetes-Related Deaths
	Rate per 1,000
TOTAL	8.8
Race and ethnicity	
American Indian or Alaska Native	3.3
Asian or Pacific Islander	5.4
Asian	6.3
Native Hawaiian and other Pacific Islander	2.5
Black or African American	8.1
White	8.9
Hispanic or Latino	7.4
Not Hispanic or Latino	8.9
Black or African American	8.1
White	9.0
Gender	
Female	8.6
Male	9.5
Education level (aged 25 to 64 years)	
Less than high school	4.7
High school graduate	7.3
At least some college	3.4
Select populations	
Age groups (not age adjusted)	
Under 45 years	2.0
45 to 64 years	7.7

Persons With Diabetes, 1997	Diabetes-Related Deaths
	Rate per 1,000
65 to 74 years	20.1
75 years and older	73.4

DNA = Data have not been analyzed. DNC = Data are not collected. DSU = Data are statistically unreliable.
Note: Age adjusted to the year 2000 standard population.

NOTE: THE TABLE ABOVE MAY HAVE CONTINUED FROM THE PREVIOUS PAGE.

5-7. Reduce deaths from cardiovascular disease in persons with diabetes.

Target: 309 deaths per 100,000 persons with diabetes.

Baseline: 343 deaths from cardiovascular disease per 100,000 persons with diabetes occurred in 1997 (age adjusted to the year 2000 standard population).

Target setting method: 10 percent improvement.

Data sources: National Vital Statistics System (NVSS), CDC, NCHS; National Health Interview Survey (NHIS), CDC, NCHS.

NOTE: THE TABLE BELOW MAY CONTINUE TO THE FOLLOWING PAGE.

Persons With Diabetes, 1997	Cardiovascular Disease Deaths
	Rate per 100,000
TOTAL	343
Race and ethnicity	
American Indian or Alaska Native	93
Asian or Pacific Islander	223
Asian	263
Native Hawaiian and other Pacific Islander	113
Black or African American	283
White	359
Hispanic or Latino	270
Not Hispanic or Latino	351
Black or African American	284
White	367
Gender	
Female	339
Male	363

Persons With Diabetes, 1997	Cardiovascular Disease Deaths
	Rate per 100,000
Education level (aged 25 to 64 years)	
Less than high school	145
High school graduate	247
At least some college	125
Select populations	
Age groups (not age adjusted)	
Under age 45 years	38
45 to 64 years	306
65 to 74 years	850
75 years and older	3,222

DNA = Data have not been analyzed. DNC = Data are not collected. DSU = Data are statistically unreliable.
Note: Age adjusted to the year 2000 standard population.
NOTE: THE TABLE ABOVE MAY HAVE CONTINUED FROM THE PREVIOUS PAGE.

Persons with diabetes experience death rates two to four times greater than non-diabetic persons, especially from cardiovascular disease. Other causes of death include renal failure, diabetic acidosis, and infection. Studies have clearly indicated that secondary prevention[70, 71, 72, 73] and tertiary prevention[74, 75, 76, 77] can reduce overall cardiac-related illness, disability, and death. Death rates and their significance, however, are complicated by how accurately and completely diabetes is recorded on death certificates.[34, 35] Thus, attention to both prevention behaviors to delay or prevent death, as well as death rates themselves, should be examined carefully.[70, 71, 72, 73, 74, 75, 76, 77, 78, 79, 80, 81]

5-8. (Developmental) Decrease the proportion of pregnant women with gestational diabetes.

Potential data source: National Vital Statistics System (NVSS), CDC, NCHS.

Studies of diabetes and pregnancy are consistent in their conclusions that proper prepregnancy and pregnancy glycemia control and careful perinatal obstetrical monitoring are associated with reduction in perinatal death and congenital abnormalities. More recently, the importance of good fetal and neonatal nutrition in general, as well as in persons with diabetes, has been emphasized.[82, 83, 84, 85, 86, 87]

5-9. (Developmental) Reduce the frequency of foot ulcers in persons with diabetes.

Potential data source: National Health and Nutrition Examination Survey (NHANES), CDC, NCHS.

5-10. Reduce the rate of lower extremity amputations in persons with diabetes.

Target: 1.8 lower extremity amputations per 1,000 persons with diabetes per year.

Baseline: 4.1 lower extremity amputations per 1,000 persons with diabetes occurred in 1997 (age adjusted to the year 2000 standard population).

Target setting method: 55 percent improvement.

Data sources: National Hospital Discharge Survey (NHDS), CDC, NCHS; National Health Interview Survey (NHIS), CDC, NCHS.

NOTE: THE TABLE BELOW MAY CONTINUE TO THE FOLLOWING PAGE.

Persons With Diabetes, 1997	Lower Extremity Amputations
	Rate per 1,000
TOTAL	4.1
Race and ethnicity	
American Indian or Alaska Native	DSU
Asian or Pacific Islander	DSU
Asian	DNC
Native Hawaiian and other Pacific Islander	DNC
Black or African American	4.8
White	2.6
Hispanic or Latino	DSU
Not Hispanic or Latino	DSU
Black or African American	DSU
White	DSU
Gender	
Female	6.0
Male	2.4
Education level (aged 25 years and older)	
Less than high school	DNC
High school graduate	DNC
At least some college	DNC

Healthy People 2010: Objectives for Improving Health

Persons With Diabetes, 1997	Lower Extremity Amputations
	Rate per 1,000
Select populations	
Age groups (not age adjusted)	
Under 65 years	6.4
65 to 74 years	8.6
75 years and older	14.2

DNA = Data have not been analyzed. DNC = Data are not collected. DSU = Data are statistically unreliable.
Note: Age adjusted to the year 2000 standard population.

NOTE: THE TABLE ABOVE MAY HAVE CONTINUED FROM THE PREVIOUS PAGE.

5-11. (Developmental) Increase the proportion of persons with diabetes who obtain an annual urinary microalbumin measurement.

Potential data source: Behavioral Risk Factor Surveillance System (BRFSS), CDC, NCCDPHP.

Scientific evidence documents that with secondary and tertiary prevention, microvascular complications of diabetes can be reduced substantially. Improved quality of life, decreased death rates, and reduced costs all can result from improved clinical and public health diabetes prevention strategies directed at microvascular and metabolic complications from diabetes. Monitoring the consequences of these strategies through reductions in mid- and end-stage microvascular complications needs to be an important component in determining the effectiveness of national diabetes activities. In both type 1 and 2 diabetes, evidence now is established firmly that microvascular and metabolic complications of diabetes can be prevented through secondary (glucose[88, 89]) and tertiary (screening and early treatment of complications[90]) prevention strategies.[91, 92, 93, 94]

Improper nutrition, obesity, and inactivity appear to be significant risk factors for the development of type 2 diabetes. (See Focus Area 19. Nutrition and Overweight and Focus Area 22. Physical Activity and Fitness.) In addition, nutrition, weight, and physical activity components are particularly critical in both glucose management and blood pressure and lipid control in persons with diabetes. These components are closely related to abilities to control both micro- and macrovascular diabetic complications. Given the discouraging trends in obesity and physical inactivity, these elements should be particularly and carefully monitored in persons with diabetes.[95, 96, 97]

5-12. Increase the proportion of adults with diabetes who have a glycosylated hemoglobin measurement at least once a year.

Target: 50 percent.

Baseline: 24 percent of adults aged 18 years and older with diabetes had a glycosylated hemoglobin measurement at least once a year (mean of data from 39 States in 1998; age adjusted to the year 2000 standard population).

Target setting method: Better than the best.

Data source: Behavioral Risk Factor Surveillance System (BRFSS), CDC, NCCDPHP.

NOTE: THE TABLE BELOW MAY CONTINUE TO THE FOLLOWING PAGE.

Adults Aged 18 Years and Older With Diabetes, 1998	Annual Glycosylated Hemoglobin Assessment
	Percent
TOTAL	24
Race and ethnicity	
American Indian or Alaska Native	29
Asian or Pacific Islander	48
Asian	DNC
Native Hawaiian and other Pacific Islander	DNC
Black or African American	21
White	25
Hispanic or Latino	22
Not Hispanic or Latino	25
Black or African American	21
White	24
Gender	
Female	24
Male	25
Education level (aged 25 years and older)	
Less than high school	13
High school graduate	19
At least some college	31

Adults Aged 18 Years and Older With Diabetes, 1998	Annual Glycosylated Hemoglobin Assessment
	Percent
Select populations	
Age groups (not age adjusted)	
18 to 44 years	29
45 to 64 years	23
65 to 74 years	13
75 years and older	11

DNA = Data have not been analyzed. DNC = Data are not collected. DSU = Data are statistically unreliable.
Note: Age adjusted to the year 2000 standard population.

NOTE: THE TABLE ABOVE MAY HAVE CONTINUED FROM THE PREVIOUS PAGE.

During the past decade, scientific investigations have established that controlling certain macrovascular risk factors, such as elevated blood lipids and blood pressure, as well as microvascular factors, such as elevated blood glucose, will result in fewer diabetes-related complications. Further, identification of early indicators of organ damage, for example, microalbuminuria, and proper treatment with angiotensin-converting enzyme-inhibitors, will reduce progression to renal failure. Diabetes-associated complications can be detected with available laboratory and clinical measures, thus indicating the need for prevention programs. Monitoring these clinical and laboratory measures can serve to identify targets for intervention programs.[98, 99, 100, 101, 102]

5-13. Increase the proportion of adults with diabetes who have an annual dilated eye examination.

Target: 75 percent.

Baseline: 47 percent of adults aged 18 years and older with diabetes had an annual dilated eye examination in 1998 (age adjusted to the year 2000 standard population).

Target setting method: Better than the best.

Data source: National Health Interview Survey (NHIS), CDC, NCHS.

NOTE: THE TABLE BELOW MAY CONTINUE TO THE FOLLOWING PAGE.

Adults Aged 18 Years and Older With Diabetes, 1998	Annual Dilated Eye Examination
	Percent
TOTAL	47
Race and ethnicity	
American Indian or Alaska Native	DSU

Adults Aged 18 Years and Older With Diabetes, 1998	Annual Dilated Eye Examination
	Percent
Asian or Pacific Islander	DSU
Asian	DSU
Native Hawaiian and other Pacific Islander	DSU
Black or African American	43
White	49
Hispanic or Latino	38
Not Hispanic or Latino	49
Black or African American	43
White	51
Gender	
Female	46
Male	47
Education level (aged 25 years and older)	
Less than high school	36
High school graduate	45
At least some college	61
Select populations	
Age groups (not age adjusted)	
18 to 44 years	44
45 to 64 years	51
65 to 74 years	58
75 years and older	60

DNA = Data have not been analyzed. DNC = Data are not collected. DSU = Data are statistically unreliable.
Note: Age adjusted to the year 2000 standard population.
NOTE: THE TABLE ABOVE MAY HAVE CONTINUED FROM THE PREVIOUS PAGE.

5-14. Increase the proportion of adults with diabetes who have at least an annual foot examination.

Target: 75 percent.

Baseline: 55 percent of adults aged 18 years and older with diabetes had at least an annual foot examination (mean value of data from 39 States in 1998; age adjusted to the year 2000 standard population).

Target setting method: Better than the best.

Data source: Behavioral Risk Factor Surveillance System (BRFSS), CDC, NCCDPHP.

Adults Aged 18 Years and Older With Diabetes, 1998	Annual Foot Examination
	Percent
TOTAL	55
Race and ethnicity	
American Indian or Alaska Native	40
Asian or Pacific Islander	57
Asian	DNC
Native Hawaiian and other Pacific Islander	DNC
Black or African American	55
White	55
Hispanic or Latino	56
Not Hispanic or Latino	54
Black or African American	54
White	54
Gender	
Female	51
Male	59
Education level (aged 25 years and older)	
Less than high school	46
High school graduate	56
At least some college	59
Select populations	
Age groups (not age adjusted)	
18 to 44 years	53
45 to 64 years	59
65 to 74 years	56
75 years and older	51

DNA = Data have not been analyzed. DNC = Data are not collected. DSU = Data are statistically unreliable.
Note: Age adjusted to the year 2000 standard population.

NOTE: THE TABLE ABOVE MAY HAVE CONTINUED FROM THE PREVIOUS PAGE.

Health practitioner behaviors, such as blood pressure monitoring or eye and foot examinations, are associated with greater identification of early indicators of end-organ damage from diabetes. These screening behaviors are necessary to initiate secondary and tertiary prevention programs and should be monitored.[103, 104, 105]

5-15. Increase the proportion of persons with diabetes who have at least an annual dental examination.

Target: 75 percent.

Baseline: 58 percent of persons aged 2 years and older with diagnosed diabetes saw a dentist at least once within the preceding 12 months in 1997 (age adjusted to the year 2000 standard population).

Target setting method: Better than the best.

Data source: National Health Interview Survey (NHIS), CDC, NCHS.

NOTE: THE TABLE BELOW MAY CONTINUE TO THE FOLLOWING PAGE.

Persons Aged 2 Years and Older With Diabetes, 1997	Annual Dental Examination
	Percent
TOTAL	58
Race and ethnicity	
American Indian or Alaska Native	DSU
Asian or Pacific Islander	56
Asian	DSU
Native Hawaiian or Pacific Islander	DSU
Black or African American	63
White	58
Hispanic or Latino	32
Not Hispanic or Latino	61
Black or African American	63
White	61
Gender	
Female	59
Male	57
Education level (aged 25 years and older)	
Less than high school	40
High school graduate	52
At least some college	65
Disability status	
Persons with disabilities	42
Persons without disabilities	66

Persons Aged 2 Years and Older With Diabetes, 1997	Annual Dental Examination
	Percent
Select populations	
Age groups (not age adjusted)	
18 to 44 years	60
45 to 64 years	50
65 to 74 years	44
75 years and older	41

DNA = Data have not been analyzed. DNC = Data are not collected. DSU = Data are statistically unreliable.
Note: Age adjusted to the year 2000 standard population.

NOTE: THE TABLE ABOVE MAY HAVE CONTINUED FROM THE PREVIOUS PAGE.

Persons with diabetes are at increased risk for destructive periodontitis and subsequent tooth loss.[106, 107] In addition, untreated periodontitis in persons with diabetes may complicate glycemic control.[108] Regular dental visits provide opportunities for prevention, early detection, and treatment of periodontal problems in persons with diabetes.

5-16. Increase the proportion of adults with diabetes who take aspirin at least 15 times per month.

Target: 30 percent.

Baseline: 20 percent of adults aged 40 years and older with diabetes took aspirin at least 15 times per month in 1988–94 (age adjusted to the year 2000 standard population).

Target setting method: Better than the best.

Data source: National Health and Nutrition Examination Survey (NHANES), CDC, NCHS.

NOTE: THE TABLE BELOW MAY CONTINUE TO THE FOLLOWING PAGE.

Adults Aged 40 Years and Older With Diabetes, 1988–94	Took Aspirin at Least 15 Times per Month
	Percent
TOTAL	20
Race and ethnicity	
American Indian or Alaska Native	DSU
Asian or Pacific Islander	DSU
Asian	DNC
Native Hawaiian and other Pacific Islander	DNC

| Adults Aged 40 Years and Older With Diabetes, 1988–94 | Took Aspirin at Least 15 Times per Month |
	Percent
Black or African American	9
White	23
Hispanic or Latino	DSU
Mexican American	8
Not Hispanic or Latino	DNA
Black or African American	8
White	25
Gender	
Female	15
Male	27
Education level	
Less than high school	16
High school graduate	24
At least some college	22

DNA = Data have not been analyzed. DNC = Data are not collected. DSU = Data are statistically unreliable.
Note: Age adjusted to the year 2000 standard population.

NOTE: THE TABLE ABOVE MAY HAVE CONTINUED FROM THE PREVIOUS PAGE.

5-17. Increase the proportion of adults with diabetes who perform self-blood-glucose-monitoring at least once daily.

Target: 60 percent.

Baseline: 42 percent of adults aged 18 years and older with diabetes performed self-blood-glucose-monitoring at least once daily (mean of data from 39 States in 1998; age adjusted to the year 2000 standard population).

Target setting method: Better than the best.

Data source: Behavioral Risk Factor Surveillance System (BRFSS), CDC, NCCDPHP.

NOTE: THE TABLE BELOW MAY CONTINUE TO THE FOLLOWING PAGE.

| Adults Aged 18 Years and Older With Diabetes, 1998 | Daily Self-Blood-Glucose-Monitoring |
	Percent
TOTAL	42
Race and ethnicity	
American Indian or Alaska Native	53
Asian or Pacific Islander	30

Adults Aged 18 Years and Older With Diabetes, 1998	Daily Self-Blood-Glucose-Monitoring
	Percent
Asian	DNC
Native Hawaiian and other Pacific Islander	DNC
Black or African American	40
White	43
Hispanic or Latino	36
Not Hispanic or Latino	43
Black or African American	37
White	45
Gender	
Female	43
Male	41
Education level (aged 25 years and older)	
Less than high school	38
High school graduate	41
At least some college	44
Select populations	
Age groups (not age adjusted)	
18 to 44 years	43
45 to 64 years	41
65 to 74 years	44
75 years and older	38

DNA = Data have not been analyzed. DNC = Data are not collected. DSU = Data are statistically unreliable.
Note: Age adjusted to the year 2000 standard population.
NOTE: THE TABLE ABOVE MAY HAVE CONTINUED FROM THE PREVIOUS PAGE.

Certain activities, ultimately chosen by individuals themselves, are essential in the proper preventive management of diabetes. Smoking cessation, use of aspirin, and self-blood-glucose-monitoring are representative of individual behaviors that should be periodically monitored because each behavior is associated with a decreased likelihood of microvascular and macrovascular complications.[109, 110, 111, 112, 113] Aspirin therapy in persons with diabetes mellitus—especially in the presence of other cardiovascular risk factors, such as high blood pressure, elevated blood lipids, etc.—has been demonstrated to reduce the likelihood of a future heart attack or stroke.[113]

Related Objectives From Other Focus Areas

1. **Access to Quality Health Services**
   1-1. Persons with health insurance
   1-2. Health insurance coverage for clinical preventive services
   1-3. Counseling about health behaviors

4. **Chronic Kidney Disease**
   4-1. End-stage renal disease
   4-2. Cardiovascular disease deaths in persons with chronic kidney failure
   4-7. Kidney failure due to diabetes
   4-8. Medical therapy for persons with diabetes and proteinuria

9. **Family Planning**
   9-3. Contraceptive use
   9-11. Pregnancy prevention education

12. **Heart Disease and Stroke**
   12-1. Coronary heart disease (CHD) deaths
   12-2. Knowledge of symptoms of heart attack and importance of calling 911
   12-7. Stroke deaths
   12-8. Knowledge of early warning symptoms of stroke
   12-9. High blood pressure
   12-10. High blood pressure control
   12-11. Action to help control blood pressure
   12-12. Blood pressure monitoring
   12-13. Mean total cholesterol levels
   12-14. High blood cholesterol levels
   12-15. Blood cholesterol screening
   12-16. LDL-cholesterol level in CHD patients

14. **Immunization and Infectious Diseases**
   14-5. Invasive pneumococcal infections
   14-29. Influenza and pneumococcal vaccination of high-risk adults

16. **Maternal, Infant, and Child Health**
   16-6. Prenatal care
   16-10. Low birth weight and very low birth weight
   16-19. Breastfeeding

19. **Nutrition and Overweight**
   19-1. Healthy weight in adults
   19-2. Obesity in adults
   19-3. Overweight or obesity in children and adolescents
   19-16. Worksite promotion of nutrition education and weight management
   19-17. Nutrition counseling for medical conditions

22. **Physical Activity and Fitness**
   22-1. No leisure- time physical activity
   22-2. Moderate physical activity
   22-3. Vigorous physical activity
   22-6. Moderate physical activity in adolescents
   22-7. Vigorous physical activity in adolescents

28. Vision and Hearing

    28-1. Dilated eye examinations

    28-5. Impairment due to diabetic retinopathy

    28-10. Vision rehabilitation services and devices

Terminology

(A listing of abbreviations and acronyms used in this publication appears in Appendix H.)

Ascertainment: The processes and systems used to collect information and data about a particular health condition, for example, written surveys, telephone calls, electronic records, etc.

Comorbidity: The presence of serious health conditions in addition to the one being examined, for example, high blood pressure in people with diabetes mellitus.

Diabetes mellitus (diabetes): A chronic disease due to either or both insulin deficiency and resistance to insulin action, and associated with hyperglycemia (elevated blood glucose levels). Over time, without proper preventive treatment, organ complications related to diabetes develop, including heart, nerve, foot, eye, and kidney damage; problems with pregnancy also occur. Diabetes is classified into four major categories:

    Type 1 diabetes: (Previously called insulin-dependent diabetes mellitus [IDDM] or juvenile-onset diabetes [JODM]) represents clinically about 5 percent of all persons with diagnosed diabetes. Its clinical onset is typically at ages under 30 years. Most often this type of diabetes represents an autoimmune destructive disease in beta (insulin-producing) cells of the pancreas in genetically susceptible individuals. Insulin therapy always is required to sustain life and maintain diabetes control.

    Type 2 diabetes: (Previously called non-insulin-dependent diabetes mellitus [NIDDM] or adult-onset diabetes [AODM]) is the most common form of diabetes in the United States and the world, especially in certain racial and ethnic groups and in elderly persons. In the United States, approximately 95 percent of all persons with diagnosed diabetes (10.5 million) and almost 100 percent of all persons with undiagnosed (5.5 million) diabetes probably have type 2 diabetes.

    Gestational diabetes mellitus (GDM): Refers to the development of hyperglycemia during pregnancy in an individual not previously known to have diabetes. Approximately 3 percent of all pregnancies are associated with GDM. GDM identifies health risks to the fetus and newborn and future diabetes in the mother and offspring.

    Other types: Include genetic abnormalities, pancreatic diseases, and medication use.

Complications: Microvascular—small vessel abnormalities in the eyes and kidneys; macrovascular—large vessel abnormalities in the heart, brain, and legs; and metabolic—abnormalities in nerves and during pregnancy.

Diabetic acidosis: A severe condition of diabetes. Due to a lack of insulin, the body breaks down fat tissue and converts the fat to very strong acids. The condition most often is associated with a very high blood sugar and happens most often in poorly controlled or newly diagnosed type 1 diabetes.

Direct costs: Costs associated with an illness that can be attributed to a medical service, procedure, medication, etc. Examples include payment for an x ray; pharmaceutical drugs, for example, insulin; surgery; or a clinic visit.

Formal diabetes education: Self-management training that includes a process of initial individual patient assessment; instruction provided or supervised by a qualified health professional; evaluation of accumulation by the diabetic patient of appropriate knowledge, skills, and attitudes; and ongoing reassessment and training.

Indirect costs: Those costs associated with an illness that occur because an individual cannot work at his or her usual job due to premature death, sickness, or disability (for example, amputation).

Prevention: Primary—stopping or delaying onset of diabetes; secondary—early identification and stopping or delaying onset of complications; tertiary—stopping disability from disease and its complications.

Thrifty gene: An idea which suggests that a "thrifty gene" is present in people likely to develop type 2 diabetes. It is speculated that thousands of years ago, people with this "thrifty gene" could store food very efficiently and thus survive long periods of starvation. Now when starvation is unusual, this thrifty gene tends to make people overweight and thus prone to diabetes.

Urinary microalbumin measurement: A laboratory procedure to detect very small quantities of protein in the urine, indicating early kidney damage.

References

[1] Clark, C. How should we respond to the worldwide diabetes epidemic? *Diabetes Care* 21:475-476, 1998.

[2] Burke, J.; Williams, K.; Gaskill, S.; et al. Rapid rise in the incidence of type 2 diabetes from 1987 to 1996: Results from the San Antonio Heart Study. *Archives of Internal Medicine* 159:1450-1457, 1999.

[3] King, H.; Aubert, R.; and Herman, H. Global burden of diabetes, 1995–2025: Prevalence, numerical estimates and projections. *Diabetes Care* 21:1414-1431, 1997.

[4] Flegal, K.; Ezzati, T.; Harris, M.; et al. Prevalence of diabetes in Mexican Americans, Cubans and Puerto Ricans from the Hispanic Health and Nutrition Examination Survey, 1982–1984. *Diabetes Care* 14:628-638, 1991.

[5] American Diabetes Association (ADA). *Diabetes 1996: Vital Statistics*. Alexandria, VA: ADA, 1996.

[6] Centers for Disease Control and Prevention (CDC). *National Diabetes Fact Sheet: National Estimates and General Information on Diabetes in the United States*. Atlanta, GA: U.S. Department of Health and Human Services (HHS), CDC, 1999.

[7] CDC. *Diabetes Surveillance, 1997*. Atlanta, GA: HHS, 1997.

[8] ADA. Economic consequences of diabetes mellitus in the U.S. in 1997. *Diabetes Care* 21:296-306, 1998.

[9] Hodgson, T., and Cohen, A. Medical care expenditures for diabetes, its chronic complications and its comorbidities. *Preventive Medicine* 29:173-186, 1999.

[10] Vinicor, F. Is diabetes a public health disorder? *Diabetes Care* 17(S1):22-27, 1994.

[11] Diabetes Control and Complications Trial Research Group. The effects of intensive treatment of diabetes on the development and progression of long-term complications in insulin-dependent diabetes mellitus. *New England Journal of Medicine* 329:977-986, 1993.

[12] Gotto, A. Cholesterol management in theory and practice. *Circulation* 96:4424-4430, 1997.

[13] American College of Physicians, ADA, and Academy of Ophthalmology. Screening guidelines for diabetic retinopathy. *Annals of Internal Medicine* 116:683-685, 1992.

[14] Levin, M. Diabetes and peripheral neuropathy. *Diabetes Care* 21:1, 1998.

[15] Steffes, M. Diabetic nephropathy: Incidence, prevalence, and treatment. *Diabetes Care* 20:1059-1060, 1997.

[16] Diabetes Control and Complications Trial Research Group. Lifetime benefits and costs of intensive therapy as practiced in the Diabetes Control and Complications Trial. *Journal of the American Medical Association* 276:1409-1415, 1996.

[17] Eastman, R.; Javitt, J.; Herman, W.; et al. Prevention strategies for non-insulin dependent diabetes mellitus: An economic perspective. In: LeRoith, D.; Taylor, S.; and Olefsky, J.; eds. *Diabetes Mellitus*. Philadelphia, PA: Lippincott-Raven Publishers, 1996, 621-630.

[18] Vinicor, F. Challenges to the translation of the Diabetes Control and Complications Trial. *Diabetes Review* 2:371-383, 1994.

[19] Brechner, R.; Cowie, C.; Howie, L.; et al. Ophthalmic examination among adults with diagnosed diabetes mellitus. *Journal of the American Medical Association* 270:1714-1718, 1993.

[20] Kraft, S.; Marrero, D.; Lazaridis, E.; et al. Primary care physicians' practice patterns and diabetic retinopathy. *Archives of Family Medicine* 6:29-37, 1997.

[21] CDC. Trends in the prevalence and incidence of self-reported diabetes mellitus—United States, 1980–1994. *Morbidity and Mortality Weekly Report* 46:1014-1018, 1997.

[22] Kuckzmarski, R. Increasing prevalence of overweight among U.S. adults: National Health and Nutrition Examination Survey 1960–1994. *Journal of the American Medical Association* 272:205-211, 1994.

[23] Christoffel, K., and Ariza, A. The epidemiology of overweight in children: Relevance for clinical care. *Pediatrics* 101:103-105, 1998.

[24] Fagot-Campagna, A.; Rios Burrows, N.; and Williamson, D. The public health epidemiology of type 2 diabetes in children and adolescents: A case study of American Indian adolescents in the Southwestern United States. *Clinica Chimica Acta* 286:81-95, 1999.

[25] Rosenbloom, A.; Joe, J.; Young, R.; et al. Emerging epidemic of type 2 diabetes in youth. *Diabetes Care* 22:345-354, 1999.

[26] HHS. *Physical Activity and Health: A Report of the Surgeon General*. Atlanta, GA: HHS, CDC, National Center for Chronic Disease Prevention and Health Promotion, 1996.

[27] Dietz, W. Critical periods in childhood for the development of obesity. *American Journal of Clinical Nutrition* 59:955-959, 1994.

[28] Vita, A.; Terry, R.; Hubert, H.; et al. Aging, health risk and cumulative disability. *New England Journal of Medicine* 338:1035-1041, 1998.

[29] Herman, W.; Thompson, T.; Visscher, W.; et al. Diabetes mellitus and its complications in an African American community: Project DIRECT. *Journal of the National Medical Association* 90:147-156, 1998.

[30] Pollard, K.M., and O'Hare, W.P. America's racial and ethnic minorities. *Population Bulletin* 54:1-48, 1999.

[31] Pearce, D.; Griffin, T.; Kelly, J.; et al. An overview of the population in Europe and North America. *Population Trends* 89:24-36, 1997.

[32] Expert Committee on the Diagnosis and Classification of Diabetes Mellitus. Report of the Expert Committee on the Diagnosis and Classification of Diabetes Mellitus. *Diabetes Care* 20:1183-1197, 1997.

[33] Eastman, R., and Vinicor, F. Science: Moving us in the right direction. *Diabetes Care* 20(7):1057-1058, 1997.

[34] Bild, D., and Stevenson, J. Frequency of recording of diabetes on U.S. death certificates: Analysis of the 1986 National Mortality Follow Back Survey. *Journal of Clinical Epidemiology* 454:275-281, 1992.

[35] Vinicor, F., and Will, J. The grim reaper and diabetes mellitus (DM): Do we know how often (s)he strikes? *Diabetes* 48:A170, 1999.

[36] Levatan, C.; Passaro, M.; Jablonski, K.; et al. Unrecognized diabetes among hospitalized patients. *Diabetes Care* 21:246-249, 1998.

[37] Glasgow, R.; Wagner, E.; Kaplan, R.; et al. If diabetes is a public health problem, why not treat it as one? A population-based approach to chronic illness. *Annals of Behavioral Medicine* 21:159-170, 1999.

[38] Pozzilli, P. Prevention of insulin-dependent diabetes. *Diabetes Metabolism Review* 12:27-136, 1996.

[39] O'Rahilly, S. Diabetes in midlife: Planting genetic time bombs. *Nature Medicine* 3:1080-1081, 1997.

[40] Neel, J. At mid-point in the molecular revolution. *Bioessays* 18:943-944, 1996.

[41] Swinburn, B. The thrifty genotype hypothesis: How does it look after 30 years? *Diabetes Medicine* 13:695-699, 1996.

[42] DPT I Study Group. The Diabetes Prevention Trial: Type 1 diabetes (DPT1): Implementation of screening and staging of relatives. *Transplant Process* 27:3377, 1995.

[43] National Institutes of Health. Non-Insulin Dependent Diabetes Primary Prevention Trial. *NIH Guide to Grants and Contracts* 22:1-20, 1993.

[44] Sussman, L. Socio-cultural concerns of diabetes mellitus. In: Haire-Joshu, D., ed. *Management of Diabetes Mellitus: Perspectives of Care Across the Life Span*. 2nd ed. St. Louis, MO: Mosby, 1996, 473-512.

[45] Hahn, R. *Sickness and Healing: An Anthropologic Perspective*. New Haven, CT: Yale University Press, 1995.

[46] Resnicow, K.; Baranowski, T.; Ahluwalia, J.; et al. Cultural sensitivity in public health: Defined and demystified. *Ethnicity & Disease* 9(1):10-21, 1999.

[47] Yen, I., and Syme, S. The social environment and health: A discussion of the epidemiologic literature. *Annual Review of Public Health* 20:287-308, 1999.

[48] Robinson, N.; Lloyd, C.; and Stevens, L. Social deprivation and mortality in adults with diabetes mellitus. *Diabetes Medicine* 15:205-212, 1998.

[49] Williamson, D., and Fast, J. Poverty and medical treatment: When public policy compromises accessibility. *Canadian Journal of Public Health* 89:120-124, 1998.

[50] Amiel, S.A. The medical cost of social deprivation—Whose job is it anyways? (Editorial). *Diabetes Medicine* 15:187, 1998.

[51] Marmot, M. Improvement of social environment to improve health. *Lancet* 351:57-60, 1998.

[52] Erickson, P.; Wilson, R.; and Shannon, I. *Years of Healthy Life.* Hyattsville, MD: National Center for Health Statistics, 1995.

[53] Murray, C., and Lopez, A. Alternative projections of mortality and disability by cause, 1990–2020: Global Burden of Disease Study. *Lancet* 349:1498-1504, 1997.

[54] Weatherall, D. *Science and the Quiet Art: The Role of Medical Research in Health Care.* New York, NY: W.W. Norton, 1995.

[55] Detsky, A., and Naglie, I. A clinician's guide to cost-effectiveness analysis. *Annals of Internal Medicine* 113:147-154, 1990.

[56] Wagner, E.; Austin, B.; and von Korff, M. Organizing care for patients with chronic illness. *Milbank Quarterly* 4:511-544, 1996.

[57] Etzweiler, D. Chronic care: A need in search of a system. *Diabetes Educator* 23:569-573, 1997.

[58] McDonald, R. The evolving care of diabetes: Models, managed care and public health. *Annals of Internal Medicine* 20:685-686, 1997.

[59] Smith, D. Toward common ground. *Diabetes Care* 20:467-468, 1997.

[60] Glasgow, R.; Strycker, L.; Hampson, S.; et al. Personal-model beliefs and social-environmental barriers related to diabetes self-care management. *Diabetes Care* 20:556-561, 1997.

[61] Golden, M. Incorporation of quality-of-life considerations into intensive diabetes management protocols in adolescents. *Diabetes Care* 21:885-886, 1998.

[62] Weed, D. Towards a philosophy of public health. *Journal of Epidemiology and Community Health* 53:99-104, 1999.

[63] Vinicor, F. The public health burden of diabetes and the reality of limits. *Diabetes Care* 21(S3):C15-18, 1998.

[64] Glasgow, R., and Osteen, V. Evaluating diabetes education—Are we measuring the most important outcomes? *Diabetes Care* 15:1423-1432, 1992.

[65] Brown, S. Studies of educational interventions and outcomes in diabetic adults: A meta-analysis revisited. *Patient Education Counseling* 16:189-215, 1990.

[66] Harris, M. NIDDM: Epidemiology and scope of the problem. *Diabetes Spectrum* 9:26-29, 1996.

[67] Harris, M.; Eastman, R.; Cowie, C.; et al. Comparison of diabetes diagnostic categories in the U.S. population according to 1997 American Diabetes Association and 1980–1985 World Health Organization Diagnostic Criteria. *Diabetes Care* 20:1859-1862, 1997.

[68] Nathan, D.; Meigs, J.; and Singer, D. The epidemiology of cardiovascular disease in type 2 diabetes mellitus: How sweet it is...or is it? *Lancet* 350:4-9, 1997.

[69] Harris, M.; Flegal, K.; Cowie, C.; et al. Prevalence of diabetes, impaired fasting glucose, and impaired glucose tolerance in U.S. adults: The Third National Health and Nutrition Examination Survey, 1988–1994. *Diabetes Care* 21:518-524, 1998.

[70] Hansson, L.; Zanchetti, A.; George-Carruthers, S.; et al. Effects of intensive blood-pressure lowering and low-dose aspirin in patients with hypertension: Principal results of

the Hypertension Optimal Treatment (HOT) Randomized Trial. *Lancet* 351:1755-1762, 1998.

[71] The UK Prospective Diabetes Study (UKPDS) Group. Tight blood pressure control and risk of macrovascular and microvascular complications in type 2 diabetes: UKPDS 38. *British Medical Journal* 317: 703-713, 1998.

[72] Lyons, T., and Jenkins, A. Lipoprotein glycation and its metabolic consequences. *Current Opinion in Lipidology* 8:174-180, 1997.

[73] Kannel, W. The worth of controlling plasma lipids. *American Journal of Cardiology* 81:1047-1049, 1998.

[74] Malmberg, K. Diabetes Mellitus, Insulin-Glucose Infusion in Acute Myocardial Infarction (DIGAMI) Study Group. Prospective randomized study of intensive insulin treatment on long term survival after acute myocardial infarction in patients with diabetes mellitus. *British Medical Journal* 14:1512-1515, 1997.

[75] Vinicor, F. Features of macrovascular disease of diabetes. In: Haire-Joshu, D., ed. *Management of Diabetes Mellitus: Perspectives of Care Across the Life Span.* 2nd ed. St. Louis, MO: Mosby, 1996, 281-308.

[76] Depre, C.; Vanoverschelde, J.; and Taegtmeyer, H. Glucose for the heart. *Circulation* 99: 578-588, 1999.

[77] Shotliff, K.; Kaushal, R.; Dove, D.; et al. Withholding thrombolysis in patients with diabetes mellitus and acute myocardial infarction. *Diabetic Medicine* 15:1028-1030, 1998.

[78] Ochi, J.; Melton, L.; Palumbo, P.; et al. A population based study of diabetes mortality. *Diabetes Care* 8:224-229, 1985.

[79] Stern, M. Diabetes and cardiovascular disease: The "common soil" hypothesis. *Diabetes* 44:369-374, 1995.

[80] Haffner, S. Management of dyslipidemia in adults with diabetes. *Diabetes Care* 21:160-178, 1998.

[81] Califf, R., and Granger, C. Hypertension and diabetes and the Fosinopril vs. Amlodipine Cardiovascular Events Trial (FACET). *Diabetes Care* 21:655-657, 1998.

[82] Lesser, K., and Carpenter, M. Metabolic changes associated with normal pregnancy and pregnancy associated with diabetes mellitus. *Seminars in Perinatalogy* 18:399-406, 1994.

[83] Kitzmiller, J.; Buchanan, T.; Kjos, S.; et al. Preconception care of diabetes, congenital malformations, and spontaneous abortions. *Diabetes Care* 514-541, 1996.

[84] ADA. Preconception care of women with diabetes. *Diabetes Care* 20(S1):40-43, 1997.

[85] Jovanovic, L. American Diabetes Association's Fourth International Workshop-Conference on Gestational Diabetes Mellitus: Summary and discussion. *Diabetes Care* 21(S2):131-137, 1998.

[86] Gold, A.; Reilly, R.; Little, J.; et al. The effect of glycemic control in the pre-conception period and early pregnancy on birth weight in women with IDDM. *Diabetes Care* 21:535-538, 1998.

[87] ADA. Preconception care of women with diabetes. *Diabetes Care* 22(S1):56-59, 1999.

[88] Reichard, P.; Nilsson, B.; and Rosenqvist, U. The effect of long-term intensified insulin treatment on the development of microvascular complications of diabetes mellitus. *New England Journal of Medicine* 329:304-309, 1993.

[89] UKPDS Group. Intensive blood-glucose control with sulphonylureas or insulin compared with conventional treatment and risk of complications in patients with type 2 diabetes (UKPDS 33). *Lancet* 352:837-853, 1998.

[90] Reichard, P.; Pihl, M.; Rosenqvist, U.; et al. Complications in IDDM are caused by elevated blood glucose levels: The Stockholm Diabetes Intervention Study (SDIS) at 10-year follow-up. *Diabetologia* 39:1483-1488, 1996.

[91] Frank, R. Etiologic mechanisms in diabetic retinopathy. In: Ryan, S.J., ed. *Retina.* Vol. 2. St. Louis, MO: Mosby, 1989, 301-326.

[92] Defronzo, R.A. Nephropathy. In: Lebovitz, H.; DeFronzo, R.A.; et al. *Therapy for Diabetes Mellitus and Related Disorders.* 2nd ed. Alexandria, VA: ADA, 1994, 257-269.

[93] Clark, C., and Lee, D. Prevention and treatment of the complications of diabetes mellitus. *New England Journal of Medicine* 332:1210-1217, 1995.

[94] Nathan, D. The pathophysiology of diabetic complications: How much does the glucose hypothesis explain? *Annals of Internal Medicine* 124:86-89, 1996.

[95] Wylie-Rosett, J. Efficacy of diet and exercise in reducing body weight and conversion to overt diabetes. *Diabetes Care* 21:334-335, 1998.

[96] Wheeler, M. A brave new world for nutrition and diabetes. *Diabetes Care* 20:109-110, 1997.

[97] Clark, D. Physical activity efficacy and effectiveness among older adults and minorities. *Diabetes Care* 20:1176-1182, 1997.

[98] Haffner, S. The Scandinavian Simvastatin Survival Study (4S) Subgroup Analysis of Diabetic Subjects: Implications for the prevention of coronary heart disease. *Diabetes Care* 20:469-471, 1997.

[99] Braatvedt, G.; Drury, P.; and Cundy, T. Assessing glycemic control in diabetes: Relationships between fructosamine and HbA$_{1C}$. *New Zealand Journal of Medicine* 110:459-462, 1997.

[100] Dinneen, S., and Gertstein, H. The association of microalbuminuria and mortality in non-insulin dependent diabetes mellitus. *Archives of Internal Medicine* 14:1413-1418, 1997.

[101] Durrington, P. Prevention of macrovascular disease: Absolute proof or absolute risk? *Diabetic Medicine* 12:561-562, 1995.

[102] Eckel, R. Natural history of macrovascular disease and classic risk factors for athersclerosis: Session summary. *Diabetes Care* 22(S3):21-24, 1999.

[103] Peters, A.; Legerreta, A.; Ossorio, R.; et al. Quality of outpatient care provided to diabetic patients: A health maintenance organization experience. *Diabetes Care* 19:601-606, 1996.

[104] Weiner, J.; Parente, S.; Garnick, D.; et al. Variation in office-based quality: Claims-based profile of care provided to Medicare patients with diabetes. *Journal of the American Medical Association* 273:1503-1508, 1995.

[105] Clark, C. Where do we go from here? *Annals of Internal Medicine* 124:184-186, 1995.

[106] Loe, H. Periodontal disease: The sixth complication of diabetes mellitus. *Diabetes Care* 16(S1):329-334, 1993.

[107] Papapanou, P. Periodontal diseases: Epidemiology. *Annals of Periodontology* 1:1-36, 1996.

[108] Taylor, G. Periodontal treatment and its effects on glycemic control. *Oral Surgery, Oral Medicine, Oral Pathology, Oral Radiology, and Endodontics* 87:311-316, 1999.

[109] Miller, C.; Probait, C.; and Acterbaerg, C. Knowledge and misconceptions about food labels among women with NIDDM. *Diabetes Educator* 23:425-432, 1997.

[110] Rubin, R., and Peyrot, M. Psychosocial problems and interventions in diabetes. *Diabetes Care* 15:1640-1657, 1992.

[111] CDC. Diabetes-specific preventive-care practices among adults in a managed care population—Colorado Behavioral Risk Factor Surveillance System. *Morbidity and Mortality Weekly Report* 46:1018-1023, 1997.

[112] CDC. Preventive-care knowledge and practices among persons with diabetes mellitus—North Carolina Behavioral Risk Factor Surveillance System, 1994–1995. *Morbidity and Mortality Weekly Report* 46:1023-1026, 1997.

[113] ADA. Aspirin therapy in diabetes. *Diabetes Care* 22(S1):45-46, 1999.

6

Disability and Secondary Conditions

Co-Lead Agencies: Centers for Disease Control and Prevention
National Institute on Disability and Rehabilitation
Research, U.S. Department of Education

Contents

Promote the health of people with disabilities, prevent secondary conditions, and eliminate disparities between people with and without disabilities in the U.S. population.

Overview

Because disability status has been traditionally equated with health status, the health and well-being of people with disabilities has been addressed primarily in a medical care, rehabilitation, and long-term care financing context. Four main misconceptions emerge from this contextual approach: (1) all people with disabilities automatically have poor health, (2) public health should focus only on preventing disabling conditions, (3) a standard definition of "disability" or "people with disabilities" is not needed for public health purposes, and (4) the environment plays no role in the disabling process. These misconceptions have led to an underemphasis of health promotion and disease prevention activities targeting people with disabilities and an increase in the occurrence of secondary conditions (medical, social, emotional, family, or community problems that a person with a primary disabling condition likely experiences).

Issues

Challenging these misconceptions will help to clarify the health status of people with disabilities and address the environmental barriers that undermine their health, well-being, and participation in life activities. A broad array of health promotion activities are relevant to all people experiencing a disability, whether they are categorized by racial or ethnic group, gender, and primary conditions or diagnoses, such as major depression, cerebral palsy, diabetes, spinal cord injury, or fetal alcohol syndrome. The similarities among people with disabilities are as important as or more important than the differences among clinical diagnostic groups. Caregiver issues also have been considered, as well as environmental barriers. Environmental factors affect the health and well-being of people with disabilities in many ways. For example, weather can hamper wheelchair mobility, medical offices and equipment may not be accessible, and shelters or fitness centers may not be staffed or equipped for people with disabilities. Compliance with the Americans with Disabilities Act (ADA) would help overcome some of these barriers. A crosscutting goal is to eliminate disparities with the nondisabled population.

The *International Classification of Functioning and Disability* (ICIDH-2), developed by the World Health Organization (WHO) with the input of numerous nations—including the United States—provides uniform language and a framework for describing functioning, health, and disability status among all people.[1] This framework clarifies definitional issues and includes environmental factors.

Trends

An estimated 54 million persons in the United States, or nearly 20 percent of the population, currently live with disabilities.[2] Data for the period 1970 to 1994 suggest that the proportion is increasing.[3] The increase in disability among all age groups indicates a growing need for public health programs serving people with disabilities.

From 1990 to 1994, disability rates increased among youth under age 18 years.[3] There was a 33 percent increase in activity limitations among girls, from 4.2 percent to 5.6 percent, and a 40 percent increase in activity limitations among boys, from 5.6 percent to 7.9 percent.

Among adults aged 18 to 44 years, there was a 16 percent increase in activity limitations, from 8.8 percent in 1990 to 10.3 percent in 1994.[3] This increase suggests that 3.1 million more people aged 18 to 44 years were limited in 1994 than in 1990.

The absolute number of adults aged 65 years and older with disabilities increased from 26.9 million in 1982 to 34.1 million in 1996. Because the total number of adults aged 65 years and older increased even faster, the proportion of those with disabilities declined from 24.9 percent in 1982 to 21.3 percent in 1994.[3] However, the rise in numbers indicates a growing need for programs and services to serve this older population.

The direct medical and indirect annual costs associated with disability are more than $300 billion, or 4 percent of the gross domestic product.[4] This total cost includes $160 billion in medical care expenditures (1994 dollars) and lost productivity costs approaching $155 billion.

The health promotion and disease prevention needs of people with disabilities are not nullified because they are born with an impairing condition or have experienced a disease or injury that has long-term consequences.[5] People with disabilities have increased health concerns and susceptibility to secondary conditions. Having a long-term condition increases the need for health promotion that can be medical, physical, social, emotional, or societal.

People who have activity limitations report having had more days of pain, depression, anxiety, and sleeplessness and fewer days of vitality during the previous month than people not reporting activity limitations.[6] Increased emotional distress, however, does not arise directly from the person's limitations. The distress is likely to stem from encounters with environmental barriers that reduce the individual's ability to participate in life activities and that undermine physical and emotional health. In view of the increased rates of disability among youth, it is particularly important to target activities and services that address all aspects of health and well-being, including promoting health, preventing secondary conditions, and removing environmental barriers, as well as providing access to medical care. For an older person with a disability, it is important to target worsening coexisting conditions that may intensify and thus threaten general well-being. For example, declining vision combined with declining hearing can greatly impair mobility, nutrition, and fitness.[7]

Disparities

Disability can be viewed as a universal phenomenon everyone experiences at some time.[8] Disability also can be viewed as representing a minority of the population, in that people with disabilities may be less visible, undercounted, and underserved.[9] As a potentially underserved group, people with disabilities would be expected to experience disadvantages in health and well-being compared with the general population. People with disabilities may experience lack of access to health services and medical care and may be considered at increased risk for various conditions.

Mental Status and Participation in Social Activities
(By disability status, United States, 1997 and 1998)

- Children reported sad, unhappy, depressed*: 17% / 31%
- Adults reported feelings interfering with activities*: 7% / 28%
- Adult participation in social activities*: 100% / 95%
- Adults reported sufficient emotional support**: 79% / 70%
- Adults reported satisfaction with life**: 96% / 87%

Percent

■ People without disabilities   □ People with disabilities

Sources: *CDC, NCHS. National Health Interview Survey (NHIS), 1997.
**CDC, NCCDPHP. Behavioral Risk Factor Surveillance System (BRFSS), 1998.

Few data systems identify people with disabilities as a subpopulation. Disparities need to be identified to plan appropriate public health programs. Despite the paucity of data, some disparities between people with and without disabilities have been noted. These disparities include excess weight, reduced physical activity, increased stress, and less frequent mammograms for women over age 55 years with disabilities.[10]

Opportunities

Health promotion programs that focus on improving functioning across a spectrum of diagnoses and a range of age groups are effective in reducing secondary conditions and outpatient physician visits among people with disabilities.[11, 12, 13] For example, a focus on improving muscle tone, flexibility, and strength can accrue benefits for mobility-impaired people in wheelchairs and mobility-impaired people with arthritis.[14] For people with communication disabilities and disorders, interventions can improve access to health-enhancement programs. People with sight impairments can have access to readable job applications, food labels, and medications. People with hearing impairments can have access to televised or videotaped exercise programs that are captioned or signed by interpreters depicted within an inset of a video screen. Often, the most effective interventions may be environmental rather than medical.

Many health promotion interventions already in place for the population at large may be easily adapted to the needs of people with disabilities. New strategies can be influenced by results from studies that describe risk factors for secondary conditions or protective factors against additional impairments. For example, the number of cases of secondary osteoporosis among able-bodied women and their range of bone mineral density deficits can be estimated by using existing Federal data sets. The degree to which women exercise and ingest calcium or estrogen supplements also can be estimated, leading to measurements of the influence of both risk and protective factors associated with osteoporosis in the able-bodied population. Because women with mobility impairments experience an elevated risk for secondary osteoporosis at earlier ages, their risk factors, including diminished bone mineral density, and their potential protective factors, including optimal calcium or estrogen supplementation and types of exercise, become critically important epidemiologic parameters.[15, 16] The results of investigations of secondary osteoporosis already influence health promotion strategies among able-bodied women. Similar investigations can augment the development of health promotion strategies among women with disabilities.

Current guidelines provide opportunity to design health promotion interventions targeting people with disabilities that accommodate ongoing evidence-based evaluation[17] and demonstrate cost-effectiveness.[18, 19] For example, clinical interventions that focus on appropriate and timely medical care can be equally accessible for people with and without disabilities. Mammography screening is recommended every 1 to 2 years, with or without an annual clinical breast examination, for able-bodied women aged 50 to 69 years.[20] This recommendation also can be adapted for women with disabilities. Clinical providers, however, must first recognize the reasons women with disabilities often refrain from seeking mammography services, such as the lack of adaptive equipment on mammography screening machines or unfamiliarity with the needs of people with disabilities expressed by clinicians. Counseling to prevent injuries among all adults also is recommended. For example, men and women with disabilities, especially those with skeletal insufficiencies or calcium deficits, are at increased risk for fractures. Adding bone mineral screening and fitness counseling during clinical encounters may be beneficial in preventing injuries. In these ways, evidence-based health promotion and disease prevention programs can be developed, implemented, and evaluated to target the health and injury disparities between people with and without disabilities.

Health promotion interventions for people with disabilities—in the community, clinical settings, or elsewhere—should include culturally and linguistically appropriate elements.

Interim Progress Toward Year 2000 Objectives

Healthy People 2000 did not have a chapter specifically establishing health objectives for people with disabilities. However, some objectives targeted people with disabilities, including leisure-time physical activity, use of community support programs by people with severe mental disorders, treatment for depression, activity limitations associated with chronic conditions and back conditions, and receipt of recommended clinical preventive services. A progress review held in January 1997 showed that none of these specific objectives relevant to people with disabilities had been met,[10] and parity with the nondisabled population will continue to be monitored.

People with disabilities reporting no leisure-time physical activity declined from the 1985 baseline of 35 percent to 29 percent in 1995, short of the target of 20 percent for 2000. In addition, the review noted several disparities: 40 percent of people with disabilities aged 20 years and older reported being overweight compared with 35 percent of the general population and short of the goal of 25 percent; 49 percent of people aged 18 years and older with disabilities reported adverse health effects from stress compared with 34 percent of the general population; and clinical preventive services showed disparities for data on tetanus boosters (56 percent versus 59 percent for the general population), Pap tests (69 percent versus 77 percent of women aged 18 years and over in 1994), and breast exams and mammograms (50 percent versus 56 percent for women aged 50 years and over).

Note: Unless otherwise noted, data are from the Centers for Disease Control and Prevention, National Center for Health Statistics, *Healthy People 2000 Review, 1998–99*.

Disability and Secondary Conditions

Goal: Promote the health of people with disabilities, prevent secondary conditions, and eliminate disparities between people with and without disabilities in the U.S. population.

Number	Objective Short Title
6-1	Standard definition of people with disabilities in data sets
6-2	Feelings and depression among children with disabilities
6-3	Feelings and depression interfering with activities among adults with disabilities
6-4	Social participation among adults with disabilities
6-5	Sufficient emotional support among adults with disabilities
6-6	Satisfaction with life among adults with disabilities
6-7	Congregate care of children and adults with disabilities
6-8	Employment parity
6-9	Inclusion of children and youth with disabilities in regular education programs
6-10	Accessibility of health and wellness programs
6-11	Assistive devices and technology
6-12	Environmental barriers affecting participation in activities
6-13	Surveillance and health promotion programs

6-1. **Include in the core of all relevant Healthy People 2010 surveillance instruments a standardized set of questions that identify "people with disabilities."**

Target: 100 percent.

Baseline: No Healthy People 2010 surveillance instruments include a standard set of questions that identify people with disabilities in 1999.

Target setting method: Total coverage.

Data source: CDC, NCEH.

The call for statistics on people with disabilities is longstanding and increasing. Various Federal agencies have attempted to collect these data in several research areas.[21] Two separate issues exist regarding data collection: (1) using different operational definitions of disability and (2) not collecting information from people with disabilities during surveys. None of the federally funded surveys attempting to collect data on people with disabilities is using the same definition of disability. This lack of standardization has made it difficult to (1) identify and include individuals with a disability, (2) measure the nature and extent of disability in the United States, (3) assess the impact of various disabilities on the person's ability to participate in society, (4) assess the extent of secondary conditions among people with disabilities, and (5) identify environmental barriers to participation and risk factors for poor health in this population.

The issue of not including people with disabilities is reflected in the initial survey design. Most studies are not designed to include, target, and analyze data on people with disabilities. People with disabilities could be included as a select population if, for example, the data collection method ensured appropriate access and outreach.

To remedy these gaps, a set of survey questions has been developed and is being tested to identify individuals with varying degrees of disability in terms of activity limitations.[22] This short set of questions may be placed in the core of all Healthy People surveillance instruments that collect demographic data to include and standardize information on people with disabilities. On the basis of standardization and inclusion in the Nation's disability data collection activities, the call for disability statistics may be satisfied. Once collected, these data will help government policymakers, consumers and advocates, researchers, and clinicians make better informed choices to promote the health status and well-being of people with disabilities.

6-2. Reduce the proportion of children and adolescents with disabilities who are reported to be sad, unhappy, or depressed.

Target: 17 percent.

Baseline: 31 percent of children and adolescents aged 4 to 11 years with disabilities were reported to be sad, unhappy, or depressed in 1997.

Target setting method: 45 percent improvement (parity with children and adolescents without disabilities in 1997).

Data source: National Health Interview Survey (NHIS), CDC, NCHS.

NOTE: THE TABLE BELOW MAY CONTINUE TO THE FOLLOWING PAGE.

Children and Adolescents Aged 4 to 11 Years, 1997	Reported To Be Sad, Unhappy, or Depressed	
	With Disabilities	Without Disabilities*
	Percent	
TOTAL	31	17
Race and ethnicity		
American Indian or Alaska Native	DSU	DSU
Asian or Pacific Islander	DSU	13
Asian	DSU	16
Native Hawaiian and other Pacific Islander	DSU	DSU
Black or African American	DSU	16
White	31	17
Hispanic or Latino	32	16
Not Hispanic or Latino	30	17
Black or African American	DSU	17
White	31	18
Gender		
Female	32	16
Male	30	18
Family income level		
Poor	37	20
Near poor	31	17
Middle/high income	27	17

Children and Adolescents Aged 4 to 11 Years, 1997	Reported To Be Sad, Unhappy, or Depressed	
	With Disabilities	Without Disabilities*
	Percent	
Geographic location		
Urban	27	17
Rural	39	16

DNA = Data have not been analyzed. DNC = Data are not collected. DSU = Data are statistically unreliable.

*The total represents the target. Data for population groups by race, ethnicity, gender, socioeconomic status, and geographic location are displayed to further characterize the issue.

NOTE: THE TABLE ABOVE MAY HAVE CONTINUED FROM THE PREVIOUS PAGE.

6-3. Reduce the proportion of adults with disabilities who report feelings such as sadness, unhappiness, or depression that prevent them from being active.

Target: 7 percent.

Baseline: 28 percent of adults aged 18 years and older with disabilities reported feelings that prevented them from being active in 1997 (age adjusted to the year 2000 standard population).

Target setting method: 75 percent improvement (parity with adults aged 18 years and older without disabilities in 1997).

Data source: National Health Interview Survey (NHIS), CDC, NCHS.

NOTE: THE TABLE BELOW MAY CONTINUE TO THE FOLLOWING PAGE.

Adults Aged 18 Years and Older, 1997	Reported Feelings That Prevent Activity	
	With Disabilities	Without Disabilities*
	Percent	
TOTAL	28	7
Race and ethnicity		
American Indian or Alaska Native	22	15
Asian or Pacific Islander	30	7
Asian	DSU	6
Native Hawaiian and other Pacific Islander	DSU	14
Black or African American	31	8
White	28	7
Hispanic or Latino	40	9
Not Hispanic or Latino	27	7

Adults Aged 18 Years and Older, 1997	Reported Feelings That Prevent Activity	
	With Disabilities	Without Disabilities*
	Percent	
Black or African American	31	8
White	27	6
Gender		
Female	30	8
Male	26	6
Family income level		
Poor	38	13
Near poor	30	10
Middle/high income	21	6
Education level (aged 25 years and older)		
Less than high school	34	10
High school graduate	29	7
At least some college	25	5
Geographical location		
Urban	29	7
Rural	26	6

DNA = Data have not been analyzed. DNC = Data are not collected. DSU = Data are statistically unreliable.

Note: Age adjusted to the year 2000 standard population.

*The total represents the target. Data for population groups by race, ethnicity, gender, socioeconomic status, and geographic location are displayed to further characterize the issue.

NOTE: THE TABLE ABOVE MAY HAVE CONTINUED FROM THE PREVIOUS PAGE.

Children and adults with disabilities and their families face issues of coping, adapting, adjusting, and learning to live well with the disability—a dynamic, on-going process. Good mental health, including refusing to internalize the social stigma of disability and developing a positive attitude and strong self-esteem, is a key ingredient to overcoming these issues.[23] Improving mental health status among people with disabilities and their families will help address psychological barriers and enhance their ability to participate fully in society.[24]

6-4. Increase the proportion of adults with disabilities who participate in social activities.

Target: 100 percent.

Baseline: 95.4 percent of adults aged 18 years and older with disabilities participated in social activities in 1997 (age adjusted to the year 2000 standard population).

Target setting method: Total participation (parity with adults aged 18 years and older without disabilities in 1997).

Data source: National Health Interview Survey (NHIS), CDC, NCHS.

NOTE: THE TABLE BELOW MAY CONTINUE TO THE FOLLOWING PAGE.

Adults Aged 18 Years and Older, 1997	Participation in Social Activity	
	With Disabilities	Without Disabilities*
	Percent	
TOTAL	95.4	100.0
Race and ethnicity		
American Indian or Alaska Native	87.4	100.0
Asian or Pacific Islander	99.6	100.0
Asian	99.5	100.0
Native Hawaiian and other Pacific Islander	100.0	100.0
Black or African American	95.0	99.8
White	95.6	100.0
Hispanic or Latino	93.9	100.0
Not Hispanic or Latino	95.5	100.0
Black or African American	95.0	99.8
White	95.7	100.0
Gender		
Female	95.2	99.9
Male	95.7	100.0
Family income level		
Poor	93.1	99.9
Near poor	95.8	99.9
Middle/high income	96.5	100.0

Adults Aged 18 Years and Older, 1997	Participation in Social Activity	
	With Disabilities	Without Disabilities*
	Percent	
Education level (aged 25 years and older)		
Less than high school	94.1	99.9
High school graduate	94.8	99.9
At least some college	96.0	100.0
Geographic location		
Urban	95.3	100.0
Rural	95.6	99.9

DNA = Data have not been analyzed. DNC = Data are not collected. DSU = Data are statistically unreliable.
Note: Age adjusted to the year 2000 standard population.
*The total represents the target. Data for population groups by race, ethnicity, gender, socioeconomic status, and geographic location are displayed to further characterize the issue.
NOTE: THE TABLE ABOVE MAY HAVE CONTINUED FROM THE PREVIOUS PAGE.

People with disabilities report significantly lower levels of social participation compared with people without disabilities.[25] Participating in social activities routinely requires personal interaction with the environment, a component of life that is vital to the well-being of all humanity. ICIDH-2, the *International Classification of Functioning and Disability,* highlights the importance of participating in social activities as a measurable outcome of living well with a disability.[1] The ICIDH-2 framework indicates that the environment should be examined as a barrier to participation.

Social participation can include activities such as volunteering, shopping, going to the movies, or attending sporting events. Targeting increased participation in regular social activities such as traveling, socializing with friends and family, attending church or community events, and voting can result in improved functional status and well-being.

6-5. Increase the proportion of adults with disabilities reporting sufficient emotional support.

Target: 79 percent.

Baseline: 71 percent of adults aged 18 years and older with disabilities reported sufficient emotional support in 1998 (data from 11 States and the District of Columbia; age adjusted to the year 2000 standard population).

Target setting method: 11 percent improvement (parity with adults aged 18 years and older without disabilities in 1998).

Data source: Behavioral Risk Factor Surveillance System (BRFSS), CDC, NCCDPHP.

Adults Aged 18 Years and Older, 1998	Reported Sufficient Emotional Support*	
	With Disabilities	Without Disabilities†
	Percent	
TOTAL	71	79
Race and ethnicity		
American Indian or Alaska Native	56	72
Asian or Pacific Islander	49	66
Asian	DSU	DSU
Native Hawaiian and other Pacific Islander	DSU	DSU
Black or African American	53	68
White	74	82
Hispanic or Latino	44	68
Not Hispanic or Latino	72	80
Black or African American	DNA	DNA
White	DNA	DNA
Gender		
Female	70	79
Male	70	78
Education level (aged 25 years and older)		
Less than high school	58	70
High school graduate	74	76
At least some college	74	83

DNA = Data have not been analyzed. DNC = Data are not collected. DSU = Data are statistically unreliable.
Note: Age adjusted to the year 2000 standard population.
*Data are from 11 States and the District of Columbia.
†The total represents the target. Data for population groups by race, ethnicity, gender, socioeconomic status, and geographic location are displayed to further characterize the issue.

Emotional support often is derived from a person's social support systems. Two hypotheses suggest that social support helps a person cope with stress and that supportive relationships are a protective factor in various life situations.[26] With the information gained by monitoring the personal perspective, the United States may better meet the needs of people with disabilities.

6-6. Increase the proportion of adults with disabilities reporting satisfaction with life.

Target: 96 percent.

Baseline: 87 percent of adults aged 18 years and older with disabilities reported satisfaction with life in 1998 (data from 11 States and the District of Columbia; age adjusted to the year 2000 standard population).

Target setting method: 10 percent improvement (parity with adults without disabilities in 1998).

Data source: Behavioral Risk Factor Surveillance System (BRFSS), CDC, NCCDPHP.

NOTE: THE TABLE BELOW MAY CONTINUE TO THE FOLLOWING PAGE.

Adults Aged 18 Years and Older, 1998	Reported Satisfaction With Life*	
	With Disabilities	Without Disabilities†
	Percent	
TOTAL	87	96
Race and ethnicity		
American Indian or Alaska Native	78	92
Asian or Pacific Islander	78	98
Asian	DSU	DSU
Native Hawaiian and other Pacific Islander	DSU	DSU
Black or African American	83	92
White	88	96
Hispanic or Latino	80	93
Not Hispanic or Latino	87	96
Black or African American	DNA	DNA
White	DNA	DNA
Gender		
Female	87	95
Male	86	96

Healthy People 2010: Objectives for Improving Health

Adults Aged 18 Years and Older, 1998	Reported Satisfaction With Life*	
	With Disabilities	Without Disabilities†
	Percent	
Education level (aged 25 years and older)		
Less than high school	84	94
High school graduate	87	95
At least some college	89	97

DNA = Data have not been analyzed. DNC = Data are not collected. DSU = Data are statistically unreliable.
Note: Age adjusted to the year 2000 standard population.
*Data are from 11 States and the District of Columbia.
†The total represents the target. Data for population groups by race, ethnicity, gender, socioeconomic status, and geographic location are displayed to further characterize the issue.
NOTE: THE TABLE ABOVE MAY HAVE CONTINUED FROM THE PREVIOUS PAGE.

Satisfaction with life is associated with the more general term "quality of life," which is a personal evaluation of one's own position in numerous dimensions of life, including physical, emotional, social, spiritual, environmental support, and level of independence.[27] Monitoring the life satisfaction of people with disabilities, as well as that of the broader population, allows an opportunity to evaluate society's progress in accommodating the needs of people with disabilities.

6-7. Reduce the number of people with disabilities in congregate care facilities, consistent with permanency planning principles.

Target and baseline:

Objective	Reduction in People With Disabilities in Congregate Care Facilities	1997 Baseline	2010 Target
		Number of Persons	
6-7a.	Persons aged 22 years and older in 16 or more bed congregate facilities	93,362	46,681
6-7b.	Persons aged 21 years and under in congregate care facilities	24,300	0

Target setting method: 50 percent improvement for 6-7a; total elimination for 6-7b.

Data source: Survey of State Developmental Disabilities Directors, University of Minnesota.

Many people with activity limitations or cognitive impairments need ongoing and long-term assistance, yet some do not require institutional care.[28] From the 1970s through the 1990s, States began reducing the size of and closing State institutions that served people with mental retardation or developmental disabilities. This social, political, and economic movement resulted in a dramatic growth in the total number of individuals served in community residential settings—from 5,000 in 1960 to 255,117 in 1996.[29, 30] This movement, coupled with increases in life expectancy and an expanding elderly population, resulted in the development of several community-based and in-home assistance programs, such as home-delivered meals, hospice care, and homemaker and home-health services. The goal to increase home and community-based care will broaden health and lifestyle choices for people with disabilities and their families.[31]

Much of this expansion in community services is funded through the Medicaid Home and Community-Based Services (HCBS) Waiver Program, a Federal-State partnership authorized in 1981 under Title XIX of the Social Security Act. Between 1990 and 1997, the HCBS Program demonstrated a 25.8 percent increase in benefits per person.[30] Despite this dramatic growth to support home and community-based care, in 1993, only 11 percent of long-term Medicaid expenditures and 5.3 percent of total Medicaid expenditures went toward community-based care.[32] The other sources of support for community-based long-term care are Medicare, Title III of the Older Americans Act, and the Social Services Block Grant.[32]

6-8. Eliminate disparities in employment rates between working-aged adults with and without disabilities.

Target: 82 percent.

Baseline: 52 percent of adults aged 21 through 64 years with disabilities were employed in 1994–95.

Target setting method: 58 percent improvement (parity with adults without disabilities in 1994–95).

Data source: Survey of Income and Program Participation (SIPP), U.S. Department of Commerce, Bureau of the Census.

Adults Aged 21 through 64 Years, 1994–95	Employment of People With Disabilities	Employment of People Without Disabilities*
	Percent	
TOTAL	52	82
Race and ethnicity		
American Indian or Alaska Native	41	77
Asian or Pacific Islander	48	78
Asian	DNC	DNC
Native Hawaiian and other Pacific Islander	DNC	DNC

Adults Aged 21 through 64 Years, 1994–95	Employment of People With Disabilities	Employment of People Without Disabilities*
	Percent	
Black or African American	37	77
White	DNA	DNA
Hispanic or Latino	45	76
Not Hispanic or Latino	DNA	DNA
Black or African American	DNA	DNA
White	57	84
Gender		
Female	46	75
Male	60	90
Education level		
Less than high school	34	69
High school graduate	54	81
At least some college	63	83

DNA = Data have not been analyzed. DNC = Data are not collected. DSU = Data are statistically unreliable.
*The total represents the target. Data for population groups by race, ethnicity, gender, and socioeconomic status are displayed to further characterize the issue.

The ability to work has implications for economic and social self-sufficiency, for full inclusion and integration into society, and for personal self-esteem. Work and disability are understood best within the context of a person's abilities and the role of accommodation, accessibility, and legal mandates. The Presidential Task Force on Employment of Adults with Disabilities emphasized the need for a coordinated and aggressive national policy to address the many components of work and disability.[33] Changes in economic policies and benefits underscore the need to continue to examine and address the structural, social, and psychological deterrents to work for some persons with disabilities.

In 1994–95, employment rates varied depending on degree of disability. For persons aged 21 through 64 years with no disability, the rate was 82 percent, whereas those with a nonsevere disability had a rate of 77 percent, and those with a severe disability had a rate of 26 percent. Analyses of rates by gender indicate similar patterns.[2] Moreover, employment patterns for persons with disabilities mirror general social patterns of employment rates for age, race, and ethnicity.[34] Education has a positive association with employment for all people, although the association is strongest for adolescents and adults with a "work disability."

6-9. Increase the proportion of children and youth with disabilities who spend at least 80 percent of their time in regular education programs.

Target: 60 percent.

Baseline: 45 percent of children and youth aged 6 to 21 years with disabilities spent at least 80 percent of their time in regular education programs in the 1995–96 school year.

Target setting method: 33 percent improvement. (Better than the best will be used when data are available.)

Data source: Data Analysis System (DANS), U.S. Department of Education, Office of Special Education.

Data for population groups currently are not analyzed.

This objective aims to improve the well-being of students with disabilities by en-couraging academic and learning opportunities and nonacademic social and emo-tional experiences that can facilitate normal growth and development, postsecondary educational attainment, independent living skills, and economic participation as adults. Serving students with disabilities in regular nonspecial education classrooms is a concern that cuts across the goals of many Federal agencies. The current target of the Office of Special Education and Rehabilitative Services is that 60 percent of children and youth with disabilities aged 6 through 21 years will be reported by the States as being served in the regular education classroom at least 80 percent of the time. In support of the target, the 1997 Amendments to the Individuals with Disabilities Education Act states that "to the maximum extent appropriate, children and youth with disabilities, including chil-dren in public or private institutions or other care facilities, are educated with children who are not disabled."[35]

6-10. (Developmental) Increase the proportion of health and wellness and treatment programs and facilities that provide full access for people with disabilities.

Potential data source: National Independent Living Centers Network.

For people with disabilities to have the opportunity for healthy lives, both physi-cally and emotionally, programs and facilities that offer wellness and treatment services must be fully accessible. Effective enforcement of the Americans with Disabilities Act can improve services for people with disabilities and help prevent secondary disabilities.

6-11. (Developmental) Reduce the proportion of people with disabilities who report not having the assistive devices and technology needed.

Potential data source: National Health Interview Survey (NHIS), CDC, NCHS.

In 1990, a one-time survey showed that 2.5 million people said they needed assistive technology that they did not have.[36] The inability to pay for such technology was the main reason given for the unmet need. Assistive technology can be critical in the lives of people with disabilities; thus, technology need, availability, and use must be studied.[37] Technology can aid the independence and self-sufficiency of people with disabilities and can enable people to work, attend school, and participate in community life. Without assistive technology, people with disabilities may become dependent and isolated.

6-12. (Developmental) Reduce the proportion of people with disabilities reporting environmental barriers to participation in home, school, work, or community activities.

Potential data source: Behavioral Risk Factor Surveillance System (BRFSS), CDC, NCCDPHP.

The focus on measuring the environmental impact on people with disabilities echoes the underlying theme of the disability rights movement and the ADA.[38] Both argue that the most important outcome for persons with disabilities—in fact, for all persons in the United States—is their full participation as active, involved, and productive members of society. Indeed, this participation is the implicit outcome for the overarching Healthy People goals to achieve a healthier life and eliminate disparities.

A special 1999 Colorado Behavioral Risk Factor Surveillance System (BRFSS) survey showed that compared to 43 percent of people without disabilities, 55 percent of adults aged 18 years and older with disabilities reported encountering environmental barriers daily or weekly and/or barriers that were very problematic.[39] Similar data will be collected from several other States.

Full participation cannot be achieved without eliminating environmental barriers found within architectural structures, technology, organizational policies and practices, and social attitudes and without moving toward universal design and non-discriminatory elements. Thus public health agencies need to measure not only the nature and extent of disability in the United States but also the extent to which environmental barriers and universal design elements impede or facilitate social participation.

6-13. Increase the number of Tribes, States, and the District of Columbia that have public health surveillance and health promotion programs for people with disabilities and caregivers.

Target and baseline:

Objective	Increase in Public Health Surveillance and Health Promotion Programs for People With Disabilities and Caregivers	1999 Baseline	2010 Target
		Number	
6-13a.	States and the District of Columbia	14	51
6-13b.	Tribes	Developmental	

Target setting method: Total coverage.

Data sources: Tribal, State, and District of Columbia reports; Office on Disability and Health, CDC.

The needs of people with disabilities and caregivers should be addressed by public health activities. In a telephone survey, 23 percent of all U.S. households included at least one caregiver.[40] While not all people with disabilities are dependent on the services of an unpaid (usually a family member) or paid caregiver, meeting the needs of those who benefit from personal assistance cannot be easily separated from the needs of people who provide assistance.[41] Whether caring for infants, children, or adults with disabilities or for the increasing number of people who become activity-limited as they grow older, the caregiver is an important health component.[42]

Related Objectives From Other Focus Areas

1. **Access to Quality Health Services**
   1-1. Persons with health insurance
   1-4. Source of ongoing care
   1-5. Usual primary care provider
   1-6. Difficulties or delays in obtaining needed health care
   1-16. Pressure ulcers among nursing home residents
2. **Arthritis, Osteoporosis, and Chronic Back Conditions**
   2-3. Personal care limitations
   2-5. Employment rate
   2-8. Arthritis education
   2-11. Activity limitations due to chronic back conditions
3. **Cancer**
   3-9. Sun exposure and skin cancer
   3-11. Pap tests
   3-12. Colorectal cancer screening
   3-13. Mammograms

4. **Chronic Kidney Disease**
   4-2. Cardiovascular disease deaths in persons with chronic kidney disease
   4-7. Kidney failure due to diabetes

5. **Diabetes**
   5-1. Diabetes education
   5-2. New cases of diabetes
   5-3. Overall cases of diagnosed diabetes
   5-4. Diagnosis of diabetes
   5-9. Foot ulcers
   5-10. Lower extremity amputations

7. **Educational and Community-Based Programs**
   7-1. High school completion
   7-3. Health-risk behavior information for college and university students
   7-6. Participation in employer-sponsored health promotion activities
   7-11. Culturally appropriate and linguistically competent community health promotion programs
   7-12. Older adult participation in community health promotion activities

9. **Family Planning**
   9-2. Birth spacing
   9-4. Contraceptive failure
   9-7. Adolescent pregnancy

12. **Heart Disease and Stroke**
   12-1. Coronary heart disease (CHD) deaths
   12-7. Stroke deaths
   12-9. High blood pressure
   12-10. High blood pressure control
   12-11. Action to help control blood pressure
   12-12. Blood pressure monitoring
   12-13. Mean total blood cholesterol levels
   12-14. High blood cholesterol levels
   12-15. Blood cholesterol screening

14. **Immunization and Infectious Diseases**
   14-22. Universally recommended vaccination of children aged 19 to 35 months
   14-24. Fully immunized young children and adolescents
   14-26. Children participating in population-based immunization registries
   14-29. Influenza and pneumococcal vaccination of high-risk adults

16. **Maternal, Infant, and Child Health**
   16-1. Fetal and infant deaths
   16-2. Child deaths
   16-3. Adolescent and young adult deaths
   16-4. Maternal deaths
   16-6. Prenatal care
   16-9. Cesarean births
   16-10. Low birth weight and very low birth weight
   16-11. Preterm births
   16-13. Infants put to sleep on their backs
   16-16. Optimum folic acid levels
   16-17. Prenatal substance exposure
   16-19. Breastfeeding

16-21. Sepsis among children with sickle cell disease

16-22. Medical homes for children with special health care needs

16-23. Service systems for children with special health care needs

17. **Medical Product Safety**

17-3.   Provider review of medications taken by patients

18. **Mental Health and Mental Disorders**

18-4.   Employment of persons with serious mental illness

18-9.   Treatment for adults with mental disorders

19. **Nutrition and Overweight**

19-1.   Healthy weight in adults

19-2.   Obesity in adults

19-3.   Overweight or obesity in children and adolescents

19-4.   Growth retardation in children

19-5.   Fruit intake

19-6.   Vegetable intake

19-7.   Grain product intake

19-8.   Saturated fat intake

19-9.   Total fat intake

19-10. Sodium intake

19-11. Calcium intake

19-12. Iron deficiency in young children and in females of childbearing age

19-13. Anemia in low-income pregnant females

19-17. Nutrition counseling for medical conditions

19-18. Food security

20. **Occupational Safety and Health**

20-1.   Work-related injury deaths

21. **Oral Health**

21-1.   Dental caries experience

21-2.   Untreated dental decay

21-3.   No permanent tooth loss

21-4.   Complete tooth loss

21-5.   Periodontal disease

21-6.   Early detection of oral and pharyngeal cancers

21-8.   Dental sealants

21-10. Use of oral health care system

21-15. Referral for cleft lip or palate

21-16. Oral and craniofacial State-based surveillance system

22. **Physical Activity and Fitness**

22-1.   No leisure-time physical activity

22-2.   Moderate physical activity

22-3.   Vigorous physical activity

22-4.   Muscular strength and endurance

22-5.   Flexibility

23. **Public Health Infrastructure**

23-4.   Data for all population groups

23-5.   Data for Leading Health Indicators, Health Status Indicators, and Priority Data Needs at Tribal, State, and local levels

23-6.   National tracking of Healthy People 2010 objectives

24. **Respiratory Diseases**
   24-1. Deaths from asthma
   24-2. Hospitalizations for asthma
   24-3. Hospital emergency department visits for asthma
   24-4. Activity limitations
   24-5. School or work days lost
   24-6. Patient education
   24-7. Appropriate asthma care
   24-8. Surveillance systems
   24-9. Activity limitations due to chronic lung and breathing problems
   24-10. Deaths from COPD

27. **Tobacco Use**
   27-1. Adult tobacco use
   27-5. Smoking cessation by adults
   27-6. Smoking cessation during pregnancy

28. **Vision and Hearing**
   28-4. Impairment in children and adolescents
   28-10. Vision rehabilitation services and devices
   28-12. Otitis media
   28-13. Rehabilitation for hearing impairment

Terminology

(A listing of abbreviations and acronyms used in this publication appears in Appendix H.)

Activity limitations: Problems in a person's performance of everyday functions such as communication, self-care, mobility, learning, and behavior.

Assistive devices and technology: Under the Assistive Technology Act of 1998 (Public Law 105-394), "any item, piece of equipment, or product system, whether acquired commercially, modified, or customized, that is used to increase, maintain, or improve the functional capabilities of individuals with disabilities."

Congregate care facilities: An out-of-home facility that provides housing for people with disabilities in which rotating staff members provide care—16 or more beds when referring to adults and any number of beds when referring to children and youth under age 21 years. Congregate care excludes foster care, adoptive homes, residential schools, correctional facilities, and nursing facilities.[30]

Disability: The general term used to represent the interactions between individuals with a health condition and barriers in their environment.

Environmental factors: The policies, systems, social contexts, and physical barriers or facilitators that affect a person's participation in activities, including work, school, leisure, and community events.

Health promotion: Efforts to create healthy lifestyles and a healthy environment to prevent medical and other secondary conditions, such as teaching people how to address their health care needs and increasing opportunities to participate in usual life activities.

ICIDH-2: *International Classification of Functioning and Disability*, the World Health Organization's conceptual and coding framework for describing a person's functioning and disability associated with his or her health condition.

People with disabilities: People identified as having an activity limitation or who use assistance or who perceive themselves as having a disability.

Permanency planning: A planning process undertaken by public and private agencies on behalf of a child with developmental disabilities and their families with the explicit goal of securing a permanent living arrangement that enhances the child's growth and development.[41]

Secondary conditions: Medical, social, emotional, mental, family, or community problems that a person with a primary disabling condition likely experiences.

References

[1] World Health Organization (WHO). *International Classification of Functioning and Disability (ICIDH-2): Beta-1 Draft for Field Trials*. Geneva, Switzerland: WHO, 1997, 11-21, 206-215, 221-225.

[2] McNeil, J.M. Americans with disabilities 1994–95. *Current Populations Report* P7061:3-6, August 1997.

[3] National Institute on Disability and Rehabilitation Research. *Trends in Disability Prevalence and Their Causes: Proceedings of the Fourth National Disability Statistics and Policy Forum, May 16, 1997, Washington, DC*. San Francisco, CA: The Disability Statistics Rehabilitation Research and Training Center, 1998.

[4] Institute of Medicine. *Enabling America: Assessing the Role of Rehabilitation Science and Engineering*. Washington, DC: National Academy Press, 1997, 2.

[5] U.S. Department of Health and Human Services (HHS). *Healthy People 2000: National Health Promotion and Disease Prevention Objectives*. Pub. No. (PHS) 91-50213. Washington, DC: HHS, Public Health Service (PHS), Office of Disease Prevention and Health Promotion (ODPHP), 1991, 39-42.

[6] Centers for Disease Control and Prevention (CDC). Health-related quality of life and activity limitation—Eight states, 1995. *Morbidity and Mortality Weekly Report* (47):134-140, 1998.

[7] Manton, K.; Corder, L.; and Stallard, E. *Chronic Disability Trends in Elderly in United States Populations 1982–1994*. Washington, DC: National Academy of Sciences, 1997, 2593-2598.

[8] Zola, I. Disability statistics, what we count and what it tells us, a personal and political analysis. *Journal of Disability Policy Studies* 4(2):10-39, 1993.

[9] Hahn, H. The political implications of disability definitions and data. *Journal of Disability Policy Studies* 4(2):42-52, 1993.

[10] HHS. *Healthy People 2000 Progress Review, People With Disabilities*. Washington, DC: HHS, PHS, ODPHP, 1997, 1-3.

[11] Seekins, T.; White, G.; Ravesloot, C.; et al. Developing and evaluating community-based health promotion programs for people with disabilities. In: *Secondary Conditions Among People With Disabilities: Current Research and Trends*. Pacific Grove, CA: Brookes-Cole Publisher, in press.

[12] Lorig, K. A workplace health education program that reduces outpatient visits. *Medical Care* 9:1044-1054, 1995.

[13] Research and Training Center on Rural Rehabilitation. *Cost Containment Through Disability Prevention: Preliminary Results of a Health Promotion Workshop for People With Physical Disabilities.* Missoula, MT: University of Montana, the Center, 1996.

[14] Lorig, K.; Lubeck, D.; Kraines, R.; et al. Outcomes of self-help education for patients with arthritis. *Arthritis Rheumatism* 28(6):680-685, 1985.

[15] National Osteoporosis Foundation. *Physician Guide to Prevention and Treatment of Osteoporosis.* Washington, DC: the Foundation, 1998.

[16] Melnikova, N; Hough, J.; and Lollar, D. Osteoporosis among women with physical disabilities: Risk factors and protective factors. Paper presented at 126th Annual Meeting of the American Public Health Association, Disability Forum Special Interest Group in Washington, DC, November 17, 1998.

[17] HHS. *Healthy People in Healthy Communities: A Guide for Community Leaders.* Washington, DC: HHS, PHS, Office of Public Health and Science (OPHS), ODPHP, 1998.

[18] HHS. *U.S. Preventive Services Task Force: Guide to Clinical Preventive Services.* 2nd ed. Washington, DC: HHS, OPHS, ODPHP, 1995, Chapter V.

[19] HHS. *Task Force on Community Preventive Services: Guide to Community Preventive Services.* Washington, DC: HHS, in press.

[20] U.S. Public Health Service. *Putting Prevention Into Practice: Clinicians Handbook of Preventive Services.* 2nd ed. McLean, VA: International Medical Publishing, Inc., 1998, Chapter 36.

[21] National Council on Disability. *Reorienting Disability Research: Letter to the United States President.* Washington, DC: the Council, 1998, 1-17.

[22] Office on Disability and Health. *1999 Behavioral Risk Factor Surveillance System Disability Module.* Atlanta, GA: CDC, 1999.

[23] Tuttle, D. *Self Esteem and Adjusting With Blindness: The Process of Responding to Life Demands.* Springfield, IL: Charles C. Thomas Publisher, 1984, 61, 145-158.

[24] Sowers, J., and Powers, L. Enhancing the participation and independence of students with severe and multiple disabilities in performing community activities. *Mental Retardation* 33(4):209-220, 1995.

[25] Kaye, S. Is the status of people with disabilities improving? *Disability Status Abstract* (21):3-4, May 1998.

[26] Novack, T., and Gage, R. Assessment of family functioning and social support. In: Cushman, L., and Scherer, M., eds. *Psychological Assessment in Medical Rehabilitation.* Washington, DC: American Psychological Association, 1995, 286-297.

[27] Patrick, D. Rethinking prevention for people with disabilities part 1: A conceptual model for promoting health. *American Journal of Health Promotion* 11(4):25-260, 1997.

[28] Swain, P. Helping disabled people: The users view. *British Medical Journal* 306(6883):990-992, 1993.

[29] Braddock, D.; Hemp, R.; Parish, S.; et al. *The State of the States in Developmental Disabilities.* 5th ed. Washington, DC: American Association on Mental Retardation, 1998, 9-10.

[30] Prouty, R., and Lakin, K. *Residential Services for Persons With Developmental Disabilities: Status and Trends Through 1997.* Minneapolis, MN: University of Minnesota, Re-

search Training Center on Community Living, Institute on Community Integration, 1998, xii, 47, 53, 58, 60, 65-67, 76, 88, 101.

[31] Kane, R. Expanding the home care concept: Blurring distinctions among home care, institutional care and other long-term care facilities. *Milbank Quarterly* 73(2):161-186, 1995.

[32] Hardwick, S.; Pack, J.; Donohoe, E.; et al. *Across the States 1994: Profiles of Long-Term Care Systems*. Washington, DC: American Association of Retired Persons, Center on Elderly People Living Alone, Public Policy Institute, 1994, 5-7.

[33] Presidential Task Force on Employment of Adults with Disabilities. *Recharting the Course: First Report*. Washington, DC: the Task Force, 1998.

[34] Stoddard, S.; Jans, L.; Ripple, J.; et al. *Chartbook on Work and Disabilities in the United States, 1998*. Washington, DC: U.S. Department of Education (DoE), National Institute on Disability and Rehabilitation, 1998.

[35] DoE. *To Assure the Free Appropriate Public Education of All Children with Disabilities: Nineteenth Annual Report to Congress on the Implementation of the Individuals with Disabilities Education Act, Section 618*. Washington, DC: DoE, 1997.

[36] Laplante, M.; Hendershot, G.; and Moss, A. Assistive technology devices and home accessibility features: Prevalence, payment, need, and trends. In: *Advance Data from Vital and Health Statistics: No. 217*. Hyattsville, MD: National Center for Health Statistics, 1992.

[37] National Council on Disability. *Study on Financing of Assistive Technology Devices and Services for Individuals With Disabilities*. Washington, DC: the Council, 1993.

[38] National Council on Disability. *Equality of Opportunity: The Making of the Americans with Disabilities Act*. Washington, DC: the Council, 1997, 9-21.

[39] Craig Hospital and the Colorado Department of Public Health and Environment. Craig Hospital Inventory of Environmental Factors. Short form (CHIEF SF). *Colorado 1999 Behavioral Risk Surveillance System Disability Study*. Englewood, CO: Craig Hospital, Denver, CO, and Colorado Department of Public Health and Environment, Survey Research Unit.

[40] National Alliance for Caregiving and the American Association of Retired Persons. *Family Caregiving in the U.S.: Findings From a National Survey*. Bethesda, MD: American Association of Retired Persons, Washington, DC, 1997, 8.

[41] Singer, G., and Irvin, L. *Support for Caregiving Families: Enabling Positive Adaptation to Disability*. Baltimore, MD: Paul H. Brooks Publishing Company, 1989, 44.

[42] Pugliese, J.M.; Ingram, T.O.; and Edwards, G. *Stability of Employment Status of Caregivers Who Have a Child With a Disability*. Birmingham, AL: United Cerebral Palsy of Greater Birmingham, Inc., 1998.

7

Educational and Community-Based Programs

Co-Lead Agencies: Centers for Disease Control and Prevention
Health Resources and Services Administration

Contents

Goal

Increase the quality, availability, and effectiveness of educational and community-based programs designed to prevent disease and improve health and quality of life.

Overview

Educational and community-based programs have played an integral role in the attainment of Healthy People 2000 objectives and will continue to contribute to the improvement of health outcomes in the United States by the year 2010. These programs, developed to reach people outside traditional health care settings, are fundamental for health promotion and quality of life.

Issues and Trends

People working together can improve individual health and create healthier communities. Although more research is needed in community health improvement, clearly, the health of communities not only depends on the health of individuals but also on whether the physical and social aspects of communities enable people to live healthy lives.[1] Health and quality of life rely on many community systems and factors, not simply on a well-functioning health and medical care system. Making changes within existing systems, such as the school system, can effectively and efficiently improve the health of a large segment of the community. Also, environmental and policy approaches, such as better street lighting and policies to fortify foods, tend to have a greater impact on the whole community than do individual-oriented approaches.[2] An increasing number of communities are using community health planning processes, such as Assessment Protocol for Excellence in Public Health (APEX/PH); Healthy Cities, Healthy Communities; and Planned Approach to Community Health (PATCH), to take ownership of their health and quality-of-life improvement process.[3]

Communities experiencing the most success in addressing health and quality-of-life issues have involved many components of their community: public health, health care, business, local governments, schools, civic organizations, voluntary health organizations, faith organizations, park and recreation departments, and other interested groups and private citizens. Communities that are eager to improve the health of specific at-risk groups have found that they are more likely to be successful if they work collaboratively within their communities and if the social and physical environments also are conducive to supporting healthy changes.

Because many health problems relate to more than one behavioral risk factor as well as to social and environmental factors, communities with effective programs also work to improve health by addressing the multiple determinants of a health problem. Among the more effective community health promotion programs are those that implement comprehensive intervention plans with multiple intervention strategies, such as educational, policy, and environmental, within various settings, such as the community, health care facilities, schools (including colleges and universities), and worksites.[1, 4, 5, 6]

Educational strategies may include efforts to increase health awareness, communication, and skill building. Policy strategies are those laws, regulations, formal and informal rules, and understandings adopted on a collective basis to guide individual and collective behavior.[2, 7, 8, 9] These include health-friendly policies designed to encourage healthful actions (for example, flex-time at worksites that enables employees to engage in physical activity, clinic hours that meet the needs of working people), and policies to discourage or limit unhealthy actions (for example, restrictions on the sale of tobacco products to minors as a way to discourage youth tobacco use). Environmental strategies are measures that alter or control the legal, social, economic, and physical environment.[10] They make the environment more supportive of health and well-being (for example, increasing the accessibility of low-fat foods in grocery stores to encourage a low-fat diet). Environmental measures also are used to discourage actions that are not supportive of health (for example, the removal of cigarette vending machines from public buildings to discourage smoking).

These educational, policy, and environmental strategies are effective when used in as many settings as appropriate.[5] Settings—schools, worksites, health care facilities, and the community—serve as channels to reach desired audiences as well as apply strategies in as broad a population as possible. These settings also provide major social structures for intervening at the policy level to facilitate healthful choices.[10]

The school setting. The importance of including health instruction in education curricula has been recognized since the early 1900s.[11] In 1997, the Institute of Medicine advised that students should receive the health-related education and services necessary for them to derive maximum benefit from their education and enable them to become healthy, productive adults.[12]

The school setting, ranging from preschool to university, is an important avenue to reach the entire population and specifically to educate children and youth. Schools have more influence on the lives of young people than any other social institution except the family and provide a setting in which friendship networks develop, socialization occurs, and norms that govern behavior are developed and reinforced. Each school day about 48 million youth in the United States attend almost 110,000 elementary and secondary schools for about 6 hours of classroom time. More than 95 percent of all youth aged 5 to 17 years are enrolled in school. Schools are second only to homes among the primary places that children spend their time and thus are one of the significant places where children may be exposed to potentially harmful environmental conditions. (See Focus Area 8. Environmental Health.) During high school, national dropout rates average 12 percent. Prior to high school, dropout is almost nonexistent.[13, 14, 15] Because healthy children learn better than children with health problems, schools also have an interest in addressing the health needs of students. Although schools alone cannot be expected to address the health and related social problems of youth, they can provide, through their climate and curriculum, a focal point for efforts to reduce health-risk behaviors and improve the health status of youth.[16]

In 1990, the key elements of school health education were identified: a documented, planned, and sequential program of health education for students in kindergarten through grade 12; a curriculum that addresses and integrates education about a range of categorical health problems and issues at developmentally appropriate ages; activities to help young persons develop the skills they will need to avoid risky behaviors; instruction provided for a prescribed amount of time at each grade level; management and coordination in each school by an education professional trained to implement the program; instruction from teachers who have been trained to teach the subject; involvement of parents, health professionals, and other concerned community members; and periodic evaluation, updating, and improvement.[17]

More than 12 million students currently are enrolled in the Nation's 3,600 colleges and universities.[18] Thus, colleges and universities are important settings for reducing health-risk behaviors among many young adults. Health clinics at the postsecondary level can help empower students to take responsibility for their own health through education, prevention, early detection, and treatment. In addition, colleges and universities can play an important role in eliminating racial and ethnic disparities and other inequalities in health outcomes by influencing how people think about these issues and providing a place where opinions and behaviors contributing to these factors can be addressed.

The worksite setting. The growing cost of health care combined with the increase of preventable acute and chronic illnesses drive the continuing need for comprehensive worksite health promotion programs. (See Focus Area 20. Occupational Safety and Health.) The worksite setting provides an opportunity to implement educational programs and policy and environmental actions that support health, which benefit managers, employees, and, ultimately, the community as a whole. These programs have become an integral part of corporate plans to reduce health care costs, improve worker morale, decrease absenteeism, and improve behaviors associated with increased worker productivity.[19] Although reductions in health risks have been achieved through many worksite health promotion programs, risk reduction for hourly and part-time workers and companies with fewer than 50 employees has lagged.[20]

The health care setting. In health care facilities, including hospitals, medical and dental clinics, and offices, health care providers often see their patients at a teachable moment. Individualized education and counseling by health care providers at such moments in these settings have been shown to have positive and clinically significant effects on behavior in persons with chronic and acute conditions.[10]

(See Focus Area 1. Access to Quality Health Services.) Providers must be cognizant of these opportunities and prepared to provide appropriate patient education. Institutions that employ providers also must be cognizant and allow sufficient time and training for patient education and counseling to occur.

The health care setting is critical to the delivery of health education and health promotion because of the dramatic change it has undergone in the past 10 years. In 1989, 18 percent[21] of the population reported they were covered by some form of managed care; in 1996 that number had risen to 29 percent, an increase of 57 percent. As of June 1999, the number had jumped to 70 percent. As of January 1, 1997, more than 4.9 million Medicare beneficiaries were enrolled in managed care plans, accounting for 13 percent of the total Medicare program and representing a 108 percent increase in managed care enrollment since 1993. As of June 30, 1998, over 16 million, or 54 percent, of Medicaid beneficiaries were enrolled in managed care programs.

Growth in enrollment in managed care plans has been accompanied by the development of the Health Plan Employer Data and Information Set (HEDIS) and a set of common data indicators to examine performance by managed care organizations (MCOs) by the National Committee on Quality Assurance (NCQA). The latest version of HEDIS requires MCOs to report on more than 50 prevention-oriented indicators.[22] With the increasing marketing importance of HEDIS to MCOs, there will be greater demands for MCO health promotion programs to address HEDIS-related issues.[23] As a result, increased attention must be devoted to examining patient satisfaction with health promotion programs in health care organizations.

The community setting. While health promotion in schools, health care centers, and worksites provides targeted interventions for specific population groups, community-based programs can reach the entire population. Broad public concern and support are vital to the functioning of a healthy community and to ensure the conditions in which people can be healthy.[24] Included in the community setting are public facilities; local government and agencies; and social service, faith, and civic organizations that provide channels to reach people where they live, work, and play. They can be strong advocates for educational, policy, and environmental changes throughout the community. Places of worship may be a particularly important setting for health promotion initiatives, and they may effectively reach some underserved populations. Approaches to prevention must account for the character of the community and ensure community participation in the process.[3] Valuable and effective health benefits of community-based approaches have been demonstrated by community interventions that have served a variety of ethnic, racial, and socioeconomic population groups.[3, 7, 25] Community-based approaches in conjunction with targeted approaches in schools, health care, and worksites increase the likelihood for success to improve personal and community health.

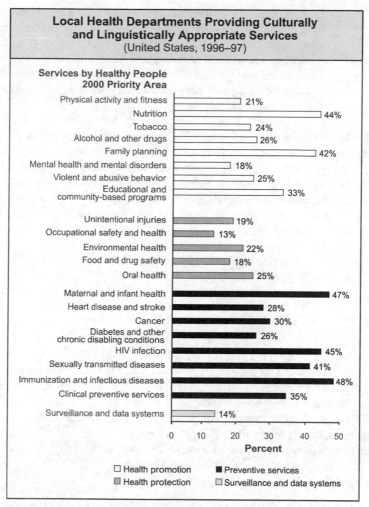

Local Health Departments Providing Culturally and Linguistically Appropriate Services
(United States, 1996–97)

Services by Healthy People 2000 Priority Area

Priority Area	Percent
Physical activity and fitness	21%
Nutrition	44%
Tobacco	24%
Alcohol and other drugs	26%
Family planning	42%
Mental health and mental disorders	18%
Violent and abusive behavior	25%
Educational and community-based programs	33%
Unintentional injuries	19%
Occupational safety and health	13%
Environmental health	22%
Food and drug safety	18%
Oral health	25%
Maternal and infant health	47%
Heart disease and stroke	28%
Cancer	30%
Diabetes and other chronic disabling conditions	26%
HIV infection	45%
Sexually transmitted diseases	41%
Immunization and infectious diseases	48%
Clinical preventive services	35%
Surveillance and data systems	14%

Legend:
☐ Health promotion ■ Preventive services
▨ Health protection ☐ Surveillance and data systems

Source: National Association of County and City Health Officials, National Profile of Local Health Departments, 1996–97.

A community health promotion program should include:

- Community participation with representation from at least three of the following community sectors: government, education, business, faith organizations, health care, media, voluntary agencies, and the public.

- Community assessment to determine community health problems, resources, and perceptions and priorities for action.

- Measurable objectives that address at least one of the following: health outcomes, risk factors, public awareness, or services and protection.

- Monitoring and evaluation processes to determine whether the objectives are reached.

■ Comprehensive, multifaceted, culturally relevant interventions that have multiple targets for change—individuals (for example, racial and ethnic, age, and socioeconomic groups), organizations (for example, worksites, schools, and faith communities), and environments (for example, local policies and regulations)—and multiple approaches to change, including education, community organization, and regulatory and environmental reforms.

Schools are natural settings for reaching children and youth whereas worksites can reach the majority of adults. Efforts to reach older adults necessarily must involve the community at large. Senior centers have been established in most communities and provide a range of services, including health promotion programs for adults aged 60 years and older. Several types of housing arrangements designed specifically for older adults also can be found in many communities, including congregate housing, life care facilities, and retirement villages. These usually offer some mix of health care, recreational programs, and other types of activities and services. Health promotion strategies, policies, and educational approaches have been developed for aging populations.[26]

Disparities

The U.S. population is composed of many diverse groups. Evidence indicates a persistent disparity in the health status of racially and culturally diverse populations as compared with the overall health status of the U.S. population. Over the next decade, the composition of the Nation will become more racially and ethnically diverse, thereby increasing the need for effective prevention programs tailored to specific community needs. Poverty, lack of adequate access to quality health services, lack of culturally and linguistically competent health services, and lack of preventive health care also are underlying factors that must be addressed. (See Focus Area 1. Access to Quality Health Services.) Given these disparities, the need for appropriate interventions is clear.

Effective prevention programs in diverse communities must be tailored to community needs and take into consideration factors concerning individuals, such as disability status, sexual orientation, and gender appropriateness, which also play a significant role in determining health outcomes, behaviors, use patterns, and attitudes across age, racial, and ethnic groups. For example, women often are the health care decisionmakers and caregivers in their families and in their communities. When provided with enabling services and health promotion and prevention information, they can make better health choices and better navigate the health care system to get the information and services they and their families need.

Opportunities

Health promotion programs need to be sensitive to the diverse cultural norms and beliefs of the people for whom the programs are intended. Achieving such sensitivity is a continuing challenge as the Nation's population becomes increasingly diverse. To ensure that interventions are culturally appropriate, linguistically competent, and appropriate for the needs of racial, ethnic, gender, sexual orientation, disability status, and age groups within the community, members of the populations served and their gatekeepers must be involved in the community assessment and planning process.

Community assessment helps to identify the cultural traditions and beliefs of the community and the education, literacy level, and language preferences necessary for the development of appropriate materials and programs. In addition, a community assessment can help identify levels of social capital and community capacity. Such assessments help identify the skills, resources, and abilities needed to manage health improvement programs in communities.[5, 27]

Educational and community-based programs must be supported by accurate, appropriate, and accessible information derived from a science base. Increasing evidence supports the efficacy and effectiveness of health education and health promotion in schools, worksites, health care facilities, and community-based programming.[8] Gaps in research include the dissemination and diffusion of effective programs, new technologies, policies, relationships between settings, and approaches to disadvantaged and special populations.[10]

Communities need to be involved as partners in conducting research ensuring that the content of the prevention efforts developed is tailored to meet the needs of the communities and populations being served. Communities also need to be involved as equal partners in research—to enhance the appropriateness and sustainability of science-based interventions and prevention programs and ensure that the lessons of research are transferred back to the community. Sustainability is necessary for successful research to be translated into programs of lasting benefit to communities.

The importance of social ecology on behavior and the successes of environmental and policy approaches to health promotion and disease prevention need further documentation. Techniques to evaluate community processes and community health improvement methods and models need to be refined and disseminated so that other communities can learn from and duplicate successful strategies. Issues of partnering and the role of collaborative efforts to increase the capacity of individuals and communities to achieve long-term outcomes and improvements in health status are not fully understood[27] and should be evaluated. Mechanisms need to be developed to share what is learned in an appropriate and timely manner with communities.

Interim Progress Toward Year 2000 Objectives

Progress toward the 14 educational and community-based program objectives in Healthy People 2000 has been mixed. Improvements have been made in the number of worksites that offer health promotion activities and in the proportion of hospitals that offer patient education programs. New information from the National College Health Risk Behavior Survey shows that college students are receiving information on health topics such as human immunodeficiency virus (HIV) and sexually transmitted disease prevention. High school completion rates have not changed from their baseline. Participation in health promotion activities by hourly workers over age 18 years exceeds the target. Baseline data are available for older adults participating in health promotion activities and on counties with programs for certain racial and ethnic populations.

Note: Unless otherwise noted, data are from the Centers for Disease Control and Prevention, National Center for Health Statistics, *Healthy People 2000 Review, 1998–99.*

Educational and Community-Based Programs

Goal: Increase the quality, availability, and effectiveness of educational and community-based programs designed to prevent disease and improve health and quality of life.

Number	Objective Short Title

School Setting

7-1	High school completion
7-2	School health education
7-3	Health-risk behavior information for college and university students
7-4	School nurse-to-student ratio

Worksite Setting

7-5	Worksite health promotion programs
7-6	Participation in employer-sponsored health promotion activities

Health Care Setting

7-7	Patient and family education
7-8	Satisfaction with patient education
7-9	Health care organization sponsorship of community health promotion activities

Community Setting and Select Populations

7-10	Community health promotion programs
7-11	Culturally appropriate and linguistically competent community health promotion programs
7-12	Older adult participation in community health promotion activities

School Setting

7-1. Increase high school completion.

Target: 90 percent.

Baseline: 85 percent of persons aged 18 to 24 years had completed high school in 1998.

Target setting method: Consistent with National Education Goals Panel—Goals 2000.

Data source: Current Population Survey, U.S. Department of Commerce, Bureau of the Census.

NOTE: THE TABLE BELOW MAY CONTINUE TO THE FOLLOWING PAGE.

Persons Aged 18 to 24 Years, 1998 (unless noted)	Completed High School
	Percent
TOTAL	85
Race and ethnicity	
American Indian or Alaska Native	85
Asian or Pacific Islander	94
Asian	94
Native Hawaiian and other Pacific Islander	DSU
Black or African American	81
White	85
Hispanic or Latino	63
Not Hispanic or Latino	DNA
Black or African American	81
White	90
Gender	
Female	87
Male	83
Family income level	
Poor	DNA
Near poor	DNA
Middle/high income	DNA

Persons Aged 18 to 24 Years, 1998 (unless noted)	Completed High School
	Percent
Disability status	
Persons with disabilities	79 (1995)
Persons without disabilities	86 (1995)

DNA = Data have not been analyzed. DNC = Data are not collected. DSU = Data are statistically unreliable.

NOTE: THE TABLE ABOVE MAY HAVE CONTINUED FROM THE PREVIOUS PAGE.

Dropping out of school is associated with delayed employment opportunities, poverty, and poor health. During adolescence, dropping out of school is associated with multiple social and health problems, including substance abuse, delinquency, intentional and unintentional injury, and unintended pregnancy. Some researchers suggest that the antecedents of drug and alcohol problems, school dropout, delinquency, and a host of other problems can be identified in the early elementary grades, long before the actual problems manifest themselves. These antecedents include low academic achievement and low attachment to school, adverse peer influence, inadequate family management and parental supervision, parental substance abuse, sensation-seeking behavior, and diminished personal capabilities. Children who perform poorly in school, are more than a year behind their modal grade, and are chronically truant are more likely to exhibit risk behaviors and experience serious problems in adolescence. Finally, risk of these outcomes is increased if children fail to form meaningful social bonds to positive adult and peer role models with whom they interact at school or in the community. If high school dropout rates are addressed as part of the Nation's health promotion and disease prevention agenda, unwarranted risks of problem behavior may be reduced and the health of young people improved.

The target of 90 percent set for this objective is consistent with the National Education Goal to increase the high school graduation rate to at least 90 percent. A National Education Objective under that goal is to eliminate the gap in high school graduation rates between racial and ethnic minority and nonminority students. In 1998, only 63 percent of Hispanic or Latino and 81 percent of African American youth aged 18 to 24 years had completed high school, compared to a completion rate of 90 percent for white, non-Hispanic youth.

7-2. Increase the proportion of middle, junior high, and senior high schools that provide school health education to prevent health problems in the following areas: unintentional injury; violence; suicide; tobacco use and addiction; alcohol and other drug use; unintended pregnancy, HIV/AIDS, and STD infection; unhealthy dietary patterns; inadequate physical activity; and environmental health.

Target and baseline:

Objective	Schools Providing School Health Education in Priority Areas	1994 Baseline	2010 Target
		Percent	
7-2a.	**All components**	28	70
	Individual components to prevent health problems in the following areas		
7-2b.	Unintentional injury	66	90
7-2c.	Violence	58	80
7-2d.	Suicide	58	80
7-2e.	Tobacco use and addiction	86	95
7-2f.	Alcohol and other drug use	90	95
7-2g.	Unintended pregnancy, HIV/AIDS, and STD infection	65	90
7-2h.	Unhealthy dietary patterns	84	95
7-2i.	Inadequate physical activity	78	90
7-2j.	Environmental health	60	80

Target setting method: 150 percent improvement for 7-2a; percentage improvement varies for individual components 7-2b through 7-2j.

Data source: School Health Policies and Programs Study (SHPPS), CDC, NCCDPHP.

7-3. Increase the proportion of college and university students who receive information from their institution on each of the six priority health-risk behavior areas.

Target: 25 percent.

Baseline: 6 percent of undergraduate students received information from their college or university on all six topics in 1995: injuries (intentional and unintentional), tobacco use, alcohol and illicit drug use, sexual behaviors that cause unintended pregnancies and sexually transmitted diseases, dietary patterns that cause disease, and inadequate physical activity.

Target setting method: Better than the best.

Data source: National College Health Risk Behavior Survey, CDC, NCCDPHP.

Undergraduates, 1995	Received Information on Six Priority Health-Risk Behavior Areas
	Percent
TOTAL	6
Race and ethnicity	
American Indian or Alaska Native	DSU
Asian or Pacific Islander	DSU
Asian	DSU
Native Hawaiian and other Pacific Islander	DSU
Black or African American	8
White	6
Hispanic or Latino	5
Not Hispanic or Latino	DNA
Black or African American	8
White	6
Gender	
Female	6
Male	6
Family income level	
Poor	DNC
Near poor	DNC
Middle/high income	DNC
Disability status	
Persons with disabilities	DNC
Persons without disabilities	DNC
Sexual orientation	DNC

DNA = Data have not been analyzed. DNC = Data are not collected. DSU = Data are statistically unreliable.

The School Health Education Study[28] conducted during the 1960s identified 10 conceptual areas that have traditionally served as the basis of health education curricula. Subsequently, six categories of behaviors have been identified as responsible for more than 70 percent of illness, disability, and death among adolescents and young adults. These categories, which should be the primary focus of school health education, are injuries (unintentional and intentional), tobacco use, alcohol and illicit drug use, sexual behaviors that cause unintended pregnancies and sexually transmitted diseases, dietary patterns that cause disease, and inadequate physical activity.[29] While unintentional and intentional injuries are grouped together, the prevention program and policy implications for each are distinct given the differences in the risk behaviors and related health outcomes. In addition to the 6 behavior categories, environmental health (recognized influence on personal and community health), mental and emotional health, personal health, and consumer health are among the 10 conceptual areas being added to track the influence of these factors between 2000 and 2010. Text about the contributions school health education can make in achieving objectives can be found in the appropriate Healthy People 2010 focus areas.

The overall goal of the National Health Education Standards for youth is to achieve health literacy.[30] It is important that youth are able to find, understand, and use information and services to enhance health. Research has shown that for health education curricula to affect priority health-risk behaviors among adolescents, effective strategies, considerable instructional time, and well-prepared teachers are required. To attain this objective, States and school districts need to support effective health education with appropriate policies, teacher training, effective curricula, and regular progress assessment. In addition, the support of families, peers, and the community at large is critical to long-term behavior change among adolescents. Health education and health promotion activities also can be conducted in postsecondary settings and reach the Nation's future leaders, teachers, corporate executives, health professionals, and public health personnel. Personal involvement in a health promotion program can educate future leaders about the importance of health and engender a commitment to prevention.

In 1995, 23 percent of undergraduate students reported receiving information on unintentional injuries, 38 percent on intentional injuries, 49 percent on alcohol and other drug use, 55 percent on unintended pregnancy, HIV/AIDS, and STD infection; 30 percent on unhealthy dietary patterns; and 36 percent on inadequate physical activity.[31]

7-4.   Increase the proportion of the Nation's elementary, middle, junior high, and senior high schools that have a nurse-to-student ratio of at least 1:750.

Target and baseline:

Objective	Increase in Schools With Nurse-to-Student Ratio of at Least 1:750	1994 Baseline	2010 Target
		Percent	
7-4a.	All middle, junior high, and senior high schools	28	50
7-4b.	Senior high schools	26	50
7-4c.	Middle and junior high schools	32	50
7-4d.	Elementary schools	Developmental	

Target setting method: 79 percent improvement for 7-4a (all schools combined); percentage improvement varies for individual components 7-4b and 7-4c.

Data source: School Health Policies and Programs Study (SHPPS), CDC, NCCDPHP. Data for elementary schools are developmental.

The importance of providing health services to students in schools is widely accepted.[12] Such services began over 100 years ago to control communicable disease and reduce absenteeism. Over the years, school health services have evolved to keep pace with changes in the health care, social, and educational systems in the United States.[32] Current models of school health services reflect an understanding that children's physical and mental health are linked to their abilities to succeed academically and socially in the school environment.[15]

School nurses serve 48 million youth in the Nation's schools. School nurses assess student health and development, help families determine when medical services are needed, and serve as a professional link with physicians and community resources. Nurses manage care and provide services to support and sustain school attendance and academic achievement. A licensed practical nurse or registered nurse is an essential component of a healthy school. The ratio of 1 school nurse per 750 students should be improved if many students with special needs are enrolled.[33] For children with disabilities, the nurse is an essential resource. These children are dependent on daily medication, nursing procedures, or special diets for normal function.

7-5. **Increase the proportion of worksites that offer a comprehensive employee health promotion program to their employees.**

Target and baseline:

Objective	Increase in Worksites Offering a Comprehensive Employer-Sponsored Health Promotion Program	1999 Baseline	2010 Target
		Percent	
7-5a.	Worksites with fewer than 50 employees	Developmental	
7-5b.	Worksites with 50 or more employees	34	75
7-5c.	Worksites with 50 to 99 employees	33	75
7-5d.	Worksites with 100 to 249 employees	33	75
7-5e.	Worksites with 250 to 749 employees	38	75
7-5f.	Worksites with 750 or more employees	50	75

Target setting method: Better than the best.

Data source: National Worksite Health Promotion Survey, Association for Worksite Health Promotion (AWHP).

7-6. **Increase the proportion of employees who participate in employer-sponsored health promotion activities.**

Target: 75 percent.

Baseline: 61 percent of employees aged 18 years and older participated in employer-sponsored health promotion activities in 1994.

Target setting method: Better than the best.

Data source: National Health Interview Survey (NHIS), CDC, NCHS.

NOTE: THE TABLE BELOW MAY CONTINUE TO THE FOLLOWING PAGE.

Employees Aged 18 Years and Older, 1994	Participated in Employer-Sponsored Health Promotion Activities
	Percent
TOTAL	61
Race and ethnicity	
American Indian or Alaska Native	DSU
Asian or Pacific Islander	50

Employees Aged 18 Years and Older, 1994	Participated in Employer-Sponsored Health Promotion Activities
	Percent
Asian	DNC
Native Hawaiian and other Pacific Islander	DNC
Black or African American	57
White	61
Hispanic or Latino	60
Not Hispanic or Latino	62
Black or African American	57
White	62
Gender	
Female	60
Male	63
Family income level	
Poor	57
Near poor	63
Middle/high income	61
Education level (aged 25 years and older)	
Less than high school	62
High school graduate	65
At least some college	60
Geographic location	
Urban	61
Rural	64
Insurance status	
Persons with insurance	DNA
Persons without insurance	DNA
Disability status	
Persons with activity limitations	56
Persons without activity limitations	62

Employees Aged 18 Years and Older, 1994	Participated in Employer-Sponsored Health Promotion Activities
	Percent
Select populations	
Employees at worksites with 50 or more employees	65
Employees at worksites with fewer than 50 employees	DSU

DNA = Data have not been analyzed. DNC = Data are not collected. DSU = Data are statistically unreliable.

NOTE: THE TABLE ABOVE MAY HAVE CONTINUED FROM THE PREVIOUS PAGE.

By 1999, 95 percent of employers with more than 50 employees reported that they offered at least one health promotion activity.[20] While the growth in worksite health promotion programming since 1985 has been remarkable, many programs lack comprehensive design or sufficient duration and therefore are potentially limited in their impact on employee health and well-being.[34] Participation rates in worksite health promotion programs generally are low. Most worksite statistics indicate that enrollees in worksite health promotion programs tend to be salaried employees whose general health is better than average. Employees working in administrative support, service, crafts, and trades often have greater health risks and higher rates of illness and injury than professional and administrative workers do. Contributing factors include differences in socioeconomic status, in the nature of the work, and in access to and extent of health insurance coverage as well as exclusion of those workers from worksite health promotion programs. This exclusion may be an unintentional result of failing to market the program effectively to the workers.[35] Optimally, worksite health promotion efforts should be part of a comprehensive occupational health and safety program.

More than 80 percent of private-sector employees work in organizations of fewer than 50 people.[36] Over the next decade, strategies need to be developed to provide workers in these settings access to health promotion programs.[37, 38] Limited purchasing power can make the provision of health promotion services difficult for worksites with only a few employees. Employers can take advantage of community agency programs and services through outsourcing and by collaborating with other small worksites to purchase services, such as employee assistance programs and health insurance for preventive health services, to increase their purchasing power and benefits offered to their employees.[38]

Collaboration between trade and professional organizations is needed to identify new opportunities for worksite health promotion. Employee involvement to define and manage worksite health promotion activities can be especially valuable to address resource constraints among smaller employers while simultaneously enhancing program success.[38]

7-7.   (Developmental) Increase the proportion of health care organizations that provide patient and family education.

Potential data source: Joint Commission on Accreditation of Healthcare Organizations (JCAHO) Survey.

7-8.   (Developmental) Increase the proportion of patients who report that they are satisfied with the patient education they receive from their health care organization.

Potential data source: Press Ganey.

7-9.   (Developmental) Increase the proportion of hospitals and managed care organizations that provide community disease prevention and health promotion activities that address the priority health needs identified by their community.

Potential data source: Annual Survey, American Hospital Association.

The concept of increased consumer protection in the health care industry, particularly in the form of a Consumers' Bill of Rights and Responsibilities, is gaining support. These protections include consumers' rights to accurate, easily understood information related to choice of a health plan—its benefits, availability of specialty care, and confidentiality of medical records. However, the right to comprehensive patient and family education is missing from this list. Two distinctive characteristics of health care settings underscore their importance to promote patient and family education: improved health is a primary objective; and health care providers generally are considered credible sources of information.[10] The interaction between these two factors helps create an environment conducive to effective patient and family education programs and activities. The positive and clinically significant effects of patient education and counseling of persons with chronic and acute conditions are well documented; however, the amount and types of health promotion and disease prevention activities offered by managed care organizations to their participating employers vary widely.[23]

On the national level, about 70 percent of employees are covered by some form of managed care. The growth of MCOs is expected to increase. For example, as of January 1, 1997, more than 4.9 million Medicare beneficiaries were enrolled in managed care plans, accounting for 13 percent of the total Medicare program and representing a 108 percent increase in managed care enrollment since 1993.[39] Another important factor is the emerging role of the National Committee on Quality Assurance and its development of the Health Plan Employer Data and Information Set (HEDIS) and set of common data indicators for examining performance of MCOs. The latest version of HEDIS requires MCOs to report on more than 50 prevention-oriented indicators, largely secondary and tertiary prevention-related issues.[22] With the increasing marketing importance of HEDIS to MCOs, there will be greater demands for health promotion to address HEDIS-related issues, potentially leaving critical programming gaps.[23] As a result, increased public attention must be devoted to examining patient satisfaction in health care organizations.

Community health promotion services provided by hospitals and MCOs are growing, as illustrated by the expansion of Federal and State managed care reform legislation directed at the creation of a core set of prevention activities across MCOs.[23] Despite the different motivations and strategic objectives of public health and managed care organizations, they share a mutual interest to improve the health of communities and specific populations within communities. Collaboration between managed care plans and public health agencies is a logical consequence of the health promotion objectives shared by these organizations.[40] Additionally, a number of Federal public health agencies are developing collaborative relationships with the managed care community on issues of clinical preventive services and prevention surveillance and research.[41]

Community Setting and Select Populations

7-10. (Developmental) Increase the proportion of Tribal and local health service areas or jurisdictions that have established a community health promotion program that addresses multiple Healthy People 2010 focus areas.

Potential data source: Special Survey, Association of State and Territorial Directors of Health Promotion and Public Health Education (ASTDHPPHE).

This objective reflects the need for comprehensive and multifaceted health promotion and community health improvement activities at the State and local levels. A 1996 review of the literature on 135 urban health promotion programs conducted between 1980 and 1995 found that a specific model for program planning and implementation was identified in only 41 percent of programs.[42] In addition, community members constituted the smallest percentage of those involved in the local effort, and very little tailoring to the population and population groups served was noted. These efforts also had a strong focus on the individual rather than the population.[42]

This objective includes activities conducted through local health departments as well as those conducted by other community-based organizations, particularly in those communities not served by a local health department. Activities such as Assessment Protocol for Excellence in Public Health (APEX/PH); Healthy Cities, Healthy Communities; and Planned Approach to Community Health (PATCH) recognize the need for community involvement and mobilization as basic methods for planning, implementing, and evaluating educational and community-based programs. Public health departments, community health centers, faith communities, civic organizations, voluntary health organizations, businesses, worksites, schools, universities, Area Health Education Centers (AHECs), and healthy city or community groups are a few of the organizations that plan and deliver such programs in the United States.

Identifying the use of established health promotion planning and identification models provides information on strategically planned and implemented programs. Single-method or noncomprehensive approaches are considered less productive.

7-11. Increase the proportion of local health departments that have established culturally appropriate and linguistically competent community health promotion and disease prevention programs.

Target and baseline:

Objective	Increase in Local Health Department Community Health Promotion and Disease Prevention Programs That Are Culturally Appropriate and Linguistically Competent	1996–97 Baseline	2010 Target
		Percent	
7-11a.	Access to quality health services	Developmental	
	Clinical preventive services	35	*
7-11b.	Arthritis, osteoporosis, and chronic back conditions	Developmental	
7-11c.	Cancer	30	50
	Diabetes and chronic disabling conditions	26	*
7-11d.	Chronic kidney disease	Developmental	
7-11e.	Diabetes	Developmental	
7-11f.	Disability and secondary conditions	Developmental	
7-11g.	Educational and community-based programs	33	50
7-11h.	Environmental health	22	50
7-11i.	Family planning	42	50
	Food and drug safety	18	*
7-11j.	Food safety	Developmental	
7-11k.	Medical product safety	Developmental	
7-11l.	Health communication	Developmental	
7-11m.	Heart disease and stroke	28	50
7-11n.	HIV	45	50
7-11o.	Immunization and infectious diseases	48	50

Objective	Increase in Local Health Department Community Health Promotion and Disease Prevention Programs That Are Culturally Appropriate and Linguistically Competent	1996–97 Baseline	2010 Target
		Percent	
7-11p.	Injury and violence prevention	Developmental	
	Unintentional injuries	19	*
	Violent and abusive behavior	25	*
7-11q.	Maternal, infant (and child) health	47	50
7-11r.	Mental health (and mental disorders)	18	50
7-11s.	Nutrition and overweight	44	50
7-11t.	Occupational safety and health	13	50
7-11u.	Oral health	25	50
7-11v.	Physical activity and fitness	21	50
7-11w.	Public health infrastructure	Developmental	
	Surveillance and data systems	14	*
7-11x.	Respiratory diseases	Developmental	
7-11y.	Sexually transmitted diseases	41	50
7-11z.	Substance abuse (alcohol and other drugs)	26	50
7-11aa.	Tobacco use	24	50
7-11bb.	Vision and hearing	Developmental	

*These are Healthy People 2000 priority areas that are not applicable to Healthy People 2010.

Target setting method: Percentage improvement varies by program.

Data source: National Profile of Local Health Departments, National Association of County and City Health Officials (NACCHO).

Over the next decade, the Nation's population will become even more diverse. Mainstream health education activities often fail to reach select populations.[43] This may contribute to select and disadvantaged communities lagging behind the overall U.S. population on virtually all health status indicators. In 1991, an estimated 78,643 excess deaths occurred among African Americans and an additional 4,485 among Hispanics or Latinos.[44] Approximately 75 percent of these excess deaths occurred in seven categories, all of which had contributing factors that can be controlled or prevented: cancer, cardiovascular disease, cirrhosis, diabetes, HIV or AIDS, homicide, and unintentional injuries. Special efforts are needed to develop and disseminate culturally and linguistically appropriate health information to overcome the cultural differences and meet the special language needs of these population groups.

7-12. Increase the proportion of older adults who have participated during the preceding year in at least one organized health promotion activity.

Target: 90 percent.

Baseline: 12 percent of adults aged 65 years and older participated during the preceding year in at least one organized health promotion activity in 1998 (age adjusted to the year 2000 standard population).

Target setting method: Better than the best.

Data source: National Health Interview Survey (NHIS), CDC, NCHS.

NOTE: THE TABLE BELOW MAY CONTINUE TO THE FOLLOWING PAGE.

Adults Aged 65 Years and Older, 1998 (unless noted)	Participated in at Least One Health Promotion Activity in Preceding Year
	Percent
TOTAL	12
Race and ethnicity	
American Indian or Alaska Native	DSU
Asian or Pacific Islander	22
Asian	22
Native Hawaiian and other Pacific Islander	DSU
Black or African American	8
White	12
Hispanic or Latino	8
Not Hispanic or Latino	12
Black or African American	8
White	12
Gender	
Female	13
Male	10
Family income level	
Poor	8
Near poor	9
Middle/high income	16

Adults Aged 65 Years and Older, 1998 (unless noted)	Participated in at Least One Health Promotion Activity in Preceding Year
	Percent
Education level	
Less than high school	6
High school	10
At least some college	20
Disability status	
Persons with activity limitations	10 (1995)
Persons without activity limitations	12 (1995)
Sexual orientation	DNC

DNA = Data have not been analyzed. DNC = Data are not collected. DSU = Data are statistically unreliable.
Note: Age adjusted to the year 2000 standard population.
NOTE: THE TABLE ABOVE MAY HAVE CONTINUED FROM THE PREVIOUS PAGE.

Adults aged 65 years or older numbered 33.9 million in 1996. They represented 12.8 percent of the U.S. population, about one in every eight persons. More than any other age group, older adults are seeking health information and are willing to make changes to maintain their health and independence. Prevention efforts should focus on modifiable risk behaviors and early diagnosis and match the leading problems by age (for example, aged 60 or 65 to 74 years, 75 to 84 years, and 85 years and older) and functional status. Programs should address these health issues through multiple strategies, including education, counseling, screening/chemoprophylaxis, environmental enhancements, and protective services. As with any successful program, those for older adults need to be tailored to the audience.

Related Objectives From Other Focus Areas

1. **Access to Quality Health Services**
   1-3. Counseling about health behaviors
2. **Arthritis, Osteoporosis, and Chronic Back Conditions**
   2-8. Arthritis education
3. **Cancer**
   3-10. Provider counseling about cancer prevention
5. **Diabetes**
   5-1. Diabetes education

Terminology

(A listing of abbreviations and acronyms used in this publication appears in Appendix H.)

Community: A specific group of people, often living in a defined geographical area, who share a common culture, values, and norms and who are arranged in a social structure according to relationships the community has developed over a period of time.[45]

Community-based program: A planned, coordinated, ongoing effort operated by a community that characteristically includes multiple interventions intended to improve the health status of members of the community.

Community capacity: The characteristics of communities that affect their ability to identify, mobilize, and address social and public health problems.[46, 47]

Community health planning or community health improvement process: Helps a community mobilize to collect and use local data; set health priorities; and design, implement, and evaluate comprehensive programs that address community health and quality of life issues.[1]

Community health promotion program: Includes all of the following: (1) community participation with representation from at least three of the following community sectors: government, education, business, faith organizations, health care, media, voluntary agencies, and the public, (2) community assessment, guided by a community assessment and planning model, to determine community health problems, resources, perceptions, and priorities for action, (3) targeted and measurable objectives to address at least one of the following: health outcomes, risk factors, public awareness, services, and protection, (4) comprehensive, multifaceted, culturally relevant interventions that have multiple targets for change, and (5) monitoring and evaluation processes to determine whether the objectives are reached.

Comprehensive worksite health promotion programs: Refers to programs that contain the following elements: (1) health education that focuses on skill development and lifestyle behavior change in addition to information dissemination and awareness building, preferably tailored to employees' interests and needs, (2) supportive social and physical work environments, including established norms for healthy behavior and policies that promote health and reduce the risk of disease, such as worksite smoking policies, healthy nutrition alternatives in the cafeteria and vending services, and opportunities for obtaining regular physical activity, (3) integration of the worksite program into the organization's administrative structure, (4) related programs, such as employee assistance programs, and (5) screening programs, preferably linked to medical care service delivery to ensure followup and appropriate treatment as necessary and to encourage adherence. Optimally, these efforts should be part of a comprehensive occupational health and safety program.[37, 48]

Culturally appropriate: Refers to an unbiased attitude and organizational policy that values cultural diversity in the population served. Reflects an understanding of diverse attitudes, beliefs, behaviors, practices, and communication patterns that could be attributed to race, ethnicity, religion, socioeconomic status, historical and social context, physical or mental ability, age, gender, sexual orientation, or generational and acculturation status. Includes an awareness that cultural differences may affect health and the effectiveness of health care delivery. Knowledge of disease prevalence in specific cultural populations, whether defined by race, ethnicity, socioeconomic status, physical or mental ability, gender, sexual orientation, age, disability, or habits.

Excess deaths: The statistically significant difference between the number of deaths expected and the number that actually occurred.

Health: A state of physical, mental, and social well-being and not merely the absence of disease and infirmity.

Health care organizations: Included are hospitals, managed care organizations, home health organizations, long-term care facilities, and community-based health care providers.

Health education: Any planned combination of learning experiences designed to predispose, enable, and reinforce voluntary behavior conducive to health in individuals, groups, or communities.[49]

Health literacy: The degree to which individuals have the capacity to obtain, process, and understand basic health information and services needed to make appropriate health decisions.[50]

Health promotion: Any planned combination of educational, political, regulatory, and organizational supports for actions and conditions of living conducive to the health of individuals, groups, or communities.[49]

Health promotion activity: Broadly defined to include any activity that is part of a planned health promotion program, such as implementing a policy to create a smoke-free workplace, developing walking trails in communities, or teaching the skills needed to prepare healthy meals and snacks.

Healthy community: A community that is continuously creating and improving those physical and social environments and expanding those community resources that enable people to mutually support each other in performing all the functions of life and in developing to their maximum potential.[51]

Healthy public policy: Characterized by an explicit concern for health and equity in all areas of policy and by an accountability for health impact. The main aim of healthy public policy is to create a supportive environment to enable people to lead healthy lives by making healthy choices possible and easier for citizens. It makes social and physical environments health enhancing.[45]

High school completion rate: Refers to the percentage of persons aged 18 to 24 years who are not currently enrolled in high school and who report that they have received a high school diploma or the equivalent, such as a General Education Development certificate.

Linguistically competent: Refers to skills for communicating effectively in the native language or dialect of the targeted population, taking into account general educational levels, literacy, and language preferences.

Local health service areas: Refers to local health jurisdictions and local health unit catchment areas.

Managed care organizations (MCOs): Refers to systems that integrate the financing and delivery of health care services to covered individuals by means of arrangements with selected providers to furnish health care services to members. Managed care includes health maintenance organizations, preferred provider organizations, and point-of-service plans.

Patient and family education: Refers to a planned learning experience using a combination of methods, such as teaching, counseling, skill building, and behavior modification, to promote patient self-management and patient and family empowerment regarding their health.

Postsecondary institutions: Includes 2- and 4-year community colleges, private colleges, and universities.

Quality of life: An expression that, in general, connotes an overall sense of well-being when applied to an individual and a pleasant and supportive environment when applied to a community. On the individual level, health-related quality of life (HRQOL) has a strong relationship to a person's health perceptions and ability to function. On the community level, HRQOL can be viewed as including all aspects of community life that have a direct and quantifiable influence on the physical and mental health of its members.[52]

School health education: Any combination of learning experiences organized in the school setting to predispose, enable, and reinforce behavior conducive to health or to prepare school-aged children to be able to cope with the challenges to their health in the years ahead.[49]

Settings (worksites, schools, health care sites, and the community): Major social structures that provide channels and mechanisms of influence for reaching defined populations and for intervening at the policy level to facilitate healthful choices and address quality-of-life issues. Conceptually, the overall community, worksites, schools, and health care sites are contained under the broad umbrella of "community." Health promotion and health education may occur within these individual settings or across settings in a comprehensive, communitywide approach.[10]

Social capital: The process and conditions among people and organizations that lead to accomplishing a goal of mutual social benefit, usually characterized by four interrelated constructs: trust, cooperation, civic engagement, and reciprocity.[49]

Social ecology: Refers to the complex interactions among people and their physical and social environments and the effects of these interactions on the emotional, physical, and social well-being of individuals and groups.[53]

References

[1] Centers for Disease Control and Prevention (CDC). *Planned Approach to Community Health: Guide for the Local Coordinator.* Atlanta, GA: U.S. Department of Health and Human Services (HHS), Public Health Service (PHS), CDC, National Center for Chronic Disease Prevention and Health Promotion (NCCDPHP), 1995.

[2] Brownson, R.C.; Koffman, D.M.; Novotny, T.E.; et al. Environmental and policy interventions to control tobacco use and prevent cardiovascular disease. *Health Education Quarterly* 22:478-498, 1995.

[3] Katz, M.F., and Kreuter, M.W. Community assessment and empowerment. In: Scutchfield, F.D., and Keck, C.W., eds. *Principles of Public Health Practice.* Albany, NY: Delmar Publishers, 1997, 147-156.

[4] Goodman, R.M.; Speers, M.A.; McLeroy, K.; et al. Identifying and defining the dimensions of community capacity to provide a basis for measurement. *Health Education & Behavior* 25(3):258-278, 1998.

[5] Steckler, A.; Allegrante, J.P.; Altman, D.; et al. Health education intervention strategies: Recommendations for future research. *Health Education Quarterly* 22:307-328, 1995.

[6] Rootman, I.; Goodstadt, M.; Hyndman, B.; et al. *Evaluation in Health Promotion Principles and Perspectives.* Copenhagen, Denmark: World Health Organization, 2000.

[7] Glanz, K.; Lankenau, B.; Foerster, S.; et al. Environmental and policy approaches to cardiovascular disease prevention through nutrition: Opportunities for state and local action. *Health Education Quarterly* 22:512-527, 1995.

[8] King, A.C.; Jeffrey, R.W.; Fridinger, F.; et al. Environmental and policy approaches to cardiovascular disease prevention through physical activity: Issues and opportunities. *Health Education Quarterly* 22:499-511, 1995.

[9] Speers, M.A., and Schmid, T.L. Policy and environmental interventions for the prevention and control of cardiovascular diseases. *Health Education Quarterly* 22:476-477, 1995.

[10] Mullen, P.D.; Evans, D.; Forster, J.; et al. Settings as an important dimension in health education/promotion policy, programs, and research. *Health Education Quarterly* 22:329-345, 1995.

[11] Commission on the Reorganization of Secondary Education. *Cardinal Principles of Secondary Education.* Bulletin 35. Washington, DC: Bureau of Education, 1918.

[12] Institute of Medicine. *Schools and Health: Our Nation's Investment.* Washington, DC: National Academy Press, 1997.

[13] National Center for Education Statistics (NCES). *Digest of Education Statistics, 1993.* Washington, DC: NCES, 1993.

[14] NCES. *Dropout Rates in the United States: 1993*. Washington, DC: U.S. Department of Education, Office of Educational Research and Improvement, 1994.

[15] National Health Education Consortium. The relationship to learning: Healthy brain development. Principles and practices of student health. *School Health* 2:262-272, 1992.

[16] Kann, L.; Collins, J.L.; Pateman, B.C.; et al. The School Health Policies and Programs Study (SHPPS): Rationale for a nationwide status report on school health programs. *Journal of School Health* 65(8):291-294, 1995.

[17] Marx, E.; Wooley, S.F.; and Northrop, D., eds. *Health is Academic: A Guide to Coordinated School Health*. New York, NY: Teachers College Press, 1998.

[18] Kominski, R., and Adams, A. *Educational Attainment in the United States: March 1993 and 1992*. Washington, DC: U.S. Bureau of the Census, 1994.

[19] Gebhardt, D.L., and Crump, C.E. Employee fitness and wellness programs in the workplace. *American Psychologist* 45:262-271, 1990.

[20] Association for Worksite Health Promotion. *1999 National Worksite Health Promotion Survey*. Northbrook, IL: the Association, 1999.

[21] National Center for Health Statistics (NCHS). *Health, United States, 1999*. With health and aging chartbook. Hyattsville, MD: NCHS, 1999.

[22] National Committee for Quality Assurance. <http://www.NCQA.org/policy/HEDIS/HEDIS.com>December 15, 1999.

[23] Chapman, L.S. Worksite health promotion in the managed care era. *The Art of Health Promotion* 1:1-7, 1998.

[24] Institute of Health Promotion Research, University of British Columbia, and British Columbia Consortium for Health Promotion Research. *Study of Participatory Research in Health Promotion. Review and Recommendations for the Development of Participatory Research in Health Promotion in Canada*. Vancouver, British Columbia: The Royal Society of Canada, 1995.

[25] Lacey, L.P.; Phillips, C.W.; Ansell, D.; et al. An urban community-based cancer prevention screen and health education intervention in Chicago. *Public Health Reports* 104(6):536-541, 1989.

[26] Hickey, T.; Speers, M.A.; and Prohaska, T.R. *Public Health and Aging*. Baltimore, MD: Johns Hopkins University Press, 1997.

[27] Kreuter, M.W.; Lezin, N.A.; and Young, L.A. Community-based collaborative mechanisms: Implications for practitioners. *Health Promotion Practice* 1(1):2000.

[28] Sliepcevich, E. *School Health Education Study: A Summary Report*. Washington, DC: School Health Education Study, 1964.

[29] Kann, L.; Kolbe, L.; and Collins, J.; eds. Measuring the health behavior of adolescents: The Youth Risk Behavior Surveillance System. *Public Health Reports* 108(Suppl.):1-67, 1993.

[30] Joint Committee on National Health Education Standards. *National Health Education Standards: Achieving Health Literacy*. Atlanta, GA: American Cancer Society, 1995.

[31] CDC. Youth risk behavior surveillance: National college health risk behavior survey—United States, 1995. *Morbidity and Mortality Weekly Report* 46(6):1-56, 1997.

[32] Lear, J.G. School-based services and adolescent health: Past, present, and future. *Adolescent Medicine: State of the Art Reviews* 7(2):163-180, 1996.

[33] Proctor, S.; Lordi, S.; and Saiger, D. *School Nursing Practice: Roles and Standards.* Scarborough, ME: National Association of School Nurses, 1993.

[34] Pelletier, K.R. A review and analysis of the health and cost-effective outcome studies of comprehensive health promotion and disease prevention programs at the worksite: 1993–95 update. *American Journal of Health Promotion* 10:380-388, 1996.

[35] HHS. *Healthy People 2000: National Health Promotion and Disease Prevention Objectives.* Pub. No. (PHS) 91-50213. Washington DC: HHS, PHS, Office of Disease Prevention and Health Promotion, 1991.

[36] NCHS. *Employer-Sponsored Health Insurance: State and National Estimates.* Hyattsville, MD: HHS, 1997.

[37] Glasgow, R.E.; McCaul, K.D.; and Fisher, K.J. Participation in worksite health promotion: A critique of the literature and recommendations for future practice. *Health Education Quarterly* 20:391-408, 1993.

[38] National Resource Center on Worksite Health Promotion. *Working for Good Health: Health Promotion and Small Business.* Washington, DC: Washington Business Group on Health, 1991.

[39] Health Care Financing Administration (HCFA). *Managed Care in Medicare and Medicaid* [fact sheet]. Washington, DC: HCFA, 1997.

[40] Halverson, P.K.; Mays, G.P.; Kaluzny, A.D.; et al. Not-so-strange bedfellows: Models of interactions between managed care plans and public health agencies. *The Milbank Quarterly* 75(1):113-138, 1997.

[41] CDC. Prevention and managed care: Opportunities for managed care organizations, purchasers of health care, and public health agencies. *Morbidity and Mortality Weekly Report* 42(Rr-14):1-12, 1995.

[42] Freudenberg, N. Health promotion in the city: A review of current practice and recommendations for new directions to improve the health of urban populations in the United States. In: *Report to the Centers for Disease Control and Prevention, Center on AIDS, Drugs, and Community Health.* New York, NY: Hunter College, City University of New York, 1997.

[43] National Heart, Lung, and Blood Institute. *Strategies for Diffusing Health Information to Minority Populations: A Profile of a Community-Based Diffusion Model.* Executive Summary. Washington, DC: HHS, 1987.

[44] NCHS. *Excess Deaths and Other Mortality Measures for Hispanic and Black Populations.* Washington, DC: HHS, 1995.

[45] World Health Organization (WHO), Division of Health Promotion, Education and Communication. *Health Promotion Glossary.* Geneva, Switzerland: WHO, 1998.

[46] McLeroy, K. Community capacity: What is it? How do we measure it? What is the role of the prevention centers and CDC? Paper presented at Sixth Annual Prevention Centers Conference, CDC, NCCDPHP in Atlanta, GA.

[47] Green, L.W., and Ottoson, J.M. *Community and Population Health.* 8th ed. New York, NY: McGraw Hill, 1999.

[48] Heaney, C.A., and Goetzel, R.Z. A review of health-related outcomes of multi-component worksite health promotion programs. *American Journal of Health Promotion* 11:290-307, 1997.

[49] Green, L.W., and Kreuter, M.W. *Health Promotion Planning: An Educational and Ecological Approach*. 3rd ed. Mountain View, CA: Mayfield Publishing Company, 1999.

[50] HHS, NIH, National Library of Medicine (NLM). Selden, C.R.; Zorn, M.; Ratzan, S.; et al.; eds. *Health Literacy, January 1990 through October 1999*. NLM Pub. No. CBM 2000-1. Bethesda, MD: NLM, 2000, vi.

[51] Duhl, L., and Hancock, T. Assessing Healthy Cities. In: *World Health Organization Healthy Cities Papers*. Copenhagen, Denmark: WHO, 1988.

[52] Moriarty, D. CDC studies community quality of life. *NACCHO NEWS* 12(3):10,13, 1996.

[53] Stokols, D. Establishing and maintaining healthy environments: Toward a social ecology of health promotion. *American Psychologist* 47(1):6-22, 1992.

8

Environmental Health

Co-Lead Agencies: Agency for Toxic Substances and Disease
                         Registry
                     Centers for Disease Control and
                         Prevention
                     National Institutes of Health

Contents

Promote health for all through a healthy environment.

According to the World Health Organization, "In its broadest sense, environmental health comprises those aspects of human health, disease, and injury that are determined or influenced by factors in the environment. This includes the study of both the direct pathological effects of various chemical, physical, and biological agents, as well as the effects on health of the broad physical and social environment, which includes housing, urban development, land-use and transportation, industry, and agriculture."[1] The term "environment" also may be used to refer to air, water, and soil. This more narrow definition ignores the manmade environment created by a society. Where and how a society chooses to grow and develop affects the quality of life by determining how long people spend traveling to work, shopping, or going to school. Where and how a society builds its houses, schools, parks, and roadways can also limit the ability of some people to move about and lead a normal life.

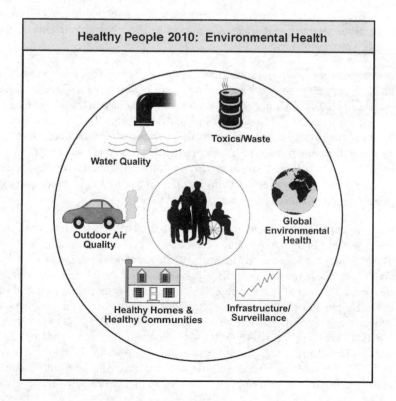

Healthy People 2010: Environmental Health

Water Quality

Toxics/Waste

Outdoor Air Quality

Global Environmental Health

Healthy Homes & Healthy Communities

Infrastructure/ Surveillance

Because the impact of the environment on human health is so great, protecting the environment has long been a mainstay of public health practice. National, State, and local efforts to ensure clean air and safe supplies of food and water, to manage sewage and municipal wastes, and to control or eliminate vector-borne illnesses have contributed a great deal to improvements in public health in the United States. Unfortunately, in spite of the billions of dollars spent to manage and clean up hazardous waste sites in the Nation each year, little money has been spent evaluating the health risks associated with chronic, low-level exposures to hazardous substances. This imbalance results in an inadequate amount of useful information to evaluate and manage these sites effectively and to evaluate the health status of people who live near the sites.[2] In the past, research in environmental epidemiology and toxicology has often been based on limited information. New knowledge about the interactions between specific genetic variations among individuals and specific environmental factors provides enormous opportunity for further developing modifications in environmental exposures that contribute to disease. Further research is needed to address these and other problems and to improve the science and management of health effects on people exposed to environmental hazards.[3]

Issues

Environmental factors play a central role in human development, health, and disease. Broadly defined, the environment, including infectious agents, is one of three primary factors that affect human health. The other two are genetic factors and personal behavior.

Human exposures to hazardous agents in the air, water, soil, and food and to physical hazards in the environment are major contributors to illness, disability, and death worldwide. Furthermore, deterioration of environmental conditions in many parts of the world slows sustainable development. Poor environmental quality is estimated to be directly responsible for approximately 25 percent of all preventable ill health in the world, with diarrheal diseases and respiratory infections heading the list.[4] Ill health resulting from poor environmental quality varies considerably among countries. Poor environmental quality has its greatest impact on people whose health status already may be at risk.

Because the effect of the environment on human health is so great, protecting the environment has been a mainstay of public health practice since 1878.[5] National, Tribal, State, and local efforts to ensure clean air and safe supplies of food and water, to manage sewage and municipal wastes, and to control or eliminate vector-borne illnesses have contributed significantly to improvements in public health in the United States. However, the public's awareness of the environment's role in health is more recent. Publication of Rachel Carson's *Silent Spring* in the early 1960s, followed by the well-publicized poor health of residents of Love Canal in western New York, a significant toxic waste site, awakened public consciousness to environmental issues. The result of these and other similar events is the so-called environmental movement that has led to the introduction into everyday life of such terms as Superfund sites, water quality, clean air, ozone, urban sprawl, and agricultural runoff.

In 1993 alone, over \$109 billion was spent on pollution abatement and control in the United States.[6] However, many hazardous sites still remain. Minimal research has been done to evaluate the health risks associated with chronic low-level exposures to hazardous substances, resulting in an inability to evaluate and manage such sites effectively and to evaluate the health status of residents living near such sites. Further environmental epidemiology and toxicology research is needed to address such problems and to improve the science and public health management of the health effects on people exposed to environmental hazards.

To address the broad range of human health issues affected by the environment, this chapter discusses six topics: outdoor air quality, water quality, toxics and waste, healthy homes and healthy communities, infrastructure and surveillance, and global environmental health issues.

Outdoor air quality. Air pollution continues to be a widespread public health and environmental problem in the United States, causing premature death, cancer, and long-term damage to respiratory and cardiovascular systems. Air pollution also reduces visibility, damages crops and buildings, and deposits pollutants on the soil and in bodies of water where they affect the chemistry of the water and the organisms living there. Approximately 113 million people live in U.S. areas designated as nonattainment areas by the U.S. Environmental Protection Agency (EPA) for one or more of the six commonly found air pollutants for which the Federal Government has established health-based standards.[7] The problem of air pollution is national—even international—in scope. Most of the U.S. population lives in expanding urban areas where air pollution crosses local and State lines and, in some cases, crosses U.S. borders with Canada and Mexico.[8, 9]

Although some progress toward reducing unhealthy air emissions has been made, a substantial air pollution problem remains, with millions of tons of toxic air pollutants released into the air each year.[10] The presence of unacceptable levels of ground-level ozone is the largest problem, as determined by the number of people affected and the number of areas not meeting Federal standards.

Motor vehicles account for approximately one-fourth of emissions that produce ozone and one-third of nitrogen oxide emissions. Particulate and sulfur dioxide emissions from motor vehicles represent approximately 20 percent and 4 percent, respectively. Some 76.6 percent of carbon monoxide emissions are produced each year by transportation sources (for example, motor vehicles).[7]

Unhealthy air is expensive. The estimated annual health costs of human exposure to all outdoor air pollutants from all sources range from \$40 billion to \$50 billion, with an associated 50,000 premature deaths.[11]

Water quality. Providing drinking water free of disease-causing agents, whether biological or chemical, is the primary goal of all water supply systems. During the first half of the 20th century the causes for most waterborne disease outbreaks were bacteria; beginning in the 1970s protozoa and chemicals became the dominant causes.[12] Most outbreaks involve only a few individuals.[13, 14, 15] In 1993, however, more than 403,000 people became sick during a single episode of waterborne cryptosporidiosis.[15]

One problem in evaluating the relationship between drinking water and infectious diseases is the lack of adequate technology to detect parasitic contamination and to determine whether the organisms detected are alive and infectious. The development of new molecular technologies to detect and monitor water contamination will enhance water quality monitoring and surveillance.

Contamination of water can come from both point (for example, industrial sites) and nonpoint (for example, agricultural runoff) sources. Biological and chemical contamination significantly reduces the value of surface waters (streams, lakes, and estuaries) for fishing, swimming, and other recreational activities. For example, during the summer of 1997, blooms of *Pfiesteria piscicida* were implicated as the likely cause of fish kills in North Carolina and Maryland. The development of intensive animal feeding operations has worsened the discharge of improperly or inadequately treated wastes,[16] which presents an increased health threat in waters used either for recreation or for producing fish and shellfish.

Toxics and waste. Critical information on the levels of exposure to hazardous substances in the environment and their associated health effects often is lacking. As a result, efficient health-outcome measures of progress in eliminating health hazards in the environment are unavailable. The identification of toxic substances and waste, whether hazardous, industrial, or municipal, that pose an environmental health risk represents a significant achievement in itself. Public health strategies are aimed at tracking the Nation's success in eliminating these substances or minimizing their effects.

Toxic and hazardous substances, including low-level radioactive wastes, deposited on land often are carried far from their sources by air, groundwater, and surface water runoff into streams, lakes, and rivers where they can accumulate in the sediments beneath the waters. Ultimate decisions about the cleanup and management of these sites must be made keeping public health concerns in mind.

The introduction and widespread use of pesticides in the American landscape continues in agricultural, commercial, recreational, and home settings. As a result, these often very toxic substances pose a potential threat to people using them, especially if they are handled, mixed, or applied inappropriately or excessively. Furthermore, children are at increased risk for pesticide poisoning because of their smaller size and because pesticides may be stored improperly or applied to surfaces that are more readily accessible by children.

Healthy homes and communities. The public's health, particularly its environmental health, depends on the interaction of many factors. To provide a healthy environment within the Nation's communities, the places people spend the most time—their homes, schools, and offices—must be considered. Potential risks include indoor air pollution; inadequate heating, cooling, and sanitation; structural problems; electrical and fire hazards; and lead-based paint hazards. More than 6 million housing units across the country meet the Federal Government's definition of substandard housing.[17]

Many factors—including air quality; lead-based paint on walls, trim, floors, ceilings, etc.; and hazardous household substances such as cleaning products and pesticides—can affect health and safety. In 1996, the American Association of Poison Control Centers reported more than 2 million poison exposures from 67 participating poison control centers. The site of exposure was a residence in 91 percent of cases.[18]

Infrastructure and surveillance. Preventing health problems caused by environmental hazards requires: (1) having enough personnel and resources to investigate and respond to diseases and injuries potentially caused by environmental hazards; (2) monitoring the population and its environment to detect hazards, exposure of the public and individuals to hazards, and diseases potentially caused by these hazards; (3) monitoring the population and its environment to assess the effectiveness of prevention programs; (4) educating the public and select populations on the relationship between health and the environment; (5) ensuring that laws, regulations, and practices protect the public and the environment from hazardous agents; (6) providing public access to understandable and useful information on hazards and their sources, distribution, and health effects; (7) coordinating the efforts of government agencies and nongovernmental groups responsible for environmental health; and (8) providing adequate resources to accomplish these tasks. Development of additional methods to measure environmental hazards in people will permit more careful assessments of exposures and health effects.

Global environmental health. Increased international travel and improvements in telecommunications and computer technology are making the world a smaller place. The term "global community" has real significance, as shared resources—air, water, and soil—draw people together. Actions in every country affect the environment and influence events around the world. Undoubtedly, the environment affects everyone's health. Sometimes benefits in one area inadvertently create worse conditions for people in different areas of the world. For example, in 1996, the United States exported more than $2.5 billion worth of pesticides.[19] Exported pesticides that are not registered, or pesticides that are restricted for use in the United States, are often used by developing countries. Their use not only endangers populations in those countries but also can contaminate food being exported from those countries to the United States. Sensitive populations, such as children and pregnant women, may be at risk from these environmental exposures. The United States can contribute to improving the health of people internationally, not only as part of a shared goal for humanity, but also because a healthy global population has positive social and economic benefits throughout the world.

Additionally, a number of countries have resources available to protect their populations from adverse health impacts, but because of inadequate information they are unable to do so. Lead abatement technology, for example, is one area where the United States can provide information to other countries. Likewise, consultation and assistance on numerous environmental health issues from lead poisoning to disaster preparedness will help reduce illness, disability, and death in countries with these problems, which can lead to a healthier global community.

The Nation should expand its efforts for improving environmental conditions to enhance the health of developing countries. It should also increase collaboration, coordination, and outreach efforts with the rest of the world to help close the gap between existing and attainable health status.

Trends

During the 1990s, progress in improving environmental health was mixed. The decline in childhood lead poisoning in the United States represents a public health success. In 1984, between 2 million and 3 million children aged 6 months to 5 years had blood lead levels (BLLs) greater than 15 µg/dL, and almost a quarter of a million had BLLs above 25 µg/dL,[20] a level that can affect vital organs and the brain. (Blood levels are measured in micrograms of lead found in a deciliter of blood.) By the early 1990s, fewer than 900,000 children had BLLs above 10µg/dL, the current standard for identifying children at risk.[21] This dramatic reduction is the result of research to identify persons at risk, professional and public education campaigns to "spread the word," broad-based screening measures to find those at risk, and effective community efforts to clean up problem areas, namely, substandard housing units. However, despite the success achieved, more remains to be done before childhood lead poisoning becomes a disease of the past. Although childhood lead poisoning occurred in all population groups, the risk was higher for persons having low income, living in older housing, and belonging to certain racial and ethnic groups. For example, among non-Hispanic black children living in homes built before 1946, 22 percent had elevated BBLs. Because the risk for lead poisoning is not spread evenly throughout the population, efforts are continuing to identify children at risk and ensure that they receive preventive interventions.[22]

Unfortunately, not all trends for environmental health issues are as encouraging. Since the mid-1980s, asthma rates in the United States have risen to the level of an epidemic.[23] Asthma and other respiratory conditions often are triggered or worsened by substances found in the air, such as tobacco smoke, ozone, and other particles or chemicals. Based on existing data, an estimated 14.9 million people in the United States had asthma in 1995,[24] including more than 5 million children aged 17 years and under.[25] Between 1980 and 1993, the overall death rate for asthma increased 57 percent, from 12.8 to 20.1 deaths per million population;[23]

for people aged 17 years and under, the death rate increased 67 percent, from 1.8 to 3.0 deaths per million population.[26] The direct economic and health care costs of asthma and other respiratory conditions can be large. In 1990, the estimated total cost of asthma was $6.2 billion; the total cost was projected to rise to $14.5 billion by the year 2000.[27] The indirect costs of asthma, measured in reduced quality of life and lost productivity, include the estimated 10 million school days each year that children miss. Lost productivity from missed work days of parents caring for children with asthma is estimated to be $1 billion—not including the cost of lost productivity from adults with asthma who miss work.[27] (See Focus Area 24. Respiratory Diseases.)

Although successes in environmental public health are possible, they are difficult to achieve. Infectious and chemical agents still contaminate food and water. Animals continue to carry diseases to human populations, and outbreaks of once-common intestinal diseases (for example, typhoid fever), although less frequent, still occur. (See Focus Area 10. Food Safety.) These outbreaks underscore the need to maintain and improve programs developed in the first half of the 20th century to ensure the safety of food and water. The challenge is to retain these basic capacities in the 21st century, with the added responsibilities for dealing with emerging hazards. The control of well-known hazards must coexist with ongoing research and the development of strategies and methods to understand and control new hazards. Another challenge is the need to help the public understand the link between human activity and the destruction of the environment.

Within the United States, significant strides toward a reduction in harmful air emissions can be achieved by individuals choosing not to drive their cars. People need to use public transit, walk, or bicycle more often. Laws can help improve street and highway design to facilitate pedestrians and bicyclists, and employers can embrace telecommuting, but the choice remains with the individual. Encouraging individuals to walk or bike also may play a role in reducing the problems of obesity and overweight individuals, which have risen to alarming levels in the U.S. population.

Urban sprawl has become an increasingly important concern in the United States for several reasons: increased outdoor air pollution in major urban areas, reduced quality of life due to the loss of free time and the stress of increased commuting time, and less green space in major metropolitan areas. Between 1983 and 1995, the average annual vehicle miles traveled increased 80 percent.[28] These conditions lead to negative health conditions, such as asthma and injuries from road rage due to traffic-related stress.[29] In addition, sprawl diminishes the amount of land available for prime recreational and agricultural uses and can bring two land uses together that do not coexist well. For example, a residential development in an area that was previously agricultural may expose residents to environmental hazards, such as pesticides, which may pose a threat to their health.

On a global scale, the U.S.-Mexico border area illustrates how human activity can contribute to damaging the environment, affecting generations to come. Over the past 30 years, this region has experienced a dramatic surge in population and industrialization. The region has had great difficulty in supporting this growth and suffers from a lack of resources and expertise to manage solid waste properly, handle and store pesticides and other hazardous materials, supply sufficient drinking water, and support other sustainable development efforts.[8] Nations need to make choices about how to deal with such regions; offering technical assistance is an option to speed knowledge transfer and reduce environmental harm.

Disparities

Studies have linked race and socioeconomic status to increased exposure to environmental hazards, and information about gene-environment interactions improves the ability to determine who has increased risk of disease from these exposures. Table 8-A and Table 8-B summarize some inequities in the United States regarding exposure to selected potential environmental hazards.

Table 8-A. Proportions of African American, Hispanic, and white populations living in air-quality nonattainment areas, 1992.[30]

| Pollutant | Demographic Breakdowns | | |
| | African Americans | Hispanics | Whites |
	Percent Living in Air-Quality Nonattainment Areas		
Particulates	16.5	34.0	14.7
Carbon monoxide	46.0	57.1	33.6
Ozone	62.2	71.2	52.5
Sulfur dioxide	12.1	5.7	7.0
Lead	9.2	18.5	6.0

Table 8-B. Proportions of certain racial and ethnic and lower socioeconomic populations in census tracts surrounding waste treatment, storage, and disposal facilities (TSDF) compared with the proportions of these groups in other census tracts, 1994.[30]

| Location of TSDFs | Demographic Breakdowns | | |
| | African Americans | Hispanics | Persons Living Below the Poverty Line |
	Percent		
Census tracts with either TSDFs or at least 50 percent of their area within 2.5 miles of a tract with TSDF	24.7	10.7	19.0
Census tracts without TSDFs	13.6	7.3	13.1

Disparities exist in the environmental exposures certain populations face and in the health status of these populations. For example, in New York City, African American, Hispanic, and low-income populations have been found to have hospitalization and death rates from asthma three to five times higher than those for all New York City residents. African American children have been found to be three times more likely than white children to be hospitalized for asthma and asthma-related conditions and four to six times more likely to die from asthma.[30] (See Focus Area 24. Respiratory Diseases.) With respect to BLL, children from certain racial and ethnic groups are disproportionately affected. While there are no studies to show rural and frontier dwellers are at increased risk to exposure to contaminated drinking water, the preponderance of this population depends on unregulated private wells for their drinking water. The U.S. Geological Survey (USGS) reports that 42.8 million persons in the United States (17 percent of the total population) were served by their own (self-supplied) water systems in 1990.[31]

Opportunities

An increase in public awareness of environmental health issues is key to achieving this chapter's goal and objectives. Education—at all levels—is a cornerstone of broad prevention efforts.

Improving the availability of environmental health data also will help meet the objectives. The Internet has increased dramatically access to environmental information. Databases such as TOXNET (at http://toxnet.nlm.nih.gov/),[32] Internet Grateful Med (at http://igm.nlm.nih.gov),[33] and TRI (the Toxics Release Inventory www.epa.gov/ceisweb1/ceishome/ceisdata/xplor-tri/explorer.htm) may provide useful information about environmental hazards or other environmental problems in communities to health care providers, policymakers, and the public. Moreover, better dissemination of global environmental health information may reduce the occurrence of disease or exposure to harmful environmental agents for U.S. citizens traveling abroad.

To be successful, programs to improve environmental health must be based on scientific evidence. The complex relationship between human health and the acute and long-term effects of environmental exposures must be studied so prevention measures can be developed. Surveillance systems to track exposures to toxic substances such as commonly used pesticides and heavy metals must be developed and maintained. To the extent possible, these systems should use biomonitoring data, which provide measurements of toxic substances in the human body. A mechanism is needed for tracking the export of pesticides restricted or not registered for use in the United States.

Environmental hazards are not limited by political boundaries. The scope of public and environmental health must be global if the Nation is to achieve good health for all persons in the United States. A global scope will help develop and achieve effective ways to prevent disease worldwide as well. The United States must work with other governments, nongovernmental organizations, and international organizations to help improve human health on a global scale.

Interim Progress Toward Year 2000 Objectives

Healthy People 2000 targets have been met for objectives dealing with outbreaks of waterborne diseases, with solid wastes, and with toxic substances released through industrial processes. Substantial progress has been made in objectives involving the proportion of people who live in counties that meet EPA air standards for air pollution, the number of States that require radon disclosures with real estate transactions, and the recycling of household hazardous waste. More moderate progress has taken place for the objectives involving radon and lead-based paint testing in homes, asthma hospitalizations, and States with laws to track environmental diseases. Mixed progress or movement away from the targets is being seen in objectives dealing with mental retardation and impaired surface waters (rivers, lakes, and estuaries). Data have been mixed or difficult to assess for the cleanup of hazardous waste sites. The target for blood lead levels in children has not been met, though some progress has been made.

Note: Unless otherwise noted, data are from the Centers for Disease Control and Prevention, National Center for Health Statistics, *Healthy People 2000 Review, 1998–99*.

Environmental Health

Goal: Promote health for all through a healthy environment.

Number   Objective Short Title

Outdoor Air Quality

8-1   Harmful air pollutants

8-2   Alternative modes of transportation

8-3   Cleaner alternative fuels

8-4   Airborne toxins

Water Quality

8-5   Safe drinking water

8-6   Waterborne disease outbreaks

8-7   Water conservation

8-8   Surface water health risks

8-9   Beach closings

8-10   Fish contamination

Toxics and Waste

8-11   Elevated blood lead levels in children

8-12   Risks posed by hazardous sites

8-13   Pesticide exposures

8-14   Toxic pollutants

8-15   Recycled municipal solid waste

Healthy Homes and Healthy Communities

8-16   Indoor allergens

8-17   Office building air quality

8-18   Homes tested for radon

8-19   Radon-resistant new home construction

8-20   School policies to protect against environmental hazards

8-21   Disaster preparedness plans and protocols

8-22   Lead-based paint testing

8-23   Substandard housing

Number	Objective Short Title

Infrastructure and Surveillance

8-24	Exposure to pesticides
8-25	Exposure to heavy metals and other toxic chemicals
8-26	Information systems used for environmental health
8-27	Monitoring environmentally related diseases
8-28	Local agencies using surveillance data for vector control

Global Environmental Health

8-29	Global burden of disease
8-30	Water quality in the U.S.–Mexico border region

Outdoor Air Quality

8-1. **Reduce the proportion of persons exposed to air that does not meet the U.S. Environmental Protection Agency's health-based standards for harmful air pollutants.**

Target and baseline:

Objective	Reduction in Air Pollutants	1997 Baseline	2010 Target
		Percent	
8-1a.	Ozone*	43	0
8-1b.	Particulate matter*	12	0
8-1c.	Carbon monoxide	19	0
8-1d.	Nitrogen dioxide	5	0
8-1e.	Sulfur dioxide	2	0
8-1f.	Lead	<1	0
		Number	
8-1g.	Total number of people	119,803,000	0

*The targets of zero percent for ozone and particulate matter are set for 2012 and 2018, respectively.

Target setting method: Consistent with the Clean Air Act (Public Law 101-549).

Data source: Aerometric Information Retrieval System (AIRS), EPA, OAR.

Note: For the purpose of this objective, EPA is counting persons living in nonattainment areas only.

Data for population groups currently are not analyzed.

Historically, EPA's air quality monitoring and National Ambient Air Quality Standards data collection have taken place in large urban centers and other areas generally considered to have the Nation's poorest air quality. As nonattainment areas become attainment areas, EPA will continue its monitoring efforts. (See Focus Area 24. Respiratory Diseases.)

8-2. Increase use of alternative modes of transportation to reduce motor vehicle emissions and improve the Nation's air quality.

Target and baseline:

Objective	Increase in Use of Alternative Modes of Transportation	1995 Baseline	2010 Target
		Percent	
8-2a.	Trips made by bicycling	0.9	1.8
8-2b.	Trips made by walking	5.4	10.8
8-2c.	Trips made by transit	1.8	3.6
8-2d.	Persons who telecommute	Developmental	

Target setting method: Consistent with the goal of the National Bicycling and Walking Study, U.S. Department of Transportation (DOT).

Data source: Nationwide Personal Transportation Survey (NPTS), U.S. Department of Transportation.

For many communities in the United States, motor vehicle emissions are the primary cause of air pollution. Increasing use of alternative modes of transportation is a comprehensive approach that each citizen can take to affect local levels of air pollution. An increase in neighborhood streets with ways to slow traffic and with more sidewalks and bike lanes, offroad pedestrian or bike routes, and bicycle and pedestrian plans and programs will aid in reaching the targets for biking, walking, and transit objectives. (See Focus Area 22. Physical Activity and Fitness.) As technology improves, telecommuting will play an increasing role in U.S. business. Many people will be able to do some or all of their work from home, thus reducing peak-period demand for transportation.

8-3. Improve the Nation's air quality by increasing the use of cleaner alternative fuels.

Target: 30 percent.

Baseline: Cleaner alternative fuels represented 2.7 percent of U.S. motor fuel consumption in 1997.

Target setting method: 10-fold improvement.

Data source: Alternatives to Traditional Transportation Fuels, U.S. Department of Energy, Energy Information Administration.

Privately owned cars, vans, and trucks; commercial fleets, trucks, and buses; and power plants are the major users of alternative fuels. Ethanol-blended fuels have been used in small engines and other nonautomotive gasoline engines since the fuels first came into the marketplace over 25 years ago. Today, all mainstream manufacturers of power equipment, motorcycles, snowmobiles, and outboard motors permit the use of ethanol blends in their products.

The primary force behind development of an alternative fuels infrastructure is the U.S. Department of Energy Clean Cities Program—a voluntary program and locally based government and industry partnership designed to promote the use of alternative fuels and alternative fuel vehicles, cleaner air in major U.S. cities, reduced dependence on imported oil, and stimulate local economic activity.[34]

Infrastructure building also is aided by development of alternative fuel vehicles by the major automobile manufacturers. Also, ethanol blends of up to 10 percent are approved under the warranties of all major auto manufacturers, domestic and foreign, marketing vehicles in the United States. In fact, some recommend the use of cleaner-burning fuels such as ethanol in their vehicle owner manuals because of ethanol's clean air benefits. Ethanol actually can enhance engine performance by increasing octane and raising oxygen, cleaning and preventing engine deposits, and acting as a gas-line antifreeze.[35]

More than a trillion miles have been driven on ethanol-blended gasolines, and ethanol-blended fuels represent more than 12 percent of U.S. motor gasoline sales. Congress established the Federal ethanol program in 1979 to stimulate rural economies and reduce the Nation's alarming dependence on imported oil through the production of a domestic, renewable energy source. The program has helped build a strong domestic energy industry. From just over 10 million gallons of production in 1979, the U.S. fuel ethanol industry has grown to more than 1.8 billion gallons of annual production capacity. Ethanol is marketed widely across the country as a high-quality octane enhancer and as an oxygenate capable of reducing air pollution and improving automobile performance.

8-4. Reduce air toxic emissions to decrease the risk of adverse health effects caused by airborne toxics.

Target: 2.0 million tons.

Baseline: 8.1 million tons of air toxics were released into the air in 1993.

Target setting method: 75 percent improvement.

Data source: U.S National Toxics Inventory, EPA.

Toxic air pollutants are those pollutants known or suspected to cause cancer or other serious health effects, such as reproductive effects or birth defects, or to cause adverse environmental effects. The degree to which a toxic air pollutant affects a person's health depends on many factors, including the quantity of pollutant the person is exposed to, the duration and frequency of exposures, the toxicity of the chemical, and the person's state of health and susceptibility. Examples of toxic air pollutants include benzene, which is found in gasoline; perchloroethylene, which is emitted from some dry cleaning facilities; and methylene chloride, which is used as a solvent and paint stripper by a number of industries.

Examples of other listed air toxics include dioxin, asbestos, toluene, and metals such as cadmium, mercury, chromium, and lead compounds.

Scientists estimate that millions of tons of toxic pollutants are released into the air each year. Some air toxics are released from natural sources such as volcanic eruptions and forest fires. Most, however, originate from manmade sources, including both mobile sources (for example, cars, buses, trucks) and stationary sources (for example, factories, refineries, power plants). Emissions from stationary sources constitute almost two-thirds of all manmade air toxics emissions. (See Focus Area 24. Respiratory Diseases.)

Water Quality

8-5. Increase the proportion of persons served by community water systems who receive a supply of drinking water that meets the regulations of the Safe Drinking Water Act.

Target: 95 percent.

Baseline: 85 percent of persons served by community water systems received drinking water that met SDWA (Public Law 93-523) regulations in 1995.

Target setting method: Consistent with EPA's strategic plan.

Data sources: Potable Water Surveillance System (PWSS) and Safe Drinking Water Information System (SDWIS), EPA.

Most people in the United States obtain their drinking water from public water supply systems. EPA has established regulations intended to ensure that community water systems supply safe drinking water to their customers. Compliance with the established regulations is one measure of the public's receipt of a safe water supply, free from disease-causing agents. In 1997, small systems (serving 25 to 3,300 people) accounted for more than 85 percent of the community water systems in the United States but served only about 10 percent of the population. These systems accounted for 91 percent of the violations of the EPA drinking water regulations.[36] According to USGS, 17 percent of the Nation's total population were served by their own water supply systems in 1990, compared with 18 percent in 1985.[31]

8-6. Reduce waterborne disease outbreaks arising from water intended for drinking among persons served by community water systems.

Target: 2 outbreaks.

Baseline: 6 outbreaks per year originated from community water systems (1987–96 average).

Target setting method: 67 percent improvement.

Data source: State Reporting Systems, CDC, NCID.

The Centers for Disease Control and Prevention (CDC) compiles the results of State investigations into waterborne disease outbreaks arising from water intended for drinking. Between 1987 and 1996, the States reported an average of 15.5 outbreaks per year, of which 6 outbreaks were identified as originating from community water supplies.[13, 14, 15] Limited existing data suggest that State and CDC surveillance systems for detecting waterborne disease outbreaks are able to detect most waterborne disease outbreaks.

8-7. Reduce per capita domestic water withdrawals.

Target: 90.9 gallons.

Baseline: 101 gallons of domestic water per capita per day were withdrawn in 1995.

Target setting method: 10 percent improvement.

Data source: U.S. Department of Interior, U.S. Geological Survey (USGS).

Historically, water management in the United States has focused on directing the country's abundant supplies of fresh water to meet the needs of users. This approach has resulted in the building of large storage reservoirs and conveyance systems, especially in the West. Increasing development costs, capital shortages, government fiscal restraint, diminishing sources of water supply, polluted water, and a growing concern for the environment have forced water managers and planners to begin to rethink traditional approaches to management and to experiment with new ones. Experts on the subject of water supply and demand agree that the West is in transition from the era of water-supply development to an era of water-demand management and conservation. As the population increases in the Eastern United States, the water quantity problems already facing the West will become apparent there as well. Estimates place the amount of water withdrawn for public supply during 1990 at about 5 percent more than during 1985.[31] Public-supply domestic deliveries averaged 105 gallons per day for each person served, the same as during 1985.[31] The per capita use remained about the same for the past decade as the result of active conservation programs that include the installation of additional meters and water-conserving plumbing fixtures.[31] Information about water use is available from USGS at http://water.usgs.gov/watuse/wudo.html.[37]

8-8. (Developmental) Increase the proportion of assessed rivers, lakes, and estuaries that are safe for fishing and recreational purposes.

Potential data source: Clean Water Act (Public Law 92-500), Section 305-b Report, EPA.

EPA reported that about 40 percent of the Nation's surface waters (streams, lakes, and estuaries) are too polluted for fishing, swimming, or other uses designated for them by States and Tribes.[38] Water quality in lakes, streams, and estuaries of the United States affects both the recreational and food production use of these waters. States and Tribes have water-quality management programs that address recreational use and fish and shellfish harvesting. EPA establishes water-quality objectives for these waters and monitors progress toward these goals. Discharging inadequately treated or inappropriate quantities of human, industrial, or agriculture wastes reduces the ability of water to provide conditions that support the growth and harvesting of fish and shellfish for human consumption. Such discharging also prevents water's use as a recreational resource.

8-9.   (Developmental) Reduce the number of beach closings that result from the presence of harmful bacteria.

Potential data source: EPA Beach Program.

During the first half of the decade, EPA plans to focus on conserving and enhancing the Nation's waters and aquatic ecosystems so that 75 percent of waters will support healthy aquatic communities.[39] Part of this effort will include developing a national beach-closing survey to monitor efforts to improve the quality of water used for recreational purposes. Although small streams, private lakes, and ponds will not be addressed by the EPA beach-closing survey (available at http://www.epa.gov/ost/beaches), this program will provide a method to evaluate progress toward improving water quality on U.S. swimming beaches. Information from the 1997 and 1998 EPA surveys has been expanded on by the Natural Resources Defense Council (NRDC) and published in its annual beach-closing report. The latest version is available from NRDC and on its Web site (http://www.nrdc.org).

8-10.   (Developmental) Reduce the potential human exposure to persistent chemicals by decreasing fish contaminant levels.

Potential data sources: U.S. Department of the Interior, U.S. Fish and Wildlife Service and USGS.

The Biomonitoring of Environmental Status and Trends (BEST) program (http://www.best.usgs.gov) is a cooperative activity of the USGS and the U.S. Fish and Wildlife Service. Designed to assess and monitor the effects of environmental contaminants on biological resources, the program measures 51 organochlorine persistent chemicals, organophosphate and carbamate insecticides, and 21 metals.

8-11. Eliminate elevated blood lead levels in children.

Target: Zero percent.

Baseline: 4.4 percent of children aged 1 to 6 years had blood lead levels exceeding 10 µg/dL during 1991–94.

Target setting method: Total elimination.

Data source: National Health and Nutrition Examination Survey (NHANES), CDC, NCHS.

NOTE: THE TABLE BELOW MAY CONTINUE TO THE FOLLOWING PAGE.

Children Aged 1 to 6 Years, 1991–94	Children With Blood Lead Levels Greater Than or Equal to 10 µg/dL			
	8-11. Residing in All Housing	Residing in Housing Built:		
		Before 1946*	1946 to 1973*	After 1973*
	Percent			
TOTAL	4.4	8.6	4.6	1.6
Race and ethnicity				
American Indian or Alaska Native	DSU	DSU	DSU	DSU
Asian or Pacific Islander	DSU	DSU	DSU	DSU
Asian	DNC	DNC	DNC	DNC
Native Hawaiian and other Pacific Islander	DNC	DNC	DNC	DNC
Black or African American	11.5	22.7	13.2	3.3
White	2.6	6.6	1.9	1.4
Hispanic or Latino	DSU	DSU	DSU	DSU
Mexican American	4.0	13.0	2.3	1.6
Not Hispanic or Latino	4.2	DNA	DNA	DNA
Black or African American	11.2	21.9	13.7	3.4
White	2.3	5.6	1.4	1.5
Gender				
Female	3.3	7.1	2.8	1.5
Male	5.5	9.6	6.6	1.7
Family income level[†]				
Low	1.9	4.1	2.0	0.4
High	1.0	0.9	2.7	0

Children Aged 1 to 6 Years, 1991–94	Children With Blood Lead Levels Greater Than or Equal to 10 µg/dL			
	8-11. Resid-ing in All Housing	Residing in Housing Built:		
		Before 1946*	1946 to 1973*	After 1973*
	Percent			
Geographic location				
Population ≥ 1 million	5.4	11.5	5.8	0.8
Population < 1 million	3.3	5.8	3.1	2.5

DNA = Data have not been analyzed. DNC = Data are not collected. DSU = Data are statistically unreliable.

*Data for "all houses" are from a separate analysis of NHANES data; data for specific periods of time provided for information purposes.

†Income categories defined using poverty-income ratio (PIR) (the ratio of total family income to the poverty threshold for the year). Low equals PIR ≤1.300; middle equals PIR 1.301 – 3.500; high equals PIR ≥3.501.

NOTE: THE TABLE ABOVE MAY HAVE CONTINUED FROM THE PREVIOUS PAGE.

Although considerable progress has been made in reducing BLLs in the Nation's children, lead poisoning remains a preventable environmental health problem in the United States. Culturally and linguistically appropriate information is needed alerting persons to the dangers of lead poisonings.

8-12. Minimize the risks to human health and the environment posed by hazardous sites.

Target: 98 percent of sites on the following lists:

8-12a.   National Priority List sites

8-12b.   Resource Conservation and Recovery Act facilities

8-12c.   Leaking underground storage facilities

8-12d.   Brownfield properties

Baseline: 1,200 National Priority List sites; 2,475 Resource Conservation and Recovery Act facilities; 370,000 leaking underground storage facilities; 1,500 brownfield properties in 1998.

Target setting method: Consistent with EPA's 1997 Strategic Plan.

Data source: Comprehensive Environmental Response and Cleanup Liability Information System (CERCLIS), EPA, OSWER.

The National Priorities List (NPL) is a published list of the most hazardous waste sites in the country eligible for extensive, long-term cleanup under the Superfund program. Sites listed on the NPL often are initially discovered by local or State agencies, businesses, EPA, the Coast Guard, or the public. If a site poses a significant risk to human health, as determined by the number and toxicity of substances discovered at the site and its capacity to affect surrounding populations, then the site is placed on the NPL. The Agency for Toxic Substances and Disease Registry (ATSDR) is the Federal health agency that issues recommendations to EPA, State health and environmental agencies, and the public concerning the elimination of public health threats at these sites. This advice often also includes recommendations to the public and the health care community concerning practices to identify and prevent exposures and adverse health effects.

The Resource Conservation and Recovery Act (RCRA) was enacted by Congress in 1976 to find a safe way to manage and dispose of the huge volumes of municipal and industrial waste generated nationwide. RCRA facilities are authorized and regulated by this act. With several amendments, the act and its subsequent regulations govern the management of nonhazardous (solid) waste, hazardous waste, and underground storage tanks (USTs). The Leaking Underground Storage Tanks Program attempts to identify and eliminate the threat to human health posed by groundwater or soil contamination from petroleum released from these tanks. The term "brownfields" denotes abandoned, idle, or underused industrial or commercial sites where expansion or redevelopment is complicated by real or perceived environmental contamination.

8-13. Reduce pesticide exposures that result in visits to a health care facility.

Target: 13,500 visits per year.

Baseline: 27,156 visits to health care facilities were due to pesticides in 1997. (A total of 129,592 pesticide exposures were documented in 1997.)

Target setting method: 50 percent improvement.

Data source: Toxic Exposure Surveillance System (TESS), American Association of Poison Control Centers.

Pesticide exposures include those involving disinfectants, fungicides, herbicides, insecticides, moth repellants, and rodenticides, as defined by EPA. The American Association of Poison Control Centers surveillance covers approximately 93 percent of the U.S. population.

8-14. (Developmental) Reduce the amount of toxic pollutants released, disposed of, treated, or used for energy recovery.

Potential data source: Toxics Release Inventory (TRI), EPA.

Reductions in toxic pollutants released, disposed of, treated, or used for energy recovery can be measured by industry's success in reducing pollution at the source—that is, not producing pollutants at all, through manufacturing process changes, shifting to less polluting ingredients, packaging changes, and other source reduction methods. For that reason, all pollutants, those released and those treated or disposed of in some manner, should be measured.

8-15. Increase recycling of municipal solid waste.

Target: 38 percent.

Baseline: 27 percent of total municipal solid waste generated was recycled in 1996 (includes composting).

Target setting method: Consistent with the EPA's 1997 Strategic Plan.

Data source: Characterization of Municipal Solid Waste, EPA.

Healthy Homes and Healthy Communities

8-16. Reduce indoor allergen levels.

Target and baseline:

Objective	Allergen	1998–99 Baseline	2010 Target
		Number of Homes (in millions)	
8-16a.	Group I dust mite allergens that exceed 2 micrograms per gram of dust in the bed	36.3	29.0
8-16b.	Group I dust mite allergens that exceed 10 micrograms per gram of dust in the bed	18.6	14.9
8-16c.	German cockroach allergens that exceed 0.1 microgram per gram of dust in the bed	4.7	3.8

Target setting method: 20 percent improvement.

Data source: National Survey of Lead and Allergens in Housing, NIEHS, and U.S. Department of Housing and Urban Development.

Indoor allergens—such as from house dust mites, cockroaches, mold, rodents, and pets—can worsen symptoms of respiratory conditions, such as asthma and allergies. These allergens are an important public health issue because most people spend the majority of their time indoors, both at home and at work. In addition, effective methods to reduce exposure to some of these allergens exist (for example, placement of impermeable covers on mattresses and pillows reduces dust mite allergen exposures in beds). (See Focus Area 24. Respiratory Diseases.)

8-17. (Developmental) Increase the number of office buildings that are managed using good indoor air quality practices.

Potential data source: Indoor Environment Division, EPA.

Healthy People 2010: Objectives for Improving Health

The air quality inside a building impacts both the comfort and health of its occupants. Pollutants are found at higher levels in indoor air as compared to outdoor air. In addition, most people spend over 90 percent of their time indoors.[40]

8-18. Increase the proportion of persons who live in homes tested for radon concentrations.

Target: 20 percent.

Baseline: 17 percent of the population lived in homes in 1998 that had been tested for radon (age adjusted to the year 2000 standard population).

Target setting method: Better than the best.

Data source: National Health Interview Survey (NHIS), CDC, NCHS.

Total Population, 1998	Persons Living in Homes Tested for Radon
	Percent
TOTAL	17
Race and ethnicity	
American Indian or Alaska Native	19
Asian or Pacific Islander	17
Asian	17
Native Hawaiian and other Pacific Islander	17
Black or African American	18
White	17
Hispanic or Latino	14
Not Hispanic or Latino	17
Black or African American	18
White	17
Gender	
Female	17
Male	17
Family income level	
Poor	15
Near poor	12
Middle/high income	18

DNA = Data have not been analyzed. DNC = Data are not collected. DSU = Data are statistically unreliable.
Note: Age adjusted to the year 2000 standard population.

8-19. Increase the number of new homes constructed to be radon resistant.

Target: 2.1 million additional new homes.

Baseline: 1.4 million new homes as of 1997.

Target setting method: 50 percent improvement.

Data source: National Association of Home Builders Research Center Survey, National Association of Home Builders.

8-20. (Developmental) Increase the proportion of the Nation's primary and secondary schools that have official school policies ensuring the safety of students and staff from environmental hazards, such as chemicals in special classrooms, poor indoor air quality, asbestos, and exposure to pesticides.

Potential data source: School Health Policies and Programs Study (SHPPS), CDC, NCCDPHP.

8-21. (Developmental) Ensure that State health departments establish training, plans, and protocols and conduct annual multi-institutional exercises to prepare for response to natural and technological disasters.

Potential data sources: Association of State and Territorial Health Officials (ASTHO); Public Health Foundation.

8-22. Increase the proportion of persons living in pre-1950s housing that has been tested for the presence of lead-based paint.

Target: 50 percent.

Baseline: 16 percent of persons living in homes built before 1950 in 1998 reported that their homes had been tested for the presence of lead-based paint (age adjusted to the year 2000 standard population).

Target setting method: Better than the best.

Data source: National Health Interview Survey (NHIS), CDC, NCHS.

Healthy People 2010: Objectives for Improving Health

Persons Living in Pre-1950s Housing, 1998	Persons Living in Homes Tested for Lead-Based Paint
	Percent
TOTAL	16
Race and ethnicity	
American Indian or Alaska Native	DSU
Asian or Pacific Islander	13
Asian	11
Native Hawaiian and other Pacific Islander	24
Black or African American	22
White	14
Hispanic or Latino	14
Not Hispanic or Latino	16
Black or African American	23
White	15
Gender	
Female	17
Male	15
Family income level	
Poor	19
Near poor	16
Middle/high income	15

DNA = Data have not been analyzed. DNC = Data are not collected. DSU = Data are statistically unreliable.
Note: Age adjusted to the year 2000 standard population.

8-23. Reduce the proportion of occupied housing units that are substandard.

Target: 3 percent.

Baseline: 6.2 percent of occupied U.S. housing units had moderate or severe physical problems in 1995.

Target setting method: 52 percent improvement.

Data source: American Housing Survey, U.S. Department of Commerce, Bureau of the Census.

Residents of substandard housing are at increased risk for fire, electrical injuries, lead poisoning, falls, rat bites, and other illnesses and injuries.

8-24. Reduce exposure to pesticides as measured by urine concentrations of metabolites.

Target and baseline:

Objective	Reduction in Pesticide Exposure as Measured by Metabolites (Pesticide)	1988–94 Baseline*	2010 Target
		Urine Concentration	
8-24a.	1-naphthol (carbaryl)	36.0 µg/g creatinine	25.2 µg/g creatinine
8-24b.	Paranitrophenol (methyl parathion and parathions)	3.8 µg/g creatinine	2.7 µg/g creatinine
8-24c.	3, 5, 6-trichloro-2-pyridinol (chlorpyrifos)	8.3 µg/g creatinine	5.8 µg/g creatinine
8-24d.	Isopropoxyphenol (propoxur)	1.6 µg/g creatinine	1.1 µg/g creatinine

*95 percent of the population had concentrations below this level.

Target setting method: 30 percent improvement.

Data source: National Health and Nutrition Examination Survey (NHANES), CDC, NCHS.

Note: Data are from a subset of NHANES data and are not nationally representative. Therefore, a population data template is not available.

Pesticides included in the table inhibit cholinesterase, an enzyme found in the human body. These pesticides are among those commonly used in the home and garden, agriculture, and industry.[41] Metabolites (or breakdown products) of pesticides are measured in urine samples obtained from persons aged 6 years and older. Urinary measurements of pesticide metabolites are an accurate way to measure recent exposure to pesticides that inhibit cholinesterase. Concentrations of pesticide metabolites in urine are corrected for kidney function and expressed in µg/g creatinine, a measure of kidney function.

8-25. (Developmental) Reduce exposure of the population to pesticides, heavy metals, and other toxic chemicals, as measured by blood and urine concentrations of the substances or their metabolites.

Objective	Exposure Item
	Heavy metals
8-25a.	Arsenic
8-25b.	Cadmium

8-25c.	Lead
8-25d.	Manganese
8-25e.	Mercury
	Pesticides
8-25f.	2, 4-D
8-25g.	o-phenylphenol
8-25h.	Permethrins
8-25i.	Diazinon
	Persistent chemicals
8-25j.	Polychlorinated biphenyls
8-25k.	Dioxins
8-25l.	Furans
	Organochlorine compounds
8-25m.	Chlordane
8-25n.	Dieldrin
8-25o.	DDT
8-25p.	Lindane

Potential data source: National Health and Nutrition Examination Survey (NHANES), CDC, NCHS.

Heavy metals, polychlorinated biphenyls (PCBs), dioxins, furans, and organochlorines are in use or have been used in the past. These compounds are known or suspected causes of cancer, birth defects, or other diseases in people.

8-26. (Developmental) Improve the quality, utility, awareness, and use of existing information systems for environmental health.

Potential data sources: Toxics Release Inventory, EPA; Environmental Defense Fund.

Other environmental health information systems include TOXLINE, Integrated Risk Information System (IRIS), Registry of Toxic Effects of Chemical Substances (RTECS®), HazDat, and Aerometric Information Retrieval System (AIRS). They can be accessed via the Internet.

8-27. Increase or maintain the number of Territories, Tribes, and States, and the District of Columbia that monitor diseases or conditions that can be caused by exposure to environmental hazards.

Target and baseline:

Objective	Disease	1997 Baseline	2010 Target
		Number of Jurisdictions	
8-27a.	Lead poisoning	51	51
8-27b.	Pesticide poisoning	20	25
8-27c.	Mercury poisoning	14	20
8-27d.	Arsenic poisoning	10	15
8-27e.	Cadmium poisoning	10	15
8-27f.	Methemoglobinemia	9	15
8-27g.	Acute chemical poisoning*	8	15
8-27h.	Carbon monoxide poisoning	7	51
8-27i.	Asthma	6	25
8-27j.	Hyperthermia	4	10
8-27k.	Hypothermia	Developmental	
8-27l.	Skin cancer	Developmental	
8-27m.	Malignant melanoma	Developmental	
8-27n.	Other skin cancer	Developmental	
8-27o.	Birth defects	Developmental	

*Includes chemicals not covered elsewhere in the table.

Note: Target and baseline data are for States and the District of Columbia. The targets will be adjusted as data for Tribes and Territories become available.

Target setting method: Total coverage or expert opinion.

Data sources: Periodic surveys, Public Health Foundation and Council of State and Territorial Epidemiologists.

8-28. (Developmental) Increase the number of local health departments or agencies that use data from surveillance of environmental risk factors as part of their vector control programs.

Potential data source: Profile of local health departments, National Association of County and City Health Officials (NACCHO).

8-29. Reduce the global burden of disease due to poor water quality, sanitation, and personal and domestic hygiene.

Target: 2,135,000 deaths.

Baseline: 2,668,200 deaths worldwide were attributable to these factors in 1990.

Target setting method: 20 percent improvement.

Data source: Global Burden of Disease, World Health Organization.

Improving access to clean water and sanitation has been cited as the single most effective means of alleviating human distress. Better water supply and sanitation may increase the average life expectancy in developing countries by 15 years. Furthermore, poor sanitation ranks as one of the highest contributing factors to the global burden of disease and injury. Diarrheal diseases, which kill nearly 3 million persons a year in developing countries, typically result from poor sanitation practices and the consumption of substandard drinking water. These diseases are mostly preventable by improving environmental services.[42, 43]

8-30. Increase the proportion of the population in the U.S.-Mexico border region that have adequate drinking water and sanitation facilities.

Target and baseline:

Objective	Type of Drinking Water and Sanitation Service	1997 Baseline	2010 Target
		Percent of Population Receiving Water Service or Treatment	
	Wastewater sewer service provided		
8-30a.	Ciudad Acuna	39	49
8-30b.	Matamoros	47	57
8-30c.	Mexicali	80	90
8-30d.	Nogales, Sonora	81	91
8-30e.	Piedras Negras	80	90
8-30f.	Reynosa	57	67
	Wastewater receiving treatment		
8-30g.	Ciudad Acuna	0	10
8-30h.	Matamoros	0	10
8-30i.	Mexicali	72	82
8-30j.	Nogales, Sonora	100	100

| 8-30k. | Piedras Negras | 0 | 10 |
| 8-30l. | Reynosa | 100 | 100 |

Target setting method: 10 percentage point improvement.

Data sources: EPA; Mexico's Comisión Nacional de Agua; State and local health departments; American Water Works Association; Rural Water Association; U.S.-Mexican Border Health Association.

Water pollution is one of the principal environmental and public health problems facing the U.S.-Mexico border area. Deficiencies in the treatment of wastewater, the disposal of untreated sewage, and inadequate operation and maintenance of treatment plants result in health risks.[8, 44] Better environmental services such as sewer service, wastewater treatment service, and safe drinking water may help achieve a balance among social and economic factors and protecting the environment in border communities and natural areas.

Related Objectives From Other Focus Areas

1. **Access to Quality Health Services**
   1-7. Core competencies in health provider training
   1-12. Single toll-free number for poison control centers
3. **Cancer**
   3-1. Overall cancer deaths
   3-2. Lung cancer deaths
   3-8. Melanoma deaths
   3.9. Sun exposure and skin cancer
   3-10. Provider counseling about cancer prevention
   3-14. Statewide cancer registries
4. **Chronic Kidney Disease**
   4-1. End-stage renal disease
6. **Disability and Secondary Conditions**
   6-12. Environmental barriers affecting participation in activities
7. **Educational and Community-Based Programs**
   7-2. School health education
   7-10. Community health promotion programs
10. **Food Safety**
    10-1. Foodborne Infections
    10-2. Outbreaks of foodborne infections
    10-5. Consumer food safety practices
11. **Health Communication**
    11-1. Households with Internet access
    11-2. Health literacy
    11-4. Quality of Internet health information sources
12. **Heart Disease and Stroke**
    12-1. Coronary heart disease (CHD) deaths

14. **Immunization and Infectious Diseases**
    14-31. Active surveillance for vaccine safety
15. **Injury and Violence Prevention**
    15-7. Nonfatal poisonings
    15-8. Deaths from poisoning
    15-10. Emergency department surveillance systems
    15-11. Hospital discharge surveillance systems
    15-12. Emergency department visits
    15-13. Deaths from unintentional injuries
    15-14. Nonfatal unintentional injuries
16. **Maternal, Infant, and Child Health**
    16-10. Low birth weight and very low birth weight
    16-11. Preterm births
    16-14. Developmental disabilities
20. **Occupational Safety and Health**
    20-1. Work-related injury deaths
    20-2. Work-related injuries
    20-7. Elevated blood lead levels from work exposure
    20-8. Occupational skin diseases or disorders
22. **Physical Activity and Fitness**
    22-14. Community walking
    22-15. Community bicycling
23. **Public Health Infrastructure**
    23-1. Public health employee access to the Internet
    23-2. Public access to information and surveillance data
    23-3. Use of geocoding in health data systems
    23-4. Data for all population groups
    23-5. Data for Leading Health Indicators, Health Status Indicators, and Priority Data Needs at State, Tribal, and local levels
    23-6. National tracking of Healthy People 2010 objectives
    23-7. Timely release of data on objectives
    23-8. Competencies for public health workers
    23-9. Training in essential public health services
    23-10. Continuing education and training by public health agencies
    23-11. Performance standards for essential public health services
    23-12. Health improvement plans
    23-13. Access to public health laboratory services
    23-14. Access to epidemiology services
    23-15. Model statutes related to essential public health services
    23-16. Data on public health expenditures
    23-17. Population-based prevention research
24. **Respiratory Diseases**
    24-1. Deaths from asthma
    24-2. Hospitalizations for asthma
    24-3. Hospital emergency department visits for asthma
    24-4. Activity limitations
    24-5. School or work days lost
    24-6. Patient education

24-7. Appropriate asthma care

24-8. Surveillance systems

27. Tobacco Use

27-9. Exposure to tobacco smoke at home among children

27-10. Exposure to environmental tobacco smoke

27-11. Smoke-free and tobacco-free schools

27-12. Worksite smoking policies

27-13. Smoke-free indoor air laws

28. Vision and Hearing

28-16. Hearing protection

28-17. Noise-induced hearing loss in children

28-21. Noise-induced hearing loss in adults

Terminology

(A listing of abbreviations and acronyms used in this publication appears in Appendix H.)

Acute chemical poisoning: Unintentional poisoning caused by chemicals that are not medicines.

Aerometric Information Retrieval System (AIRS): This system, administered by EPA, contains information about air pollution in the United States and other countries.

Algae: Small one- or many-celled plants that live in the water and do not have roots, stems, or leaves but usually contain chlorophyll.

Annual vehicle miles: The distance traveled by a passenger vehicle over a given interval of time.

Bloom: Populations of algae that have grown so large that they can be seen in water with the naked eye.

Brownfields: Abandoned, idle, or underused industrial or commercial sites that raise concern in nearby communities that any expansion or redevelopment could contaminate the environment.

Chlorophyll: The green photosynthetic pigment found chiefly in plants.

Community water system: A public water system that provides water to at least 15 service connections used by year-round residents or that regularly serves at least 25 year-round residents.

Disaster: Any event, either natural (such as hurricanes, wind storms, earthquakes, volcanic eruptions, or floods) or technological (such as the release of radiation or chemical or biologic substances), that, because of its scope or severity, overwhelms a population's ability to respond.

Domestic water use: Using water for household purposes, such as drinking, preparing food, bathing, washing clothes and dishes, flushing toilets, or watering lawns and gardens. Also called residential water use. The water may be obtained from a public supply or may be self-supplied by a homeowner (such as by a well).

Environmental epidemiology: The study of the effect on human health of physical, biological, and chemical factors in the external environment. Can include examining specific populations or communities exposed to different ambient environments to clarify the relationship between physical, biological, or chemical factors and human health.

Environmental hazards: Situations or conditions in which something in the environment, such as radiation, a chemical, or other pollutant, can cause human illness or injury.

Environmental tobacco smoke: Smoke given off by cigarettes, pipes, or cigars to which nonsmokers can be exposed.

Environmental toxicology: Scientific analysis of the relationship between exposure to hazardous substances found in the environment and adverse health effects in people.

Epidemic: The occurrence in a community or region of cases of an illness, specific health-related behavior, or other health-related events clearly in excess of normal expectancy.

Evidence based: Empirical proof that accurately validates professional guidance or recommendations or illustrates how an approach has been used successfully in the past.

Good indoor air quality practices: Operation and maintenance procedures designed to provide air quality inside a building to increase comfort and productivity and to reduce health risks for people in the building.

Greenhouse gas (GHG): A gas that absorbs radiation of specific wave lengths within the infrared spectrum of radiation released by the earth's surface and clouds so that part of the absorbed energy is trapped and the earth's surface warms up. Water vapor, carbon dioxide, nitrous oxide, methane, and ozone are the primary greenhouse gases in the earth's atmosphere.

Hazard Ranking System (HRS): The principal screening tool used by EPA to evaluate risks to public health and the environment associated with abandoned or uncontrolled hazardous waste sites. HRS calculates a score based on the potential of hazardous substances spreading from the site through the air, surface water, or ground water and on other factors, such as density and proximity of human population. This score is the primary factor in deciding whether the site should be on the National Priorities List and, if so, what ranking it should have compared to other sites on the list.

Hazardous substances: Any substance that possesses properties that can cause harm to human health and ecologic systems. A subset of these substances, toxics, or toxicants are substances not produced by a living organism that can cause harm to human health and ecologic systems.

HazDat: A scientific database maintained by the Agency for Toxic Substances and Disease Registry. Provides access to information on the release of hazardous substances from Superfund sites or from emergency events and on the effects of hazardous substances on health.

Household lead dust: Very fine particles containing lead that are usually caused by the deterioration of lead paint.

Humanitarian emergencies: Emergencies that occur as a result of disasters that destroy or have a negative effect on basic human needs, such as food, shelter, and water.

Indoor air quality (IAQ): The overall state of the air inside a building as reflected by the presence of pollutants, such as dust, fungi, animal dander, volatile organic compounds, carbon monoxide, and lead.

Indoor allergens: Fine particles in indoor air that can cause allergic reactions and respiratory problems, including dust mites and animal dander.

Infectious agents: Any organism, such as a virus, parasite, or bacterium, that is capable of invading the body, multiplying, and causing disease.

Integrated Risk Information System (IRIS): This database, maintained by EPA, contains information on health hazards from over 5,000 substances.

Metabolites: Any substance produced by biological processes in the human body. In some cases, it is not possible to measure certain substances (for example, pesticides) in the human body to determine exposure to those substances, but instead it is possible to measure the secondary substance or metabolite that is created when the human body breaks down the primary substance.

Municipal solid waste: Common garbage or trash generated by industries, businesses, institutions, and homes.

National Ambient Air Quality Standards (NAAQS): Standards set by EPA for the level of common air pollutants allowed by the Clean Air Act.

National Priorities List (NPL): EPA's list of the most serious uncontrolled or abandoned hazardous waste sites identified for possible long-term cleanup under Superfund. The list is based primarily on the score a site receives from the Hazard Ranking System. EPA updates the NPL at least yearly. A site must be on the NPL to receive funds from the Superfund Trust Fund for remedial action.

Nonattainment area: A locality where air pollution levels persistently exceed EPA's National Ambient Air Quality Standards.

Nonpoint source: The source of runoff water coming from an area such as a yard, parking lot, pasture, or other urban or agricultural area.

Ozone: Ozone occurs naturally in the stratosphere and provides a protective layer high above the earth. At ground-level, however, ambient ozone is the prime ingredient of smog. Ambient ozone refers to ozone in the troposphere—the air that people breathe—which is different from ozone in the stratosphere, the hole in the ozone layer. Ozone is not emitted directly into the air but is formed readily in the atmosphere, usually during hot summer weather, from volatile organic compounds emitted by motor vehicles, chemical plants, refineries, factories, consumer and commercial products, other industrial sources, and trees and from nitrogen oxides emitted by motor vehicles, power plants, and other sources of combustion. Changing weather patterns contribute to yearly differences in ozone concentrations from city to city.

Particulate matter: General term used for a mixture of solid particles and liquid droplets found in the air. These particles, which come in a wide range of sizes, originate from "built" and natural sources. Fine particles (PM2.5) result from fuel combustion from motor vehicles, power generation, and industrial facilities, as well as from residential fireplaces and wood stoves. Coarse particles (PM10) generally are emitted from other sources, such as vehicles traveling on unpaved roads, materials handling, and crushing and grinding operations, as well as windblown dust.

Per capita water use: The average amount of water used per person during a standard period, generally per day. In the United States, this measure usually is reported in gallons per day.

Persistent chemicals: Chemicals, such as organochlorine compounds, that remain in the environment for a long time and can accumulate in the fat of people and animals exposed to them.

Photosynthesis: Formation of carbohydrates from carbon dioxide and a source of hydrogen (as water) in the chlorophyll-containing tissues of plants exposed to light.

Point source: The source of water coming from a specific location, such as a drain pipe from a wastewater treatment plant or an industrial plant.

Poisoning: An exposure to a toxic substance that produces negative signs or symptoms.

Premature death: A death that occurs earlier than the life expectancy for most members of the population.

Protozoa: A subkingdom of the animal kingdom, including all of the so-called acellular or unicellular forms (for example, Amoeba, Giardia, and Cryptosporidium).

Radon: A colorless, naturally occurring radioactive gas found in some soils or rocks.

Radon-resistant construction: Affordable and simple techniques that, when incorporated during construction of a new home, reduce indoor radon levels by preventing radon entry and providing a means for venting radon to the outdoors.

Registry of Toxic Effects of Chemical Substances (RTECS®): Maintained by the National Institute for Occupational Safety and Health, this database contains information on the toxic effects of chemical substances. The list of substances includes drugs, food additives, preservatives, ores, pesticides, dyes, detergents, lubricants, soaps, plastics, extracts from plant and animal sources, plants or animals that are toxic by contact or consumption, and industrial intermediates and waste products from production processes.

Service connection: The point at which a customer's water supply attaches to a water utilities distribution system.

Special classrooms: Classrooms with special characteristics, such as laboratories and art rooms, in which particular environmental hazards may be found.

Substandard housing: Housing with moderate or severe physical problems in plumbing, heating, or electrical systems, upkeep and sanitation, hallways, or kitchens.

Superfund: The program operated under the legislative authority of Comprehensive Environmental Response, Compensation, and Liability Act (CERCLA) and Superfund Amendments and Reauthorization Act (SARA) that funds and carries out EPA solid waste emergency and long-term removal or remedial activities. These activities include establishing the National Priorities List, investigating sites for inclusion on the list, determining their priority, and conducting or supervising cleanup and other remedial actions or both.

Sustainable development: Growth and development within a society that is intended to meet the needs of the present without compromising the ability of future generations to meet their own needs.

Toxic Release Inventory (TRI): EPA's list of more that 600 designated chemicals that threaten health and the environment. Authorized under the Emergency Planning and Community Right-To-Know Act (EPCRA) of 1986, this system requires manufacturers to report releases of these chemicals to EPA and State governments. EPA compiles the data in an online, publicly accessible national computerized database.

TOXLINE: A collection of online information on drugs and other chemicals maintained by the National Library of Medicine.

Transit: Represents what used to be called "mass transit." The 1990 Nationwide Personal Transportation Survey (NPTS/U.S. Department of Transportation) included the following modes in its transit count: bus, subway or elevated rail, commuter rail, streetcar, and trolley. The 1995 NPTS characterizes a "trip" as travel to a destination (for example, worksite). Travel to work, for instance, that includes two stops along the way (trip chains) would constitute three "trips."

µg/dL: Micrograms per deciliter.

Urban sprawl: Unplanned and inefficient development of open land.

Vector-borne diseases: Illnesses that are transmitted to people by organisms, such as insects.

Vector control: Control of any object, organism, or thing that transmits disease from one host to another.

Waterborne disease outbreaks: Includes only outbreaks from infectious agents and chemical poisoning incidents in which two or more people experience a similar illness after consumption or use of water intended for drinking and epidemiologic evidence implicates water as the source of illness. The stipulation that at least two people be ill is waived for single cases of laboratory-confirmed, primary amebic meningoencephalitis and for single cases of chemical poisoning if water-quality data indicate contamination by the chemical.

References

[1] World Health Organization (WHO). *Indicators for Policy and Decision Making in Environmental Health.* (Draft). Geneva, Switzerland: WHO, 1997.

[2] National Research Council. *Environmental Epidemiology: Public Health and Hazardous Wastes.* Vol. 1. Washington, DC: National Academy Press, 1991.

[3] Agency for Toxic Substances and Disease Registry (ATSDR). *Priority Health Conditions—An Integrated Strategy to Evaluate the Relationship Between Illness and Exposure to Hazardous Substances.* Atlanta, GA: U.S. Department of Health and Human Services (HHS), 1993.

[4] WHO. *Fact Sheet 170.* Geneva, Switzerland: WHO, 1997.

[5] Commissioned Corps of the U.S. Public Health Service, HHS. <http://www.os.dhhs.gov/phs/corps/direct1.html#history> June 14, 2000.

[6] U.S. Bureau of Economic Analysis. *Survey of Current Business.* May 1995.

[7] U.S. Environmental Protection Agency (EPA). *National Air Quality and Trends Report.* Washington, DC: EPA, Office of Air and Radiation, 1997.

[8] EPA. *U.S.-Mexico Border XXI Program: Framework Document.* No. EPA 160. R-96-003. Washington, DC: EPA, 1996.

[9] Thurston, G.D.; Gorczynski, J.E.; Currie, J.J.; et al. The nature and origins of acid summer haze air pollution in metropolitan Toronto, Ontario. *Environmental Research* 65(2):254-270, 1994.

[10] EPA. *1997 National Toxics Inventory Report.* Washington, DC: EPA, 1997.

[11] American Lung Association. *Health Costs of Air Pollution.* 1990.

[12] Craun, G.F. Statistics of waterbourne outbreaks in the U.S. (1920–1980). In: Craun, G.F., ed. *Waterborne Disease Outbreaks in the United States.* Boca Raton, FL: CRC Press, 1986.

[13] Centers for Disease Control and Prevention (CDC). Surveillance for waterborne disease outbreaks—United States, 1991–1992. *Morbidity and Mortality Weekly Report* 42(SS-5):1-22, 1993.

[14] CDC. Surveillance for waterborne disease outbreaks—United States, 1989–1990. *Morbidity and Mortality Weekly Report* 40(SS-3):1-21, 1991.

[15] CDC. Surveillance for waterborne disease outbreaks—United States, 1993–1994. *Morbidity and Mortality Weekly Report* 45(SS-1):1-33, 1995.

[16] *Animal Waste Pollution in America: An Emerging Problem, Environmental Risks of Livestock and Poultry Production.* Minority Staff Report for Senator Tom Harkin (D-IA), Ranking Member, U.S. Senate Committee on Agriculture, Nutrition, and Forestry. 1997.

[17] U.S. Bureau of the Census. American Housing Survey for the United States in 1995. In: *Current Housing Reports.* H150/95RV. Washington, DC: U.S. Government Printing Office (GPO), 1997.

[18] Litovitz, T.L.; Smilkstein, M.; Felberg, L.; et al. 1996 Annual Report of the American Association of Poison Control Centers: Toxic Exposure Surveillance System. *American Journal of Emergency Medicine* 15:447-500, 1997.

[19] Chemical Economics Handbook. SRF International, September 1997. Retrieved April 10, 1998, from DIALOG database (#359).

[20] ATSDR. *The Nature and Extent of Childhood Lead Poisoning in Children in the United States: A Report to Congress.* Washington, DC: HHS, 1988.

[21] CDC. *Screening Young Children for Lead Poisoning: Guidance for State and Local Public Health Officials.* Atlanta, GA: CDC, 1997.

[22] CDC. Update: Blood lead levels in the United States, 1991–1994. *Morbidity and Mortality Weekly Report* 46:143, 1997.

[23] Mannino, D.M.; Homa, D.M.; Pertowski, C.A.; et al. Surveillance for asthma—United States, 1960—1995. In: CDC Surveillance Summaries, April 24, 1998. *Morbidity and Mortality Weekly Report* 47(SS-1):1-27, 1998.

[24] National Heart, Lung, and Blood Institute. *Data Fact Sheet. Asthma Statistics.* Bethesda, MD: National Institutes of Health, Public Health Service, 1999.

[25] President's Task Force on Environmental Health Risks and Safety Risks to Children. *Asthma and the Environment: A Strategy to Protect Children.* Washington, DC: the Task Force, 1998.

[26] Redd, S. Chief, Air and Respiratory Branch, National Centers for Environmental Health, CDC. Personal communication.

[27] Weiss, K.B.; Gergen, P.J.; and Hodgson, T.A. An economic evaluation of asthma in the United States. *New England Journal of Medicine* 326:862-866, 1992.

[28] Hu, P.S. *Summary of Travel Trends 1995 Nationwide Personal Transportation Survey.* Washington, DC: U.S. Department of Transportation, 1999, 13.

[29] Schmidt, C. *Environmental Health Perspectives* 106(6):1998.

[30] Institute of Medicine. *Toward Environmental Justice—Research, Education, and Health Policy Needs.* Washington, DC: National Academy Press, 1999.

[31] U.S. Geological Survey. U.S. Geological Survey: Estimated use of water in the United States in 1990. *USGS National Circular* 1081. Washington, DC: GPO, 1993.

[32] Toxnet7, National Library of Medicine, Toxicology and Environmental Health Information Program, Bethesda, MD.

[33] Internet Grateful Med, National Library of Medicine, Bethesda, MD.

[34] U.S. Department of Energy Clean Cities Program <http://www.ccities.doe.gov/>.

[35] Renewable Fuels Association <http://www.ethanolrfa.org>.

[36] EPA. *Description of FY 1993–FY 1997 PWS Statistics, Safe Drinking Water Information System (SDWIS/FED).* Washington, DC: EPA, Office of Enforcement and Compliance Assurance, 1997 data frozen April 1, 1998.

[37] Solley, W.B.; Pierce, R.R.; and Perlman, H.A. *Estimated Water Use in the United States, 1995, U.S. Geological Survey Circular 1200.* Washington, DC: U.S. Department of Interior, GPO, 1998.

[38] EPA. *National Water Quality Inventory: 1994 Report to Congress.* Washington, DC: EPA, 1994.

[39] EPA. *Strategic Plan.* Washington, DC: EPA, 1997.

[40] Spengler, J.D., and Sexton, K. Indoor air pollution: a public health perspective. *Science* 221:9-17, 1983.

[41] EPA. Pesticides Industry Sales and Usage—1994 and 1995 Market Estimates. Washington, DC: EPA, 1997.

[42] World Resources Institute. *World Resources: A Guide to the Global Environment, the Urban Environment, 1996–1997.* Oxford, United Kingdom: Oxford University Press.

[43] Murray, C.J.L., and Lopez, A.D., eds. *The Global Burden of Disease.* Cambridge, MA: Harvard University Press, 1996.

[44] WHO. *The World Health Report 1997: Conquering Suffering, Enriching Humanity.* Geneva, Switzerland: WHO, 1997.

9
Family Planning

Lead Agency: Office of Population Affairs

Contents

Goal

Improve pregnancy planning and spacing and prevent unintended pregnancy.

Overview

In an era when technology should enable couples to have considerable control over their fertility, half of all pregnancies in the United States are unintended.[1] Although between 1987 and 1994 the proportion of pregnancies that were unintended declined in the United States from 57 to 49 percent,[2] other industrialized nations report fewer unintended pregnancies,[3] suggesting that the number of unintended pregnancies can be reduced further. Family planning remains a keystone in attaining a national goal aimed at achieving planned, wanted pregnancies and preventing unintended pregnancies. Family planning services provide opportunities for individuals to receive medical advice and assistance in controlling if and when they get pregnant and for health providers to offer health education and related medical care.

The family planning objectives for Healthy People 2010 echo the recommendations contained in the 1995 Institute of Medicine report *The Best Intentions: Unintended Pregnancy and the Well-Being of Children and Families.*[4] The foremost recommendation of the report calls for the Nation to adopt a social norm in which all pregnancies are intended—that is, clearly and consciously desired at the time of conception. Emphasizing personal choice and intent, this norm speaks to planning for pregnancy, as well as to avoiding unintended pregnancy.

Unintended pregnancy rates in the United States show a decline, probably as a result of higher contraceptive use and use of more effective contraceptive methods.[2] Despite this improvement, unintended pregnancy remains a common problem, and further progress is needed.

Issues and Trends

One important determinant of pregnancy and birth rates is contraceptive use. The proportion of all females aged 15 to 44 years who currently are practicing contraception (including females who have been sterilized for contraceptive reasons and husbands or partners who have had vasectomies) rose from about 56 percent in 1982 to 60 percent in 1988 and 64 percent in 1995.[5] However, 5.2 percent of all females aged 15 to 44 years had intercourse in the past 3 months and did not use contraceptives.[5]

No one method of contraception is likely to be consistently and continuously suitable for each woman, man, or couple. Total abstinence is the only fool-proof

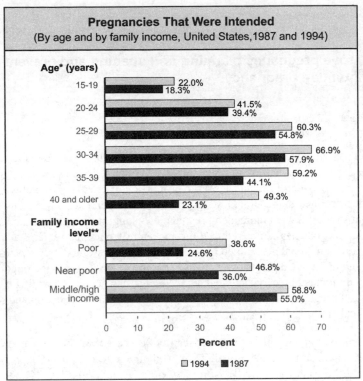

Pregnancies That Were Intended
(By age and by family income, United States,1987 and 1994)

Age* (years)

	1994	1987
15-19	22.0%	18.3%
20-24	41.5%	39.4%
25-29	60.3%	54.8%
30-34	66.9%	57.9%
35-39	59.2%	44.1%
40 and older	49.3%	23.1%

Family income level**

	1994	1987
Poor	38.6%	24.6%
Near poor	46.8%	36.0%
Middle/high income	58.8%	55.0%

Percent (0 10 20 30 40 50 60 70)

☐ 1994 ■ 1987

Sources: *Henshaw, S.K. Unintended pregnancy in the United States. *Family Planning Perspectives* 30(1):24-29, 46, 1998. **Brown, S.S., and Eisenberg, L. *The Best Intentions: Unintended Pregnancy and the Well-Being of Children and Families.* Washington, DC: National Academy Press, 1995.

method of contraception. Sterilization, the most common method of contraception in the United States, has near-perfect effectiveness and differs from other methods because it is usually permanent.[5]

Used by an estimated 10 million females, combination oral contraceptives are the most popular method of reversible contraception in the United States. Other hormonal contraceptives, such as injectables and implants, and intrauterine devices (IUDs) have the appeal of providing effective contraception without the need for daily compliance. For barrier methods, such as the condom and diaphragm, the average effectiveness is more variable. Used correctly and consistently, condoms can prevent both pregnancy and disease. Other barrier methods include the diaphragm, cervical cap, and female condom, which may reduce the risk but do not prevent sexually transmitted diseases (STDs) that primarily affect the cervix. Spermicides used alone (foams, creams, and jellies), coitus interruptus (withdrawal), and periodic abstinence (calendar rhythm) are other options; however, their effectiveness in actual use is lower than that for other methods.

Contraceptive method choices are far from ideal. Even with all financial and knowledge barriers removed, effective and consistent contraceptive use is difficult. Contraceptive research and development efforts must be expanded to bring new methods to the market, methods that combine high contraceptive efficacy and ease of use with protection against STDs and human immunodeficiency virus (HIV). Increased attention also must be given to bringing new methods to the United States, including male methods of contraception, spermicide, and microbicide alternatives. Improving the range of contraceptive choices increases the likelihood that individuals and couples will be able to find a contraceptive method that suits them. Greater choice enhances individuals' control over their fertility and reduces the risk of unintended pregnancy.

Reducing unintended pregnancies is possible and necessary. Unintended pregnancy in the United States is serious and costly and occurs frequently. Socially, the costs can be measured in unintended births, reduced educational attainment and employment opportunity, greater welfare dependency, and increased potential for child abuse and neglect. Economically, health care costs are increased. An unintended pregnancy, once it occurs, is expensive no matter what the outcome. Medically, unintended pregnancies are serious in terms of the lost opportunity to prepare for an optimal pregnancy, the increased likelihood of infant and maternal illness, and the likelihood of abortion.[4] The consequences of unintended pregnancy are not confined to those occurring in teenagers or unmarried couples. In fact, unintended pregnancy can carry serious consequences at all ages and life stages.[4]

With an unintended pregnancy, the mother is less likely to seek prenatal care in the first trimester and more likely not to obtain prenatal care at all.[6, 7] She is less likely to breastfeed[8] and more likely to expose the fetus to harmful substances, such as tobacco or alcohol.[4] The child of such a pregnancy is at greater risk of low birth weight, dying in its first year, being abused, and not receiving sufficient resources for healthy development.[9] A disproportionate share of the women bearing children whose conception was unintended are unmarried or at either end of the reproductive age span—factors that, in themselves, carry increased medical and social burdens for children and their parents. Pregnancy begun without some degree of planning often prevents individual women and men from participating in preconception risk identification and management.

For teenagers, the problems associated with unintended pregnancy are compounded, and the consequences are well documented. Teenaged mothers are less likely to get or stay married, less likely to complete high school or college, and more likely to require public assistance and to live in poverty than their peers who are not mothers. Infants born to teenaged mothers, especially mothers under age 15 years, are more likely to suffer from low birth weight, neonatal death, and sudden infant death syndrome. The infants may be at greater risk of child abuse, neglect, and behavioral and educational problems at later stages.[10] Nearly 1 million teenage pregnancies occur each year in the United States.[11] Clearly, the solution to the problem needs to be found.

Unintended pregnancy is expensive, and contraceptives save health care resources by preventing unintended pregnancy.[12] The pregnancy care cost for one woman who does not intend to be pregnant, yet is sexually active and uses no contraception, is estimated at about $3,200 annually in a managed care setting.[12, 13] Estimates of the overall cost to U.S. taxpayers for teenage childbearing range between $7 billion and $15 billion a year, mainly attributed to higher public assistance costs, foregone tax revenues resulting from changes in productivity of the teen parents, increased child welfare, and higher criminal justice costs.[14] Unintended births to teenagers, which account for about 40 percent of teenaged pregnancies, cost more than $1.3 billion in direct health expenditures each year.[15]

Induced abortion is another consequence of unintended pregnancy. Although the numbers of abortions in this country have been declining over the past 15 years,[16] approximately one abortion occurs for every three live births annually in the United States, a ratio two to four times higher than in many other Western democracies. Just as unintended pregnancy occurs across the spectrum of age and socioeconomic status, women of all reproductive ages, married or unmarried, and in all income categories obtain abortions.

Abortion results when women have unintended pregnancies, and adequate access to family planning services reduces the number of unintended pregnancies. Each year, publicly subsidized family planning services prevent an estimated 1.3 million unintended pregnancies.[17] For every $1 spent on publicly funded contraceptive services, $3 is saved in Medicaid bills for pregnancy-related health care and medical care for newborns.[17]

Disparities

Unintended pregnancies occur among females of all socioeconomic levels and all marital status and age groups, but females under age 20 years and poor and African American women are especially likely to become pregnant unintentionally.[4] More than 4 in 10 pregnancies to white and Hispanic females are unintended; 7 in 10 pregnancies to African American females are unintended. Unintended pregnancies during contraceptive use are most common among African American and Hispanic females. Poverty is strongly related to greater difficulty in using reversible contraceptive methods successfully, with these females also the least likely to have the resources necessary to access family planning services and the most likely to be affected negatively by an unintended pregnancy. For this reason, publicly subsidized family planning services are important. Yet, half of all females who are at risk for an unintended pregnancy and need publicly subsidized family planning services are not getting them.[18] Clearly, while these programs have contributed substantially to preventing unintended pregnancy, the need for services continues to outstrip resources available.

Difficulty in obtaining and paying for care is, of course, exacerbated for poor and low-income people. Several Federal programs support family planning services, with most targeting poor or low-income females. The Medicaid program is the largest, but reimbursement for family planning services is typically not available to adolescents, women without children, women who are married, and working poor women whose income may just exceed the eligibility level.

An estimated 6.6 million females receive services from subsidized family planning providers annually, slightly less than one-half of those considered to be in need of subsidized family planning services (those at risk of unintended pregnancy and with a family income less than 250 percent of the poverty level).[19] Family planning programs consisting of some 3,000 agencies with over 7,000 clinic locations provide nearly 40 percent of family planning services in the United States. Health departments represent nearly half of these locations, along with hospitals, community health centers, and other public and nonprofit organizations. Nearly two-thirds of all females served (4.2 million) obtained care at 1 of 4,200 clinics receiving funds from the Federal Title X Family Planning Program.[19]

Opportunities

A 1995 survey of the Nation's family planning agencies estimated that almost 70 percent of agencies have at least one special program of outreach education or service to meet the needs of teenagers. Fewer have special programs for hard-to-serve populations, such as homeless persons, persons with disabilities, or substance abusers.[20] Furthermore, whether those agencies target their services or simply provide care to those who happened to seek it is not known.[21] The need for family planning services among all these groups is undeniably great. In the case of substance abuse, the link between illegal drug use and infection with HIV has meant more Federal and State funding for programs designed to reach these groups. Thus, substance abusers may be more likely to be targeted by family planning agencies than other hard-to-reach populations. Some programs focus specifically on HIV prevention, whereas others offer comprehensive family planning services and related education and counseling.[21]

Language and cultural differences are significant barriers to serving non-English-speaking population groups. Providers report that they often have difficulty finding staff with appropriate language skills who also have adequate family planning skills and experience. Furthermore, simply speaking the language of the client is not sufficient; the provider also must be able to relate on a cultural level.[21] Persons of various ethnic backgrounds often are uncomfortable talking to strangers about intimate topics, such as sex and birth control, let alone undergoing a pelvic or breast exam. Some racial and ethnic groups tend to visit a doctor only when they are sick and not to seek preventive services, including family planning. Reaching such populations can be difficult.

Providing outreach, education, and clinical services to hard-to-reach populations is expensive. Frequently, these groups have more health problems than less disadvantaged family planning clients, and these health problems are not necessarily confined to family planning. One study estimated that the cost of providing services to homeless women is twice that of other women, with homeless women at such high risk of gynecological problems that they must undergo a complete exam and diagnostic workup at every visit.[21] Disabled individuals often require extra staff, equipment, and time (especially if they are clients with developmental disabilities) to ensure contraceptive compliance and to deal with side-effect issues.[21] The extra time, effort, and expense required to reach hard-to-serve groups undoubtedly discourage some family planning agencies from implementing programs for these populations.[20] Clearly, there is a need to expand services to hard-to-reach populations and to find effective strategies to overcome barriers to services experienced by individuals in these populations.

Finally, public education and information about family planning need to be expanded. Public education efforts and the media could help persons to understand better the benefits of sexual abstinence. Numerous studies and polls indicate a disturbing degree of misinformation about contraceptive methods. The modest health risks of oral contraceptives frequently are exaggerated, whereas the more considerable benefits are underestimated. Knowledge about emergency contraception is not widespread, and the relative effectiveness of various contraceptive methods often is not well understood. Moreover, the risk of unintended pregnancy in the absence of contraceptive use is underestimated, and many population groups lack accurate information on STDs and reproductive health in general.[22] The media—print, broadcast, and video—must be encouraged to help in the task of conveying accurate and balanced information on contraception, highlighting the benefits as well as the risks of contraceptives.

Access to quality contraceptive services continues to be an important factor in promoting healthy pregnancies and preventing unintended pregnancies. Although people in the United States view contraception as basic to their lives and their health care, health insurance plans traditionally have not covered family planning services. Three-fourths of U.S. women of childbearing age rely on private insurance; the extent to which they are covered for contraception can differ dramatically depending on the type of insurance.[23] Traditional plans provide the least comprehensive coverage for family planning services, while health maintenance organizations (HMOs) and newer managed care plans provide more comprehensive contraceptive coverage. Increased access through insurance coverage for family planning is important because in the absence of comprehensive coverage, many women may opt for whatever method may be covered by their health plan rather than the method most appropriate for their individual needs and circumstances. Other women may opt not to use contraception if it is not covered under their insurance plan.

Interim Progress Toward Year 2000 Objectives

Of the 12 family planning Healthy People 2000 objectives, progress has been made for 9 objectives. Substantial decreases have occurred in unintended pregnancy. The use of contraceptives among females aged 15 to 44 years at risk for unintended pregnancy has increased. The pregnancy rate for females using a contraceptive method has declined. Increases in adolescents' abstinence from sexual intercourse have occurred, as well as in their use of contraceptives. Although short of the year 2000 targets, decreases in adolescent pregnancy have been reported. Data are not available to update objectives on family planning counseling and age-appropriate preconception care counseling.

Note: Unless otherwise noted, data are from the Centers for Disease Control and Prevention, National Center for Health Statistics, *Healthy People 2000 Review, 1998–99.*

Family Planning

Goal: Improve pregnancy planning and spacing and prevent unintended pregnancy.

Number	Objective Short Title
9-1	Intended pregnancy
9-2	Birth spacing
9-3	Contraceptive use
9-4	Contraceptive failure
9-5	Emergency contraception
9-6	Male involvement in pregnancy prevention
9-7	Adolescent pregnancy
9-8	Abstinence before age 15 years
9-9	Abstinence among adolescents aged 15 to 17 years
9-10	Pregnancy prevention and sexually transmitted disease (STD) protection
9-11	Pregnancy prevention education
9-12	Problems in becoming pregnant and maintaining a pregnancy
9-13	Insurance coverage for contraceptive supplies and services

9-1. Increase the proportion of pregnancies that are intended.

Target: 70 percent.

Baseline: 51 percent of all pregnancies among females aged 15 to 44 years were intended in 1995.

Target setting method: Better than the best.

Data sources: National Survey of Family Growth (NSFG), CDC, NCHS; National Vital Statistics System (NVSS), CDC, NCHS; Abortion Provider Survey, The Alan Guttmacher Institute; Abortion Surveillance Data, CDC, NCCDPHP.

NOTE: THE TABLE BELOW MAY CONTINUE TO THE FOLLOWING PAGE.

Pregnancies Among Females Aged 15 to 44 Years, 1995	Intended Pregnancy
	Percent
TOTAL	51
Race and ethnicity	
American Indian or Alaska Native	DSU
Asian or Pacific Islander	DSU
Asian	DSU
Native Hawaiian and other Pacific Islander	DSU
Black or African American	28
White	57
Hispanic or Latino	51
Not Hispanic or Latino	51
Black or African American	DNA
White	DNA
Family income level	
Poor	39
Near poor	47
Middle/high income	59

Pregnancies Among Females Aged 15 to 44 Years, 1995	Intended Pregnancy
	Percent
Select populations	
Age groups	
15 to 19 years	22
20 to 24 years	42
25 to 29 years	60
30 to 34 years	67
35 to 39 years	59
40 to 44 years	49
Marital status	
Currently married	69
Formerly married	38
Never married	22

DNA = Data have not been analyzed. DNC = Data are not collected. DSU = Data are statistically unreliable.

NOTE: THE TABLE ABOVE MAY HAVE CONTINUED FROM THE PREVIOUS PAGE.

A significant decline in the rates of unintended pregnancy has occurred, indicating that progress toward a goal of increased intended pregnancy is possible. Between 1987 and 1994, the proportion of pregnancies that were unintended declined from 57 to 49 percent.[2] By comparison, the percentage of unintended pregnancy is much lower in some other countries—in 1994–95, it was 39 percent in Canada and 6 percent in the Netherlands.[3] Overall, females in the United States spend three-fourths of their reproductive years trying to avoid pregnancy.[17] Unintended pregnancy often is mistakenly perceived as predominantly an adolescent problem; however, unintended pregnancy is a problem among all reproductive age groups. In 1994, nearly one-half (48 percent) of females aged 15 to 44 years had at least one unintended pregnancy in their lifetime, more than one-fourth (28 percent) had one or more unplanned births, nearly one-third (30 percent) had one or more abortions, and 1 in 10 (11 percent) had both an unintended birth and an induced abortion.[2] A goal of 70 percent is ambitious and will require strategies to reduce the gaps among population groups.

9-2. Reduce the proportion of births occurring within 24 months of a previous birth.

Target: 6 percent.

Baseline: 11 percent of females aged 15 to 44 years gave birth within 24 months of a previous birth in 1995.

Target setting method: Better than the best.

Data source: National Survey of Family Growth (NSFG), CDC, NCHS.

NOTE: THE TABLE BELOW MAY CONTINUE TO THE FOLLOWING PAGE.

Females Aged 15 to 44 Years, 1995	New Birth Occurred Within 24 Months of Previous Birth
	Percent
TOTAL	11
Race and ethnicity	
American Indian or Alaska Native	DSU
Asian or Pacific Islander	DSU
Asian	DSU
Native Hawaiian and other Pacific Islander	DSU
Black or African American	14
White	10
Hispanic or Latino	14
Not Hispanic or Latino	10
Black or African American	14
White	10
Family income level (aged 20 to 44 years)	
Poor	20
Near poor	11
Middle/high income	7
Disability status	
Persons with disabilities	DNC
Persons without disabilities	DNC
Select populations	
Age groups	
15 to 19 years	9
20 to 24 years	14
25 to 29 years	10
30 to 34 years	11
35 to 39 years	10
40 to 44 years	DSU

Females Aged 15 to 44 Years, 1995	New Birth Occurred Within 24 Months of Previous Birth
	Percent
Marital status	
Currently married	11
Formerly married	13
Never married	11

DNA = Data have not been analyzed. DNC = Data are not collected. DSU = Data are statistically unreliable.

NOTE: THE TABLE ABOVE MAY HAVE CONTINUED FROM THE PREVIOUS PAGE.

Encouraging females of all ages to space their pregnancies adequately can help lower their risk of adverse perinatal outcomes. To the extent that very closely spaced pregnancies are unplanned, unintended pregnancy may increase the risk of low birth weight.[4] A recent study indicates that females who wait 18 to 23 months after delivery before conceiving their next child lower their risk of adverse perinatal outcomes, including low birth weight, preterm birth, and small-for-size gestational age.[24] Health care providers can help all new mothers understand that they can become pregnant again soon after delivery and should assist them with contraceptive education and supplies.

For adolescents, bearing a child is associated with poor outcomes for young females and their children. Giving birth to a second child while still a teen further increases these risks. The prevention of second and subsequent births to very young females is of great interest to public health. Research has shown that such births are associated with physical and mental health problems for the mother and the child.[25] Yet, analysis indicates that in the 2 years following the first birth, teenaged mothers have a second birth at about the same rate as other mothers. In 1997, nearly one in every five births to teenaged mothers was a birth of second order or higher.[26]

9-3. Increase the proportion of females at risk of unintended pregnancy (and their partners) who use contraception.

Target: 100 percent.

Baseline: 93 percent of females aged 15 to 44 years at risk of unintended pregnancy used contraception in 1995.

Target setting method: Total coverage.

Data source: National Survey of Family Growth (NSFG), CDC, NCHS.

Healthy People 2010: Objectives for Improving Health

Females Aged 15 to 44 Years at Risk of Unintended Pregnancy, 1995	Used Contraception
	Percent
TOTAL	93
Race and ethnicity	
American Indian or Alaska Native	DSU
Asian or Pacific Islander	DSU
Asian	DSU
Native Hawaiian and other Pacific Islander	DSU
Black or African American	90
White	93
Hispanic or Latino	91
Not Hispanic or Latino	93
Black or African American	90
White	93
Family income level	
Poor	92
Near poor	91
Middle/high income	93
Select populations	
Age groups	
15 to 19 years	81
20 to 24 years	91
25 to 29 years	94
30 to 34 years	94
35 to 39 years	95
40 to 44 years	93
Marital status	
Currently married	95
Formerly married	92
Never married	88

DNA = Data have not been analyzed. DNC = Data are not collected. DSU = Data are statistically unreliable.

The percentage of at-risk females using any form of contraception rose from 88 in 1982 to 93 in 1995.[27] Increasing the target to 100 percent by 2010 will be challenging and could reduce dramatically occurrences of unintended pregnancy. Poor or nonexistent contraceptive use is one of the main causes of unintended pregnancy, with unintended pregnancy occurring among two groups: females using no contraception and females whose contraceptives fail or are used improperly. In the

United States, the small proportion of females who are at risk of unintended pregnancy and use no method of contraception account for over half of all unintended pregnancies. Reducing the proportion of sexually active persons using no birth control method and increasing the effectiveness (correct and consistent use) with which persons use contraceptive methods would do much to lower the unintended pregnancy rate.[28] Just reducing the proportion of females not using contraception by half could prevent as many as one-third of all unintended pregnancies and 500,000 abortions per year.[29]

9-4. Reduce the proportion of females experiencing pregnancy despite use of a reversible contraceptive method.

Target: 7 percent.

Baseline: 13 percent of females aged 15 to 44 years experienced pregnancy despite use of a reversible contraceptive method in 1995.

Target setting method: Better than the best (retain year 2000 target).

Data sources: National Survey of Family Growth (NSFG), CDC, NCHS; Abortion Patient Survey, The Alan Guttmacher Institute.

NOTE: THE TABLE BELOW MAY CONTINUE TO THE FOLLOWING PAGE.

Females Aged 15 to 44 Years Using Reversible Contraception, 1995	Experienced Pregnancy
	Percent
TOTAL	13
Race and ethnicity	
American Indian or Alaska Native	DSU
Asian or Pacific Islander	DSU
Asian	DSU
Native Hawaiian and other Pacific Islander	DSU
Black or African American	DNC
White	DNC
Hispanic or Latino	15
Not Hispanic or Latino	DNA
Black or African American	20
White	11
Family income level	
Poor	DSU
Near poor	18
Middle/high income	10

Healthy People 2010: Objectives for Improving Health

Females Aged 15 to 44 Years Using Reversible Contraception, 1995	Experienced Pregnancy
	Percent
Disability status	
Persons with disabilities	DNC
Persons without disabilities	DNC
Select populations	
Marital/cohabiting status	
Married	9
Cohabiting	22
Unmarried, not cohabiting	14

DNA = Data have not been analyzed. DNC = Data are not collected. DSU = Data are statistically unreliable.

NOTE: THE TABLE ABOVE MAY HAVE CONTINUED FROM THE PREVIOUS PAGE.

The public health benefits of improved contraceptive practices are potentially enormous. Whether fertile females who are sexually active and do not want to get pregnant experience an unintended pregnancy is a function of their choice—and their partners' choice—of contraceptive methods and how effectively they use them. The efficacy of reversible contraceptive methods depends on consistent and appropriate usage. Unintended pregnancies experienced by females using reversible methods are primarily a result of inconsistent and/or inappropriate use.[30] Ideally, an objective would focus on consistent and correct use of a particular method. The data, however, cannot address the role that method switching may play in unintended pregnancy.

9-5. (Developmental) Increase the proportion of health care providers who provide emergency contraception.

Potential data source: The Alan Guttmacher Institute.

The *U.S. Guide to Clinical Preventive Services*[16] identifies postcoital administration of emergency contraceptive pills (ECP) after unprotected intercourse as an effective means of reducing subsequent pregnancy. ECP is estimated to reduce the risk of subsequent pregnancy by 75 percent. Yet this method, which has the public health potential of significantly reducing unintended pregnancy, is not well known and not yet widely available to the public. Surveys indicate that knowledge and use of postcoital contraception remains low among patients and clinicians alike.[29] In 1995, less than 1 percent of females in the United States reported ever having used ECP.[31]

Several developments, however, have formalized recognition within the medical community of ECP as an effective means of preventing pregnancy, including the American College of Obstetricians and Gynecologists issuance of practice guidelines for emergency oral contraception. Barriers to the more frequent use of ECP include a lack of physician awareness of the method, a lack of public awareness of the method's availability, and a lack of access by patients to a physician who will prescribe the method.[32] Increased public awareness, including culturally and linguistically competent education about ECP as well as direct access to and insurance reimbursement for ECP, would contribute significantly toward attainment of this objective.

In February 1997, the Food and Drug Administration (FDA) announced that certain regimens of combined oral contraceptives are safe and effective for ECP when initiated within 72 hours after unprotected intercourse.[33] The FDA notice was intended to encourage manufacturers to make this additional contraceptive option available.[33] One product, an emergency contraceptive kit, has been approved by FDA and is being marketed. On July 28, 1999, FDA approved the first progestin-only emergency contraceptive.

9-6. (Developmental) Increase male involvement in pregnancy prevention and family planning efforts.

Potential data source: National Survey of Family Growth (NSFG), CDC, NCHS.

There is increasing recognition of the value of male involvement in pregnancy prevention and family planning. Several related developments in public health and welfare demonstrate that male involvement is key, including culturally and linguistically appropriate programs promoting condom use and addressing HIV and STD prevention, culturally and linguistically competent services targeting men as part of managed care marketing strategies, emphasis on male responsibility in welfare, child support enforcement, and pregnancy prevention efforts. Concern about the spread of HIV and other STDs and the recognition of condoms as the most effective way of preventing transmission during intercourse have accentuated the need to change the sexual behavior of males. The need for rapid treatment of male partners of females testing positive for bacterial STDs is a critical element in slowing not only STD spread but also that of HIV.

Yet, information about how males could and should participate in pregnancy prevention programs is lacking. For many years, reproductive policy in the United States concentrated almost entirely on females. The National Survey of Adolescent Males (NSAM), begun in 1988 by the Urban Institute and repeated again in 1995, collected the first national trend data on the reproductive behavior of male teens. An Urban Institute survey of publicly funded family planning clinics found that males make up more than 10 percent of the total clientele in only 13 percent of clinics. An average of 6 percent of clients are males. Males represent an even smaller share of clients who receive family planning services subsidized by the Title X program (2 percent in 1991) or by Medicaid (2 percent in 1990).[34] Even though males do not actually get pregnant, integrating them in prevention programs makes sense. Males must be included in any efforts to address unintended pregnancy.[35]

The next National Survey of Family Growth (NSFG) is being expanded to include males, providing an avenue for institutionalizing data collection about male fertility that will be reflected in the Healthy People 2010 objectives. Over the course of Healthy People 2010, male measures for family planning objectives will shift from NSAM to NSFG. NSFG will be able to collect information from males about sexual activity, contraceptive use, pregnancies to which they contribute, and the outcomes of these pregnancies, as well as male perceptions of their and their partners' views on the intendedness of pregnancies and births. NSFG will cover a broader range of male age groups than had been covered under the NSAM, which included only males aged 15 to 19 years.

9-7. Reduce pregnancies among adolescent females.

Target: 43 pregnancies per 1,000.

Baseline: 68 pregnancies per 1,000 females aged 15 to 17 years occurred in 1996.

Target setting method: Better than the best.

Data sources: Abortion Provider Survey, The Alan Guttmacher Institute; National Vital Statistics System (NVSS), CDC, NCHS; National Survey of Family Growth (NSFG), CDC, NCHS; Abortion Surveillance Data, CDC, NCCDPHP.

NOTE: THE TABLE BELOW MAY CONTINUE TO THE FOLLOWING PAGE.

Females Aged 15 to 17 Years, 1996	Pregnancy Rate per 1,000
TOTAL	68
Race and ethnicity	
American Indian or Alaska Native	DNC
Asian or Pacific Islander	DNC
Asian	DNC
Native Hawaiian and other Pacific Islander	DNC
Black or African American	124
White	58
Hispanic or Latino	105
Not Hispanic or Latino	62
Black or African American	128
White	44
Family income level	
Poor	DSU
Near poor	DSU
Middle/high income	DSU

Females Aged 15 to 17 Years, 1996	Pregnancy
	Rate per 1,000
Disability status	
Persons with disabilities	DNC
Persons without disabilities	DNC

DNA = Data have not been analyzed. DNC = Data are not collected. DSU = Data are statistically unreliable.

NOTE: THE TABLE ABOVE MAY HAVE CONTINUED FROM THE PREVIOUS PAGE.

The teenage pregnancy rate in the United States is much higher than in many other developed countries—twice as high as in England and Wales, France, and Canada and nine times as high as in the Netherlands or Japan.[10] Teenage pregnancy remains an intense national issue, within the context of public health and welfare reform, concerning the optimum potential of the Nation's youth and the growth and development of newborns. Most adolescent childbearing occurs outside marriage, a trend that has increased markedly during the past two decades. In 1997, 78 percent of births to adolescent females (under age 20 years) were out of wedlock, compared to 44 percent two decades earlier (1977).[26]

Females under age 15 years experience about 30,000 pregnancies each year.[36] Consensus is widespread that all pregnancies in this age group are inappropriate and that ideally the target number should be zero. Nearly two-thirds of pregnancies in this age group end in induced abortion or fetal loss. Because of the relatively small numbers of events (and small sample sizes for fetal losses) involved, the resulting rates are not as stable as for older females. Almost no discernible decline in pregnancy rates for this age group occurs on an annual basis. Therefore, baseline and target data for pregnancies among adolescents under age 15 years are not included in this objective.[36]

9-8. Increase the proportion of adolescents who have never engaged in sexual intercourse before age 15 years.

Target and baseline:

Objective	Increase in Adolescents Aged 15 to 19 Years Never Engaging in Sexual Intercourse Before Age 15 Years	1995 Baseline	2010 Target
		Percent	
9-8a.	Females	81	88
9-8b.	Males	79	88

Target setting method: Better than the best.

Data sources: Females—National Survey of Family Growth (NSFG), CDC, NCHS; Males—National Survey of Adolescent Males (NSAM), Urban Institute.

Adolescents Aged 15 to 19 Years, 1995	No Intercourse Before Age 15 Years	
	9-8a. Females	9-8b. Males
	Percent	
TOTAL	81	79
Race and ethnicity		
American Indian or Alaska Native	DSU	DSU
Asian or Pacific Islander	DSU	DSU
Asian	DSU	DNC
Native Hawaiian and other Pacific Islander	DSU	DNC
Black or African American	70	50
White	83	84
Hispanic or Latino	76	73
Not Hispanic or Latino	81	79
Black or African American	69	51
White	83	86
Family income level		
Poor	DSU	DNC
Near poor	DSU	DNC
Middle/high income	DSU	DNC

DNA = Data have not been analyzed. DNC = Data are not collected. DSU = Data are statistically unreliable.

9-9. Increase the proportion of adolescents who have never engaged in sexual intercourse.

Target and baseline:

Objective	Increase in Adolescents Aged 15 to 17 Years Never Engaging in Sexual Intercourse	1995 Baseline	2010 Target
		Percent	
9-9a.	Females	62	75
9-9b.	Males	57	75

Target setting method: Better than the best.

Data sources: Females—National Survey of Family Growth (NSFG), CDC, NCHS; Males—National Survey of Adolescent Males (NSAM), Urban Institute.

Adolescents Aged 15 to 17 Years, 1995	Never Engaged in Sexual Intercourse	
	9-9a. Females	9-9b. Males
	Percent	
TOTAL	62	57
Race and ethnicity		
American Indian or Alaska Native	DSU	DSU
Asian or Pacific Islander	DSU	DSU
Asian	DSU	DNC
Native Hawaiian and other Pacific Islander	DSU	DNC
Black or African American	51	24
White	63	64
Hispanic or Latino	49	50
Not Hispanic or Latino	64	57
Black or African American	52	24
White	65	65
Family income level		
Poor	DSU	DNC
Near poor	DSU	DNC
Middle/high income	DSU	DNC

DNA = Data have not been analyzed. DNC = Data are not collected. DSU = Data are statistically unreliable.

Sexual experience, and particularly age at first intercourse, represents a critical indicator of the risk of pregnancy and STDs. Although all forms of intercourse (vaginal, oral, and anal) involve risk of disease transmission, this chapter focuses on avoiding unintended pregnancy and not on sexual behavior per se. Therefore, the relevant objectives reference heterosexual, vaginal intercourse only. Youth who begin having sex at younger ages are exposed to these risks over a longer period of time. Research has shown that youth who have early sexual experiences are more likely at later ages to have more sexual partners and more frequent intercourse.[37] Adolescents should be encouraged to delay sexual intercourse until they are physically, cognitively, and emotionally ready for mature sexual relationships and their consequences. They should receive education about intimacy; setting limits; resistance to social, media, peer, and partner pressure; the benefits of abstinence from intercourse; and prevention of pregnancy and STDs. Because many adolescents are or will be sexually active, they should receive support and assistance in developing the skills to evaluate their readiness for mature sexual relationships. Culturally and linguistically appropriate materials are needed that can capture the attention and affect the behaviors of these youth.

9-10. **Increase the proportion of sexually active, unmarried adolescents aged 15 to 17 years who use contraception that both effectively prevents pregnancy and provides barrier protection against disease.**

Target and baseline:

Objective	Increase in Contraceptive Use at First Intercourse by Sexually Active, Unmarried Adolescents Aged 15 to 17 Years	1995 Baseline	2010 Target
		Percent	
	Condom		
9-10a.	Females	67	75
9-10b.	Males	72	83
	Condom plus hormonal method		
9-10c.	Females	7	9
9-10d.	Males	8	11

Target setting method: Better than the best.

Data sources: Females—National Survey of Family Growth (NSFG), CDC, NCHS; Males—National Survey of Adolescent Males (NSAM), Urban Institute.

NOTE: THE TABLE BELOW MAY CONTINUE TO THE FOLLOWING PAGE.

Sexually Active, Unmarried Adolescents Aged 15 to 17 Years, 1995	Used Condom at First Intercourse		Used Condom Plus Hormonal Method at First Intercourse	
	9-10a. Females	9-10b. Males	9-10c. Females	9-10d. Males
	Percent			
TOTAL	67	72	7	8
Race and ethnicity				
American Indian or Alaska Native	DSU	DSU	DSU	DSU
Asian or Pacific Islander	DSU	DSU	DSU	DSU
Asian	DSU	DNC	DSU	DNC
Native Hawaiian and other Pacific Islander	DSU	DNC	DSU	DNC
Black or African American	60	60	9	12
White	72	77	6	8
Hispanic or Latino	52	64	DSU	7
Not Hispanic or Latino	71	70	7	7
Black or African American	60	61	9	11
White	75	79	6	8

Sexually Active, Unmarried Adolescents Aged 15 to 17 Years, 1995	Used Condom at First Intercourse		Used Condom Plus Hormonal Method at First Intercourse	
	9-10a. Females	9-10b. Males	9-10c. Females	9-10d. Males
	Percent			
Family income level				
Poor	DSU	DNC	DSU	DNC
Near poor	DSU	DNC	DSU	DNC
Middle/high income	DSU	DNC	DSU	DNC

DNA = Data have not been analyzed. DNC = Data are not collected. DSU = Data are statistically unreliable.

NOTE: THE TABLE ABOVE MAY HAVE CONTINUED FROM THE PREVIOUS PAGE.

Target and baseline:

Objective	Increase in Contraceptive Use at Last Intercourse by Sexually Active, Unmarried Adolescents Aged 15 to 17 Years	1995 Baseline	2010 Target
	Condom	*Percent*	
9-10e.	Females	39	49
9-10f.	Males	70	79
	Condom plus hormonal method		
9-10g.	Females	7	11
9-10h.	Males	16	20

Target setting method: Better than the best.

Data sources: Females—National Survey of Family Growth (NSFG), CDC, NCHS; Males—National Survey of Adolescent Males (NSAM), Urban Institute.

NOTE: THE TABLE BELOW MAY CONTINUE TO THE FOLLOWING PAGE.

Sexually Active, Unmarried Adolescents Aged 15 to 17 Years, 1995	Used Condom at Last Intercourse		Used Condom Plus Hormonal Method at Last Intercourse	
	9-10e. Females	9-10f. Males	9-10g. Females	9-10h. Males
	Percent			
TOTAL	39	70	7	16
Race and ethnicity				
American Indian or Alaska Native	DSU	DSU	DSU	DSU
Asian or Pacific Islander	DSU	DSU	DSU	DSU

Sexually Active, Unmarried Adolescents Aged 15 to 17 Years, 1995	Used Condom at Last Intercourse		Used Condom Plus Hormonal Method at Last Intercourse	
	9-10e. Females	9-10f. Males	9-10g. Females	9-10h. Males
	Percent			
Asian	DSU	DSU	DSU	DSU
Native Hawaiian and other Pacific Islander	DSU	DSU	DSU	DSU
Black or African American	48	78	10	19
White	38	67	6	15
Hispanic or Latino	26	59	DSU	10
Not Hispanic or Latino	42	65	9	17
Black or African American	47	78	10	18
White	40	69	8	16
Family income level				
Poor	DSU	DNC	DSU	DNC
Near poor	DSU	DNC	DSU	DNC
Middle/high income	DSU	DNC	DSU	DNC

DNA = Data have not been analyzed. DNC = Data are not collected. DSU = Data are statistically unreliable.

NOTE: THE TABLE ABOVE MAY HAVE CONTINUED FROM THE PREVIOUS PAGE.

There are two major health consequences of unprotected intercourse among youth—STDs, including HIV infection, and unintended pregnancy. Although abstinence is the most effective way for adolescents to avoid STDs and pregnancy and should be stressed as the certain way to prevent STDs and pregnancy, sexually active teens must be taught to use condoms properly, effectively, and consistently. Teenaged females and males who depend upon hormonal methods of contraception must be educated about the inability of these methods to prevent STDs. (See Focus Area 13. HIV and Focus Area 25. Sexually Transmitted Diseases.) Condom use must be promoted in conjunction with other contraceptive methods.[38]

Public health messages encourage individuals whose behavior places them at risk of exposure to STDs, HIV, and unintended pregnancy to use condoms, as well as effective pregnancy prevention methods, consistently and correctly.[39] Sexual intercourse in the teen years, especially first intercourse, often is unplanned and unprotected by contraception. Condom use at last intercourse has risen substantially and significantly among both male and female teenagers, suggesting more protection from STD transmission. Condom use at first intercourse also has risen—an important indicator of how well teenagers anticipate and plan for protection at the initiation of sexual activity. Culturally and linguistically appropriate materials are needed that can capture the attention and affect the behaviors of these youth.

While condom use has risen among most teenagers, the use of oral contraceptives has dropped dramatically, suggesting greater vulnerability to unintended pregnancy if other hormonal methods or consistent use of condoms is not practiced. Among currently sexually active females, the use of oral contraceptives at last intercourse fell from 43 percent to 25 percent between 1988 and 1995. The reductions in the use of oral contraception are evident across African American, Hispanic, and white teenagers. Some of the reduction in oral contraceptive use is counteracted by the adoption of new hormonal methods of contraception, such as hormonal implants and injectables. In 1995, 7 percent of sexually active teenaged females overall used these methods at last intercourse. They were used most widely among sexually active African American teenaged females: 16 percent reported using either a hormonal implant or an injectable at last intercourse.[40]

9-11. Increase the proportion of young adults who have received formal instruction before turning age 18 years on reproductive health issues, including all of the following topics: birth control methods, safer sex to prevent HIV, prevention of sexually transmitted diseases, and abstinence.

Target: 90 percent.

Baseline: 64 percent of females aged 18 to 24 years reported having received formal instruction on all of these reproductive health issues before turning age 18 years in 1995. (Data on males will be available in the future.)

Target setting method: Better than the best.

Data source: National Survey of Family Growth, (NSFG), CDC, NCHS.

NOTE: THE TABLE BELOW MAY CONTINUE TO THE FOLLOWING PAGE.

Females Aged 18 to 24 Years, 1995	Received Reproductive Health Instruction Prior to Age 18 Years		
	9-11. Aged 18 to 24 Years	Aged 18 to 19 Years*	Aged 20 to 24 Years*
	Percent		
TOTAL	64	80	57
Race and ethnicity			
American Indian or Alaska Native	DSU	DSU	DSU
Asian or Pacific Islander	DSU	DSU	DSU
Asian	DSU	DSU	DSU

Females Aged 18 to 24 Years, 1995	Received Reproductive Health Instruction Prior to Age 18 Years		
	9-11. Aged 18 to 24 Years	Aged 18 to 19 Years*	Aged 20 to 24 Years*
	Percent		
Native Hawaiian and other Pacific Islander	DSU	DSU	DSU
Black or African American	65	81	59
White	64	81	57
Hispanic or Latino	56	69	51
Not Hispanic or Latino	65	82	58
Black or African American	66	80	60
White	65	83	58
Family income level			
Poor	63	82	56
Near poor	58	76	52
Middle/high income	66	81	60
Sexual orientation	DNC	DNC	DNC

DNA = Data have not been analyzed. DNC = Data are not collected. DSU = Data are statistically unreliable.
*Data for females aged 18 to 19 years and 20 to 24 years are displayed to further characterize the issue.
NOTE: THE TABLE ABOVE MAY HAVE CONTINUED FROM THE PREVIOUS PAGE.

All adolescents need education that teaches the interpersonal skills they will need to withstand pressure to have sex until they are ready and that includes up-to-date information about methods to prevent pregnancy and STDs. More important, they need to receive this education before they start having sex. Ideally, such education would be developmentally appropriate, include special education students, be culturally and linguistically appropriate, be medically accurate, involve parents, and be linked into a broader context of avoiding risky health behaviors and promoting improved health. Education and knowledge, however, are not enough. Adolescents need strong reinforcement from parents, schools, the media, and other sources about the importance of making conscious, informed, responsible decisions regarding whether to have intercourse; the necessity of consistent, correct condom use to protect themselves and their partners against STDs and HIV; and the use of effective contraception to prevent unintended pregnancy. (See Focus Area 13. HIV and Focus Area 25. Sexually Transmitted Diseases.)

Becoming a sexually healthy adult is a key developmental task of adolescence. Adults can encourage adolescent sexual health by providing accurate information and education about sexuality, fostering responsible decisionmaking skills, offering support and guidance in exploring and affirming personal values, and modeling healthy sexual attitudes and behaviors. Discussions between parents and their children about sexuality and their family value system related to sexual behavior are crucial. Yet, many parents of adolescents aged 10 to 15 years in families today do not talk enough about such important topics as relationships and becoming sexually active.[41]

9-12. Reduce the proportion of married couples whose ability to conceive or maintain a pregnancy is impaired.

Target: 10 percent.

Baseline: 13 percent of married couples with wives aged 15 to 44 years had impaired ability to conceive or maintain a pregnancy in 1995.

Target setting method: 23 percent improvement.

Data source: National Survey of Family Growth (NSFG), CDC, NCHS.

NOTE: THE TABLE BELOW MAY CONTINUE TO THE FOLLOWING PAGE.

Married Couples With Wives Aged 15 to 44 Years, 1995	Impaired Fecundity
	Percent
TOTAL	13
Race and ethnicity	
American Indian or Alaska Native	DSU
Asian or Pacific Islander	DSU
Asian	DSU
Native Hawaiian and other Pacific Islander	DSU
Black or African American	14
White	13
Hispanic or Latino	13
Not Hispanic or Latino	13
Black or African American	14
White	13
Family income level (aged 20 to 44 years)	
Poor	15
Near poor	13
Middle/high income	13

Married Couples With Wives Aged 15 to 44 Years, 1995	Impaired Fecundity
	Percent
Select populations	
Parity status	
Parity 0	25
Parity 1 or more	10

DNA = Data have not been analyzed. DNC = Data are not collected. DSU = Data are statistically unreliable.

NOTE: THE TABLE ABOVE MAY HAVE CONTINUED FROM THE PREVIOUS PAGE.

A woman is classified as having impaired fecundity if it is impossible for her (or her husband or cohabiting partner) to have a baby for any reason other than a sterilizing operation, it is difficult or dangerous to carry a baby to term, or she and her partner have not used contraception and have not had a pregnancy for 3 years or longer. Impaired fecundity includes problems carrying pregnancies to term in addition to problems conceiving, whereas infertility includes only problems conceiving. By 1995, there had been a small overall decline in infertility, which was more marked in Hispanic couples.

Although infertility itself does not represent a serious public health threat, it carries significant personal, societal, and economic consequences that call for data surveillance and action. Infertility due to STDs is a preventable condition. Diagnosis and treatment of infertility are very costly, time-consuming, and invasive, and they can place immense stress on marital and family relations. Furthermore, those costs are likely to rise. The trend to delay childbearing (fecundity becomes increasingly impaired with age), the availability of fewer infants for adoption, and the development of new drugs and treatment procedures will mean that more and more couples seek expensive infertility services.

9-13. (Developmental) Increase the proportion of health insurance policies that cover contraceptive supplies and services.

Potential data source: The Alan Guttmacher Institute.

In a 1995 report, the Institute of Medicine concluded that among the reasons for high rates of unintended pregnancy in the United States was lack of contraceptive coverage by private health insurance.[4] The report noted that many privately insured females who need contraceptive care must go out of plan and pay for it themselves, use over-the-counter methods that may be less effective, or not use any method at all. It recommended increasing the proportion of health insurance policies that cover contraceptive services and supplies.

The issue of private insurance coverage for reversible contraceptive methods affects most women and their families. Both newer managed care insurance plans and traditional fee-for-service insurance plans are more likely to pay for general gynecological services than they are to cover contraceptive services or supplies.[42] Many insurance plans do not cover reversible contraceptive methods. A 1993 survey conducted by the Alan Guttmacher Institute found that half of indemnity plans and 7 percent of health maintenance organizations (HMOs) do not cover nonpermanent contraception. The survey also found that plans that do cover contraceptive services and/or supplies are often inconsistent in which methods they cover and have a pronounced bias toward covering permanent surgical methods.[43]

Related Objectives From Other Focus Areas

1. **Access to Quality Health Services**
   - 1-2. Health insurance coverage for clinical preventive services
   - 1-3. Counseling about health behaviors
   - 1-7. Core competencies in health provider training

3. **Cancer**
   - 3-3. Breast cancer deaths
   - 3-4. Cervical cancer deaths
   - 3-10. Provider counseling about cancer prevention
   - 3-11. Pap tests
   - 3-13. Mammograms

7. **Educational and Community-Based Programs**
   - 7-2. School health education
   - 7-3. Health-risk behavior information for college and university students
   - 7-9. Health care organization sponsorship of community health promotion activities
   - 7-11. Culturally appropriate and linguistically competent community health promotion programs

11. **Health Communication**
   - 11-3. Research and evaluation of communication programs
   - 11-6. Satisfaction with health care providers' communication skills

13. **HIV**
   - 13-1. New AIDS cases
   - 13-5. New HIV cases
   - 13-6. Condom use
   - 13-7. Knowledge of serostatus
   - 13-9. HIV/AIDS, STD, and TB education in State prisons
   - 13-10. HIV counseling and testing in State prisons
   - 13-12. Screening for STDs and immunization for hepatitis B
   - 13-14. HIV-infection deaths
   - 13-15. Interval between HIV infection and AIDS diagnosis
   - 13-17. Perinatally acquired HIV infection

14. **Immunization and Infectious Diseases**
   - 14-3. Hepatitis B in adults and high-risk groups
   - 14-9. Hepatitis C
   - 14-28. Hepatitis B vaccination among high-risk groups

15. **Injury and Violence Prevention**
     15-34. Physical assault by intimate partners
     15-35. Rape or attempted rape
     15-36. Sexual assault other than rape

16. **Maternal, Infant, and Child Health**
     16-3. Adolescent and young adult deaths
     16-4. Maternal deaths
     16-5. Maternal illness and complications due to pregnancy
     16-6. Prenatal care
     16-16. Optimum folic acid levels
     16-17. Prenatal substance exposure

19. **Nutrition and Overweight**
     19-12. Iron deficiency in young children and in females of childbearing age
     19-13. Anemia in low-income pregnant females
     19-14. Iron deficiency in pregnant females

25. **Sexually Transmitted Diseases**
     25-1. Chlamydia
     25-2. Gonorrhea
     25-3. Primary and secondary syphilis
     25-4. Genital herpes
     25-5. Human papillomavirus infection
     25-6. Pelvic inflammatory disease (PID)
     25-7. Fertility problems
     25-8. Heterosexually transmitted HIV infection in women
     25-9. Congenital syphilis
     25-10. Neonatal STDs
     25-11. Responsible adolescent sexual behavior
     25-12. Responsible sexual behavior messages on television
     25-13. Hepatitis B vaccine services in STD clinics
     25-14. Screening in youth detention facilities and jails
     25-15. Contracts to treat nonplan partners of STD patients
     25-16. Annual screening for genital chlamydia
     25-17. Screening of pregnant women
     25-18. Compliance with recognized STD treatment standards
     25-19. Provider referral services for sex partners

26. **Substance Abuse**
     26-19. Treatment in correctional institutions

Terminology

(A listing of abbreviations and acronyms used in this publication appears in Appendix H.)

Contraception (birth control): The means of pregnancy prevention. Methods include permanent methods (vasectomy for men and tubal ligation for women) and temporary methods (for example, hormonal implant, injectable, birth control pill, emergency contraceptive pills, intrauterine device, diaphragm, female condom, male condom, spermicidal foam/cream/jelly, sponge, cervical cap, abstinence, natural family planning, calendar rhythm, and withdrawal).

Emergency contraceptive pills (ECPs): The use of prescribed doses of birth control pills to prevent pregnancy following unprotected vaginal intercourse. The pills must be taken within 72 hours of having unprotected sex.

Family planning: The process of establishing the preferred number and spacing of one's children, selecting the means to achieve the goals, and effectively using that means.

Federal Title X Family Planning Program: A program created in 1970 as Title X at the Public Health Service Act. The program provides grants for the provision of family planning information and services.

Impaired fecundity: A broad term used to describe problems with pregnancy loss as well as problems conceiving a pregnancy.

Infertility: Failure to conceive a pregnancy after 12 months of unprotected intercourse.

Intended pregnancy: A pregnancy that a woman states was wanted at the time of conception.

Mistimed conception: Those that were wanted by the woman at some time in the future but occurred sooner than they were wanted. For example, a woman became pregnant at age 18 years but actually wanted to have her first child at age 21 years.

Parity: The number of live births a woman has had.

Unintended pregnancy: A general term that includes pregnancies a woman reports as either mistimed or unwanted at the time of conception. If an unintended pregnancy occurs and is carried to term, the birth may be a wanted one, but the pregnancy would be classified as unintended.

Unwanted conception: Those that occurred when the woman did not want any pregnancy then or in the future. For example, a woman wanted only two children but became pregnant with her third.

References

[1] National Center for Health Statistics (NCHS). *Healthy People 2000 Review, 1997*. Hyattsville, MD: Public Health Service (PHS), 1997.

[2] Henshaw, S.K. Unintended pregnancy in the United States. *Family Planning Perspectives* 30(1):24-29, 46, 1998.

[3] Delbanco, S.; Lundy, J.; Hoff, T.; et al. Public knowledge and perceptions about unplanned pregnancy and contraception in three countries. *Family Planning Perspectives* 29(2):70-75, 1997.

[4] Brown, S.S., and Eisenberg, L., eds. *The Best Intentions: Unintended Pregnancy and the Well-Being of Children and Families*. Washington, DC: National Academy Press, 1995.

[5] Piccinino, L.J., and Mosher, W.D. Trends in contraceptive use in the United States: 1982–1995. *Family Planning Perspectives* 30(1):4-10, 46, 1998.

[6] Kost, K.; Landry, D.; and Darroch, J. Predicting maternal behaviors during pregnancy: Does intention status matter? *Family Planning Perspectives* 30(2):79-88, 1998.

[7] Piccinino, L.J. Unintended pregnancy and childbearing. Reproductive health of women. In: Wilcox, L.S., and Marks, J.S., eds. *From Data to Action: CDC's Public Health Surveil-*

lance for Women, Infants and Children. Atlanta, GA: U.S. Department of Health and Human Services (HHS), PHS, Centers for Disease Control and Prevention, 1994.

[8] Dye, T.D.; Wojtowycz, M.A.; Aubry, R.H.; et al. Unintended pregnancy and breast-feeding behavior. American Journal of Public Health 87(10):1709-1711, 1997.

[9] Kost, K.; Landry, D.; and Darroch, J. The effects of pregnancy planning status on birth outcomes and infant care. Family Planning Perspectives 30(5):223-230, 1998.

[10] The Alan Guttmacher Institute. Sex and America's Teenagers. New York, NY: the Institute, 1994.

[11] Henshaw, S.K. U.S. Teenage Pregnancy Statistics. New York, NY: The Alan Guttmacher Institute, 1998.

[12] Trussell, J.; Levengue, J.; Koenig, J.; et al. The economic value of contraception: A comparison of 15 methods. American Journal of Public Health 85(4):494-503, 1995.

[13] Lee, L.R., and Stewart, F.H. Failing to prevent unintended pregnancy is costly (Editorial). American Journal of Public Health 85(4):479-480, 1995.

[14] Maynard, R.A., ed. Kids Having Kids: The Economic and Social Consequences of Teen Pregnancy. Washington, DC: Urban Institute Press, 1997.

[15] Trussell, J.; Koenig, J.; Stewart, F.; et al. Medical care cost savings from adolescents' contraceptive use. Family Planning Perspectives 29(6):248-255, 295, 1997.

[16] HHS. Guide to Clinical Preventive Services. 2nd ed. Washington, DC: HHS, 1995.

[17] Forrest, J.D., and Samara, R. Impact of publicly funded contraceptive services on unintended pregnancies and implications for Medicaid expenditures. Family Planning Perspectives 28(5):188-195, 1996.

[18] The Alan Guttmacher Institute. Contraceptive Needs and Services, 1995. New York, NY: the Institute, 1997, 7 (table A).

[19] Frost, J. Family planning clinic services in the United States, 1994. Family Planning Perspectives 28(3):92-100, 1996.

[20] Frost, J., and Bolzan, M. The provision of public-sector services by family planning agencies in 1995. Family Planning Perspectives 29(1):6-14, 1997.

[21] Donovan, P. Taking family planning services to hard-to-reach populations. Family Planning Perspectives 28(3):120-126, 1996.

[22] Mauldon, J., and Delbanco, S. Public perceptions about unplanned pregnancy. Family Planning Perspectives 29(1):25-29, 40, 1997.

[23] The Guttmacher Report on Public Policy. The Need for and Cost of Mandating Private Insurance Coverage of Contraception. Vol. 1, No. 4. New York, NY: The Alan Guttmacher Institute, 1998.

[24] Zhu, B.; Rolfs, R.; Nangle, B.; et al. Effect of the interval between pregnancies on perinatal outcomes. New England Journal of Medicine 340(8):589-594, 1999.

[25] Klerman, L. "Can intervention programs prevent subsequent births to teenage mothers? Reactions to reviews of recent research." Paper for Program on Preventing Second Births to Teenage Mothers: Demonstration Findings, sponsored by the American Enterprise Institute for Public Policy Research, March 6, 1998.

[26] Ventura, S.J.; Martin, J.A.; Curtin, S.C.; et al. Births: Final data for 1997. *National Vital Statistics Reports* 47(18), 1999.

[27] NCHS. *Healthy People 2000 Review, 1998–99*. Hyattsville, MD: PHS, 1999.

[28] Westoff, C.D. Contraceptive paths toward the reduction of unintended pregnancy and abortion. *Family Planning Perspectives* 20(1):4-13, 1988.

[29] Yuzpe, A.A.; Thurlow, H.J.; Ramzy, I.; et al. Post coital contraception—A pilot study. *Journal of Reproductive Medicine* 13:53-58, 1974.

[30] Haishan, F.; Darroch, J.E.; Hass, T.; et al. Contraceptive failure rates: New estimates from the 1995 National Survey of Family Growth. *Family Planning Perspectives* 31(2):56-63, 1999.

[31] NCHS, CDC. Unpublished tabulation from the 1995 National Survey of Family Growth.

[32] American College of Obstetricians and Gynecologists. Evidence-Based Guidelines for Clinical Issues in Obstetrics and Gynecology. *Practice Patterns* 3, December 1996.

[33] 62 *Federal Register* 8610. Prescription drug products: Certain combined oral contraceptives for use in postcoital emergency contraception. Washington, DC: U.S. Government Printing Office, February 25, 1997.

[34] Schulte, M.M., and Sonenstein, F.L. Special report. Men at family planning clinics: The new patients? *Family Planning Perspectives* 27(5):212-216, 225, 1995.

[35] Sonenstein, F.L.; Stewart, K.; Lindberg, L.D.; et al. *Involving Males in Preventing Teen Pregnancy: A Guide for Program Planners*. Washington, DC: The Urban Institute, 1997.

[36] Ventura, S.J.; Mosher, W.D.; Curtin, S.C.; et al. Trends in pregnancies and pregnancy rates by outcome: Estimates for the United States, 1976–96. *National Vital Statistics Reports* 47(29), 1999.

[37] Office of the Assistant Secretary for Planning and Evaluation (OASPE). *Trends in the Well-Being of America's Children and Youth: 1998*. Washington, DC: HHS, OASPE, 1996, 324.

[38] American College of Obstetricians and Gynecologists, Committee on Adolescent Health Care. Condom availability for adolescents, Opinion No. 154, April 1995. *International Journal of Gynaecology and Obstetrics* 49(3):347-351, June 1995.

[39] Santelli, J.; Warren, C.; Lowry, R.; et al. The use of condoms with other contraceptive methods among young men and women. *Family Planning Perspectives* 29(6):261-267, 1997.

[40] Abma, J., and Sonenstein, F. Teenage sexual behavior and contraceptive use: An update. Paper presented at the American Enterprise Institute Sexuality and American Social Policy Seminar Series, April 28, 1998.

[41] Kaiser Family Foundation and Children Now National Survey. Talking With Kids About Tough Issues. News release, March 1, 1999.

[42] Landry, D.J., and Forrest, J.D. Private physicians' provision of contraceptive services. *Family Planning Perspectives* 28(5):203-209, 1996.

[43] The Alan Guttmacher Institute. *Uneven & Unequal: Insurance Coverage and Reproductive Health Services*. New York, NY: the Institute, 1994.

10

Food Safety

Co-Lead Agencies: Food and Drug Administration
Food Safety and Inspection Service,
     U.S. Department of Agriculture

Contents

Reduce foodborne illnesses.

Overview

Foodborne illnesses impose a burden on public health and contribute significantly to the cost of health care.

From 1988 through 1992, foodborne disease outbreaks caused an annual average of more than 15,000 cases of illness in the United States.[1] The actual illness rate may be higher because a count is taken only when the microorganism that caused the illness is identified by a laboratory and reported by a physician.

When unreported cases are taken into account, an estimated 76 million illnesses, 325,000 hospitalizations, and 5,000 deaths each year may be associated with microorganisms in food.[2] Hospitalizations due to foodborne illnesses are estimated to cost over $3 billion each year.[3] The cost of lost productivity is estimated at between $20 billion and $40 billion each year.[3] In addition to acute illness, some microorganisms can cause delayed or chronic illness. Foodborne chemical contaminants may cause chronic rather than acute problems, and specific estimates of their impact on health and the economy are not available.

Since 1996, selected State and local health departments, the Centers for Disease Control and Prevention (CDC), the Food and Drug Administration (FDA), and the Food Safety and Inspection Service (FSIS) of the U.S. Department of Agriculture (USDA) have been cooperating in FoodNet to produce better national estimates of foodborne disease. The focus is on organisms that cause the highest number of foodborne illnesses and on new or emerging foodborne pathogens. Active surveillance, based on laboratory data, is being conducted at FoodNet sites.

The success of improvements in food production, processing, preparation, and storage practices can be measured through the reduction in outbreaks of disease caused by foodborne pathogens. An outbreak occurs when two or more cases of a similar illness result from eating the same food.[1] Smaller outbreaks—those with fewer cases—may be a direct result of improved food preparation practices and better epidemiologic followup once cases are identified.

Issues and Trends

Underlying forces may make foodborne illnesses more of a problem in the years to come. These include emerging pathogens; improper food preparation, storage, and distribution practices; insufficient training of retail employees; an increasingly global food supply; and an increase in the number of people at risk because of aging and compromised capacity to fight foodborne diseases.[4]

Emerging pathogens. Microorganisms continue to adapt and evolve, sometimes increasing in their ability to make an individual sick. Microorganisms previously not recognized as human pathogens or pathogens unexpectedly found in particular foods have caused outbreaks of illness. Examples are *Listeria monocytogenes, Escherichia coli* O157:H7, and *Cyclospora cayetanensis.* Known pathogens also may become resistant to drugs. For example, some strains of *Salmonella* species now are resistant to multiple important antimicrobial drugs.

The general trend toward increased resistance by microorganisms to multiple antimicrobial agents heightens public health concerns about treatment options and health care costs associated with foodborne illness. Of particular concern is the potential for transmission of antimicrobial-resistant pathogens to humans through the food supply. For these reasons, increased testing is planned to identify and monitor changes in patterns and trends of antimicrobial resistance in both human and animal populations.

Food preparation and storage practices. Most meals (71 percent) and snacks (78 percent) are prepared at home.[5] For these meals, the food-preparing consumer needs to protect against foodborne illness. Surveys show that consumers should improve the way they prepare, thaw, and store food.[6, 7]

Training of retail employees. The retail food industry has a large employee population with high rates of turnover. Language and literacy barriers and nonuniform systems for training and certifying workers pose additional challenges. Improper holding temperatures, inadequate cooking, poor personal hygiene, contaminated equipment, and foods from unsafe sources have been associated with foodborne disease outbreaks in retail food establishments. Retail food employees' use of safe food preparation and storage practices, along with use of recommended practices spelled out in the U.S. Public Health Service's *Food Code*, should reduce outbreaks.

Global food supply. An increasing amount of the food eaten in most countries originates in other countries. Diverse methods of and standards for growing and processing agricultural products and different frequencies and types of gastrointestinal infections in food workers in different regions increase the possibility of food contamination and the range of pathogens expected.

Protecting the safety of the Nation's food supply involves safeguarding against both biological and chemical contaminants in food. Chemical contaminants in food can include pesticides, toxic elements, naturally occurring toxins (for example, mycotoxins and phytotoxins), antibiotic residues in animal products, endocrine disruptor compounds, and other trace substances in food. Many questions remain unanswered about the chronic effects of exposure to these types of substances. (See Focus Area 8. Environmental Health.)

The U.S. Environmental Protection Agency (EPA) has set safety standards (tolerances) to limit the amount of pesticide residues that legally may remain in or on food or animal feed sold in the United States. Consumers and others have been concerned about the potential risk to children from pesticides. The Food Quality Protection Act of 1996 requires EPA to reassess all existing standards for pesticides by the year 2006. Under this act, EPA considers the risk from dietary exposures from all food uses of pesticides and drinking water; nonoccupational exposure, such as the use of the pesticides for lawn care; and any special sensitivities for children. FDA monitors domestic and imported foods to ensure compliance with these pesticide safety standards.[8] Under the Pesticide Data Program, USDA's Agricultural Marketing Service measures how much of certain pesticides remains in or on food.[9]

Naturally occurring toxins present a different issue. Mycotoxins cannot be avoided entirely or eliminated from human foods or animal feeds because the molds that create them occur naturally in grains and other food commodities. Risk reduction strategies, such as adherence to specific good manufacturing practices (GMPs), have been developed for aflatoxins. For other mycotoxins, FDA is using a science-based risk assessment procedure to help identify appropriate risk reduction measures.

Because representative national data systems may not be available in the first half of the decade for tracking progress on mycotoxins in foods, this subject is not covered in this focus area's objectives. Research on risk reduction and efforts to collect representative national data on mycotoxins in foods will be addressed in the coming decade.

Allergen risk. Although most foodborne illness results from a microbial or chemical contaminant in food, a food itself also can cause severe adverse reactions. In the United States food allergy is an important problem: 2 to 4 percent of children under age 6 years[10, 11] and 1 to 2 percent of adults are allergic to specific foods.[12] The foods most likely to cause allergic reactions are milk and milk products, eggs and egg products, peanuts and peanut products, tree nuts and tree nut products, soybeans and soybean products, fish and fish products, shellfish and shellfish products, cereals containing gluten, and seeds. Allergic reactions to natural rubber latex from food handlers' gloves have been reported.[13, 14]

Based on a 3-year study of anaphylaxis cases treated at an emergency department, an estimated 2,500 individuals per year in the United States experience food-induced anaphylaxis.[15, 16] Food allergy is the most frequent cause of anaphylaxis occurring outside of the hospital and the most common cause for emergency department visits for anaphylaxis.[17] Because potentially allergenic foods are present as ingredients in a variety of food products, and because even trace amounts of these allergenic foods can induce anaphylaxis, research, education, and clear food ingredient labeling information are critical for managing food allergies.

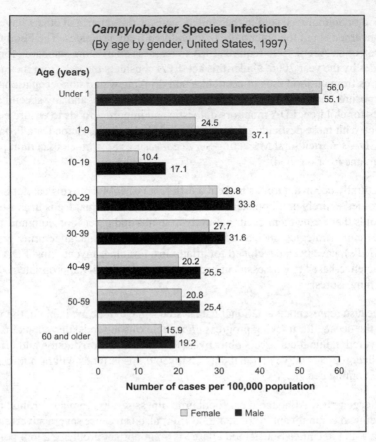

Campylobacter Species Infections
(By age by gender, United States, 1997)

Age (years)

Age	Female	Male
Under 1	56.0	55.1
1-9	24.5	37.1
10-19	10.4	17.1
20-29	29.8	33.8
30-39	27.7	31.6
40-49	20.2	25.5
50-59	20.8	25.4
60 and older	15.9	19.2

Number of cases per 100,000 population

☐ Female ■ Male

Source: CDC, NCID. Foodborne Disease Active Surveillance Network (FoodNet), unpublished data, 1997.

The Food, Drug, and Cosmetic Act requires manufacturers to list all ingredients of a packaged food, with two exemptions. Spices, flavorings, and colorings may be declared collectively without each one being named.[18] Incidental additives, such as processing aids present in a food at insignificant levels and not having a technical or functional effect in the finished food, do not have to be listed individually.[19] However, the presence of a substance that may cause an adverse reaction is considered significant and so it must be listed on the food label. FDA has advised manufacturers that, because adhering to GMPs is essential for effective reduction of adverse reactions, precautionary labeling, such as "may contain (insert name of allergenic ingredient)," should not be used in lieu of adherence to GMPs.[20]

Disparities

More than 30 million people in the United States are likely to be particularly susceptible to foodborne disease.[21] Very young, elderly, and immunocompromised persons experience the most serious foodborne illnesses. They may become ill from smaller doses of organisms and may be more likely than other persons to die of foodborne disease. For example, children under age 1 year have the highest rate of *Campylobacter* species infections (see figure). Other high-risk populations include residents in nursing homes or chronic care facilities; hospitalized, cancer, and organ transplant patients; and individuals with AIDS, with cirrhosis, on antimicrobial treatment, or with reduced stomach acid such as due to antacid medications. In cases of listeriosis and toxoplasmosis, pregnant women and their fetuses or newborns are at higher risk than other groups.

Representative data on specific U.S. populations, such as racial and ethnic groups or socioeconomic groups, are not available from FoodNet. Efforts are under way to improve reporting of this information. A report from the United Kingdom indicates a relationship between socioeconomic status and foodborne illness that may apply to the United States. It found that hospital admissions for gastrointestinal infections increased with increasing socioeconomic deprivation.[22]

Opportunities

The opportunities to reduce the burden of foodborne illness involve risk reduction and control interventions targeted at various steps from production to consumption. These strategies include Hazard Analysis and Critical Control Points programs (required starting in 1997 for seafood and in 1998 for meat and poultry processing); improved adherence to GMPs; education of food processors, preparers, and servers at all levels in the food industry and in the home; and improved investigation of outbreaks and sporadic cases of foodborne illness.

The Partnership for Food Safety Education was formed in 1997 as a part of the National Food Safety Initiative. The Partnership—composed of industry, State, and consumer organizations and government liaisons from FDA, FSIS, Cooperative State Research, Education, and Extension Service (CSREES), CDC, and EPA—cooperatively developed the FightBAC!™ Campaign with messages to reach all consumers. The messages are based on four key food safety practices:

- Clean: Wash hands and surfaces often.
- Separate: Don't cross-contaminate.
- Cook: Cook to proper temperatures.
- Chill: Refrigerate promptly.

Increased surveillance, planned as a result of the 1997 initiative and the improvements to the FoodNet program, will inform the public health community, veterinary and producer groups, and regulatory agencies of the extent of the problem of human pathogens that come from the intestines of animals. These organisms might resist drug therapy when human illness occurs. Public health experts anticipate an initial increase in the number of resistant pathogens detected due to improved surveillance. Over time, as control and educational programs are enacted, decreases should follow. Wider and more representative testing will give a better picture of the nature and extent to which antimicrobial-resistant foodborne pathogens are transmitted from animals to humans.

Interim Progress Toward Year 2000 Objectives

Of the four Healthy People 2000 food safety objectives targeted to reducing foodborne illness, only one has been met—reducing the incidence of disease caused by four key pathogens (*Salmonella* species, *Campylobacter* species, *Escherichia coli* O157:H7, and *Listeria monocytogenes*). Two objectives show solid progress—decreasing the number of outbreaks of *Salmonella* serotype Enteritidis from 77 to 44 outbreaks per year and State agency adoption (16 States) and review (23 States plus Puerto Rico and the District of Columbia) of the *Food Code* for retail-level food establishments (1999 *Food Code* data). The consumer food safety practices objective shows improvement. In fact, the target for washing cutting boards with soap has been surpassed (79 percent) if all safe practices, such as washing with bleach or using a different cutting board following use with raw meat or poultry, are considered.

Note: Data are from the Centers for Disease Control and Prevention, National Center for Health Statistics, *Healthy People 2000 Review, 1998–99,* and from the *Healthy People 2000 Progress Review, Food and Drug Safety,* September 1, 1999.

Food Safety

Goal: Reduce foodborne illnesses.

Number	Objective Short Title
10-1	Foodborne infections
10-2	Outbreaks of foodborne infections
10-3	Antimicrobial resistance of *Salmonella* species
10-4	Food allergy deaths
10-5	Consumer food safety practices
10-6	Safe food preparation practices in retail establishments
10-7	Organophosphate pesticide exposure

10-1. Reduce infections caused by key foodborne pathogens.

Target and baseline:

Objective	Reduction in Infections Caused by Microorganisms	1997 Baseline	2010 Target
		Cases per 100,000	
10-1a.	*Campylobacter* species	24.6	12.3
10-1b.	*Escherichia coli* O157:H7	2.1	1.0
10-1c.	*Listeria monocytogenes*	0.5	0.25
10-1d.	*Salmonella* species	13.7	6.8
10-1e.	*Cyclospora cayetanensis*	Developmental	
10-1f.	Postdiarrheal hemolytic uremic syndrome	Developmental	
10-1g.	Congenital *Toxoplasma gondii*	Developmental	

Target setting method: 50 percent improvement.

Data sources: Foodborne Disease Active Surveillance Network (FoodNet), CDC, NCID; FDA, CFSAN; FSIS, OPHS; and State agencies.

Potential data source: Toxoplasmosis data—National Notifiable Diseases Surveillance System (NNDSS), CDC, NCID.

NOTE: THE TABLE BELOW MAY CONTINUE TO THE FOLLOWING PAGE.

Total Population, 1997	**10-1a.** *Campylobacter* **Species**	**10-1b.** *Escherichia coli* O157:H7	**10-1c.** *Listeria monocytogenes*	**10-1d.** *Salmonella* **Species**
	Cases per 100,000			
TOTAL	24.6	2.1	0.5	13.7
Race and ethnicity				
American Indian or Alaska Native	DSU	DSU	DSU	DSU
Native Hawaiian and other Pacific Islander	DSU	DSU	DSU	DSU
Black or African American	DSU	DSU	DSU	DSU
White	DSU	DSU	DSU	DSU

Total Population, 1997	10-1a. Campylobacter Species	10-1b. Escherichia coli O157:H7	10-1c. Listeria monocytogenes	10-1d. Salmonella Species
	Cases per 100,000			
Hispanic or Latino	DSU	DSU	DSU	DSU
Not Hispanic or Latino	DSU	DSU	DSU	DSU
Black or African American	DSU	DSU	DSU	DSU
White	DSU	DSU	DSU	DSU
Gender				
Female	21.7	2.2	0.4	13.3
Male	27.5	2.0	0.5	14.0
Family income level				
Poor	DNC	DNC	DNC	DNC
Near poor	DNC	DNC	DNC	DNC
Middle/high income	DNC	DNC	DNC	DNC
Select populations				
Age groups				
Under 1 year	55.5	4.6	2.3	111.4
1 to 19 years	21.9	4.9	0.1	17.5
20 to 59 years	27.2	0.9	0.3	10.7
60 years and older	17.1	1.6	1.7	9.1

DNA = Data have not been analyzed. DNC = Data are not collected. DSU = Data are statistically unreliable.

NOTE: THE TABLE ABOVE MAY HAVE CONTINUED FROM THE PREVIOUS PAGE.

Campylobacteriosis and salmonellosis are the most frequently reported foodborne illnesses in the United States.[2] The emerging pathogens *E. coli* O157:H7 and *L. monocytogenes* cause infections that are less often reported but commonly more severe. *L. monocytogenes* is rare; however, septicemia and meningitis may result from infection with this organism, and up to 20 percent of patients may die.[2] Persons with altered or deficient immune response, such as infants and young children, older adults, pregnant women and their fetuses, and immunosuppressed persons, are at highest risk. Listeriosis in pregnant women may lead to miscarriage, stillbirth, or septicemia and meningitis in newborns.

Cyclospora cayetanensis, a parasite, was made a nationally notifiable disease (States report all cases to CDC) and added to FoodNet in 1998. Information about this emerging pathogen, such as the proportion of infections that are foodborne, is needed. Examination for *C. cayetanensis* is not universal in clinical laboratories; thus, data for this organism may be less reliable than for the other organisms.

The parasite *Toxoplasma gondii* causes toxoplasmosis and may cause miscarriage, stillbirth, or fetal abnormality. Although results of *Toxoplasma gondii* testing are not generally reported by clinicians, results from national surveys that include blood testing suggest that toxoplasmosis may be one of the most common infections associated with food. Blood tests reveal toxoplasmosis infections at a rate of 7.2 percent for children aged 6 to 10 years.[23] Preliminary data from a European study showed that a majority of toxoplasmosis cases were foodborne.[24] Another study found that food consumption and preparation practices accounted for five of the top six practices by pregnant women that were significantly associated with congenital toxoplasmosis.[25] The food practices were eating raw or undercooked minced meat products, eating raw or undercooked mutton, eating raw or undercooked pork or lamb, eating unwashed raw vegetables, and washing kitchen knives infrequently after preparation of raw meat and prior to handling another food item.[25] Changing the cat litter, although often thought to be the major cause of toxoplasmosis, ranked fifth in importance of the six practices. As with other parasitic diseases, diagnostic laboratory testing for toxoplasmosis often is not available or is done infrequently. Efforts are under way in the United States to make congenital toxoplasmosis a nationally notifiable disease, with serological data collection beginning in 2000.

10-2. Reduce outbreaks of infections caused by key foodborne bacteria.

Target and baseline:

Objective	Reduction in Infections Caused by Foodborne Bacteria	1997 Baseline	2010 Target
		Number of Outbreaks per Year	
10-2a.	*Escherichia coli* O157:H7	22	11
10-2b.	*Salmonella* serotype Enteritidis	44	22

Target setting method: 50 percent improvement.

Data source: Foodborne Disease Outbreak Surveillance System, CDC, NCID.

Outbreaks of *E. coli* O157:H7 have been associated with undercooked or raw ground beef, unpasteurized apple juice, and some types of fresh (raw) produce. The most frequent known cause of outbreaks of *Salmonella* Enteritidis is the consumption of food that contains undercooked or raw eggs.

10-3. Prevent an increase in the proportion of isolates of *Salmonella* species from humans and from animals at slaughter that are resistant to antimicrobial drugs.

Target and baseline:

Objective	Prevention of Increase in Proportion of *Salmonella* Species Resistant to Antimicrobial Drugs	1997 Baseline	2010 Target
		Percent of Isolates	
	***Salmonella* from humans that are resistant to:**		
10-3a.	Fluoroquinolones	0	0
10-3b.	Third-generation cephalosporins	0	0
10-3c.	Gentamicin	3	3
10-3d.	Ampicillin	18	18
	***Salmonella* from cattle at slaughter that are resistant to:**		
10-3e.	Fluoroquinolones	Developmental	
10-3f.	Third-generation cephalosporins	Developmental	
10-3g.	Gentamicin	Developmental	
10-3h.	Ampicillin	Developmental	
	***Salmonella* from broilers at slaughter that are resistant to:**		
10-3i.	Fluoroquinolones	Developmental	
10-3j.	Third-generation cephalosporins	Developmental	
10-3k.	Gentamicin	Developmental	
10-3l.	Ampicillin	Developmental	
	***Salmonella* from swine at slaughter that are resistant to:**		
10-3m.	Fluoroquinolones	Developmental	
10-3n.	Third-generation cephalosporins	Developmental	
10-3o.	Gentamicin	Developmental	
10-3p.	Ampicillin	Developmental	

Target setting method: No increase.

Data sources: National Antimicrobial Resistance Monitoring System: Enteric Bacteria–*Salmonella* (NARMS: Enteric Bacteria), CDC, NCID; FDA, CVM; USDA, FSIS, APHIS, and ARS; Foodborne Disease Active Surveillance Network (FoodNet), CDC, FDA, USDA, FSIS.

10-4. (Developmental) Reduce deaths from anaphylaxis caused by food allergies.

Potential data source: National Vital Statistics System (NVSS), CDC, NCHS.

10-5. Increase the proportion of consumers who follow key food safety practices.

Target: 79 percent.

Baseline: 72 percent of consumers followed key food safety practices in 1998, based on total population of adults who engaged in the practice.

Target setting method: Better than the best.

Data source: Food Safety Survey (FSS), FDA and FSIS, USDA.

NOTE: THE TABLE BELOW MAY CONTINUE TO THE FOLLOWING PAGE.

Adult Population, 1998	Followed Key Food Safety Practices
	Percent
TOTAL	72
Race and ethnicity	
American Indian or Alaska Native	DSU
Asian or Pacific Islander	DSU
Asian	DNC
Native Hawaiian and other Pacific Islander	DNC
Black or African American	70
White	73
Hispanic or Latino	DSU
Not Hispanic or Latino	72
Black or African American	DSU
White	DSU
Gender	
Female	75
Male	69
Family income level (annual)	
Less than $10,000	DSU
$10,000 to $19,999	72
$20,000 and above	72

Adult Population, 1998	Followed Key Food Safety Practices
	Percent
Education level (aged 18 years and older)	
Less than high school	DSU
High school graduate	74
At least some college	72
Disability status	
Persons with disabilities	DNC
Persons without disabilities	DNC
Select populations	
Children under age 5 years in household	
No	72
Yes	73
Age groups	
18 to 59 years	72
60 years and older	75

DNA = Data have not been analyzed. DNC = Data are not collected. DSU = Data are statistically unreliable.
Note: Adjusted to 1993 census proportions on gender, race, and education.
NOTE: THE TABLE ABOVE MAY HAVE CONTINUED FROM THE PREVIOUS PAGE.

Key food safety practices are based on the four FightBAC!™ Campaign messages: clean—wash hands and surfaces often; separate—don't cross-contaminate; cook—cook to proper temperatures; and chill—refrigerate promptly.

10-6. (Developmental) Improve food employee behaviors and food preparation practices that directly relate to foodborne illnesses in retail food establishments.

Potential data source: Retail Food Database of Foodborne Illness Risk Factors, FDA, CFSAN.

Five food safety risk factors related to employee behaviors and preparation practices have been identified by CDC as contributing to foodborne illness: improper holding temperatures, inadequate cooking, contaminated equipment, food from an unsafe source, and poor personal hygiene. "For each year from 1988 through 1992, the most commonly reported food preparation practice that contributed to foodborne disease concerned improper holding temperature; the second concerned poor personal hygiene of food handlers. Food obtained from an unsafe source was the least commonly reported factor for all 5 years. In most outbreaks caused by bacterial pathogens, the food was stored at improper holding temperatures."[1]

To help control the risk factors, the *Food Code* provides key public health interventions: use of time-temperature control, prevention of hand contact with foods as a vehicle of contamination, employee health, demonstration of knowledge by the manager, and a consumer advisory to inform consumers of their risk when eating raw or undercooked animal foods. Proper application and implementation of these interventions are crucial to combat foodborne disease.

10-7. (Developmental) Reduce human exposure to organophosphate pesticides from food.

Potential data source: Total Diet Study, FDA, CFSAN.

The Food Quality Protection Act of 1996 mandated that EPA reassess existing standards for pesticides used on food crops. Organophosphates, a group of approximately 40 closely related pesticides, have been designated as first priority in the standards reassessment. These pesticides are used on fruits and vegetables important in the diet of children.

Related Objectives From Other Focus Areas

8. **Environmental Health**
   8-5. Safe drinking water
   8-6. Waterborne disease outbreaks
   8-8. Surface water health risks
   8-10. Fish contamination
   8-24. Exposure to pesticides
   8-25. Exposure to heavy metals and other toxic chemicals
   8-29. Global burden of disease
   8-30. Water quality in the U.S.-Mexico border region
14. **Immunization and Infectious Diseases**
   14-21. Antimicrobial use in intensive care units
20. **Occupational Safety and Health**
   20-8. Occupational skin diseases or disorders
23. **Public Health Infrastructure**
   23-2. Public access to information and surveillance data

Terminology

(A listing of abbreviations and acronyms used in this publication appears in Appendix H.)

Anaphylaxis: A severe allergic reaction commonly caused by certain foods. It occurs within minutes of exposure and may include hives, itching, skin swelling, blood vessel collapse, shock, and often life-threatening respiratory distress.[26]

Cephalosporins, third generation: Potent antimicrobial drugs capable of fighting a wide variety of bacterial infections. *Salmonella* species infections in certain high-risk and severely ill patients, particularly children, often are treated with such drugs.

Emerging pathogen: An illness-causing microorganism previously unknown to be a human pathogen, a foodborne pathogen not expected to occur in particular foods, or a pathogen that has caused a dramatic increase in new cases of illness.

Food Code: A book of recommendations of the U.S. Public Health Service that FDA first published in 1993 and revises every 2 years. It consists of model requirements for safeguarding public health and ensuring food is unadulterated and honestly presented to the consumer. FDA offers the *Food Code* for adoption by local, State, Tribal, and Federal government jurisdictions for administration by the units that have compliance responsibilities for food service, retail food stores, or food vending operations.

Foodborne disease or **foodborne illness:** Infection or intoxication caused by microbial or chemical contaminants in foods. Some foodborne illnesses, such as salmonellosis and staphylococcal food poisoning, can be caused by a single helping or less of a food that contains sufficient microorganisms or toxin to cause illness. Other foodborne illnesses result from eating compounds, such as naturally occurring aflatoxin, in foods over long periods of time.

Foodborne disease outbreak: When two or more cases of a similar illness result from eating the same food.[1]

Food industry: Food producers (farmers, fishers, ranchers), food processors, food storers, food warehousers and transporters, and retail food operators.

FoodNet: The Foodborne Diseases Active Surveillance Network, a collaborative project conducted by CDC, participating States, FSIS, and FDA that began in 1996. FoodNet produces national estimates of the burden and sources of specific diseases in the United States through active surveillance and other studies. California, Connecticut, Georgia, Maryland, Minnesota, New York, Oregon, and Tennessee, representing a total population of 28 million people (approximately 10 percent of the U.S. population), are the eight FoodNet sites.[27]

Good manufacturing practices (GMPs): Criteria, including regulations, that ensure that food is fit for consumption and is manufactured under sanitary conditions. These criteria address factors that affect production of safe food, including disease control, cleanliness (personal hygiene and dress codes), education, and training.

Hazard Analysis and Critical Control Points (HACCP): A science-based and systematic approach to prevent potential food safety problems by anticipating how and where biological, chemical, or physical hazards are most likely to occur and by installing appropriate measures to prevent them from occurring. The seven principles of HACCP are hazard analysis, determination of critical control points, specification of critical limits, monitoring, corrective actions, verification, and documentation (recordkeeping).

Hemolytic uremic syndrome (HUS), postdiarrheal: A serious, sometimes fatal complication often associated with illness caused by *Escherichia coli* O157:H7 and other shiga toxin-producing *E. coli*.[28] HUS occurs mainly in children under the age of 10 years. Renal failure, hemolytic anemia, and a severe decrease in the number of blood platelets characterize HUS.

Mycotoxins: Naturally occurring toxins formed by fungi (molds) in food and in animal feed (for example, aflatoxins, fumonisins, deoxynivalenol, and patulin).

Outbreak: See foodborne disease outbreak above.

Pathogen: A microorganism that causes illness.

Retail food industry: As covered by the *Food Code*, a level within the food industry that includes but is not limited to the following establishments: vending operations, grocery stores, other retail food outlets, and food service in restaurants and institutions.

References

[1] Centers for Disease Control and Prevention (CDC). Surveillance for foodborne-disease outbreaks—United States, 1988–92. *Morbidity and Mortality Weekly Report* 45(SS-5):1-55, 1996.

[2] Mead, P.S.; Slutsker, L.; Dietz, V.; et al. Food-related illness and death in the United States. *Emerging Infectious Diseases* 5(5):607-625, 1999.

[3] Food and Drug Administration (FDA), U.S. Department of Agriculture (USDA), and U.S. Environmental Protection Agency (EPA). *Food Safety From Farm to Table: A National Food Safety Initiative. Report to the President, May 1997*. Washington, DC: FDA, USDA, EPA, 1997.

[4] U.S. Department of Health and Human Services (HHS). *Healthy People 2000 Progress Review, Food and Drug Safety*. Washington, DC: HHS, Public Health Service (PHS), Office of Disease Prevention and Health Promotion (ODPHP), 1995.

[5] Lin, B.H.; Guthrie, J.; and Frazão, E. Away-from-home foods increasingly important to quality of American diet. *Agriculture Information Bulletin* No. 749, 22, 1999.

[6] Altekruse, S.F.; Street, D.A.; Fein, S.B.; et al. Consumer knowledge of foodborne microbial hazards and food-handling practices. *Journal of Food Protection* 59:287-294, 1996.

[7] National Center for Health Statistics (NCHS). *Healthy People 2000 Review, 1998–99*. Hyattsville, MD: NCHS, 1999, 126-127.

[8] FDA. *Pesticide Program Residue Monitoring, 1997*. Washington, DC: FDA, 1998.

[9] Agricultural Marketing Service. *Pesticide Data Program—Annual Summary, Calendar Year 1997*. Washington, DC: USDA, 1997.

[10] Kayosaari, M. Food allergy in Finnish children aged 1-6 years. *Acta Paediatrica Scandinavica* 71(5):815-819, 1982.

[11] Bock, S.A. Prospective appraisal of complaints of adverse reactions to foods in children during the first three years of life. *Pediatrics* 79(5):683-688, 1987.

[12] Sampson, H.A., and Metcalf, D.D. Food allergies. *Journal of the American Medical Association* 268(20):2840-2844, 1992.

[13] Schwartz, H.J. Latex: A potential hidden "food" allergen in fast food restaurants. *Journal of Allergy and Clinical Immunology* 95(1, Part 1):139-40, 1995.

[14] Tomazic, V.J.; Shampaine, E.L.; Lamanna, A.; et al. Cornstarch powder on latex products is an allergen carrier. *Journal of Allergy and Clinical Immunology* 93(4):751-758, 1994.

[15] Yocum, M.W., and Khan, D.A. Assessment of patients who have experienced anaphylaxis: A 3-year survey. *Mayo Clinic Proceedings* 69(1):16-23, 1994.

[16] Sampson, H.A. Fatal food-induced anaphylaxis. *Allergy* 53(Suppl. 46):125-130, 1998.

[17] Kemp, S.F.; Lockey, R.F.; Wolf, B.L.; et al. Anaphylaxis. *Archives of Internal Medicine* 155(16):1749-1754, 1995.

[18] *Federal Food, Drug, and Cosmetic Act, As Amended July 1993.* Section 403 (i). Washington, DC: U.S. Government Printing Office (GPO), 1993.

[19] *Code of Federal Regulations,* Title 21, Part 101, Section 100 (a)(3). Washington, DC: GPO, 1998.

[20] FDA. Notice to Manufacturers: Label Declaration of Allergenic Substances in Foods, 1996. Letter from FDA, Center for Food Safety and Applied Nutrition, June 10, 1996.

[21] Council for Agricultural Science and Technology. *Foodborne Pathogens: Risks and Consequences.* Task Force Report No. 122, 1994.

[22] Olowokure, B.; Hawker, J.; Weinberg, J.; et al. Deprivation and hospital admission for infectious intestinal diseases. *Lancet* 353(9155):807-808, 1999.

[23] NCHS. *National Health and Nutrition Examination Survey III, 1988–94.* Washington, DC: CDC, National Center for Infectious Diseases, unpublished data.

[24] CDC. National Workshop on Toxoplasmosis: Preventing Congenital Toxoplasmosis. Atlanta, GA, September 9-10, 1998.

[25] Kapperud, G.; Jenum, P.A.; Stray-Pederson, B.; et al. Risk factors for *Toxoplasma gondii* infection in pregnancy. Results of a prospective case-control study in Norway. *American Journal of Epidemiology* 144(4):405-412, 1996.

[26] *Dorland's Illustrated Medical Dictionary.* 28th ed. Philadelphia, PA: Saunders Co., 1994, 68-69.

[27] CDC. *FoodNet 1998 Surveillance Results: Preliminary Report, March 1999.* Washington, DC: CDC, 1999.

[28] Lindsay, J.A. Chronic sequelae of foodborne disease. *Emerging Infectious Diseases* 3(4):443-452, 1997.

11

Health Communication

Lead Agency: Office of Disease Prevention and Health Promotion

Contents

Use communication strategically to improve health.

Health communication encompasses the study and use of communication strategies to inform and influence individual and community decisions that enhance health. It links the domains of communication and health and is increasingly recognized as a necessary element of efforts to improve personal and public health.[1, 2, 3] Health communication can contribute to all aspects of disease prevention and health promotion and is relevant in a number of contexts, including (1) health professional-patient relations, (2) individuals' exposure to, search for, and use of health information, (3) individuals' adherence to clinical recommendations and regimens, (4) the construction of public health messages and campaigns, (5) the dissemination of individual and population health risk information, that is, risk communication, (6) images of health in the mass media and the culture at large, (7) the education of consumers about how to gain access to the public health and health care systems, and (8) the development of telehealth applications.[3, 4, 5, 6, 7, 8, 9, 10, 11]

For individuals, effective health communication can help raise awareness of health risks and solutions, provide the motivation and skills needed to reduce these risks, help them find support from other people in similar situations, and affect or reinforce attitudes.[1] Health communication also can increase demand for appropriate health services and decrease demand for inappropriate health services. It can make available information to assist in making complex choices, such as selecting health plans, care providers, and treatments.[1] For the community, health communication can be used to influence the public agenda, advocate for policies and programs, promote positive changes in the socioeconomic and physical environments, improve the delivery of public health and health care services, and encourage social norms that benefit health and quality of life.[2]

The practice of health communication has contributed to health promotion and disease prevention in several areas. One is the improvement of interpersonal and group interactions in clinical situations (for example, provider-patient, provider-provider, and among members of a health care team) through the training of health professionals and patients in effective communication skills.[3, 4] Collaborative relationships are enhanced when all parties are capable of good communication.

Another area is the dissemination of health messages through public education campaigns that seek to change the social climate to encourage healthy behaviors, create awareness, change attitudes, and motivate individuals to adopt recommended behaviors.[6, 9, 10] Campaigns traditionally have relied on mass communica-

Attributes of Effective Health Communication

- **Accuracy**: The content is valid and without errors of fact, interpretation, or judgment.

- **Availability**: The content (whether targeted message or other information) is delivered or placed where the audience can access it. Placement varies according to audience, message complexity, and purpose, ranging from interpersonal and social networks to billboards and mass transit signs to prime-time TV or radio, to public kiosks (print or electronic), to the Internet.

- **Balance**: Where appropriate, the content presents the benefits and risks of potential actions or recognizes different and valid perspectives on the issue.

- **Consistency**: The content remains internally consistent over time and also is consistent with information from other sources (the latter is a problem when other widely available content is not accurate or reliable).

- **Cultural competence**: The design, implementation, and evaluation process that accounts for special issues for select population groups (for example, ethnic, racial, and linguistic) and also educational levels and disability.

- **Evidence base**: Relevant scientific evidence that has undergone comprehensive review and rigorous analysis to formulate practice guidelines, performance measures, review criteria, and technology assessments for telehealth applications.

- **Reach**: The content gets to or is available to the largest possible number of people in the target population.

- **Reliability**: The source of the content is credible, and the content itself is kept up to date.

- **Repetition**: The delivery of/access to the content is continued or repeated over time, both to reinforce the impact with a given audience and to reach new generations.

- **Timeliness**: The content is provided or available when the audience is most receptive to, or in need of, the specific information.

- **Understandability**: The reading or language level and format (including multimedia) are appropriate for the specific audience.

tion (such as public service announcements on billboards, radio, and television) and educational messages in printed materials (such as pamphlets) to deliver health messages. Other campaigns have integrated mass media with community-based programs. Many campaigns have used social marketing techniques.

Increasingly, health improvement activities are taking advantage of digital technologies, such as CD-ROM and the World Wide Web (Web), that can target audiences, tailor messages, and engage people in interactive, ongoing exchanges about health.[4, 11, 12] An emerging area is health communication to support community-centered prevention.[13] Community-centered prevention shifts attention from the individual to group-level change and emphasizes the empowerment of individuals and communities to effect change on multiple levels.

A set of Leading Health Indicators, which focus on key health improvement activities and are described in *Healthy People 2010: Understanding and Improving Health*, all depend to some extent on effective health communication. The promotion of regular physical activity, healthy weight, good nutrition, and responsible sexual behavior will require a range of information, education, and advocacy efforts, as will the reduction of tobacco use, substance abuse, injuries, and violence. For example, advocacy efforts to change prices and availability of tobacco and alcohol products have resulted in lower consumption levels. (See Focus Area 26. Substance Abuse and Focus Area 27. Tobacco Use.) Effective counseling and patient education for behavior change require health care providers and patients to have good communication skills. Public information campaigns are used to promote increased fruit and vegetable consumption (5-A-Day for Better Health!), higher rates of preventive screening (mammogram and colonoscopy), higher rates of clinical preventive services (immunization), and greater rates of adoption of risk-reducing behaviors (Back to Sleep and Buckle Up for Safety).

Health communication alone, however, cannot change systemic problems related to health, such as poverty, environmental degradation, or lack of access to health care, but comprehensive health communication programs should include a systematic exploration of all the factors that contribute to health and the strategies that could be used to influence these factors. Well-designed health communication activities help individuals better understand their own and their communities' needs so that they can take appropriate actions to maximize health.

Issues and Trends

The environment for communicating about health has changed significantly. These changes include dramatic increases in the number of communication channels and the number of health issues vying for public attention as well as consumer demands for more and better quality health information, and the increased sophistication of marketing and sales techniques, such as direct-to-consumer advertising of prescription drugs and sales of medical devices and medications over the Internet. The expansion of communication channels and health issues on the public agenda increases competition for people's time and attention; at the same time, people have more opportunities to select information based on their personal interests and preferences. The trend toward commercialization of the Internet suggests that the marketing model of other mass media will be applied to emerging media, which has important consequences for the ability of noncommercial and public health-oriented health communications to stand out in a cluttered health information environment.

Communication occurs in a variety of contexts (for example, school, home, and work); through a variety of channels (for example, interpersonal, small group, organizational, community, and mass media) with a variety of messages; and for a variety of reasons. In such an environment, people do not pay attention to all communications they receive but selectively attend to and purposefully seek out information.[8] One of the main challenges in the design of effective health communication programs is to identify the optimal contexts, channels, content, and reasons that will motivate people to pay attention to and use health information.

A one-dimensional approach to health promotion, such as reliance on mass media campaigns or other single-component communication activities, has been shown to be insufficient to achieve program goals. Successful health promotion efforts increasingly rely on multidimensional interventions to reach diverse audiences about complex health concerns, and communication is integrated from the beginning with other components, such as community-based programs, policy changes, and improvements in services and the health delivery system.[10, 14] Research shows that health communication best supports health promotion when multiple communication channels are used to reach specific audience segments with information that is appropriate and relevant to them.[6] An important factor in the design of multidimensional programs is to allot sufficient time for planning, implementation, and evaluation and sufficient money to support the many elements of the program. Public-private partnerships and collaborations can leverage resources to strengthen the impact of multidimensional efforts. Collaboration can have the added benefit of reducing message clutter and targeting health concerns that cannot be fully addressed by public resources or market incentives alone.

Research indicates that effective health promotion and communication initiatives adopt an audience-centered perspective, which means that promotion and communication activities reflect audiences' preferred formats, channels, and contexts.[6] These considerations are particularly relevant for racial and ethnic populations, who may have different languages and sources of information. In these cases, public education campaigns must be conceptualized and developed by individuals with specific knowledge of the cultural characteristics, media habits, and language preferences of intended audiences. Direct translation of health information or health promotion materials should be avoided. Credible channels of communication need to be identified for each major group. Television and radio serving specific racial and ethnic populations can be effective means to deliver health messages when care is taken to account for the language, culture, and socioeconomic situations of intended audiences.

An audience-centered perspective also reflects the realities of people's everyday lives and their current practices, attitudes and beliefs, and lifestyles. Some specific audience characteristics that are relevant include gender, age, education and income levels, ethnicity, sexual orientation, cultural beliefs and values, primary language(s), and physical and mental functioning. Additional considerations include their experience with the health care system, attitudes toward different types of health problems, and willingness to use certain types of health services. Particular attention should be paid to the needs of underserved audience members.

Targeting specific segments of a population and tailoring messages for individual use are two methods to make health promotion activities relevant to audiences.[15] Examples include the targeted use of mass media messages for adolescent girls at increased risk of smoking;[16] the tailoring of computer-generated nutritional information to help individuals reduce their fat intake and increase fruit and vegetable consumption;[17] and a national telephone service for Spanish speakers to obtain AIDS information as well as counseling and referrals.[18]

Interventions that account for the cultural practices and needs of specific populations have shown some success. For example, a breastfeeding promotion program among Navajo women that was based on investigations of their cultural beliefs about infant feeding practices showed increased rates of breastfeeding.[19] Similarly, an intervention that used the novela, a popular form of Latino mass media, to reach young people and their parents sought to improve parent-youth communication in Hispanic families and to influence the adolescents' attitudes about alcohol.[20]

Advances in medical and consumer health informatics are changing the delivery of health information and services and are likely to have a growing impact on individual and community health.[3, 4, 11, 21] The convergence of media (computers, telephones, television, radio, video, print, and audio) and the emergence of the Internet create a nearly ubiquitous networked communication infrastructure. This infrastructure facilitates access to an increasing array of health information and health-related support services and extends the reach of health communication efforts. Delivery channels such as the Internet expand the choices available for health professionals to reach patients and consumers and for patients and consumers to interact with health professionals and with each other (for example, in online support groups).

Compared to traditional mass media, interactive media may have several advantages for health communication efforts. These advantages include (1) improved access to personalized health information, (2) access to health information, support, and services on demand, (3) enhanced ability to distribute materials widely and update content or functions rapidly, (4) just-in-time expert decision support, and (5) more choices for consumers.[4, 21] The health impact of interactivity, customization, and enhanced multimedia is just beginning to be explored, and already interactive health communication technologies are being used to exchange information, facilitate informed decisionmaking, promote healthy behaviors, enhance peer and emotional support, promote self-care, manage demand for health services, and support clinical care.

Widespread availability and use of interactive health communication and telehealth applications create at least two serious challenges. One is related to the risks associated with consumers' use of poor quality health information to make decisions. Concerns are growing about the Web making available large amounts of information that may be misleading, inaccurate, or inappropriate, which may put consumers at unnecessary risk. Although many health professionals agree that the Internet is a boon for consumers because they have easier access to much more information than before, professionals also are concerned that the poor quality of a lot of information on the Web will undermine informed decisionmaking. These concerns are driving the development of a quality standards agenda to help health professionals and consumers find reliable Web sites and health information on the Internet. An expert panel convened by the U.S. Department of Health and Human Services describes high quality health information as accurate, current, valid, appropriate, intelligible, and free of bias.[4]

The other challenge is related to the protection of privacy and confidentiality of personal health information. The personal privacy and the confidentiality of health information are major issues for consumers, and these concerns are magnified when information is collected, stored, and made available online.[4] As the availability and variety of interactive health applications grow, consumer confidence about developers' ability or intent to ensure privacy will be challenged. In the near future, personal health information will be collected during both clinical and nonclinical encounters in disparate settings, such as schools, mobile clinics, public places, and homes, and will be made available for administrative, financial, clinical, and research purposes. Although public health and health services research may require de-identified personal health information, policies and procedures to protect privacy will need to ensure a balance between confidentiality and appropriate access to personal health information.

The trend of rapidly expanding opportunities in health communication intersects with recent demands for more rigorous evaluation of all aspects of the health care and public health delivery systems and for evidence-based practices.[22] Numerous studies of provider-patient communication support the connection among the quality of the provider-patient interaction, patient behavior, and health outcomes.[23] As the knowledge base about provider-patient interactions increases, a need becomes apparent for the development of practice guidelines to promote better provider-patient communication. Additional evidence about the process of health information-seeking and the role of health information in decisionmaking also is needed. Health communication campaigns could benefit as well from more rigorous formative research and evaluation of outcomes. Expected outcomes should be an important consideration and central element of campaign design. As health communication increasingly involves electronic media, new evaluation approaches are emerging.[4, 24, 25, 26] Given the critical role that communication plays in all aspects of public health and health care, health communication and outcomes research should become more tightly linked across all health communication domains.

Because national data systems will not be available in the first half of the decade for tracking progress, one subject of interest concerning health communication is not addressed in this focus area's objectives. Representing a research and data collection agenda for the coming decade, the topic covers persons who report being satisfied with the health information they received during their most recent search for such information. Health-conscious consumers increasingly are proactive in seeking out health information. Individuals want information about prevention and wellness as much as about medical problems. Public health and the medical community share an interest in promoting—and sustaining—informed decisions for better health. Surveys suggest that people want to get health information from a professional and that counseling by health professionals can be effective both in reducing lifestyle risks and supporting self-management of chronic diseases like diabetes. (See Focus Area 1. Access to Quality Health Services and Focus Area 7. Educational and Community-Based Programs.) However, diminished time in clinical visits and some clinicians' discomfort with open communication work against optimum information exchange. In addition, many people want information to be available when and where they need it most. Health information should be not only easily accessible but also of good quality and relevant for the needs of the person. The increasing use of the Internet as a source for health information will require greater awareness of the importance of the quality of information.

Disparities

Often people with the greatest health burdens have the least access to information, communication technologies, health care, and supporting social services. Even the most carefully designed health communication programs will have limited impact if underserved communities lack access to crucial health professionals, services, and communication channels that are part of a health improvement project.

Research indicates that even after targeted health communication interventions, low-education and low-income groups remain less knowledgeable and less likely to change behavior than higher education and income groups, which creates a knowledge gap and leaves some people chronically uninformed.[27] With communication technologies, the disparity in access to electronic information resources is commonly referred to as the "digital divide."[28] The digital divide becomes more critical as the amount and variety of health resources available over the Internet increase and as people need more sophisticated skills to use electronic resources.[29] Equitably distributed health communication resources and skills, and a robust communication infrastructure can contribute to the closing of the digital divide and the overarching goal of Healthy People 2010 to eliminate health disparities.

Even with access to information and services, however, disparities may still exist because many people lack health literacy.[30] Health literacy is increasingly vital to help people navigate a complex health system and better manage their own health. Differences in the ability to read and understand materials related to personal health as well as navigate the health system appear to contribute to health disparities. People with low health literacy are more likely to report poor health, have an incomplete understanding of their health problems and treatment, and be at greater risk of hospitalization.[31] The average annual health care costs of persons with very low literacy (reading at the grade two level or below) may be four times greater than for the general population.[32] An estimated 75 percent of persons in the United States with chronic physical or mental health problems are in the limited literacy category.[33] People with chronic conditions, such as asthma, hypertension, and diabetes, and low reading skills have been found to have less knowledge of their conditions than people with higher reading skills.[34, 35]

Although the majority of people with marginal or low literacy are white native-born Americans,[36] changing demographics suggest that low literacy is an increasing problem among certain racial and ethnic groups, non-English-speaking populations, and persons over age 65 years. One study of Medicare enrollees found that 34 percent of English speakers and 54 percent of Spanish speakers had inadequate or marginal health literacy.[37] As the U.S. population ages, low health literacy among elderly people is potentially a large problem. Nearly half of the people in the elderly population have low reading skills, and reading ability appears to decline with age. A study of patients 60 years and older at a public hospital found that 81 percent could not read and understand basic materials such as prescription labels and appointments.[38]

Opportunities

For health communication to contribute to the improvement of personal and community health during the first decade of the 21st century, stakeholders, including health professionals, researchers, public officials, and the lay public, must collaborate on a range of activities. These activities include (1) initiatives to build a robust health information system that provides equitable access, (2) development of high-quality, audience-appropriate information and support services for specific health problems and health-related decisions for all segments of the population, especially underserved persons, (3) training of health professionals in the science of communication and the use of communication technologies, (4) evaluation of interventions, and (5) promotion of a critical understanding and practice of effective health communication.

A national health information infrastructure (NHII) provides a framework that stakeholders can use to communicate with each other and to transform data into useful information on multiple levels. Efforts are under way throughout the world to develop integrated national and global health information infrastructures to support health improvements. In the United States, the National Committee on Vital and Health Statistics (NCVHS) is advising the Secretary of Health and Human Services and Congress on the health information needs of the country. The NCVHS defines NHII as all of the technologies, standards, applications, systems, values, and laws that support individual health, health care, and public health. Issues related to technical standards, privacy and confidentiality, and regulatory guidelines are being addressed by the public and private sectors.[39, 40]

The infrastructure makes it possible for people not only to use health information designed by others but also to create resources to manage their own health and to influence the health of their communities. For example, community groups could use computers to gain access to survey information about the quality of life in their neighborhoods and apply this information to create an action plan to present to local elected and public health officials. Information is a critical element of informed participation and decisionmaking, and appropriate, quality information and support services for all are empowering and democratic.

As patients and consumers become more knowledgeable about health information, services, and technologies, health professionals will need to meet the challenge of becoming better communicators and users of information technologies. Health professionals need a high level of interpersonal skills to interact with diverse populations and patients who may have different cultural, linguistic, educational, and socioeconomic backgrounds. Health professionals also need more direct training in and experience with all forms of computer and telecommunication technologies. In addition to searching for information, patients and consumers want to use technology to discuss health concerns, and health professionals need to be ready to respond. To support an increase in health communication activities, research and evaluation of all forms of health communication will be necessary to build the scientific base of the field and the practice of evidence-based health communication. Collectively, these opportunities represent important areas to make significant improvements in personal and community health.

Interim Progress Toward Year 2000 Objectives

Health Communication is a new focus area for Healthy People 2010.

Health Communication

Goal: Use communication strategically to improve health.

Number	Objective Short Title
11-1	Households with Internet access
11-2	Health literacy
11-3	Research and evaluation of communication programs
11-4	Quality of Internet health information sources
11-5	Centers for excellence
11-6	Satisfaction with health care providers' communication skills

11-1. Increase the proportion of households with access to the Internet at home.

Target: 80 percent.

Baseline: 26 percent of households had access to the Internet at home in 1998.

Target setting method: Better than the best.

Data source: Computer and Internet Use Supplement to the Current Population Survey, U.S. Department of Commerce, Bureau of the Census.

NOTE: THE TABLE BELOW MAY CONTINUE TO THE FOLLOWING PAGE.

Households, 1998	Internet Access at Home
	Percent
TOTAL	26
Race and ethnicity (head of household)	
American Indian or Alaska Native	DNA
Asian or Pacific Islander	DNA
Asian	DNC
Native Hawaiian and other Pacific Islander	DNC
Black or African American	DNA
White	DNA
Hispanic or Latino	13
Not Hispanic or Latino	DNA
American Indian or Alaska Native	19
Asian or Pacific Islander	36
Black or African American	11
White	30
Gender (head of household)	
Female	DNA
Male	DNA
Family income level	
Poor	DNA
Near poor	DNA
Middle/high income	DNA

Households, 1998	Internet Access at Home
	Percent
Education level (head of household)	
Less than high school	DNA
High school graduate	14
At least some college	DNA
Geographic location	
Urban	28
Rural	22

DNA = Data have not been analyzed. DNC = Data are not collected. DSU = Data are statistically unreliable.

NOTE: THE TABLE ABOVE MAY HAVE CONTINUED FROM THE PREVIOUS PAGE.

Many health care organizations and public service agencies use the Internet as one of their main channels for information delivery. Access to the Internet and subsequent technologies is likely to become essential to gain access to health information, contact health care organizations and health professionals, receive services at a distance, and participate in efforts to improve local and national health.[4, 11] The integration of communication media means electronic access to health information not only via computers but also with Web-enabled televisions and telephones, handheld devices, and other emerging technologies. Technical literacy, or the ability to use electronic technologies and applications, will be essential to gain access to this information.

Internet availability in the home is an important indicator of equitable access among population groups. An increasing number of people have access to the Internet at work and public facilities, such as libraries and community centers, but several limitations affect the use of online health information and support in these settings. Some employers monitor electronic mail and the types of sites visited by employees. Access in public settings may be problematic because of privacy and confidentiality concerns, and access may be needed during times when these facilities are unavailable. Because of the potentially sensitive nature of health-related uses of the Internet, access at home is essential.

Although the proportion of people with access to the Internet has risen dramatically since 1995, many segments of the population lack access, such as low-income and rural households; persons with less education; and certain racial and ethnic groups, such as African Americans and Hispanics.[28] Internet access rates vary considerably according to income. Only 11 percent of households earning $24,999 or less have access, whereas 19 percent are connected among those earning $25,000 to $34,999; 30 percent have access among those earning $35,000 to $49,999; and 52 percent of households with $50,000 or greater in income have an Internet connection.[28] Barriers to Internet access include cost, lack of services in certain communities, limited literacy, lack of familiarity with different technologies, and, especially for people with disabilities, inaccessible formats that limit appropriate and effective technology use. Initiatives to promote universal access to the Internet will involve public and private sector stakeholders, particularly government agencies and technology corporations.

11-2. (Developmental) Improve the health literacy of persons with inadequate or marginal literacy skills.

Potential data source: National Adult Literacy Survey, 2002, U.S. Department of Education.

Responses from the National Adult Literacy Survey indicate that approximately 90 million adults in the United States have inadequate or marginal literacy skills.[36] Written information is not the only way to communicate about health, but a great deal of health education and promotion are organized around the use of print materials, usually written at the 10th grade level and above. These materials are of little use to people who have limited literacy skills.[41] The result is that a very large segment of the population is denied the full benefits of health information and services.

Closing the gap in health literacy is an issue of fundamental fairness and equity and is essential to reduce health disparities. Public and private efforts need to occur in two areas: the development of appropriate written materials and improvement in skills of those persons with limited literacy. The knowledge exists to create effective, culturally and linguistically appropriate, plain language health communications. Professional publications and Federal documents provide the criteria to integrate and apply the principles of organization, writing style, layout, and design for effective communication.[41, 42] These criteria should be widely distributed and used. Many organizations such as public and medical libraries, voluntary, professional, and community groups, and schools could offer health literacy programs that target skill improvement for low-literacy and limited English proficient individuals. If appropriate materials exist and people receive the training to use them, then measurable improvements in health literacy for the least literate can occur.

11-3. (Developmental) Increase the proportion of health communication activities that include research and evaluation.

Potential data sources: Sponsored survey of *Federal Register* notices; Grantmakers in Health; National Health Council.

Effective health communication programs are built on sound research and evaluation. Meaningful research and evaluation are not afterthoughts but integral parts of initial program design. Research provides the ideas and tools to design and carry out formative, process, and outcome evaluations to improve health communication efforts, certify the degree of change that has occurred, and identify programs or elements of programs that are not working.[1, 10] Research and evaluation systematically obtain information that can be used to refine the design, development, implementation, adoption, redesign, and overall quality of a communication intervention.[43, 44]

Programs funded by Federal, philanthropic, and not-for-profit organizations could be strengthened with requirements for a minimum set of evaluation activities and specific measurements. The level of research and evaluation required should reflect the costs, scope, and potential impact (in terms of benefit or harm) of the communication activity proposed. At a minimum, programs should be expected to conduct appropriate audience testing for need, cultural and linguistic competence, comprehension, and receptivity. Requirements and specifications for evaluation could be set for grant-funded communication programs and included in requests for funding proposals and grant program guidelines as well as for programs directly funded and implemented by public or private sector organizations by including research and evaluation activities in their work plans.

11-4. (Developmental) Increase the proportion of health-related World Wide Web sites that disclose information that can be used to assess the quality of the site.

Potential data sources: Health on the Net Foundation; Health Internet Ethics (Hi-Ethics); Internet Healthcare Coalition.

With the rapidly growing volume of health information, advertising, products, and services available on World Wide Web sites, serious concerns arise regarding the accuracy, appropriateness, and potential health impact of these sites.[4, 21] People are using the Internet to look up information, purchase medications, consult remotely with providers, and maintain their personal health records. Approximately 70 million persons in the United States use the Internet for health-related reasons,[45] and the potential for harm from inaccurate information, inferior quality goods, and inappropriate services is significant. Many initiatives are under way to identify appropriate and feasible approaches to evaluate online health sites.[26] Professional associations are issuing guidelines and recommendations,[46, 47, 48] Federal agencies such as the Federal Trade Commission are actively monitoring and sanctioning owners of Web sites that are false or misleading,[49] and developers and purchasers of online health resources are being urged to adopt standards for quality assurance.[4]

To allow users to evaluate the quality and appropriateness of Internet health resources, health-related Web sites should publicly disclose the following essential information about their site:[4] (1) the identity of the developers and sponsors of the site (and how to contact them) and information about any potential conflicts of interest or biases, (2) the explicit purpose of the site, including any commercial purposes and advertising, (3) the original sources of the content on the site, (4) how the privacy and confidentiality of any personal information collected from users is protected, (5) how the site is evaluated, (6) and how the content is updated. An additional mark of quality which should be present in a Web site relates to the site's accessibility by all users. Contents of the site should be presented in a way that it can be used by people with disabilities and with low-end technology.

11-5. (Developmental) Increase the number of centers for excellence that seek to advance the research and practice of health communication.

Potential data sources: Health Communication Interest Group, American Public Health Association; Society for Social Marketing; Association of Schools of Public Health; Health Communication Divisions, International Communication Association and National Communication Association; NCI.

To enlarge the knowledge base of health communication and incorporate it into health promotion practice, a research and training infrastructure is needed to develop, model, and coordinate activities. For this purpose, centers for excellence located in academic institutions, national organizations, or research centers would be instrumental to meet scientific and practical needs. The centers would be responsible for an array of activities, such as (1) promoting the adoption of health communication theories and practices in health care, disease prevention, and health promotion initiatives, (2) developing and disseminating quality standards, (3) coordinating initiatives to develop a consensus research agenda, (4) developing systems to identify and assess health communication research, (5) evaluating communication strategies, messages, materials, and resources, (6) fostering networking and collaboration among health communicators, health educators, and other health professionals, (7) promoting health communication skills training for health professionals, and (8) promoting research and dissemination activities among specific population groups.

These centers should provide expert staff, model curricula with core competencies in health communication and media technologies, appropriately equipped media labs, research seminars, continuing education and distance learning courses, and training and placement programs to expand the pool of health communication professionals and health professionals with communication skills. The centers also could create databases that would catalog items such as formative and outcomes research studies and reports and could partner with existing governmental dissemination networks to make data publicly available. Centers for excellence in health communication could be funded through Federal grants, foundations, or private sector health care organizations.

11-6. (Developmental) Increase the proportion of persons who report that their health care providers have satisfactory communication skills.

Potential data sources: National Committee for Quality Assurance; Behavioral Risk Factor Surveillance System (BRFSS), CDC, NCCDPHP; National Health

Interview Survey (NHIS), CDC, NCHS; industry surveys (FIND/SVP, Nielsen, Jupiter Communications).

Good provider-patient communication contributes to quality care and improved health status. Patients' assessment of their providers' communication skills is important for individuals with a usual source of care as well as for those without, who may have less frequent contact with the medical care system. Studies indicate that patients find communicating with their health care providers difficult[23, 50] and report that providers do not give them enough information, even though they highly value the information and want to know more.[51] Clear, candid, accurate, culturally and linguistically competent provider-patient communication is essential for the prevention, diagnosis, treatment, and management of health concerns.[23, 52]

Effective communication underpins prevention and screening efforts at the clinical level, when providers have the opportunity to engage in one-on-one counseling and supply information that is culturally and linguistically appropriate and delivered at the person's health literacy level. Diagnoses and treatments require doctors to negotiate a common understanding with patients about what is to be done. The quality of provider-patient communication can affect numerous outcomes, including patient adherence to recommendations and health status.[53] Appropriate information and communication with a provider not only can relieve patients' anxieties but also can help patients understand their choices, allow them to participate in informed decisionmaking, and better manage their own health concerns.

Related Objectives From Other Focus Areas

1. **Access**
   1-3. Counseling about health behaviors
   1-12. Single toll-free number for poison control centers
2. **Arthritis, Osteoporosis, and Chronic Back Conditions**
   2-8. Arthritis education
3. **Cancer**
   3-10. Provider counseling about cancer prevention
4. **Chronic Kidney Disease**
   4-3. Counseling for chronic kidney failure care
5. **Diabetes**
   5-1. Diabetes education
7. **Educational and Community-Based Programs**
   7-2. School health education
   7-3. Health-risk behavior information for college and university students
   7-5. Worksite health promotion programs
   7-7. Patient and family education
   7-8. Satisfaction with patient education
   7-9. Health care organization sponsorship of community health promotion activities

Terminology

(A listing of abbreviations and acronyms used in this publication appears in Appendix H.)

Accuracy: Content that is valid and without errors of fact, interpretation, or judgment.

Advocacy: Communication directed at policymakers and decisionmakers to promote policies, regulations, and programs to bring about change.

Availability: Content (whether a targeted message or other information) that is delivered or placed where the audience can access it. Placement varies according to audience, message complexity, and purpose—from interpersonal and social networks to billboards, mass transit signs, prime-time TV, and radio and from public kiosks (print or electronic) to the Internet.

Balance: Where appropriate, content that fairly and accurately presents the benefits and risks of potential actions or recognizes different and valid perspectives on an issue.

Consistency: Content that remains internally consistent over time and also is consistent with information from other sources.

Consumer health informatics: Interactive health communication (see below) focusing on consumers.

Consumer health information: Information designed to help individuals understand their health and make health-related decisions for themselves and their families.

Cultural competence: The design, implementation, and evaluation process that accounts for special issues of select population groups (ethnic and racial, linguistic) as well as differing educational levels and physical abilities.

Decision support systems: Computer software programs designed to assist diagnostic and treatment decisions. Examples include drug alert notification systems, prompts to implement practice guidelines, and health risk appraisals.

Evidence base: Relevant scientific evidence that has undergone comprehensive review and rigorous analysis to formulate practice guidelines, performance measures, review criteria, and technology assessments[22] for telehealth applications.[4, 24]

Formative research: Assesses the nature of the problem, the needs of the target audience, and the implementation process to inform and improve program design. Formative research is conducted both prior to and during program development to adapt the program to audience needs. Common methods include literature reviews, reviews of existing programs, and surveys, interviews, and focus group discussions with members of the target audience.

Health communication: The art and technique of informing, influencing, and motivating individual, institutional, and public audiences about important health issues. The scope of health communication includes disease prevention, health promotion, health care policy, and the business of health care as well as enhancement of the quality of life and health of individuals within the community.[54]

Health education: Any planned combination of learning experiences designed to predispose, enable, and reinforce voluntary behavior conducive to health in individuals, groups, or communities.[55]

Health literacy: The degree to which individuals have the capacity to obtain, process, and understand basic health information and services needed to make appropriate health decisions.[30] (See also *Literacy.*)

Health promotion: Any planned combination of educational, political, regulatory, and organizational supports for actions and conditions of living conducive to the health of individuals, groups, or communities.

Interactive health communication: The interaction of an individual with an electronic device or communication technology to access or transmit health information or to receive guidance on a health-related issue.[21]

Internet: A worldwide interconnection of computer networks operated by government, commercial, and academic organizations and private citizens.

Literacy: The ability to read, write, and speak in English and to compute and solve problems at levels of proficiency necessary to function on the job and in society, to achieve one's goals, and develop one's knowledge and potential.[56]

Medical informatics: A field of study concerned with the broad range of issues in the management and use of biomedical information, including medical computing and the study of the nature of medical information itself.[57]

Outcome evaluation (sometimes called impact evaluation): Examines the results of a communication intervention, including changes in awareness, attitudes, beliefs, actions, professional practices, policies, costs, and institutional or social systems.

Patient communication: Information for individuals with health conditions to help them maximize recovery, maintain therapeutic regimens, and understand alternative approaches. Patient communication includes educational resources, provider-patient communication, and, increasingly, peer-to-peer communication.

Process evaluation: Monitors the administrative, organizational, or other operational characteristics of an intervention. Process evaluation includes monitoring the dissemination of communication products to intended users (whether gatekeepers or audiences) and audience members' exposure to a message. For an interactive health communication application, process evaluation may include testing how the application functions.

Reach: Information that gets to or is available to the largest possible number of people in the target population.

Reliability: Content that is credible in terms of its source and is kept up to date.

Repetition: Delivery of and access to content continued or repeated over time, both to reinforce the impact with a given audience and to reach new generations.

Risk communication: Engaging communities in discussions about environmental and other health risks and about approaches to deal with them. Risk communication also includes individual counseling about genetic risks and consequent choices.

Social marketing: The application of marketing principles and techniques to program development, implementation, and evaluation to promote healthy behaviors or reduce risky ones.[58, 59]

Tailoring: Creating messages and materials to reach one specific person based on characteristics unique to that person, related to the outcome of interest, and derived from an assessment of that individual.[15]

Targeting: Creating messages and materials intended to reach a specific segment of a population, usually based on one or more demographic or other characteristics shared by its members.[15]

Telehealth: The application of telecommunication and computer technologies to the broad spectrum of public health, medicine, and health.

Telemedicine: The use of electronic information and communication technologies to provide clinical care across distance.[24]

Timeliness: Content that is provided or available when the audience is most receptive to, or in need of, the specific information.

Underserved: Individuals or groups who lack access to health services or information relative to the national average. The underserved population may include residents of rural, remote, or inner-city areas; members of certain racial and ethnic groups; socio-economically disadvantaged persons; or people with disabilities.

Understandability: Reading or language level and format (including multimedia) appropriate for a specific audience.

World Wide Web (Web): An international virtual network composed of Internet host computers that can be accessed by graphical browsers.

References

[1] National Cancer Institute (NCI). *Making Health Communications Work*. Pub. No. NIH 89-1493. Washington, DC: U.S. Department of Health and Human Services (HHS), 1989.

[2] Piotrow, P.T.; Kincaid, D.L.; Rimon, II, J.G.; et al. *Health Communication*. Westport, CT: Praeger, 1997.

[3] Jackson, L.D., and Duffy, B.K., eds. *Health Communication Research*. Westport, CT: Greenwood, 1998.

[4] Science Panel on Interactive Communication and Health. Eng, T.R., and Gustafson, D.H., eds. *Wired for Health and Well-Being: The Emergence of Interactive Health Communication*. Washington, DC: HHS, 1999.

[5] Northouse, L.L., and Northouse, P.G. *Health Communication: Strategies for Health Professionals*. 3rd ed. Stamford, CT: Appleton & Lange, 1998.

[6] Maibach, E., and Parrott, R.L. *Designing Health Messages*. Thousand Oaks, CA: Sage Publications, 1995.

[7] Ray, E.B., and Donohew, L., eds. *Communication and Health: Systems and Applications*. Hillsdale, NJ: Lawrence Erlbaum Associates, 1990.

[8] Freimuth, V.S.; Stein, J.A.; and Kean, T.J. *Searching for Health Information: The Cancer Information Service Model*. Philadelphia, PA: University of Pennsylvania Press, 1989.

[9] Atkin, C., and Wallack, L., eds. *Mass Communication and Public Health*. Newbury Park, CA: Sage Publications, 1990.

[10] Backer, T.E.; Rogers, E.M.; and Sopory, P. *Designing Health Communication Campaigns: What Works?* Newbury Park, CA: Sage Publications, 1992.

[11] Harris, L.M., ed. Health and the new media. *Technologies Transforming Personal and Public Health*. Mahwah, NJ: Lawrence Erlbaum Associates, 1995.

[12] Street, R.L.; Gold, W.R.; and Manning, T., eds. *Health Promotion and Interactive Technology: Theoretical Applications and Future Directions*. Mahwah, NJ: Lawrence Erlbaum Associates, 1997.

[13] Finnegan, Jr., J.R., and Viswanath, K. Health and communication: Medical and public health influences on the research agenda. In: Ray, E.B., and Donohew, L., eds. *Communication and Health: Systems and Applications*. Hillsdale, NJ: Lawrence Erlbaum Associates, 1990.

[14] Simons-Morton, B.G.; Donohew, L.; and Crump, A.D. Health communication in the prevention of alcohol, tobacco, and drug use. *Health Education & Behavior* 24:544-554, 1997.

[15] Kreuter, M.W.; Strecher, V.J.; and Glassman, B. One size does not fit all: The case for tailoring print materials. *Society of Behavioral Medicine* 21:276-283, 1999.

[16] Worden, J.K.; Flynn, B.S.; Solomon, L.J.; et al. Using mass media to prevent cigarette smoking among adolescent girls. *Health Education Quarterly* 23:453-468, 1996.

[17] Brug, J.; Glanz, K.; Van Assema, P.; et al. The impact of computer-tailored feedback and iterative feedback on fat, fruit, and vegetable intake. *Health Education & Behavior* 25:517-531, 1998.

[18] Scott, S.A.; Jorgensen, C.M.; and Suarez, L. Concerns and dilemmas of Hispanic AIDS information seekers: Spanish-speaking callers to the CDC National AIDS hotline. *Health Education & Behavior* 25(4):501-516, 1998.

[19] Wright, A.L.; Naylor, A.; Wester, R.; et al. Using cultural knowledge in health promotion: Breastfeeding among the Navajo. *Health Education & Behavior* 24:625-639, 1997.

[20] Lalonde, B.; Rabinowitz, P.; Shefsky, M.L.; et al. La Esperanza del Valle: Alcohol prevention novelas for Hispanic youth and their families. *Health Education & Behavior* 24:587-602, 1997.

[21] Robinson, T.N.; Patrick, K.; Eng, T.R.; et al., for the Science Panel on Interactive Communication and Health. An evidence-based approach to interactive health communication: A challenge to medicine in the Information Age. *Journal of the American Medical Association* 280:1264-1269, 1998.

[22] Agency for Health Care Policy and Research. *Evidence-based Practice Centers*. RFP No. AHCPR-97-0001. Washington, DC: HHS, 1997.

[23] Roter, D.L., and Hall, J.A. *Doctors Talking with Patients/Patients Talking with Doctors: Improving Communication in Medical Visits*. Westport, CT: Auburn House, 1992.

[24] Committee on Evaluating Clinical Applications of Telemedicine. Field, M.J., ed. *Telemedicine: A Guide to Assessing Telecommunications for Health Care*. Washington, DC: National Academy Press, 1996.

[25] Anderson, J.G.; Aydin, C.E.; and Jay, S.J., eds. *Evaluating Health Care Information Systems*. Thousand Oaks, CA: Sage Publications, 1994.

[26] Kim, P.; Eng, T.R.; Deering, M.J.; et al. Published criteria for evaluating health-related Web sites: Review. *British Medical Journal* 318:647-649, 1999.

[27] Freimuth, V.S. The chronically uninformed: Closing the knowledge gap in health. In: Ray, E.B., and Donohew, L., eds. *Communication and Health: Systems and Applications*. Hillsdale, NJ: Lawrence Erlbaum Associates, 1990.

[28] U.S. Department of Commerce. *Falling Through the Net: Defining the Digital Divide*. Washington, DC: National Telecommunications and Information Administration, 1999. <http://www.ntia.doc.gov/ntiahome/digitaldivide/>July 29, 1999.

[29] Eng, T.R.; Maxfield, A.; Patrick, K.; et al. Access to health information and support: A public highway or a private road? *Journal of the American Medical Association* 280(15):1371-1375, 1998.

[30] HHS, National Institutes of Health, National Library of Medicine (NLM). In: Seiden, C.R.; Zorn, M.; Ratzan, S.; et al.; eds. *Health Literacy, January 1990 Through 1999*. NLM Pub. No. CBM 2000-1. Bethesda, MD: NLM, February 2000, vi.

[31] Baker, D.W.; Parker, R.M.; Williams, M.V.; et al. The relationship of patient reading ability to self-reported health and use of health services. *American Journal of Public Health* 87:1027-1030, 1997.

[32] Weiss, B.D.; Blanchard, J.S.; McGee, D.L.; et al. Illiteracy among Medicaid recipients and its relationship to health care costs. *Journal of Health Care for the Poor and Underserved* 5:99-111, 1994.

[33] Davis, T.C.; Meldrum, H.; Tippy, P.K.P.; et al. How poor literacy leads to poor healthcare. *Patient Care* 94-108, 1996.

[34] Williams, M.V.; Baker, D.W.; Parker, R.M.; et al. Relationship of functional health literacy to patients' knowledge of their chronic disease. A study of patients with hypertension and diabetes. *Archives of Internal Medicine* 158:166-172, 1998.

[35] Williams, M.V.; Baker, D.W.; Honig, E.G.; et al. Inadequate literacy is a barrier to asthma knowledge and self-care. *Chest* 114:1008-1015, 1998.

[36] Kirsch, I.; Jungeblut, A.; Jenkins, L.; et al. *Adult Literacy in America: A First Look at the Findings of the National Adult Literacy Survey.* Washington, DC: National Center for Education Statistics, U.S. Department of Education, 1993.

[37] Gazmararian, J.A.; Baker, D.W.; Williams, M.V.; et al. Health literacy among Medicare enrollees in a managed care organization. *Journal of the American Medical Association* 281:545-551, 1999.

[38] Williams, M.V.; Parker, R.M.; Baker, D.W.; et al. Inadequate functional health literacy among patients at two public hospitals. *Journal of the American Medical Association* 274:1677-1682, 1995.

[39] National Committee on Vital and Health Statistics. Assuring a health dimension for the National Information Infrastructure. 1998. <http://www.ncvhs.hhs.gov/hii-nii.htm>August 10, 1999.

[40] National Committee on Vital and Health Statistics. *Toward a National Health Information Infrastructure.* 2000. <http://www.ncvhs.hhs.gov/NHII2KReport.htm>July 28, 2000.

[41] NCI. *Clear & Simple: Developing Effective Print Materials for Low-literate Readers.* Pub. No. NIH 95-3594. Washington, DC: HHS, 1995.

[42] Doak, C.C.; Doak, L.G.; and Root, J.H. *Teaching Patients with Low Literacy Skills.* 2nd ed. Philadelphia, PA: J.B. Lippincott Company, 1996.

[43] Rossi, P.H. Twelve laws of evaluation research. In: Fisher, A.; Pavlova, M.; and Covello, V.; eds. *Evaluation and Effective Risk Communications, Workshop Proceedings.* Interagency Task Force on Environmental Cancer and Heart and Lung Disease, Committee on Public Education and Communication. EPA/600/9-90/054. Washington, DC: U.S. Environmental Protection Agency (EPA), 1991.

[44] Rossi, P.H., and Freeman, H.E. *Evaluation: A Systematic Approach.* 5th ed. Newbury Park, CA: Sage Publications, 1993.

[45] ReutersHealth. Americans seek health information on-line. <http://www.reutershealth.com>August 6, 1999.

[46] American Telemedicine Association. American Telemedicine Association issues advisory on use of medical Web sites. <http://www.atmeda.org>August 10, 1999.

[47] Hi-Ethics. Health Internet Ethics: Ethical Principles for Offering Internet Health Services to Consumers, 2000. <http://www.hiethics.org>July 28, 2000.

[48] eHealth Ethics Initiative. eHealth Code of Ethics, 2000. <http://www.ihc.net/ethics/ethics.html>July 28, 2000.

[49] U.S. Federal Trade Commission (FTC). "Operation Cure All" targets Internet health fraud. Press release. Washington, DC: FTC, June 24, 1999.

[50] Rosenberg, E.E.; Lussier, M.T.; and Beaudoin, C. Lessons for clinicians from physician-patient communication literature. *Archives of Family Medicine* 6:279-283, 1997.

[51] Laine, C.; Davidoff, F.; Lewis, C.E.; et al. Important elements of outpatient care: A comparison of patients' and physicians' opinions. *Annals of Internal Medicine* 125:640-645, 1996.

[52] Schatz, B., and O'Hanlan, K. *Anti-Gay Discrimination in Medicine: Results of a National Survey of Lesbian, Gay and Bisexual Physicians.* San Francisco, CA: American Association of Physicians for Human Rights and Gay Lesbian Medical Association, 1994.

[53] Ong, L.M.L.; de Haes, J.C.J.M.; Hoos, A.M.; et al. Doctor-patient communication: A review of the literature. *Social Science and Medicine* 40:903-918, 1995.

[54] Ratzan, S.C., ed. Health communication, challenges for the 21st century. Special issue. *American Behavioral Scientist* 38(2), 1994.

[55] Green, L.W., and Kreuter, M.W. *Health Promotion Planning: An Educational and Ecological Approach.* 3rd ed. Mountain View, CA: Mayfield Publishing Company, 1999.

[56] U.S. Congress. National Literacy Act of 1991. Public Law 102-73, 1991.

[57] Shortliffe, E.H., and Perreault, L.E., eds. *Medical Informatics.* New York, NY: Addison-Wesley, 1990.

[58] Lefebvre, R.C., and Rochlin, L. Social marketing. In: Glanz, K.; Lewis, F.M.; and Rimer, B.K.; eds. *Health Behavior and Health Education: Theory, Research, and Practice.* 2nd ed. San Francisco, CA: Jossey-Bass Publishers, 1997, 384-401.

[59] Ling, J.C.; Franklin, B.A.; Lindsteadt, J.F.; et al. Social marketing, its place in public health. *Annual Reviews of Public Health* 13:341-362, 1992.

12

Heart Disease and Stroke

Co-Lead Agencies: Centers for Disease Control and Prevention
National Institutes of Health

Contents

Goal

Improve cardiovascular health and quality of life through the prevention, detection, and treatment of risk factors; early identification and treatment of heart attacks and strokes; and prevention of recurrent cardiovascular events.

Overview

Heart disease is the leading cause of death for all people in the United States. Stroke is the third leading cause of death. Heart disease and stroke continue to be major causes of disability and significant contributors to increases in health care costs in the United States.[1]

Epidemiologic and statistical studies have identified a number of factors that increase the risk of heart disease and stroke. In addition, clinical trials and prevention research studies have demonstrated effective strategies to prevent and control these risk factors and thereby reduce illnesses, disabilities, and deaths caused by heart disease and stroke.

Issues and Trends

Coronary heart disease (CHD) accounts for the largest proportion of heart disease. About 12 million people in the United States have CHD.[1] The CHD death rate peaked in the mid-1960s and has declined in the general population over the past 35 years. This decline began in females in the 1950s and in males in the 1960s. Although absolute declines have been much greater in males than in females, rates of decline also have been greater in males, but in recent years they have been greater in females.

Since 1950, there has been a clear rise and fall in CHD death rates for each racial and gender group. Although the age-adjusted death rate for CHD continues to decline each year, declines in the unadjusted death rate and in the number of deaths have slowed because of an increase in the number of older people in the United States, who have higher rates of CHD.

High blood cholesterol is a major risk factor for CHD that can be modified. More than 50 million U.S. adults have blood cholesterol levels that require medical advice and treatment.[2] More than 90 million adults have cholesterol levels that are higher than desirable. Experts recommend that all adults aged 20 years and older have their cholesterol levels checked at least once every 5 years to help them take action to prevent or lower their risk of CHD.[3] Lifestyle changes that prevent or lower high blood cholesterol include eating a diet low in saturated fat and cholesterol, increasing physical activity, and reducing excess weight.[3]

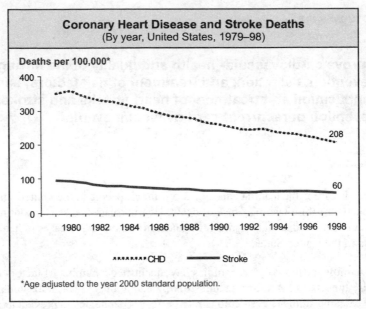

Coronary Heart Disease and Stroke Deaths
(By year, United States, 1979–98)

Deaths per 100,000*

208

60

1980 1982 1984 1986 1988 1990 1992 1994 1996 1998

CHD   Stroke

*Age adjusted to the year 2000 standard population.

Source: CDC, NCHS. National Vital Statistics System (NVSS), 1979–98.

About 4 million persons have cerebrovascular disease,[1] a major form of which is stroke. About 600,000 strokes occur each year in the United States, resulting in about 158,000 deaths. Death rates for stroke are highest in the southeastern United States. Like CHD death rates, stroke death rates have declined over the past 30 years. The decline accelerated in the 1970s for whites and African Americans. The rate of decline, however, has slowed in recent years. The overall decline has occurred mainly because of improvements in the detection and treatment of high blood pressure (hypertension).

High blood pressure is known as the "silent killer" and remains a major risk factor for CHD, stroke, and heart failure. About 50 million adults in the United States have high blood pressure. High blood pressure also is more common in older persons. Comparing the 1976–80 National Health and Nutrition Examination Survey (NHANES II) and the 1988–91 survey (NHANES III, phase 1) reveals an increase from 51 to 73 percent in the proportion of persons who were aware that they had high blood pressure.[4, 5] Nevertheless, a large proportion of persons with high blood pressure still are unaware that they have this disorder.[4, 5]

The age composition of the U.S. population changed dramatically during the 20th century and will continue to change during the 21st century. By the end of the 1990s, one in every four persons was aged 50 years or older. By 2030, about one in three will be aged 50 years or older. Most significant has been the increase in the size of the population aged 65 years and older. In addition, the percentage of persons aged 85 years and older has increased significantly. Heart disease and stroke deaths rise significantly after age 65 years, accounting for more than 40 percent of all deaths among persons aged 65 to 74 years and almost 60 percent of those aged 85 years and older. In the 1980s and 1990s, heart failure emerged as a major chronic disease for older adults.[6, 7, 8, 9] Almost 75 percent of the nearly 5 million patients with heart failure in the United States are older than 65 years.[8] Hospitalization rates for heart failure continue to increase significantly in those aged 65 years and older.[9]

Atrial fibrillation (AF) affects close to 2 million people in the United States. The number of existing cases of AF increases with age and is more common in males than in females.[10] Even though prevalence of AF is greater in males than in females, the absolute number of males and females with AF is about equal. About 70 percent of persons with AF are between age 65 and 85 years. About 15 percent of strokes occur in persons with AF.[10] Because females have a longer life expectancy than males, the actual number of cases in elderly females (older than 75 years) is greater than in elderly males. Cases of AF may continue to rise as persons live longer and as more persons survive a first heart attack.

Because national data systems will not be available in the first half of the decade for tracking progress, two subjects of interest are not addressed in this focus area's objectives. Representing a research and data collection agenda for the coming decade, the topics are related to provider counseling and increasing awareness of cardiovascular disease (CVD) as the leading cause of death for all females. The first topic covers instruction of high-risk patients and family members or significant others in preparing appropriate heart attack and stroke action plans for seeking rapid emergency care, including when to call 911 or the local emergency number. The second topic deals with increasing awareness among all females that CVD is their leading cause of death.

Disparities

In general, the heart disease death rate has been consistently higher in males than in females and higher in the African American population than in the white population. In addition, over the past 30 years the CHD death rate has declined differentially by gender and race. In the 1970s, African American females experienced the greatest decline in CHD. This steep decline leveled off in the 1980s, when rates of decline for white males and females exceeded those for African American males and females, and African American females had the lowest rate of decline.[11] In the 1980s, males had a steeper rate of decline than females. Between 1980 and 1995, the percentage declines were greater in males than in females and greater in whites than in African Americans. In 1995, the age-adjusted death rate for heart disease was 42 percent higher in African American males than in white males, 65 percent higher in African American females than in white females, and almost twice as high in males as in females.

Disparities also exist in treatment outcomes for patients who have heart attacks. Females, in general, have poorer outcomes following a heart attack than do males: 44 percent of females who have a heart attack die within a year, compared with 27 percent of males. At older ages, females who have a heart attack are twice as likely as males to die within a few weeks.[12] These differences are explained, in part, by the presence of coexisting conditions such as high blood pressure, diabetes, and congestive heart failure. After controlling for such factors, however, studies indicate an association remains between female gender and death following a heart attack. Complications are more frequent in females than in males after coronary intervention procedures, such as angioplasty or bypass surgery, are performed. Additional studies are needed to evaluate specific interventions and determine whether gender-specific interventions may be beneficial. In general, factors such as age (older), gender (female), race or ethnicity, low socioeconomic status, and prior medical conditions (previous heart attack, history of angina or diabetes) have been associated with longer prehospital delays in seeking care for symptoms of a heart attack.[13]

The male-female disparity in stroke deaths widened from the 1970s until the 1980s and then narrowed. Although stroke death rates have been decreasing, the decline among African Americans has not been as substantial as the decline in the total population. The racial differences in the number of new cases of stroke and deaths due to stroke are even greater than those found in CHD. Stroke deaths are highest in African American females born before 1950 and in African American males born after 1950. Among the racial and gender groups, declines in the stroke death rate are smallest in African American males. When adjusted for age, stroke deaths are almost 80 percent higher in African Americans than in whites and about 17 percent higher in males than in females. Moreover, age-specific stroke deaths are higher in African Americans than in whites in all age groups up to age 84 years and higher in males than in females throughout all adult age groups.

The number of existing cases of high blood pressure is nearly 40 percent higher in African Americans than in whites (an estimated 6.4 million African Americans have high blood pressure),[14] and its effects are more frequent and severe in the African American population.

Other racial and ethnic CHD and stroke data indicate that among U.S. adults aged 20 years and older, the age-adjusted (year 2000) prevalence of heart attacks is 5.2 percent for non-Hispanic white males and 2.0 percent for females; 4.3 percent for non-Hispanic black males and 3.3 percent for females; 4.1 percent for Mexican American males and 1.9 percent for females. Among American Indians aged 65 to 74 years the rates (per 1,000) of new and recurrent heart attacks are 25.1 for males and 9.1 for females. The average annual CHD incidence rate (per 1,000) in Japanese American males living in Hawaii was 4.6 for ages 45 to 49 years, 6.0 for ages 50 to 54 years, 7.2 for ages 55 to 59 years, 8.8 for ages 60 to 64 years, and 10.5 for ages 65 to 68 years.[10]

For stroke, other data show that the estimated age-adjusted (2000 standard) prevalence of stroke for persons aged 20 years and older in the United States was 2.2 percent for non-Hispanic white males and 1.5 percent for females; for non-Hispanic blacks, 2.5 percent for males and 3.2 percent for females; and for Mexican Americans, 2.3 percent for males and 1.3 percent for females. The rates (per

1,000) of new and recurrent strokes in American Indians aged 65 to 74 years are
15.2 for males and 7.9 for females. The average annual incidence rates (per 1,000)
of stroke in Japanese American males increased with advancing age from 45 to 49
years to 65 to 68 years at the initial examination: 2.1 to 8.2 for total stroke, 1.5 to
6.6 for thromboembolic stroke, and 0.4 to 1.0 for intracerebral hemorrhage.[10]

Opportunities

Primary prevention. Heart disease and stroke share several risk factors, including high blood pressure, cigarette smoking, high blood cholesterol, and overweight. Physical inactivity and diabetes are additional risk factors for heart
disease. (See Focus Area 5. Diabetes.) The lifetime risk for developing CHD is
very high in the United States: one of every two males and one of every three females aged 40 years and under will develop CHD sometime in their life. Primary
prevention, specifically through lifestyle interventions that promote heart-healthy
behaviors, is a major strategy to reduce the development of heart disease or
stroke.[15, 16, 17, 18, 19]

A number of studies have shown that lifestyle interventions can help prevent high
blood pressure and reduce blood cholesterol levels. For high blood pressure, these
interventions include increasing the level of aerobic physical activity, maintaining
a healthy weight, limiting the consumption of alcohol to moderate levels for those
who drink, reducing salt and sodium intake, and eating a reduced-fat diet high in
fruits, vegetables, and low-fat dairy food. Moreover, studies show that a diet low
in saturated fat, dietary cholesterol, and total fat—with physical activity and
weight control—can lower blood cholesterol levels.[20, 21, 22]

Overweight and obesity are growing public health problems, affecting adults, adolescents, and children. Overweight and obesity affect a large proportion of the
U.S. population—55 percent of adults. These persons are at increased risk of illness from high blood pressure, high blood cholesterol and other lipid disorders,
type 2 diabetes, CHD, stroke, and other diseases. Efforts to prevent overweight
and obesity by promoting heart-healthy behaviors—beginning in childhood—are
needed to help reverse the trend. Balancing calorie intake with physical activity is
critical. Research in the 1990s showed that a wide range of physical activities are
beneficial to health and that everyone can benefit from physical activity. Even
when physical activity is less than vigorous, it can still produce health benefits,
including a decreased risk of CHD.[23, 24, 25, 26] (See Focus Area 19. Nutrition and
Overweight.)

Nonetheless, increasing the level of physical activity remains a challenge. Furthermore, according to the 1996 surgeon general's report on physical activity and
health,[27] the percentage of people who say they engage in no leisure-time physical
activity is higher among females than males, among African Americans and Hispanics than whites, among older adults than younger adults, and among the less
affluent than the more affluent. (See Focus Area 22. Physical Activity and Fitness.)

Progress on smoking cessation will play a critical role in achieving the Healthy People 2010 objective for heart disease reduction. Smoking cessation has major and immediate health benefits for men and women of all ages. For example, people who quit smoking before age 50 years have half the risk of dying in the next 15 years, compared with people who continue to smoke.[28]

Studies have shown that risk factors for heart disease and stroke develop early in life: atherosclerosis already is present in late adolescence, diabetes in overweight children is on the rise, and hypertension can begin in the early teens.[29, 30] Tobacco use also begins in adolescence; therefore, primary prevention efforts should be expanded in elementary and secondary schools and at the college level. Nationwide mass media campaigns, community-based programs, and other communication efforts should be expanded to give groups better access to information and programs. These programs should promote heart-healthy behaviors at the community level as well as detect and treat existing risk factors.

Risk factor detection and treatment. Screening for risk factors, particularly for high blood pressure and high blood cholesterol, is an important step in identifying individuals whose risk factors may be undiagnosed and referring them to ongoing care. A host of studies has shown that dietary and pharmacologic therapy can reduce CHD and stroke risk factors, especially high blood pressure and high blood cholesterol. These interventions, coupled with other lifestyle changes, such as stopping smoking, increasing physical activity, and maintaining a healthy weight, can be even more effective in lowering the risk of a heart attack or stroke.[31, 32, 33, 34]

Research showing the importance of blood pressure to health led to the introduction by the National Heart, Lung, and Blood Institute (NHLBI) of the National High Blood Pressure Education Program (NHBPEP) in 1972.[35] NHBPEP is the first large-scale public outreach and education campaign to reduce high blood pressure. Its promotion of the detection, treatment, and control of high blood pressure has been credited with influencing the dramatic increase in the public's understanding of hypertension and its role in heart attacks and strokes, as well as related declines in deaths. The percentage of people who were able to control their high blood pressure through lifestyle changes and through antihypertensive drug therapy rose from about 16 percent in 1971–72 to about 65 percent in 1988–94.[1] About 90 percent of all adults now have their blood pressure measured at least once every 2 years. Average blood pressure levels have fallen by 10 to 12 mmHg since the advent of NHBPEP.[36] A slowly changing issue has been the recognition of systolic blood pressure as a more important predictor of CHD than diastolic blood pressure, especially in older adults.[37, 38]

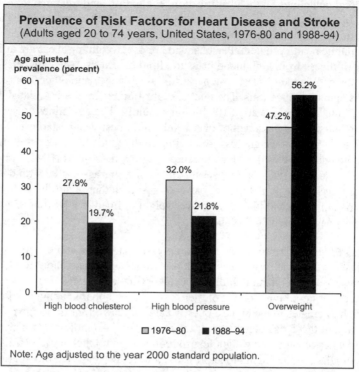

Prevalence of Risk Factors for Heart Disease and Stroke
(Adults aged 20 to 74 years, United States, 1976-80 and 1988-94)

Age adjusted
prevalence (percent)

High blood cholesterol: 27.9% (1976–80), 19.7% (1988–94)
High blood pressure: 32.0% (1976–80), 21.8% (1988–94)
Overweight: 47.2% (1976–80), 56.2% (1988–94)

□ 1976–80 ■ 1988–94

Note: Age adjusted to the year 2000 standard population.

Source: CDC, NCHS. National Health and Nutrition Examination Survey (NHANES), 1976–80 and 1988–94.

High blood cholesterol is total cholesterol of 240 mg/dL or more.
High blood pressure is average (among 3 blood pressures) of 140/90+ or taking antihypertensive medication. All pregnant women are excluded.
Overweight is body mass index (BMI) of 25 or more.

Research reported in the 1980s showed for the first time that lowering high blood cholesterol significantly reduces the risk for heart attacks and heart attack deaths. This research led to the creation of the National Cholesterol Education Program (NCEP) in 1985.[39] Clinical trials have proved that lowering cholesterol in persons with and without existing CHD reduces illness and death from CHD and even reduces overall death rates. Since NCEP was launched, the percentage of persons who have had their cholesterol checked has more than doubled, from 35 percent in 1983 to 75 percent in 1995.[40] Consumption of saturated fat, total fat, and cholesterol declined during the 1980s and 1990s, average blood cholesterol levels in adults dropped from 213 mg/dL in 1978 to 203 mg/dL in 1991 (age adjusted to 1980 population), and the prevalence of high blood cholesterol requiring medical advice and treatment fell from 36 percent to 29 percent.[39] These results reflect the impact of NCEP's population and high-risk strategies for lowering cholesterol.

The NHLBI Obesity Education Initiative, in cooperation with the National Institute of Diabetes and Digestive and Kidney Diseases, released in 1998 the first

Federal guidelines on the identification, evaluation, and treatment of overweight and obesity in adults.[41] These clinical practice guidelines are designed to help physicians in their identification and treatment of overweight and obesity, a growing public health problem. Persons who are overweight or obese are at increased risk of illness from high blood pressure, lipid disorders, type 2 diabetes, CHD, stroke, gallbladder disease, osteoarthritis, sleep apnea and other respiratory problems, and certain cancers. The total cost attributable to obesity-related diseases in the United States is nearly $100 billion annually. The guidelines present a new approach to the assessment of overweight and obesity and establish principles of safe and effective weight loss. According to the guidelines, the assessment of overweight involves three key measures—body mass index (BMI), waist circumference, and risk factors for diseases and conditions associated with obesity. The definitions in the guidelines are based on research that relates body mass index to the risk of death and illness, with overweight defined as a BMI of 25 to 29.9 and obesity as a BMI of 30 and above.[41]

As BMI levels rise, the average blood pressure and total cholesterol levels increase, and average high-density lipoprotein (HDL) (good cholesterol) levels decrease. Males in the highest obesity category have more than twice the risk of high blood pressure, high blood cholesterol, or both, compared to males of normal weight. Females in the highest obesity category have four times the risk of either or both of these risk factors, compared to normal weight females. Therefore, the guidelines recommend weight loss to reduce high total cholesterol, raise low levels of HDL, reduce high blood pressure, and reduce elevated blood glucose in overweight persons who have two or more risk factors and in obese persons. Overweight persons without other risk factors are advised to prevent further weight gain.

The clinical practice guideline on smoking cessation issued by the Agency for Health Care Policy and Research (now the Agency for Healthcare Research and Quality) clearly shows that a variety of interventions are effective and concludes that improvements in cessation will require active participation of health care systems.[42]

These national education efforts have changed the way people think about their health. More people than ever are having their blood pressure and their cholesterol levels checked and are taking action to keep them under control. Individuals are aware of preventive measures and health promotion behaviors that can reduce their risk of developing CHD- and stroke-related illnesses. In addition, improved pharmacologic therapies are available to treat and control major CHD risk factors, such as high blood pressure, high blood cholesterol, and obesity. These therapies however, may be underutilized by health care providers.

Early identification and treatment. Each year in the United States, about 1.1 million persons experience a heart attack (acute myocardial infarction [AMI]). In 1996, 476,000 persons died from heart attacks—about 51 percent were males and 49 percent were females. More than half of these deaths occurred suddenly, within

1 hour of symptom onset, outside the hospital.[1, 43] For those patients who survive a heart attack, delay in treatment can mean increased damage to the heart muscle and poorer outcomes.

The benefits of rapid identification and treatment of heart attacks are clear. Early treatment of heart attack patients reduces heart-muscle damage, improves heart muscle function, and lowers the heart attack death rate.[44, 45]

Controlled trials of clot-dissolving (thrombolytic) agents used during the acute phase of a heart attack have demonstrated the benefits of opening the affected coronary artery and reestablishing blood flow. The results from these trials have been incorporated into the current treatment model for early intervention during the acute phase of a heart attack.[44] Patients who receive clot-dissolving agents in the first and second hours after the onset of heart attack symptoms experience significant reductions in disability and death when compared to patients who are treated in the third to sixth hours.[46] Even patients who are treated between 6 and 12 hours after the onset of symptoms show modest but significant benefits when compared to patients whose treatment is delayed more than 12 hours.[47] Other acute interventions for heart attack patients include balloon angioplasty, coronary stenting, and coronary artery bypass surgery.[45, 48] The importance of early treatment has generated a growing interest in detecting the earliest warning, or "prodromal," symptoms of a heart attack, thus providing the lead time needed to treat heart attack patients as quickly and effectively as possible.[49]

As with heart attacks, deaths from stroke can be reduced or delayed by preventing and controlling risk factors and using the most effective therapies in a timely manner. Functional limitations can be minimized when patients are treated with clot-dissolving therapy within 3 hours of a thrombotic stroke.[50] As therapies have become increasingly more effective, delays in treatment initiation and lack of implementation of therapies pose major barriers to improving outcomes. Thus far, efforts to provide appropriate access to timely and optimal care to patients with acute coronary syndromes and thrombotic stroke generally are not organized into a unified, cohesive system in communities across the United States.[51]

Early access to emergency health care services is also a critical determinant of outcome for victims of out-of-hospital cardiac arrest. For out-of-hospital cardiac arrest where bystanders are present, a key factor is minimizing the time from the moment the collapse is recognized to the delivery of a short burst of electrical current. Collapse recognition occurs when a bystander notices that the affected individual is unresponsive, has slowed or stopped breathing, or lacks a detectable pulse.[51] As soon as the emergency is recognized, the bystander should call 911 or the local emergency number. Cardiopulmonary resuscitation (CPR) is critical and should begin immediately. The sooner CPR and defibrillation are given to a person in cardiac arrest or ventilation is given for respiratory arrest, the greater the chances of survival.[52] (See Focus Area 1. Access to Quality Health Services.)

Despite evidence that effective treatment depends on rapid response to the patient, only a minority of individuals who can benefit from defibrillatory shock or thrombolytic agents are treated early enough for them to work.[53] The public health challenge is to develop and maintain programs for easier identification and treatment of individuals with AMI and out-of-hospital cardiac arrest.

Counseling by health care providers could help to increase awareness of the symptoms and signs of a heart attack or stroke and the appropriate actions to take, such as accessing emergency medical services. It also can help reduce and control factors that increase the risk of a heart attack or a stroke. To focus resources where they might derive the greatest benefit, education should be, at a minimum, aimed at reducing delays in seeking treatment for those individuals who are at high risk for a future cardiovascular event—for example, those with existing CHD and multiple CHD risk factors.

Cardiovascular disease (CVD) recurrence. Patients with CHD, atherosclerotic disease of the aorta or peripheral arteries, or carotid artery disease are at high risk for heart attack and CHD death.[54, 55] About 50 percent of all heart attacks and at least 70 percent of CHD deaths occur in individuals with prior symptoms of CVD.[56, 57] The risk for heart attack and death among persons with established CHD (or other atherosclerotic disease) is five to seven times higher than among the general population.[3]

Risk factor control can greatly reduce the risk of subsequent cardiovascular problems in patients with CHD. For example, clinical trials have proved that lowering low-density lipoprotein (LDL) cholesterol levels in CHD patients dramatically reduces heart attacks, CHD and CVD deaths, and total deaths.[58, 59, 60] Clinical trials have also demonstrated that lowering blood pressure in such patients reduces CVD endpoints (such as heart disease, stroke, heart attacks, and coronary artery disease) and deaths from all causes.[61, 62, 63] Adequate control of risk factors in the 12 million adults with CHD could reduce the overall rate of heart attacks and CHD deaths in the United States by over 20 percent. Many CHD patients, however, are not getting the aggressive risk factor management they need.

Clinical trials also show that therapeutic interventions can relieve symptoms, reduce deaths, reduce the number of rehospitalizations, and improve the quality of life for older adults with heart failure. Despite the development and promotion of clinical practice guidelines, physicians are continuing to underutilize recommended therapies. As the number of older adults who experience heart failure rises (expected to double by about 2040), these guidelines will need to be incorporated into clinical practice.[64, 65]

Adherence and compliance. There currently exist a number of well-established recommendations for preventing and treating cardiovascular disease and its associated risk factors.[66, 67, 68] However, the potential benefits to be gained from applying these science-based recommendations often are not realized because of the multiple factors involved in adherence to such recommendations. The ability or willingness of the patient to carry out a treatment program successfully is of critical importance.

Experience with the long-term management of asymptomatic CHD risk factors such as hypertension indicates that a sizable number of patients do not successfully carry out their prescribed treatment regimen. The reasons vary: the patient may choose not to have the initial prescription filled, may successfully initiate therapy only to abandon it after a few weeks or months, or may comply with only part of the regimen and thus fail to achieve optimal control. Continued efforts are needed to better understand the determinants of adherence to ensure that patients stay with their prescribed therapy.[69, 70] Also, health care providers and the health care systems in which they work are critical factors in determining whether established interventions are prescribed and patients adequately educated and monitored for therapeutic response.[71, 72] Finally, support from the patient's community and greater use of technology such as the Internet also have an increasingly important role in promoting long-term adherence to lifestyle and pharmacologic regimens. Achieving long-term control of CHD risk factors requires that the same interest and attention given to initial evaluation and treatment decisions also be given to long-term management issues.

Future efforts. Population studies and public outreach are two of the most important areas of future research. Advanced technology allows researchers to screen persons noninvasively and painlessly for signs of developing atherosclerosis. Eventually, when their role in medical practice has been better delineated, noninvasive methods (such as magnetic resonance imaging and ultrasound) may be used to determine the number of persons in the population who have heart disease or are at risk of developing heart disease.

Many people know what a desirable cholesterol level is, what their blood pressure should be, and that these factors relate to a risk of heart disease and stroke. The average person can expect to live 5.5 years longer today than he or she did 30 years ago, and nearly 4 years of that gain in life expectancy can be attributed to progress against CVD, including CHD and stroke. However, much remains to be done to ensure that all segments of the population share in these benefits. Although national health data on African Americans and Hispanics have been collected since the early 1980s, data on heart disease and stroke risk factors are sparse for other population groups, including American Indians, Alaska Natives, Native Hawaiians, Asians, and Pacific Islanders. Adequate national data on all these populations will enable researchers to examine racial and ethnic differences more fully.

Public outreach and community health intervention efforts, such as those that encourage persons to lower their high blood pressure or to get their cholesterol checked or to help people stop smoking, are important parts of health care in the United States. Culturally and linguistically appropriate counseling by health care providers is important to those efforts. New coalitions between health care providers and individual communities are forming to focus on the prevention and management of chronic CVD throughout all stages of life. Emerging areas of research include the effect of socioeconomic status on health and access to care; health status in rural populations, which often have low income and education levels; and quality of life as a criterion for evaluating treatment. With the knowledge gained through these efforts, communities will be able to use well-tested health promotion, disease prevention, and early management strategies to lower their costs and begin to extend the benefits of improved health to all persons in the United States.[73]

Interim Progress Toward Year 2000 Objectives

Extensive progress has been made in reducing deaths from and risk factors for heart disease and stroke, but significant challenges remain. Between 1987 and 1996, the age-adjusted death rate for CHD declined by 22.2 percent, and for stroke, it declined by 13.2 percent. Despite these achievements, the Healthy People 2000 objectives on CHD and stroke did not reach the year 2000 targets, and the disparities between African Americans and whites were not reduced.

However, progress occurred in reducing high blood cholesterol and controlling high blood pressure. Average total cholesterol declined from 213 mg/dL in 1976–80 to 203 mg/dL in 1988–94, and the prevalence of high blood cholesterol declined from 26 percent to 19 percent, thereby achieving the year 2000 target. In the same time period, control rates among persons who have high blood pressure increased from 11 percent to 29 percent. However, levels fell short of year 2000 targets. The age-adjusted prevalence of overweight or obesity increased from 26 percent in 1976–80 to 35 percent in 1988–94.

The percentage of the population who engaged in light to moderate physical activity remained stable at around 22 percent between 1985 and 1995. Caloric intake from fat as a percentage of total calories consumed declined from 36 percent in 1976–80 to 34 percent in 1988–94, but fell short of the target of 30 percent. Smoking among adults declined steadily from the mid-1960s through the late 1980s, and has leveled off in the 1990s. In 1998, median adult smoking prevalence for all 50 States and the District of Columbia was 22.9 percent—25.3 percent for men and 21.0 percent for women.[73]

Note: Unless otherwise noted, data are from the Centers for Disease Control and Prevention, National Center for Health Statistics, Healthy People 2000 Review, 1998–99.

Heart Disease and Stroke

Goal: Improve cardiovascular health and quality of life through the prevention, detection, and treatment of risk factors; early identification and treatment of heart attacks and strokes; and prevention of recurrent cardiovascular events.

Number	Objective Short Title
Heart Disease	
12-1	Coronary heart disease (CHD) deaths
12-2	Knowledge of symptoms of heart attack and importance of calling 911
12-3	Artery-opening therapy
12-4	Bystander response to cardiac arrest
12-5	Out-of-hospital emergency care
12-6	Heart failure hospitalizations
Stroke	
12-7	Stroke deaths
12-8	Knowledge of early warning symptoms of stroke
Blood Pressure	
12-9	High blood pressure
12-10	High blood pressure control
12-11	Action to help control blood pressure
12-12	Blood pressure monitoring
Cholesterol	
12-13	Mean total blood cholesterol levels
12-14	High blood cholesterol levels
12-15	Blood cholesterol screening
12-16	LDL-cholesterol level in CHD patients

Heart Disease

12-1. Reduce coronary heart disease deaths.

Target: 166 deaths per 100,000 population.

Baseline: 208 coronary heart disease deaths per 100,000 population in 1998 (age adjusted to the year 2000 standard population).

Target setting method: 20 percent improvement.

Data source: National Vital Statistics System (NVSS), CDC, NCHS.

NOTE: THE TABLE BELOW MAY CONTINUE TO THE FOLLOWING PAGE.

Total Population, 1998	Coronary Heart Disease Deaths
	Rate per 100,000
TOTAL	208
Race and ethnicity	
American Indian or Alaska Native	126
Asian or Pacific Islander	123
Asian	DNC
Native Hawaiian and other Pacific Islander	DNC
Black or African American	252
White	206
Hispanic or Latino	145
Not Hispanic or Latino	211
Black or African American	257
White	208
Gender	
Female	165
Male	265
Education level (aged 25 to 64 years)	
Less than high school	96
High school graduate	80
At least some college	38

Total Population, 1998	Coronary Heart Disease Deaths
	Rate per 100,000
Disability status	
Persons with disabilities	DNC
Persons without disabilities	DNC

DNA = Data have not been analyzed. DNC = Data are not collected. DSU = Data are statistically unreliable.
Note: Age adjusted to the year 2000 standard population.

NOTE: THE TABLE ABOVE MAY HAVE CONTINUED FROM THE PREVIOUS PAGE.

12-2. **(Developmental) Increase the proportion of adults aged 20 years and older who are aware of the early warning symptoms and signs of a heart attack and the importance of accessing rapid emergency care by calling 911.**

Potential data source: National Health Interview Survey (NHIS), CDC, NCHS.

12-3. **(Developmental) Increase the proportion of eligible patients with heart attacks who receive artery-opening therapy within an hour of symptom onset.**

Potential data source: National Registry of Myocardial Infarction, National Acute Myocardial Infarction Project, HCFA.

12-4. **(Developmental) Increase the proportion of adults aged 20 years and older who call 911 and administer cardiopulmonary resuscitation (CPR) when they witness an out-of-hospital cardiac arrest.**

Potential data source: National Health Interview Survey (NHIS), CDC, NCHS.

12-5. **(Developmental) Increase the proportion of eligible persons with witnessed out-of-hospital cardiac arrest who receive their first therapeutic electrical shock within 6 minutes after collapse recognition.**

Potential data source: Medical Expenditure Panel Survey (MEPS), AHRQ.

12-6. Reduce hospitalizations of older adults with congestive heart failure as the principal diagnosis.

Target and baseline:

Objective	Reduction in Hospitalizations of Older Adults With Congestive Heart Failure as the Principal Diagnosis	1997 Baseline	2010 Target
		Per 1,000 Population	
12-6a.	Adults aged 65 to 74 years	13.2	6.5
12-6b.	Adults aged 75 to 84 years	26.7	13.5
12-6c.	Adults aged 85 years and older	52.7	26.5

Target setting method: Better than the best.

Data source: National Hospital Discharge Survey (NHDS), CDC, NCHS.

NOTE: THE TABLE BELOW MAY CONTINUE TO THE FOLLOWING PAGE.

Adults With Congestive Heart Failure as Principal Diagnosis, 1997	Heart Failure Hospitalizations		
	12-6a. Aged 65 to 74 Years	12-6b. Aged 75 to 84 Years	12-6c. Aged 85 Years and Older
	Rate per 1,000		
TOTAL	13.2	26.7	52.7
Race and ethnicity			
American Indian or Alaska Native	DSU	DSU	DSU
Asian or Pacific Islander	DSU	DSU	DSU
Asian	DNC	DNC	DNC
Native Hawaiian and other Pacific Islander	DNC	DNC	DNC
Black or African American	20.0	21.4	47.0
White	9.9	21.4	41.8
Hispanic or Latino	DSU	DSU	DSU
Not Hispanic or Latino	DSU	DSU	DSU
Black or African American	DSU	DSU	DSU
White	DSU	DSU	DSU

Adults With Congestive Heart Failure as Principal Diagnosis, 1997	Heart Failure Hospitalizations		
	12-6a. Aged 65 to 74 Years	12-6b. Aged 75 to 84 Years	12-6c. Aged 85 Years and Older
	Rate per 1,000		
Gender			
Female	11.5	25.0	50.2
Male	15.3	29.2	58.8
Education level			
Less than high school	DNC	DNC	DNC
High school graduate	DNC	DNC	DNC
At least some college	DNC	DNC	DNC
Disability status			
People with disabilities	DNC	DNC	DNC
People without disabilities	DNC	DNC	DNC

DNA = Data have not been analyzed. DNC = Data are not collected. DSU = Data are statistically unreliable.

NOTE: THE TABLE ABOVE MAY HAVE CONTINUED FROM THE PREVIOUS PAGE.

Stroke

12-7. Reduce stroke deaths.

Target: 48 deaths per 100,000 population.

Baseline: 60 deaths from stroke per 100,000 population occurred in 1998 (age adjusted to the year 2000 standard population).

Target setting method: 20 percent improvement.

Data source: National Vital Statistics System (NVSS), CDC, NCHS.

NOTE: THE TABLE BELOW MAY CONTINUE TO THE FOLLOWING PAGE.

Total Population, 1998	Stroke Deaths
	Rate per 100,000
TOTAL	60
Race and ethnicity	
American Indian or Alaska Native	38
Asian or Pacific Islander	51
Asian	DNC
Native Hawaiian and other Pacific Islander	DNC
Black or African American	80
White	58

Total Population, 1998	Stroke Deaths
	Rate per 100,000
Hispanic or Latino	39
Not Hispanic or Latino	60
Black or African American	82
White	58
Gender	
Female	58
Male	60
Education level (aged 25 to 64 years)	
Less than high school	22
High school graduate	17
At least some college	8
Disability status	
Persons with disabilities	DNC
Persons without disabilities	DNC

DNA = Data have not been analyzed. DNC = Data are not collected. DSU = Data are statistically unreliable.
Note: Age adjusted to the year 2000 standard population.
NOTE: THE TABLE ABOVE MAY HAVE CONTINUED FROM THE PREVIOUS PAGE.

12-8. (Developmental) Increase the proportion of adults who are aware of the early warning symptoms and signs of a stroke.

Potential data source: National Health Interview Survey (NHIS), CDC, NCHS.

Blood Pressure

12-9. Reduce the proportion of adults with high blood pressure.

Target: 16 percent.

Baseline: 28 percent of adults aged 20 years and older had high blood pressure in 1988–94 (age adjusted to the year 2000 standard population).

Target setting method: Better than the best.

Data source: National Health and Nutrition Examination Survey (NHANES), CDC, NCHS.

Adults Aged 20 Years and Older, 1988–94 (unless noted)	High Blood Pressure
	Percent
TOTAL	28
Race and ethnicity	
American Indian or Alaska Native	DSU
Asian or Pacific Islander	DSU
Asian	DNC
Native Hawaiian and other Pacific Islander	DNC
Black or African American	40
White	27
Hispanic or Latino	DSU
Mexican American	29
Not Hispanic or Latino	28
Black or African American	40
White	27
Gender	
Female	26
Male	30
Family income level	
Poor	32
Near poor	30
Middle/high income	27
Disability status	
Persons with disabilities	32 (1991–94)
Persons without disabilities	27 (1991–94)
Select populations	
Persons with diabetes	DNA
Persons without diabetes	DNA

DNA = Data have not been analyzed. DNC = Data are not collected. DSU = Data are statistically unreliable.
Note: Age adjusted to the year 2000 standard population.

12-10. Increase the proportion of adults with high blood pressure whose blood pressure is under control.

Target: 50 percent.

Baseline: 18 percent of adults aged 18 years and older with high blood pressure had it under control in 1988–94 (age adjusted to the year 2000 standard population).

Target setting method: Better than the best.

Data source: National Health and Nutrition Examination Survey (NHANES), CDC, NCHS.

NOTE: THE TABLE BELOW MAY CONTINUE TO THE FOLLOWING PAGE.

Adults Aged 18 Years and Older With High Blood Pressure, 1988–94 (unless noted)	Blood Pressure Controlled
	Percent
TOTAL	18
Race and ethnicity	
American Indian or Alaska Native	DSU
Asian or Pacific Islander	DSU
Asian	DNC
Native Hawaiian and other Pacific Islander	DNC
Black or African American	19
White	18
Hispanic or Latino	DSU
Mexican American	13
Not Hispanic or Latino	DNA
Black or African American	19
White	18
Gender	
Female	28
Male	13
Family income level	
Poor	25
Near poor	20
Middle/high income	16
Disability status (aged 20 years and older)	
Persons with disabilities	24 (1991–94)
Persons without disabilities	16 (1991–94)

Adults Aged 18 Years and Older With High Blood Pressure, 1988–94 (unless noted)	Blood Pressure Controlled
	Percent
Select populations	
Persons with diabetes	DNA
Persons without diabetes	DNA

DNA = Data have not been analyzed. DNC = Data are not collected. DSU = Data are statistically unreliable.
Note: Age adjusted to the year 2000 standard population.

NOTE: THE TABLE ABOVE MAY HAVE CONTINUED FROM THE PREVIOUS PAGE.

12-11. Increase the proportion of adults with high blood pressure who are taking action (for example, losing weight, increasing physical activity, or reducing sodium intake) to help control their blood pressure.

Target: 95 percent.

Baseline: 82 percent of adults aged 18 years and older with high blood pressure were taking action to control it in 1998 (age adjusted to the year 2000 standard population).

Target setting method: Better than the best.

Data source: National Health Interview Survey (NHIS), CDC, NCHS.

NOTE: THE TABLE BELOW MAY CONTINUE TO THE FOLLOWING PAGE.

Adults Aged 18 Years and Older With High Blood Pressure, 1998 (unless noted)	Taking Action To Control Blood Pressure
	Percent
TOTAL	82
Race and ethnicity	
American Indian or Alaska Native	DSU
Asian or Pacific Islander	76
Asian	75
Native Hawaiian and other Pacific Islander	DSU
Black or African American	86
White	80
Hispanic or Latino	74
Not Hispanic or Latino	83
Black or African American	87
White	81

Adults Aged 18 Years and Older With High Blood Pressure, 1998 (unless noted)	Taking Action To Control Blood Pressure
	Percent
Gender	
Female	83
Male	80
Family income level	
Poor	80
Near poor	79
Middle/high income	81
Disability status	
Persons with activity limitations	84 (1994)
Persons without activity limitations	76 (1994)
Geographic variation	
Urban	83
Rural	80
Select populations	
Persons with diabetes	DNA
Persons without diabetes	DNA

DNA = Data have not been analyzed. DNC = Data are not collected. DSU = Data are statistically unreliable.
Note: Age adjusted to the year 2000 standard population.
NOTE: THE TABLE ABOVE MAY HAVE CONTINUED FROM THE PREVIOUS PAGE.

12-12. Increase the proportion of adults who have had their blood pressure measured within the preceding 2 years and can state whether their blood pressure was normal or high.

Target: 95 percent.

Baseline: 90 percent of adults aged 18 years and older had their blood pressure measured in the past 2 years and could state whether it was normal or high in 1998 (age adjusted to the year 2000 standard population).

Target setting method: Better than the best.

Data source: National Health Interview Survey (NHIS), CDC, NCHS.

Adults Aged 18 Years and Older, 1998 (unless noted)	Had Blood Pressure Measured in Past 2 Years and Knew Whether It Was Normal or High
	Percent
TOTAL	90
Race and ethnicity	
American Indian or Alaska Native	89
Asian or Pacific Islander	86
Asian	86
Native Hawaiian and other Pacific Islander	86
Black or African American	92
White	90
Hispanic or Latino	84
Not Hispanic or Latino	91
Black or African American	92
White	91
Gender	
Female	92
Male	87
Education level (aged 25 years and older)	
Less than high school	84
High school graduate	90
At least some college	93
Disability status	
Persons with activity limitations	90 (1994)
Persons without activity limitations	84 (1994)

DNA = Data have not been analyzed. DNC = Data are not collected. DSU = Data are statistically unreliable.
Note: Age adjusted to the year 2000 standard population.

Cholesterol

12-13. Reduce the mean total blood cholesterol levels among adults.

Target: 199 mg/dL (mean).

Baseline: 206 mg/dL was the mean total blood cholesterol level for adults aged 20 years and older in 1988–94 (age adjusted to the year 2000 standard population).

Target setting method: Better than the best.

Data source: National Health and Nutrition Examination Survey (NHANES), CDC, NCHS.

Adults Aged 20 Years and Older, 1988–94 (unless noted)	Mean Cholesterol Level
	mg/dL
TOTAL	206
Race and ethnicity	
American Indian or Alaska Native	DSU
Asian or Pacific Islander	DSU
Asian	DNC
Native Hawaiian and other Pacific Islander	DNC
Black or African American	204
White	206
Hispanic or Latino	DSU
Mexican American	205
Not Hispanic or Latino	206
Black or African American	204
White	206
Gender	
Female	207
Male	204
Family income level	
Poor	205
Near poor	204
Middle/high income	206
Disability status	
Persons with disabilities	208 (1991–94)
Persons without disabilities	204 (1991–94)

DNA = Data have not been analyzed. DNC = Data are not collected. DSU = Data are statistically unreliable.
Note: Age adjusted to the year 2000 standard population.

Healthy People 2010: Objectives for Improving Health

12-14. Reduce the proportion of adults with high total blood cholesterol levels.

Target: 17 percent.

Baseline: 21 percent of adults aged 20 years and older had total blood cholesterol levels of 240 mg/dL or greater in 1988–94 (age adjusted to the year 2000 standard population).

Target setting method: Better than the best.

Data source: National Health and Nutrition Examination Survey (NHANES), CDC, NCHS.

NOTE: THE TABLE BELOW MAY CONTINUE TO THE FOLLOWING PAGE.

Adults Aged 20 Years and Older, 1988–94 (unless noted)	Total Blood Cholesterol Level of 240 mg/dL or Greater
	Percent
TOTAL	21
Race and ethnicity	
American Indian or Alaska Native	DSU
Asian or Pacific Islander	DSU
Asian	DNC
Native Hawaiian and other Pacific Islander	DNC
Black or African American	19
White	21
Hispanic or Latino	DNC
Mexican American	18
Not Hispanic or Latino	DNA
Black or African American	19
White	21
Gender	
Female	22
Male	19
Education level	
Less than high school	22
High school graduate	22
At least some college	19

Adults Aged 20 Years and Older, 1988–94 (unless noted)	Total Blood Cholesterol Level of 240 mg/dL or Greater
	Percent
Disability status	
Persons with disabilities	24 (1991–94)
Persons without disabilities	19 (1991–94)

DNA = Data have not been analyzed. DNC = Data are not collected. DSU = Data are statistically unreliable.
Note: Age adjusted to the year 2000 standard population.

NOTE: THE TABLE ABOVE MAY HAVE CONTINUED FROM THE PREVIOUS PAGE.

12-15. Increase the proportion of adults who have had their blood cholesterol checked within the preceding 5 years.

Target: 80 percent.

Baseline: 67 percent of adults aged 18 years and older had their blood cholesterol checked within the preceding 5 years in 1998 (age adjusted to the year 2000 standard population).

Target setting method: Better than the best.

Data source: National Health Interview Survey (NHIS), CDC, NCHS.

NOTE: THE TABLE BELOW MAY CONTINUE TO THE FOLLOWING PAGE.

Adults Aged 18 Years and Older, 1998 (unless noted)	Blood Cholesterol Checked in Past 5 Years
	Percent
TOTAL	67
Race and ethnicity	
American Indian or Alaska Native	58
Asian or Pacific Islander	68
Asian	69
Native Hawaiian and other Pacific Islander	65
Black or African American	67
White	67
Hispanic or Latino	59
Not Hispanic or Latino	68
Black or African American	67
White	70

Adults Aged 18 Years and Older, 1998 (unless noted)	Blood Cholesterol Checked in Past 5 Years
	Percent
Gender	
Female	70
Male	64
Education level (aged 25 years and older)	
Less than high school	58
High school graduate	69
At least some college	78
Disability status	
Persons with activity limitations	72 (1993)
Persons without activity limitations	66 (1993)
Geographic variation	
Urban	68
Rural	63

DNA = Data have not been analyzed. DNC = Data are not collected. DSU = Data are statistically unreliable.
Note: Age adjusted to the year 2000 standard population.
NOTE: THE TABLE ABOVE MAY HAVE CONTINUED FROM THE PREVIOUS PAGE.

12-16. (Developmental) Increase the proportion of persons with coronary heart disease who have their LDL-cholesterol level treated to a goal of less than or equal to 100 mg/dL.

Potential data source: National Health and Nutrition Examination Survey (NHANES), CDC, NCHS.

Related Objectives From Other Focus Areas

1. **Access to Quality Health Services**
    1-3. Counseling about health behaviors
    1-7. Core competencies in health provider training
    1-10. Delay or difficulty in getting emergency care
    1-11. Rapid prehospital emergency care
4. **Chronic Kidney Disease**
    4-2. Cardiovascular disease deaths in persons with chronic kidney failure
7. **Educational and Community-Based Programs**
    7-2. School health education
    7-5. Worksite health promotion programs
    7-8. Satisfaction with patient education
    7-10. Community health promotion programs

Terminology

(A listing of acronyms and abbreviations used in this publication appears in Appendix H.)

Angina (angina pectoris): A pain or discomfort in the chest that occurs when some part of the heart does not receive enough blood. Angina is a common symptom of coronary heart disease. It often recurs in a regular or characteristic pattern. However, it may first appear as a very severe episode or as frequently recurring bouts. When an established stable pattern of angina changes sharply—for example, it may be provoked by far less exercise than in the past, or it may appear at rest—it is referred to as unstable angina.

Angioplasty: A nonsurgical procedure used to treat blockages in blood vessels, particularly the coronary arteries that feed the heart. Also known as percutaneous transluminal coronary angioplasty (PTCA). An inflatable balloon or other device on a thin tube (catheter), fed through blood vessels to the point of blockage, is used to open the artery.

Anticoagulants: Drugs that delay the clotting (coagulation) of blood. When a blood vessel is plugged up by a clot and an anticoagulant is given, it tends to prevent new clots from forming or the existing clot from enlarging. An anticoagulant does not dissolve an existing blood clot.

Arrhythmia: A change in the regular beat or rhythm of the heart. The heart may seem to skip a beat, or beat irregularly, or beat very fast or very slowly.

Atherosclerosis: A type of hardening of the arteries in which cholesterol and other substances in the blood are deposited in the walls of arteries, including the coronary arteries that supply blood to the heart. In time, narrowing of the coronary arteries by atherosclerosis may reduce the flow of oxygen-rich blood to the heart.

Atrial fibrillation (AF): The most common sustained irregular heart rhythm encountered in clinical practice. AF occurs when the two small upper chambers of the heart (the atria) quiver instead of beating effectively, and blood cannot be pumped completely out of them when the heart beats, allowing the blood to pool and clot. If a piece of the blood clot in the atria becomes lodged in an artery in the brain, a stroke may result. AF is a risk factor for stroke and heart failure.

Blood pressure: The force of the blood pushing against the walls of arteries. Blood pressure is given as two numbers that measure systolic pressure (the first number, which measures the pressure while the heart is contracting) and diastolic pressure (the second number, which measures the pressure when the heart is resting between beats). Blood pressures of 140/90 mmHg or above are considered high, while blood pressures in the range of 130–139/85–89 are high normal. Less than 130/85 mmHg is normal.

Body mass index (BMI): Weight (in kilograms) divided by the square of height (in meters), or weight (in pounds) divided by the square of height (in inches) times 704.5. Because it is readily calculated, BMI is the measurement of choice as an indicator of healthy weight, overweight, and obesity.

Cardiovascular disease (CVD): Includes a variety of diseases of the heart and blood vessels, coronary heart disease (coronary artery disease, ischemic heart disease), stroke (brain attack), high blood pressure (hypertension), rheumatic heart disease, congestive heart failure, and peripheral artery disease.

Cerebrovascular disease: Affects the blood vessels supplying blood to the brain. Stroke occurs when a blood vessel bringing oxygen and nutrients to the brain bursts or is clogged by a blood clot. Because of this rupture or blockage, part of the brain does not get the flow of blood it needs, and nerve cells in the affected area die. Small stroke-like events, such as transient ischemic attacks (TIAs), which resolve in a day or less, are symptoms of cerebrovascular disease.

Cholesterol: A waxy substance that circulates in the bloodstream. When the level of cholesterol in the blood is too high, some of the cholesterol is deposited in the walls of the blood vessels. Over time, these deposits can build up until they narrow the blood vessels, causing atherosclerosis, which reduces the blood flow. The higher the blood cholesterol level, the greater is the risk of getting heart disease. Blood cholesterol levels of less than 200 mg/dL are considered desirable. Levels of 240 mg/dL or above are considered high and require further testing and possible intervention. Levels of 200–239 mg/dL are considered borderline. Lowering blood cholesterol reduces the risk of heart disease.

Congestive heart failure (or heart failure): A condition in which the heart cannot pump enough blood to meet the needs of the body's other organs. Heart failure can result from narrowed arteries that supply blood to the heart muscle and from other factors. As the flow of blood out of the heart slows, blood returning to the heart through the veins backs up, causing congestion in the tissues. Often swelling (edema) results, most commonly in the legs and ankles, but possibly in other parts of the body as well. Sometimes fluid collects in the lungs and interferes with breathing, causing shortness of breath, especially when a person is lying down.

Coronary heart disease (CHD): A condition in which the flow of blood to the heart muscle is reduced. Like any muscle, the heart needs a constant supply of oxygen and nutrients that are carried to it by the blood in the coronary arteries. When the coronary arteries become narrowed or clogged, they cannot supply enough blood to the heart. If not enough oxygen-carrying blood reaches the heart, the heart may respond with pain called angina. The pain usually is felt in the chest or sometimes in the left arm or shoulder. When the blood supply is cut off completely, the result is a heart attack. The part of the heart muscle that does not receive oxygen begins to die, and some of the heart muscle is permanently damaged.

Coronary stenting: A procedure that uses a wire mesh tube (a stent) to prop open an artery that recently has been cleared using angioplasty. The stent remains in the artery permanently, holding it open to improve blood flow to the heart muscle and relieve symptoms, such as chest pain.

HDL (high-density lipoprotein) cholesterol: The so-called good cholesterol. Cholesterol travels in the blood combined with protein in packages called lipoproteins. HDL is thought to carry cholesterol away from other parts of the body back to the liver for removal from the body. A low level of HDL increases the risk for CHD, whereas a high HDL level helps protect against CHD.

Heart attack (also called acute myocardial infarction): Occurs when a coronary artery becomes completely blocked, usually by a blood clot (thrombus), resulting in lack of blood flow to the heart muscle and therefore loss of needed oxygen. As a result, part of the heart muscle dies (infarcts). The blood clot usually forms over the site of a cholesterol-rich narrowing (or plaque) that has burst or ruptured.

Heart disease: The leading cause of death and a common cause of illness and disability in the United States. Coronary heart disease and ischemic heart disease are specific names for the principal form of heart disease, which is the result of atherosclerosis, or the buildup of cholesterol deposits in the coronary arteries that feed the heart.

High blood pressure: A systolic blood pressure of 140 mmHg or greater or a diastolic pressure of 90 mmHg or greater. With high blood pressure, the heart has to work harder, resulting in an increased risk of a heart attack, stroke, heart failure, kidney and eye problems, and peripheral vascular disease.

Ischemic heart disease: Includes heart attack and related heart problems caused by narrowing of the coronary arteries and therefore a decreased supply of blood and oxygen to the heart. Also called coronary artery disease and coronary heart disease.

LDL (low-density lipoprotein): The so-called bad cholesterol. LDL contains most of the cholesterol in the blood and carries it to the tissues and organs of the body, including the arteries. Cholesterol from LDL is the main source of damaging buildup and blockage in the arteries. The higher the level of LDL in the blood, the greater is the risk for CHD.

Lipid: Fat and fat-like substances such as cholesterol that are present in blood and body tissues.

Peripheral vascular disease: Refers to diseases of any blood vessels outside the heart and to diseases of the lymph vessels. It is often a narrowing of the blood vessels that carry blood to leg and arm muscles. Symptoms include leg pain (for example, in the calves) when walking and ulcers or sores on the legs and feet.

Stroke: A form of cerebrovascular disease that affects the arteries of the central nervous system. A stroke occurs when blood vessels bringing oxygen and nutrients to the brain burst or become clogged by a blood clot or some other particle. Because of this rupture or blockage, part of the brain does not get the flow of blood it needs. Deprived of oxygen, nerve cells in the affected area of the brain cannot function and die within minutes. When nerve cells cannot function, the part of the body controlled by these cells cannot function either.

References

[1] National Heart, Lung, and Blood Institute (NHLBI). *Morbidity and Mortality: 1998 Chartbook on Cardiovascular, Lung, and Blood Diseases.* Bethesda, MD: Public Health Service (PHS), National Institutes of Health (NIH), NHLBI, October 1998.

[2] Sempos, C.T.; Cleeman, J.I.; Carroll, M.K.; et al. Prevalence of high blood cholesterol among U.S. adults: An update based on guidelines from the second report of the National Cholesterol Education Program Adult Treatment Panel. *Journal of the American Medical Association* 269:3009-3014, 1993.

[3] Expert Panel on Detection, Evaluation, and Treatment of High Blood Cholesterol in Adults. National Cholesterol Education Program: Second report of the Expert Panel on Detection, Evaluation, and Treatment of High Blood Cholesterol in Adults (Adult Treatment Panel II). *Circulation* 89:1329-1445, 1994.

[4] The sixth report of the Joint National Committee on Prevention, Detection, Evaluation, and Treatment of High Blood Pressure. *Archives of Internal Medicine* 157(21):2413-2446, 1997.

[5] Burt, V.L.; Culter, J.A.; Higgins, M.; et al. Trends in the prevalence, awareness, treatment, and control of hypertension in the adult U.S. population. *Hypertension* 26:60-69, 1995.

[6] Centers for Disease Control and Prevention (CDC). Mortality from congestive heart failure—United States, 1980–1990. *Morbidity and Mortality Weekly Report* 43(5):77-78, 1994.

[7] Gillum, R.F. Epidemiology of heart failure in the United States. *American Heart Journal* 126:1042-1047, 1993.

[8] Lenfant, C. Fixing the failing heart. *Circulation* 95:771-772, 1997.

[9] Croft, J.B.; Giles, W.H.; Pollard, R.A.; et al. National trends in the initial hospitalizations for heart failure. *Journal of the American Geriatrics Society* 45:270-275, 1997.

[10] American Heart Association (AHA). *2000 Heart and Stroke Statistical Update.* Dallas, TX: AHA, 2000.

[11] Huston, S.L.; Lengerich, E.J.; Conlisk, E.; et al. Trends in ischemic heart disease death rates for blacks and whites—United States, 1981–1995. *Morbidity and Mortality Weekly Review* 47:945-949, 1998.

[12] Gillum, R.F.; Muscolino, M.F.; and Madans, J.A. Fatal MI among black men and women. *Annals of Internal Medicine* 127:111-118, 1997.

[13] National Heart Attack Alert Program Coordination Committee. *Working Group Report on Educational Strategies To Prevent Prehospital Delay in Patients at High Risk for Acute Myocardial Infarction.* NIH Pub. No. 97-3787. Bethesda, MD: NIH, NHLBI, 1997.

[14] Burt, V.; Whelton, P.; and Roccella, E.J. Prevalence of hypertension in the U.S. adult population. *Hypertension* 25:305-313, 1995.

[15] Stone, N.J. Primary prevention of coronary disease. *Clinical Cornerstone* 1(1):31-49, 1998.

[16] Benson, R.T., and Sacco, R.L. Stroke prevention: Hypertension, diabetes, tobacco, and lipids. *Neurologic Clinics* 18(2):309-319, 2000.

[17] Paffenbarger, Jr., R.S.; Hyde, R.T.; Wing, A.; et al. The association of changes in physical activity levels and other lifestyle characteristics with mortality among men. *New England Journal of Medicine* 328:538-545, 1993.

[18] Blair, S.N.; Kampert, J.B.; Kohl, H.W.; et al. Influences of cardiopulmonary fitness and other precurors on cardiovascular disease and all-cause mortality in men and women. *Journal of the American Medical Association* 276:205-210, 1996.

[19] American Diabetes Association (ADA). *Diabetes 1996: Vital Statistics*. Alexandria, VA: ADA, 1996.

[20] He, J.; Whelton, P.K., Appel, L.J.; et al. Long-term effects of weight loss and dietary sodium reduction on incidence of hypertension. *Hypertension* 35(2):544-549, 2000.

[21] Leiter, L.A.; Abbott, D.; Campbell, N.R.; et al. Lifestyle modifications to prevent and control hypertension. 2. Recommendations on obesity and weight loss. Canadian Hypertension Society, Canadian Coalition for High Blood Pressure Prevention and Control, Laboratory Centre for Disease Control at Health Canada, Heart and Stroke Foundation of Canada. *Canadian Medical Association Journal* 160(Suppl. 9):S7-12, 1999.

[22] Hooper, L.; Summerbell, C.D.; Higgins, J.P.; et al. Reduced or modified dietary fat for prevention of cardiovascular disease. *Cochrane Database System Review* 2:CD002137, 2000.

[23] Pate, R.R.; Pratt, M.; Blair, S.N.; et al. Physical activity and public health: A recommendation from the Centers for Disease Control and Prevention and the American College of Sports Medicine. *Journal of the American Medical Association* 273:402-407, 1995.

[24] Physical activity and cardiovascular health. NIH Consensus Development Panel on Physical Activity and Cardiovascular Health. *Journal of the American Medical Association* 276(3):241-246, 1996.

[25] Dunn, A.L.; Marcus, B.H.; Kampert, J.B.; et al. Comparison of lifestyle and structured interventions to increase physical activity and cardiorespiratory fitness: A randomized trial. *Journal of the American Medical Association* 281:327-334, 1999.

[26] Manson, J.A.; Hu, F.; Rich-Edwards, J.W.; et al. A prospective study of walking as compared with vigorous exercise in the prevention of coronary heart disease in women. *New England Journal of Medicine* 341:650-658, 1999.

[27] U.S. Department of Health and Human Services (HHS). *Physical Activity and Health: A Report of the Surgeon General*. Atlanta, GA: HHS, CDC, National Center for Chronic Disease Prevention and Health Promotion (NCCDPHP), 1996.

[28] HHS. *The Health Benefits of Smoking Cessation. A Report of the Surgeon General*. HHS Pub. No. CDC 90-8416. Atlanta, GA: HHS, PHS, CDC, NCCDPHP, Office on Smoking and Health, 1990.

[29] Freedman, D.S.; Dietz, W.H.; Srinivasan, S.R.; et al. The relation of overweight to cardiovascular risk factors among children and adolescents: The Bogalusa Heart Study. *Pediatrics* 103:1175-1182, 1999.

[30] Winkleby, M.; Robinson, T.; Sundquist, J.; et al. Ethnic variations in cardiovascular disease risk factors among children and young adults: Findings from the Third National Health and Nutrition Examination Survey (NHANES), 1988–1994. *Journal of the American Medical Association* 281(11):1006-1013, 1999.

[31] Leon, A.S.; Cornett, J.; Jacobs, Jr., D.R.; et al. Leisure time physical activity and risk of coronary heart disease and death: The Multiple Risk Factor Intervention Trial. *Journal of the American Medical Association* 258:2388-2395, 1987.

[32] O'Connor, G.T.; Hennekens, C.H.; Willett, W.H.; et al. Physical exercise and reduced risk of nonfatal myocardial infarction. *American Journal of Epidemiology* 142:1147-1156, 1995.

[33] Blair, S.N.; Kohl, III, H.W.; Barlow, C.E.; et al. Changes in physical fitness and all cause mortality: A prospective study of healthy and unhealthy men. *Journal of the American Medical Association* 273:1093-1098, 1995.

[34] Willett, W.H.; Dietz, W.H.; and Colditz, G.A. Primary care: Guidelines for healthy weight. *New England Journal of Medicine* 341:427-434, 1999.

[35] Roccella, E.J., and Horan, M.J. The National High Blood Pressure Education Program: Measuring progress and assessing its impact. *Health Psychology* (Suppl. 7):237-303, 1998.

[36] National Center for Health Statistics (NCHS). *Health, United States, 1998.* Hyattsville, MD: HHS, CDC, NCHS, 1998.

[37] Kannel, W.B.; Dawber, T.R.; and McGee, D.L. Perspectives on systolic hypertension, the Framingham Study. *Circulation* 61:1179-82, 1980.

[38] Systolic Hypertension in the Elderly Program (SHEP) Cooperative Research Group. Prevention of stroke by antihypertensive drug treatment in older persons with isolated systolic hypertension. Final results of the SHEP. *Journal of the American Medical Association* 265:3255-3264, 1991.

[39] Cleeman, J.I., and Lenfant, C. The National Cholesterol Education Program: Progress and prospects. *Journal of the American Medical Association* 280:2099-2104, 1998.

[40] NHLBI. Cholesterol Awareness Surveys. Press conference. Bethesda, MD: NHLBI, December 4, 1995.

[41] Clinical guidelines on the identification, evaluation, and treatment of overweight and obesity in adults: Evidence report. *Journal of Obesity Research* (Suppl. 2):51S-204S, 1998.

[42] HHS. *Smoking Cessation. Clinical Practice Guidelines No. 18.* HHS Pub. No. (AHCPR) 96-0692. Washington, DC: HHS, PHS, Agency for Health Care Policy and Research, 1996.

[43] Benson, V., and Marano, M.A. Current estimates from the National Health Interview Survey (NHIS), 1995. *Vital and Health Statistics* 10(199):1-428, 1998.

[44] National Heart Attack Alert Program Coordinating Committee, 60 Minutes to Treatment Working Group. Emergency Department: Rapid identification and treatment of patients with acute myocardial infarction. *Annals of Emergency Medicine* 23:311-329, 1994.

[45] Ryan, T.J.; Antman, E.M.; Brooks, N.H.; et al. 1999 update: ACC/AHA guidelines for the management of patients with acute myocardial infarction: A report of the American College of Cardiology/American Heart Association Task Force on Practice Guidelines (Committee on Management of Acute Myocardial Infarction). *Journal of the American College of Cardiology* 34:890-911, 1999.

[46] Boersma, E.; Maas, A.C.P.; Deckers, J.W.; et al. Early thrombolytic treatment in acute myocardial infarction: Reappraisal of the golden hour. *Lancet* 348:771-775, 1996.

[47] Betts, J.H. Late assessment of thrombolytic efficacy with altiplase (rt-PA) 6-24 hours after onset of acute myocardial infarction. *Australian New Zealand Journal of Medicine* 23:745-748, 1993.

[48] Global Use of Strategies to Open Occluded Coronary Arteries in Acute Coronary Syndrome's (GUSTO IIb) Angioplasty Substudy Investigators. A clinical trial comparing primary coronary angioplasty with tissue plasminogen activator for acute myocardial infarction. *New England Journal of Medicine* 336:1621-1628, 1997.

[49] Bahr, R.D. Introduction: community message in acute myocardial ischemia. *Clinician* 14:1, 1996.

[50] National Institute of Neurological Disorders and Stroke, rt-PA Stroke Study Group. Tissue plasminogen activator for acute ischemic stroke. *New England Journal of Medicine* 333(24):1581-1587, 1995.

[51] ADA. Emergency Cardiovascular Care Programs. Chain of Survival. Links in the Chain. <http://www.proed.net/ecc/chain/links.htm>June 1999.

[52] National Heart Attack Alert Program Coordinating Committee, Access to Care Subcommittee. Access to timely and optimal care of patients with acute coronary syndromes—Community planning considerations: Report by the National Heart Attack Alert Program. *Journal of Thrombosis and Thrombolysis* 6:19-46, 1998.

[53] National Heart Attack Alert Program. *Patient/Bystander Recognition and Action: Rapid Identification and Treatment of Acute Myocardial Infarction.* NIH Pub. No. 93-3303 Bethesda, MD: NHLBI, NIH, 1993.

[54] Criqui, M.H.; Langer, R.D.; Fronek, A.; et al. Mortality over a period of 10 years in patients with peripheral arterial disease. *New England Journal of Medicine* 326(6):381-386, 1992.

[55] Salonen, J.T., and Salonen, R. Ultrasonographically assessed carotid morphology and the risk of coronary heart disease. *Arteriosclerosis and Thrombosis* 11(5):1245-1249, 1991.

[56] Kannel, W.B., and Schatzkin, A. Sudden death: Lessons from subsets in population studies. *Journal of the American College of Cardiology* 5(Suppl. 6):141-149B, 1985.

[57] Kuller, L.; Perper, J.; and Cooper, M. Demographic characteristics and trends in arteriosclerotic heart disease mortality: Sudden death and myocardial infarction. *Circulation* 51(Suppl. 1):III-1-III-15, 1975.

[58] Scandinavian Simvastatin Survival Study Group. Randomized trial of cholesterol lowering in 4,444 patients with coronary heart disease: The Scandinavian Simvastat in Survival Study (4S). *Lancet* 334:1383-1389, 1994.

[59] Sacks, F.M.; Pfeffer, M.A.; Moye, L.A.; et al., for the Cholesterol and Recurrent Events Trial Investigators. The effect of pravastatin on coronary events after myocardial infarction in patients with average cholesterol levels. *New England Journal of Medicine* 335:1001-1009, 1996.

[60] Long-Term Intervention with Pravastatin in Ischaemic Disease (LIPID) Study Group. Prevention of cardiovascular events and death with pravastatin in patients with coronary heart disease and a broad range of initial cholesterol levels. *New England Journal of Medicine* 339:1349-1357, 1998.

[61] Joint National Committee on Detection, Evaluation, and Treatment of High Blood Pressure. *The Sixth Report of the Joint National Committee on Detection, Evaluation, and Treatment of High Blood Pressure.* NIH Pub. No. 98-4080. Bethesda, MD: National High Blood Pressure Education Program, NIH, NHLBI, November 1998, 24-25.

[62] Psaty, B.M.; Smith, N.L.; Siscovick, D.S.; et al. Health outcomes associated with antihypertensive therapies used as first-line agents: A systematic review and meta-analysis. *Journal of the American Medical Association* 277:739-745, 1997.

[63] MacMahon, S., and Rodgers, A. The effect of blood pressure reduction in older patients: An overview of five randomized controlled trials in elderly hypertensives. *Clinical and Experimental Hypertension* 15(6):967-978, 1993.

[64] Packer, M.; Poole-Wilson, P.A.; Armstrong, P.W.; et al. Comparative effects of low and high doses of the angiotensin-converting enzyme inhibitor, lisinopril, on morbidity and mortality in chronic heart failure. ATLAS Study Group. *Circulation* 100(23):2312-2318, 1999.

[65] Chodoff, P.; Bischof, R.O.; Nash, D.B.; et al. AHCPR guidelines on heart failure: Comparison of a family medicine and an internal medicine practice with the guidelines and an educational intervention to modify behavior. *Clinical Performance Quality Health Care* 4(4):179-185, 1996.

[66] Haynes, R.B. Improving patient compliance in management of hypertension. In: Kaplan, N.M., and Ram, C.V., eds. *Individualized Therapy of Hypertension.* New York, NY: Marcel Dekker, Inc., 1995, 257-273.

[67] Luscher, F.T.; Vetter, H.; Siegenthaler, W.; et al. Compliance in hypertension: Facts and concepts. *Journal of Hypertension* 3:3-9, 1985.

[68] Dunbar-Jacob, J., and Stunkard, A.J. Adherence to diet and drug regimen. In: Levy, R.; Rifkind, B.; and Ernst, N.; eds. *Nutrition, Lipids, and Coronary Heart Disease.* New York, NY: Raven Press, 1979, 391-423.

[69] Williams, G.H. Assessing patient wellness: New perspectives on quality of life and compliance. *American Journal of Hypertension* 11:186S-191S, 1998.

[70] Roter, D.L.; Hall, J.A.; Merisca, R.; et al. Effectiveness of interventions to improve patient compliance. A meta-analysis. *Medical Care* 36:1138-1161, 1998.

[71] Houston, N.M.; Hill, M.; Kottke, T.; et al. The multilevel compliance challenge: Recommendations for a call to action. A statement for health care professionals. *Circulation* 95:1085-1090, 1997.

[72] Stewart, M.A. Effective physician-patient communication and health outcomes: A review. *Canadian Medical Association Journal* 152:1423, 1996.

[73] CDC. State-specific prevalence of current cigarette and cigar smoking adults—United States, 1998. *Morbidity and Mortality Weekly Report* 48(45), 1999.

13

HIV

Co-Lead Agencies: Centers for Disease Control and Prevention
                     Health Resources and Services Administration

Contents

Goal

Prevent human immunodeficiency virus (HIV) infection and its related illness and death.

Overview

In 1981, a new infectious disease, AIDS, or acquired immunodeficiency syndrome, was identified in the United States.[1] Several years later, the causative agent of AIDS—human immunodeficiency virus (HIV)—was discovered. This discovery coincided with the growing recognition of AIDS in the United States as part of a global infectious disease pandemic.

Currently, HIV/AIDS has been reported in virtually every racial and ethnic population, every age group, and every socioeconomic group in every State and most large cities in the United States.[2] Initially identified among men who have sex with men on the East and West Coasts,[3] the AIDS epidemic is composed of diverse multiple subepidemics that vary by region and community. By the end of 1998, more than 680,000 cases of AIDS had been reported, and nearly 410,800 people had died from HIV disease or AIDS.[2]

Issues

Estimates of the number of people infected with HIV in the United States range from 800,000 to 900,000.[4] The HIV/AIDS subepidemics not only vary by region and community but also may vary by population, risk behavior, and geography. Elimination of disparities in the rate of infection among certain racial and ethnic groups, particularly African American and Hispanic populations, remains a challenge. Recently introduced therapies for HIV/AIDS have reduced illness, disability, and death due to HIV/AIDS; however, access to culturally and linguistically appropriate testing and care may limit progress in this area.

In the United States, HIV/AIDS remains a significant cause of illness, disability, and death, despite declines in 1996 and 1997.[5, 6] Current surveillance provides population-based HIV/AIDS data for tracking trends in the epidemic, targeting and allocating resources for prevention and treatment services, and planning and conducting program evaluation activities. Since the early 1980s, surveillance studies have identified four distinct populations and issues that have affected the epidemic in these populations:

■ Men who have sex with men, facilitated by frequent changes of sex partners in highly infected sexual networks and by high-risk sexual practices.

■ Injection drug users, facilitated by the shared use of needles and syringes contaminated with HIV-infected blood.

■ Heterosexual persons (principally in certain racial and ethnic populations), facilitated by (1) a high rate of HIV among drug-using populations that resulted in heterosexual transmission to some partners, (2) high rates of other sexually transmitted diseases (STDs) that can increase both susceptibility to and transmissibility of HIV infection, (3) high-risk sexual practices (mainly unprotected sex) associated with certain addictive substances, such as crack cocaine, and (4) sex in exchange for drugs.

■ Perinatal transmission among infants, caused by undetected or untreated HIV infection in pregnant females (although the number of perinatally infected infants has declined dramatically since the mid-1990s to a point where elimination of perinatal transmission in the United States may be possible).

The proportion of different population groups affected by HIV/AIDS has changed over time. By 1998, 83 percent of the cumulative AIDS cases had occurred in males, 16 percent in females, and 1 percent in children.[3] The response to the epidemic reflects these changes:

■ Comparing the 1980s to the 1990s, the proportion of AIDS cases in white men who have sex with men declined, whereas the proportion in females and males in other racial and ethnic populations increased, particularly among African Americans and Hispanics (see Disparities section). AIDS cases also appeared to be increasing among injection drug users and their sexual partners.[5]

■ Increases among women have occurred over time. By the mid-1980s, the majority of AIDS cases had been reported among males, with only 7 percent reported among females in 1983.[7] Reported AIDS cases in females have increased steadily since then and accounted for nearly 23 percent of the cases reported in 1998.[3]

■ Monitoring and tracking of the current HIV/AIDS epidemic remains a challenge. Even though AIDS may occur much later than infection with HIV, only AIDS cases are currently reported by all State health departments. Because tracking HIV is more accurate for tracking the status of the epidemic and because States are making progress in reporting HIV infection, it is anticipated that key baseline data about HIV will be available by the early 2000s.[4]

■ Although a test for HIV was developed and made widely available in the early to mid-1980s, the lack of available treatment until 1995, negative implications of treatment (including concerns about lack of confidentiality), and possible discrimination and stigmatization resulted in barriers to the reporting of HIV infection.

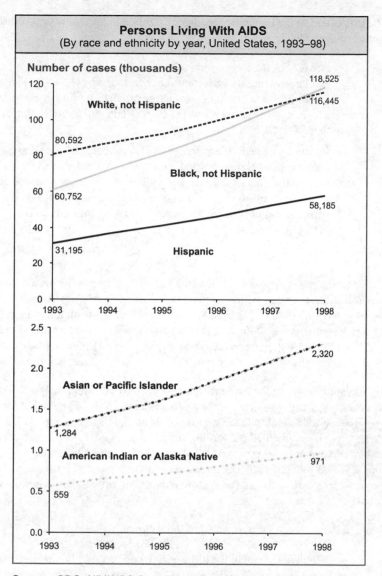

Persons Living With AIDS
(By race and ethnicity by year, United States, 1993–98)

Number of cases (thousands)

White, not Hispanic
118,525
116,445
80,592

Black, not Hispanic
60,752
58,185

Hispanic
31,195

Asian or Pacific Islander
2,320
1,284

American Indian or Alaska Native
971
559

Source: CDC. *HIV/AIDS Surveillance Report.* Vol. 11, No. 1, 1999.

The lifetime costs of health care associated with HIV, in light of recent advances in diagnostics and therapeutics, have grown from $55,000 to $155,000 or more per person.[8] These costs mean that HIV prevention efforts may be even more cost-effective and even cost-saving to society. Prevention efforts include availability of culturally and linguistically appropriate HIV counseling and testing, partner counseling, and referral systems for individuals at high risk for HIV infection; needle and syringe exchange programs; and information, education, treatment and counseling for injection drug users.

The true extent of the epidemic remains difficult to assess for several reasons, including the following:

■ Because of the long period of time from initial HIV infection to AIDS and because highly active antiretroviral therapy (HAART) has slowed the progression to AIDS, new cases of AIDS no longer provide accurate information about the current HIV epidemic in the United States.[4]

■ Because of a lack of awareness of HIV serostatus as well as delays in accessing counseling, testing, and care services by individuals who may be infected or are at risk of infection, some populations do not perceive themselves to be at risk. As a result, some HIV-infected persons are not identified and provided care until late in the course of their infection.[9]

Trends

HIV infection rates appear to have stabilized since the early 1990s at about 40,000 new infections per year, which represents a slowing from growth rates experienced in the mid-1980s.[10] At least 800,000 persons are estimated to be infected with HIV, with over 200,000 to 250,000 persons who are not aware of their infection.[11] About 335,000 persons are estimated to be in treatment with new antiretroviral treatment therapies, and another 215,000 are not currently in treatment.[5, 9, 12]

Significant changes in the epidemic have occurred over time. In 1992, AIDS became a leading cause of death among persons aged 25 to 44 years, but by 1997 had dropped to the eighth leading cause of death in this age group. In 1997, however, HIV/AIDS remained the leading cause of death only for African Americans among persons in this age group.[13, 14] Between 1992 and 1997, the number of persons reported living with AIDS increased in all groups as a result of the 1993 expanded AIDS case definition and, more recently, improved survival rates due to new HAART treatment.

Some of these changes are reflected in the following:

■ Women accounted for just under 14 percent of persons over age 13 years living with AIDS in 1992, compared with 20 percent in 1998.[2, 15]

■ By the end of 1998, the number of African Americans living with AIDS, which increased from 33 percent of the AIDS population in 1992 to 40 percent in 1998, was almost identical to the number of whites living with AIDS.[2]

■ Persons living in the South accounted for 34 percent of AIDS cases in 1992 and 39 percent in 1998. Persons living in the Northeast accounted for 28 percent in 1992 and 31 percent in 1998. The proportion living in the West declined from 24 percent to 21 percent.[2, 16]

■ By December 1998, approximately 297,136 persons were reported to be living with AIDS, compared with 269,775 in 1997.[2, 6]

In late 1982, cases of AIDS attributed to blood transfusions were first reported in the United States.[17, 18] The publication, dissemination, and implementation of specific guidelines and recommendations to prevent HIV infection among health care workers and to test donated blood for HIV[19, 20, 21, 22] have resulted in a reduction in transfusion-related AIDS and increases in safety among health workers.

Another prevention success has been the 66 percent decline in perinatal transmission from 1992 to 1997.[23] With the finding that perinatal HIV transmission rates could be reduced substantially with zidovudine therapy during pregnancy, the U.S. Public Health Service issued guidelines recommending that HIV counseling and voluntary testing become a part of routine prenatal care for all pregnant women.[23] This policy ensures that HIV-infected pregnant women have access to important health care for themselves and also have the opportunity to reduce the risk of HIV transmission to their infants. Subsequent declines in new cases of AIDS among children demonstrate that these strategies are showing success in reducing mother-to-infant HIV transmission.[24, 25]

However, initial declines in deaths from AIDS after the availability of treatments have slowed. Deaths from AIDS continued to decline throughout 1997 and 1998 (down 42 percent and 20 percent, respectively, compared to 1996), and the number of persons living with AIDS (AIDS prevalence) in 1997 and 1998 increased by 12 percent and 10 percent, respectively.[2, 16] If declines continue in newly diagnosed AIDS cases in the coming years, an increasing number of persons will be living with HIV infection. As HIV surveillance extends to additional States, so will the ability to monitor HIV cases and to direct prevention and treatment services to people with asymptomatic infection or mild illness.

Principal health determinants. Behaviors (sexual practices, substance abuse, and accessing prenatal care) and biomedical status (having other STDs) are major determinants of HIV transmission. Unprotected sexual contact, whether homosexual or heterosexual, with a person infected with HIV and sharing drug-injection equipment with an HIV-infected individual account for most HIV transmission in the United States.[26, 27] Increasing the number of people who know their HIV serostatus is an important component of a national program to slow or halt the transmission of HIV in the United States.

For persons infected with HIV, behavioral determinants also play an important role in health maintenance. Although drugs are available specifically to prevent and treat a number of opportunistic infections, HIV-infected individuals also need to make lifestyle-related behavioral changes to avoid many of these infections. The new HIV antiretroviral drug therapies for HIV infection bring with them difficulties in adhering to complex, expensive, and demanding medication schedules, posing a significant challenge for many persons infected with HIV.

Because HIV infection weakens the immune system, people with tuberculosis (TB) infection and HIV infection are at very high risk of developing active TB disease.[28]

Interventions. Interventions for combating HIV are behavioral as well as biomedical. Recent advances in antiretroviral therapy have been credited with dramatic declines in deaths associated with HIV/AIDS. However, declines in overall AIDS cases, particularly in the early epicenters of the epidemic such as San Francisco and New York City, predate the advent of antiretroviral therapies and support the belief that behavior-based prevention programs are effective. In San Francisco, for example, new cases of AIDS among men who have sex with men began dropping in 1992, suggesting that sustained, comprehensive prevention activities begun in the 1980s succeeded in reducing HIV transmission in this group.[29]

Behavioral interventions to prevent HIV vary depending on the audience for whom the program is designed, who designed it, and funds available. Effective community-level prevention strategies in the United States have included social marketing interventions to increase condom use and messages about safer sex and needle-sharing that rely on popular opinion leaders and role model stories. Effective small and large group interventions have aimed at increasing safer sex practices for high-risk HIV-infected men and women and have tended to employ cognitive behavioral and skill-building methods.[29]

Several effective individual counseling or education interventions have focused on increasing condom use and other safer sex practices for HIV-infected persons. For example, at the individual level, client-centered HIV counseling and testing appear to be effective in preventing high-risk uninfected persons from becoming infected and in helping HIV-infected persons prevent transmission to uninfected partners. Intervention venues vary and include STD clinic waiting rooms, drug treatment centers, schools, community agencies, street settings, and community settings where HIV-infected and high-risk uninfected persons congregate.[29]

While HIV testing in STD clinics is an important intervention, detection and treatment of other STDs are also an important biomedical component of an HIV prevention program that should include both behavioral and biomedical interventions. STD prevention programs must address STD concerns and their cofactor role in HIV transmission. Early STD detection and treatment are a biomedical tool for lowering the risk for sexual transmission of HIV infection. Behavioral interventions emphasize reducing the number of sex partners, knowing the serostatus of one's partner, using condoms consistently and correctly, and avoiding risky sexual behaviors.[26, 30, 31]

Disparities

In the United States, African Americans and Hispanics have been affected disproportionately by HIV and AIDS, compared to other racial and ethnic groups.

Through December 1998, 688,200 cases of AIDS had been reported among persons of all ages and racial and ethnic groups, including 304,094 cases among whites, 251,408 cases among African Americans, and 124,841 cases among Hispanics. Although 55 percent of the reported AIDS cases occurred among African Americans and Hispanics, these two population groups represent an estimated 13 percent and 12 percent, respectively, of the total U.S. population.[2]

In 1997, AIDS remained the leading cause of death for all African Americans aged 25 to 44 years—the second leading cause among African American females and the leading cause among African American males.[13] In 1996, for the first time, African Americans accounted for a larger proportion of AIDS cases than whites, and this trend has continued. The AIDS case rate among African Americans in calendar year 1998 was 66.4 per 100,000 persons, or eight times the rate for whites (8.2 per 100,000) and over twice the rate for Hispanics (28.1 per 100,000).[2]

Among women with AIDS, African Americans and Hispanics have been especially affected, accounting for nearly 77 percent of cumulative cases reported among women by 1998. Of the 109,311 AIDS cases in women reported through December 1998, 61,874 cases occurred in African American women and 21,937 occurred in Hispanic women.[2]

For young adults aged 20 to 24 years, 24,437 cumulative AIDS cases were reported through December 1998. Of this total, 10,107 (41 percent) occurred among African Americans, 8,804 (36 percent) among whites, and 5,203 (21 percent) among Hispanics. Overall, 73 percent (17,797) of the AIDS cases in this age group occurred among males and 27 (6,640) percent among females. Among African Americans in this age group, 63 percent were male, and 37 percent were female. Among Hispanics, 74 percent were male, and 26 percent were female. Because the time from initial infection with HIV to the development of AIDS is long and variable (often 8 to 10 years or more), many of these young adults likely acquired their infections while in their teens.[2]

Among teenagers aged 13 to 19 years, 3,423 cumulative AIDS cases had been reported through December 1998.[2] In this age group, 1,047 cases (31 percent) occurred among whites, 1,654 (48 percent) among African Americans, and 668 (20 percent) among Hispanics. Overall, males accounted for 61 percent of the AIDS cases in this age group, and females accounted for 39 percent. Among African American teenagers with AIDS, 46 percent were male, and 54 percent were female. Among Hispanic teens, 67 percent of those with AIDS were male, and 33 percent were female. Among white teenagers with AIDS, 79 percent were male, and 21 percent were female.[2]

The disproportionate impact of HIV/AIDS on African Americans and Hispanics underscores the importance of implementing and sustaining effective prevention efforts for these racial and ethnic populations. HIV prevention efforts must take into account not only the multiracial and multicultural nature of society, but also other social and economic factors—such as poverty, underemployment, and poor access to the health care system. These factors affect health status and disproportionately affect African American, Hispanic, Alaska Native, and American Indian populations.

Opportunities

In the 21st century, strategies for reducing HIV transmission will continue to evolve and will require shifts from current efforts.[32] Future strategies should focus on:

- Continuing to address the disproportionate impact of HIV/AIDS among certain racial and ethnic groups.

- Enhancing prevention strategies for populations that are particularly high risk, such as injection drug users, homeless persons, runaway youth, mentally ill persons, and incarcerated persons. Some of these populations are also difficult to reach.

- Increasing the number of people who learn their HIV status in order to detect HIV infection when the potential for transmission is greatest and the need for prevention, care, and treatment, including HAART, is greatest.

- Reaching high-risk seronegative people to help them to stay uninfected.

- Improving access to HAART, thereby reducing deaths and HIV-associated illness and, possibly, infection of others.

- Increasing efforts and opportunities to provide counseling to prevent transmission and reinfection for all HIV-infected individuals who are receiving medical and supportive care.

- Detecting and treating ulcerative and inflammatory STDs, especially in groups at risk for HIV infection.

- Setting the discovery of a safe and effective HIV vaccine as a reachable goal, as a result of ongoing HIV vaccine testing. The development and testing of candidate microbicides may be important in enhancing prevention efforts until a vaccine is available.

Interim Progress Toward Year 2000 Objectives

Data to assess progress are available for 13 of the 17 Healthy People 2000 HIV objectives. Two objectives have met or exceeded the year 2000 targets. The objective to lower the risk of transfusion-transmitted HIV infection exceeded its target, and the objective to protect workers from exposure to bloodborne infections was met with the Occupational Safety and Health Administration's bloodborne pathogens standard in December 1991. Data show progress toward the year 2000 targets for objectives to slow the rise in the rate of new AIDS cases, contain the rate of

HIV infection, and increase the proportion of sexually active females whose partners used condoms at last sexual intercourse. The objective to increase the proportion of HIV-positive people who know their serostatus is moving away from its
target, as are objectives for counseling, outreach, and school-based AIDS education.

Note: Unless otherwise noted, data are from the Centers for Disease Control and
Prevention, National Center for Health Statistics, *Healthy People 2000 Review, 1998–99*.

HIV

Goal: Prevent HIV infection and its related illness and death.

Number	Objective Short Title
13-1	New AIDS cases
13-2	AIDS among men who have sex with men
13-3	AIDS among persons who inject drugs
13-4	AIDS among men who have sex with men and who inject drugs
13-5	New HIV cases
13-6	Condom use
13-7	Knowledge of serostatus
13-8	HIV counseling and education for persons in substance abuse treatment
13-9	HIV/AIDS, STD, and TB education in State prisons
13-10	HIV counseling and testing in State prisons
13-11	HIV testing in TB patients
13-12	Screening for STDs and immunization for hepatitis B
13-13	Treatment according to guidelines
13-14	HIV-infection deaths
13-15	Interval between HIV infection and AIDS diagnosis
13-16	Interval between AIDS diagnosis and death from AIDS
13-17	Perinatally acquired HIV infection

13-1. Reduce AIDS among adolescents and adults.

Target: 1.0 new case per 100,000 persons.

Baseline: 19.5 cases of AIDS per 100,000 persons aged 13 years and older in 1998. Data are estimated; adjusted for delays in reporting.

Target setting method: Better than the best.

Data source: HIV/AIDS Surveillance System, CDC, NCHSTP.

Persons Aged 13 Years and Older, 1998	New AIDS Cases		
	13-1. Both Genders	Females*	Males*
	Rate per 100,000		
TOTAL	19.5	8.8	30.8
Race and ethnicity			
American Indian or Alaska Native	9.4	4.5	14.5
Asian or Pacific Islander	4.3	1.2	7.8
Asian	DNC	DNC	DNC
Native Hawaiian and other Pacific Islander	DNC	DNC	DNC
Black or African American	DNC	DNC	DNC
White	DNC	DNC	DNC
Hispanic or Latino	33.0	13.8	52.2
Not Hispanic or Latino	DNC	DNC	DNC
Black or African American	82.9	48.5	122.9
White	8.5	2.2	15.2
Family income level			
Poor	DNC	DNC	DNC
Near poor	DNC	DNC	DNC
Middle/high income	DNC	DNC	DNC
Sexual orientation	DNC	DNC	DNC

DNA = Data have not been analyzed. DNC = Data are not collected. DSU = Data are statistically unreliable.
*Data for females and males are displayed to further characterize the issue.

Historically, AIDS incidence data have served as the basis for assessing needs for prevention and treatment programs. However, because of the effect of potent antiretroviral therapies, AIDS incidence no longer can provide unbiased information on HIV incidence patterns; it is hoped that AIDS will not develop in the growing number of HIV-infected persons as they benefit from these new therapies. Persons reported with AIDS will increasingly represent persons who were diagnosed too late for them to benefit from treatments, persons who either did not seek or had no access to care, or persons who failed treatment. This objective will be modified to track HIV cases as additional States implement HIV surveillance programs as an extension of their current AIDS case surveillance systems.

13-2. Reduce the number of new AIDS cases among adolescent and adult men who have sex with men.

Target: 13,385 new cases.

Baseline: 17,847 new cases of AIDS in 1998 among males aged 13 years and older. Data are estimated; risk is redistributed; adjusted for delays in reporting.

Target setting method: 25 percent improvement.

Data source: HIV/AIDS Surveillance System, CDC, NCHSTP.

In 1998, an estimated 17,847 AIDS cases were diagnosed among men having sex with men. This was a decrease from 1997 and part of a continuing trend. The decline is a result of prevention activities and the impact of and access to potent antiretroviral therapies that are delaying progression to AIDS in many HIV-infected individuals.

However, men who have sex with men (MSM) remains a population at risk for HIV infection, and continued efforts to promote behavioral risk reduction among at-risk youth are needed. Prevention programs for adolescent and adult MSM need to focus on both HIV-infected and uninfected populations. Challenges to HIV prevention programs for MSM include (1) reaching MSM who may not identify themselves as homosexual or bisexual, (2) representing MSM from certain racial and ethnic groups in HIV prevention planning, (3) increasing knowledge about HIV risk, and (4) improving access to HIV testing and health care.[33] Serologic surveys, HIV/AIDS case surveillance, and supplemental research and evaluation studies of MSM from certain racial and ethnic groups and other HIV-infected and at-risk populations also are needed to target intervention programs.[4] This objective will be modified when additional States implement HIV infection surveillance as an extension of their current AIDS case surveillance systems.

13-3. Reduce the number of new AIDS cases among females and males who inject drugs.

Target: 9,075 cases.

Baseline: 12,099 new cases of AIDS among injection drug users aged 13 years and older (females, 3,667; males, 8,432) in 1998. Data are point estimates; risk redistributed; adjusted for delays in reporting.

Target setting method: 25 percent improvement.

Data source: HIV/AIDS Surveillance System, CDC, NCHSTP.

In 1998, an estimated 12,099 cases were diagnosed among adult men and women who injected drugs. This was a decrease from the previous year and part of a continuing trend. The decline is a result of prevention activities and the impact of potent antiretroviral therapies that are delaying progression to AIDS in many HIV-infected individuals.

Prevention measures for reducing the occurrence of AIDS associated with injection drug users (IDUs) included: (1) preventing the initiation of injecting-drug use, (2) increasing the number of IDUs in drug treatment, (3) encouraging safer injecting practices among IDUs, and (4) promoting safer sexual behavior among IDUs and their sex partners.[34, 35, 36] Persons who continue to inject drugs should be screened periodically for HIV infection and advised of measures that may reduce risks for infection.

13-4. Reduce the number of new AIDS cases among adolescent and adult men who have sex with men and inject drugs.

Target: 1,592 cases.

Baseline: 2,122 new cases of AIDS among males aged 13 years and older in 1998. Data are point estimates; risk redistributed; adjusted for delays in reporting.

Target setting method: 25 percent improvement.

Data source: HIV/AIDS Surveillance System, CDC, NCHSTP.

In 1998, an estimated 2,122 AIDS cases were diagnosed among adult and adolescent men who have sex with men and who inject drugs. This was a decrease from 1997 and part of a continuing trend. The decline is a result of prevention activities and the impact of potent antiretroviral therapies which are delaying progression to AIDS in many HIV-infected individuals.

Prevention programs for adolescent and adult MSM and IDUs need to focus on both HIV-infected and uninfected populations. Challenges to the design and implementation of HIV prevention programs among MSM and IDUs include: (1) reaching MSM who may not identify themselves as homosexual or bisexual, (2) representing MSM from certain racial and ethnic groups in HIV prevention planning, (3) increasing knowledge about HIV risk, (4) improving access to HIV testing and health care, (5) preventing the initiation of injecting-drug use, (6) increasing the number of IDUs in drug treatment, (7) encouraging safer injecting practices among IDUs, and (8) promoting safer sexual behaviors among IDUs and their sex partners.[33, 34, 35, 36] This objective will be modified when additional States implement HIV infection surveillance as an extension of their current AIDS case surveillance systems.

13-5. (Developmental) Reduce the number of cases of HIV infection among adolescents and adults.

Potential data source: HIV/AIDS Surveillance System, CDC, NCHSTP.

Recent advances in HIV treatment have slowed the progression of HIV disease for infected persons on treatment and contributed to a decline in AIDS incidence. These advances in treatment have diminished the ability of AIDS surveillance data to represent trends in HIV incidence or to represent the impact of the epidemic on the health care system. Once HIV case surveillance is implemented nationwide by 2001, the Centers for Disease Control and Prevention (CDC) will be able to report baseline data and progress toward the objective of "reducing the annual incidence of HIV infection."

13-6. Increase the proportion of sexually active persons who use condoms.

Target and baseline:

Objective	Increase in Sexually Active Persons Using Condoms	1995 Baseline	2010 Target
		Percent	
13-6a.	Females aged 18 to 44 years	23	50
13-6b.	Males aged 18 to 49 years	Developmental	

Target setting method: Better than the best.

Data source: National Survey of Family Growth (NSFG), CDC, NCHS.

NOTE: THE TABLE BELOW MAY CONTINUE TO THE FOLLOWING PAGE.

Unmarried Females 18 to 44 years, 1995	13-6a. Reported Condom Use by Partners*
	Percent
TOTAL	23
Race and ethnicity	
American Indian or Alaska Native	DSU
Asian or Pacific Islander	DSU
Asian	DNC
Native Hawaiian and other Pacific Islander	DNC
Black or African American	22
White	23

Unmarried Females 18 to 44 years, 1995	13-6a. Reported Condom Use by Partners*
	Percent
Hispanic or Latino	17
Aged 18 to 19 years	16
Aged 20 to 24 years	18
Aged 25 to 29 years	19
Aged 30 to 34 years	22
Aged 35 to 44 years	9
Not Hispanic or Latino	24
Black or African American	22
Aged 18 to 19 years	31
Aged 20 to 24 years	35
Aged 25 to 29 years	23
Aged 30 to 34 years	17
Aged 35 to 44 years	12
White	24
Aged 18 to 19 years	39
Aged 20 to 24 years	29
Aged 25 to 29 years	24
Aged 30 to 34 years	14
Aged 35 to 44 years	18
Family income level	
Poor	16
Near poor	21
Middle/high income	27
Education level (aged 25 to 44 years)	
Less than high school	7
High school	15
At least some college	25
Geographic location	
Urban	24
Rural	18
Sexual orientation	DNC

DNA = Data have not been analyzed. DNC = Data are not collected. DSU = Data are statistically unreliable.
*Data for both genders and for males currently are not collected.

NOTE: THE TABLE ABOVE MAY HAVE CONTINUED FROM THE PREVIOUS PAGE.

When used consistently and correctly, latex condoms are highly effective in preventing HIV transmission. Increased use of latex condoms is essential for slowing the spread of HIV infection. Carefully designed studies among heterosexual couples in which one partner is HIV positive and the other is not demonstrate that latex condoms provide a high level of protection against HIV.[9, 26]

Persons in some populations, especially sexually active young persons, may experience problems in obtaining access to condoms because of several factors, including cost, convenience, and embarrassment.[37, 38] The lack of readily accessible condoms may also be a significant barrier to consistent use. To eliminate this barrier, many local communities actively support programs that make condoms available to populations most vulnerable to HIV infection, including sexually active young persons.[37, 38] Research shows that providing access to condoms can increase their use among sexually active young persons.[37, 38] Research also clearly demonstrates that—despite fears to the contrary—young persons who participate in comprehensive HIV prevention programs that include approaches to ensure access to condoms are no more likely to initiate or increase sexual activity than other young persons.[37, 38]

In addition to access, the correct and consistent use of condoms is an issue for many young females, some of whom are having intercourse with older males. Young females often are limited by intimidation or threats of mistrust by their partners if they suggest condom use.[38] Knowledge of effective negotiating skills is another critical element of increased condom use.[38]

13-7. (Developmental) Increase the number of HIV-positive persons who know their serostatus.

Potential data source: HIV/AIDS Surveillance System, CDC, NCHSTP.

Advances in HIV prevention and treatment increase the importance of persons learning their HIV status.[9] Estimates are that approximately 250,000 persons in the United States are unaware they were infected with HIV in 1998.[11] HIV testing provides a critical avenue to reach persons at risk with prevention counseling and services as well as to link infected individuals with needed care and treatment services. Clearly, infected persons should be counseled about ways they can protect their own health and keep from infecting others. New treatments offer infected persons the promise of a longer, healthier life. For HIV-infected pregnant females, therapy is available to reduce the chance of transmitting HIV to their babies. Although the evidence still is not entirely clear, persons who are being treated successfully for HIV may be less likely to transmit the virus. Because the science is evolving, communicating the continuing need for infected persons, even those in treatment, to take steps to protect their partners is essential.[4]

13-8. Increase the proportion of substance abuse treatment facilities that offer HIV/AIDS education, counseling, and support.

Target: 70 percent.

Baseline: 58 percent of substance abuse treatment facilities offered HIV/AIDS education, counseling, and support in 1997.

Target setting method: 21 percent improvement.

Data source: Uniform Facility Data Set (UFDS), SAMHSA.

To date, more than one-third of all reported AIDS cases in the United States have occurred among injection drug users, their heterosexual sex partners, and children whose mothers were injection drug users or sex partners of injection drug users.[2]

Preventing drug use and providing treatment to stop drug use among persons already using drugs are the best ways to prevent drug-associated transmission of HIV. Among persons who inject drugs, reusing or sharing blood-contaminated injection equipment (particularly syringes) continues to play a substantial role in HIV transmission, as well as the transmission of hepatitis B and C and other bloodborne infections.[27]

Needle and syringe exchange programs (NSEPs) can be an effective component of comprehensive community-based HIV prevention efforts.[27] Additionally, NSEPs can provide a pathway for linking injection drug users to other important services, such as risk-reduction counseling, drug treatment, and support services.

13-9. (Developmental) Increase the number of State prison systems that provide comprehensive HIV/AIDS, sexually transmitted diseases, and tuberculosis (TB) education.

Potential data source: Survey of HIV, STD, and TB Prevention in Correctional Facilities, CDC/National Institute of Justice.

Incarceration provides an environment in which early interventions and risk-reduction behaviors can be taught and reinforced over time. It also represents an opportunity to provide the education, support, and continuity of care needed when incarcerated persons are released and return to their home communities.

13-10. (Developmental) Increase the proportion of inmates in State prison systems who receive voluntary HIV counseling and testing during incarceration.

Potential data source: Survey of HIV, STD, and TB Prevention in Correctional Facilities, CDC and National Institute of Justice.

Although not standardized, State prison systems can provide access to treatment and care for persons infected with HIV. Early access to care reduces both immediate and long-term health care costs for correctional institutions and the community. This objective focuses on State systems because, in accordance with the Federal Bureau of Prisons guidance, all Federal correctional facilities are required to provide HIV testing to all inmates at some time prior to discharge.[39] Continuing this practice is important. It is also important to provide HIV testing to inmates upon intake to allow for sufficient medical care and necessary followup. In addition, discharge planning and formal linkages with community-based HIV care should be offered to all HIV-positive inmates just prior to or upon release.

13-11. Increase the proportion of adults with tuberculosis (TB) who have been tested for HIV.

Target: 85 percent.

Baseline: 55 percent of adults aged 25 to 44 years with TB were tested for HIV in 1998.

Target setting method: Better than the best.

Data source: National TB Surveillance System, CDC, DTBE.

NOTE: THE TABLE BELOW MAY CONTINUE TO THE FOLLOWING PAGE.

Adults Aged 25 to 44 Years With TB, 1998	Tested for HIV
	Percent
TOTAL	55
Race and ethnicity	
American Indian or Alaska Native	39
Asian or Pacific Islander	29
Asian	DNC
Native Hawaiian and other Pacific Islander	DNC
Black or African American	76
White	50
Hispanic or Latino	46
Not Hispanic or Latino	58
Black or African American	76
White	58
Gender	
Female	51
Male	58

| Adults Aged 25 to 44 Years With TB, 1998 | Tested for HIV |
	Percent
Family income level	
Poor	DNC
Near poor	DNC
Middle/high income	DNC

DNA = Data have not been analyzed. DNC = Data are not collected. DSU = Data are statistically unreliable.

NOTE: THE TABLE ABOVE MAY HAVE CONTINUED FROM THE PREVIOUS PAGE.

The rapid rate of progression from infection with TB bacteria to active TB disease among HIV-positive patients with *Mycobacterium tuberculosis* has been well documented.[40, 41] When State health departments compared their TB and AIDS registries, 27 percent of the TB cases reported in 1993–94 in adults aged 25 to 44 years had a match in the AIDS registry. However, estimates based on registry matches provide only a minimum estimate of coinfection.[28]

Early detection of HIV in TB patients also allows for early intervention and treatment that may prevent or delay the development of other HIV-related illnesses and AIDS. It is possible that many persons diagnosed with TB have immune system problems caused by HIV and are unaware of their HIV status. In 1998, 55 percent of TB case reports for persons aged 15 to 44 years included information about HIV status. Among the States with information for 75 percent or more of the cases in this age group, the proportion of TB cases in HIV-infected patients ranged from 0 to 47 percent.[42] Because testing is voluntary, some patients may decline HIV testing.

13-12. (Developmental) Increase the proportion of adults in publicly funded HIV counseling and testing sites who are screened for common bacterial sexually transmitted diseases (STDs) (chlamydia, gonorrhea, and syphilis) and are immunized against hepatitis B virus.

Potential data source: HIV Counseling and Testing Data System (CTS), CDC, NCHSTP.

Data indicate that the presence of other STDs substantially increases the risk of HIV transmission by making it easier both to get and to give HIV infection.[31, 43] Treating other STDs reduces the spread of HIV. STD rates in the United States are high, and STD clinical services are inadequate in the face of a changing HIV epidemic.[44]

STD vaccines can minimize the probability of infection. While vaccines for some STDs are in various stages of development, an effective vaccine for hepatitis B is widely available. Unfortunately, hepatitis B vaccine coverage remains low, especially in high-risk groups. The main reasons are a lack of awareness among health care providers, limited opportunity to reach high-risk youth in traditional health care settings, and limited financial support for widescale implementation of this intervention.[45] Many persons requesting HIV counseling and testing, although not HIV infected, are nonetheless at high risk for acquiring sexually transmitted infections.[41, 45] Offering hepatitis B vaccine at sites screening for common STDs would take advantage of reaching high-risk persons who otherwise may not have access to immunization services.

13-13. Increase the proportion of HIV-infected adolescents and adults who receive testing, treatment, and prophylaxis consistent with current Public Health Service treatment guidelines.

Target and baseline:

Objective	Increase in HIV-Infected Persons Aged 13 Years and Older Receiving Testing, Treatment, and Prophylaxis Consistent With Current Public Health Service Guidelines	1997 Baseline	2010 Target
		Percent	
	Testing		
13-13a.	Viral load testing	Developmental	
13-13b.	Tuberculin skin testing (TST)	Developmental	
	Treatment		
13-13c.	Any antiretroviral therapy	80	95
13-13d.	Highly active antiretroviral therapy (HAART)	40	95
	Prophylaxis		
13-13e.	*Pneumocystis carinii* pneumonia (PCP) prophylaxis	80	95
13-13f.	*Mycobacterium avium* complex (MAC) prophylaxis	44	95

Note: Data from 11 cities and 9 States.

Target setting method: An improvement to the same percentage as that projected for *Pneumocystis carinii* pneumonia prophylaxis.

Data source: Adult Spectrum of Disease (ASD) Surveillance Project, CDC, NCHSTP.

Data for population groups currently are not collected.

Estimated new cases of AIDS in adults and adolescents declined by 15 percent from 1996 to 1997.[46] As new therapies continue to be developed and as people with HIV/AIDS live longer, HIV-infected persons need access to these life-enhancing treatments. Once individuals access care, they need to receive the most beneficial treatment possible. The survival benefits of antiretroviral therapy, *Pneumocystis carinii* pneumonia (PCP) and *Mycobacterium avium* complex (MAC) prophylaxis, and TB prophylaxis have been demonstrated for persons with HIV/AIDS who meet the criteria for these preventive therapies. (CD4+ testing is included as a standard of care in the Public Health Service treatment guidelines but is not included here because it already is provided to nearly 100 percent of individuals measured by this objective.)[46]

Data from HIV and AIDS case surveillance continue to reflect the disproportionate impact of the epidemic on select populations, especially females, youth, and children. Everyone needs equal access to appropriate care and treatment services necessary to maintain a healthy life.

13-14. Reduce deaths from HIV infection.

Target: 0.7 deaths per 100,000 persons.

Baseline: 4.9 deaths from HIV infection per 100,000 persons in 1998 (age adjusted to the year 2000 population).

Target setting method: Better than the best.

Data source: National Vital Statistics System, CDC, NCHS.

NOTE: THE TABLE BELOW MAY CONTINUE TO THE FOLLOWING PAGE.

Total Population, 1998	Deaths Due to HIV Infection		
	13-14. Both Genders	Females*	Males*
	Rate per 100,000		
TOTAL	4.9	2.3	7.7
Race and ethnicity			
American Indian or Alaska Native	2.3	DSU	4.0
Asian or Pacific Islander	0.8	DSU	1.4
Asian	DNC	DNC	DNC
Native Hawaiian and other Pacific Islander	DNC	DNC	DNC
Black or African American	22.1	12.2	34.0
White	2.7	0.8	4.6
Hispanic or Latino	6.7	2.8	10.7
Not Hispanic or Latino	4.7	2.2	7.3
Black or African American	22.8	12.6	35.1
White	2.1	0.5	3.8

Total Population, 1998	Deaths Due to HIV Infection		
	13-14. Both Genders	Females*	Males*
	Rate per 100,000		
Education level (aged 25 to 64 years)			
Less than high school	17.3	10.6	23.4
High school graduate	11.7	5.6	18.3
At least some college	4.3	1.1	7.5

DNA = Data have not been analyzed. DNC = Data are not collected. DSU = Data are statistically unreliable.
Note: Age adjusted to the year 2000 standard population.
*Data for females and males are displayed to further characterize the issue.
NOTE: THE TABLE ABOVE MAY HAVE CONTINUED FROM THE PREVIOUS PAGE.

The impact of new combination drug therapies first was reported in 1997 when deaths attributable to HIV infection were down 44 percent from the first 6 months of 1996, compared with the first 6 months of 1997.[4, 5, 46, 47, 48] These surveillance data suggest that not only are new therapies delaying progression from AIDS to death, but, with early diagnosis and treatment, these therapies also are helping to delay the progression from HIV infection to an AIDS diagnosis for many persons.

13-15. (Developmental) Extend the interval of time between an initial diagnosis of HIV infection and AIDS diagnosis in order to increase years of life of an individual infected with HIV.

Potential data source: HIV/AIDS Surveillance System, CDC, NCHSTP.

This objective is meant to identify which populations are not benefiting from current treatment therapies and where to direct resources. HIV-infected persons should be identified at the earliest possible opportunity and referred to appropriate medical, social, and preventive services that may preserve their health, help them avoid opportunistic illnesses, reduce sexual and drug-use behaviors that may spread HIV, and generally extend the quality of their lives. For HIV-infected persons to benefit from treatment advances, HIV counseling and testing programs must facilitate an early diagnosis of HIV infection. All persons should have equal access to appropriate care and treatment services necessary for maintaining a healthy life.

13-16. (Developmental) Increase years of life of an HIV-infected person by extending the interval of time between an AIDS diagnosis and death.

Potential data source: HIV/AIDS Surveillance System, CDC, NCHSTP.

This objective provides insight into which population groups lack or fail to respond to treatment. To sustain reductions in deaths due to HIV infection, access to treatment and care is necessary. Targeting prevention efforts at groups disproportionately affected also is important.

13-17. (Developmental) Reduce new cases of perinatally acquired HIV infection.

Potential data source: HIV/AIDS Surveillance System, CDC, NCHSTP.

Perinatal transmission of HIV accounts for virtually all new HIV infections in children. Through 1993, an estimated 15,000 HIV-infected children were born to HIV-positive women in the United States. As of June 1998, 8,280 AIDS cases had been reported in children under age 13 years in the United States. Perinatally acquired AIDS cases have been reported from 48 States, the District of Columbia, Puerto Rico, and the U.S. Virgin Islands.[2, 25]

The National Institutes of Health sponsored an AIDS clinical trial, ACTG-076, after demonstrating that the risk of perinatal HIV transmission could be reduced by as much as two-thirds with the use of zidovudine therapy. This therapy was given to HIV-positive pregnant females during pregnancy and childbirth and to their newborns for 6 weeks after birth.[24] Additional research confirmed that routine and universal counseling and voluntary testing, combined with zidovudine therapy, are highly effective in preventing HIV.[24] In addition, recently completed and ongoing research suggests that other antiretroviral agents also can reduce significantly maternal-infant HIV transmission. These additional therapeutic options should increase the opportunity to intervene to reduce perinatal HIV transmission. Substantial declines in perinatal AIDS cases have been reported. Estimated new cases of pediatric AIDS declined from 947 in 1992 to 225 in 1998.[2]

Even though these prevention efforts are proving to be effective in reducing perinatal HIV transmission, the continued number of new cases of perinatally acquired HIV infection among infants indicates an ongoing risk of perinatal transmission and underscores the need for strategies to ensure that HIV-infected females have access to and receive adequate prenatal care, timely HIV counseling, and voluntary testing; gain access to HIV-related care and services; receive chemoprophylaxis to reduce perinatal transmission; and avoid breastfeeding. In 1998, the Institute of Medicine (IOM) completed a study to assess the impact of current approaches for reducing perinatal HIV transmission. IOM recommended that the United States adopt a national policy of universal HIV testing, with patient notification, as a routine component of prenatal care.[49] The U.S. Public Health Service currently is revising its guidelines to assure voluntary screening of all pregnant women. This objective will remain developmental until all States extend their surveillance systems to include HIV.

Related Objectives From Other Focus Areas

7. **Educational and Community-Based Programs**
   7-2. School health education
9. **Family Planning**
   9-10. Pregnancy prevention and sexually transmitted disease (STD) protection
14. **Immunization and Infectious Diseases**
    14-11. Tuberculosis
    14-13. Treatment for high-risk persons with latent tuberculosis infection
20. **Occupational Safety and Health**
    20-10. Needlestick injuries
25. **Sexually Transmitted Diseases**
    25-8. Heterosexually transmitted HIV infection in women
    25-11. Responsible adolescent sexual behavior
    25-17. Screening of pregnant women

Terminology

(A listing of acronyms and abbreviations used in this publication appears in Appendix H.)

AIDS: Acquired immunodeficiency syndrome, the most severe phase of infection with the human immunodeficiency virus (HIV). Persons infected with HIV are said to have AIDS when they get certain opportunistic infections or when their CD4+ cell count drops below 200.

CD4+ cell (also known as T helper cell): A type of T cell found in the blood that is involved in protecting the body against infections. CD4+ cells normally orchestrate the immune response, signaling other cells in the immune system to perform their special disease-fighting functions.

CD4+ cell count: A measure of the number of CD4+ cells present in the blood. Because HIV infection kills CD4+ cells, CD4+ cell count is used to track the progress of HIV infection.

Cost-effective: Indicates that the cost of a particular intervention compares favorably to life-saving interventions associated with other diseases.

Cost-saving: Indicates that a particular intervention averts health care costs in excess of the cost of the intervention.

HAART (highly active antiretroviral therapy): Aggressive anti-HIV treatment usually including a combination of drugs called protease inhibitors and reverse transcriptase inhibitors whose purpose is to reduce viral load infection to undetectable levels.

HIV (human immunodeficiency virus): A virus that infects and takes over certain cells of the immune system that are important in fighting disease.

HIV antiretrovirals: Drugs, such as zidovudine (AZT) and saquinavir, designed to attack HIV and prevent it from multiplying.

***Mycobacterium avium* complex (MAC):** Bacteria that cause disease in individuals who have weakened immune systems and one of the opportunistic infections that define AIDS.

Opportunistic infections: Infections that take advantage of the opportunity offered when a person's immune system has been weakened by HIV infection. At least 25 medical conditions, including bacterial, fungal, and viral infections and certain types of cancer, are associated with HIV infection.

Pandemic: An epidemic over a large area or country.

***Pneumocystis carinii* pneumonia (PCP):** A type of pneumonia that strikes individuals who have weakened immune systems.

Prevalence: A proportion of persons in a population who are infected, at a specified point in time or over a specified period of time, with HIV.

Prophylactic: Something that guards against or prevents disease.

Prophylaxis: Measures designed to prevent the spread of disease and preserve health; protective or preventive treatment.

Protease: An enzyme that triggers the breakdown of proteins in the body. HIV's protease enzyme breaks apart long strands of viral protein into the separate proteins constituting the viral core and the enzymes it contains. HIV protease acts as new virus particles are budding off a cell membrane.

Protease inhibitor: A drug that binds to and blocks HIV protease from working, thus preventing the production of new functional viral particles.

Serostatus: The result of a blood test for the antibodies that the immune system creates to fight specific diseases.

> **Seronegative:** Indicates that a person's blood lacks antibodies to a specific infectious agent, such as HIV.

> **Seropositive:** Indicates that a person's blood contains antibodies to infections, such as HIV.

Subepidemic: The morbidity that occurs within a proportion of the population infected by the epidemic.

Universal infection control precautions: Guidelines and procedures to protect health care workers from exposure to infection from blood and other body fluids.

References

[1] Centers for Disease Control. Kaposi's sarcoma and pneumocystis pneumonia among homosexual men—New York City and California. *Morbidity and Mortality Weekly Report* 30(25):305-308, 1981.

[2] Centers for Disease Control and Prevention (CDC). *HIV/AIDS Surveillance Report* 10(2), 1998.

[3] Centers for Disease Control. Update on acquired immune deficiency syndrome (AIDS)—United States. *Morbidity and Mortality Weekly Report* 31(37):507-514, 1982.

[4] CDC. CDC guidelines for national human immunodeficiency virus case surveillance, including monitoring for human immunodeficiency virus infection and acquired immunode-ficiency syndrome. *Morbidity and Mortality Weekly Report* 48(RR-13), 1999.

[5] CDC. Update: Trends in AIDS incidence, deaths, and prevention—United States, 1996. *Morbidity and Mortality Weekly Report* 46(8):165-173, 1997.

[6] CDC. *HIV/AIDS Surveillance Report* 9(2), 1997.

[7] CDC. Current trends update: Acquired immunodeficiency syndrome (AIDS)—United States. *Morbidity and Mortality Weekly Report* 32(52):688-691, 1984.

[8] Holtgrave, D.R., and Pinkerton, S.D. Updates of cost of illness and quality of life estimates for use in economic evaluations of HIV prevention programs. *Journal of Acquired Immune Syndrome and Human Retrovirology* 16(1):54-62, 1997.

[9] Sweeney, P.A.; Fleming, P.L.; Karon, J.M.; et al. A minimum estimate of the number of living HIV-infected persons confidentially tested in the United States [Abstract 1-16]. Paper presented at the Interscience Conference on Antimicrobial Agents and Chemotherapy in Toronto, Canada, September 1997.

[10] Karon, J.M.; Rosenberg, P.S.; McQuillan, G.; et al. Prevalence of HIV infection in the United States, 1984–1992. *Journal of the American Medical Association* 276(2):126-131, 1996.

[11] CDC. HIV/AIDS Surveillance Branch, unpublished data, 1999.

[12] Bozzette, S.A.; Berry, S.H.; Duan, N.; et al. The care of HIV-infected adults in the United States, 1984–1992. *The New England Journal of Medicine* 339(26):1897-1904, 1998.

[13] Hoyert, D.L.; Kochanek, K.D.; and Murphy, S.L. Births and deaths: Final data for 1997. *National Vital Statistics Report* 47(19). Hyattsville, MD: National Center for Health Statistics, 1999.

[14] CDC. Update: Trends in AIDS incidence—United States, 1996. *Morbidity and Mortality Weekly Report* 46(37):861-867, 1997.

[15] CDC. *HIV/AIDS Surveillance Report* 5(4), 1994.

[16] CDC. *HIV/AIDS Surveillance Report*. 11(1), 1999.

[17] CDC. Update on acquired immune deficiency syndrome (AIDS) among patients with hemophilia A. *Morbidity and Mortality Weekly Report* 31(48):644-652, 1982.

[18] CDC. Possible transfusion-associated acquired immune deficiency syndrome (AIDS) —California. *Morbidity and Mortality Weekly Report* 31(48):652-654, 1982.

[19] CDC. Prevention of acquired immune deficiency syndrome (AIDS): Report of inter-agency recommendations. *Morbidity and Mortality Weekly Report* 32(8):101-104, 1983.

[20] CDC. Acquired immunodeficiency syndrome (AIDS): Precautions for health-care workers and allied professionals. *Morbidity and Mortality Weekly Report* 32(30):450-452, 1983.

[21] CDC. Provisional public health service inter-agency recommendations for screening donated blood and plasma for antibody to the virus causing acquired immunodeficiency syndrome. *Morbidity and Mortality Weekly Report* 34(1):1-5, 1985.

[22] CDC. Recommendations for preventing transmission of infection with human T-lymphotropic virus III/lymphadenopathy-associated virus in the workplace. *Morbidity and Mortality Weekly Report* 34(45):681-686, 691-696, 1985.

[23] CDC, Public Health Service Task Force. Recommendations for the use of antiretroviral drugs in pregnant women infected with HIV-1 for maternal health and for reducing perinatal HIV-1 transmission in the United States. *Morbidity and Mortality Weekly Report* 47(RR-2), 1998.

[24] Sperling, R.S.; Shapiro, D.E.; Coombs, R.W.; et al. Maternal viral load, zidovudine treatment and the risk of transmission of HIV-1 from mother-to-infant. *The New England Journal of Medicine* 335:1621-1629, 1996.

[25] CDC. Update: Perinatally acquired HIV/AIDS—United States, 1997. *Morbidity and Mortality Weekly Report* 46(46):1086-1092, 1997.

[26] CDC. Update: Barrier protection against HIV infection and other sexually transmitted diseases. *Morbidity and Mortality Weekly Report* 42(30):589-591, 1993.

[27] Institute of Medicine (IOM). The effects of needle exchange programs. In: Norman, J.; Vlahov, D.; and Moses, L.; eds. *Preventing HIV Transmission: The Role of Sterile Needles and Bleach*. Washington, DC: National Academy Press, 1995.

[28] CDC. Prevention and treatment of tuberculosis among persons with human immunodeficiency virus: Principles of therapy and revised recommendations. *Morbidity and Mortality Weekly Report* 47(RR-20), 1998.

[29] Kamb, M.L.; Fishbein, M.; Douglas, Jr., J.M.; et al. Efficacy of risk-reduction counseling to prevent human immunodeficiency virus and sexually transmitted diseases: A randomized controlled trial. Project RESPECT Study Group. *Journal of the American Medical Association* 280(13):1161-1167, 1998.

[30] CDC. HIV prevention through early detection and treatment of other sexually transmitted diseases. United States: Recommendations of the Advisory Committee for HIV and STD Prevention. *Morbidity and Mortality Weekly Report* 47(RR-12):175-219, 181, 1998.

[31] Wasserheit, J. Epidemiological synergy. Interrelationships between human immunodeficiency virus infection and other sexually transmitted diseases. *Sexually Transmitted Diseases* 19(2):61-77, 1992.

[32] Joint United Nations Programme on HIV/AIDS. *The UNAIDS Report*. Geneva, Switzerland: Joint United Nations Programme on HIV/AIDS, 1998.

[33] CDC. HIV/AIDS among racial/ethnic minority men who have sex with men—United States, 1989–1998. *Morbidity and Mortality Weekly Report* 49(1):4-11, 2000.

[34] CDC. AIDS associated with injecting-drug-use—United States, 1995. *Morbidity and Mortality Weekly Report* 40(19):392-396, 1996.

[35] Des Jarlais, D.C.; Friedman, S.R.; Sotheran, J.L.; et al. Continuity and change within an HIV epidemic: Injecting drug users in New York City, 1984–1992. *Journal of the American Medical Association* 271:121-127, 1994.

[36] Roehrich, L.; Wall, T.L.; and Sorenson, J.L. Behavorial interventions for in treatment injection drug users. In: DiClemente, R.J., and Peterson, J.L., eds. *Preventing AIDS: Theories and Methods of Behavorial Interventions*. New York, NY: Plenum Press, 1994, 189-208.

[37] CDC. Community level prevention of HIV infection among high-risk populations: The AIDS community demonstration projects. *Morbidity and Mortality Weekly Report* 45(RR-6):1-16, 1996.

[38] IOM. Factors that contribute to the hidden epidemic. In: *The Hidden Epidemic: Confronting Sexually Transmitted Diseases*. Washington, DC: National Academy Press, 1997, 69-117.

[39] Federal Bureau of Prisons. PS6190.02 infectious disease management. *BOB Program Statement*. Washington, DC: U.S. Department of Justice, 1997.

[40] Antonucci, G.; Girardi, E.; Raviglione, M.C.; et al. Gruppo Italiano di Studio Tubercolosie AIDs (GISTA). Risk factors for tuberculosis in HIV-infected persons: A prospective cohort study. *Journal of the American Medical Association* 274:143-148, 1995.

[41] Rieder, H.L.; Gauthen, G.M.; Comstock, G.W.; et al. Epidemiology of tuberculosis in the United States. *Epidemiology Review* 11:79-98, 1989.

[42] CDC. Progress toward the elimination of tuberculosis—United States, 1998. *Morbidity and Mortality Weekly Report* 48:732-736, 1999.

[43] Fleming, D.T., and Wasserheit, J.N. From epidemiological synergy to public health policy and practice: The contribution of other sexually transmitted diseases to sexual transmission of HIV infection. *Sexually Transmitted Infections* 75(1):3-17, 1999.

[44] IOM. Current STD related services. In: *The Hidden Epidemic: Confronting Sexually Transmitted Diseases*. Washington, DC: National Academy Press,1997, 175-219.

[45] CDC. *HIV counseling and testing in publicly funded sites: 1996 Annual Report*. Atlanta, GA: U.S. Department of Health and Human Services, CDC, 1998.

[46] CDC. Surveillance for AIDS refining opportunistic illnesses, 1992–1997. *Morbidity and Mortality Weekly Report* 48(SS-2), 1999.

[47] CDC. Update: Trends in AIDS incidence—United States, 1996. *Morbidity and Mortality Weekly Report* 46:861-867, 1997.

[48] Fleming, P.L.; Ward, J.W.; Karon, J.M.; et al. Declines in AIDS incidence and deaths in the United States: A signal change in the epidemic. *AIDS* 12(Suppl A):S55-S61, 1998.

[49] IOM. *Reducing the Odds: Preventing Perinatal Transmission of HIV in the United States*. Washington, DC: National Academy Press, 1999.

14

Immunization and Infectious Diseases

Lead Agency: Centers for Disease Control and Prevention

Contents

Prevent disease, disability, and death from infectious diseases, including vaccine-preventable diseases.

Overview

Infectious diseases remain major causes of illness, disability, and death. Moreover, new infectious agents and diseases are being detected, and some diseases considered under control have reemerged in recent years. In addition, antimicrobial resistance is evolving rapidly in a variety of hospital- and community-acquired infections. These trends suggest that many challenges still exist in the prevention and control of infectious diseases.

Issues

Between 1980 and 1992, the number of deaths from infectious diseases rose 58 percent in the United States.[1] Even when human immunodeficiency virus (HIV)-associated diagnoses are removed, deaths from infectious diseases still increased 22 percent during this period. (See Focus Area 13. HIV.) Considered as a group, three infectious diseases—pneumonia, influenza, and HIV infection—constituted the fifth leading cause of death in the United States in 1997.[1]

The direct and indirect costs of infectious diseases are significant. Every hospital-acquired infection adds an average of $2,100 to a hospital bill. Bloodstream infections result in an average of $3,517 in additional hospital charges per infected patient because the patient stay averages an additional 7 days. A typical case of Lyme disease diagnosed in the early stages incurs about $174 in direct medical treatment costs. Delayed diagnosis and treatment, however, can result in complications that cost from $2,228 to $6,724 per patient in direct medical costs in the first year alone.[2]

Infectious diseases also must be considered in a global context. Increases in international travel, importation of foods, inappropriate use of antibiotics on humans and animals, and environmental changes multiply the potential for worldwide epidemics of all types of infectious diseases. International cooperation and collaboration on disease surveillance, response, research, and training are essential to prevent or control these epidemics. Actions taken to improve health in one country affect the health of people worldwide.

Vaccines. Vaccines are biological substances that interact with the person's immune system to produce an immune response identical to that produced by the natural infection.

Vaccines can prevent the debilitating and, in some cases, fatal effects of infectious diseases. Vaccines help to eliminate the illness and disability of polio,[3] measles, and rubella.[4] However, the organisms that cause these diseases have not disappeared. Rather, they have receded and will reemerge if the vaccination coverage drops. The serious health burden of vaccine-preventable diseases (VPDs) is evident from the measles resurgence of 1989 to 1991, resulting in more than 55,000 cases, 11,000 hospitalizations, 120 deaths, and $100 million in direct medical care costs.[5, 6, 7, 8]

Vaccines protect more than the vaccinated individual. They also protect society. When vaccination levels in a community are high, the few who cannot be vaccinated—such as young children and persons with contraindications to vaccination—often are indirectly protected because of group immunity (in other words, they live among vaccinated persons who may offer protection from exposure to disease).

Vaccines provide significant cost benefits. Three childhood vaccines—diphtheria, tetanus toxoids, and acellular pertussis vaccine (DTaP); measles, mumps, and rubella vaccine (MMR); and *Haemophilus influenzae* type b (Hib) vaccine—result in substantial direct medical savings for each dollar spent to vaccinate children against these diseases. Varicella vaccine saves roughly 90 cents in direct medical costs for every dollar invested. Consideration of indirect savings—prevention of work loss by parents to care for ill children and prevention of death and therefore lost earnings from disability—shows that vaccines routinely recommended for children are highly cost saving. Savings range from $24 for every dollar spent on DTaP to $2 for the more recently approved Hib vaccine.[9]

Trends

Significant progress has been made in reducing indigenous (not imported) cases of VPDs. The occurrence of many VPDs is at or near record-low levels. Most diseases have been reduced by more than 95 percent from peak prevaccine levels.[10]

In 1998, overall vaccination coverage for children aged 19 to 35 months was at record-high levels.[11] Antigen-specific rates have shown striking progress since 1992.[12] For example, coverage for three or more doses of polio vaccine increased from 72 percent to 91 percent, and coverage for three or more doses of Hib vaccine increased from 28 percent to 93 percent. Significant achievements were made among racial and ethnic groups in that most of the 1996 goals for the Childhood Immunization Initiative were met for individual vaccines.[13] Since 1989, vaccination requirements have been expanded for schools and day care settings.[12] As of the 1998–99 school year, all States required vaccination against diphtheria, measles, and polio. Similarly, all States and the District of Columbia now require vaccination for children in day care.[14]

In 1996, a vaccine against hepatitis A virus (HAV) was licensed that has the potential to reduce the health burden of this disease. The vaccine is now recom-

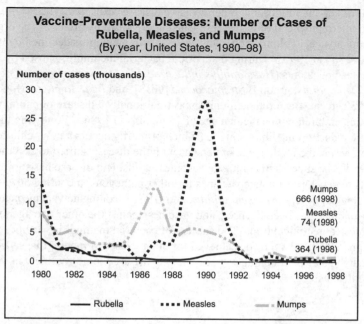

Vaccine-Preventable Diseases: Number of Cases of Rubella, Measles, and Mumps
(By year, United States, 1980–98)

Number of cases (thousands)

Mumps
666 (1998)

Measles
74 (1998)

Rubella
364 (1998)

Rubella ——— Measles ■■■■ Mumps

Source: CDC, EPO. National Notifiable Diseases Surveillance System (NNDSS), 1980–98.

mended primarily for high-risk groups. To decrease HAV transmission, universal vaccination was recommended in 1999 for children who lived in States where the rate of new cases was greater than two times the national average.[15]

Financing for childhood vaccinations has improved significantly as a result of two initiatives—Vaccines for Children and the State Children's Health Insurance Program (SCHIP)—that cover children on Medicaid, uninsured children, and American Indian and Alaska Native children. Underinsured children who receive vaccinations at federally qualified health centers also are covered. Because they promote free vaccines for children, these programs eliminate vaccine cost as a barrier to childhood vaccination. Also, the Public Health Service Act, Section 317 immunization grant program and State funds provide free vaccines for children not covered by other programs.

Vaccination rates among persons aged 65 years and older continued to increase over the decade. Influenza vaccine coverage rates were up from 33 percent in 1989 to 64 percent in 1998, and pneumococcal vaccine coverage rates were up from 15 percent to 46 percent. Despite these increases, coverage rates for certain racial and ethnic groups remain substantially below the general population.[16]

Invasive diseases invade the bloodstream and cause distant infection. The most common types of invasive disease caused by Hib are meningitis, epiglottitis, pneumonia, certain types of arthritis, and cellulitis. Conjugate vaccines—licensed in 1990 for use beginning at age 2 months—are highly effective in protecting against Hib meningitis and other invasive diseases caused by Hib. These vaccines also interrupt spread of the disease-causing organism by affecting the organism's nasopharyngeal colonization. New cases of Hib meningitis declined by 96 percent from 1987 to 1995.[17] During that period, bacterial meningitis caused by one of the five leading agents (*Haemophilus influenzae*, *Streptococcus pneumoniae*, *Neisseria meningitidis*, group B *Streptococcus* [GBS], and *Listeria monocytogenes*) fell by 55 percent. Bacterial meningitis was traditionally a disease of childhood, infecting children with a median age of 15 months in 1986.[18] Following the dramatic reduction in Hib meningitis, which primarily occurs among children under age 2 years, the median age of persons with the disease shifted to 25 years in 1995.[18] The success of conjugate vaccines against Hib disease has stimulated efforts to develop conjugate vaccines for other pathogens, including *Streptococcus pneumoniae*, *Neisseria meningitidis*, and GBS. A conjugate vaccine against *S. pneumoniae* has been licensed, and vaccines against the other two agents are being tested in clinical trials. The success of bacterial meningitis vaccines suggests comparable results may be achieved for other causes of meningitis, sepsis, and pneumonia as their conjugate vaccines become used more routinely in target populations.

Disparities

The updated *Preventing Emerging Infectious Diseases: A Strategy for the 21st Century* focuses on certain emerging infectious disease issues and on particular groups of people at risk.[19] Historically, childhood vaccination rates have been lower in certain racial and ethnic populations, compared to the white population. Vaccination rates for preschool children in racial and ethnic groups with lower vaccination rates, however, have been increasing at a more rapid rate, significantly narrowing the gap.

Efforts need to be intensified, particularly to increase vaccination coverage for children living in poverty. Substantial numbers of undervaccinated children remain in some areas, particularly the large urban areas with traditionally underserved populations, creating great concern because of the potential for outbreaks of disease.

In addition to very young children, many adults are at increased risk for VPDs. Vaccination against pneumococcal infections and influenza among persons aged 65 years and older has increased slightly for African Americans and Hispanics. The coverage in these groups, however, remains substantially below the general population. For example, influenza vaccination rates for whites were 66 percent in 1997, while for African Americans and Hispanics, rates were only 45 percent and 53 percent, respectively. In September 1997, the U.S. Department of Health and Human Services approved a plan to improve adult vaccination rates and reduce disparities among racial and ethnic groups.[20] The elimination of disparities, however, may require further interventions in particular geographic, cultural, and racial and ethnic populations.

A coordinated strategy is necessary to understand, detect, control, and prevent infectious diseases. Such a strategy will protect the gains achieved in life expectancy in the 20th century from control and prevention of infectious diseases and ensure further improvements in the 21st century.

Priority issues include antimicrobial resistance, foodborne and waterborne diseases, vector-borne and zoonotic diseases, diseases transmitted through transfusion of blood or blood products, and vaccine development and use. Some of these diseases and pathogens were unknown 20 years ago. Others are reemergent problems once thought under control. At-risk populations include persons with impaired host defenses; pregnant women and newborns; travelers, immigrants, and refugees; older adults; and other persons identified by the Advisory Committee on Immunization Practices (ACIP).

The major strategies to protect people from VPDs are the following:[21]

- Improving the quality and quantity of vaccination delivery services.
- Minimizing financial burdens for needy persons.
- Increasing community participation, education, and partnership.
- Improving monitoring of disease and vaccination coverage.
- Developing new or improved vaccines and improving vaccine use.

These strategies include a broad range of interventions for children, such as entry requirements for school and promoting the Vaccines for Children and SCHIP initiatives, in which eligible children are vaccinated in their medical home. Assessment of vaccination coverage of persons served at individual clinics and provider offices with feedback of the results to the individual providers to guide them in improving performance also is important. The exchange of information on coverage assessment among colleagues stimulates a friendly competition to achieve better vaccination levels.[22] Populations at risk of undervaccination can be reached through linkages with other programs, including Women, Infants, and Children (WIC) services.[23] State and local registries that enroll children and record their vaccinations are valuable tools for helping parents and providers to identify immunization needs of individual children, assessing coverage in individual practices, and generating communitywide estimates.[24]

In the United States, most VPDs occur among adults. Pneumococcal disease and influenza account for more than 30,000 deaths annually, most of which occur in elderly persons. Studies have consistently shown that focusing efforts to improve coverage on health care providers, as well as health care systems, is the most effective means of raising vaccine coverage in adults. For example, all health care providers should assess routinely the vaccination status of their patients. Likewise, health plans should develop mechanisms for assessing the vaccination status of their participants. Also, nursing home facilities and hospitals should ensure that policies exist to promote vaccination.

Because no vaccine is completely safe, vaccine safety research and monitoring are necessary to identify and minimize vaccine-related injuries. As programs continue to reduce the new cases of VPDs, concerns about vaccine adverse events have emerged, posing a threat to public acceptance of vaccines. Knowing the safety profile of vaccines is essential to assess accurately the risks and benefits, to formulate appropriate vaccine recommendations, and to address public concerns.

Interim Progress Toward Year 2000 Objectives

Significant progress has been made in reaching the Healthy People 2000 objectives. Reductions in indigenous cases of VPDs have been dramatic. For example, measles was reduced from a 1988 baseline of 3,396 indigenous cases to a total of only 74 in 1998. Substantial progress also has been made in reducing hepatitis B virus (HBV) transmission. The vaccine against hepatitis A provides the opportunity to reduce the burden of this disease. Achieving the year 2000 objective to reduce new cases of bacterial meningitis was entirely due to the introduction of Hib conjugate vaccines for infants.[25] In 1998, individual coverage levels for children aged 19 to 35 months were at record high levels. For example, individual coverage levels for three or more doses of polio, three or more doses of diphtheria/tetanus/acellular pertussis, one or more doses of measles/mumps/rubella, and three or more doses of Hib vaccines were each at or above 91 percent. Progress also has been made in expanding immunization requirements for schools and day care settings. Data for viral hepatitis indicate that targets for hepatitis B and C were met in the early 1990s.

Note: Unless otherwise noted, data are from the Centers for Disease Control and Prevention, National Center for Health Statistics, *Healthy People 2000 Review, 1998–99.*

Immunization and Infectious Diseases

Goal: Prevent disease, disability, and death from infectious diseases, including vaccine-preventable diseases.

Number   Objective Short Title

Diseases Preventable Through Universal Vaccination

14-1   Vaccine-preventable diseases

14-2   Hepatitis B in infants and young children

14-3   Hepatitis B in adults and high-risk groups

14-4   Bacterial meningitis in young children

14-5   Invasive pneumococcal infections

Diseases Preventable Through Targeted Vaccination

14-6   Hepatitis A

14-7   Meningococcal disease

14-8   Lyme disease

Infectious Diseases and Emerging Antimicrobial Resistance

14-9   Hepatitis C

14-10   Identification of persons with chronic hepatitis C

14-11   Tuberculosis

14-12   Curative therapy for tuberculosis

14-13   Treatment for high-risk persons with latent tuberculosis infection

14-14   Timely laboratory confirmation of tuberculosis cases

14-15   Prevention services for international travelers

14-16   Invasive early onset group B streptococcal disease

14-17   Peptic ulcer hospitalizations

14-18   Antibiotics prescribed for ear infections

14-19   Antibiotics prescribed for common cold

14-20   Hospital-acquired infections

14-21   Antimicrobial use in intensive care units

Vaccination Coverage and Strategies

Vaccine Safety

Diseases Preventable Through Universal Vaccination

14-1.   Reduce or eliminate indigenous cases of vaccine-preventable diseases.

Target and baseline:

Objective	Reduction in Vaccine-Preventable Diseases	1998 Baseline	2010 Target
		Number of Cases	
14-1a.	Congenital rubella syndrome (children under age 1 year)	7	0
14-1b.	Diphtheria (persons under age 35 years)	1	0
14-1c.	*Haemophilus influenzae* type b* (children under age 5 years)	163	0
14-1d.	Hepatitis B (persons aged 2 to 18 years)	945[†]	9
14-1e.	Measles (persons of all ages)	74	0
14-1f.	Mumps (persons of all ages)	666	0
14-1g.	Pertussis (children under age 7 years)	3,417	2,000
14-1h.	Polio (wild-type virus) (persons of all ages)	0	0
14-1i.	Rubella (persons of all ages)	364	0
14-1j.	Tetanus (persons under age 35 years)	14	0
14-1k.	Varicella (chicken pox) (persons under age 18 years)	4 million[‡]	400,000

*Includes cases with type b and unknown serotype.
[†]Estimated hepatitis B cases for 1997.[26]
[‡]Data based on average from 1990–94 for persons of all ages.

Target setting method: Total elimination for congenital rubella syndrome, diphtheria, *Haemophilus influenzae* type b, measles, mumps, polio, rubella, and tetanus; 41 percent improvement for pertussis; 99 percent improvement for hepatitis B; and 99 percent improvement for varicella.

Data sources: National Notifiable Disease Surveillance System (NNDSS), CDC, EPO; National Congenital Rubella Syndrome Registry (NCRSR), CDC, NIP—congenital rubella syndrome; Active Bacterial Core Surveillance (ABCs),

Emerging Infections Programs, CDC, NCID—*Haemophilus influenzae* type b; National Health Interview Survey (NHIS), CDC, NCHS—varicella.

Highly effective vaccines are used routinely in childhood for prevention of measles, mumps, rubella, varicella, diphtheria, tetanus, pertussis, polio, hepatitis B, and invasive Hib disease.[27] Vaccinations for these diseases have reduced reported cases of most VPDs common in childhood to record-low levels.[11, 26, 28] Measles transmission probably was interrupted multiple times in the United States since 1993.[29, 30, 31] With a high level of coverage of two doses of measles, mumps, and rubella vaccine, interruption of the spread of both rubella and mumps is feasible.[32, 33] Recent outbreaks of rubella and a number of cases of congenital rubella syndrome, however, highlight the importance of ensuring rubella immunity, particularly in women of child-bearing age and foreign-born adults.[34] Polio has been eliminated in the United States due to high vaccination coverage. Although polio is expected to be eradicated globally, surveillance for cases of the disease will continue. Because of widespread vaccination, reported cases of diphtheria are near zero.[35, 36] Tetanus toxoid is highly effective, but with the absence of group immunity, all persons must be vaccinated to achieve the goal of zero cases.[37] Pertussis among children will be reduced by increasing vaccination coverage, but the disease will continue to occur because the organism circulates among older age groups, and the vaccine is not 100 percent effective.[38, 39]

Hepatitis B virus (HBV) infection will be reduced greatly as the age groups covered by universal infant and adolescent vaccination efforts enter young adulthood, a period when the risk of HBV infection increases.

Conjugate vaccines for prevention of Hib are highly effective and have led to near elimination of invasive Hib disease.[17, 40] Further reductions in new cases are anticipated as Hib vaccine coverage increases.

The licensure of new vaccines against common diseases that are not reportable diseases, such as varicella, has created new challenges for surveillance and evaluation. Without national reporting, documenting the impact of national and State vaccination programs and measuring progress for reducing indigenous cases of disease are difficult.[41] However, with an increase in vaccination coverage and a decline in the number of new cases, varicella is expected to become a reportable condition.

14-2. Reduce chronic hepatitis B virus infections in infants and young children (perinatal infections).

Target: 400 infections.

Baseline: 1,682 chronic hepatitis B virus infections in children under age 2 years were reported in 1995.

Target setting method: 76 percent improvement.

Data sources: Perinatal Hepatitis B Prevention Program, CDC, NCID; National Vital Statistics System (NVSS), CDC, NCHS; State Perinatal Hepatitis B Prevention Programs; State Vital Statistics Systems.

Each year, 16,000 to 18,000 children in the United States are born to mothers infected with HBV.[42] Without prevention programs, about 8,000 of these infants would become infected with HBV. Ninety-five percent of the infections, however, are preventable through appropriate maternal screening and infant care.[43]

Screening pregnant women during an early prenatal visit is essential to identify those who are infected. Women at high risk should be retested late in pregnancy. In 1997, 14 States had laws or regulations to ensure such screening.

To be maximally effective, steps to prevent transmission of HBV to infants born to mothers who are infected must begin as soon as the child is born. Such infants should receive a first dose of hepatitis B vaccine within 12 hours of birth, along with hepatitis B immune globulin (HBIG), and two more doses of vaccine by age 6 months. Children need to be tested between the ages of 12 and 15 months to ensure that they are not infected and have developed immunity to the virus.

14-3. Reduce hepatitis B.

Target and baseline:

Objective	Reduction in Hepatitis B	1997 Baseline	2010 Target
	Adults	*Rate per 100,000 Population*	
14-3a.	19 to 24 years	24.0	2.4
14-3b.	25 to 39 years	20.2	5.1
14-3c.	40 years and older	15.0	3.8
	High-risk groups	*Number of Cases*	
14-3d.	Injection drug users	7,232	1,808
14-3e.	Heterosexually active persons	15,225	1,240
14-3f.	Men who have sex with men	7,232	1,808
14-3g.	Occupationally exposed workers	249	62

Target setting method: Better than the best for 14-3a, 14-3b, and 14-3c; 75 percent improvement for 14-3d, 14-3f, and 14-3g; 92 percent improvement for 14-3e.

Data sources: National Notifiable Disease Surveillance System (NNDSS), CDC, EPO; Sentinel Counties Study of Viral Hepatitis, CDC, NCID.

Select Age Groups, 1997	Hepatitis B Cases		
	14-3a. Aged 19 to 24 Years	14-3b. Aged 25 to 39 Years	14-3c. Aged 40 Years and Older
	Rate per 100,000		
TOTAL	24.0	20.2	15.0
Race and ethnicity			
American Indian or Alaska Native	16.0	20.1	10.9
Asian or Pacific Islander	42.2	30.4	33.2
Asian	DNC	DNC	DNC
Native Hawaiian and other Pacific Islander	DNC	DNC	DNC
Black or African American	48.3	32.5	27.6
White	10.4	10.2	7.4
Hispanic or Latino	16.9	16.0	18.1
Not Hispanic or Latino	25.2	20.7	14.8
Black or African American	50.6	34.1	28.4
White	10.3	10.2	7.1
Gender			
Female	24.1	15.4	9.4
Male	22.5	24.1	20.8
Family income level			
Poor	DNC	DNC	DNC
Near poor	DNC	DNC	DNC
Middle/high income	DNC	DNC	DNC

DNA = Data have not been analyzed. DNC = Data are not collected. DSU = Data are statistically unreliable.

To reduce HBV transmission in the United States by 2010, vaccination programs must be targeted to adolescents and adults in high-risk groups. The primary means of achieving high levels of vaccination coverage in groups with behavioral risk factors for HBV infection is to identify settings where these individuals can be vaccinated. Such sites include clinics that treat sexually transmitted diseases (STDs), correctional facilities (juvenile detention facilities, prisons, jails), drug treatment clinics, and community-based HIV prevention sites. The primary means of achieving high levels of vaccine coverage among household and sex contacts of the estimated 1.25 million persons in the United States with chronic HBV infection are programs that offer followup for all hepatitis B surface antigen (HBsAg)-positive persons reported to State and local health departments.

Routine infant vaccination eventually will produce a highly immune population sufficient to eliminate HBV transmission in the United States. However, high rates of acute hepatitis B continue to occur, with an estimated 65,000 cases in 1996. Most cases occur in young adult risk groups, including persons with a history of multiple sex partners, men who have sex with men, injection drug users, incarcerated persons, and household and sex contacts of persons with HBV infection. Investigation of reported cases of acute hepatitis B indicates that as many as 70 percent of these individuals previously had been seen in settings, such as drug treatment clinics, correctional facilities, or clinics for the treatment of STD, where they could have received vaccine.

14-4. Reduce bacterial meningitis in young children.

Target: 8.6 new cases per 100,000 children aged 1 through 23 months.

Baseline: 13.0 new cases of bacterial meningitis per 100,000 children aged 1 through 23 months were reported in 1998.

Target setting method: 34 percent improvement. (Better than the best will be used when data are available.)

Data source: Active Bacterial Core Surveillance (ABCs), CDC, NCID.

NOTE: THE TABLE BELOW MAY CONTINUE TO THE FOLLOWING PAGE.

Children Aged 1 Through 23 Months, 1998	New Cases of Bacterial Meningitis
	Rate per 100,000
TOTAL	13.0
Race and ethnicity	
American Indian or Alaska Native	DSU
Asian or Pacific Islander	DSU
Asian	DNC
Native Hawaiian and other Pacific Islander	DNC
Black or African American	25.9
White	11.0
Hispanic or Latino	DSU
Not Hispanic or Latino	DSU
Black or African American	DSU
White	DSU
Gender	
Female	13.0
Male	13.1

Children Aged 1 Through 23 Months, 1998	New Cases of Bacterial Meningitis
	Rate per 100,000
Family income level	
Poor	DNC
Near poor	DNC
Middle/high income	DNC

DNA = Data have not been analyzed. DNC = Data are not collected. DSU = Data are statistically unreliable.
NOTE: THE TABLE ABOVE MAY HAVE CONTINUED FROM THE PREVIOUS PAGE.

Children aged 1 month through 23 months have higher rates of meningitis than older children. New vaccines for pneumococcal disease, including pneumococcal meningitis, may help protect young children. Meningococcal conjugate vaccines are in clinical trials and may become available for widespread use before 2010, although it is not yet known whether they will be targeted to young children. Pneumococcal conjugate vaccines, modeled after the successful construction of Hib conjugate vaccines, are also in clinical trials. Before 2010, licensure and widespread use of these new products are expected.

14-5. Reduce invasive pneumococcal infections.

Target and baseline:

Objective	Reduction in Invasive Pneumococcal Infections	1997 Baseline	2010 Target
		Rate per 100,000	
	New invasive pneumococcal infections		
14-5a.	Children under age 5 years	76	46
14-5b.	Adults aged 65 years and older	62	42
	Invasive penicillin-resistant pneumococcal infections		
14-5c.	Children under age 5 years	16	6
14-5d.	Adults aged 65 years and older	9	7

Target setting method: Better than the best.

Data sources: Active Bacterial Core Surveillance (ABCs), CDC, NCID; Arctic Investigations Program (for data on pneumococcal disease rates among Alaska Natives), CDC.

Select Age Groups, 1997	New Cases of Invasive Pneumococcal Infections		New Cases of Invasive Penicillin-Resistant Pneumococcal Infections	
	14-5a. Under Age 5 Years	14-5b. Aged 65 Years and Older	14-5c. Under Age 5 Years	14-5d. Aged 65 Years and Older
	Rate per 100,000			
TOTAL	76	62	16	9
Race and ethnicity				
American Indian or Alaska Native	DSU	DSU	DSU	DSU
Asian or Pacific Islander	58	DSU	DSU	DSU
Asian	DSU	DSU	DSU	DSU
Native Hawaiian and other Pacific Islander	DSU	DSU	DSU	DSU
Black or African American	154	83	20	9
White	63	61	17	9
Hispanic or Latino	59	43	7	DSU
Not Hispanic or Latino	DSU	DSU	DSU	DSU
Black or African American	DSU	DSU	DSU	DSU
White	DNC	DNC	DNC	DNC
Gender				
Female	69	61	14	9
Male	84	62	17	9
Family income level				
Poor	DNC	DNC	DNC	DNC
Near poor	DNC	DNC	DNC	DNC
Middle/high income	DNC	DNC	DNC	DNC

DNA = Data have not been analyzed. DNC = Data are not collected. DSU = Data are statistically unreliable.

The number of invasive penicillin-resistant pneumococcal infections can be reduced by lowering the proportion of invasive pneumococcal infections due to drug-resistant strains or by decreasing invasive pneumococcal infections in general. The objectives for specific age groups address the key age groups at risk for invasive pneumococcal infections. Among children under age 5 years, promoting judicious antibiotic use may reverse the current trends toward increasing proportions of infections being caused by drug-resistant strains. For adults aged 65 years and older, licensure and widespread use of pneumococcal conjugate vaccines by

2010 could reduce dramatically all invasive pneumococcal infections, and judicious antibiotic use may have some impact on the proportion of pneumococcal infections caused by drug-resistant strains. In this age group, a much greater impact potentially is achievable through improved use of licensed 23-valent pneumococcal polysaccharide vaccine for the prevention of invasive pneumococcal disease. Increasing the use of this vaccine for elderly persons could have a beneficial impact on the rate of drug-resistant invasive pneumococcal infections.

Diseases Preventable Through Targeted Vaccination

14-6. Reduce hepatitis A.

Target: 4.5 new cases per 100,000 population.

Baseline: 11.3 new cases of hepatitis A per 100,000 population were reported in 1997.

Target setting method: Better than the best.

Data source: National Notifiable Disease Surveillance System (NNDSS), CDC, EPO.

NOTE: THE TABLE BELOW MAY CONTINUE TO THE FOLLOWING PAGE.

Total Population, 1997	New Hepatitis A Cases
	Rate per 100,000
TOTAL	11.3
Race and ethnicity	
American Indian or Alaska Native	23.1
Asian or Pacific Islander	4.6
Asian	DNC
Native Hawaiian and other Pacific Islander	DNC
Black or African American	6.0
White	8.1
Hispanic or Latino	24.2
Not Hispanic or Latino	9.8
Black or African American	6.3
White	7.3
Gender	
Female	8.1
Male	12.8

Total Population, 1997	New Hepatitis A Cases
	Rate per 100,000
Family income level	
Poor	DNC
Near poor	DNC
Middle/high income	DNC
Sexual orientation	DNC

DNA = Data have not been analyzed. DNC = Data are not collected. DSU = Data are statistically unreliable.

NOTE: THE TABLE ABOVE MAY HAVE CONTINUED FROM THE PREVIOUS PAGE.

The health status objectives for hepatitis A virus (HAV) will not be achieved until a vaccination strategy is implemented that produces high levels of immunity in children. Children have the highest rates of hepatitis A and are a primary source for new infections in the community. In 1999, the Advisory Committee on Immunization Practices (ACIP) recommended routine hepatitis A vaccination for children living in States with consistently elevated rates of hepatitis A as the approach most likely to prevent and control transmission of HAV.[15] Hepatitis A vaccine is included in the Vaccines for Children program. Incorporation of hepatitis A vaccine into the routine childhood vaccination schedule would facilitate implementation of these recommendations, but data are needed to determine the appropriate dose and timing of vaccination in the first or second year of life. Implementation of the recommendations also would be enhanced by the development of vaccines that combine HAV antigen with other antigens.

Although routine immunization of children is the approach most likely to decrease significantly the overall rates of hepatitis A in a community, it may take some time before the impact of implementing these programs is measurable. In the interim, persons in groups at high risk of HAV infection should be vaccinated routinely. These groups include:

- Illicit drug users.
- Men who have sex with men.
- Persons traveling to HAV-endemic countries (see objective 14-15).
- Persons with occupational risk of infection—that is, persons who work with HAV-infected primates or with HAV in a research laboratory. No other occupational groups have been shown to be at increased risk of exposure.
- Persons with chronic liver disease.

14-7. Reduce meningococcal disease.

Target: 1.0 new cases per 100,000 population.

Baseline: 1.3 new cases of meningococcal disease per 100,000 population were reported in 1997.

Target setting method: Better than the best.

Data sources: Active Bacterial Core Surveillance (ABCs), Emerging Infections Program Network, CDC, NCID; National Notifiable Diseases Surveillance System (NNDSS), CDC, EPO.

Total Population, 1997	New Cases of Meningococcal Disease
	Rate per 100,000
TOTAL	1.3
Race and ethnicity	
American Indian or Alaska Native	DSU
Asian or Pacific Islander	DSU
Asian	DNC
Native Hawaiian and other Pacific Islander	DNC
Black or African American	1.9
White	1.2
Hispanic or Latino	DSU
Not Hispanic or Latino	DNC
Black or African American	DNC
White	DNC
Gender	
Female	1.2
Male	1.3
Family income level	
Poor	DNC
Near poor	DNC
Middle/high income	DNC

DNA = Data have not been analyzed. DNC = Data are not collected. DSU = Data are statistically unreliable.

The polysaccharide meningococcal vaccine currently available in the United States is recommended for certain high-risk groups (people with asplenia), for laboratory personnel routinely exposed to *Neisseria meningitidis*, and for travelers to regions where meningococcal disease is hyperendemic or epidemic (the African "meningitis belt"). Routine vaccination of civilians is not recommended because of its relative ineffectiveness in children under age 2 years (among whom risk of endemic disease is highest) and its relatively short duration of protection. The vaccine is useful for controlling serogroup C meningococcal epidemics; these account, however, for less than 5 percent of the cases of meningococcal disease that occur each year in the United States. The vaccine provides no protection against serogroup B meningococci, which account for approximately one-third of the disease overall in the United States.

New meningococcal conjugate vaccines against serogroups C and Y, which account for two-thirds of current disease, now are undergoing clinical trials. Soon they should be available for incorporation into routine childhood immunization as well as for vaccination of high-risk groups, possibly including college students. Similar to Hib conjugate vaccines, new meningococcal conjugate vaccines are expected to be effective in children.

Development and licensing of new serogroup B meningococcal vaccines also will help reduce meningococcal disease.

14-8.   Reduce Lyme disease.

Target: 9.7 new cases per 100,000 population in endemic States.

Baseline: 17.4 new cases of Lyme disease per 100,000 population were reported in 1992–96.

Target setting method: 44 percent improvement. (Better than the best will be used when data are available.)

Data source: National Notifiable Disease Surveillance System (NNDSS), CDC, EPO.

NOTE: THE TABLE BELOW MAY CONTINUE TO THE FOLLOWING PAGE.

Total Population, 1992–96	New Cases of Lyme Disease
	Rate per 100,000
TOTAL	17.4
Race and ethnicity	
American Indian or Alaska Native	DSU
Asian or Pacific Islander	DSU
Asian	DNC
Native Hawaiian and other Pacific Islander	DSU
Black or African American	DSU
White	DSU

Total Population, 1992–96	New Cases of Lyme Disease
	Rate per 100,000
Hispanic or Latino	DSU
Not Hispanic or Latino	DSU
Black or African American	DSU
White	DSU
Gender	
Female	17.2*
Male	19.2*
Family income level	
Poor	DNC
Near poor	DNC
Middle/high income	DNC

DNA = Data have not been analyzed. DNC = Data are not collected. DSU = Data are statistically unreliable.
*Note: Data do not include Pennsylvania.

NOTE: THE TABLE ABOVE MAY HAVE CONTINUED FROM THE PREVIOUS PAGE.

In 1991, a standardized case definition for Lyme disease was adopted by the Council of State and Territorial Epidemiologists. Since then, the number of reported cases of Lyme disease has increased from 8,257 in 1993 to 16,455 in 1996 because of increased surveillance as well as a true increase in new cases. From 1992 through 1996, 92 percent of cases were reported from 10 endemic States. New initiatives to prevent Lyme disease include the implementation of community-based prevention programs, host-targeted acaricides to reduce the numbers of vector ticks, and appropriate use of Lyme disease vaccine.

Infectious Diseases and Emerging Antimicrobial Resistance

14-9. Reduce hepatitis C.

Target: 1 new case per 100,000 population.

Baseline: 2.4 new cases of hepatitis C per 100,000 population in selected counties were reported in 1996.

Target setting method: Better than the best.

Data source: Sentinel Counties Study of Viral Hepatitis, CDC, NCID.

Total Population, 1996	New Hepatitis C Cases
	Rate per 100,000
TOTAL	2.4
Race and ethnicity	
American Indian or Alaska Native	DNC
Asian or Pacific Islander	DSU
Asian	DNC
Native Hawaiian and other Pacific Islander	DNC
Black or African American	DSU
White	3.0
Hispanic or Latino	DSU
Not Hispanic or Latino	DSU
Black or African American	DSU
White	DSU
Gender	
Female	2.0
Male	2.8
Family income level	
Poor	DNC
Near poor	DNC
Middle/high income	DNC

DNA = Data have not been analyzed. DNC = Data are not collected. DSU = Data are statistically unreliable.
Note: Data represent rates based on estimates from selected counties.

Hepatitis C virus (HCV) is the most common chronic bloodborne viral infection in the United States.[44] This virus usually is transmitted through large or repeated percutaneous exposures to blood—for example, through sharing of equipment between injection drug users. HCV infects persons of all ages, but most new cases are among young adults aged 20 to 39 years. The highest proportion of new cases is among whites, but the highest rates of new cases are among nonwhite racial and ethnic groups.

14-10. (Developmental) Increase the proportion of persons with chronic hepatitis C infection identified by State and local health departments.

Potential data sources: State health department databases of persons with HCV infection; National Health and Nutrition Examination Survey (NHANES), CDC, NCHS.

An estimated 2.7 million persons in the United States are infected chronically with HCV. Although the annual number of newly acquired HCV infections has declined from an estimated 180,000 in the mid-1980s to an estimated 28,000 in 1995, this reservoir of chronically infected persons can transmit the virus to others, and all of them are at risk for the severe consequences of chronic liver disease. Because of the large number of people with chronic HCV infection, identification of these persons must be a major focus of a comprehensive prevention strategy. Identification of HCV-infected persons allows (1) counseling to prevent further HCV transmission, (2) vaccination against HAV and HBV to prevent additional liver damage, (3) evaluation for chronic liver disease, (4) possible antiviral therapy, and (5) counseling to avoid potential hepatotoxins, such as alcohol, that may increase the severity of HCV-related liver disease.

14-11. Reduce tuberculosis.

Target: 1.0 new case per 100,000 population.

Baseline: 6.8 new cases of tuberculosis per 100,000 population were reported in 1998.

Target setting method: Better than the best.

Data source: National TB Surveillance System, CDC, NCHSTP.

NOTE: THE TABLE BELOW MAY CONTINUE TO THE FOLLOWING PAGE.

Total Population, 1998	New Tuberculosis Cases
	Rate per 100,000
TOTAL	6.8
Race and ethnicity	
American Indian or Alaska Native	11.2
Asian or Pacific Islander	34.9
Asian	DNC
Native Hawaiian and other Pacific Islander	DNC
Black or African American	17.4
White	3.8
Hispanic or Latino	13.6
Not Hispanic or Latino	5.9
Black or African American	17.8
White	2.3
Gender	
Female	5.0
Male	8.6

Healthy People 2010: Objectives for Improving Health

Total Population, 1998	New Tuberculosis Cases
	Rate per 100,000
Family income level	
Poor	DNC
Near poor	DNC
Middle/high income	DNC

DNA = Data have not been analyzed. DNC = Data are not collected. DSU = Data are statistically unreliable.

NOTE: THE TABLE ABOVE MAY HAVE CONTINUED FROM THE PREVIOUS PAGE.

The 1989 *Strategic Plan for the Elimination of TB in the United States*[45] set a tuberculosis elimination goal of reducing TB to 1 new case per million by 2010, with an interim goal of 3.5 cases per 100,000 population by 2000. However, in the mid-1980s the trend toward TB elimination was reversed, and drug-resistant strains emerged that were even more deadly. TB cases increased by 20 percent between 1985 and 1992. Renewed efforts to combat the resurgence included improving laboratories, strengthening surveillance and expanding directly observed therapy, and expediting investigation of close contacts of TB patients. From 1993 through 1998, new cases of TB again declined, although the resurgence and related outbreaks set back TB elimination efforts by about a decade. Elimination of TB depends on significant effort and cooperation between public and private health care providers and agencies at the Federal, State, and local levels.

14-12. Increase the proportion of all tuberculosis patients who complete curative therapy within 12 months.

Target: 90 percent of patients.

Baseline: 74 percent of those tuberculosis patients reported in 1996 and started on therapy completed therapy within 12 months.

Target setting method: Better than the best.

Data source: National TB Surveillance System, CDC, NCHSTP.

NOTE: THE TABLE BELOW MAY CONTINUE TO THE FOLLOWING PAGE.

Tuberculosis Patients, 1996	Completed Curative Therapy Within 12 Months
	Percent
TOTAL	74
Race and ethnicity	
American Indian or Alaska Native	82
Asian or Pacific Islander	75
Asian	DNC

Tuberculosis Patients, 1996	Completed Curative Therapy Within 12 Months
	Percent
Native Hawaiian and other Pacific Islander	DNC
Black or African American	72
White	74
Hispanic or Latino	73
Not Hispanic or Latino	74
Black or African American	72
White	75
Gender	
Female	75
Male	73
Family income level	
Poor	DNC
Near poor	DNC
Middle/high income	DNC

DNA = Data have not been analyzed. DNC = Data are not collected. DSU = Data are statistically unreliable.

NOTE: THE TABLE ABOVE MAY HAVE CONTINUED FROM THE PREVIOUS PAGE.

The highest priority for TB control is to ensure that persons with the disease complete curative therapy. If treatment is not continued for a sufficient length of time, such persons often become ill and contagious again. Completion of therapy is essential to prevent transmission of the disease as well as to prevent outbreaks and the development and spread of drug-resistant TB.

Current therapy guidelines recommend that patients with drug-susceptible TB should complete a successful regimen within 12 months.[46] Multidrug-resistant TB presents difficult treatment problems, often requiring consultation with a TB specialist and longer treatment regimens. The measurement of completion of therapy is a long-accepted indicator of the effectiveness of community TB control efforts. Health departments traditionally have reported completion-of-therapy results to CDC and have used this information locally and statewide as an evaluation measure.

14-13. Increase the proportion of contacts and other high-risk persons with latent tuberculosis infection who complete a course of treatment.

Target: 85 percent.

Baseline: 62 percent of tuberculosis contacts and other high-risk persons who started on treatment for latent TB infection in 1997 completed treatment.

Target setting method: 27 percent improvement. (Better than the best will be used when data are available.)

Data source: Aggregate Reports for TB Reports Evaluation, CDC, NCHSTP.

Data for population groups currently are not collected.

Treatment for latent TB infection substantially reduces the risk that TB infection will progress to disease. Certain groups are at very high risk of developing TB disease once infected. Identifiable population groups at high risk for TB vary in time and geographic area, depending on unique and changing TB-related demographics.[47]

14-14. Reduce the average time for a laboratory to confirm and report tuberculosis cases.

Target: 2 days for 75 percent of cases.

Baseline: 21 days were needed for a laboratory to confirm and report 75 percent of TB cases in 1996.

Target setting method: 90 percent improvement.

Data source: Survey of State Public Health Laboratories, CDC, NCHSTP.

Commercially available nucleic acid amplification tests are capable of detecting *Mycobacterium tuberculosis* in a specimen within 48 hours of receipt. Concerns regarding sensitivity, cost, quality control, and special expertise requirements prevent widespread use of such tests. Upgrading TB laboratory capabilities and facilities, improving training in state-of-the-art mycobacteriology, and evaluating proficiency should better enable State public health laboratories to apply these new rapid tests to the diagnosis of TB.

14-15. (Developmental) Increase the proportion of international travelers who receive recommended preventive services when traveling in areas of risk for select infectious diseases: hepatitis A, malaria, and typhoid.

Potential data source: *Abstract of International Travel to and from the United States*, U.S. Department of Commerce.

The number of international travelers from the United States has increased an average of 3 percent a year for the past decade. The three diseases highlighted in this objective—hepatitis A, malaria, and typhoid—account for a large proportion of illness and disability for international travelers. Before embarking, some travelers go to a travel clinic, some visit primary care providers, and some receive no pretravel care.

An appropriate prescription of antimalarial prophylaxis medications constitutes recommended preventive services for this disease. Risk areas can be identified by referencing the malaria section in the most recent edition of *Health Information for International Travel*.

14-16. Reduce invasive early onset group B streptococcal disease.

Target: 0.5 new cases per 1,000 live births.

Baseline: 1.0 new case of invasive early onset group B streptococcal disease per 1,000 live births was reported in 1996.

Target setting method: Better than the best.

Data source: Active Bacterial Core Surveillance (ABCs), Emerging Infections Program Network, CDC, NCID.

NOTE: THE TABLE BELOW MAY CONTINUE TO THE FOLLOWING PAGE.

Live Births, 1996	New Cases of Group B Streptococcal Disease
	Rate per 1,000
TOTAL	1.0
Race and ethnicity	
American Indian or Alaska Native	DSU
Asian or Pacific Islander	DSU
Asian	DNC
Native Hawaiian and other Pacific Islander	DNC
Black or African American	1.5
White	1.0
Hispanic or Latino	DSU
Not Hispanic or Latino	DSU
Black or African American	DSU
White	DSU

Live Births, 1996	New Cases of Group B Streptococcal Disease
	Rate per 1,000
Gender	
Female	DNA
Male	DNA
Family income level	
Poor	DNC
Near poor	DNC
Middle/high income	DNC

DNA = Data have not been analyzed. DNC = Data are not collected. DSU = Data are statistically unreliable.

NOTE: THE TABLE ABOVE MAY HAVE CONTINUED FROM THE PREVIOUS PAGE.

The number of new cases of early onset group B streptococcal (GBS) disease in 1996 reflected a substantial decline from earlier years, before intervention became common practice. GBS causes bloodstream infections and meningitis in babies. Additional prevention is possible, because occurrence of the disease is more likely to reflect ineffective prevention efforts than antibiotic failures. In certain areas, rates approximating 0.5 per 1,000 births already have been achieved. Although these data may represent the background rate of nonpreventable cases, most geographic areas should be able to achieve the same low rates. The racial disparity in rates will be eliminated with more aggressive use of prevention protocols.

African Americans consistently have had higher rates of GBS diseases than other races. Implementation of GBS prevention policies is expected to eliminate the disparity. Thus, the target of 0.5 new cases per 1,000 births is one that can be obtained in all geographic areas and all racial and ethnic groups. By the year 2010, reductions in early onset disease might be the result of both improved use of intrapartum antibiotic prophylaxis and implementation of GBS conjugate vaccines currently in clinical trials.

14-17. Reduce hospitalizations caused by peptic ulcer disease in the United States.

Target: 46 hospitalizations per 100,000 population.

Baseline: 71 hospitalizations per 100,000 population occurred in 1998 (age adjusted to the year 2000 standard population).

Target setting method: Better than the best.

Data source: National Hospital Discharge Survey (NHDS), CDC, NCHS.

Total Population, 1998	Peptic Ulcer Hospitalizations
	Rate per 100,000
TOTAL	71
Race and ethnicity	
American Indian or Alaska Native	DSU
Asian or Pacific Islander	DSU
Asian	DNC
Native Hawaiian and other Pacific Islander	DNC
Black or African American	80
White	52
Hispanic or Latino	DSU
Not Hispanic or Latino	DSU
Black or African American	DSU
White	DSU
Gender	
Female	64
Male	79
Family income level	
Poor	DNC
Near poor	DNC
Middle/high income	DNC

DNA = Data have not been analyzed. DNC = Data are not collected. DSU = Data are statistically unreliable.
Note: Age adjusted to the year 2000 standard population.

Peptic ulcer disease affects up to 25 million persons in the United States and causes up to 6,500 deaths each year. Until recently, peptic ulcers were thought to be caused by stress, spicy foods, and excess stomach acid. Most patients were treated with antacids or acid-reducing medications, and recurrences were the rule after therapy was discontinued. The discovery in the 1980s that a bacterial organism, *Helicobacter pylori (H. pylori)*, causes up to 90 percent of peptic ulcers has changed the way ulcers are evaluated and managed.[48, 49] Now appropriate antibiotic regimens successfully eradicate the infection and prevent recurrence and complications such as bleeding or perforation.

Despite extensive scientific data linking peptic ulcer disease to *H. pylori*, studies indicate that many health care providers and consumers are unaware of the relationship, and many persons with ulcers do not receive appropriate therapy.[50, 51] A campaign to educate health care providers and consumers about *H. pylori* and its link to peptic ulcer disease was initiated in 1997. The Centers for Disease Control and Prevention (CDC) and Partnership *H. pylori* Educational Campaign includes partners from academic institutions, government agencies, and industry.[52] The increased awareness of the link between *H. pylori* and ulcers among health care providers and consumers is expected to lead to the increased use of appropriate antibiotics. This improved treatment, if available to those who need it, should decrease hospitalization rates—an indicator for severe illness and disability—due to peptic ulcer disease and its complications.

14-18. Reduce the number of courses of antibiotics for ear infections for young children.

Target: 88 antibiotic courses per 100 children under age 5 years.

Baseline: 108 antibiotic courses for otitis media per 100 children under age 5 years were prescribed during 1996–97 (2-year average).

Target setting method: 19 percent improvement.

Data sources: National Ambulatory Medical Care Survey (NAMCS), CDC, NCHS; National Hospital Ambulatory Medical Care Survey (NHAMCS), CDC, NCHS.

NOTE: THE TABLE BELOW MAY CONTINUE TO THE FOLLOWING PAGE.

Children Under Age 5 Years, 1996–97	Courses of Antibiotics for Ear Infections
	Rate per 100
TOTAL	108
Race and ethnicity	
American Indian or Alaska Native	DSU
Asian or Pacific Islander	DSU
Asian	DNC
Native Hawaiian and other Pacific Islander	DNC
Black or African American	84
White	116
Hispanic or Latino	DSU
Not Hispanic or Latino	DSU
Black or African American	DSU
White	DSU

Children Under Age 5 Years, 1996–97	Courses of Antibiotics for Ear Infections
	Rate per 100
Gender	
Female	107
Male	109
Family income level	
Poor	DNC
Near poor	DNC
Middle/high income	DNC

DNA = Data have not been analyzed. DNC = Data are not collected. DSU = Data are statistically unreliable.

NOTE: THE TABLE ABOVE MAY HAVE CONTINUED FROM THE PREVIOUS PAGE.

Antibiotic courses for otitis media, commonly called ear infection, can be reduced through two methods. A portion of otitis media cases—otitis media with effusion rather than acute otitis media—do not require antimicrobial treatment. A national campaign for judicious antibiotic use aims to reduce inappropriate antibiotic treatment for this portion of otitis media.[53] The leading cause of otitis media is pneumococcus. Preventing pneumococcal otitis media is expected to be possible following licensure of pneumococcal conjugate vaccines. (See Focus Area 28. Vision and Hearing.)

14-19. Reduce the number of courses of antibiotics prescribed for the sole diagnosis of the common cold.

Target: 1,268 antibiotic courses per 100,000 population.

Baseline: 2,535 antibiotic courses per 100,000 population were prescribed for the sole diagnosis of the common cold, 1996–97.

Target setting method: 50 percent improvement.

Data sources: National Ambulatory Medical Care Survey (NAMCS), CDC, NCHS; National Hospital Ambulatory Medical Care Survey (NHAMCS), CDC, NCHS.

NOTE: THE TABLE BELOW MAY CONTINUE TO THE FOLLOWING PAGE.

Total Population, 1996–97	Courses of Antibiotics for Common Cold
	Rate per 100,000
TOTAL	2,535
Race and ethnicity	
American Indian or Alaska Native	DSU

Total Population, 1996–97	Courses of Antibiotics for Common Cold
	Rate per 100,000
Asian or Pacific Islander	DSU
Asian	DNC
Native Hawaiian and other Pacific Islander	DNC
Black or African American	DSU
White	2,431
Hispanic or Latino	DSU
Not Hispanic or Latino	DSU
Black or African American	DSU
White	DSU
Gender	
Female	2,644
Male	2,421
Family income level	
Poor	DNC
Near poor	DNC
Middle/high income	DNC

DNA = Data have not been analyzed. DNC = Data are not collected. DSU = Data are statistically unreliable.
NOTE: THE TABLE ABOVE MAY HAVE CONTINUED FROM THE PREVIOUS PAGE.

The common cold does not require antimicrobial therapy. Inappropriate therapy for the common cold can be reduced by 50 percent by promoting judicious antimicrobial use, provided that caregivers and patients accept that antibiotics are ineffective in treating colds. Effective programs for the judicious use of antibiotics could help reduce the prescription of antibiotics for the common cold.

14-20. Reduce hospital-acquired infections in intensive care unit patients.

Target and baseline:

Objective	Reduction in Hospital-Acquired Infections in Intensive Care Units	1998 Baseline	2010 Target
		Infections per 1,000 Days' Use	
	Intensive care unit patients		
14-20a.	Catheter-associated urinary tract infection	5.9	5.3
14-20b.	Central line-associated blood-stream infection	5.3	4.8
14-20c.	Ventilator-associated pneumonia	11.1	10.0
	Infants weighing 1,000 grams or less at birth in intensive care		
14-20d.	Central line-associated blood-stream infection	12.2	11.0
14-20e.	Ventilator-associated pneumonia	4.9	4.4

Target setting method: 10 percent improvement. (Better than the best will be used when data are available.)

Data source: National Nosocomial Infections Surveillance System (NNIS), CDC, NCID.

> **Data for population groups currently are not collected.**

Hospital-acquired infections are a leading cause of illness and death in the United States. Each year, 36 million patients are admitted to U.S. hospitals.[54] Annually, more than 500,000 of the nearly 2 million patients stricken with a hospital-acquired infection are intensive care patients. Of the total, nearly 90,000 die. The annual cost of hospital-acquired infections is approximately $4.5 billion a year. In the past 20 years, the rate of hospital-acquired infections has increased 36 percent.

The rate of hospital-acquired infections has increased largely because hospital patients of the late 1990s on average were older and sicker than those of 20 years earlier and thus more susceptible to infection, and also because medical advances that can save or prolong lives may carry risks for infections. Because both trends are expected to continue, only a modest reduction in the number of new cases of infections can be expected; however, a small reduction will save thousands of lives.

14-21. Reduce antimicrobial use among intensive care unit patients.

Target: 120 daily doses per 1,000 patient days.

Baseline: 150 daily doses of antimicrobials per 1,000 patient days were used among intensive care unit patients in 1995.

Target setting method: 20 percent improvement.

Data source: National Nosocomial Infections Surveillance System (NNIS), CDC, NCID.

Hospital-acquired infections caused by antimicrobial-resistant pathogens can be virtually untreatable. Further, antimicrobial resistance that develops in the hospital can spread into the community and has the potential to cause a public health disaster. Excessive or inappropriate use of antimicrobials or both, which occur most frequently in intensive care units (ICUs), is the major cause of antimicrobial resistance. Research indicates that antibiotics are being used more often than hospital prescription guidelines recommend. For example, one study in the late 1990s indicated that as much as 60 percent of the hospital prescriptions for vancomycin are not in accordance with the guidelines. Decreasing the use of antimicrobials, especially in ICUs, is the critical step in reducing the public threat of antimicrobial resistance. Studies have shown that interventions in individual hospitals have achieved reductions of 20 percent or more in antimicrobial use.

Vaccination Coverage and Strategies

14-22. Achieve and maintain effective vaccination coverage levels for universally recommended vaccines among young children.

Target and baseline:

Objective	Increase in and Maintenance of Vaccination Coverage Levels Among Children Aged 19 to 35 Months	1998 Baseline	2010 Target
		Percent	
14-22a.	4 doses diphtheria-tetanus-acellular pertussis (DTaP) vaccine	84	90
14-22b.	3 doses *Haemophilus influenzae* type b (Hib) vaccine	93	90
14-22c.	3 doses hepatitis B (hep B) vaccine	87	90
14-22d.	1 dose measles-mumps-rubella (MMR) vaccine	92	90
14-22e.	3 doses polio vaccine	91	90
14-22f.	1 dose varicella vaccine	43	90

Target setting method: Consistent with the Childhood Immunization Initiative.

Data source: National Immunization Survey (NIS), CDC, NCHS and NIP.

NOTE: THE TABLE BELOW MAY CONTINUE TO THE FOLLOWING PAGE.

Children Aged 19 to 35 Months, 1998	Vaccination Coverage					
	14-22a. 4 Doses DTaP	14-22b. 3 Doses Hib	14-22c. 3 Doses Hep B	14-22d. 1 Dose MMR	14-22e. 3 Doses Polio	14-22f. 1 Dose Vari-cella
	Percent					
TOTAL	84	93	87	92	91	43
Race and ethnicity						
American Indian or Alaska Native	78	92	80	86	83	33
Asian or Pacific Islander	87	93	90	93	94	57
Asian	DNC	DNC	DNC	DNC	DNC	DNC
Native Hawaiian and other Pacific Islander	DNC	DNC	DNC	DNC	DNC	DNC
Black or African American	77	90	84	89	88	43
White	86	94	88	93	92	43
Hispanic or Latino	80	92	86	91	89	47
Not Hispanic or Latino	85	94	87	92	91	42
Black or African American	77	90	84	89	88	42
White	87	95	88	93	92	42
Gender						
Female	84	94	87	92	91	43
Male	84	93	87	92	90	43
Family income level						
Poor	81	92	86	91	90	46
Near poor	83	92	87	91	91	42
Middle/high income	89	96	89	94	92	49

Healthy People 2010: Objectives for Improving Health

Children Aged 19 to 35 Months, 1998	Vaccination Coverage					
	14-22a. 4 Doses DTaP	14-22b. 3 Doses Hib	14-22c. 3 Doses Hep B	14-22d. 1 Dose MMR	14-22e. 3 Doses Polio	14-22f. 1 Dose Vari-cella
	Percent					
Disability status						
Persons with disabilities	DNC	DNC	DNC	DNC	DNC	DNC
Persons without disabilities	DNC	DNC	DNC	DNC	DNC	DNC

DNA = Data have not been analyzed. DNC = Data are not collected. DSU = Data are statistically unreliable.

NOTE: THE TABLE ABOVE MAY HAVE CONTINUED FROM THE PREVIOUS PAGE.

Vaccination coverage levels of 90 percent are, in general, sufficient to prevent circulation of viruses and bacteria-causing vaccine-preventable diseases.[55, 56] Maintenance of high vaccination coverage levels in early childhood is the best way to prevent the spread of VPDs in childhood and to provide the foundation for controlling VPDs among adults. Diseases that affect humans only may eventually be eradicated or at least eliminated through high vaccination coverage levels.[57] These diseases include polio and measles in the near future and possibly hepatitis B later on. Although polio eradication is expected to be certified by the year 2005, vaccine coverage levels will continue to be assessed until vaccination is no longer recommended. The measles epidemic of 1989–91 demonstrated that achievement of high coverage levels at the time of school entry was insufficient to control VPD outbreaks. Although coverage levels currently are the highest ever recorded, the United States must continue to ensure that each new cohort of children is fully vaccinated with all recommended vaccine doses; as of June 22, 2000, 20 to 24 vaccine doses are recommended through age 16 years, with 16 to 20 doses by age 2 years. Any new universally recommended vaccine should be at a 90 percent coverage level within 5 years of the recommendation.

Although national coverage levels may exceed 90 percent, variation in the level of coverage among smaller areas may include subgroups of the population at substantially lower levels of protection. These subgroups or pockets of undervaccinated persons make the population vulnerable to major outbreaks of VPDs. Monitoring of coverage at smaller geographic levels within the United States helps ensure that these potential pockets of children are identified to target interventions and reduce the risk of future disease outbreaks. In addition, each State and major urban area should aim to achieve 90 percent coverage to ensure uniformly high vaccination coverage.

14-23. Maintain vaccination coverage levels for children in licensed day care facilities and children in kindergarten through the first grade.

Target and baseline:

Objective	Maintenance of Vaccination Coverage Levels for Children	1997–98 Baseline*	2010 Target
		Percent	
	Children in day care		
14-23a.	Diphtheria-tetanus-acellular per-tussis (DTaP) vaccine	96	95
14-23b.	Measles/mumps/rubella vaccines	89	95
14-23c.	Polio vaccine	96	95
14-23d.	Hepatitis B vaccine	Developmental	
14-23e.	Varicella vaccine	Developmental	
	Children in K through 1st grade		
14-23f.	Diphtheria-tetanus-acellular per-tussis (DTaP) vaccine	97	95
14-23g.	Measles/mumps/rubella vaccines	96	95
14-23h.	Polio vaccine	97	95
14-23i.	Hepatitis B vaccine	Developmental	
14-23j.	Varicella vaccine	Developmental	

*Weighted means.

Target setting method: Consistent with year 2000 target. (Better than the best will be used when data are available.)

Data source: Immunization Program Annual Reports, CDC, NIP.

> **Data for population groups currently are not collected.**

Uniformly high coverage levels are required to prevent circulation of the viruses and bacteria that cause VPDs. The target level was set to be consistent with the Healthy People 2000 objective because the achievement of that objective has resulted in the prevention of disease spread, and this objective seeks to maintain the high coverage achieved in these settings.

Entry requirements for school and day care are one of the most effective interventions the States have at their disposal to ensure that children are appropriately vaccinated. The impact of entry requirements for school and day care has been profound—more than 95 percent of children are vaccinated. Several studies support the role of entry requirements in increasing vaccination rates and decreasing the rate of new cases of measles. Strict enforcement of school vaccination requirements has been shown to play a determining role in lowering new cases of measles.[58]

14-24. Increase the proportion of young children and adolescents who receive all vaccines that have been recommended for universal administration for at least 5 years.

Target and baseline:

Objective	Increase in Coverage Levels of Universally Recommended Vaccines	1998 Baseline	2010 Target
		Percent	
14-24a.	Children aged 19 to 35 months who receive the recommended vaccines (4DTaP, 3 polio, 1 MMR, 3 Hib, 3 hep B)	73	80
14-24b.	Adolescents aged 13 to 15 years who receive the recommended vaccines	Developmental	

Target setting method: Better than the best.

Data source: National Immunization Survey (NIS), CDC, NCHS and NIP; National Health Interview Survey (NHIS), CDC, NCHS.

NOTE: THE TABLE BELOW MAY CONTINUE TO THE FOLLOWING PAGE.

Children Aged 19 to 35 Months, 1998	Vaccinations	
	14-24a. 4 DTaP, 3 Polio, 1 MMR, 3 Hib, 3 Hep B	4 DTaP, 3 Polio, 1 MMR*
	Percent	
TOTAL	73	81
Race and ethnicity		
American Indian or Alaska Native	65	75
Asian or Pacific Islander	73	82
Asian	DNC	DNC
Native Hawaiian and other Pacific Islander	DNC	DNC
Black or African American	66	74
White	74	82
Hispanic or Latino	69	77
Not Hispanic or Latino	74	81
Black or African American	67	74
White	76	83
Gender		
Female	72	81
Male	73	81

Children Aged 19 to 35 Months, 1998	Vaccinations	
	14-24a. 4 DTaP, 3 Polio, 1 MMR, 3 Hib, 3 Hep B	4 DTaP, 3 Polio, 1 MMR*
	Percent	
Family income level		
Poor	70	78
Near poor	72	80
Middle/high income	77	85
Disability status		
Persons with disabilities	DNC	DNC
Persons without disabilities	DNC	DNC

DNA = Data have not been analyzed. DNC = Data are not collected. DSU = Data are statistically unreliable.
*Data for 4 DTaP, 3 polio, and 1 MMR are displayed to further characterize the issue.
NOTE: THE TABLE ABOVE MAY HAVE CONTINUED FROM THE PREVIOUS PAGE.

Determining whether the population is protected against a VPD is best evaluated by examining the coverage level of individual vaccines (see objective 14-22). It is also important to ensure that the health care system fully vaccinates individual children, providing vaccines that have been universally recommended for at least 5 years and that are currently recommended. Changes in the immunization schedule will occur as new vaccines are added to the list of recommended vaccines and as vaccines for eradicated diseases are removed from the list.[59] For example, polio virus vaccine is not expected to be recommended by the year 2010. Although monitoring the proportion of children who have received the combination of four DTaP, three polio, and one MMR will continue for historical comparison, attention should be focused on the combination of all universally recommended vaccines.

14-25. Increase the proportion of providers who have measured the vaccination coverage levels among children in their practice population within the past 2 years.

Target and baseline:

Objective	Increase in Providers Measuring Vaccination Levels	1997 Baseline	2010 Target
		Percent	
14-25a.	Public health providers	66	90
14-25b.	Private providers	6	90

Healthy People 2010: Objectives for Improving Health

Target setting method: 36 percent improvement for public health providers; 1,400 percent improvement for private providers.

Data source: Immunization Program Annual Reports, CDC, NIP.

In 1997, 66 percent of public health department providers assessed their vaccination levels.[60] State immunization programs are collaborating with private providers to extend provider-based assessments to the private sector. With the increasing role of managed care and Health Plan Employer Data and Information Set (HEDIS) measures, private providers should have additional occasions to examine their coverage levels.

Most providers (public and private) overestimate the vaccination coverage level they are achieving with their clients.[61] Assessment of practice-based coverage levels and feedback of those data to the providers have been an effective strategy for increasing vaccination of children served by a given practice.[62, 63] Managed care organizations have begun reporting vaccination coverage levels using the HEDIS criteria as a way of evaluating quality of care.[64] Practice-based assessment also has been recommended by ACIP,[65] the National Vaccine Advisory Committee, the American Academy of Pediatrics, and the American Academy of Family Physicians,[66] as well as the Task Force for Community Preventive Services.[67] The Clinic Assessment Software Application provides a mechanism for assessing levels of vaccination coverage in a practice and could be used for tracking patients.

14-26. Increase the proportion of children who participate in fully operational population-based immunization registries.

Target: 95 percent of children under age 6 years.

Baseline: 32 percent of children under age 6 years participated in an immunization registry in 1999.

Target setting method: 197 percent improvement. (Better than the best will be used when data are available.)

Data source: Immunization Program Annual Reports, CDC, NIP.

Data for population groups currently are not collected.

A fully operational population-based registry includes capabilities to (1) protect confidential information, (2) enroll all children at the State or community level automatically at birth, (3) give providers access to complete vaccination history, (4) recommend needed vaccinations, (5) notify children who are due and overdue for vaccinations, (6) assess practice and geographic-level coverage, and (7) produce authorized immunization records. Registries may provide other important functions such as assisting in the evaluation of vaccine safety. Registries may serve other purposes as well, including VPD surveillance, vaccine efficacy monitoring, and vaccine inventory management.

Population-based immunization registries will be a cornerstone of the Nation's immunization system by 2010. Responsibility for registry development rests with State and local communities, with assistance from Federal agencies and private partners. Registries facilitate the timely vaccination of children by ensuring that the child's complete vaccination history is available to the health care provider. Registries are valuable given the mobile nature of today's population and that many persons do not see the same provider consistently. Registries also can be used to monitor the vaccination status of populations that are low income, uninsured, and at greater risk for incomplete vaccination.

Few population-based immunization registries existed at the State or community level before 1992, and limited data are available regarding their implementation. A 1999 CDC survey showed immunization registries are being developed in all States.[68] Additional efforts are under way to establish registry links between private providers and immunization partners such as managed care organizations and WIC programs. Issues such as privacy, confidentiality, and access of registry data are being addressed as registries are developed.

Participation in immunization registries will continue to increase. The development of childhood immunization registries has widespread support among parents and providers,[69] and the required technology is becoming less expensive and simpler. Registries are part of the current trend to computerize medical data in the United States. To be successful, registries must be integrated seamlessly into the current provider environment and create no additional burdens.

14-27. Increase routine vaccination coverage levels for adolescents.

Target and baseline:

Objective	Increase in Vaccination Coverage Levels for Adolescents Aged 13 to 15 Years	1997 Baseline*	2010 Target
		Percent	
14-27a.	3 or more doses of hepatitis B	48	90
14-27b.	2 or more doses of measles, mumps, rubella	89	90
14-27c.	1 or more doses of tetanus-diphtheria booster	93	90
14-27d.	1 or more doses of varicella (excluding children who have had varicella)	45	90

*Data primarily are based on parental recall; provider verification has not occurred.

Target setting method: Consistent with target levels established under Childhood Immunization Initiative.

Data source: National Health Interview Survey (NHIS), CDC, NCHS.

Adolescents Aged 13 Through 15 Years, 1997	14-27a. 3 or More Doses Hep B	14-27b. 2 or More Doses MMR	14-27c. 1 or More Doses Tetanus-Diphtheria Booster	14-27d. 1 or More Doses Varicella
	Percent			
TOTAL	48	89	93	45
Race and ethnicity				
American Indian or Alaska Native	DSU	DSU	DSU	DSU
Asian or Pacific Islander	46	90	92	DSU
Asian	DSU	87	90	DSU
Native Hawaiian and other Pacific Islander	DSU	DSU	DSU	DSU
Black or African American	59	88	93	49
White	46	89	93	44
Hispanic or Latino	55	88	91	58
Not Hispanic or Latino	47	89	93	42
Black or African American	59	88	93	49
White	44	89	93	40
Gender				
Female	49	91	94	41
Male	47	88	91	49
Family income level				
Poor	52	87	93	43
Near poor	48	90	91	52
Middle/high income	43	89	93	45
Geographic location				
Urban	50	90	94	46
Rural	43	87	90	43
Disability status				
Persons with disabilities	DNA	DNA	DNA	DNA
Persons without disabilities	DNA	DNA	DNA	DNA

DNA = Data have not been analyzed. DNC = Data are not collected. DSU = Data are statistically unreliable.

Illness and disability caused by vaccine-preventable diseases, such as hepatitis B, measles, and varicella, continue among adolescents.[26] While primary health care providers are vital to ensuring that infants and younger children are up to date on their vaccinations, they have an equally important role in ensuring comprehensive vaccination for adolescents.[70] Any new universally recommended vaccine for adolescents should be at a 90 percent coverage level within 5 years of the recommendation. An estimated 79 percent of adolescents and children visit a health care provider annually.[71] Providers such as nurses, nurse practitioners, pediatricians, family physicians, general practitioners, and emergency medicine specialists deliver most of the primary health care received by adolescents.[72] Strategies should specifically target these providers to increase vaccination among adolescents, especially hard-to-reach and at-risk adolescents in urban and rural areas.

School entry requirements ensure high vaccination levels. Much of the experience to date in implementing adolescent vaccination comes from school-based hepatitis B demonstration projects.[73] To encourage school participation in an adolescent vaccination program, a partnership between schools and local health departments is essential.

Managed care organizations also have an increasingly important role in the delivery of health care services, including vaccinations, to adolescents. Measures for assessing immunization recommendations for adolescents have been incorporated into HEDIS 3.0.[64] Such standards should greatly assist in implementing immunization recommendations for adolescents in the managed care setting.

14-28. Increase hepatitis B vaccine coverage among high-risk groups.

Target and baseline:

Objective	Increase in Hepatitis B Vaccine Coverage in High-Risk Groups	1995 Baseline	2010 Target
		Percent	
14-28a.	Long-term hemodialysis patients	35	90
14-28b.	Men who have sex with men	9	60
14-28c.	Occupationally exposed workers	71	98

Target setting method: 157 percent improvement for long-term hemodialysis patients; 567 percent improvement for men who have sex with men; 38 percent improvement for occupationally exposed workers.

Data sources: Young Men's Survey, CDC, NCHSTP; Annual Survey of Chronic Hemodialysis Centers, CDC, NCID, and HCFA; periodic vaccine coverage surveys, CDC, NCID.

Hepatitis B vaccination has been recommended for persons with risk factors for hepatitis B virus infection since the vaccine was first licensed in 1981. These risk groups include the following: hemodialysis patients, men who have sex with men, incarcerated persons, health care and public safety workers who have exposure to blood in the workplace, persons with a history of sexually transmitted diseases or multiple sex partners, injection drug users, and household and sex contacts of HBV-infected persons. While data currently are not collected for inmates in long-term correctional facilities, it is recommended that prison officials should consider undertaking screening and vaccination programs directed at inmates with histories of high-risk behaviors.

14-29. Increase the proportion of adults who are vaccinated annually against influenza and ever vaccinated against pneumococcal disease.

Target and baseline:

Objective	Increase in Adults Vaccinated	1998* Baseline (unless noted)	2010 Target
		Percent	
	Noninstitutionalized adults aged 65 years and older		
14-29a.	Influenza vaccine	64	90
14-29b.	Pneumococcal vaccine	46	90
	Noninstitutionalized high-risk adults aged 18 to 64 years		
14-29c.	Influenza vaccine	26	60
14-29d.	Pneumococcal vaccine	13	60
	Institutionalized adults (persons in long-term or nursing homes)[†]		
14-29e.	Influenza vaccine	59 (1997)	90
14-29f.	Pneumococcal vaccine	25 (1997)	90

*Age adjusted to the year 2000 standard population.

[†]National Nursing Home Survey estimates include a significant number of residents who have an unknown vaccination status. See *Tracking Healthy People 2010* for further discussion of the data issues.

Target setting method: Better than the best.

Data sources: National Health Interview Survey (NHIS), CDC, NCHS—noninstitutionalized populations; National Nursing Home Survey (NNHS), CDC, NCHS—institutionalized populations.

Select Age Groups, 1998 (unless noted)	Annual Influenza and One-Time Pneumococcal Vaccination					
	Noninstitutionalized Adults Aged 65 Years and Older		Noninstitutionalized High-Risk Adults Aged 18 to 64 Years		Institutionalized Adults Aged 18 Years and Older	
	14-29a. Influenza	14-29b. Pneumococcal Disease	14-29c. Influenza	14-29d. Pneumococcal Disease	14-29e. Influenza (1997)	14-29f. Pneumococcal Disease (1997)
	Percent					
TOTAL	64	46	26	13	59	25
Race and ethnicity						
American Indian/ Alaska Native	DSU	DSU	29	25	DSU	DSU
Asian or Pacific Islander	68	36	30	DSU	DSU	DSU
Asian	67	36	31	DSU	DNC	DNC
Native Hawaiian and other Pacific Islander	DSU	DSU	DSU	DSU	DNC	DNC
Black or African American	46	26	23	14	DNA	DNA
White	65	48	27	13	DNA	DNA
Hispanic or Latino	51	23	24	11	61	23
Not Hispanic or Latino	64	47	26	13	DNA	DNA
Black or African American	47	26	23	14	61	22
White	66	50	27	13	62	24
Gender						
Female	63	46	28	13	DNA	DNA
Male	64	47	24	13	DNA	DNA
Education level (age 25 years and older)						
Less than high school	58	40	24	14	DNC	DNC
High school graduate	66	48	26	14	DNC	DNC
At least some college	67	52	31	14	DNC	DNC

Healthy People 2010: Objectives for Improving Health

Select Age Groups, 1998 (unless noted)	Annual Influenza and One-Time Pneumococcal Vaccination					
	Noninstitutionalized Adults Aged 65 Years and Older		Noninstitutionalized High-Risk Adults Aged 18 to 64 Years		Institutionalized Adults Aged 18 Years and Older	
	14-29a. Influenza	14-29b. Pneumococcal Disease	14-29c. Influenza	14-29d. Pneumococcal Disease	14-29e. Influenza (1997)	14-29f. Pneumococcal Disease (1997)
	Percent					
Disability status (1997)						
Persons with disabilities	66	47	28	16	DNA	DNA
Persons without disabilities	62	40	23	9	DNA	DNA
Select populations (not age adjusted)						
Age groups (1997)						
18 to 49 years	NA	NA	20	8	59	24
50 to 64 years	NA	NA	40	19	62	23
65 to 74 years	61	40	NA	NA	62	28
75 to 84 years	66	46	NA	NA	61	26
85 years and older	67	42	NA	NA	66	30
Persons with high-risk conditions (not age adjusted) (1997)						
Persons with diabetes	68	44	27	15	DNA	DNA
Persons with heart disease	71	51	25	11	DNA	DNA
Persons with lung disease	73	65	25	13	DNA	DNA
Persons with lung disease (excluding asthma)	74	66	26	14	DNA	DNA
Persons with kidney disease	71	46	21	13	DNA	DNA

Select Age Groups, 1998 (unless noted)	Annual Influenza and One-Time Pneumococcal Vaccination					
	Noninstitutionalized Adults Aged 65 Years and Older		Noninstitutionalized High-Risk Adults Aged 18 to 64 Years		Institutionalized Adults Aged 18 Years and Older	
	14-29a. Influenza	14-29b. Pneumococcal Disease	14-29c. Influenza	14-29d. Pneumococcal Disease	14-29e. Influenza (1997)	14-29f. Pneumococcal Disease (1997)
	Percent					
Persons with liver disease	71	43	26	10	DNA	DNA
Persons with cancer	71	51	25	10	DNA	DNA

DNA = Data have not been analyzed. DNC = Data are not collected. DSU = Data are statistically unreliable. NA = Not applicable.

Note: Age adjusted to the year 2000 standard population.

NOTE: THE TABLE ABOVE MAY HAVE CONTINUED FROM THE PREVIOUS PAGE.

Federal initiatives have highlighted the need to focus vaccination resources on adults.[74] Vaccination is an effective strategy to reduce illness and deaths due to pneumococcal disease and influenza. Current levels of coverage among adults vary widely among age, risk, and racial and ethnic groups. Any new universally recommended vaccine for adults should be at a 60 percent coverage level within 5 years of recommendation. Influenza and pneumococcal vaccines are covered by Medicare; thus vaccinating greater numbers of adults aged 65 years and older is feasible. High-risk adults aged 18 to 64 years may not have insurance coverage for influenza and pneumococcal vaccines.

With the aging of the U.S. population, increasing numbers of adults will be at risk for these major causes of illness and death. Persons with high-risk conditions (that is, heart disease, diabetes, and chronic respiratory disease[75, 76]) remain at increased risk for these diseases, as do persons living in institutional settings.

Continuing education of providers and the community is needed to increase awareness of and demand for adult vaccination services. Interventions such as standing orders for vaccination, provider reminders and feedback, and patient notifications and reminders have been effective in increasing adult vaccination levels.[22, 77] Guidelines and tools for implementing these interventions are available through *Put Prevention Into Practice*, a national campaign to improve delivery of clinical preventive services.[78] Measurement and feedback about vaccination providers' performance in delivering vaccines enhance coverage rates. Providers should be given feedback on their performance in a timely manner. Measurement and feedback can result in improvements in vaccine coverage either by changing provider knowledge, attitudes, and behavior or by stimulating changes in the vaccine delivery system—for example, reminders and standing orders—or some combination.

In addition, opportunities for vaccination outside of primary care and other traditional health care settings could be increased to reach adults who do not routinely access primary care. For example, over 90 million emergency department visits are made in the United States annually. Emergency department vaccination is likely to increase vaccination rates among select populations difficult to vaccinate through office-based programs. In any nontraditional site, a method for tracking and communicating vaccinations is needed so that vaccination information may be shared with patients' primary care providers.[79]

Vaccine Safety

14-30. Reduce vaccine-associated adverse events.

14-30a. Eliminate vaccine-associated paralytic polio (VAPP).

Target: Zero cases.

Baseline: 5 VAPP cases occurred in 1997.

Target setting method: Total elimination.

Data source: National Notifiable Disease Surveillance System (NNDSS), CDC, EPO.

14-30b. Reduce febrile seizures following pertussis vaccines.

Target: 75 febrile seizures.

Baseline: 152 febrile seizures followed pertussis vaccines in 1998.

Target setting method: 50 percent improvement.

Data sources: Vaccine Adverse Event Reporting System (VAERS) and Vaccine Safety Datalink (VSD), CDC, NIP.

Because no natural reservoirs for wild poliomyelitis exist, vaccine-associated paralytic polio (VAPP) is caused by the oral polio vaccine (OPV). With global polio eradication targeted for 2000, use of OPV should decrease and then stop, resulting in zero cases of VAPP. From 1980 to 1998, no indigenous cases of paralytic poliomyelitis caused by wild polio virus transmission have occurred in the United States. However, 141 cases of VAPP have been reported in this same period, averaging 8 or 9 cases per year. Persons with VAPP experience the full range of illness and disability as well as loss of social function associated with being partially or fully paralyzed. Due to the progress in global poliomyelitis eradication and to the reduction of the burden of VAPP in the United States, ACIP recommended that beginning in 2000, only intravenous polio vaccine (IPV) will be used for routine immunization.[80] In general, IPV is as effective as OPV and should be sufficient at preventing polio in the United States.

Controlled clinical trials indicate that whole cell pertussis (wP) vaccines cause seizures at a frequency of 1 per 1,750 doses.[38, 81, 82] The majority of these seizures are febrile seizures without any residual deficit. Nevertheless, such seizures—frightening patients and parents alike—frequently result in emergency department or other medical visits as well as costly diagnostic evaluations to rule out possible neurologic disorders. Recently licensed acellular pertussis (aP) vaccines are less likely to cause fever or seizures; data show seizure frequency of up to 1 per 14,280 doses.[38] With the increasing use of aP vaccines, the number of pertussis vaccine-associated febrile seizures should be reduced by 50 percent.

14-31. Increase the number of persons under active surveillance for vaccine safety via large linked databases.

Target: 13 million persons.

Baseline: 6 million persons were under active surveillance for vaccine safety via large linked databases in 1999.

Target setting method: 117 percent improvement.

Data source: Vaccine Safety Datalink, CDC, NIP.

A high standard of safety is expected of vaccines since they are recommended for millions of healthy people, including infants. Vaccine safety monitoring to identify and minimize vaccine-related reactions is necessary to help ensure safety because no vaccine is completely safe. Knowledge of vaccine safety is essential to assess accurately the risks and benefits in formulating vaccine use recommendations. For example, the Institute of Medicine has reported that of 76 adverse events assessed, 66 percent had inadequate or no evidence available to accept or reject vaccine as a cause of the adverse reactions.[83, 84]

In collaboration with several health maintenance organizations, CDC has linked anonymous vaccination and medical records in a large database.[85] This system is used to study vaccine safety, especially for evaluating new concerns arising from the Vaccine Adverse Event Reporting System (VAERS) and other sources. These databases also are used for monitoring vaccine safety, conducting active surveillance of VPDs, carrying out vaccine safety and immunogenicity trials, evaluating vaccine economics, and assessing vaccine coverage.

Related Objectives From Other Focus Areas

1. Access to Quality Health Services
- 1-1. Persons with health insurance
- 1-2. Health insurance coverage for clinical preventive services
- 1-3. Counseling about health behaviors
- 1-4. Source of ongoing care
- 1-5. Usual primary care provider
- 1-6. Difficulties or delays in obtaining needed health care
- 1-7. Core competencies in health provider training
- 1-8. Racial and ethnic representation in health professions
- 1-9. Hospitalization for ambulatory-care-sensitive conditions
- 1-14. Special needs of children
- 1-15. Long-term care services

7. Educational and Community-Based Programs
- 7-2. School health education
- 7-4. School nurse-to-student ratio
- 7-5. Worksite health promotion programs
- 7-6. Participation in employer-sponsored health promotion activities
- 7-7. Patient and family education
- 7-8. Satisfaction with patient education
- 7-9. Health care organization sponsorship of community health promotion activities
- 7-10. Community health promotion programs
- 7-11. Culturally appropriate and linguistically competent community health promotion programs
- 7-12. Older adult participation in community health promotion activities

8. Environmental Health
- 8-5. Safe drinking water
- 8-6. Waterborne disease outbreaks
- 8-29. Global burden of disease
- 8-30. Water quality in the U.S.-Mexico border region

10. Food Safety
- 10-1. Foodborne infections
- 10-2. Outbreaks of foodborne infections
- 10-3. Antimicrobial resistance of *Salmonella* species
- 10-5. Consumer food safety practices
- 10-6. Safe food preparation practices in retail establishments

11. Health Communication
- 11-1. Households with Internet access
- 11-2. Health literacy
- 11-3. Research and evaluation of communication programs
- 11-4. Quality of Internet health information sources
- 11-5. Centers for excellence
- 11-6. Satisfaction with health care providers' communication skills

13. HIV

13-9. HIV/AIDS, STD, and TB education in State prisons

13-11. HIV testing in TB patients

13-12. Screening for STDs and immunization for hepatitis B

16. Maternal, Infant, and Child Health

16-22. Medical homes for children with special health care needs

23. Public Health Infrastructure

23-1. Public health employee access to the Internet

23-2. Public access to information and surveillance data

23-3. Use of geocoding in health data systems

23-4. Data for all population groups

23-5. Data for Leading Health Indicators, Health Status Indicators, and Priority Data Needs at State, Tribal, and local levels

23-6. National tracking of Healthy People 2010 objectives

23-7. Timely release of data on objectives

23-8. Competencies for public health workers

23-9. Training in essential public health services

23-10. Continuing education and training by public health agencies

23-11. Performance standards for essential public health services

23-12. Health improvement plans

23-14. Access to epidemiology services

23-15. Model statutes related to essential public health services

23-17. Population-based prevention research

25. Sexually Transmitted Diseases

25-13. Hepatitis B vaccine services in STD clinics

Terminology

(A list of abbreviations and acronyms used in this publication appears in Appendix H.)

Advisory Committee on Immunization Practices (ACIP): Federally chartered advisory committee with the goals of providing advice to the CDC Director on decreasing disease through the use of vaccines and other biological products and on improving the safety of their use.

Colonization: The establishment of a colony or growth of an organism in a patient, typically in a nonsterile anatomic site such as the skin, nasal mucosa, or colon.

Common cold: Defined based on International Classification of Disease (ICD)-9 diagnostic codes 460.0, 461.0, 465.0, 465.8, 465.9, and 472.0.

Complete curative therapy: Full course of recommended treatment.

Comprehensive primary care: All aspects of routine health care (preventive, diagnostic, and therapeutic) delivered by a trained health care provider.

Conjugate vaccine: A type of inactivated vaccine composed of fractions of bacteria linked to a protein. This linkage makes the vaccine more potent.

Distant infection: The spread of infection in a patient from one anatomic site to another site in the body, such as through the blood stream from the lungs to the liver or brain.

Emerging infectious diseases: Diseases of infectious origin whose occurrence in humans has increased within the past two decades or threatens to increase in the near future. Recognition of an emerging disease occurs because the disease is present in the population for the first time, the disease has been detected for the first time, or links between an infectious agent and a chronic disease or syndrome have only recently been identified.

Group B *Streptococcus* (GBS): A normal germ found in the intestines and on the genitals of about one out of five pregnant women. GBS is usually not harmful to the woman carrying the germ but it can cause dangerous infections in the blood, spinal fluid, and lungs of babies born to these women.

> **Early onset of group B streptococcal disease:** Illness onset at less than 7 days of age.

> **Invasive group B streptococcal disease:** Isolation of group B *Streptococcus* from a normally sterile site, such as blood or cerebrospinal fluid.

Group immunity: The immunity of a group or community. Immunity based on the resistance to infection among a high proportion of individual members of the group.

Hospital-acquired infection: Any infection that a patient acquires as a result of medical treatment while in the hospital.

Invasive pneumococcal infection: Isolating the bacteria *Streptococcus pneumoniae* from a normally sterile site, including blood, cerebrospinal fluid, or pleural fluid.

Latent TB infection: The state of being infected with the organism *Mycobacterium tuberculosis* but without signs or symptoms of active TB disease.

Multiple sex partners: More than one partner in the prior 6 months.

National Notifiable Disease Surveillance System (NNDSS): Tracking system that State health departments use to report cases of selected diseases to CDC. (See Reportable disease).

Patient day: A day or part of a day for which a patient was hospitalized.

Penicillin resistant: Having a minimum inhibitory concentration (MIC) equal to or greater than 2 µg/ml. Strains with "intermediate" susceptibility are not included in this category.

Reemerging infectious diseases: Reappearance of a known infection after a decline in occurrence. Reemergence of "old" infectious agents can be the result of lapses in public health measures, changes in human behavior that increase person-to-person transmission of infectious agents, changes in food handling or eating habits, or changes in the way humans interact with their environment.

Reportable disease: A disease for which there are legal requirements for reporting and notification to public health authorities. In the United States, requirements for reporting diseases are mandated by State laws or regulations, and the list of reportable diseases in each State differs.

Surveillance regions: The nine regions of the United States used for influenza surveillance purposes.

Vaccine Adverse Event Reporting System (VAERS). A passive surveillance system that monitors vaccine safety by collecting and analyzing reports of adverse events following immunization from vaccine manufacturers, private practitioners, State and local public health clinics, parents, and individuals who receive vaccines. CDC and the Food and Drug Administration work together to implement VAERS.

Vaccines: Biological substances used to stimulate the development of antibodies and thus confer active immunity against a specific disease or number of diseases.

Vector-borne disease: Viral and bacterial diseases transmitted to humans by arthropods, primarily mosquitoes, ticks, and fleas.

Zoonotic disease: Viral and bacterial diseases transmitted to humans by arthropods, primarily mosquitoes, ticks, and fleas.

References

[1] Hoyert, D.L.; Kochanek, K.D.; and Murphy, S.L. Deaths: Final data for 1997. *National Vital Statistics Reports* 19(47):1999.

[2] Meltzer, M.I.; Dennis, D.T.; and Orloski, K.A. The cost effectiveness of vaccinating against Lyme disease. *Emerging Infectious Diseases* 5(3):321-328, 1999. <http://www.cdc.gov/ncidod/eid/vol5no3/meltzer.htm>December 14, 1999.

[3] Centers for Disease Control and Prevention (CDC). Summary of notifiable diseases—United States, 1994. *Morbidity and Mortality Weekly Report* 43(53), 1995.

[4] National Communicable Disease Center (NCDC). *Rubella Surveillance No. 1.* Atlanta, GA: NCDC, 1969.

[5] Atkinson, W.; Wolfe, C.; Humiston, S.G.; et al.; eds. *Epidemiology and Prevention of Vaccine-Preventable Diseases.* Atlanta, GA: U.S. Department of Health and Human Services (HHS), CDC, 2000.

[6] Atkinson, W.L.; Orenstein, W.A.; and Krugman, S. The resurgence of measles in the United States, 1989–90. *Annual Review of Medicine* 43:451-463, 1992.

[7] Gindler, J.S.; Atkinson, W.L.; Markowitz, L.E.; et al. The epidemiology of measles in the United States in 1989–1990. *Pediatric Infectious Disease Journal* 11(10):841-846, 1992.

[8] National Vaccine Advisory Committee. The measles epidemic: The problems, barriers and recommendations. *Journal of the American Medical Association* 266(11):1547-1552, 1991.

[9] Ekwueme, D.U.; et. al. Economic evaluation of use of diphtheria, tetanus, and acellular pertussis vaccine (DTaP) or diphtheria, tetanus and whole-cell pertussis vaccine (DTwP) in the United States, 1997. *Archives of Pediatric and Adolescent Medicine.* (in press) August 2000.

[10] CDC. Achievements in public health, 1900–1999: Impact of vaccines universally recommended for children—United States, 1990–1998. *Morbidity and Mortality Weekly Report* 48(12):243-248, 1999.

[11] CDC. Notice to readers: National vaccination coverage levels among children aged 19–35 months—United States, 1998. *Morbidity and Mortality Weekly Report* 48(37):829-830, 1999.

[12] National Center for Health Statistics (NHCS). *Healthy People 2000 Review, 1998–99.* Hyattsville, MD: Public Health Service (PHS), 1999, 195-205.

[13] CDC. Vaccination coverage by race/ethnicity and poverty level among children aged 19–35 months—United States, 1996. *Morbidity and Mortality Weekly Report* 46(41):963-968, 1997.

[14] CDC. *State Immunization Requirements, 1998–1999.* Washington, DC: U.S. Government Printing Office, 1999, 1-27.

[15] CDC. Prevention of hepatitis A through active or passive immunization: Recommendations of the Advisory Committee on Immunization Practices (ACIP). *Morbidity and Mortality Weekly Report* 48(RR-12):1-37, 1999.

[16] CDC, NCHS. National Health Interview Survey, unpublished data.

[17] CDC. Progress toward elimination of *Haemophilus influenzae* type b disease among infants and children—United States, 1987–1995. *Morbidity and Mortality Weekly Report* 45(42):901-906, 1996.

[18] Schuchat, A.; Robinson, A.K.; and Wenger, J.D. Bacterial meningitis in the United States in 1995. *New England Journal of Medicine* 337:970-976,1997.

[19] CDC. *Preventing Emerging Infectious Diseases Threat: A Strategy for the 21st Century.* Atlanta, GA: HHS, PHS, 1998. <http://www.cdc.gov/ncidod/emergplan>October 12, 1999.

[20] HHS. *Adult Immunization Action Plan, Report of the Workgroup on Adult Immunization.* Washington, DC: HHS, 1997. <http://www.cdc.gov/od/nvpo/adult.htm>November 23, 1999.

[21] CDC. Reported vaccine-preventable disease—United States, 1993, and the Childhood Immunization Initiative. *Morbidity and Mortality Weekly Report* 43(4):57-60, 1994.

[22] Shefer, A.; Briss, P.; Rodewald, L.; et al. Improving immunization coverage rates: An evidence-based review of the literature. *Epidemiologic Reviews* 21(1), 1999.

[23] Hoekstra, E.J.; LeBaron, C.W.; Megaloeconomou, Y.; et al. Impact of a large-scale immunization initiative in the Special Supplemental Nutrition Program for Women, Infants, and Children (WIC). *Journal of the American Medical Association* 280(13):1143-1147, 1998.

[24] Abramson, J.S.; O'Shea, T.M.; Ratledge, D.L.; et al. Development of a vaccine tracking system to improve the rate of age-appropriate primary immunization in children of lower socioeconomic status. *Journal of Pediatrics* 126(4):583-586, 1995.

[25] CDC. Progress toward eliminating *Haemophilus influenzae* type b disease among infants and children—United States, 1987–1997. *Morbidity and Mortality Weekly Report* 47(46):993-998,1998.

[26] CDC. Summary of notifiable diseases—United States 1997. *Morbidity and Mortality Weekly Report* 46(54):1-87, 1998.

[27] CDC. Prevention of varicella: Recommendations of the Advisory Committee on Immunization Practices (ACIP). *Morbidity and Mortality Weekly Report* 45(RR-11):1-25, 1996.

[28] CDC. National, State and urban area vaccination coverage levels among children aged 19–35 months—United States, 1997. *Morbidity and Mortality Weekly Report* 47(26):547-554, 1998.

[29] Rota, J.S.; Heath, J.L.; Rota, R.A.; et al. Molecular epidemiology of measles virus: Identification of pathways of transmission and implications for measles elimination. *Journal of Infectious Diseases* 173(1):32-37, 1996.

[30] CDC. Measles—United States, 1996, and the interruption of indigenous transmission. *Morbidity and Mortality Weekly Report* 46(11):242-246, 1997.

[31] CDC. Epidemiology of measles—United States, 1998. *Morbidity and Mortality Weekly Report* 48(34):749-753, 1999.

[32] Wharton, M. Mumps. In: Wallace, R.B.; Duebbeling, B.N.; Last, J.M.; et al.; eds. *Public Health and Preventive Medicine.* 14th ed. Stamford, CT: Appleton & Lange, 1998, 93-95.

[33] CDC. Measles, mumps and rubella—vaccine use and strategies for elimination of measles, rubella—and congenital rubella syndrome and control of mumps: Recommendations of the Advisory Committee on Immunization Practices (ACIP). *Morbidity and Mortality Weekly Report* 47(RR-8):1-57, 1998.

[34] CDC. Rubella and congenital rubella syndrome—United States, 1994–1997. *Morbidity and Mortality Weekly Report* 46(16):350-354, 1997.

[35] Bisgard, K.M.; Hardy, I.R.B.; Popovic, T.; et al. Respiratory diphtheria in the United States, 1980–1995. *American Journal of Public Health* 88(5):787-791, 1998.

[36] CDC. Toxigenic *Corynebacterium diphtheriae*—Northern Plains Indian Community, August–October 1996. *Morbidity and Mortality Weekly Report* 46(22):506-510, 1997.

[37] Bardenheier, B.; Prevots, D.R.; Khetsuriani, N.; et al. Tetanus surveillance—United States, 1995–1997. *Morbidity and Mortality Weekly Report* 47(SS-2):1-13, 1998.

[38] CDC. Pertussis vaccination: Use of acellular pertussis vaccines among infants and young children. *Morbidity and Mortality Weekly Report* 46(RR-7):1-25, 1997.

[39] Guris, D.; Strebel, P.M.; Tachdjian, R.; et al. Effectiveness of the pertussis vaccination program as determined by use of the screening method—United States, 1992–1994. *Journal of Infectious Diseases* 176(2):456-463, 1997.

[40] Bisgard, K.M.; Kao, A.; Leake, J.; et al. The epidemiology of *Haemophilus influenzae* invasive disease in the United States, 1994–1995: Near disappearance of vaccine-preventable childhood disease. *Emerging Infectious Diseases* 4(2):229-237, 1998.

[41] CDC. Varicella-related deaths among adults—United States, 1997. *Morbidity and Mortality Weekly Report* 46(19):409-412, 1997.

[42] CDC. *Hepatitis Surveillance Report.* No. 56. Atlanta, GA: CDC, 1996.

[43] CDC. Hepatitis B virus: A comprehensive strategy for eliminating transmission in the United States through universal childhood vaccination: Recommendations of the Advisory Committee on Immunization Practices (ACIP). *Morbidity and Mortality Weekly Report* 40(RR-13):1-19, 1991.

[44] CDC. Recommendations for prevention and control of hepatitis C virus (HCV) infection and HCV-related chronic disease. *Morbidity and Mortality Weekly Report* 47(RR-19):1-39, 1998.

[45] CDC. A strategic plan for the elimination of tuberculosis in the United States. *Morbidity and Mortality Weekly Report* 38(S-3):1-25, 1989.

[46] American Thoracic Society and CDC. Treatment of tuberculosis and tuberculosis infection in adults and children. *American Journal of Respiratory Care Medicine* 149:1359-1374, 1994.

[47] CDC. Screening for tuberculosis and tuberculosis infection in high-risk populations. *Morbidity and Mortality Weekly Report* 44(RR-11):9-13, 1995.

[48] Marshall, B., and Warren, J.R. Unidentified curved bacilli on gastric epithelium in active chronic gastritis. *Lancet* 1:1273-1275, 1983.

[49] CDC. Knowledge about causes of peptic ulcer disease—United States. *Morbidity and Mortality Weekly Report* 45(42):985-987, 1997.

[50] American Digestive Health Foundation and Opinion Research Corporation. *Familiarity With H. pylori Among Adults With Digestive Disorders and Their Views Toward Diagnostic and Treatment Options.* Bethesda, MD: the Foundation and the Corporation, 1995.

[51] Breuer, T.; Malaty, H.M.; Goodman, K.; et al. Has the scientific evidence about *Helicobacter pylori* infection in gastrointestinal diseases reached the practicing physicians in the U.S.? *American Journal of Gastroenterology* 91:1905, 1996.

[52] CDC. National Center for Infectious Diseases, Division of Bacterial and Mycotic Diseases, Atlanta, GA, 1999.

[53] Powell, S.E.; Marcy, S.M.; Phillips, W.R.; et al. Otitis media—principles of judicious use of antimicrobial agents. *Pediatrics* 101:165-171, 1998.

[54] Institute of Medicine (IOM). *To Err Is Human: Building a Safer Health System.* Kohn, L.T.; Corrigan, J.M.; and Donaldson, M.S.; eds. Washington, DC: Committee on Quality of Health Care in America, IOM, 2000.

[55] Redd, S.C.; Markowitz, L.E.; and Katz, S.L. Measles Vaccine. In: Plotkin, S.A., and Orenstein, W.A., eds. *Vaccines.* 3rd ed. Philadelphia, PA: W.B. Saunders Company, 1999, 222-226.

[56] Orenstein, W.H.; Hinman, A.R.; and Rodewald, L.E. Public health considerations in the United States. In: Plotkin, S.A., and Orenstein, W.A., eds. *Vaccines.* 3rd ed. Philadelphia, PA: W.B. Saunders Company, 1999, 1006-1032.

[57] Dowdle, W.R., and Hopkins, D.R., eds. *The Eradication of Infectious Diseases: Dahlem Workshop Report.* Chichester, NY: John Wiley and Sons, 1997, 1-218.

[58] CDC. School immunization requirements for measles—United States, 1981. *Morbidity and Mortality Weekly Report* 30:158-160, 1981.

[59] CDC. Notice to readers: Recommended childhood immunization schedule—United States, 2000. *Morbidity and Mortality Weekly Report* 49(2):35-38, 47, 2000.

[60] CDC, National Immunization Program, Immunization Services Division. *Annual Immunization Assessment Progress—Percentage of Sites Assessed Nationwide in 1997* [chart]. Atlanta, GA: CDC, 1997. <http://www.cdc.gov/nip/afix/pres/prog/97perc.gif> November 23, 1999.

[61] Watt, J.; Kahane, S.; Smith, N.; et al. The difference between measured and estimated vaccination coverage among private physicians in California. Paper presented at Ambulatory Pediatric Association in New Orleans, LA, May 1998.

[62] LeBaron, C.W.; Chaney, M.; Baughman, A.L.; et al. Impact of measurement and feedback on vaccination coverage in public clinics, 1988–1994. *Journal of the American Medical Association* 277(8):631-635, 1997.

[63] Dini, E.F.; Chaney, M.; Moolenaar, R.L.; et al. Information as intervention: How Georgia used vaccination coverage data to double public sector vaccination coverage in seven years. *Journal of Public Health Management and Practice* 2(1):45-49, 1996.

[64] National Committee for Quality Assurance (NCQA). The Health Plan Employer Data and Information Set (HEDIS) 3.0/1998, Vol. 2, Technical Specifications. Washington, DC: NCQA, 1997, 38-48.

[65] CDC. Recommendations of the Advisory Committee on Immunization Practices. Programmatic strategies to increase vaccination rates—assessment and feedback of pro-

vider-based vaccination coverage information. *Morbidity and Mortality Weekly Report* 45(10):219-220, 1996.

[66] CDC. *Standards for Pediatric Immunization Practices.* Washington, DC: U.S. Government Printing Office, 1993.

[67] Briss, P.A.; et al. Reviews of evidence regarding interventions to improve vaccination coverage in children, adolescents, and adults. *American Journal of Preventive Medicine* 18(1s):97-140, 2000.

[68] CDC. Progress in the development of immunization registries—United States, 1999. *Morbidity and Mortality Weekly Report* 49(13):274-278, 2000.

[69] Sharp, K.; Edgar, T.; and Fowler, K. *Findings of Focus Group Research on Immunization Registries.* Rockville, MD: Westat, 1998. <http://www.cdc.gov/nip/registry /i_fgmenu.htm>October 1999.

[70] CDC. Immunization of adolescents: Recommendations of the Advisory Committee on Immunization Practices, the American Academy of Pediatrics, the American Academy of Family Physicians, and the American Medical Association. *Morbidity and Mortality Weekly Report* 45(RR-13):1-16, 1996.

[71] Benson, V., and Marano, M.A. Current estimates from the National Health Interview Survey, 1995. NCHS. *Vital and Health Statistics* 10(199), 1998.

[72] NCHS. *Health—United States, 1994.* Hyattsville, MD: PHS, 1995.

[73] Unti, L., and Woodruff, B.A. A review of adolescent school-based hepatitis B vaccination projects: A report prepared for the Centers for Disease Control and Prevention, Hepatitis Branch. Washington, DC: HHS, PHS, October 1996.

[74] Fedson, D.S. Adult immunization: Summary of the National Vaccine Advisory Committee report. *Journal of the American Medical Association* 272(14):1133-1137, 1994.

[75] CDC. Prevention and control of influenza: Recommendations of the Advisory Committee on Immunization Practices. *Morbidity and Mortality Weekly Report* 47(RR-6):1-26, 1998.

[76] CDC. Prevention of pneumococcal disease: Recommendations of the Advisory Committee on Immunization Practices. *Morbidity and Mortality Weekly Report* 46(RR-8):1-24, 1997.

[77] Gyorkos, T.W.; Tannenbaum, T.N.; Abrahamowicz, M.; et al. Evaluation of the effectiveness of immunization delivery methods. *Canadian Journal of Public Health* 85:S14-S30, 1994.

[78] HHS. Implementing preventive care. In: *The Clinician's Handbook of Preventive Services.* 2nd ed. Washington, DC: HHS, PHS, Office of Public Health and Science, Office of Disease Prevention and Health Promotion, 1998.

[79] CDC. Adult immunization programs in nontraditional settings: Quality standards and guidance for program evaluation. *Morbidity and Mortality Weekly Report* 49(RR-01):1-13, 2000.

[80] CDC. Notice to Readers: Recommendations of the Advisory Committee on Immunization Practices: Revised recommendations for routine poliomyelitis vaccination. *Morbidity and Mortality Weekly Report* 48(27):590, 1999.

[81] Cody, C.L.; Baraff, L.J.; Cherry, J.D.; et al. Nature and rates of adverse reactions associated with DTP and DT immunizations in infants and children. *Pediatrics* 68:650-660, 1981.

[82] CDC. Diphtheria, tetanus, and pertussis: Recommendations for vaccine use and other preventive measures. Recommendations of the Advisory Committee on Immunization Practices. *Morbidity and Mortality Weekly Report* 40(RR-10):1-28, 1991.

[83] Stratton, K.R.; Howe, C.J.; and Johnston, Jr., R.B. *Adverse Events Associated with Childhood Vaccines—Evidence Bearing on Causality.* Washington, DC: National Academy Press, 1994.

[84] Howson, C.P.; Howe, C.J.; and Fineberg, F.V. *Adverse Effects of Pertussis and Rubella Vaccines.* Washington, DC: National Academy Press, 1991.

[85] Chen, R.T.; Glasser, J.W.; Rhodes, P.H.; et al. The Vaccine Safety Datalink Project: A new tool for improving vaccine safety monitoring in the United States. *Pediatrics* 99:765-773, 1997.

Volume II

- **Objectives for Improving Health Part B: Focus Areas 15-28**

- **Appendices**

U.S. Department of Health and Human Services
November 2000

15

Injury and Violence Prevention

Lead Agency: Centers for Disease Control and Prevention

Contents

Goal

Reduce injuries, disabilities, and deaths due to unintentional injuries and violence.

Overview

The risk of injury is so great that most persons sustain a significant injury at some time during their lives.[1] Nevertheless, this widespread human damage too often is taken for granted, in the erroneous belief that injuries happen by chance and are the result of unpreventable "accidents." In fact, many injuries are not "accidents," or random, uncontrollable acts of fate; rather, most injuries are predictable and preventable.[2]

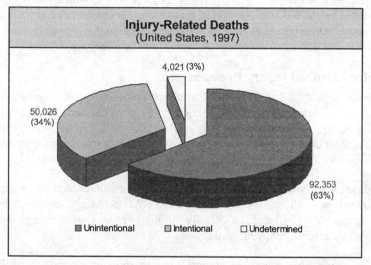

Injury-Related Deaths
(United States, 1997)

4,021 (3%)

50,026 (34%)

92,353 (63%)

■ Unintentional   ▨ Intentional   ☐ Undetermined

Source: CDC, NCHS. National Vital Statistics System (NVSS), 1997.

Issues and Trends

Injury Prevention

In 1997, 146,400 persons in the United States died from injuries due to a variety of causes such as motor vehicle crashes, firearms, poisonings, suffocations, falls, fires, and drownings. About 400 persons die from injuries each day, including 55 children and teenagers. One death out of every 17 in the United States results from injury.[3] Of these deaths, 63 percent are classified as unintentional and 34 percent as intentional. Unintentional injury deaths include approximately 42,000 resulting from motor vehicle crashes per year. In 1997, of approximately 50,000 intentional injury deaths, almost 31,000 were classified as suicide and nearly 20,000 as homicide.[1] In 1997, injuries accounted for 20 percent more years of potential life lost (YPLL) than cancer did (1,990 per 100,000 compared to 1,500 per 100,000).[4]

For ages 1 through 44 years, deaths from injuries far surpass those from cancer—the overall leading natural cause of death at these ages—by about three to one. Injuries cause more than two out of five deaths (43 percent) of children aged 1 through 4 years and result in four times the number of deaths due to birth defects, the second leading cause of death for this age group. For ages 15 to 24 years, injury deaths exceed deaths from all other causes combined from ages 5 through 44 years. For ages 15 to 24 years, injuries are the cause of nearly four out of five deaths. After age 44 years, injuries account for fewer deaths than other health problems, such as heart disease, cancer, and stroke. However, despite the decrease in the proportion of deaths due to injury, the death rate from injuries is actually higher among older persons than among younger persons.

Injuries often are classified on the basis of events and behaviors that preceded them as well as the intent of the persons involved. For example, many injuries are preceded by alcohol consumption in amounts or circumstances that increase risk of injury.[5] Although the events leading to an intentional injury and an unintentional injury differ, the outcomes and extent of the injury are similar.

Unintentional Injury Prevention

More persons aged 1 to 34 years die as a result of unintentional injuries than any other cause of death. Across all ages, 92,353 persons died in 1997 as a result of unintentional injuries. Motor vehicle crashes account for approximately half the deaths from unintentional injuries; other unintentional injuries rank second, and falls rank third, followed by poisonings, suffocations, and drownings.[6]

Additional millions of persons are incapacitated by unintentional injuries, with many suffering lifelong disabilities. These events occur disproportionately among young and elderly persons. In 1995, 29 million persons visited emergency departments as a result of unintentional injuries.[7]

Although the greatest impact of injury is in human suffering and loss of life, the financial cost is staggering. Included in the costs associated with injuries are the costs of direct medical care and rehabilitation as well as lost income and productivity. By the late 1990s, injury costs were estimated at more than $441 billion annually, an increase of 42 percent over the 1980s.[8] As with other health problems, it costs far less to prevent injuries than to treat them. For example:

- Every child safety seat saves $85 in direct medical costs and an additional $1,275 in other costs.
- Every bicycle helmet saves $395 in direct medical costs and other costs.

- Every smoke detector saves $35 in direct medical costs and an additional $865 in other costs.

- Every dollar spent on poison control centers saves $6.50 in medical costs.[9]

Several themes become evident when examining reports on injury prevention and control, including acute care, treatment, and rehabilitation. First, unintentional injury comprises a group of complex problems involving many different sectors of society. No single force working alone can accomplish everything needed to reduce the number of injuries. Improved outcomes require the combined efforts of many fields, including health, education, transportation, law, engineering, and safety sciences. Second, many of the factors that cause unintentional injuries are closely associated with violent and abusive behavior. Injury prevention and control addresses both unintentional and intentional injuries.

Violence and Abuse Prevention

Violence in the United States is pervasive and can change quality of life. Reports of children killing children in schools are shocking and cause parents to worry about the safety of their children at school. Reports of gang violence make persons fearful for their safety. Although suicide rates began decreasing in the mid-1990s, prior increases among youth aged 10 to 19 years and adults aged 65 years and older have raised concerns about the vulnerability of these population groups. Intimate partner violence and sexual assault threaten people in all walks of life.

Violence claims the lives of many of the Nation's young persons and threatens the health and well-being of many persons of all ages in the United States. On an average day in America, 53 persons die from homicide, and a minimum of 18,000 persons survive interpersonal assaults, 84 persons complete suicide, and as many as 3,000 persons attempt suicide.[10] (See Focus Area 18. Mental Health and Mental Disorders.)

Youth continue to be involved as both perpetrators and victims of violence. Elderly persons, females, and children continue to be targets of both physical and sexual assaults, which are frequently perpetrated by individuals they know. Examples of general issues that impede the public health response to progress in this area include the lack of comparable data sources, lack of standardized definitions and definitional issues, lack of resources to establish adequately consistent tracking systems, and lack of resources to fund promising prevention programs.

Because national data systems will not be available in the first half of the decade for tracking progress, one subject of interest, maltreatment of elderly persons, is not addressed in this focus area's objectives. The maltreatment of persons aged 60 years and older is a topic for research and data collection for the coming decade.

Disparities

While every person is at risk for injury, some groups appear to experience certain types of injuries more frequently. American Indians or Alaska Natives have disproportionately higher death rates from motor vehicle crashes, residential fires, and drownings. In addition, their death rates are about 1.75 times higher than the death rate for the overall U.S. population. Higher death rates from unintentional injury also occur among African Americans.[1]

Certain racial and ethnic groups experience more unintentional injuries and deaths than whites. Unintentional injuries are the second leading cause of death for American Indian males and the third leading cause of death for American Indian females. More than 1,000 American Indians die from injuries, and 10,000 more are hospitalized for injuries each year. The age-adjusted injury death rate for American Indians is three times higher than that of all other persons in the United States. Among American Indians, 46 percent of the YPLL is a result of injury, which is five times greater than the YPLL due to a next highest cause, heart disease (8 percent). Among the factors that contribute to these increased rates for American Indians are rural or isolated living, minimal emergency medical services, and great distances to sophisticated trauma care.[11]

African American, Hispanic, and American Indian children are at higher risk than white children for home fire deaths.[12] Adults aged 65 years and older are at increased risk of death from fire because they are more vulnerable to smoke inhalation and burns and are less likely to recover. Sense impairment (such as blindness or hearing loss) may prevent older adults from noticing a fire, and mobility impairment may prevent them from escaping its consequences. Older adults also are less likely to have learned fire safety behavior and prevention information, because they grew up at a time when little fire safety was taught in schools, and most current educational programs target children.

In every age group, drowning rates are almost two to four times greater for males than for females.[13] In 1997, the overall drowning rate for African Americans was 50 percent greater than that for whites; however, the rate was not higher for all age groups. For example, among children aged 1 through 4 years, the drowning rate for whites was slightly higher than the rate for African Americans. For children aged 5 to 19 years, African American children are twice as likely to drown as white children.[14]

Homicide victimization is especially high among African American and Hispanic youth. In 1995, African American males and females aged 15 to 24 years had homicide rates (74.4 per 100,000) that were more than twice the rate of their Hispanic counterparts (34.1 per 100,000) and nearly 14 times the rate of their white non-Hispanic counterparts (5.4 per 100,000).[15]

Trends in suicide among blacks aged 10 to 19 years in the United States during 1980–95 indicate that suicidal behavior among all youth has increased; however, rates for black youth have shown a greater increase.[16]

Healthy People 2010: Objectives for Improving Health

Although black youth historically have lower suicide rates than have whites, during 1980–95, the suicide rate for black youth aged 10 to 19 years increased from 2.1 to 4.5 per 100,000 population. As of 1995, suicide was the third leading cause of death among blacks aged 15 to 19 years.[17]

Opportunities

To reduce the number and severity of injuries, prevention activities must focus on the type of injury—drowning, fall, fire or burn, firearm, or motor vehicle.[18] For example, a nonfatal spinal cord injury produces the same outcome whether it was caused by an unintentional motor vehicle crash or an attempted suicide.

Understanding injuries allows for development and implementation of effective prevention interventions. Some interventions can reduce injuries from both unintentional and violence-related episodes. For instance, efforts to promote proper storage of firearms in homes can help reduce the risk of assaultive, intentional self-inflicted, and unintentional shootings in the home.[19] Higher taxes on alcoholic beverages are associated with lower death rates from motor vehicle crashes and lower rates for some categories of violent crime, including rape.[20, 21]

Many injuries and injury-related deaths occur in some population groups (such as younger children from birth to age 4 years) where the intentionality of the injury is unknown and requires more detailed investigation. As these cases are examined, interventions can be developed to address ways injuries occur—for instance, unintentional poisonings in children or hangings among teenagers—that are emerging in society as growing public health concerns.

Poverty, discrimination, lack of education, and lack of employment opportunities are important risk factors for violence and must be addressed as part of any comprehensive solution to the epidemic of violence. Strategies for reducing violence should begin early in life, before violent beliefs and behavioral patterns can be adopted.

Many potentially effective culturally and linguistically competent intervention strategies for violence prevention exist, such as parent training, mentoring, home visitation, and education.[22] Evaluation of ongoing programs is a major component to help identify effective approaches for violence prevention. The public health approach to violence prevention is multidisciplinary, encouraging experts from scientific disciplines, organizations, and communities to work together to find solutions to violence in the Nation.

Many school-aged children suffer disabling and fatal injuries each year. As educational programs for school children are developed and proven effective in preventing injuries, these programs should be included in quality health education curricula at the appropriate grade level. Education should aim at reducing risks of injury directly and at preparing children to be knowledgeable adults. (See Focus Area 7. Educational and Community-Based Programs.)

A total of 45 objectives addressed injury prevention in Healthy People 2000. Twenty-six objectives were specific for unintentional injuries, and 19 objectives were specific for violence prevention. By the end of the decade, targets had been met for 11 objectives. Unintentional injury objectives showing achievement were unintentional injury hospitalizations, residential fire deaths, nonfatal head injuries, spinal cord injuries, nonfatal poisonings, and pedestrian deaths. Violence prevention objectives that met their targets were homicide, suicide, weapon carrying by adolescents, conflict resolution in schools, and child death review systems.

Progress was made for 13 objectives. Much of the progress made in unintentional injury objectives was with motor vehicle fatalities and use of vehicle occupant restraints. Those unintentional injury objectives showing progress were unintentional injury deaths, motor vehicle deaths, motor vehicle crash deaths, motor vehicle occupant protection systems, helmet use by motorcyclists and bicyclists, safety belt use laws, alcohol-related motor vehicle deaths, and drownings. Violence prevention objectives showing progress were firearm-related deaths, partner abuse, rape and attempted rape, physical fighting among adolescents aged 14 to 17 years, and the number of States with firearm storage laws.

There were six objectives with no progress or movement away from the Healthy People 2000 targets. In unintentional injury, the hospitalization rate for hip fractures remains above baseline levels, indicating no progress toward the year 2000 target. Data from five violence prevention objectives also show movement away from the year 2000 target. Those objectives relate to child abuse and neglect, assault injuries, suicide attempts among adolescents aged 14 to 17 years, battered women turned away from shelters, and suicide prevention protocols in jails.

Note: Unless otherwise noted, data are from the Centers for Disease Control and Prevention, National Center for Health Statistics, *Healthy People 2000 Review, 1998–99.*

Injury and Violence Prevention

Goal: Reduce injuries, disabilities, and deaths due to unintentional injuries and violence.

Number	Objective Short Title

Injury Prevention

15-1	Nonfatal head injuries
15-2	Nonfatal spinal cord injuries
15-3	Firearm-related deaths
15-4	Proper firearm storage in homes
15-5	Nonfatal firearm-related injuries
15-6	Child fatality review
15-7	Nonfatal poisonings
15-8	Deaths from poisoning
15-9	Deaths from suffocation
15-10	Emergency department surveillance systems
15-11	Hospital discharge surveillance systems
15-12	Emergency department visits

Unintentional Injury Prevention

15-13	Deaths from unintentional injuries
15-14	Nonfatal unintentional injuries
15-15	Deaths from motor vehicle crashes
15-16	Pedestrian deaths
15-17	Nonfatal motor vehicle injuries
15-18	Nonfatal pedestrian injuries
15-19	Safety belts
15-20	Child restraints
15-21	Motorcycle helmet use
15-22	Graduated driver licensing
15-23	Bicycle helmet use
15-24	Bicycle helmet laws
15-25	Residential fire deaths
15-26	Functioning smoke alarms in residences
15-27	Deaths from falls

Injury Prevention

15-1. Reduce hospitalization for nonfatal head injuries.

Target: 45 hospitalizations per 100,000 population.

Baseline: 60.6 hospitalizations for nonfatal head injuries per 100,000 population occurred in 1998 (age adjusted to the year 2000 standard population).

Target setting method: Better than the best.

Data source: National Hospital Discharge Survey (NHDS), CDC, NCHS.

NOTE: THE TABLE BELOW MAY CONTINUE TO THE FOLLOWING PAGE.

Total Population, 1998	Hospitalizations for Nonfatal Head Injuries
	Rate per 100,000
TOTAL	60.6
Race and ethnicity	
American Indian or Alaska Native	DSU
Asian or Pacific Islander	DSU
Asian	DNC
Native Hawaiian and other Pacific Islander	DNC
Black or African American	58.4
White	46.0
Hispanic or Latino	DSU
Not Hispanic or Latino	DSU
Black or African American	DSU
White	DSU
Gender	
Female	42.8
Male	77.9
Education level	
Less than high school	DNC
High school graduate	DNC
At least some college	DNC

Total Population, 1998	Hospitalizations for Nonfatal Head Injuries
	Rate per 100,000
Select populations	
Males aged 15 to 24 years (not age adjusted)	117.6
Persons aged 75 years and older (not age adjusted)	174.9

DNA = Data have not been analyzed. DNC = Data are not collected. DSU = Data are statistically unreliable.
Note: Age adjusted to the year 2000 standard population.

NOTE: THE TABLE ABOVE MAY HAVE CONTINUED FROM THE PREVIOUS PAGE.

15-2. Reduce hospitalization for nonfatal spinal cord injuries.

Target: 2.4 hospitalizations per 100,000 population.

Baseline: 4.5 hospitalizations for nonfatal spinal cord injuries per 100,000 population occurred in 1998 (age adjusted to the year 2000 standard population).

Target setting method: 46 percent improvement. (Better than the best will be used when data are available.)

Data source: National Hospital Discharge Survey (NHDS), CDC, NCHS.

NOTE: THE TABLE BELOW MAY CONTINUE TO THE FOLLOWING PAGE.

Total Population, 1998	Hospitalizations for Nonfatal Spinal Cord Injuries
	Rate per 100,000
TOTAL	4.5
Race and ethnicity	
American Indian or Alaska Native	DSU
Asian or Pacific Islander	DSU
Asian	DNC
Native Hawaiian and other Pacific Islander	DNC
Black or African American	DSU
White	3.4
Hispanic or Latino	DSU
Not Hispanic or Latino	DSU
Black or African American	DSU
White	DSU

Total Population, 1998	Hospitalizations for Nonfatal Spinal Cord Injuries
	Rate per 100,000
Gender	
Female	DSU
Male	7.6
Education level	
Less than high school	DNC
High school graduate	DNC
At least some college	DNC

DNA = Data have not been analyzed. DNC = Data are not collected. DSU = Data are statistically unreliable.
Note: Age adjusted to the year 2000 standard population.

NOTE: THE TABLE ABOVE MAY HAVE CONTINUED FROM THE PREVIOUS PAGE.

The physical and emotional toll associated with head and spinal cord injuries can be significant for the survivors and their families. Persons with existing disabilities from head and spinal cord injuries are at high risk for further secondary disabilities. Prevention efforts should target motor vehicle crashes, falls, firearm injury, diving, and water safety.

Among pedalcyclists killed, most died from head injuries. Similarly, the common cause of death among motorcyclists is catastrophic head injury. Death rates from head injuries have been shown to be twice as high among cyclists in States lacking helmet laws or having laws that apply only to young riders, compared with States where laws apply to all riders.

Falls account for 87 percent of all fractures among adults aged 65 years and older and are the second leading cause of both spinal cord injury and brain injury for this age group.[23, 24] Falls also cause the majority of deaths and severe injuries from head trauma among children under age 14 years. Falls account for 90 percent of the most severe playground-related injuries treated in hospital emergency departments (mostly head injuries and fractures) and one-third of reported fatalities. Head injuries are involved in about 75 percent of all reported fall-related deaths associated with playground equipment.

Many diving-related incidents also result in spinal cord injury. Diving-related injury first becomes an issue during adolescence. Injuries to males outnumber injuries to females. Diving injuries account for one of eight spinal cord injuries, with half of those injuries resulting in quadriplegia.[25]

15-3. Reduce firearm-related deaths.

Target: 4.1 deaths per 100,000 population.

Baseline: 11.3 deaths per 100,000 population were related to firearm injuries in 1998 (age adjusted to the year 2000 standard population).

Target setting method: Better than the best.

Data source: National Vital Statistics System (NVSS), CDC, NCHS.

Total Population, 1998	Firearm-Related Deaths
	Rate per 100,000
TOTAL	11.3
Race and ethnicity	
American Indian or Alaska Native	11.3
Asian or Pacific Islander	4.2
Asian	DNC
Native Hawaiian and other Pacific Islander	DNC
Black or African American	20.3
White	10.0
Hispanic or Latino	9.7
Cuban	11.0
Mexican	9.8
Puerto Rican	8.4
Not Hispanic or Latino	11.3
Black or African American	21.0
White	9.6
Gender	
Female	3.3
Male	20.1
Education level (aged 25 to 64 years)	
Less than high school	21.4
High school graduate	17.7
At least some college	7.0
Select firearm-related deaths	
Homicides	4.3
Suicides	6.5
Unintentional deaths	0.5

DNA = Data have not been analyzed. DNC = Data are not collected. DSU = Data are statistically unreliable.
Note: Age adjusted to the year 2000 standard population.

15-4. Reduce the proportion of persons living in homes with firearms that are loaded and unlocked.

Target: 16 percent.

Baseline: 19 percent of the population lived in homes with loaded and unlocked firearms in 1998 (age adjusted to the year 2000 standard population).

Target setting method: Better than the best.

Data source: National Health Interview Survey (NHIS), CDC, NCHS.

Total Population, 1998	Loaded, Unlocked Firearms in Home
	Percent
TOTAL	19
Race and ethnicity	
American Indian or Alaska Native	25
Asian or Pacific Islander	DSU
Asian	DSU
Native Hawaiian and other Pacific Islander	DSU
Black or African American	28
White	18
Hispanic or Latino	17
Not Hispanic or Latino	19
Black or African American	28
White	18
Gender	
Female	16
Male	21
Education level (aged 25 years and older)	
Less than high school	22
High school graduate	17
At least some college	21

DNA = Data have not been analyzed. DNC = Data are not collected. DSU = Data are statistically unreliable.
Note: Age adjusted to the year 2000 standard population.

15-5. Reduce nonfatal firearm-related injuries.

Target: 8.6 injuries per 100,000 population.

Baseline: 24.0 nonfatal firearm-related injuries per 100,000 population occurred in 1997.

Target setting method: Better than the best.

Data source: National Electronic Injury Surveillance System (NEISS), Consumer Product Safety Commission (CPSC).

Total Population, 1997	Nonfatal Firearm-Related Injuries
	Rate per 100,000
TOTAL	24.0
Race and ethnicity	
American Indian or Alaska Native	DSU
Asian or Pacific Islander	DSU
Asian	DSU
Native Hawaiian and other Pacific Islander	DSU
Black or African American	DNA
White	DNA
Hispanic or Latino	39.0
Not Hispanic or Latino	DNA
Black or African American	92.0
White	8.7
Gender	
Female	5.3
Male	43.5
Education level	
Less than high school	DNC
High school graduate	DNC
At least some college	DNC
Select populations	
Males aged 15 to 24 years	143.8

DNA = Data have not been analyzed. DNC = Data are not collected. DSU = Data are statistically unreliable.

The United States has the highest rates of lethal childhood violence than every other industrialized country.[26] The increase in the total homicide rate from 1979 through 1993 resulted solely from increases in firearm-related homicides.[27] Fatalities, however, are only part of the problem. For each of the 32,436 persons killed by a gunshot wound in the United States in 1997, approximately 2 more were treated for nonfatal wounds in hospital emergency departments.[28]

Healthy People 2010: Objectives for Improving Health

15-6. (Developmental) Extend State-level child fatality review of deaths due to external causes for children aged 14 years and under.

Potential data source: Inter-Agency Council on Child Abuse and Neglect (ICAN) National Database, FBI Uniform Crime Report, U.S. Department of Justice.

Death resulting from injury is one of the most profound public health issues facing children in the United States today. In 1997, nearly 19,000 children aged 19 years and under were victims of injury—33 percent from violence and 67 percent from unintentional injury.[29]

In examination of these trends in childhood injury-related cause of death, information has typically come from one of several sources (vital statistics, protective service records, and the FBI Uniform Crime Report), each with specific limitations. In response to the increasing trend of violence against children and the lack of a comprehensive data source on violent childhood deaths, the Child Fatality Review Team (CFRT) process was developed in 1978 in California.

The goal of the CFRTs is the prevention of childhood fatalities. Their responsibility is to review so-called "suspicious" or "preventable" childhood fatalities. Minimal or core standards for CFRTs must include representatives from criminal justice, health, and social services. After integrating information from multiple sources, review teams strive to determine if the cause and manner of death were recorded accurately and to suggest prevention initiatives for all relevant agencies. Simply reviewing fatalities is not helpful unless recommendations for prevention also are included and plans are made for periodic followup to ensure that recommendations are being acted on.

Focusing on children aged 14 years and under will include most "unexplained" childhood deaths and is considered a more reasonable goal to achieve. However, States should continue to improve their CFRT systems. Teams with adequate resources are encouraged to extend their review to all causes of death for all children aged 18 years and under as their ultimate goal. CFRTs also should include culturally appropriate members.

15-7. Reduce nonfatal poisonings.

Target: 292 nonfatal poisonings per 100,000 population.

Baseline: 348.4 nonfatal poisonings per 100,000 population occurred in 1997 (age adjusted to the year 2000 standard population).

Target setting method: Better than the best.

Data source: National Hospital Ambulatory Medical Care Survey (NHAMCS), CDC, NCHS.

Total Population, 1997 (unless noted)	Nonfatal Poisonings
	Rate per 100,000
TOTAL	348.4
Race and ethnicity	
American Indian or Alaska Native	DSU
Asian or Pacific Islander	DSU
Asian	DSU
Native Hawaiian and other Pacific Islander	DSU
Black or African American	464.5
White	340.6
Hispanic or Latino	DSU
Not Hispanic or Latino	DSU
Black or African American	DSU
White	DSU
Gender	
Female	410.9
Male	281.6
Education level	
Less than high school	DNC
High school graduate	DNC
At least some college	DNC
Select types of poisonings (not age adjusted)	
Assault or attempted homicides	6.0 (1996)
Intentional suicide attempts	63.0 (1996)
Unintentional poisonings	268.0 (1996)
Select populations (not age adjusted)	
Children aged 4 years and under	460.0

DNA = Data have not been analyzed. DNC = Data are not collected. DSU = Data are statistically unreliable.
Note: Age adjusted to the year 2000 standard population.

15-8. Reduce deaths caused by poisonings.

Target: 1.5 deaths per 100,000 population.

Baseline: 6.8 deaths per 100,000 population were caused by poisonings in 1998 (age adjusted to the year 2000 standard population).

Target setting method: Better than the best.

Data source: National Vital Statistics System (NVSS), CDC, NCHS.

Total Population, 1998	Poisoning Deaths
	Rate per 100,000
TOTAL	6.8
Race and ethnicity	
American Indian or Alaska Native	8.1
Asian or Pacific Islander	1.6
Asian	DNC
Native Hawaiian and other Pacific Islander	DNC
Black or African American	7.9
White	6.9
Hispanic or Latino	5.9
Cuban	4.3
Mexican	5.1
Puerto Rican	12.0
Not Hispanic or Latino	6.8
Black or African American	8.2
White	6.9
Gender	
Female	4.1
Male	9.6
Education level (aged 25 to 64 years)	
Less than high school	18.5
High school graduate	15.2
At least some college	6.2
Select poisoning deaths	
Unintentional deaths	4.0
Suicides	1.9
Homicides	0*

DNA = Data have not been analyzed. DNC = Data are not collected. DSU = Data are statistically unreliable.
Note: Age adjusted to the year 2000 standard population.
*Value is greater than zero but less than 0.05.

Children are at significantly greater risk from poisoning death and exposure than adults because children are more likely to ingest potentially harmful chemicals. In 1995, 80 children aged 14 years and under died from poisoning. Children aged 4 years and under accounted for nearly half of these deaths. In 1996, more than 1.1 million unintentional poisonings among children aged 5 years and under were reported to U.S. poison control centers. Approximately 90 percent of all poison exposures occur at a residence.[30]

In 1996, 29 children aged 5 years and under died from exposure to medicines and household products. Among children aged 5 years and under, 60 percent of poisoning exposures come from nonpharmaceutical products such as cosmetics, cleaning substances, plants, foreign bodies, toys, pesticides, and art supplies; 40 percent come from pharmaceuticals. Immediately calling a poison control center can reduce the likelihood of severe poisoning, decrease the cost of a poisoning incident, and prevent the need for a hospital emergency department (ED) visit.

The total annual cost of poisoning-related injury and death exceeds $7.6 billion among children aged 14 years and under. Children aged 4 years and under account for $5.1 billion, or two-thirds, of these costs. Medical expenses associated with a poisoning exposure average $925 per case. The average cost of hospital treatment for a poisoning exposure is $8,700.[31]

15-9. Reduce deaths caused by suffocation.

Target: 3.0 deaths per 100,000 population.

Baseline: 4.1 deaths per 100,000 population were caused by suffocation in 1998 (age adjusted to the year 2000 standard population).

Target setting method: Better than the best.

Data source: National Vital Statistics System (NVSS), CDC, NCHS.

NOTE: THE TABLE BELOW MAY CONTINUE TO THE FOLLOWING PAGE.

Total Population, 1998	Suffocation Deaths
	Rate per 100,000
TOTAL	4.1
Race and ethnicity	
American Indian or Alaska Native	7.6
Asian or Pacific Islander	3.5
Asian	DNC
Native Hawaiian and other Pacific Islander	DNC
Black or African American	4.2
White	4.1
Hispanic or Latino	3.1
Not Hispanic or Latino	4.2
Black or African American	4.4
White	4.1
Gender	
Female	2.4
Male	6.0

Total Population, 1998	Suffocation Deaths
	Rate per 100,000
Education level (aged 25 to 64 years)	
Less than high school	6.5
High school graduate	5.1
At least some college	2.2
Select suffocation deaths	
Homicides	0.2
Suicides	2.1
Unintentional deaths	1.7

DNA = Data have not been analyzed. DNC = Data are not collected. DSU = Data are statistically unreliable.
Note: Age adjusted to the year 2000 standard population.

NOTE: THE TABLE ABOVE MAY HAVE CONTINUED FROM THE PREVIOUS PAGE.

In 1997, 10,650 persons died from suffocation. In the same year, 934 children aged 14 years and under died from suffocation. Of these children, 64 percent were aged 4 years and under.[32] Approximately 5,000 children aged 14 years and under are treated in hospital EDs for aspirating and ingesting toys and toy parts each year. The majority of childhood suffocations, strangulations, and chokings occur in the home. The total annual cost of airway obstruction injury among children aged 14 years and under exceeds $1.5 billion. Children aged 4 years and under account for more than 60 percent of these costs. It is estimated that as many as 900 infants whose deaths are attributed to sudden infant death syndrome (SIDS) each year are found in potentially suffocating environments, frequently on their stomachs, with their noses and mouths covered by soft bedding.[33]

15-10. Increase the number of States and the District of Columbia with statewide emergency department surveillance systems that collect data on external causes of injury.

Target: All States and the District of Columbia.

Baseline: 12 States had statewide ED surveillance systems that collected data on external causes of injury in 1998.

Target setting method: Total coverage.

Data source: External Cause of Injury Survey, American Public Health Association (APHA).

15-11. Increase the number of States and the District of Columbia that collect data on external causes of injury through hospital discharge data systems.

Target: All States and the District of Columbia.

Baseline: 23 States collected data on external causes of injury through hospital discharge data systems in 1998.

Target setting method: Total coverage.

Data source: External Cause of Injury Survey, American Public Health Association (APHA).

15-12. Reduce hospital emergency department visits caused by injuries.

Target: 126 hospital emergency department visits per 1,000 population.

Baseline: 131 hospital emergency department visits per 1,000 population were caused by injury in 1997 (age adjusted to the year 2000 standard population).

Target setting method: Better than the best.

Data source: National Hospital Ambulatory Medical Care Survey (NHAMCS), CDC, NCHS.

NOTE: THE TABLE BELOW MAY CONTINUE TO THE FOLLOWING PAGE.

Total Population, 1997	Injury-Related Hospital Emergency Department Visits
	Rate per 1,000
TOTAL	131
Race and ethnicity	
American Indian or Alaska Native	DSU
Asian or Pacific Islander	DSU
Asian	DSU
Native Hawaiian and other Pacific Islander	DSU
Black or African American	182
White	127
Hispanic or Latino	DSU
Not Hispanic or Latino	DSU
Black or African American	DSU
White	DSU

Total Population, 1997	Injury-Related Hospital Emergency Department Visits
	Rate per 1,000
Gender	
Female	116
Male	146
Education level	
Less than high school	DNC
High school graduate	DNC
At least some college	DNC

DNA = Data have not been analyzed. DNC = Data are not collected. DSU = Data are statistically unreliable.
Note: Age adjusted to the year 2000 standard population.

NOTE: THE TABLE ABOVE MAY HAVE CONTINUED FROM THE PREVIOUS PAGE.

Emergency department (ED) patient records and hospital discharge systems are an important source of public health surveillance and an integral part of the vision of electronically linked health information systems that can serve multiple purposes. Because of the volume and case mix of patients they treat, EDs are well positioned to provide data on cause and severity of injuries. Access to such data can help with the development of population-based public health interventions.

Unintentional Injury Prevention

15-13. Reduce deaths caused by unintentional injuries.

Target: 17.5 deaths per 100,000 population.

Baseline: 35.0 deaths per 100,000 population were caused by unintentional injuries in 1998 (age adjusted to the year 2000 standard population).

Target setting method: Better than the best.

Data source: National Vital Statistics System (NVSS), CDC, NCHS.

NOTE: THE TABLE BELOW MAY CONTINUE TO THE FOLLOWING PAGE.

Total Population, 1998	Unintentional Injury Deaths
	Rate per 100,000
TOTAL	35.0
Race and ethnicity	
American Indian or Alaska Native	59.9
Asian or Pacific Islander	17.6

Total Population, 1998	Unintentional Injury Deaths
	Rate per 100,000
Asian	DNC
Native Hawaiian and other Pacific Islander	DNC
Black or African American	39.5
White	34.8
Hispanic or Latino	30.2
Cuban	22.5
Mexican	32.1
Puerto Rican	28.8
Not Hispanic or Latino	35.1
Black or African American	40.7
White	34.6
Gender	
Female	22.1
Male	49.4
Education level (aged 25 to 64 years)	
Less than high school	54.5
High school graduate	41.5
At least some college	17.4
Select populations	
American Indian or Alaska Native males	83.6
Black or African American males	60.8
Hispanic males	46.2
White males	48.7

DNA = Data have not been analyzed. DNC = Data are not collected. DSU = Data are statistically unreliable.
Note: Age adjusted to the year 2000 standard population.

NOTE: THE TABLE ABOVE MAY HAVE CONTINUED FROM THE PREVIOUS PAGE.

15-14. (Developmental) Reduce nonfatal unintentional injuries.

Potential data source: National Hospital Ambulatory Medical Care Survey, Emergency Department Component, CDC, NCHS.

15-15. Reduce deaths caused by motor vehicle crashes.

Target and baseline:

Objective	Reduction in Deaths Caused by Motor Vehicle Crashes	1998 Baseline	2010 Target
15-15a.	Deaths per 100,000 population	15.6*	9.2
15-15b.	Deaths per 100 million vehicle miles traveled	1.6	0.8

*Age adjusted to the year 2000 standard population.

Target setting method: Better than the best for 15-15a; 50 percent improvement for 15-15b. (Better than the best will be used when data are available.)

Data sources: National Vital Statistics System (NVSS), CDC, NCHS; Fatality Analysis Reporting System (FARS), DOT, NHTSA.

NOTE: THE TABLE BELOW MAY CONTINUE TO THE FOLLOWING PAGE.

Total Population, 1998 (unless noted)	Motor Vehicle Crash Deaths	
	15-15a. Rate per 100,000	15-15b. Rate per 100 Million VMT
TOTAL	15.6	1.6
Race and ethnicity		
American Indian or Alaska Native	30.4	DNC
Asian or Pacific Islander	9.3	DNC
Asian	DNC	DNC
Native Hawaiian and other Pacific Islander	DNC	DNC
Black or African American	16.8	DNC
White	15.6	DNC
Hispanic or Latino	14.7	DNC
Cuban	10.9	DNC
Mexican	16.5	DNC
Puerto Rican	10.8	DNC
Not Hispanic or Latino	15.6	DNC
Black or African American	17.3	DNC
White	15.5	DNC
Gender		
Female	10.1	DNA
Male	21.6	DNA

Total Population, 1998 (unless noted)	Motor Vehicle Crash Deaths	
	15-15a. Rate per 100,000	15-15b. Rate per 100 Million VMT
Education level (aged 25 to 64 years)		
Less than high school	25.8	DNC
High school graduate	20.2	DNC
At least some college	8.9	DNC
Select populations		
Children aged 14 years and under (not age adjusted)	4.4	DNA
Persons aged 15 to 24 years (not age adjusted)	26.4	DNA
Persons aged 70 years and older (not age adjusted)	25.5	DNA
Motorcyclists	NA	21.0 (1997)

DNA = Data have not been analyzed. DNC = Data are not collected. DSU = Data are statistically unreliable. NA = not applicable.

Note: Data for 15-15a. are age adjusted to the year 2000 standard population.

NOTE: THE TABLE ABOVE MAY HAVE CONTINUED FROM THE PREVIOUS PAGE.

15-16. Reduce pedestrian deaths on public roads.

Target: 1.0 pedestrian death per 100,000 population.

Baseline: 1.9 pedestrian deaths per 100,000 population occurred on public roads in 1998.

Target setting method: 50 percent improvement. (Better than the best will be used when data are available.)

Data source: Fatality Analysis Reporting System (FARS), DOT, NHTSA.

NOTE: THE TABLE BELOW MAY CONTINUE TO THE FOLLOWING PAGE.

Total Population, 1998	Pedestrian Deaths on Public Roads
	Rate per 100,000
TOTAL	1.9
Race and ethnicity	
American Indian or Alaska Native	DNC
Asian or Pacific Islander	DNC
Asian	DNA
Native Hawaiian and other Pacific Islander	DNC

Healthy People 2010: Objectives for Improving Health

Total Population, 1998	Pedestrian Deaths on Public Roads
	Rate per 100,000
Black or African American	DNA
White	DNA
Hispanic or Latino	DNC
Not Hispanic or Latino	DNC
Black or African American	DNC
White	DNC
Gender	
Female	1.2
Male	2.7
Education level	
Less than high school	DNC
High school graduate	DNC
At least some college	DNC
Select populations	
Persons aged 70 years and older	3.9

DNA = Data have not been analyzed. DNC = Data are not collected. DSU = Data are statistically unreliable.

NOTE: THE TABLE ABOVE MAY HAVE CONTINUED FROM THE PREVIOUS PAGE.

15-17. Reduce nonfatal injuries caused by motor vehicle crashes.

Target: 933 nonfatal injuries per 100,000 population.

Baseline: 1,181 nonfatal injuries per 100,000 population were caused by motor vehicle crashes in 1998.

Target setting method: 21 percent improvement. (Better than the best will be used when data are available.)

Data source: General Estimates System (GES), DOT, NHTSA.

NOTE: THE TABLE BELOW MAY CONTINUE TO THE FOLLOWING PAGE.

Total Population, 1998 (unless noted)	Nonfatal Motor Vehicle Crash Injuries
	Rate per 100,000
TOTAL	1,181
Race and ethnicity	
American Indian or Alaska Native	DNC
Asian or Pacific Islander	DNC
Asian	DNC

Total Population, 1998 (unless noted)	Nonfatal Motor Vehicle Crash Injuries
	Rate per 100,000
Native Hawaiian and other Pacific Islander	DNC
Black or African American	DNC
White	DNC
Hispanic or Latino	DNC
Not Hispanic or Latino	DNC
Black or African American	DNC
White	DNC
Gender	
Female	DNA
Male	DNA
Education level	
Less than high school	DNC
High school graduate	DNC
At least some college	DNC
Select populations	
Persons aged 16 to 20 years	3,116 (1997)
Persons aged 21 to 24 years	2,496 (1997)

DNA = Data have not been analyzed. DNC = Data are not collected. DSU = Data are statistically unreliable.

NOTE: THE TABLE ABOVE MAY HAVE CONTINUED FROM THE PREVIOUS PAGE.

15-18. Reduce nonfatal pedestrian injuries on public roads.

Target: 19 nonfatal injuries per 100,000 population.

Baseline: 26 nonfatal pedestrian injuries per 100,000 population occurred on public roads in 1998.

Target setting method: 28 percent improvement. (Better than the best will be used when data are available.)

Data source: General Estimates System (GES), DOT, NHTSA.

NOTE: THE TABLE BELOW MAY CONTINUE TO THE FOLLOWING PAGE.

Total Population, 1998	Nonfatal Pedestrian Injuries on Public Roads
	Rate per 100,000
TOTAL	26
Race and ethnicity	
American Indian or Alaska Native	DNC

Total Population, 1998	Nonfatal Pedestrian Injuries on Public Roads
	Rate per 100,000
Asian or Pacific Islander	DNC
Asian	DNC
Native Hawaiian and other Pacific Islander	DNC
Black or African American	DNC
White	DNC
Hispanic or Latino	DNC
Not Hispanic or Latino	DNC
Black or African American	DNC
White	DNC
Gender	
Female	DNA
Male	DNA
Education level	
Less than high school	DNC
High school graduate	DNC
At least some college	DNC
Select populations	
Persons aged 5 to 9 years	42
Persons aged 10 to 15 years	44
Persons aged 16 to 20 years	38

DNA = Data have not been analyzed. DNC = Data are not collected. DSU = Data are statistically unreliable.
NOTE: THE TABLE ABOVE MAY HAVE CONTINUED FROM THE PREVIOUS PAGE.

15-19. Increase use of safety belts.

Target: 92 percent.

Baseline: 69 percent of the total population used safety belts in 1998.

Target setting method: 33 percent improvement. (Better than the best will be used when data are available.)

Data sources: National Occupant Protection Use Survey (NOPUS), DOT, NHTSA; Youth Risk Behavior Surveillance System (YRBSS), CDC, NCCDPHP.

Total Population, 1998 (unless noted)	Safety Belt Use
	Percent
TOTAL	69
Race and ethnicity	
American Indian or Alaska Native	DNC
Asian or Pacific Islander	DNC
Asian	DNC
Native Hawaiian and other Pacific Islander	DNC
Black or African American	DNA
White	DNA
Hispanic or Latino	DNC
Not Hispanic or Latino	DNC
Black or African American	DNC
White	DNC
Gender	
Female	DNA
Male	DNA
Education level	
Less than high school	DNC
High school graduate	DNC
At least some college	DNC
Select populations	
9th through 12th grade students	84 (1999)

DNA = Data have not been analyzed. DNC = Data are not collected. DSU = Data are statistically unreliable.

15-20. Increase use of child restraints.

Target: 100 percent.

Baseline: 92 percent of motor vehicle occupants aged 4 years and under used child restraints in 1998.

Target setting method: Total coverage.

Data source: National Occupant Protection Use Survey (NOPUS), Controlled Intersection Study, DOT, NHTSA.

> **Data for population groups currently are not collected.**

15-21. Increase the proportion of motorcyclists using helmets.

Target: 79 percent.

Baseline: 67 percent of motorcycle operators and passengers used helmets in 1998.

Target setting method: 18 percent improvement. (Better than the best will be used when data are available.)

Data sources: National Occupant Protection Use Survey (NOPUS), DOT, NHTSA; Youth Risk Behavior Surveillance System (YRBSS), CDC, NCCDPHP.

Motorcycle Operators and Passengers, 1998 (unless noted)	Helmet Use
	Percent
TOTAL	67
Race and ethnicity	
American Indian or Alaska Native	DNC
Asian or Pacific Islander	DNC
Asian	DNC
Native Hawaiian and other Pacific Islander	DNC
Black or African American	DNC
White	DNC
Hispanic or Latino	DNC
Not Hispanic or Latino	DNC
Black or African American	DNC
White	DNC
Gender	
Female	DNC
Male	DNC
Education level	
Less than high school	DNC
High school graduate	DNC
At least some college	DNC
Select populations	
9th through 12th grade students	62 (1999)

DNA = Data have not been analyzed. DNC = Data are not collected. DSU = Data are statistically unreliable.

15-22. Increase the number of States and the District of Columbia that have adopted a graduated driver licensing model law.

Target: All States and the District of Columbia.

Baseline: 23 States had a graduated driver licensing model law in 1999.

Target setting method: Total coverage.

Data source: U.S. Licensing Systems for Young Drivers, Insurance Institute for Highway Safety.

Motor vehicle crashes remain a major public health problem. They are the leading cause of death for persons in the United States aged 5 to 29 years. In 1998, 41,471 persons died in motor vehicle crashes.[34] Thirty-eight percent of these deaths occurred in alcohol-related crashes.[34] The motor vehicle death rate per 100,000 persons is especially high among persons aged 16 to 24 years and persons aged 75 years and older. Safety belts, when worn correctly, are the most effective way for occupants to reduce the risk of death and serious injury in a motor vehicle crash on public roads (including those on Indian Reservations). As of December 1998, the national safety belt use rate was 69 percent.

In 1998, 69,000 pedestrians were injured, and 5,220 were killed in traffic crashes in the United States. On average, a pedestrian is killed in a motor vehicle crash every 101 minutes, and one is injured every 8 minutes.[35]

In 1998, persons aged 70 years and older made up 9 percent of the population but accounted for 14 percent of all traffic fatalities and 18 percent of all pedestrian fatalities. Compared with the fatality rate for drivers aged 25 through 69 years, the rate for drivers in the oldest group is nine times higher.[36]

Older persons also are more susceptible than younger persons to medical complications following motor vehicle crash injuries. Thus, they are more likely to die from their injuries.[36]

Fewer persons aged 70 years and older are licensed to drive, compared to younger persons, and they drive fewer miles per licensed driver. Persons in this older age group, however, have higher rates of fatal crashes per mile driven, per 100,000 persons, and per licensed driver than any other group except young drivers (aged 16 to 24 years).

Pedestrians account for about 13 percent of motor vehicle deaths. The problem of pedestrian deaths and injuries is worse among young children and older adults. Children are more likely to be injured, while older adults are more likely to die in pedestrian crashes.[35]

As of December 1997, 49 States had safety belt laws. Eleven States had primary enforcement laws, and the remaining 38 States had secondary enforcement laws.[37] In 1998, the average observed belt use rate by States with secondary enforcement laws was 62 percent, compared to 79 percent in States with primary enforcement laws.[37]

Among children aged 1 to 14 years, crash injuries are the leading cause of death. In 1998, 2,549 children aged 14 years and under died in motor vehicle crashes.[34] The use of age-appropriate restraint systems can reduce this problem. Because all States have child restraint laws, more children now ride restrained. However, loopholes in the laws exempt many children from coverage under either safety belt or child restraint use laws. Another problem is the persistence of incorrect use of child restraints and safety belts.[38]

Motorcycles are less stable and less visible than cars, and they have high-performance capabilities. When motorcycles crash, their riders lack the protection of an enclosed vehicle, so they are more likely to be injured or killed. The number of deaths on motorcycles per mile traveled is about 16 times the number of deaths in cars. Wearing a motorcycle helmet reduces the chances of dying in a motorcy-cle crash by 29 percent and reduces the chances of brain injury by 67 percent. An unhelmeted rider is 40 percent more likely to suffer a fatal head injury, compared with a helmeted rider. In 1998, 2,284 motorcyclists died in crashes.[39]

Teenagers accounted for 10 percent of the U.S. population in 1997 and 15 percent of the motor vehicle deaths. In 1998, 3,427 drivers aged 15 to 20 years were killed, and an additional 348,000 were injured in motor vehicle crashes.[40] Gradu-ated licensing laws allow a young driver to gain driving experience at incremental levels. Graduated licensing is a system for phasing in on-road driving that allows beginners to obtain their initial experience under lower risk conditions.

The National Committee on Uniform Traffic Laws and Ordinances (NCUTLO) has developed a model law that calls for a minimum of 6 months in the learner stage and a minimum of 6 months in the intermediate license stage with night driving restrictions. Twenty-three States have all the core provisions of the model graduated licensing model law developed by NCUTLO. The NCUTLO model also requires applicants for intermediate and full licenses to have no safety belt or zero tolerance violations and to be conviction-free during the mandatory holding periods.

15-23. (Developmental) Increase use of helmets by bicyclists.

Potential data sources: Consumer Product Safety Commission; Behavioral Risk Factor Surveillance System (BRFSS), CDC; World Health Organization Study of Health Behavior in School Children.

15-24. Increase the number of States and the District of Columbia with laws requiring bicycle helmets for bicycle riders.

Target: All States and the District of Columbia.

Baseline: 10 States had laws requiring bicycle helmets for bicycle riders under age 15 years in 1999.

Target setting method: Total coverage.

Data source: National Safe Kids Campaign.

Head injuries are the most serious type of injury sustained by pedalcyclists of all ages. In 1998, 761 bicyclists were killed in crashes involving motor vehicles, and an additional 53,000 were injured in traffic crashes. Almost one-third (30 percent) of the pedalcyclists killed in traffic crashes in 1998 were between age 5 and 15 years. The proportion of pedalcyclist fatalities among persons aged 25 to 64 years was 1.7 times higher in 1997 than in 1987 (46 percent and 27 percent, respectively).[41] More bicyclists were killed on major roads than on local roads (59 percent compared with 36 percent) in 1997.[42]

Bicycle helmets reduce the risk of bicycle-related head injury by 85 percent.[43] Although no States have bicycle laws that apply to all riders, 15 States have laws that apply to young bicyclists under age 18 years.[44] In addition, several localities have ordinances that require some or all bicyclists to wear helmets. Helmets are important for riders of all ages, especially because older bicyclists represent two-thirds of bicycle deaths.[43]

15-25. Reduce residential fire deaths.

Target: 0.2 deaths per 100,000 population.

Baseline: 1.2 deaths per 100,000 population were caused by residential fires in 1998 (age adjusted to the year 2000 standard population).

Target setting method: Better than the best.

Data source: National Vital Statistics System (NVSS), CDC, NCHS.

NOTE: THE TABLE BELOW MAY CONTINUE TO THE FOLLOWING PAGE.

Total Population, 1998	Residential Fire Deaths
	Rate per 100,000
TOTAL	1.2
Race and ethnicity	
American Indian or Alaska Native	2.1
Asian or Pacific Islander	0.3
Asian	DNC
Native Hawaiian and other Pacific Islander	DNC

Healthy People 2010: Objectives for Improving Health

Total Population, 1998	Residential Fire Deaths
	Rate per 100,000
Black or African American	3.0
White	1.0
Hispanic or Latino	0.9
Cuban	DSU
Mexican	0.9
Puerto Rican	1.2
Not Hispanic or Latino	1.2
Black or African American	3.0
White	1.0
Gender	
Female	0.9
Male	1.6
Education level (aged 25 to 64 years)	
Less than high school	2.0
High school graduate	1.2
At least some college	0.4
Select populations	
Persons aged 4 years and under (not age adjusted)	1.6
Persons aged 65 years and older (not age adjusted)	3.2
Black or African American	3.0
Females	2.2
Males	4.0

DNA = Data have not been analyzed. DNC = Data are not collected. DSU = Data are statistically unreliable.
Note: Age adjusted to the year 2000 standard population.
NOTE: THE TABLE ABOVE MAY HAVE CONTINUED FROM THE PREVIOUS PAGE.

15-26. Increase functioning residential smoke alarms.

Target and baseline:

Objective	Increase in Functioning Residential Smoke Alarms	1998 Baseline	2010 Target
		Percent	
15-26a.	Total population living in residences with functioning smoke alarm on every floor	88	100
15-26b.	Residences with a functioning smoke alarm on every floor	87	100

*Age adjusted to the year 2000 standard population.

Target setting method: Total coverage.

Data source: National Health Interview Survey (NHIS), CDC, NCHS.

NOTE: THE TABLE BELOW MAY CONTINUE TO THE FOLLOWING PAGE.

Total Population, 1998	15-26a. Live in Residences With Functioning Smoke Alarm on Every Floor
	Percent
TOTAL	88
Race and ethnicity	
American Indian or Alaska Native	84
Asian or Pacific Islander	90
Asian	91
Native Hawaiian and other Pacific Islander	88
Black or African American	86
White	88
Hispanic or Latino	81
Not Hispanic or Latino	88
Black or African American	86
White	89
Gender	
Female	88
Male	87

Total Population, 1998	15-26a. Live in Residences With Functioning Smoke Alarm on Every Floor
	Percent
Education level (aged 25 years and older)	
Less than high school	81
High school graduate	88
At least some college	90

DNA = Data have not been analyzed. DNC = Data are not collected. DSU = Data are statistically unreliable.
Note: Age adjusted to the year 2000 standard population.
NOTE: THE TABLE ABOVE MAY HAVE CONTINUED FROM THE PREVIOUS PAGE.

In 1997, 3,220 deaths occurred as a result of residential fires. Residential property loss caused by these fires was roughly $4.4 billion. In 1995, the cost of all fire-related deaths and injuries, including deaths and injuries to firefighters, was estimated at $15.8 billion.[45]

Fires are the second leading cause of unintentional injury death among children. Compared to the total population, children aged 4 years and under have a fire death rate more than twice the national average. About 800 children aged 14 years and under die by fire each year, and 65 percent of these children are under age 5 years. Children are disproportionately affected because they react less effectively to fire than adults, and they also generally sustain more severe burns at lower temperatures than adults. Two-thirds of fire-related deaths and injuries among children under age 5 years occur in homes without functioning smoke alarms.[46]

Functioning smoke alarms on every level and in every sleeping area of a home can provide residents with sufficient warning to escape from nearly all types of fires. Therefore, functioning smoke alarms can be highly effective in preventing fire-related deaths. If a fire occurs, homes with smoke alarms are roughly half as likely to have a death occur as homes without smoke alarms.[46]

15-27. Reduce deaths from falls.

Target: 3.0 deaths per 100,000 population.

Baseline: 4.7 deaths per 100,000 population were caused by falls in 1998 (age adjusted to the year 2000 standard population).

Target setting method: Better than the best.

Data source: National Vital Statistics System (NVSS), CDC, NCHS.

Total Population, 1998	Deaths From Falls
	Rate per 100,000
TOTAL	4.7
Race and ethnicity	
American Indian or Alaska Native	4.4
Asian or Pacific Islander	3.4
Asian	DNC
Native Hawaiian and other Pacific Islander	DNC
Black or African American	3.1
White	4.9
Hispanic or Latino	3.7
Cuban	3.3
Mexican	3.6
Puerto Rican	3.4
Not Hispanic or Latino	4.7
Black or African American	3.2
White	4.9
Gender	
Female	3.5
Male	6.4
Education level (aged 25 to 64 years)	
Less than high school	2.9
High school graduate	2.4
At least some college	1.2
Select populations	
Persons aged 65 to 84 years (not age adjusted)	17.2
Persons aged 85 years and older (not age adjusted)	107.9

DNA = Data have not been analyzed. DNC = Data are not collected. DSU = Data are statistically unreliable.
Note: Age adjusted to the year 2000 standard population.

15-28. Reduce hip fractures among older adults.

Target and baseline:

Objective	Reduction in Hip Fractures	1998 Baseline	2010 Target
		Rate per 100,000	
15-28a.	Females aged 65 years and older	1,055.8	416
15-28b.	Males aged 65 years and older	592.7	474

Target setting method: Better than the best for 15-28a; 20 percent improvement for 15-28b. (Better than the best will be used when data are available.)

Data source: National Hospital Discharge Survey (NHDS), CDC, NCHS.

Adults Aged 65 Years and Older, 1998	Hip Fracture	
	15-28a. Females	15-28b. Males
	Rate per 100,000	
TOTAL	1,055.8	592.7
Race and ethnicity		
American Indian or Alaska Native	DSU	DSU
Asian or Pacific Islander	DSU	DSU
Asian	DNC	DNC
Native Hawaiian and other Pacific Islander	DNC	DNC
Black or African American	417.6	DSU
White	874.2	459.6
Hispanic or Latino	DSU	DSU
Not Hispanic or Latino	DSU	DSU
Black or African American	DSU	DSU
White	DSU	DSU
Education level (aged 25 to 64 years)		
Less than high school	DNC	DNC
High school graduate	DNC	DNC
At least some college	DNC	DNC

DNA = Data have not been analyzed. DNC = Data are not collected. DSU = Data are statistically unreliable.

In 1995, falls became the leading cause of injury deaths among adults aged 65 years and older. In 1997, 9,023 adults over age 65 years died as a result of falls.[47] Falls are the most common cause of injuries and hospital admissions for trauma among elderly persons. Since most fractures are the result of falls, understanding factors that contribute to falling is essential to designing effective intervention strategies. For all ages combined, alcohol use has been implicated in 35 to 63 percent of deaths from falls. For persons aged 65 years and older, 60 percent of fatal falls occur in the home, 30 percent occur in public places, and 10 percent occur in health care institutions.[48]

The most serious fall-related injury is hip fracture. Approximately 212,000 hip fractures occur each year in the United States among adults aged 65 years and older; 75 to 80 percent of all hip fractures are sustained by females.[49] The impact of these injuries on the quality of life is enormous. Half of all elderly adults hospitalized for hip fracture cannot return home or live independently after the fracture. The total direct cost of all fall injuries for adults aged 65 years and older in 1994 was $20.2 billion.[50] Factors that contribute to falls include difficulties in gait and balance, neurological and musculoskeletal disabilities, psychoactive medications, dementia, and visual impairment.[51] Environmental hazards such as slippery surfaces, uneven floors, poor lighting on stairs, loose rugs, unstable furniture, grab bars in bathrooms, and objects on floors also may play a role.

15-29. Reduce drownings.

Target: 0.9 drownings per 100,000 population.

Baseline: 1.6 drownings per 100,000 population occurred in 1998 (age adjusted to the year 2000 standard population).

Target setting method: Better than the best.

Data source: National Vital Statistics System (NVSS), CDC, NCHS, CPSC.

NOTE: THE TABLE BELOW MAY CONTINUE TO THE FOLLOWING PAGE.

Total Population, 1998	Drownings
	Rate per 100,000
TOTAL	1.6
Race and ethnicity	
American Indian or Alaska Native	3.1
Asian or Pacific Islander	1.5
Asian	DNC
Native Hawaiian and other Pacific Islander	DNC
Black or African American	2.3
White	1.5
Hispanic or Latino	1.5
Cuban	DSU
Mexican	1.5
Puerto Rican	1.0

Total Population, 1998	Drownings
	Rate per 100,000
Not Hispanic or Latino	1.6
Black or African American	2.4
White	1.5
Gender	
Female	0.6
Male	2.7
Education level (aged 25 to 64 years)	
Less than high school	2.6
High school graduate	1.7
At least some college	0.9
Geographic location	
Urban (metropolitan statistical area)	1.4
Rural (nonmetropolitan statistical area)	2.1
Select populations	
Males aged 15 to 34 years (not age adjusted)	3.4
Black or African American males	4.2
Age groups	
Children aged 4 years and younger (not age adjusted)	2.9
Adolescents aged 10 to 14 years	1.0
Adolescents aged 15 to 19 years	2.2
Young adults aged 20 to 24 years	2.2

DNA = Data have not been analyzed. DNC = Data are not collected. DSU = Data are statistically unreliable.
Note: Age adjusted to the year 2000 standard population.

NOTE: THE TABLE ABOVE MAY HAVE CONTINUED FROM THE PREVIOUS PAGE.

In 1997, drownings accounted for over 4,000 deaths in the United States.[52] In 1998, 8,061 crashes involving recreational boats resulted in 4,612 injuries and 815 (574 drownings) deaths.[53] Drowning is the second leading cause of injury-related death for children and adolescents aged 1 to 19 years, accounting for 1,502 deaths in 1995.[54]

Most deaths involving diving occur among persons aged 15 to 39 years, with the largest proportion (14.8 percent) occurring among persons aged 30 to 39 years. Many diving-related incidents result in spinal cord injury. Alcohol use is involved in about 50 percent of deaths associated with water recreation.[53]

Backyard swimming pools and spas represent the greatest risk to preschoolers, particularly those 18 to 30 months of age. Of the 600 annual drowning deaths of children from birth to 5 years of age, more than 300 occur in residential swimming pools. Annually, approximately 2,300 nonfatal injuries sustained in residential swimming pools occur in this age group.[25]

15-30. Reduce hospital emergency department visits for nonfatal dog bite injuries.

Target: 114 hospital emergency department visits per 100,000 population.

Baseline: 151.4 hospital emergency department visits per 100,000 population were for nonfatal dog bite injuries in 1997 (age adjusted to the year 2000 standard population).

Target setting method: Better than the best.

Data source: National Hospital Ambulatory Medical Care Survey (NHAMCS), CDC, NCHS.

Total Population, 1997	Hospital Emergency Department Visits for Nonfatal Dog Bite Injuries
	Rate per 100,000
TOTAL	151.4
Race and ethnicity	
American Indian or Alaska Native	DSU
Asian or Pacific Islander	DSU
Asian	DNC
Native Hawaiian and other Pacific Islander	DNC
Black or African American	115.1
White	164.2
Hispanic or Latino	DSU
Not Hispanic or Latino	DSU
Black or African American	DSU
White	DSU
Gender	
Female	150.8
Male	152.0
Education level	
Less than high school	DNC
High school graduate	DNC
At least some college	DNC

DNA = Data have not been analyzed. DNC = Data are not collected. DSU = Data are statistically unreliable.
Note: Age adjusted to the year 2000 standard population.

Between 500,000 and 4 million persons in the United States are bitten by dogs every year.[55] Children are among the most vulnerable, and almost half of all people are estimated to have been bitten by a dog during childhood. Among children, more than half of bites have been to the head, face, or neck. Because of the risk to large parts of the population, especially children, effective prevention strategies are needed to reduce the painful and costly burden of dog bites. More knowledge is needed through a combination of enhanced and coordinated dog bite reporting systems, expanded population-based surveys, and implementation and evaluation of prevention trials. Particularly for the more severe episodes, information needs to be obtained regarding high-risk situations, high-risk dogs, and elements of successful interventions.

15-31. (Developmental) Increase the proportion of public and private schools that require use of appropriate head, face, eye, and mouth protection for students participating in school-sponsored physical activities.

Potential data source: School Health Policies and Programs Study (SHPPS), CDC, NCCDPHP.

Trauma to the head, face, eyes, and mouth occurs frequently during school-sponsored physical activities. Schools with recreation and sports programs can reduce traumas by requiring students to use appropriate protective gear.

Violence and Abuse Prevention

15-32. Reduce homicides.

Target: 3.0 homicides per 100,000 population.

Baseline: 6.5 homicides per 100,000 population occurred in 1998 (age adjusted to the year 2000 standard population).

Target setting method: Better than the best.

Data sources: National Vital Statistics System (NVSS), CDC, NCHS; FBI Uniform Crime Reports, U.S. Department of Justice.

NOTE: THE TABLE BELOW MAY CONTINUE TO THE FOLLOWING PAGE.

Total Population, 1998	Homicides
	Rate per 100,000
TOTAL	6.5
Race and ethnicity	
American Indian or Alaska Native	9.1
Asian or Pacific Islander	3.5
Asian	DNC

Total Population, 1998	Homicides
	Rate per 100,000
Native Hawaiian and other Pacific Islander	DNC
Black or African American	22.6
White	4.0
Hispanic or Latino	8.8
Cuban	8.3
Mexican	9.0
Puerto Rican	7.9
Not Hispanic or Latino	6.2
Black or African American	23.4
White	3.1
Gender	
Female	3.1
Male	10.0
Education level (aged 25 to 64 years)	
Less than high school	17.1
High school graduate	9.9
At least some college	2.7
Select populations (not age adjusted)	
Children under 1 year	8.1
Children aged 1 to 4 years	2.6
Children aged 10 to 14 years	1.5
Adolescents aged 15 to 19 years	11.7
Persons aged 15 to 34 years	13.0
Intimate partners aged 14 to 45 years (spouse, ex-spouse, boyfriend, girlfriend)	DNC
Black or African Americans aged 15 to 34 years	48.2
Females	13.3
Males	84.9
Hispanic males aged 15 to 34 years	33.5

DNA = Data have not been analyzed. DNC = Data are not collected. DSU = Data are statistically unreliable.
Note: Age adjusted to the year 2000 standard population.

NOTE: THE TABLE ABOVE MAY HAVE CONTINUED FROM THE PREVIOUS PAGE.

Homicide was the cause of death for 19,491 persons in United States (7.2 per 100,000 population) in 1997.[56] Homicide is the second leading cause of death for young persons aged 15 to 24 years and the leading cause of death for African Americans in this age group.[57] Homicide rates are dropping among all groups, but the decreases are not as dramatic among youth, who already exhibit the highest rates. In 1997, 6,146 young persons aged 15 to 24 years were victims of homicide, amounting to almost 17 youth homicide victims per day in the United States.[58] Of all homicide victims in 1997, 37 percent were under age 24 years.[59] The homicide rate among males aged 15 to 24 years in the United States is 10 times higher than in Canada, 15 times higher than in Australia, and 28 times higher than in France or Germany.[60]

15-33. Reduce maltreatment and maltreatment fatalities of children.

15-33a. Reduce maltreatment of children.

Target: 10.3 per 1,000 children under age 18 years.

Baseline: 12.9 child victims of maltreatment per 1,000 children under age 18 years were reported in 1998.

Target setting method: 20 percent improvement. (Better than the best will be used when data are available.)

Data source: National Child Abuse and Neglect Data System (NCANDS), Administration on Children, Youth and Families, Administration for Children and Families (ACF), Children's Bureau.

Data for population groups currently are not analyzed.

15-33b. Reduce child maltreatment fatalities.

Target: 1.4 per 100,000 children under age 18 years.

Baseline: 1.6 child maltreatment fatalities per 100,000 children under age 18 years occurred in 1998.

Target setting method: 12 percent improvement. (Better than the best will be used when data are available.)

Data source: National Child Abuse and Neglect Data System (NCANDS), Administration on Children, Youth, and Families, Administration for Children and Families (ACF), Children's Bureau.

Data for population groups currently are not analyzed.

The 1997 Child Maltreatment report from the States to the National Child Abuse and Neglect Data System found there were approximately 984,000 victims of maltreatment, a decrease from more than 1 million victims in 1996 in the 50 States, the District of Columbia, Puerto Rico, the Virgin Islands, and Guam. The rate of child victims was 13.9 per 1,000 children in the general population in 1997, which is slightly higher than the rate of 13.4 victims per 1,000 children in 1990. There were an estimated 1,196 fatalities due to child maltreatment in the 50 States and the District of Columbia. The findings regarding the types of maltreatment were as follows: 55.9 percent neglect, 24.6 percent physical abuse, 12.5 percent sexual abuse, and 6.1 percent emotional abuse. It is also important to note that 58.8 percent of the substantiated or indicated reports of maltreatment were from professional sources: legal, medical, social service, or education professionals. Based on data from 39 States, 75.4 percent of the perpetrators were the victim's parents, 10.2 percent were relatives, and 1.9 percent were individuals in other caretaking relationships.[61]

Information needs to be collected about new cases and causes of maltreatment. National surveys of new cases are needed to describe the magnitude of the problem. In addition, existing interventions and their impact need to be evaluated. Some long-term studies on home-visitation programs for young mothers have shown potential for preventing child abuse and neglect.

15-34. Reduce the rate of physical assault by current or former intimate partners.

Target: 3.3 physical assaults per 1,000 persons aged 12 years and older.

Baseline: 4.4 physical assaults per 1,000 persons aged 12 years and older by current or former intimate partners occurred in 1998.

Target setting method: Better than the best.

Data source: National Crime Victimization Survey (NCVS), U.S. Department of Justice, Bureau of Justice Statistics.

NOTE: THE TABLE BELOW MAY CONTINUE TO THE FOLLOWING PAGE.

Persons Aged 12 Years and Older, 1998	Physical Assault by Current and/or Former Intimate Partners
	Rate per 1,000
TOTAL	4.4
Race and ethnicity	
American Indian or Alaska Native	DSU
Asian or Pacific Islander	DSU
Asian	DNC
Native Hawaiian and other Pacific Islander	DSU
Black or African American	5.1
White	4.3

Persons Aged 12 Years and Older, 1998	Physical Assault by Current and/or Former Intimate Partners
	Rate per 1,000
Hispanic or Latino	3.4
Not Hispanic or Latino	4.4
Black or African American	DNA
White	DNA
Gender	
Female	7.2
Male	1.3
Education level	
Less than high school	DNA
High school graduate	DNA
At least some college	DNA
Sexual orientation	DNC

DNA = Data have not been analyzed. DNC = Data are not collected. DSU = Data are statistically unreliable.

NOTE: THE TABLE ABOVE MAY HAVE CONTINUED FROM THE PREVIOUS PAGE.

15-35. Reduce the annual rate of rape or attempted rape.

Target: 0.7 rapes or attempted rapes per 1,000 persons.

Baseline: 0.8 rapes or attempted rapes per 1,000 persons aged 12 years and older occurred in 1998.

Target setting method: Better than the best.

Data source: National Crime Victimization Survey (NCVS), U.S. Department of Justice, Bureau of Justice Statistics.

NOTE: THE TABLE BELOW MAY CONTINUE TO THE FOLLOWING PAGE.

Persons Aged 12 Years and Older, 1998	Rape or Attempted Rape
	Rate per 1,000
TOTAL	0.8
Race and ethnicity	
Other (Asian/Pacific Islander and American Indian/Alaska Native)	DNA
Native Hawaiian and other Pacific Islander	DNC
Black or African American	DSU
White	0.8

Persons Aged 12 Years and Older, 1998	Rape or Attempted Rape
	Rate per 1,000
Hispanic or Latino	DSU
Not Hispanic or Latino	0.8
Black or African American	DSU
White	DSU
Gender	
Female	1.4
Male	DSU
Education level	
Less than high school	DNA
High school graduate	DNA
At least some college	DNA
Sexual orientation	DNC
Select populations	
Age groups	
Adolescents aged 12 to 15 years	DSU
Adolescents aged 16 to 19 years	DSU
Young adults aged 20 to 24 years	3.4

DNA = Data have not been analyzed. DNC = Data are not collected. DSU = Data are statistically unreliable.

NOTE: THE TABLE ABOVE MAY HAVE CONTINUED FROM THE PREVIOUS PAGE.

15-36. Reduce sexual assault other than rape.

Target: 0.4 sexual assaults other than rape per 1,000 persons aged 12 years and older.

Baseline: 0.6 sexual assaults other than rape per 1,000 persons aged 12 years and older occurred in 1998.

Target setting method: Better than the best.

Data source: National Crime Victimization Survey (NCVS), DOJ, BJS.

NOTE: THE TABLE BELOW MAY CONTINUE TO THE FOLLOWING PAGE.

Persons Aged 12 Years and Older, 1998	Sexual Assault Other Than Rape
	Rate per 1,000
TOTAL	0.6
Race and ethnicity	
Other (Asian/Pacific Islander and American Indian/Alaska Native)	DSU

Persons Aged 12 Years and Older, 1998	Sexual Assault Other Than Rape
	Rate per 1,000
Native Hawaiian and other Pacific Islander	DSU
Black or African American	DSU
White	0.5
Hispanic or Latino	DSU
Not Hispanic or Latino	0.7
Black or African American	DNA
White	DNA
Gender	
Female	1.1
Male	DSU
Education level	
Less than high school	DNA
High school graduate	DNA
At least some college	DNA
Sexual orientation	DNC

DNA = Data have not been analyzed. DNC = Data are not collected. DSU = Data are statistically unreliable.

NOTE: THE TABLE ABOVE MAY HAVE CONTINUED FROM THE PREVIOUS PAGE.

Both females and males experience family and intimate violence and sexual assault. Perpetrators can be the same or opposite sex. Male victimization of females is more common in intimate partner violence and sexual assault.

In 1995, almost 5,000 females in the United States were murdered. In those cases for which the Federal Bureau of Investigation had data on the relationship between the offender and the victim, 85 percent were killed by someone they knew. Nearly half of the females who knew the perpetrators were murdered by a husband, ex-husband, or boyfriend.[62] In 1994, more than 500,000 females were seen in hospital EDs for violence-related injuries, and 37 percent of those females were there for injuries inflicted by spouses, ex-spouses, or nonmarital partners.[63] Although most assault victims survive, they suffer physically and emotionally.

Violence against women is primarily partner violence. A national survey conducted from November 1995 to May 1996 estimates that approximately 1.5 million females and 834,700 males are raped and/or physically assaulted by an intimate partner annually in the United States. Seventy-six percent of the females who were raped and/or physically assaulted since age 18 years were assaulted by a current or former husband, cohabiting partner, or date, compared with 18 percent of the males. Females are significantly more likely than males to be injured during an assault: 32 percent of the females and 16 percent of the males who were raped since age 18 years were injured during their most recent rape; 39 percent of the females and 25 percent of the males who were physically assaulted since age 18 years were injured during their most recent assault. About one in three females who were injured during a rape or physical assault required medical care.[64]

Estimates of abuse rates during pregnancy also are a concern. A 1996 literature review indicted that estimated proportions of women experiencing IPV during pregnancy ranged between 0.9 percent and 20.1 percent. The majority were between 4 and 8 percent. The proportion of pregnant women who had experienced IPV at any time in the past ranged between 9.7 percent and 29.7 percent.[65]

Males who are physically violent toward their partners are more likely to be sexually violent toward them and are more likely to use violence toward children.[66] The perpetration of IPV is most common in adults who, as children or adolescents, witnessed IPV or became the targets of violence from their caregivers.[66]

Survey data from 1994 indicate that 407,190 females aged 12 years and older were victims of rape, attempted rape, or sexual assault.[67] Other surveys indicate that the problem is underestimated.[68] For example, the National Women's Study, in conjunction with estimates based on the U.S. Census, suggests that 12.1 million females in the United States have been victims of forcible rape sometime in their lives. According to this study, 0.7 percent or approximately 683,000 of adult females experienced a forcible rape in the past year.[69]

Teen dating violence is a concern that may stem from childhood abuse or other experiences with violence. Battering in teen relationships is very different from IPV that occurs between adults. The issue of teen dating violence requires national attention and prevention efforts that need to continue focusing on adolescent violence within the larger context of family violence.

The nature of IPV and sexual violence makes such problems difficult to study. Consequently, much remains unknown about the factors that increase or decrease the likelihood that males will behave violently toward females, the factors that endanger or protect females from violence, and the physical and emotional consequences of such violence for females and their children.

15-37. Reduce physical assaults.

Target: 13.6 physical assaults per 1,000 persons aged 12 years older.

Baseline: 31.1 physical assaults per 1,000 persons aged 12 years and older occurred in 1998.

Target setting method: Better than the best.

Data source: National Crime Victimization Survey (NCVS), U.S. Department of Justice, Bureau of Justice Statistics.

Persons Aged 12 Years and Older, 1998	Physical Assaults
	Rate per 1,000
TOTAL	31.1
Race and ethnicity	
American Indian or Alaska Native	99.4
Asian or Pacific Islander	13.7
Asian	DNC
Native Hawaiian and other Pacific Islander	DNC
Black or African American	33.8
White	31.0
Hispanic or Latino	25.9
Not Hispanic or Latino	31.4
Black or African American	DNA
White	DNA
Gender	
Female	25.1
Male	DSU
Education level	
Less than high school	DNA
High school graduate	DNA
At least some college	DNA
Select populations	
Adolescents aged 12 to 15 years	70.5
Adolescents aged 16 to 19 years	76.8
Young adults aged 20 to 24 years	56.0

DNA = Data have not been analyzed. DNC = Data are not collected. DSU = Data are statistically unreliable.

15-38. Reduce physical fighting among adolescents.

Target: 32 percent.

Baseline: 36 percent of adolescents in grades 9 through 12 engaged in physical fighting in the previous 12 months in 1999.

Target setting method: Better than the best.

Data source: Youth Risk Behavior Surveillance System (YRBSS), CDC, NCCDPHP.

Adolescents in Grades 9 Through 12, 1999	Fighting in Past 12 Months
	Percent
TOTAL	36
Race and ethnicity	
American Indian or Alaska Native	DSU
Asian or Pacific Islander	DSU
Asian	DSU
Native Hawaiian and other Pacific Islander	DSU
Black or African American	41
White	34
Hispanic or Latino	40
Not Hispanic or Latino	35
Black or African American	41
White	33
Gender	
Female	27
Male	44
Parents' education level	
Less than high school	DNC
High school graduate	DNC
At least some college	DNC
Select populations	
9th grade	41
10th grade	38
11th grade	31
12th grade	30

DNA = Data have not been analyzed. DNC = Data are not collected. DSU = Data are statistically unreliable.

15-39. Reduce weapon carrying by adolescents on school property.

Target: 4.9 percent.

Baseline: 6.9 percent of students in grades 9 through 12 carried weapons on school property during the past 30 days in 1999.

Target setting method: Better than the best.

Data source: Youth Risk Behavior Surveillance System (YRBSS), CDC, NCCDPHP.

Students in Grades 9 Through 12, 1999	Weapon Carrying on School Property in Past 30 Days
	Percent
TOTAL	6.9
Race and ethnicity	
American Indian or Alaska Native	DSU
Asian or Pacific Islander	DSU
Asian	DSU
Native Hawaiian and other Pacific Islander	DSU
Black or African American	6.1
White	7.0
Hispanic or Latino	7.9
Not Hispanic or Latino	6.8
Black or African American	5.0
White	6.4
Gender	
Female	2.8
Male	11.0
Parents' education level	
Less than high school	DNC
High school graduate	DNC
Some college	DNC
Select populations	
9th grade	7.2
10th grade	6.6
11th grade	7.0
12th grade	6.2

DNA = Data have not been analyzed. DNC = Data are not collected. DSU = Data are statistically unreliable.

In 1998, physical assault victimization among adolescents took place twice as often as in the general population of persons aged 12 years and older. Assaults were significantly higher among males. While the total assaults for blacks and whites and Hispanics and non-Hispanics were similar, aggravated assault was higher for blacks than whites (11.9 versus 7.0 per 1,000), and simple assault was higher for non-Hispanics than Hispanics (23.9 versus 19.5 per 1,000). Assaults were higher for those with lower household incomes; rates of assault victimization decreased from 54.2 per 1,000 persons in households with annual incomes of less than $7,500 to less than 30 per 1,000 persons in households with annual incomes greater than $35,000.[70]

In 1999, 36 percent of students in grades 9 through 12 had been in a physical fight one or more times during the 12 months preceding the survey.[71] Overall, male students were significantly more likely than female students to have been in a physical fight. This gender difference was identified for white and Hispanic students and for each grade. Overall, Hispanic students (40 percent) were significantly more likely than white students (33 percent) to have been in a physical fight. Female and male students in grade 9 were significantly more likely than female and male students in grade 11 to have been in a physical fight. Black female students were more likely than white female students to report this behavior, and male students in grade 9 were much more likely than male students in grade 12 to report this behavior. Nationwide, 4.0 percent of students had been treated by a doctor or nurse for injuries sustained in a physical fight one or more times during the 12 months preceding the survey.[71]

Nationwide, 6.9 percent of students carried a weapon (for example, a gun, knife, or club) on school property one or more times during the 30 days preceding the survey. Overall, male students were significantly more likely than female students to have carried a weapon on school property. This significant gender difference was identified for white and Hispanic students and each grade. Overall, Hispanic students were significantly more likely than black students to have carried a weapon on school property. Black female students were significantly more likely than white female students to have carried a weapon on school property, and Hispanics and white male students were significantly more likely than black male students to report this behavior.[71]

Violence prevention programs for youth need to focus on strategies that reduce involvement in physical fighting and discourage weapon carrying on school property. Strategies to reduce weapon carrying on school property, physical fighting, and resulting injuries among youth should begin early in life and must be tailored to youth of widely varying social, economic, cultural, and ethnic backgrounds.[72] As with other areas of violence and abuse, carefully controlled studies to evaluate the effectiveness of various strategies and interventions are needed. Physicians and other health professionals are in a position to provide effective primary prevention messages to youth and their families. Also, ED workers treating adolescents with fight-related injuries can practice secondary interventions, as they do with victims of child abuse, sexual assault, or attempted suicide.

Related Objectives From Other Focus Areas

1. **Access to Quality Health Services**
   - 1-3. Counseling about health behaviors
   - 1-11. Rapid prehospital emergency care
   - 1-12. Single toll-free number for poison control centers
7. **Educational and Community-Based Programs**
   - 7-3. Health-risk behavior information for college and university students
8. **Environmental Health**
   - 8-13. Pesticide exposures
   - 8-24. Exposure to pesticides
   - 8-25. Exposure to heavy metals and other toxic chemicals
18. **Mental Health and Mental Disorders**
   - 18-1. Suicide
   - 18-2. Adolescent suicide attempts
20. **Occupational Safety and Health**
   - 20-1. Work-related injury deaths
   - 20-2. Work-related injuries
   - 20-5. Work-related homicides
   - 20-6. Work-related assaults
26. **Subtance Abuse**
   - 26-1. Motor vehicle crash deaths and injuries
   - 26-5. Alcohol-related hospital emergency department visits
   - 26-6. Adolescents riding with a driver who has been drinking
   - 26-7. Alcohol- and drug-related violence
   - 26-24. Administrative license revocation laws
   - 26-25. Blood alcohol concentration (BAC) levels for motor vehicle drivers

Terminology

(A listing of abbreviations and acronyms used in this publication appears in Appendix H.)

Age-adjusted injury rate: An injury rate calculated to reflect a standard age distribution.

Attempted rape: Includes males and females, heterosexual and homosexual rape, and verbal threats of rape.

Graduated licensing laws: Require young drivers to progress through phases of restricted driving before they are allowed to get their unrestricted licenses. Such restrictions include a mandatory supervised driving period, night driving curfews, limits on teen passengers riding with a beginning driver, and a lower blood alcohol concentration (BAC) level for teens than for adults.

Homicide: Fatal injury intentionally caused to one human being by another.

Impaired driving: Driving while under the influence of alcohol or drugs.

Injury: Unintentional or intentional damage to the body resulting from acute exposure to thermal, mechanical, electrical, or chemical energy or from the absence of such essentials as heat or oxygen.

Intimate partner(s): Refers to spouses, ex-spouses, boyfriends, girlfriends, and former boyfriends and girlfriends (includes same-sex partners). Intimate partners may or may not be cohabitating and need not be engaging in sexual activities.

Intimate partner violence: Actual or threatened physical or sexual violence or psychological and emotional abuse by an intimate partner.

Motorcyclist: Includes both operator and rider (passenger).

NCUTLO: National Committee on Uniform Traffic Laws and Ordinances.

Pedalcyclists: Riders of bicycles and tricycles.

Premature death: Dying before life expectancy is reached.

Primary enforcement: A stipulation of a safety belt use law that allows law enforcement officials to stop a driver solely on the basis of a safety belt law violation.

Rape: Forced sexual intercourse, including both psychological coercion and physical force. Forced sexual intercourse means vaginal, anal, or oral penetration by the offender(s) and includes incidents of penetration by a foreign object. Also included are attempted rapes, male and female victims, and heterosexual and homosexual rape.

Risk factor: A characteristic that has been demonstrated statistically to be associated with a particular injury.

Secondary enforcement: A stipulation of a safety belt use law that allows law enforcement officials to address a safety belt use law violation only after a driver has been stopped for some other purpose.

Sexual assault: A wide range of victimizations separate from rape and attempted rape. Included are attacks or attempted attacks of unwanted sexual contact between the victim and the offender that may or may not involve force; includes grabbing or fondling. Verbal threats also are included.

Suffocation: Includes inhalation and ingestion of food or other objects; accidental mechanical suffocation; suicide and self-inflicted injury by hanging, strangulation, and suffocation; assault by hanging and strangulation; and hanging, strangulation, or suffocation undetermined whether accidental or purposely inflicted.

Target population: The group of persons (usually those at high risk) whom program interventions are designed to reach.

Trauma registry: A collection of data on patients who receive hospital care for certain types of injuries, such as blunt or penetrating trauma or burns. Such collections are designed primarily to ensure quality care in individual institutions and trauma systems but also provide useful data for the surveillance of injury and death.

Unintentional injury: A type of injury that occurs without purposeful intent.

Vehicle miles traveled (VMT): The miles of travel by all types of motor vehicles as determined by the States on the basis of actual traffic counts and established estimating procedures.

Violence: The intentional use of physical force or power, threatened or actual, against another person or against oneself or against a group of people, that results in or has a high likelihood of resulting in injury, death, psychological harm, maldevelopment, or deprivation.

Vulnerable populations: Refers to children, elderly persons, and persons with disabilities.

Years of potential life lost (YPLL): A statistical measure used to determine premature death. YPLL is calculated by subtracting an individual's age at death from a predetermined life expectancy. The Centers for Disease Control and Prevention generally uses 75 years of age for this purpose (for example, a person who died at aged 35 years would have a YPLL of 40).

References

[1] Centers for Disease Control and Prevention (CDC), National Center for Health Statistics (NCHS). Deaths: Final data for 1997. *National Vital Statistics Reports* 47(19), June 1999.

[2] Houk, V.; Brown, S.T.; and Rosenberg, M. One fine solution to the injury problem. *Public Health Reports* 102:5, 1987.

[3] Baker, S.P.; O'Neill, B.; Ginsburg, M.J.; et al. *The Injury Fact Book*. 2nd ed. New York, NY: Oxford University Press, 1992.

[4] CDC. *Health, United States, 1999*. Hyattsville, MD: U.S. Department of Health and Human Services (HHS), 1999.

[5] HHS, National Institutes of Health (NIH), National Institute on Alcohol Abuse and Alcoholism (NIAAA). *Ninth Special Report to the U.S. Congress on Alcohol and Health from the Secretary of Health and Human Services*. NIH Pub. No. 97-4017. Washington, DC: HHS, 1997.

[6] HHS, CDC, National Center for Injury Prevention and Control (NCIPC). Ten Leading Causes of Injury Deaths. Atlanta, GA: HHS, CDC, NCIPC, 1997.

[7] Schappert, S.M. Ambulatory care visits to physician offices, hospital outpatient departments and emergency departments: U.S., 1995. *Vital and Health Statistics* 13(29):1-38, 1997.

[8] National Safety Council. *Accident Facts*. 1995 ed. Itaska, IL: the Council, 1995.

[9] National Safe Kids Campaign. *Childhood Injury Factsheet*. Itaska, IL: the Campaign, 1997.

[10] Moscicki, E.K.; O'Carroll, P.W.; Rae, D.S.; et al. Suicide ideation and attempts: The Epidemiologic Catchement Area Study. In: *Report of the Secretary's Task Force on Youth Suicide*. Vol. 4. Washington, DC: HHS, 1989.

[11] Indian Health Service (IHS), Injury Prevention Program. *Injuries Among Native Americans and Alaska Natives*. Rockville, MD: IHS, 1997.

[12] U.S. Fire Administration. *Curious Kids Set Fires*. Washington, DC: Federal Emergency Management Agency, 1990.

[13] CDC, NCHS. Deaths: Final data for 1997. *National Vital Statistics Reports* 47(10):1-104, 1999.

[14] Livingson, I.L., ed. *Handbook of Black American Health: The Mosaic of Conditions, Issues, Policies, and Prospects*. Westport, CT: Greenwood Press, 1994.

[15] Anderson, R.N.; Kockanck, K.D.; and Murphey, S.L. Report of final mortality statistics, 1995. *Monthly Vital Statistics Report* 45(Suppl. 2):11, 1997.

[16] CDC. Suicide Among Black Youths—United States, 1980–1995. *Morbidity and Mortality Monthly Report* 47(10):193, 1998.

[17] HHS, CDC. *Ten Leading Causes of Death, 1995*. Atlanta, GA: HHS, 1997.

[18] McLoughlin, E.; Annest, J.L.; Fingerhut, L.A.; et al. Recommended framework for presenting injury mortality data. *Morbidity and Mortality Weekly Report* 46(RR-14), 1997.

[19] Cummings, P.; Grossman, D.C.; Rivara, F.P.; et al. State gun safe storage laws and child mortality due to firearms. *Journal of the American Medical Association* 278(13), 1997.

[20] Chaloupka, F.J.; Saffer, H.; and Grossman, M. Alcohol control policies and motor-vehicle fatalities. *Journal of Legal Studies* 22:161-186, 1993.

[21] Cook, P.J., and Moore, M.J. Economic perspectives on reducing alcohol-related violence. In: Martin, S.E., ed. *Alcohol and Interpersonal Violence: Fostering Multidisplinary Perspectives.* Based on a workshop on alcohol-related violence sponsored by NIAAA, May 14-15, 1992. NIH Pub. No. 93-3496. Rockville, MD: NIH, 1993.

[22] NCIPC. *Best Practices for Preventing Violence by Children and Adolescents: A Source Book.* Atlanta, GA: CDC, 1999 (in press).

[23] NCHS. National Vital Statistics System, unpublished data, 1999.

[24] Kraus, K.F.; Black, M.A.; Hessol, N.; et al. The incidence of acute brain injury and serious impairment in a defined population. *American Journal of Epidemiology* 119:186-201, 1984.

[25] American Academy of Pediatrics. *Injury Prevention and Control for Children and Youth.* 3rd ed. Elk Grove Village, IL: the Academy, 1997.

[26] CDC. Rates of homicide, suicide, and firearm-related death among children—26 industrialized countries, 1950–1993. *Morbidity and Mortality Weekly Report* 46(5):101, 1995.

[27] Fingerhut, L.A.; Ingram, D.D; and Feldman, J.J. Firearm and nonfirearm homicide among persons 15 to 19 years of age: Differences by level of urbanization. United States 1979–89. *Journal of the American Medical Association* 267(22):3048-3053, 1992.

[28] CDC. Nonfatal and fatal firearm-related injuries—United States, 1993–1997. *Morbidity and Mortality Weekly Report* 48(45):1029-1034, 1999.

[29] NCHS. *Vital Statistics Mortality Data, Underlying Cause of Death, 1962–97.* Hyattsville, MD: HHS, 1999.

[30] Litovitz, T.L.; Smilkstein, M.S.; Felberg, L.; et al. 1996 annual report of the American Association of Poison Control Centers Toxic Exposure Surveillance System. *American Journal of Emergency Medicine* 15(5):447-500, 1997.

[31] National Safe Kids Campaign. *Poisoning Fact Sheet.* Washington, DC: the Campaign, 1997.

[32] HHS, NCHS, National Vital Statistics System, 1997, Washington, DC.

[33] National Safe Kids Campaign. *Airway Obstruction Fact Sheet.* Washington, DC: the Campaign, 1998.

[34] National Highway Traffic Safety Administration (NHTSA). *Fatality Analysis Reporting System (FARS), 1998.* Washington, DC: NHTSA, 1998.

[35] NHTSA. *Traffic Safety Facts 1998: Pedestrians.* Washington, DC: NHTSA, 1998.

[36] NHTSA. *Traffic Safety Facts 1998: Older Populations.* Washington, DC: NHTSA, 1998.

[37] Advocates for Highway and Auto Safety (AHAS). *Safety Belt Fact Sheet*. Washington, DC: AHAS, 1998.

[38] NHTSA. *Traffic Safety Facts 1997: Children*. Washington, DC: NHTSA, 1997.

[39] NHTSA. *Traffic Safety Facts 1998: Motorcycles*. Washington, DC: NHTSA, 1998.

[40] NHTSA. *Traffic Safety Facts 1998: Young Drivers*. Washington, DC: NHTSA, 1998.

[41] NHTSA. *Traffic Safety Facts 1998: Pedalcyclists*. Washington, DC: NHTSA, 1998.

[42] Insurance Institute for Highway Safety. *Facts 1996 Fatalities: Bicycles*. Arlington, VA: the Institute, 1997.

[43] CDC. Injury-control recommendations: Bicycle helmets. *Morbidity and Mortality Weekly Report* 44(RR-1), 1995.

[44] National Safe Kids Campaign. *State Bike Helmet Legislation*. Washington, DC: the Campaign, 1998.

[45] Karter, M.J. *Fire Loss in the United States, 1998*. Quincy, MA: National Fire Protection Association, 1999.

[46] Hall, J.R. *The U.S. Fire Problem and Overview Report. Leading Causes and Other Patterns and Trends*. Quincy, MA: National Fire Protection Association.

[47] NCHS. *Mortality Data Tapes*. Hyattsville, MD: NCHS, 1998.

[48] Hingson, R., and Howland, J. Alcohol and non-traffic intentional injuries. *Addiction* 88(7):877-883, 1993.

[49] Cummings, S.R.; Rubin, S.M.; and Black, D. The future of hip fractures in the United States. Numbers, costs, and potential effects of postmenopausal estrogen. *Clinical Orthopedics* 252:163-166, 1990.

[50] Englander, F.; Hodson, T.J.; and Teregrossa, R.A. Economic dimensions of slip and fall injuries. *Journal of Forensic Science* 41(5):746-773, 1996.

[51] Tinetti, M.E., and Speechley, M. Prevention of falls among the elderly. *New England Journal of Medicine* 320(16)1055-1059, 1989.

[52] NCHS. *National Mortality Data*. Hyattsville, MD: NCHS, 1997.

[53] U.S. Department of Transportation (DOT). *Boating Statistics 1998*. Pub. No. COMDTPUB P16754.12. Washington, DC: DOT, 1999.

[54] NCHS. *Mortality Data Tapes*. Hyattsville, MD: NCHS, 1996.

[55] Sacks, J.J.; Lockwood, R.; Hornreich, J.; et al. Fatal dog attacks, 1989–94. *Pediatrics* 97:891-895, 1996.

[56] NCHS. *Mortality Data Tapes*. Hyattsville, MD: NCHS.

[57] Singh, G.K.; Kochanek, K.D.; and MacDorman, M.F. Advance report of final mortality statistics, 1994. *Monthly Vital Statistics Report* 45(3S), 1996.

[58] NCHS. *Mortality Data Tapes*. Hyattsville, MD: NCHS, 1994.

[59] NCHS. *Vital Statistics System for Numbers of Deaths, Bureau of the Census population estimates*. Washington, DC: CDC, March 2000.

[60] World Health Organization (WHO). *World Health Statistics Annual, 1994*. Geneva, Switzerland: WHO, 1995.

[61] HHS, Administration on Children, Youth, and Families. *Child Maltreatment 1997: Reports from the States to the National Child Abuse and Neglect Data System*. Washington, DC: U.S. Government Printing Office (GPO), 1999.

[62] Federal Bureau of Investigation. *Crime in the United States: 1996*. Washington, DC: GPO, 1997.

[63] Bureau of Justice Statistics (BJS). *Violence-Related Injuries Treated in Hospital Emergency Departments*. Washington, DC: U.S. Department of Justice (DOJ), 1997.

[64] Tjaden, P., and Thoennes, N. *Prevalence, Incidence, and Consequences of Violence Against Women: Findings From the National Violence Against Women Survey*. Pub. No. NCJ 172837. Washington, DC: National Institute of Justice and CDC, 1998.

[65] Gazmararian, J.A.; Lazorick, S.; Spitz, A.M.; et al. Prevalance of violence against pregnant women. *Journal of the American Medical Association* 275:1915-1920, 1996.

[66] Hotaling, G.T., and Sugarman, D.,B. An analysis of risk markers in husband to wife violence: The current state of knowledge. *Violence and Victims* 1:101-124, 1986.

[67] DOJ, BLS. *Crime Victimization in the United States, 1994*. Washington, DC: BJS, 1997.

[68] Bachman, R., and Taylor, B. The measurement of family violence and rape by the redesigned national crime victimization survey. *Justice Quarterly* 11:701-714, 1994.

[69] Kilpatrick, D.G.; Edmunds, C.N.; and Seymour, A.L. *Rape in America: A Report to the Nation*. Arlington, VA: National Victim Center, 1992, 2.

[70] DOJ. *Statistics. Criminal Victimization 1998: Changes 1997–98 With Trends, 1993–98*. Pub. No. NCJ-176353. Washington, DC: DOJ, 1999.

[71] CDC. Youth Risk Behavior Surveillance—United States, 1999. *Morbidity and Mortality Weekly Report* 49(SS5), June 9, 2000.

[72] NCIPC. *Best Practices for Preventing Violence by Children and Adolescents: A Source Book*. Atlanta, GA: NCIPC, November 1999 (in press).

16

Maternal, Infant, and Child Health

Co-Lead Agencies: Centers for Disease Control and Prevention
                     Health Resources and Services Administration

Contents

Improve the health and well-being of women, infants, children, and families.

Overview

The health of mothers, infants, and children is of critical importance, both as a reflection of the current health status of a large segment of the U.S. population and as a predictor of the health of the next generation. This focus area addresses a range of indicators of maternal, infant, and child health—those primarily affecting pregnant and postpartum women (including indicators of maternal illness and death) and those that affect infants' health and survival (including infant mortality rates; birth outcomes; prevention of birth defects; access to preventive care; and fetal, perinatal, and other infant deaths).

Infant mortality is an important measure of a nation's health and a worldwide indicator of health status and social well-being. As of 1995, the U.S. infant mortality rates ranked 25th among industrialized nations.[1] In the past decade, critical measures of increased risk of infant death, such as new cases of low birth weight (LBW) and very low birth weight (VLBW), actually have increased in the United States. In addition, the disparity in infant mortality rates between whites and specific racial and ethnic groups (especially African Americans, American Indians or Alaska Natives, Native Hawaiians, and Puerto Ricans) persists. Although the overall infant mortality rate has reached record low levels, the rate for African Americans remains twice that of whites.[2]

Issues and Trends

In 1997, 28,045 infants died before their first birthday, for an overall rate of 7.2 deaths per 1,000 live births. This rate has declined steadily over the past 20 years; in 1975, the infant mortality rate was over 15 per 1,000 live births.[2] In 1997, two-thirds of all infant deaths took place during the first 28 days of life (the neonatal period). The overall neonatal mortality rate in 1997 was 4.8 per 1,000 live births.[2] The remaining one-third of infant deaths took place during the postneonatal period from an infant's 29th day of life until the first birthday. The U.S. postneonatal mortality rate in 1997 was 2.4 deaths per 1,000 live births.[2]

Four causes account for more than half of all infant deaths: birth defects, disorders relating to short gestation and unspecified LBW, sudden infant death syndrome (SIDS), and respiratory distress syndrome. The leading causes of neonatal death in 1997 were birth defects, disorders related to short gestation and LBW, respiratory distress syndrome, and maternal complications of pregnancy. After the first month of life, SIDS is the leading cause of infant death, accounting for about one-third of

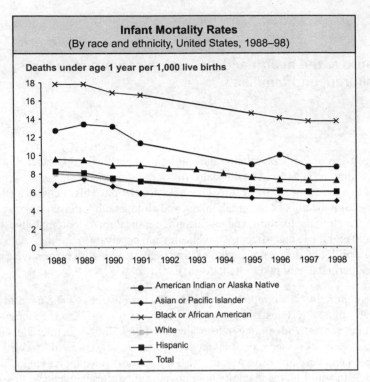

Infant Mortality Rates
(By race and ethnicity, United States, 1988–98)

Deaths under age 1 year per 1,000 live births

Legend:
- American Indian or Alaska Native
- Asian or Pacific Islander
- Black or African American
- White
- Hispanic
- Total

Source: CDC, NCHS. National Vital Statistics System (NVSS). Data for 1998 are preliminary; 1992–94 linked live birth-infant death files are not available.

Note: Data for white and Hispanic overlap from 1991 to 1998.

all deaths during this period. Maternal age also is a risk factor for infant death. Mortality rates are highest among infants born to young teenagers (aged 16 years and under) and to mothers aged 44 years and older.

The death of fetuses before birth is another important indicator of perinatal health. In 1996, nearly 7 fetal deaths were reported for every 1,000 live births and fetal deaths combined, representing a slight decline from the fetal mortality rate of 7.6 per 1,000 in 1987.[2] Fetal death sometimes is associated with pregnancies complicated by such risk factors as problems with amniotic fluid levels and maternal blood disorders.[3] Early, comprehensive, and risk-appropriate care to manage such conditions has contributed to reductions in fetal mortality rates.

Short gestation and LBW are among the leading causes of neonatal death, accounting for 20 percent of neonatal deaths. In 1998, a total of 11.6 percent of births were preterm, and 7.6 percent were LBW.[4] Included in these statistics were VLBW infants weighing less than 1,500 grams (3.3 pounds). The rate of VLBW births was 1.4 percent in 1998. The VLBW rate has increased slightly since 1990 among whites and other population groups including African Americans, Puerto Ricans, and American Indians.[1]

LBW is associated with long-term disabilities, such as cerebral palsy, autism, mental retardation, vision and hearing impairments, and other developmental disabilities. (See Focus Area 6. Disability and Secondary Conditions and Focus Area 28. Vision and Hearing.) Despite the low proportion of pregnancies resulting in LBW babies, expenditures for the care of LBW infants total more than half of the costs incurred for all newborns. In 1988, the cost of a normal, healthy delivery averaged $1,900, whereas hospital costs for LBW infants averaged $6,200.[5]

The general category of LBW infants includes both those born too early (preterm infants) and those who are born at full term but who are too small, a condition known as intrauterine growth retardation (IUGR). Maternal characteristics that are risk factors associated with IUGR include maternal LBW, prior LBW birth history, low prepregnancy weight, cigarette smoking, multiple births, and low pregnancy weight gain. Cigarette smoking is the greatest known risk factor.[6]

VLBW usually is associated with preterm birth. Relatively little is known about risk factors for preterm birth, but the primary risk factors are prior preterm birth and spontaneous abortion, low prepregnancy weight, and cigarette smoking.[6] These risk factors account for only one-third of all preterm births.

The use of alcohol, tobacco, and illegal substances during pregnancy is a major risk factor for LBW and other poor infant outcomes. Alcohol use is linked to fetal death, LBW, growth abnormalities, mental retardation, and fetal alcohol syndrome (FAS).[7] Overall rates of alcohol use during pregnancy have increased during the 1990s, and the proportion of pregnant women using alcohol at higher and more hazardous levels has increased substantially. Smoking during pregnancy is linked to LBW, preterm delivery, SIDS, and respiratory problems in newborns. In addition to the human cost of these conditions, the economic cost of services to substance-exposed infants is great: health expenditures related to FAS are estimated to be from $75 million to $9.7 billion each year.[7] Over $500 million a year is spent on medical expenses for infants exposed to cocaine in utero.[8] Smoking-attributable costs of complicated births in 1995 were estimated at $1.4 billion (11 percent of costs for all complicated births, based on smoking prevalence during pregnancy of 19 percent) and $2.0 billion (15 percent for all complicated births, based on smoking prevalence during pregnancy of 27 percent).[9]

Finally, breastfeeding is an important contributor to overall infant health because human breast milk presents the most complete form of nutrition for infants; therefore, the American Academy of Pediatrics recommends that infants be breastfed for approximately the first 6 months of life.[10] (The American Academy of Pediatrics recommends that women who test positive for human immunodeficiency virus (HIV) not breastfeed to help prevent transmission of the virus to their infants.)[11] Breastfeeding rates have increased over the years, particularly in early infancy. However, breastfeeding rates among women of all races decrease substantially by 5 to 6 months postpartum. The 1998 rates at 5 to 6 months were only 31 percent among white women, 19 percent among African American women, and 28 percent among Hispanic women.[12]

Also important to child health are the prevention and treatment of disabilities in children. Twelve percent of all children under age 18 years have a disability (defined as a limitation in one or more functional areas). In 1994, 10.6 percent of all children aged 5 to 17 years had limitations in learning ability, 6 percent had limitations in communication, 1.3 percent had limitations in mobility, and 0.9 percent had limitations in personal care.[13] The burden of childhood disability is compounded because affected children live with their disabling conditions many more years than do persons acquiring disability later in life. In 1992, asthma and mental retardation were the most common disabling conditions, accounting for 40 percent of all activity limitations.[14] Other major disabling conditions in childhood include speech impairment, hearing impairment, cerebral palsy, epilepsy, and leg impairment. (See Focus Area 6. Disability and Secondary Conditions and Focus Area 28. Vision and Hearing.)

The objectives in this focus area cover the broad array of childhood conditions and genetic disorders. Examples of preventable birth defects are spina bifida and other neural tube defects (NTDs). The occurrence of these disorders could be reduced by more than half if women consumed adequate folic acid before and during pregnancy.[15]

All States require newborns to be screened for genetic conditions, such as phenylketonuria (PKU) and hypothyroidism; the majority of States also require screening for sickle cell disease. Although not necessarily preventable, these conditions are susceptible to intervention after delivery. For example, nutritional interventions in infancy can prevent mental retardation in children with PKU, penicillin can prevent infection in children with sickle cell disease, and hormone replacement can prevent mental retardation in children with hypothyroidism. Thus, adequate screening of newborns is the first step toward prevention of illness, disability, and death.

In addition to infant deaths and health conditions, the effect of pregnancy and childbirth on women is an important indicator of women's health. In 1997, a total of 327 maternal deaths were reported by vital statistics.[16] While this number is small, maternal death remains significant because a high proportion of these deaths are preventable and because of the impact of women's premature death on families. The maternal mortality ratio among African American women consistently has been three to four times that of white women. Ectopic pregnancy is an important cause of pregnancy-related illness and disability in the United States and the leading cause of maternal death in the first trimester. The risk of ectopic pregnancy increases with age; women of all races aged 35 to 44 years are at more than three times the risk of ectopic pregnancy than are women aged 15 to 24 years.[17] Preeclampsia and eclampsia also are important causes of maternal death.

Other causes of maternal death are hemorrhage, embolism, infection, and anesthesia-related complications.

The rates of many of these indicators have shown improvement over the past decade. The rate of infant mortality declined more than 27 percent between 1987 and 1997. The rate of fetal mortality declined 8 percent between 1987 and 1995.[1] Other indicators show less progress. The LBW rate increased 10 percent between 1987 and 1998.[1] The rate of FAS has risen steeply, especially among African Americans.[18] In addition, the maternal mortality rate has not declined since 1982, nor has the disparity between African American and white women.[2, 19]

Despite these unfavorable trends, evidence is encouraging about increases in women's use of health practices that can help their own health and that of their infants. The percentage of pregnant women who start prenatal care early increased 9.2 percent between 1987 and 1998. The percentage of mothers who breastfeed their newborns also went up 18.5 percent between 1988 and 1998, with greater gains among African American and Hispanic women. Other maternal health practices have shown less improvement: in 1992–94, the proportion of women of childbearing age reporting consumption of the recommended level of folic acid (400 micrograms) was 21 percent.

Disparities

Many of these conditions and risk factors disproportionately affect certain racial and ethnic groups. The disparities between white and nonwhite groups in infant death, maternal death, and LBW are wide and, in many cases, are growing. Specifically:

■ The 1997 infant mortality rate among African American infants was 2.3 times that of white infants. Although infant mortality rates have declined within both racial groups, the proportional discrepancy between African Americans and whites remains largely unchanged.[16]

■ The rate of maternal mortality among African Americans is 20.3 per 100,000 live births, nearly four times the white rate of 5.1 per 100,000. African American women continue to be three to four times more likely than white women to die of pregnancy and its complications. The maternal death differential between African Americans and whites is highest for pregnancies that did not end in live birth (ectopic pregnancy, spontaneous and induced abortions, and gestational trophoblastic disease).[19]

■ Rates of LBW for white women have risen from 5.7 percent of births in 1990 to 6.5 percent in 1998. Among African Americans, the LBW rate has declined slightly in the 1990s but remains twice as high as that of whites—13 percent in 1998. African Americans also are more likely to have other risk factors, such as young maternal age, high birth order (that is, having many live births), less education, and inadequate prenatal care. Puerto Ricans also are especially likely to have LBW infants.[4]

■ American Indians or Alaska Natives and African Americans account for a disproportionate share of FAS deaths. In 1990, the rates of FAS among American Indians or Alaska Natives and African Americans were 5.2 and 1.4 per 1,000 live births, respectively, compared with 0.4 per 1,000 among the population as a whole.[18]

African American and Hispanic women also are less likely than whites to enter prenatal care early. For both African American and white women, the proportion entering prenatal care in the first trimester rises with maternal age until the late thirties, then begins to decline. For example, in 1998, 57 percent of African American women under age 18 years began care early, compared with 66 percent of white women of the same age. Among women aged 18 to 24 years, 68 percent of African Americans received care in their first trimester, compared to 76 percent of white women. Among women aged 25 to 39 years, 79 percent of African American women entered care early, compared with 89 percent of white women.[4]

Women in certain racial and ethnic groups also are less likely than white women to breastfeed their infants. In the early postpartum period, 45 percent of African American mothers and 66 percent of Hispanic mothers breastfed in 1998, compared with 68 percent of white women. These differences persist at 5 to 6 months postpartum, when 19 percent of African American women, 28 percent of Hispanic women, and 31 percent of white women breastfed.[12]

Opportunities

Many of the risk factors mentioned can be mitigated or prevented with good preconception and prenatal care. First, preconception screening and counseling offer an opportunity to identify and mitigate maternal risk factors before pregnancy begins. Examples include daily folic acid consumption (a protective factor) and alcohol use (a risk factor). During preconceptional counseling, healthcare providers also can refer women for medical and psychosocial or support services for any risk factors identified. Counseling needs to be culturally appropriate and linguistically competent. Prenatal visits offer an opportunity to provide information about the adverse effects of substance use, including alcohol and tobacco during pregnancy, and serve as a vehicle for referrals to treatment services. The use of timely, high-quality prenatal care can help to prevent poor birth outcomes and improve maternal health by identifying women who are at particularly high risk and taking steps to mitigate risks, such as the risk of high blood pressure or other maternal complications. Interventions targeted at prevention and cessation of substance use during pregnancy may be helpful in further reducing the rate of preterm delivery and low birth weight.[20, 21, 22] Further promotion of folic acid intake can help to reduce the rate of NTDs.[23, 24]

Other actions taken after birth can significantly improve infants' health and chances of survival. Breastfeeding has been shown to reduce rates of infection in infants and to improve long-term maternal health.[25, 26, 27, 28, 29, 30, 31, 32, 33, 34, 35, 36, 37, 38] SIDS may be preventable as well; studies show that putting infants to sleep on their backs can help to prevent SIDS.[39]

Interim Progress Toward Year 2000 Objectives

Of the 17 maternal and infant health objectives included in Healthy People 2000, progress has been made toward the target in 8 objectives, and movement has been away from the target in 5 objectives. Notable gains have been made in the areas of infant death, fetal death, cesarean birth (particularly repeat cesareans), breastfeeding, early use of prenatal care, hospitalization for complications of pregnancy, abstinence from tobacco use during pregnancy, and screening for fetal abnormalities and genetic disorders. However, no progress or movement in the wrong direction has occurred in the areas of maternal death, FAS, and LBW. For the other objectives, progress has been mixed, or data remain unavailable. Child health objectives were not included in the Maternal and Infant focus area in Healthy People 2000.

Note: Unless otherwise noted, data are from the Centers for Disease Control and Prevention, National Center for Health Statistics, *Healthy People 2000 Review, 1998–99*.

Maternal, Infant, and Child Health

Goal: Improve the health and well-being of women, infants, children, and families.

Number   Objective Short Title

Fetal, Infant, Child, and Adolescent Deaths

16-1   Fetal and infant deaths

16-2   Child deaths

16-3   Adolescent and young adult deaths

Maternal Deaths and Illnesses

16-4   Maternal deaths

16-5   Maternal illness and complications due to pregnancy

Prenatal Care

16-6   Prenatal care

16-7   Childbirth classes

Obstetrical Care

16-8   Very low birth weight infants born at level III hospitals

16-9   Cesarean births

Risk Factors

16-10   Low birth weight and very low birth weight

16-11   Preterm births

16-12   Weight gain during pregnancy

16-13   Infants put to sleep on their backs

Developmental Disabilities and Neural Tube Defects

16-14   Developmental disabilities

16-15   Spina bifida and other neural tube defects

16-16   Optimum folic acid levels

Prenatal Substance Exposure

16-17   Prenatal substance exposure

16-18   Fetal alcohol syndrome

Breastfeeding, Newborn Screening, and Service Systems

Fetal, Infant, Child, and Adolescent Deaths

16-1. Reduce fetal and infant deaths.

Target and baseline:

Objective	Reduction in Fetal and Infant Deaths	1997 Baseline	2010 Target
		Per 1,000 Live Births Plus Fetal Deaths	
16-1a.	Fetal deaths at 20 or more weeks of gestation	6.8	4.1
16-1b.	Fetal and infant deaths during perinatal period (28 weeks of gestation to 7 days or more after birth)	7.5	4.5

Target setting method: Better than the best.

Data source: National Vital Statistics System (NVSS), CDC, NCHS.

NOTE: THE TABLE BELOW MAY CONTINUE TO THE FOLLOWING PAGE.

Live Births Plus Fetal Deaths, 1997	16-1a. Fetal Deaths at 20 or More Weeks of Gestation	16-1b. Fetal and Infant Deaths During Perinatal Period
	Rate per 1,000	
TOTAL	6.8	7.5
Mother's race and ethnicity		
American Indian or Alaska Native	6.7	7.9
Asian or Pacific Islander	4.8	4.6
Asian	4.2	4.6
Native Hawaiian and other Pacific Islander	6.2	7.3
Black or African American	12.5	13.4
White	5.8	6.4
Hispanic or Latino	5.9	6.5
Not Hispanic or Latino	DNA	7.2
Black or African American	9.6	12.7
White	5.2	6.0

Live Births Plus Fetal Deaths, 1997	16-1a. Fetal Deaths at 20 or More Weeks of Gestation	16-1b. Fetal and Infant Deaths During Perinatal Period
	Rate per 1,000	
Gender		
Female	DNA	DNA
Male	DNA	DNA
Mother's education level		
Less than high school	6.5	DNA
High school graduate	6.7	DNA
At least some college	4.8	DNA
Mother's disability status		
Mothers with disabilities	DNC	DNC
Mothers without disabilities	DNC	DNC
Select populations		
Mother's age groups		
Under 15 years	14.2	DNA
15 to 19 years	7.8	DNA
20 to 24 years	6.4	DNA
25 to 29 years	6.0	DNA
30 to 34 years	6.3	DNA
35 years and older	8.9	DNA
Fetal weight		
>2,499 g	1.3	DNA
1,500 to 2,499 g	16.8	DNA
<1,500 g	213.1	DNA

DNA = Data have not been analyzed. DNC = Data are not collected. DSU = Data are statistically unreliable.

NOTE: THE TABLE ABOVE MAY HAVE CONTINUED FROM THE PREVIOUS PAGE.

Target and baseline:

Objective	Reduction in Infant Deaths	1998 Baseline	2010 Target
		Rate per 1,000 Live Births	
16-1c.	All infant deaths (within 1 year)	7.2	4.5
16-1d.	Neonatal deaths (within the first 28 days of life)	4.8	2.9
16-1e.	Postneonatal deaths (between 28 days and 1 year)	2.4	1.2

Target setting method: Better than the best.

Data source: National Vital Statistics System (NVSS), CDC, NCHS.

NOTE: THE TABLE BELOW MAY CONTINUE TO THE FOLLOWING PAGE.

Live Births, 1998	16-1c. All Infant Deaths (<1 year)	16-1d. Neonatal Deaths (<28 days)	16-1e. Postneona- tal Deaths (28 to 364 days)
	Rate per 1,000		
TOTAL	7.2	4.8	2.4
Mother's race and ethnicity			
American Indian or Alaska Native	9.3	5.0	4.3
Asian or Pacific Islander	5.5	3.9	1.7
Asian	5.0	3.6	1.3
Native Hawaiian and other Pacific Islander	10.0	6.7	3.3
Black or African American	13.8	9.4	4.4
White	6.0	4.0	2.0
Hispanic or Latino	5.8	3.9	1.9
Not Hispanic or Latino	7.5	5.0	2.5
Black or African American	13.9	9.4	4.5
White	6.0	3.9	2.0
Gender			
Female	6.5	4.4	2.2
Male	7.8	5.2	2.6
Mother's education level			
Less than high school	9.1	5.2	3.8
High school graduate	7.7	5.1	2.6
At least some college	5.3	3.8	1.5
Mother's disability status			
Mothers with disabilities	DNC	DNC	DNC
Mothers without disabilities	DNC	DNC	DNC
Select populations			
Mother's age groups			
Under 15 years	18.4	12.6	5.8
15 to 19 years	10.0	6.1	3.9
20 to 24 years	7.8	4.8	3.0
25 to 29 years	6.3	4.3	2.0

Live Births, 1998	16-1c. All Infant Deaths (<1 year)	16-1d. Neonatal Deaths (<28 days)	16-1e. Postneonatal Deaths (28 to 364 days)
	Rate per 1,000		
30 to 34 years	6.0	4.4	1.6
35 years and older	7.1	5.2	1.9
Fetal weight			
>2,499 g	2.6	0.9	1.7
1,500 to 2,499 g	16.5	9.6	6.8
<1,500 g	250.0	221.5	28.5

DNA = Data have not been analyzed. DNC = Data are not collected. DSU = Data are statistically unreliable.

NOTE: THE TABLE ABOVE MAY HAVE CONTINUED FROM THE PREVIOUS PAGE.

Target and baseline:

Objective	Reduction in Infant Deaths Related to Birth Defects	1998 Baseline	2010 Target
		Rate per 1,000 Live Births	
16-1f.	All birth defects	1.6	1.1
16-1g.	Congenital heart defects	0.53	0.38

Target setting method: Better than the best.

Data source: National Vital Statistics System (NVSS), CDC, NCHS.

NOTE: THE TABLE BELOW MAY CONTINUE TO THE FOLLOWING PAGE.

Live Births, 1998 (unless noted)	16-1f. All Infant Deaths From All Birth Defects	16-1g. All Infant Deaths From Congenital Heart Defects
	Rate per 1,000	
TOTAL	1.6	0.53
Mother's race and ethnicity		
American Indian or Alaska Native	1.7	0.67
Asian or Pacific Islander	1.5	0.50
Asian	1.5	0.48
Native Hawaiian and other Pacific Islander	DSU	DSU
Black or African American	1.8	0.60
White	1.5	0.51

Live Births, 1998 (unless noted)	16-1f. All Infant Deaths From All Birth Defects	16-1g. All Infant Deaths From Congenital Heart Defects
	Rate per 1,000	
Hispanic or Latino	1.5	0.47
Not Hispanic or Latino	1.6	0.54
Black or African American	1.8	0.61
White	1.5	0.53
Gender		
Female	1.6 (1995)	DNA
Male	1.8 (1995)	DNA
Mother's education level		
Less than high school	1.8	0.58
High school graduate	1.6	0.58
At least some college	1.4	0.45
Disability status (of infant)		
Persons with disabilities	DNC	DNC
Persons without disabilities	DNC	DNC

DNA = Data have not been analyzed. DNC = Data are not collected. DSU = Data are statistically unreliable.

NOTE: THE TABLE ABOVE MAY HAVE CONTINUED FROM THE PREVIOUS PAGE.

16-1h. Reduce deaths from sudden infant death syndrome (SIDS).

Target: 0.25 deaths per 1,000 live births.

Baseline: 0.72 deaths per 1,000 live births were from SIDS in 1998.

Target setting method: Better than the best.

Data source: National Vital Statistics System (NVSS), CDC, NCHS.

NOTE: THE TABLE BELOW MAY CONTINUE TO THE FOLLOWING PAGE.

Live Births, 1998	16-1h. SIDS Deaths
	Rate per 1,000
TOTAL	0.72
Mother's race and ethnicity	
American Indian or Alaska Native	1.52
Asian or Pacific Islander	0.39
Asian	0.27
Native Hawaiian and other Pacific Islander	DSU

Live Births, 1998	16-1h. SIDS Deaths
	Rate per 1,000
Black or African American	1.38
White	0.60
Hispanic or Latino	0.37
Not Hispanic or Latino	0.80
Black or African American	1.40
White	0.66
Gender	
Female	DNA
Male	DNA
Mother's education level	
Less than high school	1.30
High school graduate	0.79
At least some college	0.38
Disability status (of infant)	
Persons with disabilities	DNC
Persons without disabilities	DNC

DNA = Data have not been analyzed. DNC = Data are not collected. DSU = Data are statistically unreliable.
NOTE: THE TABLE ABOVE MAY HAVE CONTINUED FROM THE PREVIOUS PAGE.

Infant death is a critical indicator of the health of a population. It reflects the over-all state of maternal health as well as the quality and accessibility of primary health care available to pregnant women and infants. Despite steady declines in the 1980s and 1990s, the rate of infant mortality in the United States remains among the highest in the industrialized world.[1] Moreover, the rate of decline in infant mortality has slowed since the 1970s, when major advances in neonatal care contributed to steep reductions in the neonatal mortality rate. However, the rapid decline in this rate slowed during the 1980s. In the early 1990s, the introduction of synthetic surfactant contributed to declines in neonatal mortality rates through decreased new cases of intraventricular hemorrhage and decreased severity of respiratory disease in preterm, very small infants.[40, 41]

The health of infants depends in large part on their health in utero. A fetus with severe defects or growth problems may not be delivered alive. Because only live births are counted in infant mortality rates, perinatal and fetal mortality rates provide a more complete picture of perinatal health than does the infant mortality rate alone.

Fetal death often is associated with maternal complications of pregnancy, such as problems with amniotic fluid levels and blood disorders. Rates of fetal mortality are 35 percent greater than average in women who use tobacco during pregnancy and 77 percent higher in women who use alcohol.[3] Fetal mortality rates also are high when birth defects, such as anencephalus, renal agenesis, and hydrocephalus, are present.[3] The baseline fetal mortality rate of 6.8 per 1,000 represents only a 6.7 percent reduction since 1990, an average rate of decline of 1.3 percent per year. The fetal mortality rate among African Americans was 12.7 per 1,000 in 1995, 1.8 times that of the population as a whole. Moreover, this gap has widened since 1990. The rate among African Americans declined by only 4.5 percent over this period, a decline of less than 1 percent per year.[3] Targeting prenatal risk screening and intervention to high-risk groups, particularly African American women, is critical to reducing this gap.

The perinatal mortality rate includes both deaths of live-born infants through the first 7 days of life and fetal deaths after 28 weeks of gestation. This rate is a useful overall measure of perinatal health and the quality of health care provided to pregnant women and newborns. The rate of perinatal mortality has declined by 40 percent since 1980.[1] The gap between African Americans and whites has increased, however, with the rate among African Americans now more than twice that of whites.[1]

The infant mortality rate is made up of two components: neonatal mortality (death in the first 28 days of life) and postneonatal mortality (death from the infants' 29th day but within the first year). The leading causes of neonatal death include birth defects, disorders related to short gestation and LBW, and pregnancy complications. Of these, the most likely to be preventable are those related to preterm birth and LBW, which represent approximately 20 percent of neonatal deaths. Postneonatal death reflects events experienced in infancy, including SIDS, birth defects, injuries, and homicide. Birth defects, many of which are unlikely to be preventable given current scientific knowledge, account for approximately 17 percent of postneonatal deaths; the remainder are likely to stem from preventable causes.

SIDS is the leading cause of postneonatal death among all racial and ethnic groups, representing nearly one-third of all cases of postneonatal death. Moreover, the rate of SIDS among African Americans is 1.4 per 1,000 live births, twice that of whites. Therefore, a reduction in the rate of death from SIDS, particularly among African Americans, would contribute greatly to reducing the overall infant mortality rate and particularly to closing the racial gap in postneonatal death. The 2010 target should be achievable with continued education. (See objective 16-13 for further discussion of interventions that can help to prevent SIDS).

Rates of death from birth defects can be reduced either by preventing the occurrence of the defect itself or by providing the necessary care to prevent death. In the case of NTDs, the birth defects themselves can be prevented (see objectives 16-17 and 16-18). Death from birth defects that are not so easily prevented, such as heart problems, can be reduced with access to appropriate medical care. (Respiratory distress syndrome, another leading cause of infant death, is not a birth defect but a consequence of prematurity.)

A particular issue in the reduction of infant death is the reduction of disparities among select populations, particularly as defined by race and ethnicity, maternal age, and infant birth weight. The gap between whites and African Americans in infant death is large and has not diminished since 1990.

16-2. Reduce the rate of child deaths.

Target and baseline:

Objective	Reduction in Deaths of Children	1998 Baseline	2010 Target
		Rate per 100,000	
16-2a.	Children aged 1 to 4 years	34.6	18.6
16-2b.	Children aged 5 to 9 years	17.7	12.3

Target setting method: Better than the best.

Data source: National Vital Statistics System (NVSS), CDC, NCHS.

NOTE: THE TABLE BELOW MAY CONTINUE TO THE FOLLOWING PAGE.

Children, 1998	16-2a. Deaths of Children Aged 1 to 4 Years	16-2b. Deaths of Children Aged 5 to 9 Years
	Rate per 100,000	
TOTAL	34.6	17.7
Race and ethnicity		
American Indian or Alaska Native	59.2	22.3
Asian or Pacific Islander	18.7	12.4
Asian	DNC	DNC
Native Hawaiian and other Pacific Islander	DNC	DNC
Black or African American	61.6	29.0
White	30.1	15.7
Hispanic or Latino	30.4	15.7
Not Hispanic or Latino	35.3	18.0
Black or African American	64.7	30.6
White	29.4	15.3

Children, 1998	16-2a. Deaths of Children Aged 1 to 4 Years	16-2b. Deaths of Children Aged 5 to 9 Years
	Rate per 100,000	
Gender		
Female	31.4	15.3
Male	37.6	20.0
Family income level		
Poor	DNC	DNC
Near poor	DNC	DNC
Middle/high income	DNC	DNC
Disability status		
Persons with disabilities	DNC	DNC
Persons without disabilities	DNC	DNC

DNA = Data have not been analyzed. DNC = Data are not collected. DSU = Data are statistically unreliable.
NOTE: THE TABLE ABOVE MAY HAVE CONTINUED FROM THE PREVIOUS PAGE.

The deaths of children after infancy also present a public health concern and an opportunity for prevention. In 1997, 13,562 children aged 1 to 14 years died, representing a death rate of 25.1 per 100,000 children in that age group. The leading cause of death for children of all ages is injury, which accounts for 13.1 deaths per 100,000 preschool children (aged 1 to 4 years) and 8.7 deaths per 100,000 school-aged children (aged 5 to 14 years). Among children aged 1 to 4 years, the leading injury-related causes of death are motor vehicle crashes, drownings, and fires and burns. Among those aged 5 to 14 years, the leading causes of death include motor vehicle crashes and firearms (including unintentional deaths, homicides, and suicides). These deaths are, for the most part, preventable. Other leading causes of death among children that are less likely to be preventable include birth defects (representing 3.8 deaths per 100,000 children aged 1 to 4 years and 1.2 deaths per 100,000 children aged 5 to 14 years), malignant neoplasms (representing 2.9 deaths per 100,000 children aged 1 to 4 years and 2.7 deaths per 100,000 children aged 5 to 14 years), and diseases of the heart (representing 1.4 deaths per 100,000 children aged 1 to 4 years and 0.8 deaths per 100,000 children aged 5 to 14 years).[16]

16-3. Reduce deaths of adolescents and young adults.

Target and baseline:

Objective	Reduction in Deaths of Adolescents and Young Adults	1998 Baseline	2010 Target
		Rate per 100,000	
16-3a.	Adolescents aged 10 to 14 years	22.1	16.8
16-3b.	Adolescents aged 15 to 19 years	70.6	39.8
16-3c.	Young adults aged 20 to 24 years	95.3	49.0

Target setting method: Better than the best.

Data source: National Vital Statistics System (NVSS), CDC, NCHS.

NOTE: THE TABLE BELOW MAY CONTINUE TO THE FOLLOWING PAGE.

Adolescents and Young Adults, 1998	16-3a. Deaths of Adolescents Aged 10 to 14 Years	16-3b. Deaths of Adolescents Aged 15 to 19 Years	16-3c. Deaths of Young Adults Aged 20 to 24 Years
	Rate per 100,000		
TOTAL	22.1	70.6	95.3
Race and ethnicity			
American Indian or Alaska Native	26.7	90.5	146.1
Asian or Pacific Islander	17.9	39.9	49.1
Asian	DNC	DNC	DNC
Native Hawaiian and other Pacific Islander	DNC	DNC	DNC
Black or African American	29.9	97.2	160.3
White	20.8	66.6	84.9
Hispanic or Latino	19.1	67.6	99.6
Not Hispanic or Latino	22.6	70.7	94.0
Black or African American	31.3	100.8	165.8
White	20.8	65.3	80.2
Gender			
Female	17.2	40.8	46.5
Male	26.9	98.7	142.3
Family income level			
Poor	DNC	DNC	DNC
Near poor	DNC	DNC	DNC
Middle/high income	DNC	DNC	DNC

Adolescents and Young Adults, 1998	16-3a. Deaths of Adolescents Aged 10 to 14 Years	16-3b. Deaths of Adolescents Aged 15 to 19 Years	16-3c. Deaths of Young Adults Aged 20 to 24 Years
	Rate per 100,000		
Disability status			
Persons with disabilities	DNC	DNC	DNC
Persons without disabilities	DNC	DNC	DNC

DNA = Data have not been analyzed. DNC = Data are not collected. DSU = Data are statistically unreliable.

NOTE: THE TABLE ABOVE MAY HAVE CONTINUED FROM THE PREVIOUS PAGE.

The deaths of young adolescents, older adolescents, and young adults are more likely to be due to external causes than to congenital diseases. There were 4,261 deaths among adolescents aged 10 to 14 years in 1998, for a mortality rate of 22.1 per 100,000. The leading cause of death for adolescents in this age group was motor vehicle crashes at 5.4 deaths per 100,000 or 24.3 percent of the total mortality. Other unintentional injuries (such as falls, drownings, and poisonings) caused 3.5 deaths per 100,000 (15.9 percent); homicides caused 1.5 deaths per 100,000 (6.8 percent); suicides caused 1.6 deaths per 100,000 (7.4 percent); and AIDS caused 0.1 deaths per 100,000 (0.6 percent). Fifty-five percent of the total deaths in this age group, therefore, can be attributed to unnecessary (that is, preventable) causes. Other causes of death for this age group that are less amenable to prevention strategies given current scientific knowledge include malignant neoplasms, which caused 2.7 deaths per 100,000 (12.3 percent); birth defects, which caused 0.9 deaths per 100,000 (4.1 percent); diseases of the heart, which caused 0.9 deaths per 100,000 (4.0 percent); and a combination of other causes, which caused 5.5 deaths per 100,000 (25 percent).[16, 42]

There were 13,788 deaths in 1998 among adolescents aged 15 to 19 years, for a death rate of 70.6 per 100,000. The leading cause of death for adolescents in this age group was motor vehicle crashes at 28.4 deaths per 100,000 or 37.4 percent of total deaths. Other unintentional injuries (such as falls, drownings, and poisonings) caused 7.3 deaths per 100,000 (10.4 percent); homicides caused 11.8 deaths per 100,000 (16.8 percent); suicides caused 8.9 deaths per 100,000 (12.6 percent); and AIDS caused 0.1 deaths per 100,000 (0.2 percent). Consequently, a majority (77 percent) of the total deaths in this age group can be attributed to unnecessary (that is, preventable) causes. The remaining 23 percent of deaths among adolescents aged 15 to 19 years resulted mostly from malignant neoplasms, which caused 3.7 deaths per 100,000 (5.2 percent); diseases of the heart, which caused 2.1 deaths per 100,000 (3.0 percent); birth defects, which caused 1.1 deaths per 100,000 (1.6 percent); and a combination of other causes, which caused 9.1 deaths per 100,000 (12.9 percent).

Young adults aged 20 to 24 years had a death rate of 95.3 per 100,000 in 1998—a rate 331 percent higher than adolescents aged 10 to 14 years and 35 percent higher than adolescents aged 15 to 19 years. The leading cause of death for persons aged 20 to 24 years was motor vehicle crashes at 27.5 deaths per 100,000 or 28.9 percent of the total deaths. Other unintentional injuries (such as falls, drownings, and poisonings) caused 10.7 deaths per 100,000 (11.2 percent); homicides caused 18.1 deaths per 100,000 (19 percent); suicides caused 13.6 deaths per 100,000 (14.2 percent); and AIDS caused 1.0 deaths per 100,000 (1.4 percent). Consequently, a majority (74 percent) of the total deaths in this age group can be attributed to unnecessary (that is, preventable) causes. The remaining 26 percent of deaths among young adults aged 20 to 24 years resulted mostly from malignant neoplasms, which caused 5.5 deaths per 100,000 (5.8 percent); diseases of the heart, which caused 3.6 deaths per 100,000 (3.8 percent); birth defects, which caused 1.3 deaths per 100,000 (1.4 percent); and a combination of other causes, which caused 13.9 deaths per 100,000 (14.6 percent).

The data on deaths, however, do not adequately reflect consequences of sexual behaviors established as individuals in this age group become sexually mature. Illustratively, it is likely that most of the new HIV infections that are diagnosed each year occur among those between age 13 and 21 years. Further, about 3 million new and sexually transmitted disease infections (STDs) in addition to HIV occur among teenagers each year. In addition, about 1 million teenagers become pregnant each year. (See Focus Area 13. HIV and Focus Area 25. Sexually Transmitted Diseases.)

Maternal Deaths and Illnesses

16-4.   Reduce maternal deaths.

Target: 3.3 maternal deaths per 100,000 live births.

Baseline: 7.1 maternal deaths per 100,000 live births occurred in 1998.

Target setting method: Better than the best.

Data source: National Vital Statistics System (NVSS), CDC, NCHS.

NOTE: THE TABLE BELOW MAY CONTINUE TO THE FOLLOWING PAGE.

Live Births, 1998	Maternal Deaths
	Rate per 100,000
TOTAL	7.1
Mother's race and ethnicity	
American Indian or Alaska Native	DSU
Asian or Pacific Islander	DSU
Asian	DSU
Native Hawaiian and other Pacific Islander	DSU

Live Births, 1998	Maternal Deaths
	Rate per 100,000
Black or African American	17.1
White	5.1
Hispanic or Latino	5.7
Not Hispanic or Latino	7.5
Black or African American	17.4
White	4.9
Mother's education level	
Less than high school	DNA
High school graduate	DNA
At least some college	DNA
Mother's disability status	
Mothers with disabilities	DNC
Mothers without disabilities	DNC
Select populations	
Mother's age groups	
Under 20 years	DSU
20 to 24 years	5.0
25 to 29 years	6.7
30 to 34 years	7.5
35 years and older	14.5

DNA = Data have not been analyzed. DNC = Data are not collected. DSU = Data are statistically unreliable.

NOTE: THE TABLE ABOVE MAY HAVE CONTINUED FROM THE PREVIOUS PAGE.

16-5. Reduce maternal illness and complications due to pregnancy.

Target and baseline:

Objective	Reduction in Maternal Illness and Complications	1998 Baseline	2010 Target
		Per 100 Deliveries	
16-5a.	Maternal complications during hospitalized labor and delivery	31.2	24
16-5b.	Ectopic pregnancies	Developmental	
16-5c.	Postpartum complications, including postpartum depression	Developmental	

Target setting method: Better than the best.

Data source: National Hospital Discharge Survey, CDC, NCHS.

Potential data source: National Hospital Discharge Survey (NHDS), CDC, NCHS.

NOTE: THE TABLE BELOW MAY CONTINUE TO THE FOLLOWING PAGE.

Deliveries, 1998	16-5a. Maternal Complications During Hospitalized Labor and Delivery
	Rate per 100 Deliveries
TOTAL	31.2
Race and ethnicity	
American Indian or Alaska Native	DSU
Asian or Pacific Islander	DSU
Asian	DNC
Native Hawaiian and other Pacific Islander	DNC
Black or African American	37.7
White	30.3
Hispanic or Latino	DSU
Not Hispanic or Latino	DSU
Black or African American	DSU
White	DSU
Family income level	
Poor	DNC
Near poor	DNC
Middle/high income	DNC
Select populations	
Mother's age group	
Under 15 years	DSU
15 to 19 years	34.4
20 to 24 years	30.4
25 to 29 years	29.7
30 to 34 years	31.1
35 years and older	32.7

DNA = Data have not been analyzed. DNC = Data are not collected. DSU = Data are statistically unreliable.

In 1997, 327 maternal deaths were reported by vital statistics, the major causes of which were hemorrhage, ectopic pregnancy, pregnancy-induced hypertension, embolism, infection, and other complications of pregnancy and childbirth.[43] The overall maternal mortality rate has fluctuated between approximately 7 and 8 per 100,000 live births since 1982.[44] Moreover, the gap between African Americans and whites remains, with the maternal mortality rate among African Americans 3.6 times that of whites in 1997. The rates among African Americans have been at least three to four times higher than those of whites since 1940. The rate among African Americans also has not declined, fluctuating between about 18 and 22 per 100,000 live births.[44]

Pregnancy and delivery can lead to serious physical and mental health problems for women. In the past, maternal illness and complications were monitored through objectives relating to the ratio of antenatal hospitalizations for pregnancy complications to the total number of deliveries. This ratio has become a less useful measure, however, as rates of antenatal hospitalization in general have declined due to managed care and its emphasis on outpatient treatment.[45] Therefore, attention should be focused on the major causes of maternal illness and complications, particularly those most likely to be associated with maternal death, such as ectopic pregnancy. Pelvic inflammatory disease caused by chlamydia and gonorrhea is the leading cause of preventable tubal scarring that can result in ectopic pregnancy. (See Focus Area 25. Sexually Transmitted Diseases.) The outcomes of interest should include not only prenatal illness and complications and complications during labor and delivery but also postpartum complications. Postpartum depression, for example, is disabling for a new mother and can compromise her ability to care for her infant.

Prenatal Care

16-6. Increase the proportion of pregnant women who receive early and adequate prenatal care.

Target and baseline:

Objective	Increase in Maternal Prenatal Care	1998 Baseline	2010 Target
		Percent of Live Births	
16-6a.	Care beginning in first trimester of pregnancy	83	90
16-6b.	Early and adequate prenatal care	74	90

Target setting method: Better than the best.

Data source: National Vital Statistics System (NVSS), CDC, NCHS.

Live Births, 1998	Maternal Prenatal Care	
	16-6a. First Trimester	16-6b. Early and Adequate
	Percent	
TOTAL	83	74
Mother's race and ethnicity		
American Indian or Alaska Native	69	57
Asian or Pacific Islander	83	74
Asian	86	76
Native Hawaiian and other Pacific Islander	75	67
Black or African American	73	67
White	85	76
Hispanic or Latino	74	66
Not Hispanic or Latino	85	76
Black or African American	73	67
White	88	79
Mother's education level		
Less than high school	68	61
High school graduate	81	74
At least some college	91	82
Mother's disability status		
Mothers with disabilities	DNC	DNC
Mothers without disabilities	DNC	DNC
Select populations		
Mother's age groups		
Under 15 years	48	48
15 to 19 years	69	64
20 to 24 years	78	70
25 to 29 years	86	77
30 to 34 years	89	79
35 years and older	88	79

DNA = Data have not been analyzed. DNC = Data are not collected. DSU = Data are statistically unreliable.

NOTE: THE TABLE ABOVE MAY HAVE CONTINUED FROM THE PREVIOUS PAGE.

Prenatal care includes three major components: risk assessment, treatment for medical conditions or risk reduction, and education. Each component can contribute to reductions in perinatal illness, disability, and death by identifying and mitigating potential risks and helping women to address behavioral factors, such as smoking and alcohol use, that contribute to poor outcomes. Prenatal care is more likely to be effective if women begin receiving care early in pregnancy. Since 1990, the proportion of infants whose mothers entered prenatal care in the first trimester increased 8.8 percent, from 76 percent to 83 percent. Among African Americans, this proportion grew 19 percent and among Hispanics, 22 percent.[1] Thus, increases in early entry into prenatal care have been concentrated in those populations whose perinatal illness and disability rates and mortality rates are highest and who are most likely to have low incomes. These increases are likely due, in part, to increased access to Medicaid coverage for pregnancy-related services and improved outreach by Medicaid programs.[46] In addition, the likelihood of early entry into prenatal care rises with age. The risk of poor birth outcomes is greatest among the youngest mothers (aged 15 years and under). Clearly, therefore, continued work is needed to educate women, particularly young women, about the need to begin prenatal care early in pregnancy.

Prenatal care should begin early and continue throughout pregnancy, according to accepted standards of periodicity. For example, the American College of Obstetricians and Gynecologists recommends that women receive at least 13 prenatal visits during a full-term pregnancy.[47] Therefore, assessment of the adequacy of the care pregnant women receive must include monitoring not only the month of initiation of prenatal care but also the adequacy of the care they receive throughout pregnancy. The Adequacy of Prenatal Care Utilization Index (APNCU) measures two dimensions of care: the adequacy of initiation of care and the adequacy of the use of prenatal services once care has begun (by comparing actual use to the recommended number of visits based on the month of initiation of care and the length of the pregnancy).[48] These dimensions are combined to classify each woman's prenatal care history as inadequate, intermediate, adequate, or adequate-plus. The baseline rates presented above include all women who received either adequate or adequate-plus care.

Overall, nearly three-quarters of women receive adequate prenatal care. However, this proportion varies across racial and ethnic groups. Certain groups, such as American Indians or Alaska Natives and Samoans, are particularly likely to receive less-than-adequate prenatal care. The likelihood of receipt of adequate prenatal care rises with maternal age, with fewer than half of pregnant women aged 15 years and under receiving adequate care.[42] Prevention of unwanted pregnancy in adolescents and education of women about the need for early, continuous prenatal care are essential.

16-7. (Developmental) Increase the proportion of pregnant women who attend a series of prepared childbirth classes.

Potential data sources: National Pregnancy and Health Survey, NIH, NICHD; National Survey of Family Growth (NSFG) or National Health Interview Survey (NHIS), CDC, NCHS.

As part of comprehensive prenatal care, a formal series of prepared childbirth classes conducted by a certified childbirth educator is recommended for all women by the Expert Panel on the Content of Prenatal Care.[49] These classes can help reduce women's pain[50] and anxiety[51] as they approach childbirth, making delivery a more pleasant experience and preparing women for what they will face as they give birth. A full series of sessions is recommended for women who have never attended. A refresher series of one or two classes is recommended for women who attended during a previous pregnancy. At a minimum, the childbirth classes should include information regarding the physiology of labor and birth, exercises and self-help techniques for labor, the role of support persons, family roles and adjustments, and preferences for care during labor and birth. The classes also should include an opportunity for the mother and her partner to have questions answered about providers, prenatal care, and other relevant issues, as well as to receive information regarding birth settings and cesarean childbirth. Attendance is recommended during the third trimester of pregnancy so that information learned will be used relatively soon after presentation. Classes should begin at the 31st or 32nd week and be completed no later than 38 weeks. The refresher class should be completed at any time between 36 and 38 weeks.

Obstetrical Care

16-8. Increase the proportion of very low birth weight (VLBW) infants born at level III hospitals or subspecialty perinatal centers.

Target: 90 percent.

Baseline: 73 percent of VLBW infants were born at level III hospitals or subspecialty perinatal centers in 1996–97.

Target setting method: 25 percent improvement. (Better than the best will be used when data are available.)

Data source: Title V Reporting System, HRSA, MCHB.

Data for population groups currently are not analyzed.

Much research has demonstrated the benefits of delivering high-risk infants in settings that have the technological capacity to care for them. Specifically, research has shown that VLBW infants have lower death rates when they are delivered at level III hospitals, which are equipped to care for very small infants.[52, 53, 54] To ensure that high-risk pregnant women have access to appropriate levels of obstetric care, many States have implemented perinatal regionalization strategies and protocols for the transfer of high-risk women to level III facilities. Evidence, however, indicates that these systems may be eroding as health care networks and financing systems change.[52, 55] The proportion of VLBW infants who are delivered in the level III obstetric hospitals best equipped to provide appropriate neonatal care should be measured to monitor the continuing effectiveness of these systems and the appropriateness of the level of care delivered to high-risk pregnant women and infants.

16-9. Reduce cesarean births among low-risk (full term, singleton, vertex presentation) women.

Target and baseline:

Objective	Reduction in Cesarean Births	1998 Baseline	2010 Target
		Percent of Live Births	
16-9a.	Women giving birth for the first time	18	15
16-9b.	Prior cesarean birth	72	63

Target setting method: Better than the best.

Data source: National Vital Statistics System (NVSS), CDC, NCHS.

NOTE: THE TABLE BELOW MAY CONTINUE TO THE FOLLOWING PAGE.

Cesarean Births to Low-Risk Women, 1998	Cesarean Birth	
	16-9a. Women Giving Birth for the First Time	16-9b. Prior Cesarean Birth
	Percent	
TOTAL	18	72
Mother's race and ethnicity		
American Indian or Alaska Native	16	68
Asian or Pacific Islander	18	70
Asian	19	72
Native Hawaiian and other Pacific Islander	17	65
Black or African American	21	73
White	18	72
Hispanic or Latino	18	76
Not Hispanic or Latino	18	71
Black or African American	21	73
White	18	71
Mother's education level		
Less than high school	14	72
High school graduate	18	73
At least some college	20	71

Cesarean Births to Low-Risk Women, 1998	Cesarean Birth	
	16-9a. Women Giving Birth for the First Time	16-9b. Prior Cesarean Birth
	Percent	
Mother's disability status		
Mothers with disabilities	DNC	DNC
Mothers without disabilities	DNC	DNC
Select populations		
Mother's age groups		
Under 15 years old	13	DSU
15 to 19 years	12	67
20 to 24 years	16	70
25 to 29 years	20	71
30 to 34 years	24	72
35 years and older	32	75

DNA = Data have not been analyzed. DNC = Data are not collected. DSU = Data are statistically unreliable.

NOTE: THE TABLE ABOVE MAY HAVE CONTINUED FROM THE PREVIOUS PAGE.

During the 1980s, rates of cesarean births rose steadily, with a peak rate of 25 percent of deliveries reported in 1988. Since then, the rate has been slowly decreasing, with the majority of the decline attributable to a reduction in the rates of primary cesarean births. In 1989, the rate of vaginal births among women who had a previous cesarean birth was 19 percent; in 1995 it increased to 28 percent.[56] The improvements are likely to be attributable to use of such strategies as clearer guidelines for trials of labor and labor management, continual labor support, and focused attention on physician practice patterns.[57] Expert opinion called for use of risk-adjusted rates of cesarean births (that is, rates standardized by patient characteristics) to monitor progress over time.[58] (The targets presented here apply to the population as a whole and are not intended to be used as practice outcome objectives for individual physicians or institutions, as the medical needs of the patients in each practice will vary.) In addition to monitoring rates of cesarean births, the outcomes of these deliveries (for both the mother and the infant) should be watched closely to assure that changes in the mode of delivery do not put women or their infants at risk.

16-10. Reduce low birth weight (LBW) and very low birth weight (VLBW).

Target and baseline:

Objective	Reduction in Low and Very Low Birth Weight	1998 Baseline	2010 Target
		Percent	
16-10a.	Low birth weight (LBW)	7.6	5.0
16-10b.	Very low birth weight (VLBW)	1.4	0.9

Target setting method: Better than the best.

Data source: National Vital Statistics System (NVSS), CDC, NCHS.

NOTE: THE TABLE BELOW MAY CONTINUE TO THE FOLLOWING PAGE.

Live Births, 1998 (unless noted)	16-10a. Low Birth Weight	16-10b. Very Low Birth Weight
	Percent	
TOTAL	7.6	1.4
Mother's race and ethnicity		
American Indian or Alaska Native	6.8	1.2
Asian or Pacific Islander	7.4	1.1
Asian	7.2	1.1
Native Hawaiian and other Pacific Islander	6.5	1.4
Black or African American	13.0	3.1
White	6.5	1.1
Hispanic or Latino	6.4	1.1
Not Hispanic or Latino	7.8	1.5
Black or African American	13.2	3.1
White	6.6	1.1
Gender		
Female	8.1 (1997)	1.4 (1997)
Male	7.0 (1997)	1.4 (1997)
Mother's education level		
Less than high school	9.0	1.6
High school graduate	7.9	1.5
At least some college	6.5	1.3

Live Births, 1998 (unless noted)	16-10a. Low Birth Weight	16-10b. Very Low Birth Weight
	Percent	
Mother's disability status		
Mothers with disabilities	DNC	DNC
Mothers without disabilities	DNC	DNC
Select populations		
Mother's age groups		
Under 15 years	13.1	3.3
15 to 19 years	9.5	1.8
20 to 24 years	7.5	1.4
25 to 29 years	6.7	1.3
30 to 34 years	7.0	1.4
35 years and older	8.7	1.7

DNA = Data have not been analyzed. DNC = Data are not collected. DSU = Data are statistically unreliable.

NOTE: THE TABLE ABOVE MAY HAVE CONTINUED FROM THE PREVIOUS PAGE.

LBW is the risk factor most closely associated with neonatal death; thus, improvements in infant birth weight can contribute substantially to reductions in the infant mortality rate. Of all infants born at low birth weight, the smallest (those weighing less than 1,500 grams) are at highest risk of dying in their first year. However, some researchers have proposed that further improvement in the survival of VLBW infants is nearly impossible, and reduction in the underlying rate of VLBW births is the only avenue toward reduction of neonatal mortality rates.[59] Another important issue is the long-term effects of LBW on affected infants who survive their first year, as these infants are more likely to experience long-term developmental and neurologic disabilities than are infants of normal birth weight.[60, 61] Recent increases in LBW are due largely to preterm delivery related to increases in multiple gestation.

Smoking accounts for 20 to 30 percent of all LBW births in the United States. The effect of smoking on LBW rates appears to be attributable to intrauterine growth retardation rather than to preterm delivery.[6] VLBW is primarily associated with preterm birth, which may be associated with the use of illicit drugs during pregnancy.

16-11. Reduce preterm births.

Target and baseline:

Objective	Reduction in Preterm Births	1998 Baseline	2010 Target
		Percent	
16-11a.	Total preterm births	11.6	7.6
16-11b.	Live births at 32 to 36 weeks of gestation	9.6	6.4
16-11c.	Live births at less than 32 weeks of gestation	2.0	1.1

Target setting method: Better than the best.

Data source: National Vital Statistics System (NVSS), CDC, NCHS.

NOTE: THE TABLE BELOW MAY CONTINUE TO THE FOLLOWING PAGE.

Live Births, 1998	16-11a. Total Preterm Births	16-11b. 32 to 36 Weeks of Gestation	16-11c. Less Than 32 Weeks of Gestation
	Percent		
TOTAL	11.6	9.6	2.0
Mother's race and ethnicity			
American Indian or Alaska Native	12.2	10.2	2.0
Asian or Pacific Islander	10.4	8.9	1.4
Asian	9.7	8.4	1.3
Native Hawaiian and other Pacific Islander	11.9	9.7	2.0
Black or African American	17.5	13.4	4.1
White	10.5	8.9	1.6
Hispanic or Latino	11.4	9.7	1.7
Not Hispanic or Latino	11.7	9.6	2.0
Black or African American	17.6	13.4	4.1
White	10.2	8.7	1.5
Gender			
Female	DNA	DNA	DNA
Male	DNA	DNA	DNA

Healthy People 2010: Objectives for Improving Health

Live Births, 1998	16-11a. Total Preterm Births	16-11b. 32 to 36 Weeks of Gestation	16-11c. Less Than 32 Weeks of Gestation
	Percent		
Mother's education level			
Less than high school	13.7	11.2	2.4
High school graduate	12.0	9.9	2.1
At least some college	10.3	8.7	1.6
Mother's disability status			
Mothers with disabilities	DNC	DNC	DNC
Mothers without disabilities	DNC	DNC	DNC
Select populations			
Mother's age groups			
Under 15 years	22.0	16.2	5.8
15 to 19 years	13.8	11.1	2.7
20 to 24 years	11.5	9.6	1.9
25 to 29 years	10.6	8.9	1.7
30 to 34 years	10.8	9.1	1.8
35 years and older	12.9	10.8	2.2

DNA = Data have not been analyzed. DNC = Data are not collected. DSU = Data are statistically unreliable.
NOTE: THE TABLE ABOVE MAY HAVE CONTINUED FROM THE PREVIOUS PAGE.

Approximately two-thirds of LBW infants and 98 percent of VLBW infants are born preterm. In addition, preterm birth is the leading cause of those neonatal deaths not associated with birth defects. Survival rates of infants have been shown to increase as gestational age advances, even among very preterm infants.[62, 63] Therefore, reduction in preterm delivery holds the greatest promise for overall reduction in infant illness, disability, and death. Because the specific causes of preterm delivery are unclear, research is needed before tailored interventions can be developed.[64, 65] Preterm birth is associated with a number of modifiable risk factors, including the use of alcohol, tobacco, or other drugs during pregnancy[66, 67] and low prepregnancy weight or low weight gain during pregnancy.[68, 69] Other important risk factors for preterm birth are vaginal infections[70, 71, 72] and domestic violence.[73]

Rates of preterm delivery in the United States increased over the last three decades of the 20th century.[4, 68] Between 1989 and 1996, this increase was due largely to an increase in multiple gestation. The gap between African American and white infants persists as well, for reasons that are largely unexplained[74] and that have been shown to be independent of other known risk factors.[66, 75] Risk factors that

African American women may disproportionately experience include short inter-pregnancy intervals[76] and exposure to psychosocial stress.[75, 77]

16-12. (Developmental) Increase the proportion of mothers who achieve a recommended weight gain during their pregnancies.

Potential data source: National Vital Statistics System (NVSS), CDC, NCHS.

Current evidence indicates that gestational weight gain, particularly during the second and third trimesters, is an important determinant of fetal growth. Inade-quate weight gain during pregnancy is associated with an increased risk of IUGR, LBW, and infant death.[78, 79, 80] Maternal weight gain is susceptible to intervention and represents an avenue for prevention of poor birth outcomes. The Institute of Medicine's 1990 guidelines for weight gain in pregnancy recommend a graduated level of weight gain based on a woman's prepregnancy body mass index (BMI) (that is, the ratio of her weight to her height).[78] Under these guidelines, a woman with normal BMI should gain 25 to 35 pounds during pregnancy. Those with be-low-normal BMI should gain 28 to 40 pounds. Overweight women should gain 15 to 25 pounds.

In 1988, approximately three-quarters of married women who delivered at full term gained the recommended weight during pregnancy.[18] Two groups of women who continue to gain less than the recommended level of weight during preg-nancy—teenagers and African American women—also are at particularly high risk for having LBW infants and other adverse pregnancy outcomes.

16-13. Increase the percentage of healthy full-term infants who are put down to sleep on their backs.

Target: 70 percent.

Baseline: 35 percent of healthy full-term infants were put down to sleep on their backs in 1996.

Target setting method: Better than the best.

Data source: National Infant Sleep Position Study, NIH, NICHD.

NOTE: THE TABLE BELOW MAY CONTINUE TO THE FOLLOWING PAGE.

Infants, 1996	Put Down To Sleep on Their Backs
	Percent
TOTAL	35
Mother's race and ethnicity	
American Indian or Alaska Native	DNA

16-16. Increase the proportion of pregnancies begun with an optimum folic acid level.

Target and baseline:

Objective	Increase in Pregnancies Begun With Optimum Folic Acid Level	1991–94 Baseline	2010 Target
		Percent	
16-16a.	Consumption of at least 400 µg of folic acid each day from fortified foods or dietary supplements by nonpregnant women aged 15 to 44 years	21	80
		Number	
16-16b.	Median RBC folate level among non-pregnant women aged 15 to 44 years	160 ng/ml	220 ng/ml

Target setting method: Better than the best.

Data source: National Health and Nutrition Examination Survey (NHANES), CDC, NCHS.

NOTE: THE TABLE BELOW MAY CONTINUE TO THE FOLLOWING PAGE.

Nonpregnant Women Aged 15 to 44 Years, 1991–94	16-16a. Adequate Folic Acid	16-16b. Median RBC Folate Level
	Percent	ng/ml
TOTAL	21	160
Race and ethnicity		
American Indian or Alaska Native	DSU	DSU
Asian or Pacific Islander	DSU	DSU
Asian	DNC	DNC
Native Hawaiian and other Pacific Islander	DNC	DNC
Black or African American	17	125
White	22	169
Hispanic or Latino	DSU	DSU
Mexican American	13	158
Not Hispanic or Latino	22	159
Black or African American	18	123
White	23	170

Nonpregnant Women Aged 15 to 44 Years, 1991–94	16-16a. Adequate Folic Acid	16-16b. Median RBC Folate Level
	Percent	ng/ml
Education level		
Less than high school	12	145
High school graduate	19	148
At least some college	28	179
Disability status		
Persons with disabilities	20	169
Persons without disabilities	23	159

DNA = Data have not been analyzed. DNC = Data are not collected. DSU = Data are statistically unreliable.

NOTE: THE TABLE ABOVE MAY HAVE CONTINUED FROM THE PREVIOUS PAGE.

NTDs, including spina bifida, occur when the fetal neural tube fails to close fully, interrupting development of the central nervous system. Approximately 50 percent of pregnancies affected with NTDs may be prevented with adequate consumption of folic acid from 1 month before conception through the first 3 months of pregnancy.[23] In 1992, the U.S. Public Health Service (PHS) recommended that all women of childbearing age consume 400 micrograms of folic acid daily.[24] For women who already have had an NTD-affected pregnancy, PHS recommends that women consult with a health care professional about taking a much larger amount of folic acid—4,000 micrograms (4.0 milligrams)—when planning a pregnancy.[24] In 1998, the Institute of Medicine further recommended that to reduce the risk of an NTD-affected pregnancy, all women capable of becoming pregnant should consume 400 micrograms of folic acid daily, from fortified foods or supplements or a combination of the two, in addition to consuming folate-rich foods, such as orange juice, green vegetables, and beans.[85]

Most grain products (including enriched flour, breads, breakfast cereals, rice, and pasta) now are fortified with folic acid. However, the amount of folic acid that some segments of the reproductive-aged population might receive through their diet may not adequately meet the PHS recommendation of 400 micrograms daily. Thus, women capable of becoming pregnant need to review their dietary options, eat a diet that includes folate-rich foods, and target consumption of folic acid-fortified food as well as take a folic acid-containing supplement.

16-17. Increase abstinence from alcohol, cigarettes, and illicit drugs among pregnant women.

Target and baseline:

Objective	Increase in Reported Abstinence in Past Month From Substances by Pregnant Women*	1996–97 Baseline (unless noted)	2010 Target
		Percent	
16-17a.	Alcohol	86	94
16-17b.	Binge drinking	99	100
16-17c.	Cigarette smoking[†]	87 (1998)	99
16-17d.	Illicit drugs	98	100

*Pregnant women aged 15 to 44 years.

[†]Smoking during pregnancy for all women giving birth in 1998 in 46 States, the District of Columbia, and New York City.

Target setting method: Better than the best for 16-17a and 16-17c; complete elimination for 16-17b and 16-17d.

Data sources: National Household Survey on Drug Abuse, SAMHSA for 16-17a, 16-17b, and 16-17d; National Vital Statistics System, CDC, NCHS for 16-17c.

NOTE: THE TABLE BELOW MAY CONTINUE TO THE FOLLOWING PAGE.

Pregnant Women Aged 15 to 44 Years, 1996–97 (unless noted)	16-17a. Alcohol Absti-nence, Past Month	16-17b. No Binge Drinking, Past Month	16-17c. No Ciga-rette Smoking, 1998*	16-17d. No Drugs, Past Month
	Percent			
TOTAL	86	99	87	98
Race and ethnicity				
American Indian or Alaska Native	DNA	DNA	80	DNA
Asian or Pacific Islander	DNA	DNA	97	DNA
Asian	DNC	DNC	98	DNC
Native Hawaiian and other Pacific Islander	DNC	DNC	84	DNC
Black or African American	DNA	DNA	91	DNA
White	DNA	DNA	86	DNA

Pregnant Women Aged 15 to 44 Years, 1996–97 (unless noted)	16-17a. Alcohol Abstinence, Past Month	16-17b. No Binge Drinking, Past Month	16-17c. No Cigarette Smoking, 1998*	16-17d. No Drugs, Past Month
	Percent			
Hispanic or Latino	93	99	96	99
Not Hispanic or Latino	DNA	DNA	86	DNA
Black or African American	83	99	90	95
White	85	99	84	98
Education level (aged 18 to 44 years)				
Less than high school	79	99	78	92
High school graduate	91	99	83	100
At least some college	DNA	98	94	DNA
College graduate	DNA	DNA	DNA	DNA
Disability status				
Persons with disabilities	DNC	DNC	DNC	DNC
Persons without disabilities	DNC	DNC	DNC	DNC

DNA = Data have not been analyzed. DNC = Data are not collected. DSU = Data are statistically unreliable.
*Smoking during pregnancy for all women giving birth in 1998 in 46 States, the District of Columbia, and New York City.

NOTE: THE TABLE ABOVE MAY HAVE CONTINUED FROM THE PREVIOUS PAGE.

A range of effects, including spontaneous abortion, LBW, and preterm delivery, have been associated with prenatal use of licit and illicit drugs, including alcohol, tobacco, cocaine, and marijuana.[86, 87, 88, 20, 21, 22] As discussed above, tobacco is associated with LBW and spontaneous abortion.[86] Heavy alcohol use is associated with FAS,[87] and even moderate alcohol use has demonstrated effects on preterm delivery.[88] The use of cocaine during pregnancy is associated with premature birth and impaired fetal growth.[8, 20, 21, 22] In addition, women who use cocaine are at especially high risk of infectious diseases, including hepatitis B and HIV. Exposure to marijuana in utero may be associated with LBW, preterm birth, and neurobehavioral functioning. However, isolating the effects of marijuana use on newborns is difficult because users of the drug often use alcohol and tobacco as well.[86]

Self-reported use of illicit drugs, such as cocaine and marijuana, is quite rare, with 98 percent of pregnant women reporting abstaining from these drugs. Rates of abstinence from harmful substances during pregnancy appear to be declining slowly. The use of alcohol during pregnancy, despite the established health risk, exemplifies this trend. In 1996–97, 86 percent of pregnant women abstained from alcohol use, an increase of 9 percent from the 1988 baseline. Rates of frequent drinking (at least seven drinks per week or at least five drinks on any occasion in the past month) among pregnant women have begun to decline, with only 1.3 percent of pregnant women reporting recent binge drinking in 1996–97, compared to 2.9 percent in 1994–95.[89] Unintentional alcohol exposure is particularly likely to occur early in pregnancy, before a woman knows she is pregnant. In addition to the objectives presented here, objectives in Focus Area 26. Substance Abuse, address alcohol consumption among women of reproductive age and tobacco use by pregnant women.

16-18. (Developmental) Reduce the occurrence of fetal alcohol syndrome (FAS).

Potential data source: Fetal Alcohol Syndrome Network (FASNet), CDC, NCEH.

FAS is one of the leading preventable causes of mental retardation and a leading cause of birth defects, including growth deficiency and microcephaly. Affected children also are likely to show infantile irritability, poor coordination, hypotonia, and attention deficit/hyperactivity disorder.[88, 90] The diagnosis of FAS is based on three criteria: prenatal or postnatal growth retardation or both, central nervous system impairment, and characteristic facial malformations. Abnormalities of other organs and systems, however, have been noted in combination with these characteristics.[91] Estimates of the cases of FAS vary from 0.2 to 1.0 per 1,000 live births.[92, 93, 94] In addition to FAS, studies have documented more subtle growth and neurodevelopmental deficits among children whose mothers drank alcohol during pregnancy. Alcohol-related birth defects and alcohol-related neurodevelopmental disorders are thought to occur three to four times more often than diagnosed cases of FAS.[94] Because of these lifelong effects, and because a safe level of alcohol consumption during pregnancy has not been identified, the American Academy of Pediatrics and the American College of Obstetricians and Gynecologists recommend that women who are pregnant or are planning a pregnancy abstain from the use of alcohol.[95, 96]

Despite broad agreement on the importance of FAS, consistent diagnosis of the syndrome at birth has been difficult to achieve. Thus, accurately estimating the number or proportion of infants affected by FAS is challenging for a number of reasons: the difficulty of evaluating an infant's central nervous system, lack of training among clinicians, inconsistent diagnostic criteria, clinicians' tendency to avoid associating their patients with the stigma of alcohol problems, and failures of mothers to report alcohol intake during gestation.[7]

16-19. Increase the proportion of mothers who breastfeed their babies.

Target and baseline:

Objective	Increase in Mothers Who Breastfeed	1998 Baseline	2010 Target
		Percent	
16-19a.	In early postpartum period	64	75
16-19b.	At 6 months	29	50
16-19c.	At 1 year	16	25

Target setting method: Better than the best.

Data source: Mothers' Survey, Abbott Laboratories, Inc., Ross Products Division.

NOTE: THE TABLE BELOW MAY CONTINUE TO THE FOLLOWING PAGE.

Mothers, 1998	Breastfed		
	16-19a. Early Postpartum	**16-19b.** 6 Months	**16-19c.** 1 Year
	Percent		
TOTAL	64	29	16
Race and ethnicity			
American Indian or Alaska Native	DNC	DNC	DNC
Asian or Pacific Islander	DNC	DNC	DNC
Asian	DNC	DNC	DNC
Native Hawaiian and other Pacific Islander	DNC	DNC	DNC
Black or African American	45	19	9
White	68	31	17
Hispanic or Latino	66	28	19
Not Hispanic or Latino	DNC	DNC	DNC
Black or African American	DNC	DNC	DNC
White	DNC	DNC	DNC
Education level			
Less than high school	48	23	17
High school graduate	55	21	12
At least some college	55	21	12
College graduate	78	40	22

Mothers, 1998	Breastfed		
	16-19a. Early Postpartum	16-19b. 6 Months	16-19c. 1 Year
	Percent		
Disability status			
Persons with disabilities	DNC	DNC	DNC
Persons without disabilities	DNC	DNC	DNC

DNA = Data have not been analyzed. DNC = Data are not collected. DSU = Data are statistically unreliable.

NOTE: THE TABLE ABOVE MAY HAVE CONTINUED FROM THE PREVIOUS PAGE.

Breast milk is widely acknowledged to be the most complete form of nutrition for infants, with a range of benefits for infants' health, growth, immunity, and development. The benefits of breastfeeding include decreased new cases or severity of diarrhea,[25, 26, 27, 28, 36] respiratory infections,[29, 30] and ear infections,[26, 31, 32] among others, and reduced cost to the family.[33, 34] In addition, breastfeeding has been shown to improve maternal health, with demonstrated effects, including reduction in postpartum bleeding,[35] earlier return to prepregnancy weight,[36] reduced risk of premenopausal breast cancer,[37] and reduced risk of osteoporosis,[38] continuing long after the postpartum period. In general, the American Academy of Pediatrics considers breastfeeding to be "the ideal method of feeding and nurturing infants."[10]

Universal breastfeeding is not recommended in the United States. Women who use illicit drugs, who have active, untreated tuberculosis, or who test positive for HIV, as well as those who use certain prescribed drugs, should not breastfeed.[11, 97] In general, however, increasing the rate of breastfeeding, particularly among low-income and certain racial and ethnic populations less likely to begin breastfeeding in the hospital or to sustain it throughout the infant's first year, is an important public health goal.

Rates of breastfeeding are highest among college-educated women and women aged 35 years and older. The lowest rates of breastfeeding are found among those whose infants are at highest risk of poor health and development: those aged 21 years and under and those with low educational levels. However, many of these groups have shown the greatest increase in breastfeeding rates since 1989. Rates of breastfeeding among African American women during the postpartum period increased 65 percent, and rates of African American women breastfeeding at 6 months grew 81 percent between 1988 and 1997. Breastfeeding rates among women aged 20 years and under at both periods also increased substantially, as did those among women with a grade-school education.[12] While these improvements are encouraging, education of new mothers and their partners; education of health providers; changes in routine maternity ward practices; social support, including support from employers; and greater media portrayal of breastfeeding as the normal method of infant feeding are needed to increase breastfeeding rates among those at highest risk.

16-20. (Developmental) Ensure appropriate newborn bloodspot screening, followup testing, and referral to services.

16-20a. Ensure that all newborns are screened at birth for conditions mandated by their State-sponsored newborn screening programs, for example, phenylketonuria and hemoglobinopathies.

16-20b. Ensure that followup diagnostic testing for screening positives is performed within an appropriate time period.

16-20c. Ensure that infants with diagnosed disorders are enrolled in appropriate service interventions within an appropriate time period.

Potential data source: Title V Performance Measures, HRSA, MCHB, National Newborn Screening and Genetic Resource Center.

Newborn screening (NBS) programs began in the early 1960s with the development of a screening test for phenylketonuria (PKU) and a system for blood sample collection on filter paper and transportation of that sample. Since then, all States and some territories of the United States have included NBS as part of their preventive public health system. NBS programs in the United States were the first population-based screening programs for genetic conditions and signaled the integration of genetic testing into public health programs. The mass screening of 4 million infants per year in the United States has been heralded as a successful program that is cost effective and reduces illness, disability, and death associated with inherited conditions. The universal acceptance of newborn screening for specified conditions since 1960 attests to the undeniable benefits that flow from testing and appropriate treatment and intervention.

The array of screening tests performed by each State varies and is changing constantly. All State programs now include screening for PKU and congenital hypothyroidism. More than 40 programs screen for sickle cell disease, and almost all screen for galactosemia. Others include congenital adrenal hyperplasia, homocystinuria, maple syrup urine disease, biotinidase deficiency, and tyrosinemia. A few States also include cystic fibrosis, additional metabolic disorders, and some other conditions such as congenital infections. Virtually all States treat or refer for treatment those with a confirmed diagnosis. However, some disorders are more uniformly screened for than others, and followup testing and early initiation of preventive treatment are uneven. For example, screening for PKU and congenital hypothyroidism is virtually universal, although reporting is not.[98, 99] Screening and followup for galactosemia, sickle cell disease, and other hemoglobinopathies have been less consistent.[98, 99] Sickle cell disease can lead to severe illness and early death, and galactosemia leads to an increased risk of death from overwhelming infection in early infancy, failure to thrive, vomiting, liver disease, and mental retardation in untreated survivors.[100] Therefore, it is vital that screening be universally available, that screening be of the highest quality, that diagnostic testing be provided for those newborns who screen positive, and that followup treatment be offered to children with diagnosed disorders.[101, 102, 103]

16-21. (Developmental) Reduce hospitalization for life-threatening sepsis among children aged 4 years and under with sickling hemoglobinopathies.

Potential data source: National Hospital Discharge Survey (NHDS), CDC, NCHS.

Significant illness, disability, and death are associated with sickle cell disease because of increased susceptibility to severe bacterial infections—meningitis, pneumonia, and septicemia—all major causes of death among children with the disorder.[104, 105, 106] Life-threatening episodes of sepsis from pneumococcus and other organisms are well-recognized complications of sickle cell disease in children. The efficacy of daily oral penicillin prophylaxis in preventing infection among young children with sickle cell disease has been demonstrated.[104] Sepsis rates have been shown to be clearly improved by prophylactic therapy in the U.S. penicillin trial, but concerns about actual use of penicillin in large populations and about penicillin-resistant organisms necessitate continued monitoring of sepsis rates in large populations.

16-22. (Developmental) Increase the proportion of children with special health care needs who have access to a medical home.

Potential data source: Title V Reporting System, HRSA, MCHB.

Historically, services for children with special health care needs have been difficult for families to access and for providers to coordinate. Families must navigate a variety of organizations and providers and often face geographic and financial barriers to care. Primary care providers in the community are not always comfortable providing care to children with complex needs, nor do they have time to coordinate the variety of resources families need. A lack of knowledge—of comprehensive needs and corresponding community-based resources and of payment mechanisms—presents a challenge for both families and providers. Poor communication between families and providers and cross-cultural misunderstandings are additional concerns for both families and providers.

Care for children with special health care needs should be provided and coordinated through a "medical home" that is accessible, family-centered, continuous, comprehensive, coordinated, compassionate, and culturally competent and linguistically appropriate. Physicians and parents share responsibility for ensuring that children and their families have access to all the medical and nonmedical services needed to help them achieve their maximum potential. The attributes of such a medical home are defined below:

- Accessible care is care that is provided in the child's community, in which all insurance, including Medicaid, is accepted and changes in insurance status are accommodated.

- Family-centered care recognizes that the family is the principal care-giver and the center of strength and support for children. Family-centered services share unbiased and complete information with families on an ongoing basis.

- Continuous care assures that the same primary pediatric health care professionals are available from infancy through adolescence and provide assistance with transitions (to home, school, and adult services).

- Comprehensive health care is available 24 hours a day, 7 days a week, and addresses preventive, primary, and tertiary needs.

- Coordinated care links families to support, educational, and community-based services, and information is centralized.

- Compassionate caregivers express concern for the well-being of the child and family.

- Culturally appropriate and linguistically competent care recognizes, values, and respects the family's cultural background.[107, 108, 109, 110, 111]

16-23. Increase the proportion of Territories and States that have service systems for children with special health care needs.

Target: 100 percent.

Baseline: 15.7 percent of Territories and States met Title V for service systems for children with special health care needs in FY 1997.

Target setting method: Total coverage.

Data source: Title V Block Grant Application Form 13, HRSA, MCHB.

Children with special health care needs and their families often require a range of services.[112] Health services, for example, include health education and health promotion; preventive and primary care, including routine screening for impairments of vision, hearing, speech, and language, and assessment of physical and psychosocial milestones; specialized diagnostic and therapeutic services; and habilitation and rehabilitation services. Early intervention services are necessary as well, as are educational, vocational, and mental health services and support services for children and their families. Enabling services, such as transportation and child care, are necessary to ensure access to care. Transition services are needed to assist in the progression from adolescent health care to adult services and from school to work.

Families continuously face the challenge of obtaining and coordinating the primary and special services their children require. Differing eligibility criteria, duplication and gaps in services, inflexible funding sources, and poor coordination among service sectors are some of the barriers consistently reported. Many of these issues can be resolved only through the concerted effort of a system of services—the broad array of public and private entities serving children and families in the Nation's communities. These service systems should ensure access to a source of insurance for primary and specialty care and enabling services, an identified medical home, and care coordination. Families and their care professionals should participate in the design and implementation of these service systems.[113] This collaborative partnership will strengthen the ability of families to care for their children with special needs and will enable children with complex conditions to live at home with their families.

Related Objectives From Other Focus Areas

1. **Access to Quality Health Services**
   1-1. Persons with health insurance
   1-2. Health insurance coverage for clinical preventive services
   1-4. Source of ongoing care
   1-5. Usual primary care provider
   1-6. Difficulties or delays in obtaining needed health care
   1-9. Hospitalization for ambulatory-care-sensitive conditions
   1-12. Single toll-free number for poison control centers
   1-13. Trauma care systems
   1-14. Special needs of children

5. **Diabetes**
   5-8. Gestational diabetes

6. **Disability and Secondary Conditions**
   6-2. Feelings and depression among children with disabilities
   6-7. Congregate care of children and adults with disabilities
   6-9. Inclusion of children and youth with disabilities in regular education programs

7. **Educational and Community-Based Programs**
   7-1. High school completion
   7-2. School health education
   7-4. School nurse-to-student ratio

8. **Environmental Health**
   8-11. Elevated blood lead levels in children
   8-20. School policies to protect against environmental hazards
   8-22. Lead-based paint testing

9. **Family Planning**
   9-2. Birth spacing
   9-7. Adolescent pregnancy
   9-8. Abstinence before age 15 years
   9-9. Abstinence among adolescents aged 15 to 17 years
   9-10. Pregnancy prevention and sexually transmitted disease (STD) protection
   9-11. Pregnancy prevention education

21. **Oral Health**
   21-1. Dental caries experience
   21-2. Untreated dental decay
   21-8. Dental sealants
   21-9. Community water fluoridation
   21-10. Use of oral health care system
   21-13. School-based health centers with oral health component
   21-14. Health centers with oral health service components
   21-15. Referral for cleft lip or palate
   21-16. Oral and craniofacial State-based surveillance system

22. **Physical Activity and Fitness**
   22-6. Moderate physical activity in adolescents
   22-7. Vigorous physical activity in adolescents
   22-8. Physical education requirement in schools
   22-9. Daily physical education in schools
   22-10. Physical activity in physical education class
   22-11. Television viewing
   22-12. School physical activity facilities

24. **Respiratory Diseases**
   24-1. Deaths from asthma
   24-2. Hospitalizations for asthma
   24-3. Hospital emergency department visits for asthma
   24-5. School or work days lost

25. **Sexually Transmitted Diseases**
   25-9. Congenital syphilis
   25-10. Neonatal STDs
   25-11. Responsible adolescent sexual behavior
   25-12. Responsible sexual behavior messages on television
   25-14. Screening in youth detention facilities and jails
   25-17. Screening of pregnant women

26. **Substance Abuse**
   26-6. Adolescents riding with a driver who has been drinking
   26-9. Substance-free youth
   26-10. Adolescent and adult use of illicit substances
   26-14. Steroid use among adolescents
   26-15. Inhalant use among adolescents
   26-16. Peer disapproval of substance abuse
   26-17. Perception of risk associated with substance abuse

27. **Tobacco Use**
   27-2. Adolescent tobacco use
   27-3. Initiation of tobacco use
   27-4. Age at first use of tobacco
   27-6. Smoking cessation during pregnancy
   27-7. Smoking cessation by adolescents
   27-11. Smoke-free and tobacco-free schools
   27-14. Enforcement of illegal tobacco sales to minors laws
   27-15. Retail license suspension for sales to minors
   27-17. Adolescent disapproval of smoking

Terminology

(A listing of abbreviations and acronyms used in this publication appears in Appendix H.)

Anencephalus: Congenital absence of all or a major part of the brain.

Birth defect: An abnormality in structure, function, or body metabolism that is present at birth, such as cleft lip or palate, phenylketonuria, or sickle cell disease.

Breastfeeding: Exclusive use of human milk or use of human milk with a supplemental bottle of formula. "Exclusive breastfeeding" refers to the use of only human milk, supplemented by solid food when appropriate but not supplemented by formula.

Children with special health care needs: Children who have or are at risk for a chronic physical, developmental, behavioral, or emotional condition and who also require health care and related services of a type or amount beyond that required by children generally.

Congenital anomaly: See birth defect.

Developmental disabilities: A broad spectrum of impairments characterized by developmental delay or limitation or both in personal activity, such as mental retardation, cerebral palsy, epilepsy, hearing and other communication disorders, and vision impairment. The more severe developmental disabilities require special interdisciplinary care.

Eclampsia/Preeclampsia: A condition that occurs in the second half of pregnancy, characterized by hypertension, edema, and proteinuria. When convulsions and coma are associated, it is called eclampsia.

Ectopic pregnancy: A gestation elsewhere than in the uterus, often occurring in the fallopian tube. An ectopic pregnancy cannot develop normally and causes fainting, abdominal pain, and vaginal bleeding.

Fetal alcohol syndrome (FAS): A cluster of structural and functional abnormalities found in infants and children as a result of alcohol consumption by the mother during pregnancy and characterized by growth retardation, facial malformations, and central nervous system dysfunction.

Fetal death: The death of a fetus in utero after 20 weeks or more of gestation. The fetal death rate is the number of fetal deaths in a population divided by the total number of live births and fetal deaths in the same population during the same time period.

Genetic disorders: The group of health conditions that result primarily from alterations in a gene or combination of genes.

Gestational trophoblastic disease: A type of cancer associated with pregnancy in which a grape-like mole develops in the womb.

Hydrocephalus: A condition marked by dilation of the cerebral ventricles accompanied by cerebrospinal fluid within the skull.

Hypotonia: A condition of diminished tone of the skeletal muscles, with diminished resistance of muscles to passive stretching.

Infant death: Death of an infant less than 1 year old. Neonatal death is the death of an infant less than 28 days after birth; postneonatal death is the death of an infant between 28 days and 1 year after birth.

Infant mortality rate: The number of deaths of infants less than 1 year old (obtained from death certificates) per 1,000 live births in a population (obtained from birth certificates).

Intrapartum period: Period extending from the onset of labor through the completion of delivery.

Intrauterine growth retardation (IUGR): The failure of a fetus to maintain its expected growth potential at any stage of gestation. Infants with IUGR may be born at full term but are smaller than expected.

Level III hospital: A facility for high-risk deliveries and neonates that can provide care to very small infants, including mechanical ventilation and neonatal surgery and special care for transferred patients and for which a full-time neonatologist serves as the director.

Live birth: The complete expulsion or extraction from its mother of an infant, irrespective of the duration of pregnancy, which after such separation, breathes or shows any other evidence of life, such as the beating of the heart, pulsation of the umbilical cord, or definite movement of voluntary muscles, whether or not the umbilical cord has been cut or the placenta is attached. Each infant from such a birth is considered live born.

Low birth weight (LBW): Weight at birth of less than 2,500 grams (about 5.5 pounds).

Maternal death: Death of a woman while pregnant or within 42 days of the end of pregnancy, irrespective of the duration or site of the pregnancy, from any cause related to or aggravated by the pregnancy or its management but not from accidental or incidental causes.

Maternal mortality rate: (also referred to as the maternal mortality ratio) Represents the number of maternal deaths for every 100,000 live births.

Medical home: Medical care for infants and children that is accessible, continuous, comprehensive, family-centered, coordinated, and compassionate.

Neonatal period: The first 28 days of life.

Neural tube defects (NTDs): A set of birth defects that result from failure of the neural tube to close in utero. Two of the most common NTDs are anencephaly (absence of the majority of the brain) and spina bifida (incomplete development of the back and spine).

Occurrence: As the term is used in this chapter, occurrence is the incidence of new cases among live births per year that are caused primarily by prenatal factors. In the spina bifida and other neural tube defects objective, identification is in the first year of life, and occurrence is reported as the number of cases per 10,000 live births per year. In the fetal alcohol syndrome objective, some children who have the condition at birth are not identified until age 4 or 5 years; occurrence is reported as a number per 10,000 live births. In the developmental disabilities objective, children with specified conditions such as mental retardation are not always identified until about age 7 or 8 years even though the conditions are usually caused by prenatal events; occurrence in these objectives is reported as a number per 10,000 children aged 8 years.

Perinatal death: Includes fetal deaths after 28 weeks of gestation and infant deaths within the first 7 days of birth.

Postneonatal period: The period from an infant's 29th day of life until the first birthday.

Postpartum period: The 6-week period immediately following birth.

Preeclampsia: (see eclampsia).

Prenatal care: Pregnancy-related health care services provided to a woman between conception and delivery. The American College of Obstetricians and Gynecologists recommends at least 13 prenatal visits in a normal 9-month pregnancy: one each month for the first 28 weeks of pregnancy, one every 2 weeks until 36 weeks, and then weekly until birth.

Preterm birth: Birth occurring before 37 weeks of pregnancy.

Renal agenesis: Associated with duplicated vagina and uterus.

Sudden infant death syndrome (SIDS): Sudden, unexplained death of an infant from an unknown cause.

Surfactant: A surface-active agent that prevents the lungs from filling with water by capillary action.

Synthetic surfactant: An artificial substance that prevents a newborn's lungs from filling with water.

Teratogenic: Causing malformations of an embryo or fetus.

Very low birth weight (VLBW): Weight at birth of less than 1,500 grams (about 3.3 pounds).

References

[1] National Center for Health Statistics (NCHS). *Health, United States, 1999.* Hyattsville, MD: U.S. Department of Health and Human Services, 1999.

[2] Ventura, S.J.; Anderson, R.N.; Martin, J.A.; et al. Births and deaths: Preliminary data for 1997. *National Vital Statistics Report* 47(4):1-42, 1999.

[3] Hoyert, D.L. Medical and life-style risk factors affecting fetal mortality, 1989–90. *Vital and Health Statistics 20 Data National Vital Statistics System* 31:1-32, 1996.

[4] Ventura, S.J.; Martin, J.A.; Curtin, S.C.; et al. Births: Final data for 1997. *National Vital Statistics Report* 48(3), 2000.

[5] Lewit, E.M.; Baker, L.S.; Hope, C.; et al. The direct cost of low birth weight. *Future Child* 5(1):35-56, 1995.

[6] Camas, O.R.; Cheung, L.W.Y.; and Lieberman, E. The role of lifestyle in preventing low birth weight. *Future Child* 5(1):121-138, 1995.

[7] Stratton, K.; Howe, C.; Battaglia, F.; eds. *Fetal Alcohol Syndrome: Diagnosis, Epidemiology, Prevention, and Treatment.* Washington, DC: National Academy Press, 1996.

[8] Chasnoff, I.J.; Burns, W.J.; Schnoll, S.H.; et al. Cocaine use in pregnancy. *New England Journal of Medicine* 313:666-669, 1985.

[9] Centers for Disease Control and Prevention (CDC). Medical-care expenditures attributable to cigarette smoking during pregnancy—United States, 1995. *Morbidity and Mortality Weekly Report* 46(44):1048-1050, 1997.

[10] American Academy of Pediatrics (AAP), Work Group on Breastfeeding. Breastfeeding and the use of human milk. *Pediatrics* 100(6):1035-1039, 1997.

[11] AAP, Committee on Pediatric AIDS. Human milk, breastfeeding, and transmission of human immunodeficiency virus in the United States. *Pediatrics* 96:977-979, 1995.

[12] Ross Products Division, Abbott Laboratories, Inc. Mothers' Survey, Columbus, OH: the Company, 1999.

[13] Hogan, D.P.; Msall, M.E.; Rogers, M.L.; et al. Improved disability population estimates of functional limitation among children aged 5-17. *Maternal and Child Health Journal* 1(4):203-216, 1997.

[14] LaPlante, M.P., and Carlson, D. Disability in the United States: Prevalence and causes, 1992. *Disability Statistics Report*. Washington, DC: U.S. Department of Education, 1996.

[15] Czeik, A.E., and Dudas, J. Prevention of the first occurrence of neural tube defects by periconceptional vitamin supplementation. *New England Journal of Medicine* 327:1832-1835, 1992.

[16] Hoyert, D.L.; Kockanck, K.D.; and Murph, S.L. Deaths: Final data for 1997. *National Vital Statistics Report* 47(19), 1999.

[17] CDC. Ectopic pregnancy in the United States, 1990–92. *Morbidity and Mortality Weekly Report* 44(3):46-48, 1995.

[18] NCHS. *Healthy People 2000 Review, 1997*. Hyattsville, MD: Public Health Service, 1997, 131-132.

[19] CDC. Differences in maternal mortality among black and white women, United States. *Morbidity and Mortality Weekly Report* 44(2):6-7, 13-14, 1995.

[20] AAP, Committee on Substance Abuse. Drug-exposed infants. *Pediatrics* 96(2):364-367, 1995.

[21] Chasnoff, I.J.; Griffith, D.R.; MacGregor, S.; et al. Temporal patterns of cocaine use in pregnancy: Perinatal outcome. *Journal of the American Medical Association* 261:1741-1744, 1989.

[22] Bigol, N.; Fuchs, M.; Diaz, V.; et al. Teratogenicity of cocaine in humans. *Journal of Pediatrics* 110:93-96, 1987.

[23] Rayburn, W.F.; Stanley, J.R.; and Garrett, M.E. Periconceptional folate intake and neural tube defects. *Journal of the American College of Nutrition* 15(2):121-125, 1996.

[24] CDC. Use of folic acid for prevention of spina bifida and other neural tube defects: 1983–1991. *Morbidity and Mortality Weekly Report* 40:513-516, 1991.

[25] Howie, P.W.; Forsyth, J.S.; Ogston, S.A.; et al. Protective effect of breast feeding against infection. *British Medical Journal* 300:11-16, 1990.

[26] Kovar, M.G.; Serdula, M.K.; Marks, J.S.; et al. Review of the epidemiologic evidence for an association between infant feeding and infant health. *Pediatrics* 74:S615-S638, 1984.

[27] Popkin, B.M.; Adair, L.; Akin, J.S.; et al. Breast-feeding and diarrheal morbidity. *Pediatrics* 86:874-882, 1990.

[28] Beaudry, M.; Dufour, R.; and Marcoux, S. Relation between infant feeding and infections during the first 6 months of life. *Journal of Pediatrics* 126:191-197, 1995.

[29] Frank, A.L.; Taber, L.H.; Glezen, W.P.; et al. Breast-feeding and respiratory virus infection. *Pediatrics* 70:239-245, 1982.

[30] Wright, A.L.; Holberg, C.J.; Taussig L.M.; et al. Relationship of infant feeding to recurrent wheezing at age 6 years. *Archives of Pediatric and Adolescent Medicine* 149:758-763, 1995.

[31] Saarinen, U.M. Prolonged breast feeding as prophylaxis for recurrent otitis media. *Acta Paediatric Scandinavica* 71:567-571, 1982.

[32] Duncan, B.; Ey, J.; Holberg, C.J.; et al. Exclusive breast-feeding for at least 4 months protects against otitis media. *Pediatrics* 91:867-872, 1993.

[33] Montgomery, D., and Splett, P. Economic benefit of breast-feeding infants enrolled in WIC. *Journal of the American Dietetic Association* 97:379-385, 1997.

[34] Tuttle, C.R., and Dewey, K.G. Potential cost savings for Medi-Cal, AFDC, food stamps, and WIC programs associated with increasing breast-feeding among low-income Hmong women in California. *Journal of the American Dietetic Association* 6:885-890, 1996.

[35] Chua, S.; Arulkumaran, S.; Lim, I.; et al. Influence of breastfeeding and nipple stimulation on postpartum uterine activity. *British Journal of Obstetrics and Gynecology* 101:804-805, 1994.

[36] Dewey, K.G.; Heinig, M.J.; and Nommsen, L.A. Maternal weight-loss patterns during prolonged lactation. *American Journal of Clinical Nutrition* 58:162-166, 1993.

[37] Newcomb, P.A.; Storer, B.E.; Longnecker, M.P.; et al. Lactation and a reduced risk of premenopausal breast cancer. *New England Journal of Medicine* 330:81-87, 1994.

[38] Melton, L.J.; Bryant, S.C.; Wahner, H.W.; et al. Influence of breastfeeding and other reproductive factors on bone mass later in life. *Osteoporosis International* 3:76-83, 1993.

[39] Willinger, M.; Hoffman, H.J.; and Hartford, R.B. Infant sleep position and risk for sudden infant death syndrome: Report of meeting held January 13 and 14, 1994, National Institutes of Health, Bethesda, MD. *Pediatrics* 93(5):814-819, 1994.

[40] Palta, M.; Weinstein, M.R.; McGuinness, G.; et al. A population study. Mortality and morbidity after availability of surfactant therapy. Newborn Lung Project. *Archives of Pediatric and Adolescent Medicine* 148(12):1295-1301, 1994.

[41] Schoendorf, K.C., and Kiely, J.L. Birth weight and age-specific analysis of the 1990 U.S. infant mortality drop. Was it surfactant? *Archives of Pediatric and Adolescent Medicine* 151(2):129-134, 1997.

[42] NCHS, CDC. National Vital Statistics System, unpublished data, 1999.

[43] Berg, C.; Atrash, H.; Koonin, L.; et al. Pregnancy-related mortality in the United States, 1987–1990. *Obstetrics and Gynecology* 88:161-167, 1996.

[44] CDC. Maternal mortality—United States, 1982–1996. *Morbidity and Mortality Weekly Report* 47(34):705-707, 1998.

[45] Bennet, T.A.; Kotelchuck, M.; Cox, C.E.; et al. Pregnancy-associated hospitalizations in the United States in 1991 and 1992: A comprehensive view of maternal morbidity. *American Journal of Obstetrics and Gynecology* 178:346-356, 1998.

[46] Grad, R., and Hill, I.T. Financing maternal and child health care in the United States. In: Kotch, J.B.; Blakely, C.; Brown, S.; et al.; eds. *A Pound of Prevention: The Case for Universal Maternity Care in the U.S.* Washington, DC: American Public Health Association, 1992.

[47] American College of Obstetricians and Gynecologists (ACOG). *Manual of Standards in Obstetric-Gynecologic Practice.* 2nd ed. Chicago, IL: ACOG, 1965.

[48] Kotelchuck, M. An evaluation of the Kessner Adequacy of Prenatal Care Index and a proposed Adequacy of Prenatal Care Utilization Index. *American Journal of Public Health* 84:1414-1420, 1994.

[49] Expert Panel on the Content of Prenatal Care. *Caring for Our Future: The Content of Prenatal Care.* Washington, DC: Public Health Service, 1989.

[50] Charles, A.G.; Norr, K.L.; Block, C.R.; et al. Obstetric and psychological effects of psychoprophylactic preparation for childbirth. *American Journal of Obstetrics and Gynecology* 131(1):44-52, 1978.

[51] Genest, M. Preparation for childbirth, evidence for efficacy. A review. *Journal of Obstetric, Gynecologic, and Neonatal Nursing* 10(2):82-85, 1981.

[52] Powell, S.L.; Holt, V.L.; Hickok, D.E.; et al. Recent changes in delivery site of low-birth-weight infants in Washington: Impact on birth weight-specific mortality. *American Journal of Obstetrics and Gynecology* 173(5):1585-1592, 1995.

[53] Kirby, R.S. Perinatal mortality: The role of hospital of birth. *Journal of Perinatology* 16(1):43-49, 1996.

[54] Paneth, N.; Kiely, J.L.; Wallenstein, S.; et al. The choice of place of delivery: Effect of hospital level on mortality in all singleton births in New York City. *American Journal of Disabilities in Children* 141(1):60-64, 1987.

[55] McCormick, M.C., and Richardson, D.K. Access to neonatal intensive care. *Future Child* 5(1):162-175, 1995.

[56] Curtin, S.C. Rates of cesarean birth and vaginal birth after previous cesarean, 1991–95. *Monthly Vital Statistics Report* 45(Suppl. 3)(11):1-12, 1997.

[57] Main, E.K. Reducing cesarean birth rates with data-driven quality improvement activities. *Pediatrics* 103:374-383, 1999.

[58] ACOG, Task Force on Cesarean Delivery. *Considerations in Evaluating the Incidence of Cesarean Delivery.* Washington DC: ACOG, in press

[59] Philip, A.G. Neonatal mortality rate: Is further improvement possible? *Journal of Pediatrics* 126(3):427-433, 1995.

[60] Hack, M.; Klein, N.K.; and Taylor, H.G. Long-term developmental outcomes of low birth weight infants. *Future Child* 5(1):176-196, 1995.

[61] Schendel, D.E.; Stockbauer, J.W.; Hoffman, H.J.; et al. Relation between very low birth weight and developmental delay among preschool children without disabilities. *American Journal of Epidemiology* 146(9):740-749, 1997.

[62] Kramer, W.B.; Saade, G.R.; Goodrum, L.; et al. Neonatal outcome after active perinatal management of the very premature infant between 23 and 27 weeks gestation. *Journal of Perinatology* 17(6):439-443, 1997.

[63] Lefebvre, F.; Glorieux, J.; and St-Laurent-Gagnon, T. Neonatal survival and disability rate at age 18 months for infants born between 23 and 28 weeks of gestation. *American Journal of Obstetrics and Gynecology* 174(3):833-838, 1996.

[64] Adams, M.M.; Sarno, A.P.; Harlass, F.E.; et al. Risk factors for preterm delivery in a healthy cohort. *Epidemiology* 6(5):525-532, 1995.

[65] Harlow, B.L.; Frigoletto, F.D.; Cramer, D.W.; et al. Determinants of preterm delivery in low-risk pregnancies. The RADIUS Study Group. *Journal of Clinical Epidemiology* 49(4):441-448, 1996.

[66] Virji, S.K., and Cottington, E. Risk factors associated with preterm deliveries among racial groups in a national sample of married mothers. *American Journal of Perinatology* 8(5):347-353, 1991.

[67] Lundsberg, L.S.; Bracken, M.B.; and Saftlas, A.F. Low-to-moderate gestational alcohol use and intrauterine growth retardation, low birthweight, and preterm delivery. *Annals of Epidemiology* 7(7):498-508, 1997.

[68] Goldenberg, R.L. Prenatal care and pregnancy outcome. In: Kotch, J.B.; Blakely, C.H.; Brown, S.B.; et al.; eds. *A Pound of Prevention: The Case for Universal Maternity Care in the U.S.* Washington, DC: American Public Health Association, 1992.

[69] Carmichael, S.; Abrams, B.; and Selvin, S. The association of pattern of maternal weight gain with length of gestation and risk of spontaneous preterm delivery. *Paediatric Perinatology and Epidemiology* 11(4):392-406, 1997.

[70] Goldenberg, R.L.; Andrews, W.W.; Yuan, A.C.; et al. Sexually transmitted diseases and adverse outcomes of pregnancy. *Clinics in Perinatology* 24(1):23-41, 1997.

[71] Hillier, S.; Nugent, R.; Eschenbach, D.; et al. Association between bacterial vaginosis and preterm delivery of low-birth-weight infant. *New England Journal of Medicine* 333:1737-1742, 1995.

[72] Meis, P.H.; Goldenberg, R.L.; Mercer, G.; et al. The preterm prediction study: Significance of vaginal infections. *American Journal of Obstetrics and Gynecology* 173(4):1231-1235, 1995.

[73] Berenson, A.B.; Wieman, C.M.; Wilkinson, G.S.; et al. Perinatal morbidity associated with violence experienced by pregnant women. *American Journal of Obstetrics and Gynecology* 170(6):1760-1766, 1994.

[74] Dewey, K.G.; Heinig, M.J.; and Nommsen-Rivers, L.A. Differences in morbidity between breast-fed and formula-fed infants. *Pediatrics* 126:696-702, 1995.

[75] Copper, R.L.; Goldenberg, R.L.; Das, A.; et al. The preterm prediction study: Maternal stress is associated with spontaneous preterm birth at less than 35 weeks gestation. National Institute of Child Health and Human Development Maternal–Fetal Medicine Units Network. *American Journal of Obstetrics and Gynecology* 175(5):1286-1292, 1996.

[76] Rawlings, J.S.; Rawlings, V.B.; and Read, J.A. Prevalence of low birth weight and preterm delivery in relation to the interval between pregnancies among white and black women. *New England Journal of Medicine* 332(2):69-74, 1995.

[77] Orr, S.T.; James, S.A.; Miller, C.A.; et al. Psychosocial stressors and low birthweight in an urban population. *American Journal of Preventive Medicine* 12(6):459-466, 1996.

[78] Institute of Medicine (IOM), National Academy of Sciences, Subcommittee on Nutritional Status and Weight Gain During Pregnancy. *Nutrition During Pregnancy*. Washington, DC: National Academy Press, 1990.

[79] Hickey, C.A.; Cliver, S.P.; McNeal, S.F.; et al. Prenatal weight gain patterns and birth weight among nonobese black and white women. *Obstetrics and Gynecolology* 88(4, Part 1):490-496, 1996.

[80] Siega-Riz, A.M.; Adair, L.S.; and Hobel, C.J. Institute of Medicine maternal weight gain recommendations and pregnancy outcome in a predominantly Hispanic population. *Obstetrics and Gynecology* 84(4):565-573, 1994.

[81] Willinger, M.; Hoffman, H.J.; Wu, K.T.; et al. Factors associated with the transition to non-prone sleep positions of infants in the United States. The National Infant Sleep Position Study. *Journal of the American Medical Association* 280:329-335, 1998.

[82] Oyen, N.; Markestad, T.; Skjærven, R.; et al. Combined effects of sleeping position and prenatal risk factors in sudden infant death syndrome: The Nordic Epidemiological SIDS Study. *Pediatrics* 100(4):613-621, 1997.

[83] Martin, R.J.; DiFiore, J.M.; Korenke, C.B.; et al. Vulnerability of respiratory control in healthy preterm infants placed supine. *Journal of Pediatrics* 127(4):609-614, 1995.

[84] AAP, AAP Task Force on Infant Sleep Position and SIDS. *Changing Concepts of Sudden Infant Death Syndrome: Implications for Infant Sleeping Environment and Sleep Position*. Elk Grove Village, IL: AAP, 2000.

[85] IOM, Standing Committee on Scientific Evaluation of Dietary Reference Intakes. *Dietary Reference Intakes for Thiamine, Riboflavin, Niacin, Vitamin B-6, Folate, Vitamin B-12, Pantothenic Acid, Biotin, and Choline*. Washington, DC: National Academy Press, 1998.

[86] Zuckerman, B. Marijuana and cigarette smoking during pregnancy: Neonatal effects. In: Chasnoff, I., ed. *Drugs, Alcohol, Pregnancy, and Parenting*. Boston, MA: Kluwer Academic Publishers, 1988.

[87] Jones, K.L. Fetal alcohol syndrome. *Pediatric Review* 8:122-126, 1986.

[88] Lundsberg, L.S.; Bracken, M.B.; and Saftlas, A.F. Low-to-moderate gestational alcohol use and intrauterine growth retardation, low birth weight, and preterm delivery. *Annals of Epidemiology* 7(7):498-508, 1997.

[89] Substance Abuse and Mental Health Services Administration. National Household Survey on Drug Abuse, Main Findings, 1997. April 1999, 8.

[90] Streissguth, A.P. The behavioral teratology of alcohol: Performance, behavioral, and intellectual deficits in prenatally exposed children. In: West, J.R., ed. *Alcohol and Brain Development*. New York, NY: Oxford University Press, 1986, 3-44.

[91] Weiner, L., and Morse, B.A. FAS: Clinical perspectives and prevention. In: Chasnoff, I.J., ed. *Drugs, Alcohol, Pregnancy, and Parenting*. Boston, MA: Kluwer Academic Publishers, 1988, 127-148.

[92] CDC. Update: Trends in fetal alcohol syndrome—United States, 1979–1993. *Morbidity and Mortality Weekly Report* 44(13):245-251.

[93] Abel, E. L. Update on incidence of fetal alcohol syndrome. *Neurotoxicology and Teratology* (17)4:437-443, 1995.

[94] Sampson, P.D.; Streissguth, A.P.; Bookstein, F.L.; et al. Incidence of fetal alcohol syndrome and prevalence of alcohol-related neurodevelopmental disorders. *Teratology* 56(5):317-326, 1997.

[95] AAP, Committee on Substance Abuse, and Committee on Children with Disabilities. Fetal alcohol syndrome and fetal alcohol effects. *Pediatrics* 1993; 91(5):1004-1006.

[96] ACOG. *Technical Bulletin No. 195: Substance Abuse in Pregnancy*. Washington, DC: ACOG, 1994.

[97] AAP, Committee on Drugs. The transfer of drugs and other chemicals into human milk. *Pediatrics* 93:137-150, 1994.

[98] Council of Regional Networks for Genetic Services (CORN). Newborn Screening Committee, *National Newborn Screening Report—1993.* Atlanta, GA: CORN, 1998.

[99] CORN, Newborn Screening Committee. *National Newborn Screening Report—1993.* Atlanta, GA: CORN, 1998.

[100] AAP, Committee on Genetics. 1989 newborn screening fact sheets. *Pediatrics* 83(3):449-464, 1989.

[101] AAP, Committee on Genetics. Issues in newborn screening. *Pediatrics* 89(2):345-349, 1992.

[102] AAP, Section on Endocrinology, and Committee on Genetics and American Thyroid Committee on Public Health. Newborn screening for congenital hypothyroidism: Recommended guidelines. *Pediatrics* 91(6):1203-1209, 1993.

[103] CORN, Newborn Screening Committee. *Guidelines for the Newborn Screening System: Follow-Up of Children, Diagnosis, Management, and Evaluation.* Atlanta, GA: CORN, 1999.

[104] Gaston, M.H.; Verter, J.I.; Woods, G.; et al. Prophylaxis with oral penicillin in children with sickle cell anemia: A randomized trial. *New England Journal of Medicine* 314:1593-1599, 1986.

[105] Davis, H.; Schoendorf, K.C.; Gergen, P.J.; et al. National trends in the mortality of children with sickle cell disease, 1968 through 1992. *American Journal of Public Health* 87:1317-1322, 1997.

[106] CDC. Mortality among children with sickle cell disease identified by newborn screening during 1990–1994—California, Illinois, and New York. *Morbidity and Mortality Weekly Report* 47:169-172, 1998.

[107] AAP, Ad Hoc Task Force on Definition of the Medical Home. The medical home. *Pediatrics* 90(5):774, 1992.

[108] Sia, C.J., and Peter, M.I. The medical home comes of age. *Hawaii Medical Journal* 47(9):409-410, 1988.

[109] AAP, Committee on Child Health Financing. *Managed Care and Children With Special Health Care Needs: Creating a Medical Home.* Elk Grove Village, IL: AAP, 1998.

[110] AAP. *The Medical Home and Early Intervention: Linking Services for Children With Special Needs.* Elk Grove Village, IL: AAP, 1999.

[111] Brewer, Jr., E.J.; Stewart, J.; McPherson, M.; et al. Family-centered, community-based, coordinated care for children with special health care needs. *Pediatrics* 83(6):1055-1060, 1989.

[112] McPherson, M.; Arango, P.; Fox, H.; et al. A new definition of children with special health care needs. *Pediatrics* 102(1):137-139, 1998.

[113] AAP, Committee on Children with Disabilities. Managed care and children with special health care needs: A subject review. *Pediatrics* 102(3):657-660, 1998.

17

Medical Product Safety

Lead Agency: Food and Drug Administration

Contents

Goal

Ensure the safe and effective use of medical products.

Overview

Issues and Trends

Medical products—which include drugs, biological products, and medical devices—provide great public benefit. Although marketed medical products are required to be safe, this safety requirement does not mean they have zero risk. A safe product has reasonable risks, given the magnitude of the benefit expected from the product and the alternatives to its use. Thus the choice to use a medical product involves balancing its benefits with the potential risks of using it. The comparative evaluation—which involves weighing the benefits (positive effects) and risks (potential harm) of various medical options for treatment, prophylaxis, prevention, or diagnosis—is an essential part of determining product safety. Evaluation is done during research and development on new medical products or procedures (such as surgery) or by a regulatory authority deliberating the approval or withdrawal of a product or some intermediate action, by a physician on behalf of a patient, or by the patient. Such weighing, whether implicit or explicit, is at the heart of decisionmaking in medicine and health care.

The United States has an elaborate system to maintain this benefit-risk balance by making sure that products are developed, tested, manufactured, labeled, prescribed, dispensed, and used in a way that maximizes benefit and minimizes risk. This complex system involves several key players: manufacturers that develop and test medical products and submit applications for marketing approval to the Food and Drug Administration (FDA); FDA, which has an extensive premarketing review and approval process and uses a series of postmarketing programs to gather data on and assess risks; the health care delivery system; and patients, who rely on the health care system and providers for needed interventions and protection from injury. Regrettably, however, this elaborate benefit-risk system and its subsystems lack the integration needed to ensure optimal public health and safety.

Sources of risk. It is widely accepted that enormous benefits can be gained from using medical products. Yet while most are well tolerated, producing only minimal side effects or a low rate of adverse events, some products can be very toxic, producing a high rate of complications from side effects.[1] It is estimated that millions of adverse events associated with the use of medical products occur each year; many of these are serious and may result in death.[2]

Federal oversight of a medical product's benefits versus risks continues well beyond the initial marketing of a product. Once a medical product is approved for marketing, the safety of the product continues to be monitored by FDA, which collects and analyzes reports of product experience. As more products are approved for marketing, postmarketing surveillance becomes increasingly important. Through a program called MEDWATCH, FDA's Medical Products Reporting and Safety Information Program, health care professionals, patients, and consumers can report serious adverse events and problems associated with medical products to FDA, the manufacturer, or both. MEDWATCH also accepts reports of medication errors or potential errors. MEDWATCH partners include health professionals, consumers, and other appropriate health-related organizations or commercial interests that actively disseminate information on the critical importance of monitoring and reporting serious adverse events and product problems, along with information on how to report directly to FDA. These partners also provide a multiplier effect, by which MEDWATCH partners rapidly disseminate new FDA-related product safety information back to their membership.

The growing complexity of medical technology, coupled with economic pressures and organizational changes within health care institutions, increases the potential for unanticipated and unintended consequences in using medical devices. These developments demand that postmarket surveillance move from passive surveillance to a proactive strategy that includes understanding how organizations encounter medical devices, how problems are perceived and reported, and which characteristics of the health care system contribute to a given event. A safer patient environment can be created if increased efforts are made to identify product failures and errors before patients are injured.

Beyond the individual level of risk management (for example, patients and health care providers), managing risk must be targeted at the organization level. For example, user facilities such as hospitals, long-term care facilities, ambulatory surgical, outpatient treatment, and outpatient diagnostic centers are required to report errors related to medical devices. By law, these facilities are required to report any death to FDA and to the manufacturer of the device within 10 working days. Any serious illness or injury also must be reported by the user facility to the manufacturer within 10 working days, or, if the manufacturer is unknown, the report should be sent to FDA. Further, FDA encourages user facilities to report product or device malfunctions (for example, intravenous catheter defects) that do not result in death or serious injury directly to the manufacturer.

Efforts to manage risk at the community, national, and global levels present the most difficult public health challenges. The introduction of hepatitis B surface antigen screening and the change to an all-volunteer blood donor population in the mid-1970s resulted in substantial reductions in transfusion-transmitted viral hepatitis.[3] This success, however, was overshadowed by the unexpected emergence of a new blood-borne pathogen, human immunodeficiency virus (HIV). Since its initial recognition in the early 1980s, more than 8,000 persons have been diagnosed with transfusion-associated acquired immunodeficiency syndrome (AIDS), and approximately half of the U.S. hemophiliac population has been infected with HIV.[4] The HIV epidemic remains a potent reminder of the Nation's vulnerability to emerging agents and the tragic repercussions they can exact on those who depend on life-saving blood and blood products.

FDA has primary responsibility for ensuring blood safety. Improvements in donor screening, serologic testing, and viral inactivation procedures have made the U.S. blood supply one of the safest in the world. Nevertheless, many additional steps can be implemented by FDA, industry, consumers, and blood donor volunteers to go further. Since 1998, the U.S. Department of Health and Human Services (HHS) has coordinated the efforts of the Centers for Disease Control and Prevention (CDC), the National Institutes of Health (NIH), and FDA, with cooperation from other government agencies, in a Blood Action Plan. Consumer and donor confidence are important factors in maintaining a safe blood supply, and Healthy People 2010 objectives reflect those concerns and incorporate a science-based approach to expanding the blood supply and enhancing its safety.

Management of medical product risk. In general, the sources of medical product risks can be thought of as falling into four categories: (1) product defects, (2) known side effects, both avoidable and unavoidable, (3) medication or device errors, and (4) remaining uncertainties.[5] Because each type of risk has a different source, effective management of each is likely to be different.

Product defects. Historically, product defects have been an important source of medical product-associated injuries. In the case of pharmaceuticals, product defects usually include the lack of potency and the lack of purity of drugs. A significant portion of resources currently is devoted to regulating product quality. Research, surveillance, quality systems also called *current good manufacturing practices*, and inspections form the cornerstone of FDA efforts to minimize product defects.

Known side effects. When using a drug or other medical product, a patient runs the risk of experiencing reactions resulting from the product's interaction with the body. For pharmaceuticals, these reactions are commonly termed *side effects*. They usually are identified in a product's package insert as possible risks. Known side effects are the source of the majority of injuries and deaths resulting from product use.

Some known side effects often are predictable and avoidable. To avoid them, the health care practitioner must select the best treatment and plan appropriate measures to manage the risks to the patient. For example, when prescribing certain prescription medications that are renal toxic (toxic to the kidneys), practitioners need to ensure that their patients are well hydrated or calculate dose adjustments to reduce the risk of toxicity or kidney failure. A medical practitioner can choose the wrong therapy for a specific condition (for example, using antibiotics for viral infections). Alternatively, a practitioner may prescribe the appropriate therapy but fail to individualize the therapy or monitor the patient for signs of toxicity. Examples of avoidable side effects include the consequences of known drug-drug interactions or prescribing an inappropriate dosage for elderly persons.

In many cases, known side effects are unavoidable because they can occur even if a product is used appropriately. Although estimates vary, the overall human and economic costs of unavoidable side effects are high.[6] The risk of experiencing such side effects is the inevitable price of the benefits of treatment. Examples of common, predictable, usually unavoidable side effects include superinfection following antimicrobial chemotherapy, fatigue and depression from interferon use, and bone marrow suppression from chemotherapy. For the successful management of these risks, both the practitioner and patient must be fully aware of the risks involved in treatment, agree to the treatment, and provide careful patient monitoring to detect early symptoms of known side effects.

Medication or device errors. A medication or device error involves the incorrect use of a prescribed product or incorrect operation or placement of a medical device. Errors also involve unintended substitution of the wrong product for the prescribed product. Errors can occur, for example, when a confusing product name results in the wrong product being dispensed or when inattention results in an overdose of an intended drug. Substantial numbers of injuries and deaths occur annually because of medication or device errors.[7] In general, medication and device errors are believed to result from problems intrinsic to the health care system. That is, these errors often are the result of a sequence of errors within the health care system. For example, a physician's poor handwriting on the prescription pad and unclear or confusing prescription drug labeling result in pharmacists' misreading prescriptions and labeling and filling prescriptions with the wrong medications. Such errors are not totally preventable, but they can be minimized through enhancements aimed at integrating the overall health care system.

Remaining uncertainties. Given current scientific and medical knowledge, it is not possible to learn everything about the effects of a medical product. For example, new information about long-marketed products may become available. Therefore, a degree of uncertainty always exists about both the benefits and risks of medical products, including unexpected side effects, long-term effects, effects of off-label use, and effects in populations not studied before marketing.

Managing risk and medical product safety is a matter of continuously developing information. A comprehensive risk management system requires risk communication. Thus, effective risk communication demands that risk information be translated into words and formats that are readily understood by practitioners, caregivers, and patients. For example, U.S. Pharmacopeia (USP) and FDA have adopted the National Coordinating Council for Medication Error Reporting and Prevention (NCC MERP) Taxonomy for Medication Errors in order to report, track, and benchmark medication error data in a standardized format for hospitals nationwide. In this risk communication strategy, FDA and USP are expected to provide a nationally projected measure of errors grouped according to categories established by the NCC MERP.

Because national data systems will not be available in the first half of the decade for tracking progress, three subjects of interest are not addressed in the Healthy People 2010 Medical Product Safety objectives. Representing a research and data collection agenda for the coming decade, the topics are related to record practices of health care professionals, plasma manufacturing, and data analysis. The first topic covers health care professionals who record their patient's use of botanicals, dietary supplements, and other alternative products to identify the risks of using these products in combination with conventional drugs and biologics. The second topic addresses the development and application of effective methods for complete inactivation or removal of pathogens from plasma, blood, and blood products. The third involves the proportion of new medical products that have had pre- and postmarketing clinical data analyzed for gender differences.

Disparities

Certain groups are particularly vulnerable to poor health outcomes because they are exposed to both socioeconomic and age-related physiological stress factors that interact synergistically. People aged 65 years and older, for example, take the greatest number and quantity of medications.[8] Of elderly patients taking three or more prescription drugs for chronic conditions, more than one-third are rehospitalized within 6 months of discharge from a hospital, with 20 percent of those readmissions due to drug problems.[9] Twenty-eight percent of hospitalizations of older people are due to noncompliance with drug therapy and adverse events.[10] Adverse drug events rank fifth among the top preventable threats to the health of older people in the United States, after congestive heart failure, breast cancer, hypertension, and pneumonia.[11] Moreover, 32,000 adults aged 65 years and older suffer hip fractures each year as a result of falls associated with the use of psychotropic drugs, which are used to treat the patients' underlying medical condition.[12] A growth in these numbers is expected, given the increasing number and potency of drug products being marketed and the increasing percentage of the population that are elderly.

Data collection systems do not exist that would allow analysis of disparities in adverse events among different population groups. Because there is a need to look at select populations, which are diverse in race, ethnicity, socioeconomic status, and area of residence, it is likely that data will be needed from many provider organizations.

Another example of a common variable that predisposes individuals to vulnerability and poor health outcomes is literacy. Literacy disparities are of concern because low-literacy patients cannot be "empowered" consumers.[13] Further, patients who do not understand health professionals' instructions will not receive good-quality care. Finally, because health literacy problems are concentrated in populations that depend on public programs for their medical care, an education effort may be required to inform public assistance patients about how to understand the proper use of their medicines. To reach all people effectively, information must be provided in a variety of formats and reading levels. (See Focus Area 7. Educational and Community-Based Programs and Focus Area 11. Health Communication.)

Although medical products provide benefits, they also can cause injury and harm. FDA and other participants (for example, pharmaceutical manufacturers, health care providers, consumers, and patients) act in ways to maximize the benefits and minimize the risks associated with using medical products.[4] Often, these actions are insufficiently integrated. A common goal of maximizing benefits and minimizing risks could be greatly advanced if the participants work together within an integrated framework. An integrated benefit-risk management framework, if adopted, would contribute to improving risk communication and risk confrontation.

Risk communication. The health care industry has experienced tremendous growth and demand in building an infrastructure driven by technology. For example, elaborate information technology (IT) software programs, which link to huge databases, allow access to a vast amount of valuable information for pharmacists and other health care professionals, health care organizations, and consumers. The information in these systems is used to improve patient care, design better health care methods, improve operations, and enhance organizational planning. Many groups benefit from sharing information between different components of health care, including patients, providers, insurance companies, medical equipment companies, pharmaceutical companies, hospitals, and data processing and health research corporations. Technology is available to integrate the different components of health care, but its use today is minimal except in select health care settings. Therefore, it would be advantageous to encourage upgrades to present technology systems and links to other integrated technology systems to improve patient care, always keeping in mind, of course, patient confidentiality.

Evolving automation offers the possibility of placing the entire patient record into an electronic format. Electronic formats offer the possibility of automatically and instantaneously checking any new therapy for incompatibilities with the products, appropriate indications and dosing range, and the patient's current therapies and contraindications (for example, allergies or reduced hepatic or renal function). Electronic formats also offer the possibility of looking at diagnoses and seeing whether patients (or in cases of children, their parents) have been exposed to existing therapies in the past.

Further, as IT systems become more advanced and sophisticated, there is a growing need to ensure and protect patient confidentiality. Health plans, providers, and pharmacy benefit managers have long recognized the importance of maintaining the confidentiality of patient-identifiable medical information. There is a vast potential for information sharing between different components of health care if the confidentiality issues can be overcome. Legislation to protect patients from the inappropriate disclosure of their medical information will be essential to the development of systems that are designed to protect their health and welfare.

One final consideration for effective risk communication is to provide information about medical products that is useful for patients, consumers, and practitioners.

(See Focus Area 11. Health Communication.) Effective risk communication requires information presented in words and formats readily understood by practitioners, caregivers, and patients. This information must be disseminated in a timely fashion and incorporated into clinical practice that is aimed at altering behaviors. Since March 1999, Federal regulations have required over-the-counter (OTC) drug manufacturers to follow a specific format for the labeling of OTC drugs.[14] The format is intended to assist consumers in reading and understanding OTC drug product labeling so that they can use these products safely and effectively.

Risk confrontation. Determining the acceptable level of risk should occur in a larger context.[15] This activity is characterized as risk confrontation, defined as community-based problem solving that actively involves stakeholders in the decisionmaking process.[16] This definition implies that social and community values are at least as important as the technical judgments of professionals and should be included in the determination of acceptable risk.

Science provides only a statistical assessment of risk; it cannot determine its acceptability. Affected communities may differ from regulatory agencies in how they value either risks or benefits. They also may judge differently the amount of uncertainty that is tolerable. Advocacy groups for patients with various diseases, most notably AIDS and cancer, have shown over the past several years that it is impossible to assess accurately the acceptability of risks in light of the potential benefits without the input of the affected community. Although some advocates for patients with life-threatening illnesses are willing to accept a high degree of risk to gain the benefits of new products, other advocacy groups, such as those against mandatory vaccination, feel that no risk is acceptable.

To obtain community input, FDA has engaged in multiple outreach efforts with external stakeholders, soliciting their ideas, opinions, and concerns regarding the safe use of medical products. In the context of determining risk, for example, fostering open public discussions is critical to enhancing participants' practical understanding and illuminating practice choices in the risk decision process. A carefully prepared summary of scientific information will not give participants in the risk decision the understanding they need if that information is not relevant to the decision to be made. It is not sufficient to get the science right; an informed decision also requires getting the right science, that is, directing the scientific effort to the issues most pertinent to the decision.

The Healthy People 2000 objective on linked computer systems has been met. In 1995, 98 percent of pharmacies were using computers. Data for providers who review medications for older patients and for the proportion of patients who receive verbal and written information for new prescriptions from prescribers and dispensers show progress. The proportion of adverse event drug reports voluntarily sent to FDA that are regarded as serious has declined slightly and is moving away from the target.

Note: Unless otherwise noted, data are from the Centers for Disease Control and Prevention, National Center for Health Statistics, *Healthy People 2000 Review, 1998–99*.

Medical Product Safety

Goal: Ensure the safe and effective use of medical products.

Number	Objective Short Title
17-1	Monitoring of adverse medical events
17-2	Linked, automated information systems
17-3	Provider review of medications taken by patients
17-4	Receipt of useful information about prescriptions from pharmacies
17-5	Receipt of oral counseling about medications from prescribers and dispensers
17-6	Blood donations

17-1. **(Developmental) Increase the proportion of health care organizations that are linked in an integrated system that monitors and reports adverse events.**

17-1a. Health care organizations that are linked in an integrated system that monitors and reports adverse events associated with medical therapies.

17-1b. Health care organizations that are linked in an integrated system that monitors and reports adverse events associated with medical devices.

Potential data sources: Office of Postmarketing Drug Risk Assessment (OPDRA), MEDWATCH, and Manufacturer and User Device Experience (MAUDE) Database, FDA.

Collaboration between Federal authorities and researchers with pharmacoepidemiologic databases can be helpful in monitoring suspected associations between specific drug exposures and specific adverse events and in estimating such risk. Linked databases could provide immediate access to existing data sources with the capability of providing assessments of study feasibility, responding to specific drug safety questions within a few weeks, and providing a complete analysis of those questions deemed feasible within a few months. Databases should be able to provide exposure data on new molecular entities (those approved within the past 5 years in the United States), to perform feasibility studies of multiple drugs or multiple outcomes, to identify adverse drug events that occur infrequently (that is, at rates lower than can be detected in clinical trials), and to provide data and preliminary analyses within a very short time frame (2 to 4 weeks, depending on the problem).

To identify unknown events more rapidly, there must be an enhanced program of communication for health professionals nationwide that builds on the work of MEDWATCH, encouraging the recognition of unique and rare events. To evaluate and quantify newly identified events, there must be a significant population base under close electronic surveillance for indicators of adverse reactions. A relatively large number of persons (estimated around 20 million) is necessary because so many persons are lost to followup when they move from one provider organization to another. If medical records are ultimately transferred from one provider to another, a number smaller than 20 million may suffice to allow outcomes to be linked with earlier therapies. A system must be available for accessing the original patient record while maintaining confidentiality.

Staff-model health maintenance organizations (HMOs) are providing health care services to a greater proportion of patients and, therefore, would be a good target for linked data systems capable of picking up rare adverse events and signals in patient populations. HMOs and other health care providers capable of producing complete patient records should be particularly targeted to participate in this development. At present, there is no standard format for these records. HMOs may have different systems at each site, or, where organizations have come together to form a single large organization, each remnant of the original organizations may have preserved its own medical record system. HMOs might be encouraged to see safety surveillance data as a product, which could be purchased by the Federal Government and industry after appropriate protection of patient privacy. Alternatively, large employers or government agencies might use their purchasing power to demand safety surveillance as a deliverable under managed care contracts.

The Safe Medical Device Acts of 1990 and 1992 mandate reporting of device-related deaths to FDA and device-related deaths and serious injuries to manufacturers. The program has shown only limited success. Research on the program indicates that the quantity and quality of data received could be enhanced through training and education for end users of medical devices regarding how to report device-related deaths and serious injuries to manufacturers, additional assurance of the protection of data submitted, and regular, timely feedback. The research also suggested that a medical surveillance network could improve the protection of patients and device users by reducing the likelihood of medical device-related adverse events. The system should collect high-quality data on adverse medical events, analyze the data to identify newly emerging device problems and changes in device use, disseminate data on such problems in a timely manner to concerned parties, and apply the knowledge gained from the reported data to the device approval process and to prevention and control programs.

17-2. (Developmental) Increase the use of linked, automated systems to share information.

17-2a. By health care professionals in hospitals and comprehensive, integrated health care systems.

17-2b. By pharmacists and other dispensers.

Potential data sources: National Survey of Pharmacy Practice in Acute Care and Survey of Managed Care and Ambulatory Care Pharmacy Practice in Integrated Health Systems, American Society of Hospital Pharmacists (ASHP).

Automated information systems enable pharmacists in hospitals, HMOs, and U.S. Department of Veterans Affairs (VA) settings to review a patient's medical record, pharmaceutical history, allergies and contraindications to medications, blood chemistries and microbiological drug sensitivities, and treatment schedule files. These systems help administrative personnel in various work settings to process prescription claims and payments, measure the quality of health care, perform cost analyses, provide drug information, perform pharmacoeconomic analyses, and purchase pharmaceutical products.

Dispensers of prescription medications use linked systems to provide warnings about dosing errors and potential adverse events among medications dispensed by different sources to individual patients. In 1993, 95 percent of pharmacies used computer systems.[17] Advances in computer technology should facilitate information sharing in a way that helps health care professionals and researchers link drug products and outcomes in order to benefit individual patients and to discover previously unknown adverse reactions.

Computerization of the medication use process can help prevent prescribing, dispensing, and administration errors. The documented value of direct order entry continues to be confirmed.[18] A recent study demonstrated that replacing handwritten medication orders with a computerized physician order entry system led to a 54 percent reduction in serious medication errors.[19] In addition, the National Patient Safety Foundation at the American Medical Association (AMA) has identified direct computerized order entry as one of the best practices for preventing adverse drug events.[18]

17-3.   (Developmental) Increase the proportion of primary care providers, pharmacists, and other health care professionals who routinely review with their patients aged 65 years and older and patients with chronic illnesses or disabilities all new prescribed and over-the-counter medicines.

Potential data sources: Survey on Prescription Drug Issues and Usage, AARP; Physician Survey Under the Medication Error Reduction Initiative.

Adults aged 65 years and older account for less than 15 percent of the population, but they use about one-third of all retail prescriptions.[8] This population also purchases at least 40 percent of all nonprescription medicines.[8] Further, older adults are more likely to suffer from multiple chronic diseases and, as a result, may routinely visit multiple physicians, each of whom may be unaware of other medicines that have been prescribed.

In 1998, an AMA House of Delegates report urged physicians to incorporate medication reviews as part of routine office-based practice. The report also encouraged physicians to discuss compliance with the drug regimen with their patients and to inquire about the beneficial or adverse effects of drug therapy during followup office visits. AMA's House of Delegates report suggests that physician medication reviews are critically important in long-term therapy.[20]

17-4.   (Developmental) Increase the proportion of patients receiving information that meets guidelines for usefulness when their new prescriptions are dispensed.

Potential data source: Patient/Consumer Medication Information Survey, FDA.

A 1992 survey conducted by FDA of the amount of information received by consumers found that 14 percent of people received information about prescription drugs from prescribers and 32 percent from pharmacists.[21] These percentages do not reflect the usefulness of the information received because no content analyses were performed on the informational materials reported in the survey. Congress enacted legislation in 1996 that called on the private sector to develop a plan whereby 95 percent of persons would receive useful written information with their prescriptions by 2006. HHS approved guidelines in the Action Plan for the Provision of Useful Prescription Medicine Information in January 1997. In accordance with the plan, patient information materials were to be evaluated in 1999 and 2000. (See Focus Area 28. Vision and Hearing.)

17-5. Increase the proportion of patients who receive verbal counseling from prescribers and pharmacists on the appropriate use and potential risks of medications.

Target and baseline:

Objective	Increase in Patients Receiving Oral Counseling From:	1998 Baseline	2010 Target
		Percent	
17-5a.	Prescribers	24	95
17-5b.	Pharmacists	14	95

Target setting method: 296 percent improvement for prescribers and 579 percent improvement for pharmacists. (Better than the best will be used when data are available.)

Data source: National Survey of Prescription Drug Information Provided to Patients, FDA.

> Data for population groups currently are not analyzed.

Patients and their caregivers should be fully informed about the appropriate use and the risks of newly prescribed prescription medicines. The physician (or other prescribing health care professional) should initially discuss this information with the patient. The next opportunity for verbal counseling arises at the pharmacy. In both settings, written information about the medicine may be conveyed but is most effective when supplemental to verbal counseling. Elements of verbal counseling should include not only how much and how often to take the medication but also appropriate risk information, including precautions to take and the relevant side effects of the medication.

Participants in a 1997 national symposium on verbal counseling, sponsored by national pharmacy and pharmacist organizations, gave the highest rankings to the following reasons for such low counseling levels: patients do not understand what and why they need to know about their medicines, patients do not demand or expect counseling services from the pharmacists, and patients and payors do not see the value of counseling.[21] These findings suggest that a high number of pharmacists believe that patients do not understand what and why they need to know about their medications and, therefore, do not provide needed counseling. Since 1997, the American Pharmaceutical Association has maintained a policy stating that pharmacists should provide drug-related information to their patients in face-to-face oral consultations, supplemented by written or printed material or any other means best suited to an individual patient's needs.[22]

The National Council on Patient Information and Education (NCPIE) advocates that health care professionals anticipate consumers' desire for medication information but also recognize their possible reluctance to ask questions. NCPIE has developed several educational campaigns to facilitate question-asking behaviors by consumers and support information-giving behaviors by health care professionals.

17-6. Increase the proportion of persons who donate blood, and in so doing ensure an adequate supply of safe blood.

Target: 8 percent.

Baseline: 5 percent of the total population donated blood in 1994.

Target setting method: 60 percent improvement.

Data source: American Association of Blood Banks.

> **Data for population groups currently are not collected.**

FDA assumes primary responsibility for the safety of the Nation's blood supply. Blood availability, however, is restricted by, among other factors, the number of donors who qualify to give blood. Approximately 5 percent of the population in the United States donates blood once or twice a year. Recruitment of a larger percentage of the population would increase the availability of blood and blood products. Public awareness of the benefits that blood and blood products provide to cancer patients and others in need could serve to elicit a more generous response. Educational campaigns that address underlying public fears regarding the safety of blood donation procedures could also help. Increasing the donor pool would benefit the overall health of the Nation and remove donor incentives that border on remuneration.

Related Objectives From Other Focus Areas

1. **Access to Quality Health Care**
   1-3. Counseling about health behaviors
3. **Cancer**
   3-10. Provider counseling about cancer prevention
   3-12. Colorectal cancer screening
4. **Chronic Kidney Disease**
   4-8. Medical therapy for persons with diabetes and proteinuria
5. **Diabetes**
   5-17. Self-blood-glucose-monitoring
7. **Educational and Community-Based Programs**
   7-7. Patient and family education
   7-8. Satisfaction with patient education
   7-9. Health care organization sponsorship of community health promotion activities

Terminology

(A listing of abbreviations and acronyms used in this publication appears in Appendix H.)

Adverse drug experience (ADE): Any adverse event (defined below) associated with the use of a drug in humans, whether or not considered drug related. ADEs include the following: an adverse event occurring in the course of the use of a drug product in professional practice; an adverse event occurring as a result of a drug overdose, whether accidental or intentional; an adverse event occurring as a result of abusing a drug; an adverse event occurring from drug withdrawal; and any failure of a drug's expected pharmacological action.

Adverse event: Undesirable result from the use of a medical product. Terms used to describe such an event include adverse drug reaction (ADR), adverse experience, and adverse effect. For the purposes of Healthy People 2010, the term *adverse event* is used in most cases to avoid confusion.

Consumer: An individual who consumes or acquires medical products, such as nonprescription (over-the-counter) medicines or nonprescription medical devices, and prescription medicines.

Medical device: An instrument, apparatus, implement, machine, implant, or other similar or related article intended for use in the diagnosis of disease or other conditions or in the cure, mitigation, treatment, or prevention of disease.

Medical product: Any prescription and nonprescription drug, device, or biological product intended for use in the diagnosis of disease or other conditions or in the cure, mitigation, treatment, or prevention of the disease.

Medication or device error: A preventable event that may cause a medication or device to be used inappropriately and thus may harm a patient. Harm can occur while the medical product is being used by a health care professional, patient, or consumer.

Off-label use: Uses other than those for which the product is approved.

Patient: An individual who is under medical care or treatment.

Pharmacoepidemiologic database: A computerized database for capturing and manipulating data associated with the collection, analysis, and communication of drug or other therapeutic product risk information.

Risk assessment: Estimation and evaluation of risk.

Risk communication: Interactive process of exchanging risk information.

Superinfection: A new infection complicating the course of antimicrobial therapy by an organism different from that which caused the initial infection. The new infection results from invasion by bacteria or fungi resistant to the antimicrobial in use.

U.S. Pharmacopeia (USP): Organization that promotes the public health by establishing and disseminating officially recognized standards of quality and authoritative information for the use of medicines and other health care technologies.

References

[1] Lazarou, J.H; Pomeranz, B.; and Corey, P.N. Incidence of adverse drug reactions in hospitalized patients. A meta-analysis of prospective studies. *Journal of the American Medical Association* 279(15):1200-1205, 1998.

[2] Institute of Medicine. *To Err Is Human: Building a Safer Health System.* Kohn, L.T., ed. Washington, DC: National Academy Press, 1999.

[3] U.S. Department of Health and Human Services (HHS), Centers for Disease Control and Prevention (CDC). Public Health Service inter-agency guidelines for screening donors of blood, plasma, organs, tissues, and semen for evidence of hepatitis B. *Morbidity and Mortality Weekly Report* 40(RR-4): 1-17, 1999.

[4] CDC. *HIV/AIDS Surveillance Report* 11(1):12, 1999.

[5] Food and Drug Administration (FDA) Task Force on Risk Management. *Managing the Risks from Medical Product Use: Creating a Risk Management Framework.* Rockville, MD: FDA, May 1999.

[6] Johnson, J.A., and Bootan, L.J. Drug-related morbidity and mortality: A cost-of-illness model. *Archives of Internal Medicine* 155:1949-1956, 1995.

[7] Bates, D.W.; Cullen, D.J.; Laird, N.; et al. Incidence of adverse drug events and potential adverse drug events: Implications for prevention. *Journal of the American Medical Association* 274:29-34,1995.

[8] U.S. General Accounting Office (GAO). *Prescription Drugs and the Elderly.* AO/HEHS-95-152. Washington, DC: GAO, 1995.

[9] Bero, L.A.; Lipton, H.L.; and Bird, J.A. Characterization of geriatric drug-related hospital readmissions. *Medical Care* 29(10):989-1003, 1991.

[10] Col, N.; Fanale, J.E.; and Kronholm, P. The role of medication noncompliance and adverse drug reactions in hospitalizations of the elderly. *Archives of Internal Medicine* 150(4):841-845, 1990.

[11] Fink, A.; Siu, A.L.; Brook, R.H.; et al. Assuring the quality of health care for older persons. An expert panel's priorities. *Journal of the American Medical Association* 258(14):1905-1908, 1987.

[12] Ray, W.A.; Griffin, M.R.; Schaffner, W.; et al. Psychotropic drug use and the risk of hip fracture. *New England Journal of Medicine* 316(7):363-369, 1987.

[13] Ad Hoc Committee on Health Literacy for the Council on Scientific Affairs, American Medical Association. Health literacy: Report of the Council on Scientific Affairs. *Journal of the American Medical Association* 281(6):552-557, 1999.

[14] Federal Register. *Over the Counter Labeling for Drug Manufacturers.* Federal Register 64(51):13253-13303. Washington, DC, 1999.

[15] National Research Council, Committee on Risk Perception and Communication. *Improving Risk Communication.* Washington, DC: National Academy Press, 1989.

[16] Leviton, L.C.; Needlemen, C.E.; and Shapiro, M.A. *Confronting Public Health Risks: A Decision Maker's Guide.* Thousand Oaks, CA: Sage Publications, 1998.

[17] Association for Health System-Pharmacists (AHSP). AHSP guidelines on adverse drug reaction monitoring and reporting. *American Journal of Health-System Pharmacy* 52:417-419, 1995.

[18] Goldsmith, M.F. National Patient Safety Foundation Studies Systems. *Journal of the American Medical Association* 278:1561, 1997.

[19] Bates, D.W.; Leape, L.L.; Cullen, D.J.; et al. Effect of computerized physician order entry and a team intervention on prevention of serious medication errors. *Journal of the American Medical Association* 280(15):1311-1316, 1998.

[20] Council of Scientific Affairs. American Medical Association (AMA) Report to (I-98). *Physician Education of Their Patients About Prescription Medicines.* Chicago, IL: AMA, 1998.

[21] Morris, L.A.; Tabak, E.R.; and Gondek, K. Counseling patients about prescribed medication: 12-year trends. *Medical Care* 35(10):996-1007, 1997.

[22] Scott, D.M., and Wessels, M.J. Impact of OBRA '90 on pharmacists' patients counseling practices. *Journal of the American Pharmaceutical Association* NS37:401-406, July 1997.

18

Mental Health and Mental Disorders

Co-Lead Agencies: National Institutes of Health
Substance Abuse and Mental Health Services
Administration

Contents

Improve mental health and ensure access to appropriate, quality mental health services.

Overview

Mental health is a state of successful performance of mental function, resulting in productive activities, fulfilling relationships with other people, and the ability to adapt to change and to cope with adversity. Mental health is indispensable to personal well-being, family and interpersonal relationships, and contribution to community or society. *Mental disorders* are health conditions that are characterized by alterations in thinking, mood, or behavior (or some combination thereof), which are associated with distress and/or impaired functioning and spawn a host of human problems that may include disability, pain, or death. *Mental illness* is the term that refers collectively to all diagnosable mental disorders.

Issues

Mental disorders generate an immense public health burden of disability. The World Health Organization, in collaboration with the World Bank and Harvard University, has determined the "burden of disability" associated with the whole range of diseases and health conditions suffered by peoples throughout the world. A striking finding of the landmark *Global Burden of Disease* study is that the impact of mental illness on overall health and productivity in the United States and throughout the world often is profoundly underrecognized. In established market economies such as the United States, mental illness is on a par with heart disease and cancer as a cause of disability.[1] Suicide—a major public health problem in the United States—occurs most frequently as a consequence of a mental disorder.

Mental disorders occur across the lifespan, affecting persons of all racial and ethnic groups, both genders, and all educational and socioeconomic groups. In the United States approximately 40 million people aged 18 to 64 years, or 22 percent of the population, had a diagnosis of mental disorder alone (19 percent) or of a co-occurring mental and addictive disorder in the past year.[2, 3, 4] At least one in five children and adolescents between age 9 and 17 years has a diagnosable mental disorder in a given year.[5] Mental and behavioral disorders and serious emotional disturbances (SEDs) in children and adolescents can lead to school failure, alcohol or illicit drug use, violence, or suicide.[6, 7, 8] About 5 percent of children and adolescents are extremely impaired by mental, behavioral, and emotional disorders.[9] In later life, the majority of people aged 65 years and older cope constructively with the changes associated with aging and maintain mental health, yet an estimated 25 percent of older people (8.6 million) experience specific mental disorders, such as depression, anxiety, substance abuse, and dementia, that are not part

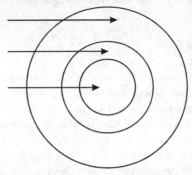

**Proportion of Adults Aged 18 Years and Older
With Mental Illness**
(By level of severity*)

Percent

23.9% Adults with any 12-month
DSM-III-R mental disorder

5.4% Adults with SMI

2.6% Adults with SPMI

*A mental disorder is any disorder coded in the *Diagnostic and Statistical Manual of Mental Disorders, III, Revised* (DSM-III-R), American Psychiatric Association, 1987.

SMI = Serious mental illness as coded in the DSM-III-R
SPMI = Serious and persistent mental illness as coded in the DSM-III-R

Source: Kessler, R.C.; Berglund, P.A.; Zbao, S.; et al. The 12-month prevalence and correlates of serious mental illness. *Mental Health, United States, 1998*. DHHS Publication Number (SMA) 99-8235. Rockville, MD: HHS, PHS, SAMHSA, CMHS, 1999.

of normal aging. Alzheimer's disease strikes 8 to 15 percent of people over age 65 years,[10] with the number of cases in the population doubling every 5 years of age after age 60 years. Alzheimer's disease is thought to be responsible for 60 to 70 percent of all cases of dementia and is one of the leading causes of nursing home placements.[11]

Mental disorders vary in severity and in their impact on people's lives. Mental disorders—such as schizophrenia, major depression and manic depressive or bipolar illness, and obsessive-compulsive disorder and panic disorder—can be enormously disabling.

■ *Schizophrenia* will affect more than 2 million people in the United States in 1 year.[3] The disorder tends to follow a long-term course, although the severity of symptoms may wax and wane. With modern treatments, increasing numbers of persons with schizophrenia can and do view recovery as an achievable goal.

■ *Affective disorders*, which encompass major depression and manic depressive illness, constitute a second category of severe mental illness. The World Health Organization found major depression to be the leading cause of disability among adults in developed nations such as the United States.[1] About 6.5 percent of women and 3.3 percent of men will have major depression in any year. Manic depressive illness affects around 1 percent of adults, with comparable rates of occurrence in men and women. A high rate of suicide is associated with such mood disorders.[12]

■ *Anxiety disorders* encompass several discrete conditions, including panic disorder, obsessive-compulsive disorder, posttraumatic stress disorder, and phobia. More common than other mental disorders, anxiety disorders affect as many as 19 million people in the United States annually.[13]

Modern treatments for mental disorders are highly effective, with a variety of treatment options available for most disorders; there is no "one size fits all" treatment. Similarly, there exists today a diverse array of treatment settings, and a person may have the option of selecting a setting based on health care coverage, the clinical needs associated with a particular type or stage of illness, and personal preference.

Prevention scientists have developed, tested, and structured preventive interventions against depression, conduct disorder, and other adverse outcomes in high-risk groups of children. When applied with fidelity, preventive interventions can decrease risk of onset or delay onset of a disorder.

Rates for the most severe forms of mental disorders have been estimated to be between 2.6 and 2.8 percent of adults aged 18 years and older during any one year.[13, 14] Despite the effectiveness of treatment and the many paths to obtaining a treatment of choice, only 25 percent of persons with a mental disorder obtain help for their illness in the health care system. In comparison, 60 to 80 percent of persons with heart disease seek and receive care.[15] More critically, 40 percent of all people who have a severe mental illness do not seek treatment from either general medical or specialty mental health providers. Indeed, the majority of persons with mental disorders do not receive mental health services. Of those aged 18 years and older getting help, about 15 percent receive help from mental health specialists.[3] Of young people aged 9 to 17 years who have a mental disorder, 27 percent receive treatment in the health sector.[16] However, an additional 20 percent of children and adolescents with mental disorders use mental health services only in their schools.[17]

The direct costs of diagnosing and treating mental disorders totaled approximately $69 billion[17] in 1996. Lost productivity and disability insurance payments due to illness or premature death accounted for an additional $74.9 billion.[17] Crime, criminal justice costs, and property loss contributed another $6 billion to the total cost of mental illness. People with mental illnesses are overrepresented in jail populations; many do not receive treatment.[18] Of the $69 billion spent for diagnosing and treating mental disorders, nearly 70 percent was for the services of mental health specialty providers, with most of the remainder for general medical services providers. The majority—53 percent—of mental health treatment was

**Proportion of Youth Aged 9 to 17 Years
With Emotional Disturbances**
(By level of severity)

Percent

20% Youth with any diagnosable disorder

9-13% Youth with a serious emotional disturbance, with substantial functional impairment

5-9% Youth with a serious emotional disturbance, with extreme functional impairment

Source: Friedman, R.M.; Katz-Leavy, J.W.; Manderscheid, R.W.; et al. Prevalence of serious emotional disturbance: An update. *Mental Health, United States, 1996.* DHHS Publication Number (SMA) 96-3098. Rockville, MD: HHS, PHS, SAMHSA, CMHS, 1996.

paid for by public sector sources, including the States and local governments as well as Medicaid and Medicare and other Federal programs; 47 percent of expenditures were from private sources. Of expenditures from private sources, almost 60 percent were from private insurance.[17] The remainder came from out-of-pocket payments, including insurance copayments, with a small amount from sources such as foundations.

Trends

Research on the brain and behavior in mental illness and mental health is moving at a rapid pace. An increasingly strong consumers' movement in the mental health field is adding urgency to the tasks of translating new knowledge into clinical practices and refining service delivery systems to use new and emerging information optimally for patient/consumer needs. Consumer and family organizations, which formed out of concern over frequent fragmentation of mental health services and lack of accessibility to such services, have assumed a substantial role in supporting development of mental health services. Diverse groups share overlapping goals, including overcoming stigma and preventing discrimination toward persons with mental illness, promoting self-help groups, and promoting recovery from mental illness.[18]

The co-occurrence of addictive disorders among persons with mental disorders is gaining increasing attention from mental health professionals. Among adults aged 18 years and older with a lifetime history of any mental disorder, 29 percent have a history of an addictive disorder; of those with an alcohol disorder, 37 percent have had a mental disorder; and among those with other drug disorders, 53 percent have had a mental disorder.[17] Having both mental and addictive disorders within the same year is a particularly significant clinical treatment issue, complicating treatment for each disorder. About 3 percent of the population aged 18 years and older has been identified as having co-occurring mental and addictive disorders in 1 year.[3, 14] Of those with a serious mental illness, 15 percent have both types of disorder in 1 year, and of those with a severe and persistent mental illness, 27 percent have both mental and addictive disorders.[14] Co-occurring, or comorbid, mental and addictive disorders are estimated to affect 50 to 60 percent of homeless persons.[19] Comorbid mental and addictive disorders also are evident in children and adolescents.[20] Especially at risk for alcohol use problems are boys diagnosed with so-called externalizing disorders such as conduct problems, oppositional-defiant disorder, and attention deficit/hyperactivity disorder (ADHD).[21] From public health promotion and disease prevention perspectives, it is noteworthy that children and adolescents with mental illnesses often do not become substance abusers until after the mental illness becomes apparent.[22] This time lag creates a window of opportunity when prevention of substance abuse in these children may be possible.[20]

As the life expectancy of individuals continues to grow longer, the sheer number—although not necessarily the proportion—of persons experiencing mental disorders of late life will expand. This trend will present society with unprecedented challenges in organizing, financing, and delivering effective preventive and treatment services for mental health in this population. As recognition continues to grow that depression and certain cognitive losses are treatable disorders and not inevitable concomitants of aging, diagnostic precision in later life and provision of targeted treatment are increasingly urgent.

Health care in the United States continues to undergo fundamental structural changes that require creative and flexible responses from service providers, administrators, researchers, and policymakers alike. Two prominent forces of change are Federal and State efforts to improve access to health care, including mental health care, and the rapid growth and impact of managed care. In 1998, the Mental Health Parity Act (P.L. 104-204) was implemented to help increase access to care. (The term "parity" or "mental health parity" refers generally to insurance coverage for mental health services that includes the same benefits and restrictions as coverage for other health services.) Although the Federal Mental Health Parity Act is quite limited in reducing insurance coverage discrepancies between physical and mental disorders, 53 percent of the U.S. population is now covered by State mental health parity laws.

Disparities

Although mental illnesses, for the most part, are equal opportunity disorders, there are some marked differences in how they present themselves and how they are prevented, diagnosed, and treated by gender, racial and ethnic group, and age.[17]

Differences between men and women are evident in the number of cases of particular mental disorders. For example, major depression affects approximately twice as many women as men.[23] Women who are poor, have little formal schooling, and are on welfare or are unemployed are more likely to experience depression than women in the general population. Anxiety, panic, and phobic disorders affect two to three times as many women as men.[24, 25, 26]

Risk for engaging in suicidal behaviors also differs by gender. A history of physical or sexual abuse appears to be a serious risk factor for suicide attempts in both women and men.[27, 28] Women attempt suicide more often than men,[29] but men's risk of completed suicide is on average four and one half times higher than women's.[30] This suicide gender gap begins in adolescence and grows through middle and later life.[31]

Specific mental disorders affect men and women at particular stages of life. Schizophrenia occurs more often in young men than in women and usually has its onset in the late teen and early adult years. Eating disorders, affecting up to 2 percent of the population, arise predominantly—but not exclusively—in adolescent and young adult women (90 percent of all cases); the median age of onset is 17 years.[2] Eating disorders often persist into adulthood and have among the highest death rates of any mental disorder.[32] Alzheimer's disease affects equal numbers of women and men, although women's longer average life spans mean that more women than men have Alzheimer's disease at any point in time.[33]

Mental disorders, in aggregate, are as common later in life as they are at other ages, although rates for specific mental disorders vary depending on age and gender.[34] In any one-year period, the number of cases of major depression in people aged 65 years and older is approximately 1 percent, which is about half the rate among persons aged 45 to 64 years.[35] Depression rates are much higher, however, among older people who experience a physical health problem—12 percent for persons hospitalized for problems such as hip fractures or heart disease.[36] Depression rates for older persons in nursing homes range from 15 to 25 percent.[37] The number of cases of dementias, such as Alzheimer's disease and other severe losses of mental abilities, are as high as 12 percent among persons aged 65 years and older.[38] By age 85 years, the rate grows to 25 percent.[39]

In contrast, rates of primary psychotic disorders drop with age;[40] thus, schizophrenia and persistent paranoid disorders affect fewer than 0.5 percent of older adults.[41] Although fewer old persons attempt suicide than do young persons,[42] the rate of completed suicide is highest among elderly men, who account for about 80 percent of suicides among persons aged 65 years and older.[43] Moreover, elderly white men have a suicide rate six times the national average.[44]

Caution is needed, however, when discussing differences among racial and ethnic groups in the rates of mental illness. Studies of the number of cases of mental health problems among racial and ethnic populations, while increasing in number, remain limited and often inconclusive. Discussion of the rates of existing cases must consider differences in how persons of different cultures and racial and ethnic groups perceive mental illness. Behavioral problems that Western medicine views as signs of mental illness may be assessed differently by individuals in various racial and ethnic groups. With this caution in mind, along with the recognition that sample sizes for racial and ethnic groups may be limited, examination of existing large-scale studies for mental health trends among racial and ethnic groups remains important.

Mental disorders are not only the cause of limitations of various life activities but also can be a secondary problem among people with other disabilities. Depression and anxiety, for example, are seen more frequently among people with disabilities than those without disabilities.[45]

Opportunities

Promising universal and targeted preventive interventions, implemented according to scientific recommendations, have great potential to reduce the risk for mental disorders and the burden of suffering in vulnerable populations. Also, social and behavioral research is beginning to explore the concept of *resilience* to identify strengths that may promote health and healing. It is generally assumed that resilience involves the interaction of biological, psychological, and environmental processes. With increased understanding of how to identify and promote resilience, it will be possible to design effective programs that draw on such internal capacity.

There is increasing awareness and concern in the public health sector regarding the impact of stress, its prevention and treatment, and the need for enhanced coping skills. Stress may be experienced by any person and provides a clear demonstration of mind-body interaction. Coping skills, acquired throughout the lifespan, are positive adaptations that affect the ability to manage stressful events. Additional research can help quantify the public health burden of stress and identify ways to prevent or alleviate it through environmental or individual strategies.

Progress in fundamental science and an emphasis on translating new knowledge into clinical applications can strengthen opportunities for future clinical and service system innovations. Research-based treatments afford an unprecedented opportunity to achieve a major reduction in the burden of disease associated with mental illness. With enhancements of clinical services and service systems, recovery is an achievable objective of mental health clinical interventions.

Evidence that mental disorders are legitimate and highly responsive to appropriate treatment promises to be a potent antidote to stigma. Stigma creates barriers to providing and receiving competent and effective mental health treatment and can lead to inappropriate treatment, unemployment, and homelessness. The elimination of stigma associated with mental disorders will in turn encourage more individuals to seek needed mental health care.

Four Healthy People 2000 objectives focus on individual behavior in coping with the symptoms of mental disorders: controlling stress, seeking help with personal and emotional problems, obtaining treatment for depression, and using community support programs for severe and persistent disorders. The least progress was achieved on objectives indicative of chronic stress exposure; that is, controlling stress and seeking treatment for depression showed the least progress. Objectives that involve seeking help for personal and emotional problems that result from disabilities, particularly those associated with severe and persistent mental disorders, showed the most progress. Five Healthy People 2000 objectives focus on the development of service delivery mechanisms for early recognition of symptoms and interventions, as well as reductions in the negative consequences of mental disorders. A slight decline in the proportion of nurse practitioners who typically inquire about the parent-child relationship has been documented (from 55 percent to 51 percent). In addition, large declines have taken place in nurse practitioners who typically inquire about their adult patients' cognitive, emotional, or behavioral functioning (from 35 percent to 19 percent for cognitive functioning and from 40 percent to 26 percent for emotional or behavioral functioning). Some offsetting increases in treatment and referral activity are reported (from 20 percent to 22 percent for cognitive problems, from 23 percent to 33 percent for emotional/behavioral problems).

Six Healthy People 2000 objectives focus on the distress and dysfunction that accompany the cognitive, emotional, and behavioral symptoms of mental disorders. The age-adjusted suicide rate in the total population has slightly declined and by 1997 already had met the target level; the rate for white men aged 65 years and older, who began the decade at highest risk for suicide (44.4 per 100,000), had declined below the year 2000 target in 1994 (38.9 per 100,000) and had declined further by 1997 (35.5 per 100,000).

Note: Unless otherwise noted, data are from the Centers for Disease Control and Prevention, National Center for Health Statistics, *Healthy People 2000 Review 1998–99.*

Mental Health and Mental Disorders

Goal: Improve mental health and ensure access to appropriate, quality mental health services.

Number   Objective Short Title

Mental Health Status Improvement

18-1   Suicide

18-2   Adolescent suicide attempts

18-3   Serious mental illness (SMI) among homeless adults

18-4   Employment of persons with SMI

18-5   Eating disorder relapses

Treatment Expansion

18-6   Primary care screening and assessment

18-7   Treatment for children with mental health problems

18-8   Juvenile justice facility screening

18-9   Treatment for adults with mental disorders

18-10   Treatment for co-occurring disorders

18-11   Adult jail diversion programs

State Activities

18-12   State tracking of consumer satisfaction

18-13   State plans addressing cultural competence

18-14   State plans addressing elderly persons

Mental Health Status Improvement

18-1. Reduce the suicide rate.

Target: 5.0 suicides per 100,000 population.

Baseline: 11.3 suicides per 100,000 population occurred in 1998 (age adjusted to the year 2000 standard population).

Target setting method: Better than the best.

Data source: National Vital Statistics System (NVSS), CDC, NCHS.

NOTE: THE TABLE BELOW MAY CONTINUE TO THE FOLLOWING PAGE.

Total Population, 1998	Suicides
	Rate per 100,000
TOTAL	11.3
Race and ethnicity	
American Indian or Alaska Native	12.6
Asian or Pacific Islander	6.6
Asian	DNC
Native Hawaiian and other Pacific Islander	DNC
Black or African American	5.8
White	12.2
Hispanic or Latino	6.3
Not Hispanic or Latino	11.8
Black or African American	6.0
White	12.8
Gender	
Female	4.3
Male	19.2
Education level (aged 25 to 64 years)	
Less than high school	17.9
High school graduate	19.2
At least some college	10.0

Total Population, 1998	Suicides
	Rate per 100,000
Age (not age adjusted)	
10 to 14 years	1.6
15 to 19 years	8.9
20 to 24 years	13.6

DNA = Data have not been analyzed. DNC = Data are not collected. DSU = Data are statistically unreliable.
Note: Age adjusted to the year 2000 standard population.

NOTE: THE TABLE ABOVE MAY HAVE CONTINUED FROM THE PREVIOUS PAGE.

18-2. Reduce the rate of suicide attempts by adolescents.

Target: 12-month average of 1 percent.

Baseline: 12-month average of 2.6 percent of adolescents in grades 9 through 12 attempted suicide in 1999.

Target setting method: Better than the best.

Data source: Youth Risk Behavior Surveillance System (YRBSS), CDC, NCCDPHP.

NOTE: THE TABLE BELOW MAY CONTINUE TO THE FOLLOWING PAGE.

Students in Grades 9 Through 12, 1999	Suicide Attempts
	Percent
TOTAL	2.6
Race and ethnicity	
American Indian or Alaska Native	DSU
Asian or Pacific Islander	DSU
Asian	DSU
Native Hawaiian and other Pacific Islander	DSU
Black or African American	3.1
White	2.2
Hispanic or Latino	3.0
Not Hispanic or Latino	2.6
Black or African American	2.9
White	1.9
Gender	
Female	3.1
Male	2.1

Students in Grades 9 Through 12, 1999	Suicide Attempts
	Percent
Parents' education level	
Less than high school	DNC
High school graduate	DNC
At least some college	DNC
Sexual orientation	DNC

DNA = Data have not been analyzed. DNC = Data are not collected. DSU = Data are statistically unreliable.
NOTE: THE TABLE ABOVE MAY HAVE CONTINUED FROM THE PREVIOUS PAGE.

Suicide is a complex behavior that can be prevented in many cases by early recognition and treatment of mental disorders. It was the ninth leading cause of death in the United States in 1996 and the third leading killer of young persons between age 15 and 24 years.[46, 47, 48, 49] At least 90 percent of all people who kill themselves have a mental or substance abuse disorder, or a combination of disorders. However, most persons with a mental or substance abuse disorder do not kill themselves; thus other factors contribute to suicide risk. In addition to mental and substance abuse disorders, risk factors include prior suicide attempt, stressful life events, and access to lethal suicide methods. Suicide is difficult to predict; therefore, preventive interventions focus on risk factors. Thus, reduction in access to lethal methods and recognition and treatment of mental and substance abuse disorders are among the most promising approaches to suicide prevention. More targeted approaches should consider risk factors most salient and appropriate for select populations.

18-3. Reduce the proportion of homeless adults who have serious mental illness (SMI).

Target: 19 percent.

Baseline: 25 percent of homeless adults aged 18 years and older had SMI in 1996.

Target setting method: 24 percent improvement. (Better than the best will be used when data are available.)

Data source: Projects for Assistance in Transition from Homelessness (PATH) Annual Application, SAMHSA, CMHS.

> Data for population groups currently are not collected.

Approximately one-quarter of homeless persons in the United States have a serious mental illness (SMI).[50] New approaches developed over the past 10 years provide ways to lower the number of persons who are homeless and who also have SMI. Using persistent patient outreach and engagement strategies, service providers are helping homeless persons with SMI connect with mainstream treatment systems.[51, 52]

Treatment alone, however, is not enough. Once permanent housing is located, appropriate mental health and social supports can help persons with mental illness remain off the street. Much of this support occurs in the form of case management, particularly if it is responsive both to emerging mental health issues and to the skills a person needs to function and thrive in the community.

18-4. Increase the proportion of persons with serious mental illness (SMI) who are employed.

Target: 51 percent.

Baseline: 43 percent of persons aged 18 years and older with SMI were employed in 1994.

Target setting method: 19 percent improvement. (Better than the best will be used when data are available.)

Data source: National Health Interview Survey (NHIS), CDC, NCHS.

Data for population groups currently are not analyzed.

Rehabilitation is an essential part of care for adults with serious mental illness. To promote independent living, rehabilitation programs often evaluate and place these persons in jobs. Rehabilitation programs also provide continuing support and help ensure that the placement is working well. Research shows that working provides both economic and personal benefits for persons with SMI that extend beyond a paycheck and workplace companionship.[53] Employment also improves self-esteem and independence; it helps a person to manage his or her own illness and return to community life.[54, 55] A majority of persons with SMI want to be employed and rank employment as a primary personal goal.[56] Helping persons with mental illness secure employment can reduce the use of mental health services and reduce the number of persons who receive Federal and State disability payments.[56]

18-5. (Developmental) Reduce the relapse rates for persons with eating disorders including anorexia nervosa and bulimia nervosa.

Potential data source: Prospective studies of patients with anorexia or bulimia nervosa, NIH, NIMH.

Anorexia nervosa is the most severe eating disorder, characterized by extreme and often life-threatening[57] weight loss associated with a distorted body image and a pathological fear of gaining weight. In cases of severe weight loss, hospital treatment often is needed. Studies suggest that from 30 to 50 percent of patients treated successfully in the hospital become ill again within 1 year of leaving the hospital.[58, 59] Efforts are under way to develop and test specific interventions that can prevent relapse in these patients. For instance, a particular kind of psychotherapy—called cognitive-behavioral treatment—has been found to lower relapse rates in persons with anorexia nervosa.[60] Treatments using medications also have been tried, both alone and in combination with talking therapy. Preliminary reports suggest that it might be possible to decrease the chance of relapse, resulting in better long-term prospects for persons with severe anorexia nervosa.

Bulimia nervosa is an eating disorder that involves eating a lot of food (binge eating) and then eliminating it (purging), whether through self-induced vomiting or through the use of diuretics or other medications. Effective short-term treatments exist for this serious mental health problem. When "remission" is defined as being symptom-free of binge eating and purging for at least 4 weeks, about 25 percent of those in remission had a relapse in less than 3 months. Around 9 months after remission, fewer than half (49 percent) of the persons remained symptom-free.[61] Risk for relapse seems to drop after 4 years of being symptom-free.[62]

Treatment Expansion

18-6. (Developmental) Increase the number of persons seen in primary health care who receive mental health screening and assessment.

Potential data source: Primary Care Data System/Federally Qualified Health Centers, HRSA.

The general medical and primary care sector consists of health care professionals such as internists, pediatricians, and nurse practitioners in office-based practice, clinics, acute medical and surgical hospitals, and nursing homes. Close to 6 percent of the adult U.S. population use the general medical sector for mental health care, with an average of about 4 mental health visits per year—far lower than the average of 14 visits per year found in the specialty medical sector.[3, 4] The general medical sector has long been identified as the initial point of contact for many adults with mental disorders; for some, these providers may be their only source of mental health services. This attention to mental state in primary care can promote early detection and intervention for mental health problems.

18-7. (Developmental) Increase the proportion of children with mental health problems who receive treatment.

Potential data source: National Household Survey on Drug Abuse (NHSDA), SAMHSA, OAS.

For many children aged 18 years and under, lifelong mental disorders may start in childhood or adolescence. For many other children, normal development is disrupted by biological, environmental, and psychosocial factors, which impair their mental health, interfere with education and social interactions, and keep them from realizing their full potential as adults.

Expanding effective services for children, particularly for those with serious emotional disturbance, depends on promoting effective collaboration across critical areas of support: families, social services, health, mental health, juvenile justice, and schools. Better services and collaboration for children with serious emotional disturbance and their families will result in greater school retention, decreased contact with the juvenile justice system, increased stability of living arrangements, and improved educational, emotional, and behavioral development.[63, 64]

18-8. (Developmental) Increase the proportion of juvenile justice facilities that screen new admissions for mental health problems.

Potential data source: Inventory of Mental Health Services in Juvenile Justice Facilities, SAMHSA.

It is estimated that over 100,000 youth are placed in juvenile justice facilities annually.[65] Although exact numbers of youths with mental disorders among those entering this system are not available, the proportion is considerably higher than in the general population. Not surprisingly, problems of suicide, self-injurious behavior, and other disorders are significant among youths in the juvenile justice system.[66] Screening activities, including parent or caregiver interviews, should be conducted by qualified mental health personnel.[66] This approach can help ensure that all youths entering the juvenile justice system who also have a treatable mental health problem are identified and receive appropriate treatment.

18-9. Increase the proportion of adults with mental disorders who receive treatment.

Target and baseline:

Objective	Increase in Adults With Mental Disorders Receiving Treatment	1997 Baseline (unless noted)	2010 Target
		Percent	
18-9a.	Adults aged 18 to 54 years with serious mental illness	47 (1991)	55
18-9b.	Adults aged 18 years and older with recognized depression	23	50
18-9c.	Adults aged 18 years and older with schizophrenia	60 (1984)	75
18-9d.	Adults aged 18 years and older with generalized anxiety disorder	38	50

Target setting method: 17 percent improvement for 18-9a. (Better than the best will be used when data are available.) Better than the best for 18-9b, 18-9c, and 18-9d.

Data sources: Epidemiologic Catchment Area (ECA) Program, NIH, NIMH; National Household Survey on Drug Abuse (NHSDA), SAMHSA, OAS; National Comorbidity Survey, SAMHSA, CMHS; NIH, NIMH.

Adults Aged 18 Years and Older With Mental Disorders, 1997 (unless noted)	Received Treatment			
	18-9a. Serious Mental Illness (aged 18 to 54 years) (1991)	18-9b. Recognized Depression	18-9c. Schizophrenia (1984)	18-9d. Generalized Anxiety Disorder
	Percent			
TOTAL	47	23	60	38
Race and ethnicity				
American Indian or Alaska Native	DNA	DSU	DSU	DSU
Asian or Pacific Islander	DNA	DSU	DSU	DSU
Asian	DNA	DNC	DSU	DNC
Native Hawaiian and other Pacific Islander	DNA	DNC	DSU	DNC
Black or African American	DNA	16	DNC	26
White	DNA	24	DNC	39
Hispanic or Latino	DNA	20	42	DSU
Not Hispanic or Latino	DNA	DNC	DNC	40
Black or African American	DNA	DNA	41	DNA
White	DNA	DNA	63	DNA
Gender				
Female	DNA	24	63	32
Male	DNA	21	51	49
Education level				
Less than high school	DNA	22	48	48
High school graduate	DNA	19	71	34
At least some college	DNA	28	66	32
Sexual orientation	DNC	DNC	DNC	DNC

DNA = Data have not been analyzed. DNC = Data are not collected. DSU = Data are statistically unreliable.

Serious mental illness. Untreated mental illnesses have human and economic costs associated with them[67, 68] Lost productivity due to illness, premature death, criminal justice interaction process, and property loss are all part of these costs. Ninety percent of those who complete suicide have a diagnosed mental illness.[3] Helping persons with mental illnesses access appropriate scientifically based treatments is essential.

Depression. At some time or another, virtually all adults will experience a tragic or unexpected loss or a serious setback and times of profound sadness, grief, or distress. Major depressive disorder, however, differs both quantitatively and qualitatively from normal sadness or grief, which is typically less pervasive and generally more time-limited. Moreover, some of the symptoms of severe depression, such as anhedonia (the inability to experience pleasure), hopelessness, and loss of mood reactivity (the ability to feel a mood uplift in response to something positive) only rarely accompany normal sadness. Suicidal thoughts and psychotic symptoms such as delusions or hallucinations virtually always signify a pathological state.[69] Depression disrupts the lives of depressed persons and their families and reduces economic productivity. Depression also can result in suicide and has an especially severe impact on women.[12, 23] Treatment can alleviate each of these problems. Available medications and psychological treatments, alone or in combination, can help 80 percent of those with depression.[70]

Depression also has a deleterious impact on the economy, costing the United States over $40 billion each year, both in diminished productivity and in use of health care resources. In the workplace, depression is a leading cause of absenteeism and diminished productivity.[71] Although only a minority seek professional help to relieve a mood disorder, depressed people are significantly more likely than others to visit a physician for some other reason.[72]

Schizophrenia is characterized by profound disruption in cognition and emotion, affecting the most fundamental human attributes: language, thought, perception, affect, and sense of self. Symptoms frequently include hearing internal voices or experiencing other sensations not connected to an obvious source (hallucinations) and assigning unusual significance or meaning to normal events or holding fixed false beliefs. No single symptom is definitive for diagnosis; rather, the diagnosis encompasses a pattern of signs and symptoms, in conjunction with impaired occupational or social functioning. The disorder affects 0.5 to 1 percent of the population over the course of a lifetime. Onset generally occurs during young adulthood (mid-20s for men, late-20s for women), although earlier and later onset do occur.[73]

Anxiety disorders, which include generalized anxiety disorder, are not only common in the United States, but they are ubiquitous across human cultures.[3, 4, 74] Twenty-four percent of the population will experience an anxiety disorder, many with overlapping substance abuse disorders.[17, 75, 76] The longitudinal course of anxiety disorders is characterized by relatively early ages of onset, chronicity, relapsing or recurrent episodes of illness, and periods of disability.[77, 78, 79, 80] Panic disorder and agoraphobia are associated with increased risks of attempted and completed suicide.[24, 81]

18-10. (Developmental) Increase the proportion of persons with co-occurring substance abuse and mental disorders who receive treatment for both disorders.

Potential data sources: National Health Interview Survey (NHIS), CDC, NCHS; National Household Survey on Drug Abuse (NHSDA), SAMHSA, OAS; Replication of National Comorbidity Survey, NIH, NIMH.

Co-occurring mental and addictive disorders are more common than previously recognized. In general, 19 percent of the adult U.S. population have a mental disorder alone (in 1 year); 3 percent have both mental and addictive disorders; and 6 percent have addictive disorders alone. Consequently, about 28 to 30 percent of the population have either a mental or addictive disorder.[3, 4] The lifetime rates of co-occurrence of mental disorders and addictive disorders are strikingly high. About one in five persons in the United States experience a mental disorder in the course of a year. Nearly one in three adults who have a mental disorder in their lifetime also experiences a co-occurring substance abuse (alcohol or other drugs) disorder, which complicates treatment. Individuals with co-occurring disorders are more likely to experience a chronic course and to use services than are those with either type of disorder alone. Clinicians, program developers, and policymakers need to be aware of these high rates of comorbidity. While an integrated approach may be indicated for persons with SMI and co-occurring addictive disorders, how public health service systems can best address issues of treating the full range of persons with co-occurring mental and substance-related disorders remains a challenge. Treatment protocols continue to be refined as research findings and promising practices are disseminated to programs and practitioners.

18-11. (Developmental) Increase the proportion of local governments with community-based jail diversion programs for adults with serious mental illness (SMI).

Potential data source: National Survey of Jail Mental Health Diversion Programs, SAMHSA.

Nearly 700,000 persons with active symptoms of serious mental illness are admitted to jails each year. They constitute about 7 percent of the jail population.[82] Individuals with SMI were overrepresented in jails compared to their numbers in the general population. Some people arrested for nonviolent crimes could be better served if diverted from the jail system to a community-based mental health treatment program.[83] Key components of a model diversion program are: (1) identifying specific program elements for diversion with accompanying resources and identified staff, (2) a specific target population, (3) a goal of avoiding or decreasing the time of incarceration, and (4) a way to link target population members with community-based mental health services.[83]

18-12. Increase the number of States and the District of Columbia that track consumers' satisfaction with the mental health services they receive.

Target: 50 States and the District of Columbia.

Baseline: 36 States tracked consumers' satisfaction with the mental health services they received in 1999.

Target setting method: Total coverage.

Data source: Mental Health Statistics Improvement Program, SAMHSA.

The health care industry increasingly is using consumer opinion to gain information on service needs and changes. Patient satisfaction studies are becoming standard practice for many health care organizations. Health care executives have indicated that consumers have a major impact on the development of health care products.[84] Nearly 90 percent of health care executives reported that they have expanded both the number and type of services based on consumer preference. The Mental Health Statistics Improvement Program has pioneered the development of a consumer-oriented mental health report card that includes a consumer survey designed to address questions of access, appropriateness, quality, and outcome of care.

18-13. (Developmental) Increase the number of States, Territories, and the District of Columbia with an operational mental health plan that addresses cultural competence.

Potential data source: National Technical Assistance Center for State Mental Health Systems, National Association of State Mental Health Program Directors, National Research Institute; SAMHSA, CMHS.

To work effectively, health care providers need to understand the differences in how various populations in the United States perceive mental health and mental illness and treatment services. These factors affect whether people seek mental health care, how they describe their symptoms, the duration of care, and the outcomes of the care received. Research has shown that various select populations use mental health services differently. They may not seek mental health services in the formal system, drop out of care, or seek care at much later stages of illness, driving the service cost higher.[85, 86, 87] This pattern of use appears to be the result of a community-based mental health service system that is not culturally relevant, responsive, or accessible to select populations.[87, 88, 89, 90] Hospitals have become the primary mental health treatment site for a disproportionate number of African Americans.[91, 92, 93, 94]

18-14. Increase the number of States, Territories, and the District of Columbia with an operational mental health plan that addresses mental health crisis interventions, ongoing screening, and treatment services for elderly persons.

Target: 50 States and the District of Columbia.

Baseline: 24 States had an operational mental health plan that addressed mental health crisis interventions, ongoing screening, and treatment services for elderly persons in 1997.

Target setting method: Total coverage.

Data source: National Technical Assistance Center for State Mental Health Systems, National Association of State Mental Health Program Directors, National Research Institute; SAMHSA, CMHS.

The Nation is growing older; the number and proportion of the population aged 65 years and older will grow rapidly after 2010. As the Nation ages, the mental health needs of elderly persons must be addressed because their needs will continue to grow. Mood disorders affect between 2 and 4 percent of community-living elderly persons.[37] Elderly persons with clinically significant depressive symptoms range from 10 to 15 percent of the U.S. population.[95] State mental health authorities and localities should become increasingly engaged in meeting the mental health needs of this growing population.

Related Objectives From Other Focus Areas

1. **Access to Quality Health Services**
   1-1. Persons with health insurance
   1-2. Health insurance coverage for clinical preventive services
   1-3. Counseling about health behaviors
   1-4. Source of ongoing care
   1-5. Usual primary care provider
   1-6. Difficulties or delays in obtaining needed health care
   1-7. Core competencies in health provider training
   1-8. Racial and ethnic representation in health professions
   1-10. Delay or difficulty in getting emergency care
   1-11. Rapid prehospital emergency care
   1-12. Single toll-free number for poison control centers
   1-13. Trauma care systems
   1-14. Special needs of children
   1-15. Long-term care services
2. **Arthritis, Osteoporosis, and Chronic Back Conditions**
   2-4. Help in coping
3. **Cancer**
   3-10. Provider counseling about cancer prevention

6. **Disability and Secondary Conditions**
   6-1. Standard definition of people with disabilities in data sets
   6-2. Feelings and depression among children with disabilities
   6-3. Feelings and depression interfering with activities among adults with disabilities
   6-4. Social participation among adults with disabilities
   6-5. Sufficient emotional support among adults with disabilities
   6-6. Satisfaction with life among adults with disabilities
   6-7. Congregate care of children and adults with disabilities
   6-8. Employment parity
   6-9. Inclusion of children and youth with disabilities in regular education programs
   6-10. Accessibility of health and wellness programs
   6-11. Assistive devices and technology
   6-12. Environmental barriers affecting participation in activities
   6-13. Surveillance and health promotion programs

7. **Educational and Community-Based Programs**
   7-1. High school completion
   7-2. School health education
   7-3. Health-risk behavior information for college and university students
   7-4. School nurse-to-student ratio
   7-5. Worksite health promotion programs
   7-6. Participation in employer-sponsored health promotion activities
   7-7. Patient and family education
   7-9. Health care organization sponsorship of community health promotion activities
   7-10. Community health promotion programs
   7-11. Culturally appropriate and linguistically competent community health promotion programs
   7-12. Older adult participation in community health promotion activities

9. **Family Planning**
   9-1. Intended pregnancy
   9-2. Birth spacing
   9-3. Contraceptive use
   9-4. Contraceptive failure
   9-5. Emergency contraception
   9-6. Male involvement in pregnancy prevention
   9-7. Adolescent pregnancy
   9-8. Abstinence before age 15 years
   9-9. Abstinence among adolescents aged 15 to 17 years
   9-10. Pregnancy prevention and sexually transmitted disease (STD) protection
   9-11. Pregnancy prevention education
   9-13. Insurance coverage for contraceptive supplies and services

11. **Health Communication**
    11-1. Households with Internet access
    11-2. Health literacy
    11-3. Research and evaluation of communication programs

23-12. Health improvement plans

23-13. Access to public health laboratory services

23-14. Access to epidemiology services

23-16. Data on public health expenditures

23-17. Population-based prevention research

25. Sexually Transmitted Diseases

25-3. Primary and secondary syphilis

25-8. Heterosexually transmitted HIV infection in women

25-9. Congenital syphilis

25-10. Neonatal STDs

25-11. Responsible adolescent sexual behavior

25-12. Responsible sexual behavior messages on television

25-14. Screening in youth detention facilities and jails

25-15. Contracts to treat nonplan partners of STD patients

25-17. Screening of pregnant women

25-18. Compliance with recognized STD treatment standards

25-19. Provider referral services for sex partners

26. Substance Abuse

26-7. Alcohol- and drug-related violence

26-8. Lost productivity

26-9. Substance-free youth

26-10. Adolescent and adult use of illicit substances

26-11. Binge drinking

26-12. Average annual alcohol consumption

26-13. Low-risk drinking among adults

26-14. Steroid use among adolescents

26-15. Inhalant use among adolescents

26-16. Peer disapproval of substance abuse

26-17. Perception of risk associated with substance abuse

26-18. Treatment gap for illicit drugs

26-22. Hospital emergency department referrals

26-23. Community partnerships and coalitions

Terminology

(A listing of abbreviations and acronyms used in this publication appears in Appendix H.)

Anxiety disorders: Anxiety disorders have multiple physical and psychological symptoms, but all have in common feelings of apprehension, tension, or uneasiness. Among the anxiety disorders are panic disorder, agoraphobia, obsessive-compulsive disorder, posttraumatic stress disorder, and generalized anxiety disorder.

Case management: Practice in which the service recipient is a partner in his or her recovery and self-management of mental illness and life.

Co-occurring/comorbidity: In general, the existence of two or more illnesses—whether physical or mental—at the same time in a single individual. In this chapter, comorbidity specifically means the existence of a mental illness and a substance abuse disorder or a mental and a physical illness in the same person at the same time.

Consumer: Any person using mental health services.

Cultural competence: In this chapter, a group of skills, attitudes, and knowledge that allows persons, organizations, and systems to work effectively with diverse racial, ethnic, and social groups.

Depression: A state of low mood that is described differently by people who experience it. Commonly described are feelings of sadness, despair, emptiness, or loss of interest or pleasure in nearly all things. Depression also can be experienced in other disorders such as bipolar disorder (manic-depressive disorder).

Diagnosable mental illness: Includes all people with a mental illness in a specified population group, whether or not they have received a formal diagnosis from a medical or mental health professional.

Homeless person: A person who lacks housing. The definition also includes a person living in transitional housing or a person who spends most nights in a supervised public or private facility providing temporary living quarters.

Juvenile justice facility: Includes detention centers, shelters, reception or diagnostic centers, training schools, ranches, forestry camps or farms, halfway houses and group homes, and residential treatment centers for young offenders.

Mental health services: Diagnostic, treatment, and preventive care that helps improve how persons with mental illness feel both physically and emotionally as well as how they interact with other persons. These services also help persons who have a strong risk of developing a mental illness.

Mental illness: The term that refers collectively to all diagnosable mental disorders. *Mental disorders* are health conditions characterized by alterations in thinking, mood, or behavior (or some combination thereof) that are all mediated by the brain and associated with distress or impaired functioning or both. Mental disorders spawn a host of human problems that may include personal distress, impaired functioning and disability, pain, or death. These disorders can occur in men and women of any age and in all racial and ethnic groups. They can be the result of family history, genetics, or other biological, environmental, social, or behavioral factors that occur alone or in combination.

Parity, mental health parity: Equivalent benefits and restrictions in insurance coverage for mental health services and for other health services.

Resilience: Manifested competence in the context of significant challenges to adaptation or development.

Schizophrenia: A mental disorder lasting for at least 6 months, including at least 1 month with two or more active-phase symptoms. Active-phase symptoms include delusions, hallucinations, disorganized speech, and grossly disorganized or catatonic behavior. Schizophrenia is accompanied by marked impairment in social or occupational functioning.

Screening for mental health problems: A brief formal or informal assessment to identify persons who have mental health problems or are likely to develop such problems. The screening process helps determine whether a person has a problem and, if so, the most appropriate mental health services for that person.

Serious emotional disturbance (SED): A diagnosable mental disorder found in persons from birth to age 18 years that is so severe and long lasting that it seriously interferes with functioning in family, school, community, or other major life activities.

Serious mental illness (SMI): A diagnosable mental disorder found in persons aged 18 years and older that is so long lasting and severe that it seriously interferes with a person's ability to take part in major life activities.

References

[1] Murray, C.J.L., and Lopez, A.D. *The Global Burden of Disease*. Cambridge, MA: Harvard University Press, 1996.

[2] Regier, D.A.; Narrow, W.; and Rae, D.S. Unpublished National Institute of Mental Health (NIMH) analyses, 1999.

[3] Regier, D.A.; Narrow, W.; Rae, D.S.; et al. The de facto U.S. mental and addictive disorders service system. Epidemiologic Catchment Area prospective 1-year prevalence rates of disorders and services. *Archives of General Psychiatry* 50:85-94, 1993.

[4] Kessler, R.C.; McGonagle, K.A.; Zhao, S.; et al. Lifetime and 12-month prevalence of DSM-III-R psychiatric disorders in the U.S. *Archives of General Psychiatry* 51:8-19, 1994.

[5] Shaffer, D.; Fisher, P.; Dulcan, M.K.; et al. The NIMH Diagnostic Interview Schedule for Children, version 2.3 (DSIC 2.3): Description, acceptability, prevalence rates and performance in the Methods for the Epidemiology of Child and Adolescent Mental Disorders Study. *Journal of the American Academy of Child and Adolescent Psychiatry* 35:865-877, 1996.

[6] Brandenberg, N.; Friedman, R.; and Silver, S. The epidemiology of childhood psychiatric disorders: Prevalence findings from recent studies. *Journal of the American Academy of Child and Adolescent Psychiatry* 29:76-83, 1990.

[7] Taylor, E.; Chadwick, O.; Heptinstall, E.; et al. Hyperactivity and conduct problems as risk factors for adolescent development. *Journal of the American Academy of Child and Adolescent Psychiatry* 35:1213-1226, 1996.

[8] Foley, H.A.; Carlton, C.O.; and Howell, R.J. The relationship of attention deficit hyperactivity disorder and conduct disorders to juvenile delinquency: Legal implications. *Bulletin of the American Academy of Psychiatry Law* 24:333-345, 1996.

[9] Friedman, R.M.; Katz-Levey, J.W.; Manderschied, R.W.; et al. Prevalence of serious emotional disturbance in children and adolescents. In: Manderscheid, R.W., and Sonnenschein, M.A., eds. *Mental Health, United States, 1996*. Rockville, MD: Center for Mental Health Services (CMHS), 1996, 71-78.

[10] Ritchie, K., and Kildea, D. Is senile dementia "age-related" or "ageing related"?— evidence from meta analysis of dementia prevalence in the oldest old. *Lancet* 346:931-934, 1995.

[11] Lebowitz, B.D.; Pearson, J.L.; and Cohen, G.D. *Clinical Geriatric Psychopharmacology*. Baltimore, MD: Williams & Wilkins, 1998.

[12] Robins, L.N.; Locke, B.Z.; and Regier, D.A. An overview of psychiatric disorders in America. In: Robins, L.N., and Regier, D.A., eds. *Psychiatric Disorders in America: The Epidemiologic Catchment Area Study*. New York, NY: Free Press, 1991.

[13] National Advisory Mental Health Council. Health care reform for Americans with severe mental illnesses: Report of the National Advisory Mental Health Council. *American Journal of Psychiatry* 150:1447-1465, 1993.

[14] Kessler, R.C.; Berglund, P.A.; Zhao, S.; et al. The 12-month prevalence and correlates of serious mental illness. In: Manderscheid, R.W., and Sonnenschein, M.A., eds. *Mental Health, United States, 1996*. DHHS Publication No. (SMA) 96-3098. Rockville, MD: CMHS, 1996.

[15] National Center for Health Statistics (NCHS), Centers for Disease Control and Prevention (CDC). Prevalence of chronic circulatory conditions. *Vital and Health Statistics* 10(94), 1992.

[16] Howard, K.I.; Cornille, T.A.; Lyons, J.S.; et al. Patterns of mental health service utilization. *Archives of General Psychiatry* 53:696-703, 1996.

[17] HHS. *Mental Health: A Report of the Surgeon General—Executive Summary*. Rockville, MD: HHS, SAMHSA, CMHS, NIH, NIMH, 1999.

[18] Frese, F.J. Advocacy, recovery, and the challenges of consumerism for schizophrenia. *Psychiatric Clinics of North America* 21:233-249, 1998.

[19] Interagency Council on the Homeless. *Outcasts on Main Street*. HHS Pub. No. ADM 92-1904. Rockville MD: Alcohol, Drug Abuse, and Mental Health Services Administration, 1992.

[20] Kessler, R.C.; Nelson, C.B.; McGonagle, K.A.; et al. The epidemiology of co-occurring addictive and mental disorders: Implications for prevention and service utilization. *American Journal of Orthopsychiatry* 66:21-23, 1996.

[21] Winkle, M. A retrospective measure of childhood behavior problems and its use in predicting adolescent problem behaviors. *Journal of Studies in Alcohol* 54:421-422, 1993.

[22] Christie, K.A.; Burke, Jr., J.D.; Regier, D.A.; et al. Epidemiologic evidence for early onset of mental disorders and higher risk of drug abuse in young adults. *American Journal of Psychiatry* 145:971-975, 1988.

[23] Weissman, M.M., and Klerman, J.K. Depression: Current understanding and changing trends. *Annual Review of Public Health* 13:319-339, 1992.

[24] American Psychiatric Association. Practice guidelines for the treatment of patients with panic disorder. *American Journal of Psychiatry* 155(Suppl. 12):1-34, 1998.

[25] Brawman-Mintzer, O., and Lydiard, R.B. Generalized anxiety disorder: Issues in epidemiology. *Journal of Clinical Psychiatry* 57(Suppl. 7):3-8, 1996.

[26] Regier, D.A.; Farmer, M.E.; Rae, D.S.; et al. One-month prevalence of mental disorders in the United States and sociodemographic characteristics: The Epidemiologic Catchment Area study. *Acta Psychiatrica Scandinavia* 88:35-47, 1993.

[27] Van der Kolk, B.A., and Perry, J.L. Childhood origins of self-destructive behavior. *American Journal of Psychiatry* 148:1665-1671, 1991.

[28] NCHS, CDC. *Vital Statistics of the United States*. Hyattsville, MD: NCHS, 1991, Tables 1-9.

[29] Moscicki, E.K. Gender differences in completed and attempted suicide. *Annals of Epidemiology* 4:152-158, 1994.

[30] CDC. Scientific Data, Surveillance, and Injury Statistics. <http://www.cdc.gov/ncipc/osp/mortdata.htm>May 25, 1999.

[31] NCHS, CDC. *Vital Statistics of the United States*. Hyattsville, MD: NCHS, 1991, Tables 1-9.

[32] Herzog, D.B., and Copeland, P.N. Medical progress: Eating disorders. *New England Journal of Medicine* 313:295-303, 1985.

[33] CDC. *Priorities for Women's Health*. Atlanta, GA: CDC, 1993.

[34] McIntosh, J.L.; Pearson, J.L.; and Lebowitz, B.D. Mental disorders of elderly men. In: Kosberg, J.I., and Kaye, L.W., eds. *Elderly Men: Special Problems and Professional Challenges*. New York, NY: Springer Publishing Company, 1997, 193-215.

[35] Weissman, M.M.; Bruce, M.L.; Leaf, P.J.; et al. Affective disorders. In: Robbins, L.N., and Regier, D.A., eds. *Psychiatric Disorders in America*. New York, NY: Free Press, 1991, 53-80.

[36] Koening, H.G., and Blazer, D.G. Mood disorders and suicide. In: Birren, J.E.; Sloane, R.B.; and Cohen, G.D.; eds. *Handbook of Mental Health and Aging*. 2nd ed. San Diego, CA: Academic Press, 1992, 379-407.

[37] NIH Consensus Development Panel on Depression in Late Life. Diagnosis and treatment of depression in late life. *Journal of the American Medical Association* 268:1018-1024, 1992.

[38] Evans, D.A.; Funkenstein, H.H.; Albert, M.S.; et al. Prevalence of Alzheimer's disease in a community population of older persons: Higher than previously reported. *Journal of the American Medical Association* 262:2551-2556, 1989.

[39] Jorm, A.F.; Korten, A.E.; and Henderson, A.S. The prevalence of dementia: A quantitative integration of the literature. *Acta Psychiatrica Scandinavia* 76:465-479, 1987.

[40] Zubenko, G.S.; Mulsant, B.H.; Sweet, R.A.; et al. Mortality of elderly patients with psychiatric disorders. *American Journal of Psychiatry* 154(10):1360-1368, 1997.

[41] Myers, J.K.; Weissman, M.M.; Tischler, G.L.; et al. Six month prevalence of psychiatric disorders in three communities. *Archives of General Psychiatry* 41:959-967, 1984.

[42] Moscicki, E.K.; O'Carroll, P.; Rae, D.S.; et al. Suicide attempts in the Epidemiologic Catchment Area Study. *The Yale Journal of Biology and Medicine* 61:259-268, 1998.

[43] CDC. Suicide among older persons—United States, 1980–1992. *Morbidity and Mortality Weekly Report* 45(1):3-6, 1996.

[44] CDC. Suicide Deaths and Rates Per 100,000. <http://www.cdc.gov/ncipc/data/us9794/Suic.htm>November 23, 1999.

[45] CDC. Health related quality of life and activity limitation: Eight States, 1995. *Morbidity and Mortality Weekly Report* 47(7):134-140, 1998.

[46] Montano, C.B. Recognition and treatment of depression in a primary care setting. *Journal of Clinical Psychiatry* 55:18-34, 1994.

[47] NCHS, CDC. *Health, United States, 1996*. Hyattsville, MD: PHS, 1997.

[48] NIMH Suicide Research Consortium. *Suicide Facts*. Rockville, MD: NIMH, 1997.

[49] CDC. Ten leading causes of death by age group, 1996. <http://www.cdc.gov/ncipc/osp/leadcaus/101c96.htm>November 23, 1999.

[50] Tessler, R., and Dennis, D. *A Synthesis of NIMH-Funded Research Concerning Persons Who Are Homeless and Mentally Ill*. DHHS Pub. No. 94-303014. Rockville, MD: NIMH, 1989.

[51] Lam, J.A., and Rosenheck, R. Street outreach for homeless persons with serious mental illness: Is it effective? *Medical Care* 37:894-907, 1999.

[52] Lehman, A., and Codray, D. Prevalence of alcohol, drug, and mental disorders among the homeless: One more time. *Contemporary Drug Problems* 20:355-383, 1993.

[53] Bell, M.D., and Lysaker, P.H. Clinical benefits of paid work activity in schizophrenia: 1-year follow up. *Schizophrenia Bulletin* 23:317-328, 1997.

[54] Arns, P.G., and Linney, J.A. Work, self, and life satisfaction for persons with severe and persistent mental disorders. *Psychosocial Rehabilitation Journal* 17:63-79, 1993.

[55] Fabian, E. Supported employment and the quality of life: Does a job make a difference? *Rehabilitation Counseling Bulletin* 2:84-87, 1992.

[56] Rogers, E.S.; Sciarappa, K.; and MacDonald, W.K. A benefit-cost analysis of a supported employment model for persons with psychiatric disability. *Evaluation and Program Planning* 18:105-115,1995.

[57] Herzog, D.B., and Copeland, P.N. Medical progress: Eating disorders. *New England Journal of Medicine* 313:295-303, 1985.

[58] Eckert, E.D.; Halmi, K.A.; Marchi, P.; et al. Ten-year follow-up of anorexia nervosa: Clinical course and outcome. *Psychological Medicine* 25:143-156, 1995.

[59] Strober, M.; Freeman, R.; and Morrell, W. The long-term course of severe anorexia nervosa in adolescents. Survival analysis of recovery, relapse, and outcome predictors over 10-15 years in a prospective study. *International Journal of Eating Disorders* 22:339-360, 1997.

[60] Pike, K.M. Long-term course of anorexia nervosa: Response, relapse, remission, and recovery. *Clinical Psychology Review* 18:447-475, 1998.

[61] Field, A.E.; Herzog, D.B.; Keller, M.B.; et al. Distinguishing recovery from remission in a cohort of bulimic women: How should asymptomatic periods be described? *Journal of Clinical Epidemiology* 50:1339-1345, 1997.

[62] Keel, P.K., and Mitchell, J.E. Outcome of bulimia nervosa. *American Journal of Psychiatry* 154:313-321, 1997.

[63] Greenberg, M.T.; Domitrovich, C.; and Bumbarger, B. *Preventing Mental Disorders in School-Aged Children: A Review of the Effectiveness of Prevention Programs.* Rockville, MD: HHS, PHS, SAMHSA, CMHS, 1999.

[64] Woodruff, D.S.; Osher, D.; Hoffman, C.C.; et al. The role of education in a system of care: Effectively serving children with emotional or behavioral disorders. In: *Systems of Care: Promising Practices in Children's Mental Health, 1998 Series.* Vol. III. Rockville, MD: HHS, PHS, SAMHSA, CMHS, 1999.

[65] Otto, R.K. Prevalence of mental disorders among youth in the juvenile justice system. In: *Responding to the Mental Health Needs of Youth in the Juvenile Justice System.* Washington, DC: National Coalition for the Mentally Ill in the Criminal Justice System, 1992.

[66] Cocozza, J.J. Identifying the needs of juveniles with co-occurring disorders. *Corrections Today,* December 1997.

[67] Wells, K.; Stewart, A.; Hays, R.; et al. The functioning and well-being of depressed patients: Results from the Medical Outcomes Study. *Journal of the American Medical Association* 262:914-919, 1989.

[68] Dohrenwend, B.S.; Dohrenwend, B.P.; Link, B.; et al. Social functioning of psychiatric patients in contrast with community cases in the general population. *Archives of General Psychiatry* 40:1174-1182, 1983.

[69] Moscicki, E.K. Identification of suicide risk factors using epidemiologic studies. *Psychiatric Clinics of North America* 20:3, 499-517, 1997.

[70] NIMH. Depression Facts, 1999. <http://www.nimh.nih.gov/depression/index.htm>November 23, 1999.

[71] Greenberg, P.E.; Stiglin, L.E.; Finkelstein, S.N.; et al. The economic burden of depression. *Journal of Clinical Psychiatry* 54:425-426, 1993.

[72] Katon, W.J. Will improving detection of depression in primary care lead to improved depressive outcomes? *General Hospital Psychiatry* 17:1-2, 1995.

[73] Häfner, H., and an der Heiden, W. Epidemiology of schizophrenia. *Canadian Journal of Psychiatry* 42:139-151, 1997.

[74] Weissman, M.M.; Bland, R.C.; Canino, G.J.; et al. The cross-national epidemiology of panic disorder. *Archives of General Psychiatry* 54:305-309, 1997.

[75] Magee, W.J.; Eaton, W.W.; Wittchen, H.U.; et al. Agoraphobia, simple phobia, and social phobia in the National Comorbidity Survey. *Archives of General Psychiatry* 53:159-168, 1996.

[76] Goldberg, D.P., and Lecrubier, Y. Form and frequency of mental disorders across centres. In: Ustun T.B., and Sartorius, N., eds. *Mental Illness in General Health Care: An International Study.* New York, NY: John Wiley & Sons, 1995, 323-334.

[77] Liebowitz, M.R. Panic disorder as a chronic illness. *Journal of Clinical Psychiatry* 58(Suppl.)13:5-8, 1997.

[78] Gorman, J.M., and Coplan, J.D. Comorbidity of depression and panic disorder. *Journal of Clinical Psychiatry* 57(Suppl. 10):34-41, 42-43, 1996.

[79] Keller, M.B., and Hanks, D.L. The natural history and heterogeneity of depressive disorders: Implications for rational antidepressant therapy. *Journal of Clinical Psychiatry* 55(Suppl. A):25-31; discussion 32-3, 98-100, 1994.

[80] Marcus, S.C.; Olfson, M.; Pincus, H.A.; et al. Self-reported anxiety, general medical conditions, and disability bed days. *American Journal of Psychiatry* 154:1766-1768, 1997.

[81] Hornig, C.D., and McNally, R.J. Panic disorder and suicide attempt. A reanalysis of data from the Epidemiologic Catchment Area Study. *British Journal of Psychiatry* 167:76-79, 1995.

[82] Morris, S.M.; Steadman, H.J.; and Veysey, B.M. Mental health services in United States jails: A survey of innovative practices. *Criminal Justice and Behavior* 24:3-19, 1997.

[83] Steadman, H.J.; Morris, S.M.; and Dennis, D. The diversion of mentally ill persons from jails to community-based services: A profile of programs. *American Journal of Public Health* 12:1630-1635, 1995.

[84] KPMG Peat Marwick LLP and Northwestern University. *New Voices: Consumerism in Health Care.* Chicago, IL: KPMG, 1998.

[85] Davis, K. *Exploring the Intersection Between Cultural Competency and Managed Behavioral Care Policy Implications for State and County Mental Health Agencies.* Alexandria, VA: National Technical Assistance Center for State Mental Health Planning (NTAC), 1997.

[86] Lefley, H.P. Culture and chronic mental illness. *Hospital and Community Psychiatry* 41:277-286, 1990.

[87] Munoz, F.U., and Endo, R., eds. *Perspectives on Minority Group Mental Health.* Washington, DC: University Press of America, 1982.

[88] Martinez, K. Cultural sensitivity in family therapy gone awry. *Hispanic Journal of Behavioral Sciences* 16:75-89, 1994.

[89] Mason, J.L. Developing culturally competent organizations. *Focal Point: The Bulletin of Research and Training Center on Family Support and Children's Mental Health* 8:1-8, 1994.

[90] Miller, S.O.; O'Neal, G.S.; and Scott, C.A.; eds. *Primary Prevention Approaches to the Development of Mental Health Services for Ethnic Minorities: Challenges to Social Work Education and Practice.* New York, NY: Council on Social Work Education, 1982.

[91] Snowden, L., and Hoschuh, J. Ethnic differences in emergency psychiatric care and hospitalization in a program for the severely mentally ill. *Community Mental Health Journal* 28, 1992.

[92] Snowden, L., and Cheung, F. Use of inpatient services by members of ethnic groups. *American Psychologist* 45:347-355, 1990.

[93] Schffler, R.M., and Miller, A.B. Demand analysis of service use among ethnic subpopulations. *Inquiry* 26:202-215, 1989.

[94] Manderscheid, R.W., and Sonnenschein, M.A. *Mental Health, United States, 1985.* Rockville, MD: NIMH, 1987.

[95] Blazer, D., and Williams, C.D. The epidemiology of dysphoria and depression in an elderly population. *American Journal of Psychiatry* 137:439-444, 1980.

19
Nutrition and Overweight

Co-Lead Agencies: Food and Drug Administration
                   National Institutes of Health

Contents

Promote health and reduce chronic disease associated with diet and weight.

Issues and Trends

Nutrition is essential for growth and development, health, and well-being. Behaviors to promote health should start early in life with breastfeeding[1] and continue through life with the development of healthful eating habits. Nutritional, or dietary, factors contribute substantially to the burden of preventable illnesses and premature deaths in the United States.[2] Indeed, dietary factors are associated with 4 of the 10 leading causes of death: coronary heart disease (CHD), some types of cancer, stroke, and type 2 diabetes.[3] These health conditions are estimated to cost society over $200 billion each year in medical expenses and lost productivity.[4] Dietary factors also are associated with osteoporosis, which affects more than 25 million persons in the United States and is the major underlying cause of bone fractures in postmenopausal women and elderly persons.[5]

Many dietary components are involved in the relationship between nutrition and health. A primary concern is consuming too much saturated fat and too few vegetables, fruits, and grain products that are high in vitamins and minerals, carbohydrates (starch and dietary fiber), and other substances that are important to good health. The 2000 *Dietary Guidelines for Americans* recommend that, to stay healthy, persons aged 2 years and older should follow these ABCs for good health: **A**im for fitness, **B**uild a healthy base, and **C**hoose sensibly. To aim for fitness, aim for a healthy weight and be physically active each day. To build a healthy base, let the Pyramid guide food choices; choose a variety of grains daily, especially whole grains; choose a variety of fruits and vegetables daily; and keep food safe to eat. To choose sensibly, choose a diet that is low in saturated fat and cholesterol and moderate in total fat; choose beverages and foods to moderate intake of sugars; choose and prepare foods with less salt; and if consuming alcoholic beverages, do so in moderation.[6] The Food Guide Pyramid, introduced in 1992, is an educational tool that conveys recommendations about the number of servings from different food groups each day and other principles of the *Dietary Guidelines for Americans*.[7] [Note: In text that follows in this chapter, *Dietary Guidelines for Americans* will refer to the 2000 *Dietary Guidelines for Americans* unless otherwise noted.]

The *Dietary Guidelines for Americans* also emphasize the need for adequate consumption of iron-rich and calcium-rich foods.[6] Although some progress has been made since the 1970s in reducing the prevalence of iron deficiency among low-

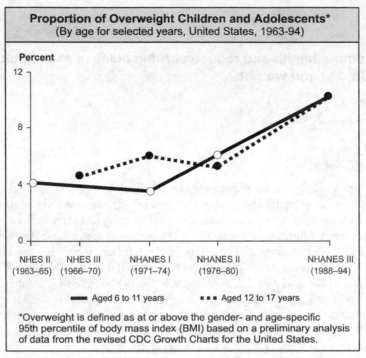

Proportion of Overweight Children and Adolescents*
(By age for selected years, United States, 1963-94)

Percent

Aged 6 to 11 years   ■ ■ ■ Aged 12 to 17 years

*Overweight is defined as at or above the gender- and age-specific
95th percentile of body mass index (BMI) based on a preliminary analysis
of data from the revised CDC Growth Charts for the United States.

Source: Adapted from Troiano, R.P., and Flegal, K.M. Data as reported
in: Overweight children and adolescents: Description, epidemiology, and
demographics. *Pediatrics* 101:497-504, 1998.

income children,[8] much more is needed to improve the health of children of all
ages and of women who are pregnant or are of childbearing age. Since the start of
this decade, consumption of calcium-rich foods, such as milk products, has generally decreased and is especially low among teenaged girls and young women.[9]
Because important sources of calcium also can include other foods with calcium—occurring naturally or through fortification—as well as dietary supplements, the current emphasis is on tracking total calcium intake from all sources, as
demonstrated by an objective in this focus area. In addition, in recent years there
has been a concerted effort to increase the folic acid intake of females of childbearing age through fortification and other means to reduce the risk of neural tube
defects.[10, 11] (See Focus Area 16. Maternal, Infant, and Child Health.)

In general, however, excesses and imbalances of some food components in the
diet have replaced once commonplace nutrient deficiencies. Unfortunately, there
has been an alarming increase in the number of overweight and obese persons.[12, 13]
Overweight results when a person eats more calories from food (energy) than he
or she expends, for example, through physical activity. This balance between energy intake and output is influenced by metabolic and genetic factors as well as
behaviors affecting dietary intake and physical activity; environmental, cultural,
and socioeconomic components also play a role.

When a body mass index (BMI) cut-point of 25 is used, nearly 55 percent of the U.S. adult population was defined as overweight or obese in 1988–94, compared to 46 percent in 1976–80.[12, 14, 15] In particular, the proportion of adults defined as obese by a BMI of 30 or greater has increased from 14.5 percent to 22.5 percent.[12] A similar increase in overweight and obesity also has been observed in children above age 6 years in both genders and in all population groups.[16]

Many diseases are associated with overweight and obesity. Persons who are overweight or obese are at increased risk for high blood pressure, type 2 diabetes, coronary heart disease, stroke, gallbladder disease, osteoarthritis, sleep apnea, respiratory problems, and some types of cancer. The health outcomes related to these diseases, however, often can be improved through weight loss or, at a minimum, no further weight gain. Total costs (medical costs and lost productivity) attributable to obesity alone amounted to an estimated $99 billion in 1995.[17]

Disparities

Disparities in health status indicators and risk factors for diet-related disease are evident in many segments of the population based on gender, age, race and ethnicity, and income. For example, overweight and obesity are observed in all population groups, but obesity is particularly common among Hispanic, African American, Native American, and Pacific Islander women. Furthermore, despite concerns about the increase in overweight and certain excesses in U.S. diets, segments of the population also suffer from undernutrition, including persons who are socially isolated and poor. Over the years, the recognition of the consequences of food insecurity (limited access to safe, nutritious food) has led to the development of national measures and surveys to evaluate food insecurity and hunger and to the ability to assess disparities among different population groups. With food security and other measures of undernutrition, such as growth retardation and iron deficiency, disparities are evident based not only on income but also on race and ethnicity.

In addition, there are concerns about the nutritional status of persons in hospitals, nursing homes, convalescent centers, and institutions; persons with disabilities, including physically, mentally, and developmentally disabled persons in community settings; children in child care facilities; persons living on reservations; persons in correctional facilities; and persons who are homeless. National data about these population groups are currently unavailable or limited. Data also are insufficient to target the fastest growing segment of the population, old and very old persons who live independently.

Opportunities

Establishing healthful dietary and physical activity behaviors needs to begin in childhood. Educating school-aged children about nutrition is important to help establish healthful eating habits early in life.[18, 19] Research suggests that parents who understand proper nutrition can help children in preschool choose healthful foods, but they have less influence on the choices of school-aged children.[20] Thus, the impact of nutrition education on health may be more effective if targeted directly at school-aged children. Unfortunately, a survey done in 1994 showed that only 69 percent of States and 80 percent of school districts required nutrition education for students in at least some grades from kindergarten through 12th grade.[21]

A well-designed curriculum that effectively addresses essential nutrition education topics can increase students' knowledge about nutrition, help shape appropriate attitudes, and help develop the behavioral skills students need to plan, prepare, and select healthful meals and snacks.[18, 22, 23] Curricula that encourage specific, healthful eating behaviors and provide students with the skills needed to adopt and maintain those behaviors have led to favorable changes in student dietary behaviors and cardiovascular disease risk factors.[18, 22, 23] In order to enhance the effectiveness of these lessons, however, nutrition course work should be part of the core curriculum for the professional preparation of teachers of all grades and should be emphasized in continuing education activities for teachers.

Topics considered to be essential at the elementary, middle, junior high, and senior high school levels include using the Food Guide Pyramid; learning the benefits of healthful eating; making healthful food choices for meals and snacks; preparing healthy meals and snacks; using food labels; eating a variety of foods; eating more fruits, vegetables, and grains; eating foods low in saturated fat and total fat more often; eating more calcium-rich foods; balancing food intake and physical activity; accepting body size differences; and following food safety practices.[18, 24] In addition, the following topics are considered to be essential at the middle, junior high, and senior high school levels: the *Dietary Guidelines for Americans;* eating disorders; healthy weight maintenance; influences on food choices such as families, culture, and media; and goals for dietary improvement.[18]

Nutrition education should be taught as part of a comprehensive school health education program, and essential nutrition education topics should be integrated into science and other curricula to reinforce principles and messages learned in the health units. Nutrition education is addressed within a school health education objective. (See Focus Area 7. Educational and Community-Based Programs.) In addition, students must have access to healthful food choices to enhance further the likelihood of adopting healthful dietary practices. For these reasons, monitoring students' eating practices at school is important.

Although health promotion efforts should begin in childhood, they need to continue throughout adulthood. In particular, public education about the long-term health consequences and risks associated with overweight and how to achieve and maintain a healthy weight is necessary. While many persons attempt to lose weight, studies show that within 5 years a majority regain the weight.[25] To maintain weight loss, healthful dietary habits must be coupled with decreased sedentary behavior and increased physical activity and become permanent lifestyle changes. (See Focus Area 22. Physical Activity and Fitness.) Additionally, changes in the physical and social environment may help persons maintain the necessary long-term lifestyle changes for both diet and physical activity.

Policymakers and program planners at the national, State, and community levels can and should provide important leadership in fostering healthful diets and physical activity patterns among people in the United States. The family and others, such as health care practitioners, schools, worksites, institutional food services, and the media, can play a key role in this process. For example, registered dietitians and other qualified health care practitioners can improve health outcomes through efforts focused on nutrition screening, assessment, and primary and secondary prevention.

Food-related businesses also can help consumers achieve healthful diets by providing nutrition information for foods purchased in supermarkets, fast-food outlets, restaurants, and carryout operations. For example, the introduction of a new food label in 1993 has resulted in nutrition information on most processed packaged foods, along with credible health and nutrient content claims and standardized serving sizes.[26] While efforts were made in the 1990s to increase the availability of nutrition information, reduced-fat foods, and other healthful food choices in supermarkets, significant challenges remain on these fronts for away-from-home foods purchased at food service outlets. The importance of addressing these challenges is suggested by recent data indicating that nearly 40 percent of a family's food budget is spent on away-from-home food, including food from restaurants and fast-food outlets.[27] One analysis found that away-from-home foods are generally higher in saturated fat, total fat, cholesterol, and sodium and lower in dietary fiber, iron, and calcium than at-home foods.[27] Away-from-home sites include restaurants, fast-food outlets, school cafeterias, vending machines, and other food service outlets. This study also suggested that persons either eat larger amounts when they eat out, eat higher calorie foods, or both.

Many of the Healthy People 2010 objectives that address nutrition and overweight in the United States measure in some way the Nation's progress toward implementing the recommendations of the *Dietary Guidelines for Americans*. The recommendations for food and nutrient intake are not intended to be met every day but rather on average over a span of time. Although the Healthy People 2010 dietary intake objectives address the proportion of the population that consumes a specified level of certain foods or nutrients, it is also important to track and report the average amount eaten by different population groups to help interpret progress on these objectives. Other objectives target aspects of undernutrition, including iron deficiency, growth retardation, and food security.

In summary, several actions are recognized as fundamental in achieving this focus area's objectives:

- Improving accessibility of nutrition information, nutrition education, nutrition counseling and related services, and healthful foods in a variety of settings and for all population groups.

- Focusing on preventing chronic disease associated with diet and weight, beginning in youth.

- Strengthening the link between nutrition and physical activity in health promotion.

- Maintaining a strong national program for basic and applied nutrition research to provide a sound science base for dietary recommendations and effective interventions.

- Maintaining a strong national nutrition monitoring program to provide accurate, reliable, timely, and comparable data to assess status and progress and to be responsive to unmet data needs and emerging issues.

- Strengthening State and community data systems to be responsive to the data users at these levels.

- Building and sustaining broad-based initiatives and commitment to these objectives by public and private sector partners at the national, State, and local levels.

Interim Progress Toward Year 2000 Objectives

Of the 27 nutrition objectives, targets for 5 have been met, including 2 related to the availability of reduced-fat foods and prevalence of growth retardation.[28] The majority of the objectives have shown some progress, including those related to total fruit, vegetable, and grain product intake and total fat and saturated fat intake; availability of nutrition labeling on foods; breastfeeding; nutrition education in schools; and availability of worksite nutrition and weight management programs. For certain other objectives, such as consumer actions to reduce salt intake and home-delivered meals to elderly persons, there has been little or no progress. And for others, such as intake of calcium-rich food and overweight and obesity, movement has been away from the targets. In particular, the proportion of adults and children who are overweight or obese has increased substantially, and this represents one of the biggest challenges for Healthy People 2010.

Note: Unless otherwise noted, data are from the Centers for Disease Control and Prevention, National Center for Health Statistics, *Healthy People 2000 Review, 1998–99.*

Nutrition and Overweight

Goal: Promote health and reduce chronic disease associated with diet and weight.

Number   Objective Short Title

Weight Status and Growth

19-1   Healthy weight in adults

19-2   Obesity in adults

19-3   Overweight or obesity in children and adolescents

19-4   Growth retardation in children

Food and Nutrient Consumption

19-5   Fruit intake

19-6   Vegetable intake

19-7   Grain product intake

19-8   Saturated fat intake

19-9   Total fat intake

19-10   Sodium intake

19-11   Calcium intake

Iron Deficiency and Anemia

19-12   Iron deficiency in young children and in females of
            childbearing age

19-13   Anemia in low-income pregnant females

19-14   Iron deficiency in pregnant females

Schools, Worksites, and Nutrition Counseling

19-15   Meals and snacks at school

19-16   Worksite promotion of nutrition education and weight management

19-17   Nutrition counseling for medical conditions

Food Security

19-18   Food security

Weight Status and Growth

19-1. Increase the proportion of adults who are at a healthy weight.

Target: 60 percent.

Baseline: 42 percent of adults aged 20 years and older were at a healthy weight (defined as a body mass index [BMI] equal to or greater than 18.5 and less than 25) in 1988–94 (age adjusted to the year 2000 standard population).

Target setting method: Better than the best.

Data source: National Health and Nutrition Examination Survey (NHANES), CDC, NCHS.

NOTE: THE TABLE BELOW MAY CONTINUE TO THE FOLLOWING PAGE.

Adults Aged 20 Years and Older, 1988–94 (unless noted)	Healthy Weight		
	19-1. Both Genders	Females*	Males*
	Percent		
TOTAL	42	45	38
Race and ethnicity			
American Indian or Alaska Native	DSU	DSU	DSU
Asian or Pacific Islander	DSU	DSU	DSU
Asian	DNC	DNC	DNC
Native Hawaiian and other Pacific Islander	DNC	DNC	DNC
Black or African American	34	29	40
White	42	47	37
Hispanic or Latino	DSU	DSU	DSU
Mexican American	30	31	30
Not Hispanic or Latino	43	47	39
Black or African American	34	29	40
White	43	49	38

Adults Aged 20 Years and Older, 1988–94 (unless noted)	Healthy Weight		
	19-1. Both Genders	Females*	Males*
	Percent		
Age			
20 to 39 years	51	55	48
40 to 59 years	36	40	31
60 years and older	36	37	33
Family income level†			
Lower income (≤130 percent of poverty threshold)	38	33	44
Higher income (>130 percent of poverty threshold)	43	48	37
Disability status			
Persons with disabilities	32 (1991–94)	35 (1991–94)	30 (1991–94)
Persons without disabilities	41 (1991–94)	45 (1991–94)	36 (1991–94)
Select populations			
Persons with arthritis	36 (1991–94)	37 (1991–94)	34 (1991–94)
Persons without arthritis	43 (1991–94)	47 (1991–94)	40 (1991–94)
Persons with diabetes	26	DNA	DNA
Persons without diabetes	43	DNA	DNA
Persons with high blood pressure	27	29	26
Persons without high blood pressure	46	50	42

DNA = Data have not been analyzed. DNC = Data are not collected. DSU = Data are statistically unreliable.

Note: Age adjusted to the year 2000 standard population.

*Data for females and males are displayed to further characterize the issue.

†A household income below 130 percent of poverty threshold is used by the Food Stamp Program.

NOTE: THE TABLE ABOVE MAY HAVE CONTINUED FROM THE PREVIOUS PAGE.

19-2.   Reduce the proportion of adults who are obese.

Target: 15 percent.

Baseline: 23 percent of adults aged 20 years and older were identified as obese (defined as a BMI of 30 or more) in 1988–94 (age adjusted to the year 2000 standard population).

Target setting method: Better than the best.

Data source: National Health and Nutrition Examination Survey (NHANES), CDC, NCHS.

Adults Aged 20 Years and Older, 1988–94 (unless noted)	Obesity		
	19-2. Both Genders	Females*	Males*
	Percent		
TOTAL	23	25	20
Race and ethnicity			
American Indian or Alaska Native	DSU	DSU	DSU
Asian or Pacific Islander	DSU	DSU	DSU
Asian	DNC	DNC	DNC
Native Hawaiian and other Pacific Islander	DNC	DNC	DNC
Black or African American	30	38	21
White	22	24	21
Hispanic or Latino	DSU	DSU	DSU
Mexican American	29	35	24
Not Hispanic or Latino	22	25	20
Black or African American	30	38	21
White	22	23	20
Age (not age adjusted)			
20 to 39 years	18	21	15
40 to 59 years	28	30	25
60 years and older	24	26	21
Family income level†			
Lower income (≤130 percent of poverty threshold)	29	35	21
Higher income (>130 percent of poverty threshold)	22	23	20
Disability status			
Persons with disabilities	30 (1991–94)	38 (1991–94)	21 (1991–94)
Persons without disabilities	23 (1991–94)	25 (1991–94)	22 (1991–94)

Adults Aged 20 Years and Older, 1988–94 (unless noted)	Obesity		
	19-2. Both Genders	Females*	Males*
	Percent		
Select populations			
Persons with arthritis	30	33	27
Persons without arthritis	21	23	19
Persons with diabetes	41	DNA	DNA
Persons without diabetes	22	DNA	DNA
Persons with high blood pressure	38	47	33
Persons without high blood pressure	18	20	16

DNA = Data have not been analyzed. DNC = Data are not collected. DSU = Data are statistically unreliable.

Note: Age adjusted to the year 2000 standard population.

*Data for females and males are displayed to further characterize the issue.

†A household income below 130 percent of poverty threshold is used by the Food Stamp Program.

NOTE: THE TABLE ABOVE MAY HAVE CONTINUED FROM THE PREVIOUS PAGE.

19-3. Reduce the proportion of children and adolescents who are overweight or obese.

Target and baseline:

Objective	Reduction in Overweight or Obese Children and Adolescents*	1988–94 Baseline	2010 Target
		Percent	
19-3a.	Children aged 6 to 11 years	11	5
19-3b.	Adolescents aged 12 to 19 years	11	5
19-3c.	Children and adolescents aged 6 to 19 years	11	5

*Defined as at or above the gender- and age-specific 95th percentile of BMI based on the revised CDC Growth Charts for the United States.

Target setting method: Better than the best.

Data source: National Health and Nutrition Examination Survey (NHANES), CDC, NCHS.

Children and Adolescents Aged 6 to 19 Years, 1988–94 (unless noted)	Overweight or Obese		
	19-3a. Children Aged 6 to 11 Years	19-3b. Adolescents Aged 12 to 19 Years	19-3c. Children and Adolescents Aged 6 to 19 Years
	Percent		
TOTAL	11	11	11
Race and ethnicity			
American Indian or Alaska Native	DSU	DSU	DNA
Asian or Pacific Islander	DSU	DSU	DNA
Asian	DNC	DNC	DNC
Native Hawaiian and other Pacific Islander	DNC	DNC	DNC
Black or African American	15	13	14
White	11	11	11
Hispanic or Latino	DSU	DSU	DSU
Mexican American	17	14	15
Not Hispanic or Latino	11	10	11
Black or African American	15	13	14
White	10	10	10
Gender			
Female	11	10	10
Male	12	11	12
Family income level*			
Lower income (≤130 percent of poverty threshold)	11	16	13
Higher income (>130 percent of poverty threshold)	11	8	10
Disability status			
Persons with disabilities	DSU (1991–94)	DSU (1991–94)	DSU (1991–94)
Persons without disabilities	13 (1991–94)	11 (1991–94)	12 (1991–94)

DNA = Data have not been analyzed. DNC = Data are not collected. DSU = Data are statistically unreliable.
*A household income below 130 percent of poverty threshold is used by the Food Stamp Program.

Maintenance of a healthy weight is a major goal in the effort to reduce the burden of illness and its consequent reduction in quality of life and life expectancy. The selection of a BMI cut-point to establish the upper limit of the healthy weight range is based on the relationship of overweight or obesity to risk factors for chronic disease or premature death. A BMI of less than 25 has been accepted by numerous groups as the upper limit of the healthy weight range, since chronic disease risk increases in most populations at or above this cut-point.[14, 15, 29] The lower cut-point for the healthy weight range (BMI of 18.5) was selected to be consistent with national and international recommendations.[14, 15] Problems associated with excessive thinness (BMI less than 18.5) include menstrual irregularity, infertility, and osteoporosis. There is some concern that the increased focus on overweight may result in more eating disorders, such as bulimia and anorexia nervosa. (See Focus Area 18. Mental Health and Mental Disorders.) However, no evidence currently exists that suggests the increased focus on overweight has resulted in additional cases of eating disorders.

Overweight and obesity are caused by many factors. These factors reflect the contributions of inherited, metabolic, behavioral, environmental, cultural, and socioeconomic components. As weight increases, so does the prevalence of health risks. Simple, health-oriented definitions of overweight and obesity should be based on the amount of excess body fat at which health risks to individuals begin to increase. No such definitions currently exist. Most current clinical studies assessing the health effects of overweight rely on a measurement of body weight adjusted for height. BMI is the choice for many researchers and health professionals. While the relation of BMI to body fat differs by age and gender, it provides valid comparisons across racial and ethnic groups.[30] However, BMI does not provide information concerning body fat distribution, which has been identified as an independent predictor of health risk.[15, 29] Thus, until a better surrogate for body fat is developed, BMI often will be used to screen for overweight and obese individuals. Health risks also increase as waist measurement increases, and thus waist measurement also can be a useful indicator.[6]

Interpretations of data about overweight and obesity have differed because criteria for these terms have varied over time, from study to study, and from one part of the world to another. National and international organizations now support the use of a BMI of 30 or greater to identify obesity.[14, 15] These BMI cut-points are only a guide to the identification and treatment of overweight and obese individuals and allow for the comparison across populations and over time. However, the health risks associated with overweight and obesity are part of a continuum and do not conform to rigid cut-points.

Overweight and obesity affect a large proportion of the U.S. population—55 percent of adults. Between 1976 and 1994, the number of cases of obesity alone increased more than 50 percent—from 14.5 percent of the adult population to 22.5 percent. Approximately 25 percent of U.S. adult females and 20 percent of U.S. adult males are obese.[12] Because weight management is difficult for most persons, the Healthy People 2010 target of no more than 15 percent of adults aged 20 years and older having a BMI of 30 or more is ambitious. Nonetheless, the potential benefits from reduction in overweight and obesity are of considerable public health importance and deserve particular emphasis and attention. A concerted public effort will be needed to prevent further increases of overweight and obesity. Health care providers, health plans, and managed care organizations need to be alert to the development of overweight and obesity in their clients and should provide information concerning the associated risks. These groups need to provide guidance to help consumers address this health problem. To lose weight and keep it off, overweight persons will need long-term lifestyle changes in dietary and physical activity patterns that they can easily incorporate into their lives.

Patterns of healthful eating behavior need to begin in childhood and be maintained throughout adulthood. These patterns can be encouraged through nutrition education at schools and worksites that takes into account cultural and other factors influencing diet. Persons should be aware of the impact that away-from-home eating can have on weight management. In order to address physical activity needs, changes in the physical environment—such as access to walkways and bicycle paths—and the social environment—through social support and safe communities—will be needed to achieve long-term success.

There is much concern about the increasing prevalence of obesity in children and adolescents. Overweight and obesity acquired during childhood or adolescence may persist into adulthood and increase the risk for some chronic diseases later in life. Teenaged boys lose some fat accumulated before puberty during adolescence, but fat deposition continues in girls. Thus, without measures of sexual maturity, measures of body fat and body weight are difficult to interpret in children and adolescents. Therefore, the objective to reduce the prevalence of overweight and obesity among children and adolescents has a target set at no more than 5 percent and uses the gender- and age-specific 95th percentile of BMI from the revised Centers for Disease Control and Prevention (CDC) Growth Charts for the United States. Interventions need to recognize that obese children also may experience psychological stress. The reduction of BMI in children and adolescents should be achieved by emphasizing physical activity and a properly balanced diet so that healthy growth is maintained. Additional research is needed to better define the prevalence and health consequences of overweight and obesity in children and adolescents and the implications of such findings for these persons as they become the next generation of adults.

19-4.   Reduce growth retardation among low-income children under age 5 years.

Target: 5 percent.

Baseline: 8 percent of low-income children under age 5 years were growth retarded in 1997 (defined as height for age below the fifth percentile in the age-gender appropriate population using the 1977 NCHS/CDC growth charts;[31] preliminary data; not age adjusted).

Target setting method: Better than the best.

Data source: Pediatric Nutrition Surveillance System, CDC, NCCDPHP.

Low-Income Children Under Age 5 Years, 1997	Growth Retardation			
	19-4. Under Age 5 Years	Under Age 1 Year*	Aged 1 Year*	Aged 2 to 4 Years*
	Percent			
TOTAL	8	10	9	6
Race and ethnicity				
American Indian or Alaska Native	8	9	7	9
Asian or Pacific Islander	9	9	11	8
Asian	DNC	DNC	DNC	DNC
Native Hawaiian and other Pacific Islander	DNC	DNC	DNC	DNC
Black or African American	DNC	DNC	DNC	DNC
White	DNC	DNC	DNC	DNC
Hispanic or Latino	7	7	8	5
Not Hispanic or Latino	DNC	DNC	DNC	DNC
Black or African American	9	15	10	5
White	8	10	9	6
Gender				
Female	8	10	8	6
Male	8	10	10	6
Disability status				
Children with disabilities	DNC	DNC	DNC	DNC
Children without disabilities	DNC	DNC	DNC	DNC

DNA = Data have not been analyzed. DNC = Data are not collected. DSU = Data are statistically unreliable.
Note: Preliminary data; not age adjusted.
*Data for specific age groups under 5 years are displayed to further characterize the issue.

Retardation in linear growth in preschool children serves as an indicator of overall health and development and also may reflect the adequacy of a child's diet. Full growth potential may not be reached because of less than optimal nutrition, infectious diseases, chronic diseases, or poor health care. Inadequate maternal weight gain during pregnancy and other prenatal factors that influence birth weight also affect the prevalence of growth retardation among infants and young children.

Growth retardation is not a problem for the majority of young children in the United States. By definition, approximately 5 percent of healthy children are expected to be below the fifth percentile of height for age due to normal biologic variation. If more than 5 percent of a population group is below the fifth percentile, this suggests that full growth potential is not being reached by some children in that group. Among some age and ethnic groups of low-income children under age 5 years in the United States, up to 15 percent are below the fifth percentile. While progress has been made in reducing the prevalence of growth retardation among low-income Hispanic and Asian or Pacific Islander children, it remains especially high for African American children in the first year of life.

Interventions to improve children's linear growth potential include better nutrition; improvements in the prevention, diagnosis, and treatment of infectious and chronic diseases; and provision and use of adequate health services. Although the response of a population to interventions for growth retardation may not be as rapid as for iron deficiency or underweight, achievement of the objective by the year 2010 in all racial and ethnic, socioeconomic, and age groups should be possible. Special attention should be given to homeless children and those with special health care needs.

Food and Nutrient Consumption

19-5. Increase the proportion of persons aged 2 years and older who consume at least two daily servings of fruit.

Target: 75 percent.

Baseline: 28 percent of persons aged 2 years and older consumed at least two daily servings of fruit in 1994–96 (age adjusted to the year 2000 standard population).

Target setting method: Better than the best.

Data source: Continuing Survey of Food Intakes by Individuals (CSFII) (2-day average), USDA.

NOTE: THE TABLE BELOW MAY CONTINUE TO THE FOLLOWING PAGE.

Persons Aged 2 Years and Older, 1994–96	Two or More Daily Servings of Fruit
	Percent
TOTAL	28
Race and ethnicity	
American Indian or Alaska Native	DSU
Asian or Pacific Islander	DSU
Asian	DNC
Native Hawaiian and other Pacific Islander	DNC
Black or African American	DNA
White	DNA

Persons Aged 2 Years and Older, 1994–96	Two or More Daily Servings of Fruit
	Percent
Hispanic or Latino	32
Mexican American	29
Other Hispanic	30
Not Hispanic or Latino	
Black or African American	24
White	27
Gender and age	
Female	
2 years and older	26
2 to 5 years (not age adjusted)	43
6 to 11 years (not age adjusted)	26
12 to 19 years (not age adjusted)	23
20 to 39 years (not age adjusted)	20
40 to 59 years (not age adjusted)	26
60 years and older (not age adjusted)	35
Male	
2 years and older	29
2 to 5 years (not age adjusted)	46
6 to 11 years (not age adjusted)	27
12 to 19 years (not age adjusted)	22
20 to 39 years (not age adjusted)	23
40 to 59 years (not age adjusted)	28
60 years and older (not age adjusted)	39
Household income level*	
Lower income (≤130 percent of poverty threshold)	23
Higher income (>130 percent of poverty threshold)	29
Disability status	
Persons with disabilities	DNC
Persons without disabilities	DNC

DNA = Data have not been analyzed. DNC = Data are not collected. DSU = Data are statistically unreliable.

Note: Age adjusted to the year 2000 standard population.

*A household income below 130 percent of poverty threshold is used by the Food Stamp Program.

NOTE: THE TABLE ABOVE MAY HAVE CONTINUED FROM THE PREVIOUS PAGE.

19-6. Increase the proportion of persons aged 2 years and older who consume at least three daily servings of vegetables, with at least one-third being dark green or orange vegetables.

Target: 50 percent.

Baseline: 3 percent of persons aged 2 years and older consumed at least three daily servings of vegetables, with at least one-third of these servings being dark green or orange vegetables in 1994–96 (age adjusted to the year 2000 standard population).

Target setting method: Better than the best.

Data source: Continuing Survey of Food Intakes by Individuals (CSFII) (2-day average), USDA.

NOTE: THE TABLE BELOW MAY CONTINUE TO THE FOLLOWING PAGE.

Persons Aged 2 Years and Older, 1994–96	Servings of Vegetables		
	19-6. Meet Both Recommen-dations	3 or More Daily Servings*	One-Third or More Servings From Dark Green or Orange Vegetables*
	Percent		
TOTAL	3	49	8
Race and ethnicity			
American Indian or Alaska Native	DSU	DSU	DSU
Asian or Pacific Islander	DSU	DSU	DSU
Asian	DNC	DNC	DNC
Native Hawaiian and other Pacific Islander	DNC	DNC	DNC
Black or African American	DNA	DNA	DNA
White	DNA	DNA	DNA
Hispanic or Latino	2	47	6
Mexican American	2	50	5
Other Hispanic	DSU	44	6
Not Hispanic or Latino	DNA	DNA	DNA
Black or African American	DNA	43	14
White	DNA	50	8

Persons Aged 2 Years and Older, 1994–96	Servings of Vegetables		
	19-6. Meet Both Recommendations	3 or More Daily Servings*	One-Third or More Servings From Dark Green or Orange Vegetables*
	Percent		
Gender and age			
Female			
2 years and older	4	41	10
2 to 5 years (not age adjusted)	DSU	23	9
6 to 11 years (not age adjusted)	DSU	24	7
12 to 19 years (not age adjusted)	2	38	7
20 to 39 years (not age adjusted)	4	43	10
40 to 59 years (not age adjusted)	4	49	11
60 years and older (not age adjusted)	6	43	13
Male			
2 years and older	3	57	7
2 to 5 years (not age adjusted)	DSU	23	8
6 to 11 years (not age adjusted)	DSU	27	6
12 to 19 years (not age adjusted)	DSU	55	4
20 to 39 years (not age adjusted)	3	68	4
40 to 59 years (not age adjusted)	4	64	9
60 years and older (not age adjusted)	6	57	11
Household income level[†]			
Lower income (≤130 percent of poverty threshold)	3	42	8
Higher income (>130 percent of poverty threshold)	4	50	8

Persons Aged 2 Years and Older, 1994–96	Servings of Vegetables		
	19-6. Meet Both Recommendations	3 or More Daily Servings*	One-Third or More Servings From Dark Green or Orange Vegetables*
	Percent		
Disability status			
Persons with disabilities	DNC	DNC	DNC
Persons without disabilities	DNC	DNC	DNC

DNA = Data have not been analyzed. DNC = Data are not collected. DSU = Data are statistically unreliable.
Note: Aged adjusted to the year 2000 standard population.
*Data for number and type of daily servings are displayed to further characterize the issue.
†A household income below 130 percent of poverty threshold is used by the Food Stamp Program.

NOTE: THE TABLE ABOVE MAY HAVE CONTINUED FROM THE PREVIOUS PAGE.

19-7. Increase the proportion of persons aged 2 years and older who consume at least six daily servings of grain products, with at least three being whole grains.

Target: 50 percent.

Baseline: 7 percent of persons aged 2 years and older consumed at least six daily servings of grain products, with at least three being whole grains in 1994–96 (age adjusted to the year 2000 standard population).

Target setting method: Better than the best.

Data source: Continuing Survey of Food Intakes by Individuals (CSFII) (2-day average), USDA.

Persons Aged 2 Years and Older, 1994–96	Servings of Grains		
	19-7. Meet Both Recommendations	6 or More Daily Servings*	3 or More Servings From Whole Grain*
	Percent		
TOTAL	7	51	7
Race and ethnicity			
American Indian or Alaska Native	DSU	DSU	DSU
Asian or Pacific Islander	DSU	DSU	DSU
Asian	DNC	DNC	DNC
Native Hawaiian and other Pacific Islander	DNC	DNC	DNC
Black or African American	DNA	DNA	DNA
White	DNA	DNA	DNA
Hispanic or Latino	4	46	4
Mexican American	3	46	4
Other Hispanic	4	46	4
Not Hispanic or Latino	DNA	DNA	DNA
Black or African American	3	40	4
White	7	54	8
Gender and age			
Female			
2 years and older	4	39	5
2 to 5 years (not age adjusted)	4	40	5
6 to 11 years (not age adjusted)	2	46	2
12 to 19 years (not age adjusted)	6	49	6
20 to 39 years (not age adjusted)	4	40	5
40 to 59 years (not age adjusted)	4	38	5
60 years and older (not age adjusted)	4	28	6

Persons Aged 2 Years and Older, 1994–96	Servings of Grains		
	19-7. Meet Both Recommendations	6 or More Daily Servings*	3 or More Servings From Whole Grain*
	Percent		
Male			
2 years and older	9	64	10
2 to 5 years (not age adjusted)	5	50	6
6 to 11 years (not age adjusted)	5	60	5
12 to 19 years (not age adjusted)	9	77	9
20 to 39 years (not age adjusted)	10	70	11
40 to 59 years (not age adjusted)	10	64	11
60 years and older (not age adjusted)	11	54	12
Household income level†			
Lower income (≤130 percent of poverty threshold)	4	44	5
Higher income (>130 percent of poverty threshold)	7	53	8
Disability status			
Persons with disabilities	DNC	DNC	DNC
Persons without disabilities	DNC	DNC	DNC

DNA = Data have not been analyzed. DNC = Data are not collected. DSU = Data are statistically unreliable.

Note: Age adjusted to the year 2000 standard population.

*Data for number and type of daily servings are displayed to further characterize the issue.

†A household income below 130 percent of poverty threshold is used by the Food Stamp Program.

NOTE: THE TABLE ABOVE MAY HAVE CONTINUED FROM THE PREVIOUS PAGE.

The *Dietary Guidelines for Americans* recommend that Americans choose a variety of grains daily, especially whole grains, and a variety of fruits and vegetables daily.[6] In the United States, persons of all ages eat fewer than the recommended number of servings of grain products, vegetables, and fruits.[28] Vegetables (including legumes, such as beans and peas), fruits, and grains are good sources of vitamins and minerals, carbohydrates (starch and dietary fiber), and other substances that are important for good health. Some evidence from clinical studies suggests that water-soluble fibers from foods such as oat bran, beans, and certain fruits are associated with lower blood glucose and blood lipid levels.[32] Dietary patterns with higher intakes of vegetables (including legumes), fruits, and grains are associated with a variety of health benefits, including a decreased risk for some types of cancer.[32, 33, 34, 35, 36, 37]

The *Dietary Guidelines for Americans* recommend three to five servings from various vegetables and vegetable juices and two to four servings from various fruits and fruit juices, depending on calorie needs. Consumers can select from a plentiful supply of fresh, frozen, dried, and canned products throughout the year to obtain five or more servings of fruits and vegetables daily. The *Dietary Guidelines for Americans* recommend that persons choose dark green leafy vegetables, orange vegetables and fruits, and dry beans and peas often. In 1994–96, the average daily intake of fruits and vegetables was five servings, but only about 7 to 10 percent of vegetable servings were dark green or deep yellow (orange), and only about 5 to 6 percent were legumes.[38] In contrast, fried potatoes accounted for about one-third (32 percent) of vegetable servings consumed by youth aged 2 to 19 years. Consumption of fruits and vegetables also is tracked at the State level and is discussed in *Tracking Healthy People 2010*.

The *Dietary Guidelines for Americans* recommend 6 to 11 daily servings of grain products, depending on calorie needs, with several of these from whole-grain foods. Although grain product consumption increased during the 1990s, consumption of whole-grain products remains very low. In 1994–96, for the population aged 2 years and older, the average daily intake of grain products was nearly seven servings, but only about 14 to 15 percent of grain servings were whole grain.[38] The guidelines also recommend that grain products be prepared with little added saturated fat and moderate or low amounts of added sugars; however, considerable amounts of fats and sugars are contributed to U.S. diets by baked products such as cookies, cakes, and doughnuts.[39, 40] No State-level data on grain intakes are available for adults, adolescents, and children.

19-8. Increase the proportion of persons aged 2 years and older who consume less than 10 percent of calories from saturated fat.

Target: 75 percent.

Baseline: 36 percent of persons aged 2 years and older consumed less than 10 percent of daily calories from saturated fat in 1994–96 (age adjusted to the year 2000 standard population).

Target setting method: Better than the best.

Data source: Continuing Survey of Food Intakes by Individuals (CSFII) (2-day average), USDA.

Persons Aged 2 Years and Older, 1994–96	Less than 10 Percent of Calories From Saturated Fat
	Percent
TOTAL	36
Race and ethnicity	
American Indian or Alaska Native	DSU
Asian or Pacific Islander	DSU
Asian	DNC
Native Hawaiian and other Pacific Islander	DNC
Black or African American	DNA
White	DNA
Hispanic or Latino	39
Mexican American	37
Other Hispanic	40
Not Hispanic or Latino	DNA
Black or African American	31
White	35
Gender and age	
Female	
2 years and older	39
2 to 5 years (not age adjusted)	23
6 to 11 years (not age adjusted)	23
12 to 19 years (not age adjusted)	34
20 to 39 years (not age adjusted)	41
40 to 59 years (not age adjusted)	42
60 years and older (not age adjusted)	47
Male	
2 years and older	32
2 to 5 years (not age adjusted)	23
6 to 11 years (not age adjusted)	25
12 to 19 years (not age adjusted)	27
20 to 39 years (not age adjusted)	32
40 to 59 years (not age adjusted)	33
60 years and older (not age adjusted)	42

Persons Aged 2 Years and Older, 1994–96	Less than 10 Percent of Calories From Saturated Fat
	Percent
Household income level*	
Lower income (≤130 percent of poverty threshold)	33
Higher income (>130 percent of poverty threshold)	36
Disability status	
Persons with disabilities	DNC
Persons without disabilities	DNC

DNA = Data have not been analyzed. DNC = Data are not collected. DSU = Data are statistically unreliable.
Note: Age adjusted to the year 2000 standard population.
*A household income below 130 percent of poverty threshold is used by the Food Stamp Program.

NOTE: THE TABLE ABOVE MAY HAVE CONTINUED FROM THE PREVIOUS PAGE.

19-9. Increase the proportion of persons aged 2 years and older who consume no more than 30 percent of calories from total fat.

Target: 75 percent.

Baseline: 33 percent of persons aged 2 years and older consumed no more than 30 percent of daily calories from total fat in 1994–96 (age adjusted to the year 2000 standard population).

Target setting method: Better than the best.

Data source: Continuing Survey of Food Intakes by Individuals (CSFII) (2-day average), USDA.

NOTE: THE TABLE BELOW MAY CONTINUE TO THE FOLLOWING PAGE.

Persons Aged 2 Years and Older, 1994–96	No More Than 30 Percent of Calories From Total Fat
	Percent
TOTAL	33
Race and ethnicity	
American Indian or Alaska Native	DSU
Asian or Pacific Islander	DSU
Asian	DNC
Native Hawaiian and other Pacific Islander	DNC

Persons Aged 2 Years and Older, 1994–96	No More Than 30 Percent of Calories From Total Fat
	Percent
Black or African American	DNA
White	DNA
Hispanic or Latino	36
Mexican American	33
Other Hispanic	38
Not Hispanic or Latino	DNA
Black or African American	26
White	33
Gender and age	
Female	
2 years and older	36
2 to 5 years (not age adjusted)	35
6 to 11 years (not age adjusted)	34
12 to 19 years (not age adjusted)	36
20 to 39 years (not age adjusted)	38
40 to 59 years (not age adjusted)	33
60 years and older (not age adjusted)	40
Male	
2 years and older	30
2 to 5 years (not age adjusted)	33
6 to 11 years (not age adjusted)	30
12 to 19 years (not age adjusted)	30
20 to 39 years (not age adjusted)	29
40 to 59 years (not age adjusted)	28
60 years and older (not age adjusted)	34
Household income level*	
Lower income ($\leq$130 percent of poverty threshold)	30
Higher income (>130 percent of poverty threshold)	34

Persons Aged 2 Years and Older, 1994–96	No More Than 30 Percent of Calories From Total Fat
	Percent
Disability status	
Persons with disabilities	DNC
Persons without disabilities	DNC

DNA = Data have not been analyzed. DNC = Data are not collected. DSU = Data are statistically unreliable.
Note: Age adjusted to the year 2000 standard population.
*A household income below 130 percent of poverty threshold is used by the Food Stamp Program.

NOTE: THE TABLE ABOVE MAY HAVE CONTINUED FROM THE PREVIOUS PAGE.

Both the *Dietary Guidelines for Americans* and the National Cholesterol Education and Prevention Program recommend a diet that contains less than 10 percent of calories from saturated fat and no more than 30 percent of calories from total fat.[6, 33, 41] This can be achieved by obtaining most calories from plant foods (grains, fruits, vegetables) that have little added fat. Such a healthful diet also can include low-fat and lean foods from the milk group and the meat group. The increase of overweight and obesity in the United States indicates that more attention needs to be paid to serving size and total calorie content because a low-fat content does not, automatically, signify a lower calorie content.

The role of fat in the diet is complicated because different types of fatty acids have different effects on health. Evidence to date is complicated, but certain messages appear clear: persons in the United States consume too much dietary fat in general, and too much of the fat consumed is from saturated fatty acids—the type associated with an increased risk for heart disease. (See Focus Area 12. Heart Disease and Stroke.)

Strong evidence from human and animal studies shows that diets low in saturated fatty acids and cholesterol are associated with low risks and rates of coronary heart disease. Saturated fatty acids are the major dietary factors that raise blood low-density lipoprotein (LDL) cholesterol levels, increasing the risk for heart disease. Increasing evidence suggests that *trans*-fatty acids also can increase LDL-cholesterol levels.[42] Monounsaturated and polyunsaturated fatty acids do not raise blood cholesterol. Omega-3 polyunsaturated fatty acids, which are found in some fish such as salmon, tuna, and mackerel, are being studied to determine whether they offer protection against heart disease.[6]

A 1989 National Research Council report[33] indicated that diets high in total fat were associated with a higher risk of several cancers, especially cancer of the colon, prostate, and breast, but noted that findings were inconsistent. (See Focus Area 3. Cancer.) A 1996 review of the evidence showed that the relationship between the amount and type of fat and the risk of cancer continues to be uncertain.[43] To help clarify the relationship between total dietary fat and the risk of cancer, a randomized clinical trial called the Women's Health Initiative has been started. Set to conclude in 2003, it is a multicenter trial designed to test several risk factors for chronic disease in U.S. females.[44] A major emphasis is to reduce fat to 25 percent of dietary calories to determine whether a low-fat diet has any effect on breast cancer risk.

The proportion of calories in the U.S. diet provided by total fat is about 33 percent, saturated fat is about 11 percent, and *trans*-fat is about 2.6 percent.[45] The primary sources of saturated fat are meats and dairy products that contain fat. Thus, nonfat and low-fat dairy products and lean meats are choices that can help reduce saturated fat intake. *Trans*-fatty acids are formed when vegetable oil is hydrogenated to solidify the oils and increase the shelf life and flavor stability of the fats and the foods that contain them. Margarines that have been formulated to contain no *trans*-fats are available in most U.S. grocery stores. Other dietary sources of *trans*-fat are restaurant and fast-food fats (including frying fats), baked products, and some snack foods, such as chips.

The major vegetable sources of monounsaturated fatty acids include nuts, avocados, olive oil, canola oil, and high-oleic forms of safflower and sunflower seed oil. The major sources of polyunsaturated fatty acids are vegetable oils, including soybean oil, corn oil, and high-linoleic forms of safflower and sunflower seed oil and a few nuts, such as walnuts. Substituting monounsaturated and polyunsaturated fatty acids for saturated fatty acids can help lower health risks.

The proportion of all meals and snacks from away-from-home sources increased by more than two-thirds between 1977–78 and 1995, from 16 percent of all meals and snacks in 1977–78 to 27 percent of all meals and snacks in 1995.[27] Away-from-home food tends to have a higher saturated fat content, and persons tend to consume more calories when eating away from home than at home.[27] In 1995, the average total fat and saturated fat content of away-from-home foods, expressed as a percentage of calories, was 38 percent and 13 percent, respectively, compared with 32 percent and 11 percent for at-home foods.[27] Meals and snacks eaten by children at school had the highest saturated fat density of all food outlets. Thus, to help assess fat and saturated fat intake, as well as develop strategies to help children reduce the amount of fat they consume, additional tracking of saturated fat and total fat intake from foods eaten away from home as well as at home is important.

19-10. Increase the proportion of persons aged 2 years and older who consume 2,400 mg or less of sodium daily.

Target: 65 percent.

Baseline: 21 percent of persons aged 2 years and older consumed 2,400 mg or less of sodium daily (from foods, dietary supplements, tap water, and salt use at the table) in 1988–94 (age adjusted to the year 2000 standard population).

Target setting method: Better than the best.

Data source: National Health and Nutrition Examination Survey (NHANES), CDC, NCHS.

NOTE: THE TABLE BELOW MAY CONTINUE TO THE FOLLOWING PAGE.

Persons Aged 2 Years and Older, 1988–94 (unless noted)	Consume 2,400 mg of Sodium or Less
	Percent
TOTAL	21
Race and ethnicity	
American Indian or Alaska Native	DSU
Asian or Pacific Islander	DSU
Asian	DNC
Native Hawaiian and other Pacific Islander	DNC
Black or African American	25
White	20
Hispanic or Latino	DSU
Mexican American	25
Not Hispanic or Latino	21
Black or African American	25
White	20
Gender and age	
Female	
2 years and older	32
2 to 5 years (not age adjusted)	64
6 to 11 years (not age adjusted)	26
12 to 19 years (not age adjusted)	29
20 years and older	30
Male	
2 years and older	9
2 to 5 years (not age adjusted)	50
6 to 11 years (not age adjusted)	16
12 to 19 years (not age adjusted)	4
20 years and older	6
Family income level*	
Lower income (≤130 percent of poverty threshold)	25
Higher income (>130 percent of poverty threshold)	20

Persons Aged 2 Years and Older, 1988–94 (unless noted)	Consume 2,400 mg of Sodium or Less
	Percent
Disability status (aged 20 years and older)	
Persons with disabilities	18 (1991–94)
Persons without disabilities	16 (1991–94)
Select populations	
Females with high blood pressure	32
Females without high blood pressure	29
Males with high blood pressure	7
Males without high blood pressure	5

DNA = Data have not been analyzed. DNC = Data are not collected. DSU = Data are statistically unreliable.

Note: Age adjusted to the year 2000 standard population.

*A household income below 130 percent of poverty threshold is used by the Food Stamp Program.

NOTE: THE TABLE ABOVE MAY HAVE CONTINUED FROM THE PREVIOUS PAGE.

The *Dietary Guidelines for Americans* recommend choosing and preparing foods with less salt (salt consists of both sodium and chloride). Most studies in diverse populations have shown that salt intake is linked to increasing levels of blood pressure.[6, 46, 47, 48] (See Focus Area 12. Heart Disease and Stroke.) Persons who consume less salt or sodium have a lower risk of developing high blood pressure.[6] Data also show that high sodium intake may increase the amount of calcium excreted in the urine and therefore increase the body's need for calcium.[49] Eating less salt may decrease the loss of calcium from bone.[6]

Most persons in the United States consume more sodium than is needed, and reduction of sodium or salt or both to no more than 2,400 mg sodium or 6 g salt per day is recommended by some authorities.[33, 46] Data from the Continuing Survey of Food Intakes by Individuals show that, even without including salt added at the table, both home foods and away-from-home foods provide excessive amounts of sodium.[27] Higher sodium intakes also tend to be associated with higher calorie intakes; for example, males, who consume more calories than females, also consume more sodium.[27]

Sodium occurs naturally in foods. However, most dietary salt or sodium is added to foods during processing or preparation, with smaller amounts added at the discretion of the consumer in the form of table salt or use of condiments such as soy sauce.[50, 51] Thus, both the sodium content of foods and estimates of the amount of salt added have been used to assess dietary sodium consumption. Other contributing sources of sodium are water, dietary supplements, and medications such as antacids.

19-11. Increase the proportion of persons aged 2 years and older who meet dietary recommendations for calcium.

Target: 75 percent.

Baseline: 46 percent of persons aged 2 years and older were at or above approximated mean calcium requirements (based on consideration of calcium from foods, dietary supplements, and antacids) in 1988–94 (age adjusted to the year 2000 standard population).

Target setting method: Better than the best.

Data source: National Health and Nutrition Examination Survey (NHANES), CDC, NCHS.

NOTE: THE TABLE BELOW MAY CONTINUE TO THE FOLLOWING PAGE.

Persons Aged 2 Years and Older, 1988–94 (unless noted)	Met Calcium Recommendations
	Percent
TOTAL	46
Race and ethnicity	
American Indian or Alaska Native	DSU
Asian or Pacific Islander	DSU
Asian	DNC
Native Hawaiian and other Pacific Islander	DNC
Black or African American	30
White	49
Hispanic or Latino	DSU
Mexican American	44
Not Hispanic or Latino	46
Black or African American	30
White	50
Gender and age	
Female	
2 years and older	36
2 to 8 years (not age adjusted)	79
9 to 19 years (not age adjusted)	19
20 to 49 years (not age adjusted)	40
50 years and older (not age adjusted)	27
Male	
2 years and older	56
2 to 8 years (not age adjusted)	89

Persons Aged 2 Years and Older, 1988–94 (unless noted)	Met Calcium Recommendations
	Percent
9 to 19 years (not age adjusted)	52
20 to 49 years (not age adjusted)	64
50 years and older (not age adjusted)	35
Family income level*	
Lower income (≤130 percent of poverty threshold)	39
Higher income (>130 percent of poverty threshold)	48
Disability status (aged 20 years and older)	
Persons with disabilities	44 (1991–94)
Persons without disabilities	44 (1991–94)

DNA = Data have not been analyzed. DNC = Data are not collected. DSU = Data are statistically unreliable.
Note: Age adjusted to the year 2000 standard population.
*A household income below 130 percent of poverty threshold is used by the Food Stamp Program.

NOTE: THE TABLE ABOVE MAY HAVE CONTINUED FROM THE PREVIOUS PAGE.

Calcium is essential for the formation and maintenance of bones and teeth.[32] The recommendations for adequate daily intakes of calcium are 500 mg for children aged 1 to 3 years, 800 mg for children aged 4 to 8 years, 1,300 mg for adolescents aged 9 to 18 years, 1,000 mg for adults aged 19 to 50 years, and 1,200 mg for adults aged 51 years and older.[52] Approximated mean calcium requirements are defined as 77 percent of the recommendations by the Institute of Medicine for adequate intakes of calcium.[52, 53] The bone mass achieved at full growth (peak bone mass) appears to be related to intake of calcium during childhood and adolescence.[33] Opinion is divided as to the age at which peak bone mass is achieved, although most of the accumulation of bone mineral occurs in humans by about age 20 years. After persons reach their adult height, a period of consolidation of bone density continues until approximately age 30 to 35 years. A high peak bone mass is thought to be protective against fractures in later life.

Osteoporosis is a complex disorder caused by many contributing factors. (See Focus Area 2. Arthritis, Osteoporosis, and Chronic Back Conditions.) Regular exercise and a diet with enough calcium help maintain good bone health and reduce the risk of osteoporosis later in life. However, the ideal level of calcium intake for development of peak bone mass is unknown. For the most part, young children appear to meet the approximate calcium requirements. In contrast, the majority of adolescent and adult females do not meet the average requirements. This is in part because of their lower food consumption, as well as the lower consumption of milk products relative to soft drinks in U.S. diets.[54] For example, in the period 1994–96, the amount of soft drinks consumed was about twice that consumed in the late 1970s and surpassed consumption of fluid milk. Thus, an increase in consumption of various sources of calcium is recommended for nearly all groups and especially for teenaged girls and women. In postmenopausal females—the group at highest risk for osteoporosis—estrogen replacement therapy under medical supervision is the most effective means to reduce the rate of bone loss and risk of fractures.[32]

The relationship between dietary calcium and blood pressure is uncertain. Results from studies that have used calcium supplements show a small reduction in systolic blood pressure in hypertensive individuals, with no significant reduction in diastolic blood pressure.[55] Among persons with normal blood pressure, there is no significant difference in blood pressure with calcium supplements.[56]

Dietary sources of calcium include milk and milk products such as cheese and yogurt, canned fish with soft bones such as sardines, dark green leafy vegetables such as kale and mustard or turnip greens, tofu made with calcium, tortillas made from lime-processed corn, calcium-enriched grain products, and other calcium-fortified foods and beverages.[6] In some locations, water is a source of calcium, but in amounts that cannot readily be determined. With current food selection practices, use of dairy products may constitute the difference between getting enough calcium in one's diet or not. Nonfat and low-fat dairy products are choices that help reduce the intake of saturated fat while still providing calcium, vitamin D, and other nutrients important for bone health. For those who have lactose intolerance, a range of lactose-reduced dairy products can provide calcium. Persons who do not (or cannot) consume and absorb adequate levels of calcium from dairy food sources may consider use of calcium-fortified foods, while persons with clinical evidence of inadequate intake should receive professional advice on the proper type and dosage of calcium supplements. Calcium supplements come in different forms, including calcium-containing antacids.

Fluid milk (but not yogurt or cheese) is an excellent source of vitamin D, which is essential for calcium utilization. Vitamin D also is synthesized in the skin upon exposure to sunlight.

19-12. Reduce iron deficiency among young children and females of childbearing age.

Target and Baseline:

Objective	Reduction in Iron Deficiency*	1988–94 Baseline	2010 Target
		Percent	
19-12a.	Children aged 1 to 2 years	9	5
19-12b.	Children aged 3 to 4 years	4	1
19-12c.	Nonpregnant females aged 12 to 49 years	11	7

*Iron deficiency is defined as having abnormal results for two or more of the following tests: serum ferritin concentration, erythrocyte protoporphyrin, or transferrin saturation. Refer to *Tracking Healthy People 2010* for threshold values.

Target setting method: Better than the best.

Data source: National Health and Nutrition Examination Survey (NHANES), CDC, NCHS.

NOTE: THE TABLE BELOW MAY CONTINUE TO THE FOLLOWING PAGE.

Select Populations, 1988–94 (unless noted)	Iron Deficiency		
	19-12a. Aged 1 to 2 Years	19-12b. Aged 3 to 4 Years	19-12c. Females of Childbearing Age
	Percent		
TOTAL	9	4	11
Race and ethnicity			
American Indian or Alaska Native	DSU	DSU	DSU
Asian or Pacific Islander	DSU	DSU	DSU
Asian	DNC	DNC	DNC
Native Hawaiian and other Pacific Islander	DNC	DNC	DNC
Black or African American	10	2	15
White	8	3	10
Hispanic or Latino	DSU	DSU	DSU
Mexican American	17	6	19

Low-Income Pregnant Females, Third Trimester, 1996	Anemia
	Percent
Hispanic or Latino	25
Not Hispanic or Latino	DNA
Black or African American	44
White	24
Disability status	
Females with disabilities	DNC
Females without disabilities	DNC

DNA = Data have not been analyzed. DNC = Data are not collected. DSU = Data are statistically unreliable.
NOTE: THE TABLE ABOVE MAY HAVE CONTINUED FROM THE PREVIOUS PAGE.

19-14. (Developmental) Reduce iron deficiency among pregnant females.

Potential data source: National Health and Nutrition Examination Survey (NHANES), CDC, NCHS.

The terms anemia, iron deficiency, and iron deficiency anemia often are used interchangeably but are not equivalent. Iron deficiency ranges from depleted iron stores without functional or health impairment to iron deficiency with anemia, which affects the functioning of several organ systems. Iron deficiency anemia is more likely than iron deficiency without anemia to cause preterm births, low birth weight, and delays in infant and child development.[57, 58, 59] Iron deficiency (with and without anemia) in adolescent females has been associated with decreased verbal learning and memory.[60] The prevalence of iron deficiency anemia among children aged 1 to 2 years and 3 to 4 years and females aged 12 to 49 years in 1988 to 1994 was 3 percent, less than 1 percent, and 4 percent, respectively.

Anemia can be caused by many factors other than iron deficiency, including other nutrient deficiencies, infection, inflammation, and hereditary anemias. Anemia is used for monitoring risk of iron deficiency at the State and local levels because of the low cost and feasibility of measuring hemoglobin or hematocrit in the clinic setting.[61] Anemia is a good predictor of iron deficiency when the prevalence of iron deficiency is high, such as during the third trimester of pregnancy. It is not a good predictor of iron deficiency when the prevalence of iron deficiency is expected to be low, such as among white, non-Hispanic children aged 3 to 4 years in the United States. In that case, the majority of anemia is due to other causes.[8] However, changes in the prevalence of anemia over time at State and local levels can be used to evaluate the effectiveness of programs to decrease the prevalence of iron deficiency.

Iron deficiency and anemia among young children declined during the 1970s in association with increased iron intake.[8] Although the prevalence of iron deficiency

Select Populations, 1988–94 (unless noted)	Iron Deficiency		
	19-12a. Aged 1 to 2 Years	19-12b. Aged 3 to 4 Years	19-12c. Females of Childbearing Age
	Percent		
Not Hispanic or Latino	DNA	DNA	DNA
Black or African American	10	2	15
White	6	1	8
Family income level*			
Lower income (≤130 percent of poverty threshold)	12	5	16
Higher income (>130 percent of poverty threshold)	7	3	9
Disability status (aged 20 to 49 years)			
Persons with disabilities	DNC	DNC	4 (1991–94)
Persons without disabilities	DNC	DNC	12 (1991–94)

DNA = Data have not been analyzed. DNC = Data are not collected. DSU = Data are statistically unreliable.
*A household income below 130 percent of poverty threshold is used by the Food Stamp Program.

NOTE: THE TABLE ABOVE MAY HAVE CONTINUED FROM THE PREVIOUS PAGE.

19-13. Reduce anemia among low-income pregnant females in their third trimester.

Target: 20 percent.

Baseline: 29 percent of low-income pregnant females in their third trimester wei anemic (defined as hemoglobin <11.0 g/dL) in 1996.

Target setting method: Better than the best.

Data source: Pregnancy Nutrition Surveillance System, CDC, NCCDPHP.

NOTE: THE TABLE BELOW MAY CONTINUE TO THE FOLLOWING PAGE.

Low-Income Pregnant Females, Third Trimester, 1996	Anemia
	Percent
TOTAL	29
Race and ethnicity	
American Indian or Alaska Native	31
Asian or Pacific Islander	26
Asian	DNC
Native Hawaiian and other Pacific Islander	DNC
Black or African American	DNC
White	DNC

among low-income children continued to decline from 1976–80 to 1988–94, the prevalence of iron deficiency among all young children remained the same, and the prevalence of iron deficiency among females of childbearing age actually increased.[9] From 1979 to 1996, the prevalence of third trimester anemia among low-income pregnant females did not change.[62, 63]

Iron deficiency is highest among toddlers and among certain racial, ethnic, and low-income children.[64] Iron deficiency can be prevented among young children by teaching families about child nutrition, including promoting breastfeeding of infants, with exclusive breastfeeding for 4 to 6 months; the use of iron-fortified formulas when formulas are used; delayed introduction of cow's milk until age 12 months; and age-appropriate introduction of iron-rich solid foods, such as iron-fortified infant cereals and pureed meats, and foods that enhance iron absorption such as vitamin C-rich fruits, vegetables, or juices.[61]

Nonpregnant females of childbearing age are at increased risk for iron deficiency because of iron loss during menstruation coupled with inadequate intake of iron.[61] Pregnant females are also at increased risk because of the increased iron requirements of pregnancy.[61, 63] Consequently, a Healthy People 2010 objective has been established to reduce the prevalence of anemia among low-income pregnant females in their third trimester. Although groups other than low-income females are considered at risk for iron deficiency during pregnancy, no nationally representative data exist on the prevalence of iron deficiency or iron deficiency anemia among pregnant females.

National data indicate that only one-fourth of all females of childbearing age (12 to 49 years) meet the U.S. recommended dietary allowance for iron (15 mg) through their diets.[65] Iron deficiency among females of childbearing age may be prevented by periodic anemia screening and appropriate treatment and by counseling them about better eating practices, such as selecting iron-rich foods, taking iron supplements during pregnancy, increasing consumption of foods that enhance iron absorption (for example, orange juice and other citrus products), and discouraging consumption of iron inhibitors (for example, coffee and tea) with iron-rich foods.[61] Some good sources of iron include ready-to-eat cereals with added iron; enriched and whole grain breads; lean meats; turkey dark meat; shellfish; spinach; and cooked dry beans, peas, and lentils.

19-15. (Developmental) Increase the proportion of children and adolescents aged 6 to 19 years whose intake of meals and snacks at school contributes to good overall dietary quality.

Potential data sources: Continuing Survey of Food Intakes by Individuals (CSFII), USDA; National Food and Nutrition Survey, USDA and CDC; National Health and Nutrition Examination Survey (NHANES), CDC, NCHS.

Students today have increased food options at school. Although students may understand that good nutrition and good health are connected, that understanding may not be reflected in their food choices and meal patterns. The U.S. Department of Agriculture (USDA) has established standards requiring schools to plan menus that meet the 1995 *Dietary Guidelines for Americans*, but these standards do not apply to à la carte foods; to foods sold in snack bars, school stores, and vending machines; or to foods students bring from home. Students' food choices are influenced by the total eating environment created by schools. This includes the types of foods available throughout the school, point-of-choice nutrition information in the cafeteria and around the school, nutrition education provided in the classroom, and nutrition promotions that reach families and affect the choices of foods brought to school.

Improving the quality of students' dietary intake in the school setting is important because, for many children, meals and snacks consumed at school make a major contribution to their total daily consumption of food and nutrients. National food consumption data collected in 1994 and 1995 show that school foods had the highest saturated fat density of all food outlets.[27] School foods also had higher than recommended levels of sodium—as did other away-from-home foods and at-home foods. Nonetheless, these analyses also showed positive aspects of foods obtained from school. School foods had the highest calcium density of all sources and the highest dietary fiber density of all away-from-home sources. The establishment of an environment that supports a good overall diet would enable school nutrition and food services, in conjunction with students, their families, and other school employees, to make an important contribution to short- and long-term disease prevention and health promotion. In addition, such an environment would foster learning readiness (for example, by encouraging students to consume substantial breakfasts).[66, 67, 68]

19-16. Increase the proportion of worksites that offer nutrition or weight management classes or counseling.

Target: 85 percent.

Baseline: 55 percent of worksites with 50 or more employees offered nutrition or weight management classes or counseling at the worksite or through their health plans in 1998–99.

Target setting method: 55 percent improvement.

Data source: National Worksite Health Promotion Survey, Association for Worksite Health Promotion (AWHP).

Worksites, 1998–99	Offer Nutrition or Weight Management Classes or Counseling		
Worksite Size	Worksite or Health Plan	Worksite	Health Plan
	Percent		
Total (50 or more employees)	55	28	39
50 to 99 employees	48	21	39
100 to 249 employees	51	29	37
250 to 749 employees	59	44	42
750 or more employees	83	70	50

Worksite programs can reach large numbers of employees with information, activities, and services that encourage the adoption of healthy dietary and physical activity behaviors.[69] (See Focus Area 7. Educational and Community-Based Programs and Focus Area 22. Physical Activity and Fitness.) Employer-sponsored programs can be offered onsite or in partnership with community organizations. Examples of such programs include weight management classes, physical activity programs, lunchtime seminars, self-help programs, cooking demonstrations and classes, healthy food service and vending machine selections, point-of-purchase nutrition information, and flexible health benefits that include nutrition-related services.

A recent study of worksite health promotion programs found that specific interventions at the worksite resulted in employees choosing to reduce the amount of fat calories they consumed and eating more fruits, vegetables, and dietary fiber.[70] Worksite health promotion programs may reduce health care costs, including employer costs for insurance programs, disability benefits, and medical expenses.[71, 72]

If possible, nutrition education and weight management programs at the worksite should be part of a comprehensive health promotion program. In addition, employers could reimburse health promotion activities and provide company time for employees to participate in the programs.[73]

Worksite programs should be made available to the family members of employees and company retirees as well as current employees. Also, these programs should be offered in a culturally and linguistically competent manner and any educational materials provided should be culturally and linguistically appropriate.

19-17. Increase the proportion of physician office visits made by patients with a diagnosis of cardiovascular disease, diabetes, or hyperlipidemia that include counseling or education related to diet and nutrition.

Target: 75 percent.

Baseline: 42 percent of physician office visits made by patients with a diagnosis of cardiovascular disease, diabetes, or hyperlipidemia included ordering or providing counseling or education on diet and nutrition in 1997 (age adjusted to the year 2000 standard population).

Target setting method: Better than the best.

Data source: National Ambulatory Medical Care Survey (NAMCS), CDC, NCHS.

NOTE: THE TABLE BELOW MAY CONTINUE TO THE FOLLOWING PAGE.

Persons With Specific Conditions, 1997	Physician Office Visits That Include Ordering or Providing Diet and Nutrition Counseling or Education			
	19-17. Any of the Three Conditions	Hyper-lipide-mia*	Cardio-vascular Dis-ease*	Diabe-tes*
	Percent			
TOTAL	42	65	36	48
Race and ethnicity				
American Indian or Alaska Native	DSU	DSU	DSU	DSU
Asian or Pacific Islander	DSU	DSU	DSU	DSU
Asian	DNC	DNC	DNC	DNC
Native Hawaiian and other Pacific Islander	DNC	DNC	DNC	DNC
Black or African American	46	DSU	40	54
White	41	64	35	47
Hispanic or Latino	DSU	DSU	DSU	DSU
Not Hispanic or Latino	DSU	DSU	DSU	DSU
Black or African American	DSU	DSU	DSU	DSU
White	DSU	DSU	DSU	DSU

Persons With Specific Conditions, 1997	Physician Office Visits That Include Ordering or Providing Diet and Nutrition Counseling or Education			
	19-17. Any of the Three Conditions	Hyper-lipide-mia*	Cardio-vascular Dis-ease*	Diabe-tes*
	Percent			
Gender				
Female	39	55	34	46
Male	44	73	38	49
Age				
20 to 44 years	45	75	37	49
45 to 64 years	41	62	36	47
65 years and older	33	44	32	45
Family income level†				
Lower income (≤130 percent of poverty threshold)	DNC	DNC	DNC	DNC
Higher income (>130 percent of poverty threshold)	DNC	DNC	DNC	DNC
Disability status				
Persons with disabilities	DNC	DNC	DNC	DNC
Persons without disabilities	DNC	DNC	DNC	DNC

DNA = Data have not been analyzed. DNC = Data are not collected. DSU = Data are statistically unreliable.
Note: Age adjusted to the year 2000 standard population.
*Data for separate conditions are displayed to further characterize the issue.
†A household income below 130 percent of poverty threshold is used by the Food Stamp Program.

NOTE: THE TABLE ABOVE MAY HAVE CONTINUED FROM THE PREVIOUS PAGE.

Primary care providers are well positioned in the health care system to provide preventive services, including nutrition screening and assessment, referral, and counseling. For example, they can screen for age-specific and diagnosis-related nutrition risk factors as a part of routine patient contact. The public views physicians—and registered dietitians in particular—as credible sources of nutrition information.[74] Dietary assessment, counseling, and followup by physicians and qualified nutrition professionals are effective in reducing patient dietary fat intake and serum cholesterol.[75, 76, 77, 78] For many physicians, referring patients to qualified nutrition professionals for nutrition assessment, education, counseling on behavioral change, diet modification, and specialized nutrition therapies represents appropriate clinical practice.

Nutrition counseling by registered dietitians and other qualified nutrition professionals has been found to be cost effective for patients with hyperlipidemia[79, 80] and type 2 diabetes mellitus.[81] Nutrition services also are a critical component of improved health outcomes for many other diseases and conditions, including obesity, gastrointestinal and hepatic disease, renal disease, cancer, HIV/AIDS, pressure ulcers, burns and trauma, eating disorders, and prenatal care. A 1997 study that evaluated the cost of covering medical nutrition therapy under Medicare part B projected savings to the program of $11 million in 2001 and $65 million in 2004.[82, 83] (See Focus Area 3. Cancer, Focus Area 4. Chronic Kidney Disease, Focus Area 13. HIV, and Focus Area 16. Maternal, Infant, and Child Health.)

Food Security

19-18. Increase food security among U.S. households and in so doing reduce hunger.

Target: 94 percent.

Baseline: 88 percent of all U.S. households were food secure in 1995.

Target setting method: 6 percentage point improvement (50 percent decrease in food insecurity; consistent with the U.S. pledge to the 1996 World Food Summit).

Data sources: Food Security Supplement to the Current Population Survey, U.S. Department of Commerce, Bureau of the Census; National Food and Nutrition Survey (beginning in 2001), HHS and USDA.

NOTE: THE TABLE BELOW MAY CONTINUE TO THE FOLLOWING PAGE.

U.S. Households, 1995	Food Secure
	Percent
TOTAL	88
Race and ethnicity	
American Indian or Alaska Native	78
Asian or Pacific Islander	91
Asian	DSU
Native Hawaiian and other Pacific Islander	DSU
Black or African American	76
White	90
Hispanic or Latino	75
Mexican American	73

U.S. Households, 1995	Food Secure
	Percent
Not Hispanic or Latino	89
Black or African American	76
White	91
Lower income level (≤130 percent of poverty threshold)*	
All	69
With children (under age 18 years)	59
With elderly persons (aged 65 years and over)	85
Higher income level (>130 percent of poverty threshold)*	
All	94
With children (under age 18 years)	91
With elderly persons (aged 65 years and over)	98
Disability status	
Persons with disabilities	DNC
Persons without disabilities	DNC
Select populations	
Household characteristics	
With children	83
With elderly persons	94

DNA = Data have not been analyzed. DNC = Data are not collected. DSU = Data are statistically unreliable.
*A household income below 130 percent poverty threshold is used by the Food Stamp Program.

NOTE: THE TABLE ABOVE MAY HAVE CONTINUED FROM THE PREVIOUS PAGE.

Food security means that people have access at all times to enough food for an active, healthy life. It implies that people have nutritionally adequate and safe foods and sufficient household resources to ensure their ability to acquire adequate, acceptable foods in socially acceptable ways—that is, through regular marketplace sources and not through severe coping strategies like emergency food sources, scavenging, and stealing. Hunger in this context refers to the uneasy or painful sensation caused by a lack of food.

While the vast majority of persons in the United States are food secure and have not experienced resource-constrained hunger, both food insecurity and hunger have remained a painful fact of life for too many people.[84, 85] The specific concern is with food insecurity and hunger resulting from inadequate household resources. Other sources of food insecurity (such as illness, child abuse and neglect, or loss of function or mobility) are not included in this definition. Food insecurity and hunger may coexist with malnutrition, but they are not the same thing or even necessarily closely associated. Food insecurity and hunger, however, are believed to have harmful health and behavioral impacts in their own right.[86] These are of particular concern for pregnant women, children, elderly persons, and other nutritionally vulnerable groups.[87]

The United States is committed to increasing food security by working with local leaders as outlined in the U.S. Action Plan on Food Security, through USDA's Community Food Security Initiative, and the Maternal and Child Health Bureau's Healthy Start.[88, 89]

Related Objectives From Other Focus Areas

1. **Access to Quality Health Services**
   1-3. Counseling about health behaviors
2. **Arthritis, Osteoporosis, and Chronic Back Conditions**
   2-9. Cases of osteoporosis
3. **Cancer**
   3-1. Overall cancer deaths
   3-3. Breast cancer deaths
   3-5. Colorectal cancer deaths
   3-10. Provider counseling about cancer prevention
4. **Chronic Kidney Disease**
   4-3. Counseling for chronic kidney failure care
5. **Diabetes**
   5-1. Diabetes education
   5-2. New cases of diabetes
   5-6. Diabetes-related deaths
7. **Educational and Community-Based Programs**
   7-2. School health education
   7-5. Worksite health promotion programs
   7-6. Participation in employer-sponsored health promotion activities
   7-10. Community health promotion programs
   7-11. Culturally appropriate and linguistically competent community health promotion programs
10. **Food Safety**
    10-4. Food allergy deaths
    10-5. Consumer food safety practices
11. **Health Communication**
    11-4. Quality of Internet health information sources
12. **Heart Disease and Stroke**
    12-1. Coronary heart disease (CHD) deaths
    12-7. Stroke deaths
    12-9. High blood pressure
    12-11. Action to help control blood pressure
    12-13. Mean total blood cholesterol levels
    12-14. High blood cholesterol levels
16. **Maternal, Infant, and Child Health**
    16-10. Low birth weight and very low birth weight
    16-12. Weight gain during pregnancy

Terminology

(A listing of abbreviations and acronyms used in this publication appears in Appendix H.)

Anemia: A condition in which the hemoglobin in red blood cells falls below normal. Anemia most often results from iron deficiency but also may result from deficiencies of folic acid, vitamin B12, or copper, or from chronic disease, certain conditions, or chronic blood loss.

Body mass index (BMI): Weight (in kilograms) divided by the square of height (in meters), or weight (in pounds) divided by the square of height (in inches) times 704.5. Because it is readily calculated, BMI is the measurement of choice as an indicator of healthy weight, overweight, and obesity.

Calorie: Unit used for measuring the energy produced by food when metabolized in the body.

Cholesterol: A waxy substance that circulates in the bloodstream. When the level of cholesterol in the blood is too high, some of the cholesterol is deposited in the walls of the blood vessels. Over time, these deposits can build up until they narrow the blood vessels, causing atherosclerosis, which reduces the blood flow. The higher the blood cholesterol level, the greater is the risk of getting heart disease. Blood cholesterol levels of less than 200 mg/dL are considered desirable. Levels of 240 mg/dL or above are considered high and require further testing and possible intervention. Levels of 200-239 mg/dL are considered borderline. Lowering blood cholesterol reduces the risk of heart disease.

HDL (high-density lipoprotein) cholesterol: The so-called good cholesterol. Cholesterol travels in the blood combined with protein in packages called lipoproteins. HDL is thought to carry cholesterol away from other parts of the body back to the liver for removal from the body. A low level of HDL increases the risk for CHD, whereas a high HDL level is protective.

LDL (low-density lipoprotein) cholesterol: The so-called bad cholesterol. LDL contains most of the cholesterol in the blood and carries it to the tissues and organs of the body, including the arteries. Cholesterol from LDL is the main source of damaging buildup and blockage in the arteries. The higher the level of LDL in the blood, the greater is the risk for CHD.

Complex carbohydrate: Starch and dietary fiber.

Coronary heart disease (CHD): The type of heart disease due to narrowing of the coronary arteries.

Dietary fiber: Plant food components, including plant cell walls, pectins, gums, and brans that cannot be digested.

***Dietary Guidelines for Americans*:** A report published by the U.S. Department of Agriculture and U.S. Department of Health and Human Services that explains how to eat to maintain health. The guidelines form the basis of national nutrition policy and are revised every 5 years. This chapter refers mostly to the 2000 guidelines.

Fats/fatty acids: Fats and fatty acids are hydrocarbon chains ending in a carboxyl group at one end that bond to glycerol to form fat. Fatty acids are characterized as saturated, monounsaturated, or polyunsaturated depending on how many double bonds are between the carbon atoms. Fatty acids supply energy and promote absorption of fat-soluble vitamins. Some fatty acids are "essential," because they cannot be made by the body.

>   **Saturated fatty acids:** Fatty acids with no double bonds between carbon atoms. Levels of saturated fatty acids are especially high in meat and dairy products that contain fat. Saturated fatty acids are linked to increased blood cholesterol levels and a greater risk for heart disease.

>   ***Trans*-fatty acids:** Alternate forms of naturally occurring unsaturated fatty acids produced in fats as a result of hydrogenation, such as when vegetable oil becomes margarine or shortening. *Trans*-fatty acids also occur in milk fat, beef fat, and lamb fat. These fatty acids have been associated with increased blood cholesterol levels.

>   **Unsaturated fatty acids:** Fatty acids with one or more double bonds between carbon atoms. These fatty acids do not raise blood cholesterol levels.

>   **Polyunsaturated:** Fatty acids with more than one double bond between carbon atoms.

>   **Monounsaturated:** Fatty acids with one double bond between carbon atoms.

Food Guide Pyramid: A graphic depiction of U.S. Department of Agriculture's current food guide that includes five major food groups in its "base" (grains, vegetables, fruits, milk products, and meats, and meat substitutes) and a "tip" depicting the relatively small contribution that discretionary fat and added sugars should make in U.S. diets. The Food Guide Pyramid provides information on the choices within each group and the recommended number of servings.

Food security: Access by all people at all times to enough food for an active, healthy life. It includes at a minimum (1) the ready availability of nutritionally adequate and safe foods, and (2) an assured ability to acquire acceptable foods in socially acceptable ways.

Food insecurity: Limited or uncertain availability of nutritionally adequate and safe foods or limited and uncertain ability to acquire acceptable foods in socially acceptable ways.

HDL-cholesterol: See cholesterol.

Hunger: The uneasy or painful sensation caused by a lack of food.

Hypertension: High blood pressure.

Hypertriglyceridemia: Elevated levels of triglycerides in the blood.

Iron deficiency: Lack of adequate iron in the body to support and maintain functioning. It can lead to iron deficiency anemia, a reduction in the concentration of hemoglobin in the red blood cells due to a lack of iron supply to the bone marrow.

LDL-cholesterol: See cholesterol.

Linear growth: Increase in length or height.

Medical nutrition therapy: Use of specific nutrition counseling and interventions, based on an assessment of nutritional status, to manage a condition or treat an illness or injury.

Metabolism: The sum total of all the chemical reactions that go on in living cells.

Nutrition: The set of processes by which nutrients and other food components are taken in by the body and used.

Obesity: A condition characterized by excessive body fat.

Osteoporosis: A bone disease characterized by a reduction in bone mass and a deterioration of the bone structure leading to bone fragility.

Overweight: Excess body weight.

Physical activity: Bodily movement that substantially increases energy expenditure.

Registered dietitian: A food and nutrition expert who has met the minimum academic and professional requirements to receive the credential "RD." Many States and Commonwealths also have licensing laws for dietitians and nutrition practitioners.

Sedentary behavior: A pattern of behavior that is relatively inactive, such as a lifestyle characterized by a lot of sitting.

Type 2 diabetes: The most common form of diabetes, which results from insulin resistance and abnormal insulin action. Type 2 diabetes was previously referred to as noninsulin-dependent diabetes mellitus (NIDDM) and adult-onset diabetes.

References

[1] American Academy of Pediatrics, Work Group on Breastfeeding. Breastfeeding and the use of human milk. *Pediatrics* 100(6):1035-1039, 1997.

[2] Frazao, E. The high costs of poor eating patterns in the United States. In: Frazao, E., ed. *America's Eating Habits: Changes and Consequences.* Washington, DC: U.S. Department of Agriculture (USDA), Economic Research Service (ERS), AIB-750, 1999.

[3] National Center for Health Statistics (NCHS). Report of final mortality statistics, 1995. *Monthly Vital Statistics Report* 45(11):Suppl. 2, June 12, 1997.

[4] Frazao, E. The American diet: A costly problem. *Food Review* 19:2-6, 1996.

[5] National Institutes of Health (NIH). *NIH Consensus Statement: Optimal Calcium Intake.* 12(4), 1994.

[6] USDA and U.S. Department of Health and Human Services (HHS). *Dietary Guidelines for Americans.* 5th ed. USDA Home and Garden Bulletin No. 232. Washington, DC: USDA, 2000.

[7] USDA. *The Food Guide Pyramid.* USDA Home and Garden Bulletin No. 252. Washington, DC: USDA, 1992.

[8] Yip, R. The changing characteristics of childhood iron nutritional status in the United States. In: Filer, Jr., L.J., ed. *Dietary Iron: Birth to Two Years.* New York, NY: Raven Press, Ltd., 1989, 37-61.

[9] NCHS. *Healthy People 2000 Review, 1998–99.* DHHS Pub. No. (PHS) 99-1256. Hyattsville, MD: Public Health Service (PHS), 1997.

[10] HHS. Recommendations for the use of folic acid to reduce the number of cases of spina bifida and other neural tube defects. *Morbidity and Mortality Weekly Report* 41:1-7, 1992.

[11] Lewis, C.J.; Crane, N.T.; Wilson, D.B.; et al. Estimated folate intakes: Data updated to reflect food fortification, increased bioavailability, and dietary supplement use. *American Journal of Clinical Nutrition* 70:198-207, 1999.

[12] Flegal, K.M.; Carroll, M.D.; Kuczmarski, R.J.; et al. Overweight and obesity in the United States: Prevalence and trends, 1960–1994. *International Journal of Obesity* 22(1):39-47, 1998.

[13] Kuczmarski, R.J.; Carroll, M.D.; Flegal, K.M.; et al. Varying body mass index cutoff points to describe overweight prevalence among U.S. adults: NHANES III (1988–1994). *Obesity Research* 5(6):542-548, 1997.

[14] World Health Organization (WHO). *Obesity: Preventing and Managing the Global Epidemic. Report of a WHO Consultation on Obesity, Geneva, 3-5 June 1997*. Geneva, Switzerland: WHO, 1998.

[15] NIH. Clinical guideline on the identification, evaluation and treatment of overweight and obesity in adults—The evidence report. *Obesity Research* 6(Suppl. 2):51S-209S, 1998.

[16] Troiano, R.P., and Flegal, K.M. Overweight children and adolescents: Description, epidemiology, and demographics. *Pediatrics* 101:497-504, 1998.

[17] Wolf, A.M., and Colditz, G.A. Current estimates of the economic cost of obesity in the United States. *Obesity Research* 6(2):97-106, 1998.

[18] Centers for Disease Control and Prevention (CDC). Guidelines for school health programs to promote lifelong healthy eating. *Morbidity and Mortality Weekly Report* 45(RR-9):1-33, 1996.

[19] Kelder, S.H.; Perry, C.L.; Klepp, K.I.; et al. Longitudinal tracking of adolescent smoking, physical activity, and food choice behaviors. *American Journal of Public Health* 84(7):1121-1126, 1994.

[20] Variyam, J.N.; Blaylock, J.; Lin, B.H.; et al. Mother's nutrition knowledge and children's dietary intakes. *American Journal of Agricultural Economics* 81(2), May 1999.

[21] Collins, J.L.; Small, M.L.; Kann, L.; et al. School health education. *Journal of School Health* 65(8):302-311, 1995.

[22] Contento, I.; Balch, G.I.; Bronner, Y.L.; et al. Nutrition education for school-aged children. *Journal of Nutrition Education* 27(6):298-311, 1995.

[23] Lytle, L., and Achterberg, C. Changing the diet of America's children: What works and why? *Journal of Nutrition Education* 27(5):250-260, 1995.

[24] USDA, Food and Nutrition Service (FNS). *Team Nutrition Strategic Plan*. Washington, DC: FNS, 1998.

[25] NIH Technology Assessment Conference Panel. Methods for voluntary weight loss and control. Consensus development conference, March 30 to April 1, 1992. *Annals of Internal Medicine* 119(7.2):764-770, 1993.

[26] Wilkening, V.L. FDA's regulations to implement the NLEA. *Nutrition Today* 13-20, 1993.

[27] Lin, B.H.; Guthrie, J.; and Frazao, E. Nutrient contribution of food away from home. In: Frazao, E., ed. *America's Eating Habits: Changes and Consequences*. Washington, DC: USDA, ERS, AIB-750, 1999.

[28] Crane, N.T.; Hubbard, V.S.; and Lewis, C.J. National nutrition objectives and the Dietary Guidelines for Americans. *Nutrition Today* 33:49-58, 1998.

[29] WHO Expert Committee. *Physical Status: The Use and Interpretation of Anthropometry. Report of a WHO Expert Committee*. WHO Technical Report Series: 854. Geneva, Switzerland: WHO, 1995.

[30] Gallagher, D.; Visser, M.; Sepulveda, D.; et al. How useful is body mass index for comparison of body fatness across age, sex, and ethnic groups. *American Journal of Epidemiology* 143(3):228-239, 1996.

[31] CDC. *Pediatric Nutrition Surveillance, 1997*. Full report. Atlanta, GA: HHS, CDC, 1998.

[32] PHS. *The Surgeon General's Report on Nutrition and Health*. DHHS Pub. No. (PHS) 88050210. Washington, DC: HHS, 1988.

[33] National Research Council. *Diet and Health: Implications for Reducing Chronic Disease Risk*. Washington, DC: National Academy Press, 1989.

[34] HHS, Food and Drug Administration (FDA). Notice of final rule: Food labeling; health claims and label statements; dietary fiber and cardiovascular disease. *Federal Register* 2552-2605, January 5, 1993.

[35] HHS, FDA. Notice of final rule: Food labeling; health claims and label statements; dietary fiber and cancer. *Federal Register* 2537-2552, January 5, 1993.

[36] Chief Medical Officer's Committee on Medical Aspects of Food. *Nutritional Aspects of the Development of Cancer*. London, England: Stationery Office, 1998.

[37] World Cancer Research Fund, in association with American Institute for Cancer Research. *Food, Nutrition and the Prevention of Cancer: A Global Perspective*. Washington, DC: the Fund, 1997.

[38] USDA, Agricultural Research Service (ARS). Unpublished data from the 1994–96 Continuing Survey of Food Intakes by Individuals, February 1998.

[39] Morton, J.F., and Guthrie, J.F. Changes in children's total fat intakes and their food sources of fat, 1989–91 versus 1994–95: Implications for diet quality. *Family Economics and Nutrition Review* 11(3):44-57, 1998.

[40] Guthrie, J.F., and Morton, J.F. Food sources of added sweeteners in the diets of Americans. *Journal of the American Dietetic Association* 100(1):43-48, 51, 2000.

[41] National Heart, Lung, and Blood Institute (NHLBI). *The Report of the Expert Panel on Population Strategies for Blood Cholesterol Reduction. National Cholesterol Education Program of the National Heart, Lung, and Blood Institute*. Washington, DC: HHS, 1990.

[42] Lichtenstein, A.H.; Ausman, L.M.; Jalbert, S.M.; et al. Effects of different forms of dietary hydrogenated fats on serum lipoprotein cholesterol levels. *New England Journal of Medicine* 340(25):1933-1940, 1999.

[43] Ip, C., and Carroll, K., eds. Proceedings of the workshop on individual fatty acids and cancer. Washington, DC, June 4-5, 1996. *American Journal of Clinical Nutrition* 66(Suppl. 6):1505S-1586S, 1997.

[44] Freedman, L.S.; Prentice, R.L.; Clifford, C.; et al. Dietary fat and breast cancer: Where are we? *Journal of the National Cancer Institute* 85(10):764-765, 1993.

[45] Allison, D.B.; Egan, S.K.; Barraj, L.M.; et al. Estimated intakes of *trans* fatty and other fatty acids in the U.S. population. *Journal of the American Dietetic Association* 99(2):166-174, 1999.

[46] NHLBI. *Sixth Report of the Joint National Committee on Prevention, Detection, Evaluation, and Treatment of High Blood Pressure*. DHHS Pub. No. 98-4080. Washington, DC: HHS, 1997.

[47] Elliott, P.; Stamler, J.; Nichols, R.; et al., for the Intersalt Cooperative Research Group. Intersalt revisited: Further analyses of 24 hour sodium excretion and blood pressure within and across populations. *British Medical Journal* 312:1249-1253, 1966.

[48] Stamler, J.; Stamler, R.; and Neaton, J.D. Blood pressure, systolic and diastolic, and cardiovascular risks: U.S. population data. *Archives of Internal Medicine* 153(5):598-615, 1993.

[49] Kurtz, T.W.; Al-Bander, H.A.; and Morris, R.C. "Salt sensitive" essential hypertension in men: Is the sodium ion alone important? *New England Journal of Medicine* 317(17):1043-1048, 1987.

[50] Mattes, R., and Donnelly, D. Relative contributions of dietary sodium sources. *Journal of the American College of Nutrition* 10(4):383-393, 1991.

[51] James, W.P.T.; Ralph, A.; and Sanchez-Castillo, C.P. The dominance of salt in manufactured food in the sodium intake of affluent societies. *Lancet* 1(8530):426-429, 1987.

[52] Institute of Medicine. *Dietary Reference Intakes for Calcium, Phosphorus, Magnesium, Vitamin D, and Fluoride*. Washington, DC: National Academy Press, 1997.

[53] Life Sciences Research Office, Federation of American Societies for Experimental Biology. Prepared for the Interagency Board for Nutrition Monitoring and Related Research. *Third Report on Nutrition Monitoring in the United States*. Vol. I. Washington, DC: U.S. Government Printing Office, 1995, 104-105.

[54] Tippett, K., and Cleveland, L. How current diets stack up: Comparison with the dietary guidelines. In: Frazao, E., ed. *America's Eating Patterns: Changes and Consequences*. Washington, DC: USDA, ERS, AIB-750, 1999.

[55] Bucher, H.C.; Cook, R.J.; Guyatt, G.; et al. Effects of dietary calcium supplementation on blood pressure. A meta-analysis of randomized controlled trials. *Journal of the American Medical Association* 275:1016-1022, 1996.

[56] Allender, P.S.; Cutler, J.A.; Follman, D.; et al. Dietary calcium and blood pressure: A meta-analysis of randomized clinical trials. *Annals of Internal Medicine* 124(9):825-829, 1996.

[57] Idjradinata, P., and Pollitt, E. Reversal of developmental delays in iron-deficient anaemic infants treated with iron. *Lancet* 341(8836):1-4, 1993.

[58] Lozoff, B.; Jimenez, E.; and Wolf, A.W. Long-term developmental outcome of infants with iron deficiency. *New England Journal of Medicine* 325(10):687-694, 1991.

[59] Scholl, T.O.; Hediger, M.L.; Fischer, R.L.; et al. Anemia vs iron deficiency: Increased risk of preterm delivery in a prospective study. *American Journal of Clinical Nutrition* 55(5):985-998, 1992.

[60] Bruner, A.B.; Joffe, A.; Duggan, A.K.; et al. Randomized study of cognitive effects of iron supplementation in non-anaemic iron-deficient adolescent girls. *Lancet* 348(9033):992-996, 1996.

[61] CDC. Recommendations to prevent and control iron deficiency in the United States. *Morbidity and Mortality Weekly Report* 47(RR-3):1-29, 1998.

[62] Perry, G.S.; Yip, R.; and Zyrkowski, C. Nutritional risk factors among low-income pregnant U.S. women: The Centers for Disease Control and Prevention (CDC) Pregnancy Nutrition Surveillance System, 1979 through 1993. *Seminars in Perinatology* 19(3):211-221, 1995.

[63] CDC. *Pregnancy Nutrition Surveillance, 1996.* Full report. Atlanta, GA: HHS, CDC, 1998.

[64] Looker, A.C.; Dallman, P.R.; Carroll, M.D.; et al. Prevalence of iron deficiency in the United States. *Journal of the American Medical Association* 277:973-976, 1997.

[65] USDA, ARS. Data tables: Results from USDA's 1994–96 Continuing Survey of Food Intakes by Individuals and 1994–96 Diet and Health Knowledge Survey. Riverdale, MD: USDA, ARS, Beltsville Human Nutrition Research Center, December 1997. <http://www.barc.usda.gov/bhnrc/foodsurvey/home.htm>January 14, 1998.

[66] Devaney, B., and Stewart, E. *Eating Breakfast: Effects of the School Breakfast Program.* Washington, DC: USDA, FNS, 1998.

[67] Murphy, J.M.; Pagano, M.E.; Nachmani, J.; et al. The relationship of school breakfast to psychosocial and academic functioning: Cross-sectional and longitudinal observations in an inner-city school sample. *Archives of Pediatric and Adolescent Medicine* 152(9):899-907, 1998.

[68] Pollitt, E. Does breakfast make a difference at school? *Journal of the American Dietetic Association* 95(10):1134-1139, 1995.

[69] PHS. *Worksite Nutrition: A Guide to Planning, Implementation, and Evaluation.* 2nd ed. Washington, DC: American Dietetic Association (ADA) and Office of Disease Prevention and Health Promotion, PHS, HHS, 1993.

[70] Sorensen, G.; Stoddard, A.; Hunt, M.K.; et al. The effects of a health promotion-health protection intervention on behavior change: The WellWorks Study. *American Journal of Public Health* 88(11):1685-1690, 1998.

[71] Goetzel, R.Z.; Jacobson, B.H.; Aldana, S.G.; et al. Health care costs of worksite health promotion participants and non-participants. *Journal of Occupational and Environmental Medicine* 40(4):341-346, 1998.

[72] Shephard, R.J. Employee health and fitness—State of the art. *Preventive Medicine* 12(5):644-653, 1983.

[73] Felix, M.R.; Stunkard, A.J.; Cohen, R.Y.; et al. Health promotion at the worksite. I. A process for establishing programs. *Preventive Medicine* 14(1):99-108, 1985.

[74] ADA. *The American Dietetic Association 1997 Nutrition Trends Survey.* Chicago, IL: ADA, 1997.

[75] Caggiula, A.W.; Christakis, G.; Farrand, M.; et al. The Multiple Risk Factor Intervention Trial (MRFIT). IV. Intervention on blood lipids. *Preventive Medicine* 10(4):443-475, 1987.

[76] Geil, P.B.; Anderson, J.W.; and Gustafson, N.J. Women and men with hypercholesterolemia respond similarly to an American Heart Association step 1 diet. *Journal of the American Dietetic Association* 95(4):436-441, 1995.

[77] Gambera, P.J.; Schneeman, B.O.; and Davis, P.A. Use of the Food Guide Pyramid and U.S. Dietary Guidelines to improve dietary intake and reduce cardiovascular risk in active-duty Air Force members. *Journal of the American Dietetic Association* 95(11):1268-1273, 1995.

[78] Hebert, J.R.; Ebbeling, C.B.; Ockene, I.S.; et al. A dietitian-delivered group nutrition program leads to reductions in dietary fat, serum cholesterol, and body weight: The Worcester Area Trial for Counseling in Hyperlipidemia (WATCH). *Journal of the American Dietetic Association* 99(5):544-552, 1999.

[79] McGehee, M.M.; Johnson, E.Q.; Rasmussen, H.M.; et al. Benefits and costs of medical nutrition therapy by registered dietitians for patients with hypercholesterolemia. *Journal of the American Dietetic Association* 95:1041-1043, 1995.

[80] Sikand, G. Medical nutrition therapy lowers serum cholesterol and saves medication costs in men with hypercholesterolemia. *Journal of the American Dietetic Association* 98:889-894, 1998.

[81] Franz, M.J.; Splett, P.L.; Monk, A.; et al. Cost-effectiveness of medical nutrition therapy provided by dietitians for persons with non-insulin dependent diabetes mellitus. *Journal of the American Dietetic Association* 95(9):1018-1024, 1995.

[82] Sheils, J.F.; Rubin, R.; and Stapleton, D.C. The estimated costs and savings of medical nutrition therapy: The Medicare population. *Journal of the American Dietetic Association* 99(4):428-435, 1999.

[83] Johnson, R.K. The Lewin Group Study—What does it tell us and why does it matter? *Journal of the American Dietetic Association* 99(4):426-427, 1999.

[84] Bickel, G.; Andrews, M.; and Carlson, S. The magnitude of hunger: In a new national measure of food security. *Topics in Clinical Nutrition* 13(4):15-30, 1998.

[85] Food Research and Action Center. *Community Childhood Hunger Identification Project: A Survey of Childhood Hunger in the United States.* Vol. 1. Washington, DC: the Center, 1995.

[86] Kendall, A.; Olson, C.M.; and Frongillo, Jr., E.A. Validation of the Radimer/Cornell measures of hunger and food insecurity. *Journal of Nutrition* 125(11):2793-2801, 1995.

[87] Foreign Agricultural Service (FAS), USDA. *U.S. Action Plan on Food Security: Solutions to Hunger.* Washington, DC: USDA, FAS, 1999.

[88] USDA. *USDA's Community Food Security Initiative Action Plan.* USDA Community Food Security Initiative, August 1999.

[89] Health Resources and Services Administration (HRSA), Maternal and Child Health Bureau. *Community Outreach, The Healthy Start Initiative: A Community-Driven Approach to Infant Mortality Reduction.* Vol. IV. Washington, DC: HRSA, 1996.

20

Occupational Safety and Health

Lead Agency: Centers for Disease Control and Prevention

Contents

Goal

Promote the health and safety of people at work through prevention and early intervention.

Overview

The toll of workplace injuries and illnesses is significant. Every 5 seconds a worker is injured in the United States.[1,2] Every 10 seconds a worker is temporarily or permanently disabled.[1,2] Each day, an average of 137 persons die from work-related diseases,[3,4] and an additional 17 die from injuries on the job.[5] Although youth (adolescents aged 17 years and under) represent only 2 percent of the total workforce, each year 74,000 require treatment in hospital emergency departments for work-related injuries, and 70 die of those injuries.[6] In 1996, an estimated 11,000 workers were disabled each day due to work-related injuries.[7] In 1996, the National Safety Council estimated that on-the-job injuries alone cost society $121 billion, representing the sum of lost wages, lost productivity, administrative expenses, health care, and other costs. The 1992 combined U.S. economic burden for occupational illnesses and injuries was an estimated $171 billion.[8]

Work-related injuries and illnesses include any injuries or illnesses incurred by persons engaged in work-related activities while on or off the worksite. This includes injuries and illnesses that occur during apprenticeships and vocational training, while working in family businesses, and even while volunteering as fire-fighters or emergency medical services (EMS) providers.

Issues

The Nation is poised to make significant improvements in the quality of life for all working people in the United States. The National Occupational Research Agenda (NORA), developed by the National Institute for Occupational Safety and Health (NIOSH) in partnership with more than 500 outside organizations and individuals, was released in April 1996 as a framework to guide occupational safety and health research into the 21st century. NORA partners include representatives from labor, industry, academia, State governments, and national professional organizations. The NORA process resulted in a consensus on the top 21 research priorities for occupational safety and health (see table).[9]

One of the 21 specific priority areas identified by the NORA process is intervention effectiveness research, a type of research aimed at finding out which prevention strategies effectively protect worker safety and health. This research will evaluate the impact of occupational prevention interventions, programs, and policies on safety and health outcomes across a broad spectrum of industries. Although measurable improvements in worker safety and health have been achieved, only a few interventions have been evaluated systematically.

Category	NORA Priority Research Areas
Disease and Injury	Allergic and Irritant Dermatitis Asthma and Chronic Obstructive Pulmonary Disease Fertility and Pregnancy Abnormalities Hearing Loss Infectious Diseases Low Back Disorders Musculoskeletal Disorders of the Upper Extremities Traumatic Injuries
Work Environment and Workforce	Emerging Technologies Indoor Environment Mixed Exposures Organization of Work Special Populations at Risk
Research Tools and Approaches	Cancer Research Methods Control Technology and Personal Protective Equipment Exposure Assessment Methods Health Services Research Intervention Effectiveness Research Risk Assessment Methods Social and Economic Consequences of Workplace Illness and Injury Surveillance Research Methods

Source: NIOSH. *National Occupational Research Agenda*. Pub. No. 96-115. Cincinnati, OH: NIOSH, 1996.

Managers of public and private sector occupational safety and health programs face increasing demands to document program cost-effectiveness and impact on worker health. The lack of evidence about intervention effectiveness stymies the introduction of new programs and threatens the continuation of ongoing programs. Corporate safety and health programs, regulatory requirements and voluntary consensus standards, workers' compensation policies and loss-control programs, engineering controls, and educational campaigns are among the types of interventions that need to be developed, implemented, and evaluated. In addition to promoting worker safety and health, intervention programs can lead to increased productivity and save on long-term operating costs.

Because national data systems will not be available in the first half of the decade for tracking progress, five subjects of interest are not addressed in this focus area's objectives. These topics represent a research and data collection agenda for the coming decade and are related to a variety of activities. The first topic covers improvement in national workplace injury and illness surveillance by increasing the number of States that code work-relatedness of injuries and illnesses in a variety of data systems, including cancer registries, trauma registries, risk factor surveys, and health facility data (for example, hospital emergency department visits, clinic visits, hospital discharge records). The second addresses the reduction of exposures that result in workers having blood lead concentrations of 10 µg/dL or greater of whole blood. The third involves increasing the proportion of health care facilities that appropriately protect workers by instituting effective prevention practices to reduce latex allergy (for example, low-protein, powder-free gloves; nonlatex gloves). The fourth is related to increasing the proportion of health care settings, correctional facilities, and homeless shelters that appropriately protect workers by implementing effective tuberculosis control programs (for example, administrative controls, work practice and engineering controls, employee training and skin testing, and where necessary personal respiratory protection). The fifth relates to increasing the proportion of agricultural tractors fitted with rollover protective structures.

Trends

A number of data systems and estimates exist to describe the nature and magnitude of occupational injuries and illnesses. These data systems have advantages as well as limitations. However, no national occupational chronic disease or death reporting system currently exists. Therefore, scientists, public health professionals, and policymakers must rely on estimates of the magnitude of occupational disease generated from a number of data sources and published epidemiologic (or population-based) studies. Although these compiled estimates generally are thought to underestimate the true extent of occupational disease, they are considered to provide the best available data. Such compilations indicate that an estimated 50,000 to 70,000 workers die each year from work-related diseases.

Data from the National Traumatic Occupational Fatalities Surveillance System (NTOF), based on death certificates from across the United States, demonstrate a general decrease in occupational death over the 16-year period from 1980 through 1995. The numbers and rates of fatal injuries from 1990 through 1995 remained relatively stable—at over 5,000 deaths per year and about 4.3 deaths per 100,000 workers. Motor vehicle-related fatalities at work, the leading cause of death for U.S. workers since 1980, accounted for 23 percent of deaths during the 16-year period. Workplace homicides became the second leading cause of death in 1990, surpassing machine-related deaths. Although the rankings of individual industry divisions have varied across the years, the largest number of traumatic occupational deaths consistently are found in construction, transportation and public utilities, and manufacturing. Industries with the highest traumatic occupational fatality rates per 100,000 workers are mining, agriculture, forestry and fishing, and construction.[10]

Rates of nonfatal injuries and illnesses have declined from a rate of 8.7 per 100 full-time workers in 1980 to 7.1 per 100 full-time workers in 1997.[11]

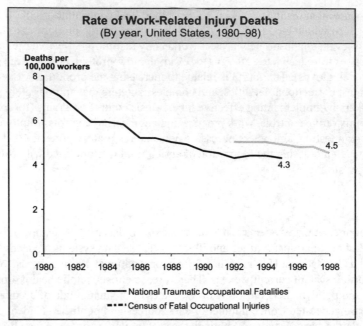

Rate of Work-Related Injury Deaths
(By year, United States, 1980–98)

Deaths per
100,000 workers

4.5

4.3

——— National Traumatic Occupational Fatalities
■ ■ ■ ■ Census of Fatal Occupational Injuries

Sources: DOL, BLS. Census of Fatal Occupational Injuries (CFOI), 1992–98. CDC, NIOSH. National Traumatic Occupational Fatalities Surveillance System (NTOF), 1980–95.

Disparities

Data systems that can routinely monitor disparities among population groups related to occupational injury and illness are not in place. NIOSH is working with partners and stakeholders in the occupational safety and health community to identify and address surveillance needs, including the need to track disparities.

Little is known about factors such as gender, genetic susceptibility, culture, and literacy that may increase the risk for occupational disease and injury. Occupational safety and health experts who worked to develop NORA agreed by consensus that many high-risk populations have been underserved by the occupational safety and health research community, resulting in important unanswered questions about the profile of hazards these workers face, the number of cases of work-related injuries and illnesses, the mechanisms of these injuries and illnesses, and the optimal approach to preventing them. As a result, special populations at risk is one of 21 NORA priority research areas that will examine the challenges faced by different groups in the increasingly diverse workforce.

Opportunities

The growing U.S. workforce, projected to be 147 million by the year 2005, also is changing. The population is increasingly diverse and more rapidly exposed to innovative work restructuring and new technologies. Evidence suggests that the way work is organized may directly affect worker health. Work organization broadly addresses the health effects of conditions of employment. It also encompasses special characteristics related to the overall economy, including the demands for productivity; the increasing presence in the workforce of adolescents aged 16 to 17 years (2.1 percent increase projected each year from 1992 to 2005), women (47 percent of the workforce in 1997), racially and ethnically diverse workers, and older workers (the aging of baby boomers); and the ongoing evolution from an industrial to a service economy.

The NORA strategic plan will ensure that research addresses the new, emerging work environment of the 21st century. Research translation, education, and outreach will ensure that labor, industry, academia, and national professional organizations have current information on how best to design prevention programs to protect worker safety and health.

Interim Progress Toward Year 2000 Objectives

For work-related injury deaths and nonfatal injuries, progress has been made toward meeting Healthy People 2000 objectives, including meeting several subobjectives (for construction and mining). The objective for reducing cases of hepatitis B infection among occupationally exposed workers has been exceeded, but the related goal for immunizing workers for hepatitis B fell short of the 2000 target. For several objectives, the Nation appears to be moving in the wrong direction—a situation that can be attributed, in part, to several confounding factors, including improved surveillance, reporting changes, and improved diagnosis. Finally, a few Healthy People 2000 objectives cannot be tracked reliably for progress, and some objectives have low relative value for monitoring improved outcomes in worker safety and health (for instance, safety belt policies at work do not equate automatically with safety belt use). These objectives have been revised, replaced, or dropped from Healthy People 2010 objectives.

Note: Unless otherwise noted, data are from the Centers for Disease Control and Prevention, National Center for Health Statistics, *Healthy People 2000 Review, 1998–99.*

Occupational Safety and Health

Goal: Promote the health and safety of people at work through prevention and early intervention.

Number	Objective Short Title
20-1	Work-related injury deaths
20-2	Work-related injuries
20-3	Overexertion or repetitive motion
20-4	Pneumoconiosis deaths
20-5	Work-related homicides
20-6	Work-related assaults
20-7	Elevated blood lead levels from work exposure
20-8	Occupational skin diseases or disorders
20-9	Worksite stress reduction programs
20-10	Needlestick injuries
20-11	Work-related, noise-induced hearing loss

20-1. Reduce deaths from work-related injuries.

Target and baseline:

Objective	Reduction in Deaths From Work-Related Injuries	1998 Baseline	2010 Target
		Deaths per 100,000 Workers Aged 16 Years and Older	
20-1a.	All industry	4.5	3.2
20-1b.	Mining	23.6	16.5
20-1c.	Construction	14.6	10.2
20-1d.	Transportation	11.8	8.3
20-1e.	Agriculture, forestry, and fishing	24.1	16.9

Target setting method: Better than the best for 20-1a; 30 percent improvement for 20-1b, 20-1c, 20-1d, and 20-1e. (Better than the best will be used when data are available.)

Data source: Census of Fatal Occupational Injuries (CFOI), DOL, BLS.

NOTE: THE TABLE BELOW MAY CONTINUE TO THE FOLLOWING PAGE.

Workers Aged 16 Years and Older, 1998	Deaths From Work-Related Injuries				
	20-1a. All Industry	20-1b. Mining	20-1c. Con-struction	20-1d. Trans-portation	20-1e. Agricul-ture, Forestry, and Fishing
	Rate per 100,000				
TOTAL	4.5	23.6	14.6	11.8	24.1
Race and ethnicity					
American Indian or Alaska Native	DSU	DSU	DSU	DSU	DSU
Asian or Pacific Islander	DSU	DSU	DSU	DSU	DSU
Asian	DNC	DNC	DNC	DNC	DNC
Native Hawaiian and other Pacific Islander	DNC	DNC	DNC	DNC	DNC
Black or African American	3.9	DNA	DNA	DNA	DNA
White	4.5	DNA	DNA	DNA	DNA

Workers Aged 16 Years and Older, 1998	Deaths From Work-Related Injuries				
	20-1a. All Industry	20-1b. Mining	20-1c. Con-struction	20-1d. Trans-portation	20-1e. Agricul-ture, Forestry, and Fishing
	Rate per 100,000				
Hispanic or Latino	5.2	DNA	DNA	DNA	DNA
Not Hispanic or Latino	DNA	DNA	DNA	DNA	DNA
Black or African American	DNA	DNA	DNA	DNA	DNA
White	DNA	DNA	DNA	DNA	DNA
Gender					
Female	0.8	DNA	DNA	DNA	DNA
Male	7.7	DNA	DNA	DNA	DNA
Family income level					
Poor	DNC	DNC	DNC	DNC	DNC
Near poor	DNC	DNC	DNC	DNC	DNC
Middle/high income	DNC	DNC	DNC	DNC	DNC
Disability status					
Persons with disabilities	DNC	DNC	DNC	DNC	DNC
Persons without disabilities	DNC	DNC	DNC	DNC	DNC

DNA = Data have not been analyzed. DNC = Data are not collected. DSU = Data are statistically unreliable.

NOTE: THE TABLE ABOVE MAY HAVE CONTINUED FROM THE PREVIOUS PAGE.

An average of 17 workers die from work-related injuries each day. These deaths are preventable. Public health efforts and resources can be targeted more effectively toward work-related injury prevention efforts, especially in those industries where the risk is greatest.

The NORA traumatic injury team has identified a number of research needs and priorities to address this issue. Specifically, the reduction of work-related injury deaths will require focused efforts to more fully identify and prioritize problems (injury surveillance), quantify and prioritize risk factors (analytic injury research), identify existing or develop new strategies to prevent occupational injuries (prevention and control), implement the most effective injury control measures (communication, dissemination, and technology transfer), and monitor the results of intervention efforts (evaluation). This approach will require the cooperation of many groups and agencies to provide the needed educational and outreach efforts, engineering controls, and enforcement of workplace safety regulations.

20-2. Reduce work-related injuries resulting in medical treatment, lost time from work, or restricted work activity.

Target and baseline:

Objective	Reduction in Work-Related Injuries Resulting in Medical Treatment, Lost Time From Work, or Restricted Activity	1998 Baseline (unless noted)	2010 Target
		Injuries per 100 Full-Time Workers Aged 16 Years and Older	
20-2a.	All industry	6.2	4.3
20-2b.	Construction	8.7	6.1
20-2c.	Health services	7.9 (1997)	5.5
20-2d.	Agriculture, forestry, and fishing	7.6	5.3
20-2e.	Transportation	7.9 (1997)	5.5
20-2f.	Mining	4.7	3.3
20-2g.	Manufacturing	8.5	6.0
20-2h.	Adolescent workers	4.8 (1997)	3.4

Target setting method: 30 percent improvement. (Better than the best will be used when data are available.)

Data sources: Annual Survey of Occupational Injuries and Illnesses, DOL, BLS; National Electronic Injury Surveillance System (NEISS), CPSC.

> **Data for population groups currently are not collected.**

In 1997, nearly 6.1 million workers suffered injuries that resulted in either lost time from work, medical treatment, or restricted work activity. This is a rate of 6.6 cases per 100 full-time workers and clearly represents a public health and occupational safety and health problem of significant proportions. Prevention efforts must be heightened to reduce the tremendous burden of these injuries on individual workers as well as society.

20-3. Reduce the rate of injury and illness cases involving days away from work due to overexertion or repetitive motion.

Target: 338 injuries per 100,000 full-time workers.

Baseline: 675 injuries per 100,000 full-time workers due to overexertion or repetitive motion were reported in 1997.

Target setting method: 50 percent improvement. (Better than the best will be used when data are available.)

Data source: Annual Survey of Occupational Injuries and Illnesses, DOL, BLS.

Data for population groups currently are not collected.

For occupational injuries and illnesses resulting in days away from work, in 1997 approximately 507,500 cases (32 percent of all cases) involved overexertion or repetitive motion. Included within this total were 297,300 injuries due to overexertion in lifting (52 percent affected the back) and 75,200 injuries or illnesses due to repetitive motion, including typing or key entry, repetitive use of tools, and repetitive placing, grasping, or moving of objects other than tools.[12] The rates per 100,000 workers were 588 (overexertion) and 87 (repetitive motion), respectively.

Research evidence suggests an association between musculoskeletal disorders and certain work-related physical factors when levels of exposure are high, especially in combination with exposure to more than one physical factor (for example, repetitive lifting of heavy objects in extreme or awkward postures). More than 3 million persons are employed in the industries with the highest numbers of cases involving days away from work because of overexertion in lifting and repetitive motion.[13] The number of workers affected can be reduced by continuing to focus national attention on prevention of this problem.

Strategies for reducing illness and injury due to overexertion or repetitive motion include increasing the number of States involved in control and evaluation activities and surveillance of musculoskeletal disorders; better support for State and community action to prevent and control musculoskeletal disorders; extending technical support and available engineering technology to industrial and service sectors to improve recognition and control of ergonomic hazards; establishing health care management strategies, as well as developing and validating standardized diagnostic criteria for early detection and treatment of musculoskeletal disorders for preventing impairment and disability; instituting ergonomic approaches at the design stage of work processes to factors that can lead to musculoskeletal problems; and increasing public awareness through media campaigns (for example, billboards and commercials) about the magnitude and severity of the problem, the need for early reporting, and early intervention to reduce disability as well as providing education about interventions.

20-4. Reduce pneumoconiosis deaths.

Target: 1,900 deaths.

Baseline: 2,928 pneumoconiosis deaths among persons aged 15 years and older occurred in 1997.

Target setting method: 10 percent fewer than the number of pneumoconiosis deaths projected for 2010 based on a 15-year trend (1982–97).

Data source: National Surveillance System for Pneumoconiosis Mortality (NSSPM), CDC, NIOSH.

Pneumoconiosis deaths are preventable through effective control of worker exposure to occupational dusts. The ultimate public health goal is to eliminate all pneumoconiosis among the Nation's current and former workers. Although progress toward this goal has been made in recent decades, the continuing occurrence of new cases of pneumoconiosis highlights the mistaken conclusion of many who have declared this a disease of the past. It will be important to maintain attention to and, as appropriate, enhance control of occupational exposures to hazardous dusts. Pneumoconiosis deaths will be measured by tracking death counts rather than age-adjusted deaths rates, emphasizing the preventability of each death.

An effective prevention strategy to reduce deaths from all types of pneumoconiosis will necessitate a broad range of approaches. Disease, disability, and hazard surveillance, both at the Federal and State levels, is required to monitor progress toward prevention and to identify new and persisting high-risk problem areas. Effective dissemination of pneumoconiosis surveillance and prevention information will raise awareness and motivate preventive actions for high-risk worker populations. Informational materials specifically designed to target regulators, employers, employees, industrial hygiene professionals, health care professionals, legislators, and the public also will contribute to elimination of pneumoconiosis.

20-5.   Reduce deaths from work-related homicides.

Target: 0.4 deaths per 100,000 workers.

Baseline: 0.5 deaths per 100,000 workers aged 16 years and older were work-related homicides in 1998.

Target setting method: 20 percent improvement. (Better than the best will be used when data are available.)

Data source: Census of Fatal Occupational Injuries (CFOI), DOL, BLS.

Data for population groups are not collected routinely.

An average of 20 workers die each week as a result of workplace homicides in the United States. The jobs where employees are at risk of being murdered in the workplace share a number of common factors, including interacting with the public, handling exchanges of money, working alone or in small numbers, and working late night or early morning hours. Workplace factors can be modified to reduce or eliminate the effects of these risk factors. Workers, employers, and others can launch workplace violence prevention efforts as a part of all comprehensive workplace safety and health initiatives.

Reducing the number of workplace homicides will require improved surveillance and analytic epidemiologic research as well as effectiveness research to assess engineering and other control strategies in various high-risk work settings. Additional education and outreach efforts also are necessary to inform workers, employers, occupational safety and health professionals, and others of the nature and magnitude of this problem and steps that can be taken to reduce the risk of workplace homicide.

20-6. Reduce work-related assaults.

Target: 0.60 assaults per 100 workers.

Baseline: 0.85 assaults per 100 workers aged 16 years and older were work-related during 1987–92.

Target setting method: 29 percent improvement. (Better than the best will be used when data are available.)

Data source: National Crime Victimization Survey, DOJ, BJS.

> Data for racial and ethnic population groups currently are not analyzed. Data for other population groups currently are not collected.

Each year between 1992 and 1996, more than 2 million persons were victims of a violent crime while they were at work or on duty. (For additional information regarding improved surveillance, see objective 20-5.)

20-7. Reduce the number of persons who have elevated blood lead concentrations from work exposures.

Target: Zero persons per 1 million.

Baseline: 93 per million persons aged 16 to 64 years had blood lead concentrations of 25 μg/dL or greater in 1998 (25 States).

Target setting method: Total elimination.

Data source: Adult Blood Lead Epidemiology and Surveillance Program, CDC, NIOSH.

> Data for population groups currently are not collected.

Twenty-five of the 27 States in NIOSH's Adult Blood Lead Epidemiology and Surveillance (ABLES) Program reported 10,501 adults (aged 16 to 64 years) with blood lead levels of 25 μg/dL or greater in 1998. Industries in which workers have been occupationally exposed to lead include battery manufacturing, nonferrous foundries, radiator repair shops, lead smelters, construction, demolition, and firing ranges. Workers in sheltered workshops (where mentally and physically challenged adults work) also are at risk for lead exposures. Lead taken home from the workplace also can harm children and spouses. Lead exposures can occur in avocations such as making pottery and stained glass, casting ammunition and fishing weights, and renovating and remodeling projects.

In the 1978 general industry standard, the Occupational Safety and Health Administration (OSHA) advised that the maximum acceptable blood lead level was 40 µg/dL and that males and females planning to have children should limit their exposure to maintain a blood lead level less than 30 µg/dL (29 CFR 1910.1025).[14] Research studies on lead toxicity in humans indicate that compliance with the current OSHA lead standard should prevent the most severe symptoms of lead poisoning and some adverse reproductive effects in exposed workers. Nonetheless, the current OSHA standards fail to protect occupationally exposed males and females or their unborn children from all the adverse effects of lead, hence the 25 µg/dL cutoff in this objective.

The target can be achieved by continuing the efforts under way for the prevention of adult lead exposures, including interventions by States participating in NIOSH's ABLES Program, Council of State and Territorial Epidemiologists (CSTE) lead initiatives, OSHA's strategic initiative to reduce adult lead exposures, and voluntary industry initiatives such as those of the Lead Industries Association Incorporated and the Battery Council International.

20-8. Reduce occupational skin diseases or disorders among full-time workers.

Target: 47 new cases per 100,000.

Baseline: 67 new cases of occupational skin diseases or disorders per 100,000 full-time workers aged 16 years and older occurred in 1997.

Target setting method: 30 percent improvement. (Better than the best will be used when data are available.)

Data source: Annual Survey of Occupational Injuries and Illnesses, DOL, BLS.

Data for population groups currently are not collected.

In 1997, occupational skin diseases or disorders (OSDs) constituted 13.5 percent of all occupational illnesses reported to the Bureau of Labor Statistics (BLS), making OSDs the most common nontrauma-related occupational illness. Research on allergic and irritant dermatitis, the most common OSD, was identified as a NORA priority. In 1997, BLS data estimated a new case rate for OSDs of 67 per 100,000 workers, or 57,900 cases in the U.S. workforce. Because of survey limitations, the number of actual OSDs is estimated to be 10 to 50 times higher than the number reported by BLS.

The greatest number of cases of OSDs is seen in manufacturing, but the highest rate for diagnosis of new cases is seen in agriculture, forestry, and fishing. In the 1988 National Health Interview Survey (NHIS), the rate of new cases was 1.7 percent for occupational contact dermatitis (OCD) occurring in the preceding year. Projecting these results to the working population in the United States resulted in an estimate of 1.87 million persons with OCD. An analysis of workers' compensation claims reported an average annual claims rate for OSDs ranging from 12 to

108 per 100,000 employees. The total annual cost of OSDs is estimated to range from $222 million to $1 billion.

OSDs are preventable. Strategies for the prevention of OSDs include identifying allergens and irritants, substituting chemicals that are less irritating or allergenic, establishing engineering controls to reduce exposure, using personal protective equipment such as gloves and special clothing, using barrier creams, emphasizing personal and occupational hygiene, establishing educational programs to increase awareness in the workplace, and providing health screening. A combination of several interventions, which included providing advice on personal protective equipment and educating the workforce about skin care and exposures, have proved to be beneficial for workers. Primary and secondary prevention programs that include health promotion or public awareness campaigns and education or disease awareness programs can successfully be directed toward workers in high-risk industries.

20-9. Increase the proportion of worksites employing 50 or more persons that provide programs to prevent or reduce employee stress.

Target: 50 percent.

Baseline: 37 percent of worksites with 50 or more employees provided worksite stress reduction programs in 1992.

Target setting method: 35 percent improvement.

Data source: National Survey of Worksite Health Promotion Activities, OPHS, ODPHP.

Job stress has been identified as a significant risk factor for a number of health problems, including cardiovascular disease, musculoskeletal disorders, and workplace injuries. Research indicates that up to one-third of all workers report high levels of stress on the job. Worksite programs to reduce stress tend to adopt either stress management (for example, helping workers cope with current levels of stress) or primary prevention (for example, altering sources of stress through job redesign). Although many of these programs have been found to be effective in reducing levels of stress, additional knowledge is needed regarding which occupations are especially prone to the effects of stress, which aspects of organizational change in today's workplace pose the greatest risk of job stress, and what interventions are most useful to control these risks. The NORA Work Organization Team is committed to identifying factors that contribute to job stress and psychological strain as well as the prevention of these disorders. Definitive research is needed to clarify the relationship between psychosocial stressors associated with work organization and safety and health concerns, including job stress. Responsibility for implementing worksite programs lies with industry and industry associations, although worker representatives and labor groups should be involved in the design and implementation of worksite stress-reduction programs.

The baseline has been set using a 1992 survey that collected worksite data from the private sector and may not reflect accurately the practices of public sector organizations. The proportion of people who reported participating in stress management programs in the private and public sectors was 40 percent according to the 1994 NHIS data and may indicate that more worksite programs are offered in the public sector. NIOSH currently is planning data collection efforts to better understand stress prevention activities in both public and private workplace settings.

20-10. Reduce occupational needlestick injuries among health care workers.

Target: 420,000 annual needlestick exposures.

Baseline: 600,000 occupational needlestick exposures to blood occurred among health care workers in 1996.

Target setting method: 30 percent improvement. (Better than the best will be used when data are available.)

Data sources: National Surveillance System for Health Care Workers, CDC, NCID, NCHSTP, NIP, NIOSH.

Needlestick injuries are a serious concern for the approximately 8 million health care workers in the United States, because they pose the greatest risk of occupational transmission of bloodborne viruses, for example, human immunodeficiency virus (HIV), hepatitis B, and hepatitis C.[15] Approximately 600,000 to 800,000 needlestick injuries occur annually, mostly among nursing staff; however, laboratory staff, physicians, housekeepers, and other health care workers also are injured.[16, 17] As of June 1999, a cumulative total of 55 documented cases and 136 possible cases of occupational transmission of HIV have occurred among health care workers.[18] In 1995, an estimated 800 health care workers became infected with the hepatitis B virus (HBV).[19] The number of health care workers who have acquired the hepatitis C virus (HCV) from an occupational exposure is unknown; however, approximately 2 to 4 percent of the 36,000 acute HCV infections in 1996 were thought to be in health care workers after an occupational exposure.[20, 21, 22] Also, the emotional impact of a needlestick can be severe and long lasting, even when a serious disease is not transmitted.

Although the new cases of HCV infection decreased in the 1990s, 36,000 persons in the United States still are infected each year (1996), and approximately 3.9 million persons currently are infected with HCV.[23] Of these infected persons, an estimated 2 to 4 percent are health care workers occupationally exposed to blood due to needlestick injuries. HIV also can be transmitted in this fashion.

Many of these exposures are preventable with currently available technology. Two studies that evaluated safety devices, ongoing surveillance of occupational injuries, and consultation with experts in occupational safety and injury prevention indicate that at least a 30 percent reduction can be achieved with new technologies and changes in technique. The use of engineering controls is an important priority in sharps injury prevention efforts. However, implementation of devices with safety features is only one component of a comprehensive program to achieve significant declines in sharps injuries. Such an approach includes modification of hazardous work practices, administrative changes to address needle hazards in the environment, safety education and awareness, and feedback on safety improvements.

20-11. (Developmental) Reduce new cases of work-related, noise-induced hearing loss.

Potential data source: Annual Survey of Occupational Injuries and Illnesses, DOL, BLS.

Related Objectives From Other Focus Areas

14. Immunization and Infectious Diseases
14-3.   Hepatitis B in adults and high-risk populations
14-28. Hepatitis B vaccination among high-risk groups

27. Tobacco Use
27-12. Worksite smoking policies
27-13. Smoke-free indoor air laws

28. Vision and Hearing
28-8.   Occupational eye injury
28-16. Hearing protection

Terminology

(A listing of abbreviations and acronyms used in this publication appears in Appendix H.)

Acoustic trauma: Hearing loss that is caused by a one-time exposure to a very loud noise, such as a gun shot or blast overpressure. A portion of the hearing loss may be temporary, but a portion will be permanent.

Asbestosis: A type of occupational dust disease of the lung caused by microscopic asbestos fibers.

Blood lead level (BLL): The concentration of lead in a sample of blood. This concentration usually is expressed in micrograms per deciliter (µg/dL) or micro moles per liter (µmol/L). One µg/dL is equal to 0.048 µmol/L.

Byssinosis: A type of occupational dust disease of the lung most often caused by cotton dust.

Coal workers' pneumoconiosis: A type of occupational dust disease of the lung caused by coal mine dust.

Ergonomic hazards: Factors or exposures that may adversely affect health and are related to the interaction between persons and their total working environment, including the organization of work, tools, equipment, and the social and behavioral elements of the workplace. These hazards also can apply to work performance capabilities and limitations of workers.

Hyperacusis: Abnormal sensitivity to everyday sound levels or noises, often sensitivity to higher pitched sounds, in the presence of essentially normal hearing and often accompanied by tinnitus. Hyperacusis often follows exposures to intense high-level sounds, such as overpressures from automobile air bag deployments or gun fire.

Musculoskeletal disorders: Conditions that involve the soft tissues of the body, including muscles, tendons, nerves, cartilage, and other supporting structures. The term usually refers to conditions of the large joints, including the neck, shoulder, elbow, hand and wrist, back, and knee.

National Occupational Research Agenda (NORA): A collaboration of the National Institute for Occupational Safety and Health (NIOSH) and its public and private partners to provide a framework to guide occupational safety and health research through the next decade.

Natural rubber latex allergy: An immediate hypersensitivity reaction to one or more natural rubber latex proteins that can result in a wide spectrum of signs and symptoms, including skin rashes; hives or wheals; flushing; itching; nasal, eye, or sinus problems; asthma; and, rarely, anaphylaxis (shock).

Noise-induced hearing loss: Hearing loss caused by repeated exposures to sounds at various loudness levels over an extended period of time. The resulting permanent hearing loss is the cumulation of many temporary hearing losses and is insidious, often unnoticed by the sufferer until listening and communication are impaired.

Occupational dusts: Dusts associated with industrial processes and other work activities.

Occupational skin disease or disorder (OSD): An abnormal skin condition caused by exposure to factors associated with employment. Examples include contact dermatitis, eczema, or rash caused by primary irritants and sensitizers or poisonous plants; oil acne; chrome ulcers; and chemical burns or inflammations.

Pneumoconiosis: A major category of lung disease caused by breathing in certain types of occupational dusts. The dust deposited in the lung can result in inflammation and scarring, with associated respiratory symptoms, reduced lung function, and disability. A number of types of dust (for example, asbestos, silica, or coal mine dust) are known to cause pneumoconiosis.

Repetitive motion injury: As reported to the Bureau of Labor Statistics (BLS), a disorder due to repetitive motion or musculoskeletal disorders of the upper extremity associated with workplace exposures to a combination of repetitive, forceful exertions and constrained or extreme postures. The term "repetitive motion injury" is no longer favored and has been replaced by "work-related musculoskeletal disorder" by the International Committee on Occupational Health (ICOH) Musculoskeletal Subcommittee. Back disorders are separately reported to the BLS as "disorders due to overexertion."

Silicosis: A type of occupational dust disease of the lung caused by crystalline silica dust.

Work-related injury (fatal or nonfatal): Any injury incurred by a worker while on or off the worksite but engaged in work-related activities. Work-related injuries may be unintentional or intentional (that is, homicide and assault). The term includes apprenticeships, vocational training, working in a family business, and work as a volunteer firefighter or emergency medical services (EMS) provider. Injuries incurred during work-related travel are included; injuries incurred during routine commuting to or from work are not included.

Work-related musculoskeletal disorder: A condition involving the soft tissues of the body, including muscles, tendons, nerves, cartilage, and other supporting structures, that is caused by exposure to work-related factors. The term usually refers to conditions of the large joints, including the neck, shoulder, elbow, hand and wrist, back, and knee.

References

[1] Bureau of Labor Statistics (BLS). Work injuries and illnesses by selected characteristics, 1993. *BLS News* Publication 95-142, April 26, 1995.

[2] BLS. Workplace injuries and illnesses in 1994. *BLS News* Publication 95-508, December 15, 1995.

[3] Centers for Disease Control and Prevention (CDC). National Occupational Research Agenda. *Morbidity and Mortality Weekly Report* 45:445-446, 1996.

[4] CDC. Clarification. *Morbidity and Mortality Weekly Report* 45:495, 1996.

[5] BLS. *National Census of Fatal Occupational Injuries, 1998.* USDL 99-208, August 4, 1999.

[6] National Institute for Occupational Safety and Health (NIOSH). Unpublished data from National Electronic Injury Surveillance System, 1999.

[7] National Safety Council. *Accident Facts, 1998.* Itasca, IL: the Council, 1999.

[8] Leigh, J.P.; Markowitz, S.B.; Fahs, M.; et al. Occupational injury and illness in the United States: Estimates of costs, morbidity, and mortality. *Archives of Internal Medicine* 157(14):1557-1568, 1997.

[9] NIOSH. *National Occupational Research Agenda.* Pub. No. 96-115. Cincinnati, OH: NIOSH, 1996.

[10] NIOSH. National Traumatic Occupational Fatalities Surveillance System. Morgantown, WV: NIOSH, 1999.

[11] BLS. Workplace Injuries and Illnesses in 1997. <http://www.bls.gov/osh_nwrl.htm>April 20, 2000.

[12] BLS. Case & Demographic Characteristics for Workplace Injuries and Illnesses Involving Days Away From Work—1997. <http://www. bls.gov/oshc_d97.htm#C>April 20, 2000.

[13] NIOSH. *Musculoskeletal Disorders and Workplace Factors—A Critical Review of Epidemiologic Evidence for Work-Related Musculoskeletal Disorders of the Neck, Upper Extremity, and Lower Back.* Pub. No. 97-141. Washington, DC: NIOSH, 1997.

[14] U.S. Department of Labor, Occupational Safety and Health Administration. Final standard for occupational exposure to lead. *Federal Register* 43:52952-53014, 1978.

[15] NIOSH. *Alert: Preventing Needlestick Injuries in Health Care Settings.* Pub. No. 2000-108. Cincinnati, OH: NIOSH, 1999.

[16] Henry, K.; Campbell, S.; Jackson, B.; et al. Long-term follow-up of health care workers with work-site exposure to human immunodeficiency virus. [Letter to the editor]. *Journal of the American Medical Association* 263(15):1765-1766, 1995.

[17] EPINet. Exposure prevention information network data reports. Charlottesville, VA: University of Virginia, International Health Care Worker Safety Center, 1999.

[18] CDC. U.S. HIV and AIDS cases reported through December 1998. *HIV/AIDS Surveillance Report* 10(2):26, 1998.

[19] CDC. Unpublished data.

[20] Alter, M.J. Epidemiology of hepatitis C in the west. *Seminars in Live Diseases* 15(1):5-14, 1995.

[21] Alter, M.J. The epidemiology of acute and chronic hepatitis C. *Clinical Liver Disease* 1(3):559-569, 1997.

[22] CDC. Unpublished data.

[23] McQuillan, G.M.; Alter, M.J.; Lambert, S.B.; et al. A population-based serologic study of hepatitis C virus infection in the United States. In: Rizzetto, M.; Purcell, R.H.; Gerin, J.L.; et al.; eds. *Viral Hepatitis and Liver Disease* 266-270, 1997.

21

Oral Health

Co-Lead Agencies: Centers for Disease Control and Prevention
Health Resources and Services Administration
Indian Health Service
National Institutes of Health

Contents

Goal

Prevent and control oral and craniofacial diseases, conditions, and injuries and improve access to related services.

Overview

Oral health is an essential and integral component of health throughout life. No one can be truly healthy unless he or she is free from the burden of oral and craniofacial diseases and conditions.[1] Millions of people in the United States experience dental caries, periodontal diseases, and cleft lip and cleft palate, resulting in needless pain and suffering; difficulty in speaking, chewing, and swallowing; increased costs of care; loss of self-esteem; decreased economic productivity through lost work and school days; and, in extreme cases, death.[2] Further, oral and pharyngeal cancers, which primarily affect adults over age 55 years, result in significant illnesses and disfigurement associated with treatment, substantial cost, and more than 8,000 deaths annually.[3]

Poor oral health and untreated oral diseases and conditions can have a significant impact on quality of life. Millions of people in the United States are at high risk for oral health problems because of underlying medical or handicapping conditions, ranging from very rare genetic diseases to more common chronic diseases such as arthritis and diabetes.[4] Oral and facial pain affects a substantial proportion of the general population.[2, 5]

Issues

Dental caries is the single most common chronic disease of childhood, occurring five to eight times as frequently as asthma, the second most common chronic disease in children.[1] Despite the reduction in cases of caries in recent years, more than half of all children have caries by the second grade, and, by the time students finish high school, about 80 percent have caries.[6] Unless arrested early, caries is irreversible.

Early childhood caries (ECC) affects the primary teeth of infants and young children aged 1 to 6 years.[7] The exact cause of ECC is unknown, but factors such as large family size, nutritional status of the mother and the infant, and the transfer of infectious organisms from caregiver to infant are under study.[8, 9] Infant feeding practices in which children are put to bed with formula or other sweetened drinks or sweetened pacifiers, especially if a child falls asleep while feeding, have been associated with ECC.[10] Some professional associations recommend that a child should first visit a dentist at age 1 year.[11]

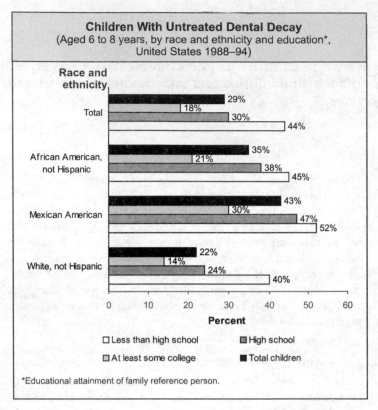

Children With Untreated Dental Decay
(Aged 6 to 8 years, by race and ethnicity and education*,
United States 1988–94)

Race and ethnicity

Total
29%
18%
30%
44%

African American, not Hispanic
35%
21%
38%
45%

Mexican American
43%
30%
47%
52%

White, not Hispanic
22%
14%
24%
40%

Percent
0 10 20 30 40 50 60

☐ Less than high school   ▨ High school
☐ At least some college   ■ Total children

*Educational attainment of family reference person.

Source: CDC, NCHS. National Health and Nutrition Examination Survey (NHANES), 1988–94.

Since the early 1970s, the cases of dental caries in permanent teeth have declined dramatically among school-aged children.[1] This decline is the result of various preventive regimens such as community water fluoridation and increased use of toothpastes and rinses that contain fluoride. Dental caries, however, remains a significant problem in some populations, particularly certain racial and ethnic groups and poor children.[12] National data indicate that 80 percent of dental caries in the permanent teeth found in children is concentrated in 25 percent of the child and adolescent population.[13] Increased use of dental sealants, toothbrushing with fluoridated toothpaste, community water fluoridation, and sound dietary practices are needed to reduce tooth decay.

Data from the third National Health and Nutrition Examination Survey (NHANES III) indicated that 30 percent of all adults had untreated dental decay; 85 percent had ever experienced dental caries. More than 37 percent of dentate persons aged 65 years or older in the United States had at least one decayed or filled root surface.[14] If current trends continue, the baby boomer generation will lose fewer teeth as they age but will have more teeth that are at risk for dental caries throughout life.

Oral and pharyngeal cancers comprise a diversity of malignant tumors that affect the oral cavity and pharynx; virtually all of these tumors are squamous cell carcinomas. Some 31,000 new cases of oral and pharyngeal cancers were expected to be diagnosed in 1999, and approximately 8,100 persons were expected to die from the disease.[3] Oral and pharyngeal cancers occur more frequently than leukemia, Hodgkin's disease, and cancers of the brain, cervix, ovary, liver, pancreas, bone, thyroid gland, testes, and stomach. Oral and pharyngeal cancers are the 7th most common cancers found among white males (4th most common among black men) and the 14th most common among U.S. women. The 5-year survival rate for oral and pharyngeal cancers is only 53 percent,[15] and most of these cancers are diagnosed at late stages.[16] Only 13 percent of U.S. adults aged 40 years or older reported having had an oral cancer examination in the past year,[17] which is the recommended interval.[18]

Cleft lip and cleft palate are among the more common birth defects in the United States. These congenital defects occur in about 1 per 1,000 live births.[19, 20] States should have an effective, efficient mechanism in place for identifying, recording, and referring for treatment infants with these conditions. Primary prevention of these craniofacial anomalies involves minimizing exposure to known causes of malformations and, where indicated, providing genetic counseling.

Oral diseases and conditions may have a significant impact on general health; some poor general health conditions also may affect oral health status. Chemotherapy for cancer may cause inflammation and infection of oral mucous tissues. Head and neck radiotherapy and medications taken for many chronic conditions can affect the salivary glands, resulting in decreases in or loss of salivary flow, which, in turn, contribute to the ability to chew and speak and to dental decay.[1] Studies point to associations between periodontal diseases and low birth weight and premature births,[21, 22, 23] as well as between periodontitis and heart disease and stroke.[24, 25, 26] The initiation and progression of periodontal infections are affected by systemic factors and habits,[27] including tobacco use, uncontrolled diabetes, stress, and genetic factors.

For patients with special risks, invasive dental procedures may result in infective endocarditis;[28] infections of artificial knee, hip, and shoulder joints; and complications associated with organ and bone marrow transplantation. Oral complications associated with human immunodeficiency virus (HIV) infection also can have a significant impact on overall health, resulting in loss of appetite, painful mouth sores, weight loss, hospitalization, and potentially life-threatening fungal infections.[1]

Many persons in the United States do not receive essential dental services.[29] Through increased access to appropriate and timely care, individuals can enjoy improved oral health. Barriers to care include cost; lack of dental insurance, public programs, or providers from underserved racial and ethnic groups; and fear of dental visits. Additionally, some people with limited oral health literacy may not be able to find or understand information and services.

To promote oral health and prevent oral diseases, oral health literacy among all groups is necessary. In addition, oral health services—preventive and restorative—should be available, accessible, and acceptable to all persons in the United States. In areas where different languages, culture, and health care beliefs would otherwise be barriers to care, a cadre of clinically and culturally competent providers must be available to provide care.

Of the 16,926 undergraduate dental students enrolled in U.S. dental schools in 1996–97, fewer than 1,000 were African American, and fewer than 1,000 were Hispanic.[30] Native Americans continue to constitute less than 1 percent of the total undergraduate dental enrollment.[30] Strategic measures are needed to increase the number of individuals from certain racial and ethnic groups who seek careers in dentistry and public health, now and in the future. With the current health disparities and projected demographic changes in the U.S. population, such measures are needed for all aspects of oral health: education, research, health promotion, and clinical services within the private and public sectors.

One subject of oral health interest, daily brushing with a fluoride-containing toothpaste, is not addressed because data for tracking progress will not be available during the first half of the decade (2000-2005).

Trends

Cases of dental caries in the permanent teeth of school-aged children have been declining in the United States since the early 1970s.[1] The proportion of untreated dental caries in permanent dentition of school-aged children also has been declining overall but has increased in the primary dentition among children aged 6 to 8 years.[31, 32] Fewer adults are having teeth extracted because of dental decay or periodontal disease, and the percentage of persons who have lost all of their natural teeth has been declining steadily.[1]

The percentage of school-aged children with dental sealants has risen in recent years as the public and private sectors increasingly use the procedure, dental insurance pays for dental sealants, and parents request sealants for their children.[32] No increase, however, has occurred among children in low-income populations.

Community water fluoridation grew rapidly from its inception in 1945 until about 1980; since then, the proportion of the U.S. population living in communities with fluoridated water supplies has remained at 60 to 62 percent.[33] About 100 million persons still lack the benefits of community water fluoridation.

Over the past 20 years, deaths from oral and pharyngeal cancers have declined by about 25 percent, and new cases have declined by 10 percent, but the 5-year survival rate has remained unchanged. African American men, however, have experienced increases in both death rates and new case rates.[15]

Spending for dental services in the United States has risen steadily but has remained fairly constant as a proportion of personal health care spending—about 5 percent in 1997.[1] Dental insurance coverage has not increased. Only 44 percent of persons in the United States have some form of private dental insurance (most with limited coverage and with high copayments), 9 percent have public dental insurance (Medicaid and Children's Health Insurance Program), 2 percent have other dental insurance, and 45 percent have no dental insurance.[34]

Disparities

As with general health, oral health status tends to vary in the United States on the basis of sociodemographic factors. For example, the level of untreated dental caries among African American children aged 6 to 8 years (36 percent) and Hispanic children (43 percent) is greater than for white children (26 percent);[6] as few as 3 percent of poor children have dental sealants compared to the national average (23 percent).[6] Further, the 5-year survival rate is lower for oral and pharyngeal cancers among African Americans than whites (34 percent versus 56 percent);[16] adults with less than a high school education (5 percent) and those with a high school education (10 percent) were less likely than those with some college (19 percent) to have had an oral cancer examination in the past year;[17] adults with some college (15 percent) have 2 to 2.5 times less destructive periodontal disease than those with high school (28 percent) and with less than high school (35 percent) levels of education.[6] Among persons aged 65 years and older, 39 percent of persons with less than a high school education were edentulous (had lost all their natural teeth) in 1997, compared with 13 percent of persons with at least some college.[35]

Promotion of oral health requires self-care and professional care as well as population-based initiatives. Several national surveys show that the proportion of the U.S. population that annually makes at least one dental visit and the average number of visits made vary significantly by age, race, dental status, level of education, and family income[6, 35, 36] For example, the Medical Expenditure Panel Survey in 1996[36] indicated that about 44 percent of the total population over age 2 visited a dentist in the past year; 50 percent of non-Hispanic whites, 30 percent of Hispanics, and 27 percent of non-Hispanic blacks had a visit while 55 percent of those with some college and only 24 percent of those with less than a high school education had a past-year visit. Approximately twice as many adults with teeth had a dental visit compared to adults without teeth.[35]

Opportunities

An increased focus on oral health by Federal, State, and professional organizations that occurred at the end of the 1990s should help achieve improvements in oral health and quality of life for individuals and communities. If initiatives, partnerships, and collaborations flourish in this environment of heightened interest, then oral health literacy will increase, access to preventive and restorative services for persons in need will improve, surveillance of oral diseases or conditions will be enhanced, and appropriate research will explore new ways to improve oral health for everyone in the United States.

Recent legislation in three States requires the widespread implementation of water fluoridation, which should lead to more communities with optimally fluoridated water. By the end of the 20th century, dental caries was limited in many children to pit and fissure tooth surfaces, for which dental sealants are ideal. Opportunities to encourage the dental profession to adopt and implement this preventive technology and for dental insurance companies to pay for sealants must be promoted. Every opportunity must be taken to educate the public about the value of sealants for children shortly after their permanent molars erupt. Opportunities must be expanded to target certain preventive procedures to poor, largely inner-city and rural children in school-based or school-linked programs.

Reducing deaths from oral and pharyngeal cancers and improving the early detection of both types of cancer require immediate attention. Efforts must be made to continue the momentum begun in the 1990s that focused on reducing the number of new cases of oral and pharyngeal cancers and improving survival.[37, 38] Specifically, dental personnel need to provide comprehensive oral cancer examinations on a routine basis for persons aged 40 years and older or who are otherwise at high risk. Dental personnel also need to provide counseling to patients to stop tobacco use and limit alcohol use, both of which are associated with oral and pharyngeal cancers.

The 21st century may provide the opportunity to reduce the burden of birth defects, such as cleft lip and cleft palate. As local and State surveillance systems of developmental anomalies are created or expanded, opportunities should be explored to integrate cleft lip and cleft palate into those systems. If studies confirm the beneficial effects of folic acid in preventing cleft lip and cleft palate, then programs incorporating the use of folic acid should be implemented and monitored.

In general, access to primary preventive and early intervention services must be improved, and barriers to the dental care system should be removed. Many persons of all ages are receiving professional services in the oral health care system, but more emphasis must be placed on vulnerable populations who need professional care.

Interim Progress Toward Year 2000 Objectives

More than half the 17 Healthy People 2000 oral health objectives show progress, and 1 was met. One objective has moved away from the target, and two have shown mixed results. Data since baseline are not available for four of the objectives. The objective of reducing deaths from oral and pharyngeal cancers was met. Dental decay has declined in persons aged 15 years nearly to its target, although less progress has occurred in children aged 6 to 8 years. Similar trends are apparent in those two age groups for untreated dental decay. Elderly persons show improvement in edentulousness, but the number of persons aged 35 to 44 years who had never lost a tooth from caries or periodontal disease fails to show improvement. An increased proportion of children are receiving dental sealants, but further improvement is needed. Little change has occurred in the proportion of the U.S. population served by fluoridated water systems.

Note: Unless otherwise noted, data are from the Centers for Disease Control and Prevention, National Center for Health Statistics, *Healthy People 2000 Review, 1998–99.*

Oral Health

Goal: Prevent and control oral and craniofacial diseases, conditions, and injuries and improve access to related services.

Number	Objective Short Title
21-1	Dental caries experience
21-2	Untreated dental decay
21-3	No permanent tooth loss
21-4	Complete tooth loss
21-5	Periodontal diseases
21-6	Early detection of oral and pharyngeal cancers
21-7	Annual examinations for oral and pharyngeal cancers
21-8	Dental sealants
21-9	Community water fluoridation
21-10	Use of oral health care system
21-11	Use of oral health care system by residents in long-term care facilities
21-12	Dental services for low-income children
21-13	School-based health centers with oral health component
21-14	Health centers with oral health service components
21-15	Referral for cleft lip or palate
21-16	Oral and craniofacial State-based surveillance system
21-17	Tribal, State, and local dental programs

21-1. Reduce the proportion of children and adolescents who have dental caries experience in their primary or permanent teeth.

21-1a. Reduce the proportion of young children with dental caries experience in their primary teeth.

Target: 11 percent.

Baseline: 18 percent of children aged 2 to 4 years had dental caries experience in 1988–94.

Target setting method: Better than the best.

Data sources: National Health and Nutrition Examination Survey (NHANES), CDC, NCHS; Oral Health Survey of Native Americans, 1999, IHS; California Oral Health Needs Assessment of Children, Dental Health Foundation, 1993–94.

Throughout childhood and adolescence, many opportunities exist for the primary prevention of dental decay. The earliest opportunity to prevent dental decay occurs during prenatal counseling about diet, oral hygiene practices, appropriate uses of fluorides, and the transmission of bacteria from parents to children. Early childhood caries, sometimes referred to as baby bottle tooth decay or nursing caries, can be a devastating condition, often requiring thousands of dollars and a hospital visit with general anesthesia for treatment.[8, 9] The pain, psychological trauma, health risks, and costs associated with restoration of these carious teeth for children affected by ECC can be substantial.[10] Dental care for pregnant females, counseling, reinforcement of health promoting behaviors with caregivers of children, and intervention by dental and other professionals to improve parenting practices (use of fluorides, use of professional services, and diet) provide the best available means of preventing this serious oral disease.

The average number of decayed and filled teeth among 2- to 4-year-olds has remained unchanged over the past 25 years.[1] Children whose parents or caregivers have less than a high school education or whose parents and caregivers are Hispanic, American Indians, or Alaska Natives appear to be at markedly increased risk for developing ECC.[4]

21-1b. Reduce the proportion of children with dental caries experience in their primary and permanent teeth.

Target: 42 percent.

Baseline: 52 percent of children aged 6 to 8 years had dental caries experience in 1988–94.

Target setting method: Better than the best.

Data sources: National Health and Nutrition Examination Survey (NHANES), CDC, NCHS; Oral Health Survey of Native Americans, 1999, IHS; California Oral Health Needs Assessment of Children, 1993–94, Dental Health Foundation; Hawai'i Children's Oral Health Assessment, 1999, State of Hawaii Department of Health.

Children aged 6 to 8 years are at an important stage of dental development. They still have the majority of their primary teeth, and their permanent first molars and incisors are erupting into their mouths. Maintaining optimal oral health for these children is important for their current functional oral health and for their long-term health. Between the time the first permanent molars erupt into the mouth and before vulnerable pits and fissures are infected, children should be assessed for their need for dental sealants.

21-1c. Reduce the proportion of adolescents with dental caries experience in their permanent teeth.

Target: 51 percent.

Baseline: 61 percent of adolescents aged 15 years had dental caries experience in 1988–94.

Target setting method: Better than the best.

Data sources: National Health and Nutrition Examination Survey (NHANES), CDC, NCHS; Oral Health Survey of Native Americans, 1999, IHS; California Oral Health Assessment of Children, 1993–94, Dental Health Foundation.

Caries experience is cumulative, thus higher among adolescents than among young children. Effective personal preventive measures—for example, tooth brushing with fluoride toothpastes—need to be applied throughout adolescence, as children become more independent in their oral hygiene and dietary habits. Regular dental visits provide an opportunity to assess oral hygiene and dietary practices and to place sealants on vulnerable permanent teeth that erupt during this life stage (including second permanent molars at around age 12 years).

NOTE: THE TABLE BELOW MAY CONTINUE TO THE FOLLOWING PAGE.

Children and Adolescents, Selected Ages, 1988–94 (unless noted)	Dental Caries Experience		
	21-1a. Aged 2 to 4 Years	21-1b. Aged 6 to 8 Years	21-1c. Aged 15 Years
	Percent		
TOTAL	18	52	61
Race and ethnicity			
American Indian or Alaska Native	76* (1999)	90* (1999)	89* (1999)
Asian or Pacific Islander	DSU	DSU	DSU
Asian	34[†] (1993–94)	90[†] (1993–94)	DSU[†] (1993–94)

Children and Adolescents, Selected Ages, 1988–94 (unless noted)	Dental Caries Experience		
	21-1a. Aged 2 to 4 Years	21-1b. Aged 6 to 8 Years	21-1c. Aged 15 Years
	Percent		
Native Hawaiian and other Pacific Islander	DNC	79[‡] (1999)	DNC
Black or African American	24	50	70
White	15	51	60
Hispanic or Latino	DSU	DSU	DSU
Mexican American	27	68	57
Not Hispanic or Latino	17	49	62
Black or African American	24	49	69
White	13	49	61
Gender			
Female	19	54	63
Male	18	50	60
Education level (head of household)			
Less than high school	29	65	59
High school graduate	18	52	63
At least some college	12	43	61
Disability status			
Persons with disabilities	DNC	DNC	DNC
Persons without disabilities	DNC	DNC	DNC
Select populations			
3rd grade students	NA	60	NA

DNA = Data have not been analyzed. DNC = Data are not collected. DSU = Data are statistically unreliable. NA = Not applicable.

*Data are for IHS service areas.

[†]Data are for California.

[‡]Data are for Hawaii.

NOTE: THE TABLE ABOVE MAY HAVE CONTINUED FROM THE PREVIOUS PAGE.

21-2. Reduce the proportion of children, adolescents, and adults with untreated dental decay.

21-2a. Reduce the proportion of young children with untreated dental decay in their primary teeth.

Target: 9 percent.

Baseline: 16 percent of children aged 2 to 4 years had untreated dental decay in 1988–94.

Target setting method: Better than the best.

Data sources: National Health and Nutrition Examination Survey (NHANES), CDC, NCHS; Oral Health Survey of Native Americans, 1999, IHS; California Oral Health Needs Assessment of Children, 1993–94, Dental Health Foundation.

Primary teeth should be retained until they come out naturally and are replaced by the permanent teeth. Healthy retained primary teeth enhance self-image; decayed or missing primary teeth may cause a child to be self-conscious and reluctant to smile. Children need to eat nutritious foods to develop normally. The pain and infection of rampant dental disease compromise their ability to eat well. Moreover, early tooth loss caused by dental decay can result in impaired speech development, failure to thrive, absence from and inability to concentrate in school, and reduced self-esteem.

Children aged 2 to 4 years are least likely to have been seen by a dentist, whereas a much larger proportion have been taken to a health provider for medical care or counseling.[39] Thus these latter providers should be trained to examine and identify major oral diseases of toddlers and refer those with problems for necessary care.

21-2b. Reduce the proportion of children with untreated dental decay in primary and permanent teeth.

Target: 21 percent.

Baseline: 29 percent of children aged 6 to 8 years had untreated dental decay in 1988–94.

Target setting method: Better than the best.

Data sources: National Health and Nutrition Examination Survey (NHANES), CDC, NCHS; Oral Health Survey of Native Americans, 1999, IHS; California Oral Health Needs Assessment of Children, 1993–94, Dental Health Foundation; Hawai'i Children's Oral Health Assessment, 1999, State of Hawaii Department of Health.

To avoid pain and discomfort, decayed primary teeth need to be restored, particularly molars in children aged 6 to 8 years. Retention of primary molars until they fall out normally (age 10 to 12 years) allows adequate dental arch space for the eruption of succeeding permanent premolars and avoids the tipping forward of first permanent molars, possibly creating serious orthodontic problems. Carious permanent teeth should be repaired promptly so that fillings may be kept small and as much natural tooth as possible conserved. Often, fillings have to be replaced several times during life; each time, additional tooth structure has to be removed, weakening the tooth. Preventing the initial cavity by appropriate use of fluorides and sealants is preferable to restoring the tooth after disease has occurred.

21-2c. Reduce the proportion of adolescents with untreated dental decay in their permanent teeth.

Target: 15 percent.

Baseline: 20 percent of adolescents aged 15 years had untreated dental decay in 1988–94.

Target setting method: Better than the best.

Data sources: National Health and Nutrition Examination Survey (NHANES), CDC, NCHS; Oral Health Survey of Native Americans, 1999, IHS; California Oral Health Needs Assessment of Children, 1993–94, Dental Health Foundation.

By age 15 years, all permanent teeth other than third molars have erupted, and vulnerable chewing surfaces of permanent second molars have been exposed to cariogenic factors for 2 or 3 years. Further, by this age, approximately 75 percent of adolescents have experienced dental decay.[6]

21-2d. Reduce the proportion of adults with untreated dental decay.

Target: 15 percent.

Baseline: 27 percent of adults aged 35 to 44 years had untreated dental decay in 1998–94.

Target setting method: Better than the best.

Data sources: National Health and Nutrition Examination Survey (NHANES), CDC, NCHS; Oral Health Survey of Native Americans, 1999, IHS.

Approximately 30 percent of adults have untreated dental decay.[6] Untreated dental decay can lead to extensive dental treatment and can be quite costly. If decay is left unheeded, an individual can experience pain, abscess, and extraction of the tooth.

Among adults aged 35 to 44 years, twice as many blacks or African Americans (46 percent) as whites (23 percent) have tooth decay. More than three times as many persons with less than a high school education (51 percent) have untreated dental decay than adults with some college education (16 percent).[6] Dental decay is just as preventable in adults as it is in children. Access to community water fluoridation benefits adults as well as children. Access to other preventive interventions is critical, as well as access to dental treatment to restore the tooth.

Children, Adolescents, and Adults, Selected Ages, 1988–94 (unless noted)	Untreated Dental Decay			
	21-2a. Aged 2 to 4 Years	21-2b. Aged 6 to 8 Years	21-2c. Aged 15 Years	21-2d. Aged 35 to 44 Years
	Percent			
TOTAL	16	29	20	27
Race and ethnicity				
American Indian or Alaska Native	67* (1999)	69* (1999)	67* (1999)	67* (1999)
Asian or Pacific Islander	DSU	DSU	DSU	DSU
Asian[†]	30[†] (1993–94)	71[†] (1993–94)	DSU[†] (1993–94)	DNC
Native Hawaiian and other Pacific Islander	DNC	39[‡] (1999)	DNC	DNC
Black or African American	22	36	29	46
White	11	26	19	24
Hispanic or Latino	DSU	DSU	DSU	DSU
Mexican American	24	43	27	34
Not Hispanic or Latino	14	26	19	DNA
Black or African American	22	35	28	47
White	11	22	18	23
Gender				
Female	16	32	22	25
Male	16	25	17	29
Education level (head of household)				
Less than high school	26	44	29	51
High school graduate	16	30	18	34
At least some college	9	25	15	16
Disability status				
Persons with disabilities	DNC	DNC	DNC	DNA
Persons without disabilities	DNC	DNC	DNC	DNA
Select populations				
3rd grade students	NA	33	NA	NA

DNA = Data have not been analyzed. DNC = Data are not collected. DSU = Data are statistically unreliable.
NA = Not applicable.

*Data are for IHS service areas.

[†]Data are for California.

[‡]Data are for Hawaii.

21-3. Increase the proportion of adults who have never had a permanent tooth extracted because of dental caries or periodontal disease.

Target: 42 percent.

Baseline: 31 percent of adults aged 35 to 44 years had never had a permanent tooth extracted because of dental caries or periodontal disease in 1988–94.

Target setting method: Better than the best.

Data sources: National Health and Nutrition Examination Survey (NHANES), CDC, NCHS; Oral Health Survey of Native Americans, 1999, IHS.

NOTE: THE TABLE BELOW MAY CONTINUE TO THE FOLLOWING PAGE.

Persons Aged 35 to 44 Years, 1988–94	No Tooth Extractions
	Percent
TOTAL	31
Race and ethnicity	
American Indian or Alaska Native	23* (1999)
Asian or Pacific Islander	DSU
Asian	DNC
Native Hawaiian and other Pacific Islander	DNC
Black or African American	12
White	34
Hispanic or Latino	DSU
Mexican American	36
Not Hispanic or Latino	DNA
Black or African American	12
White	36
Gender	
Female	32
Male	30
Education level	
Less than high school	15
High school graduate	21
At least some college	41

Persons Aged 35 to 44 Years, 1988–94	No Tooth Extractions
	Percent
Disability status	
Persons with disabilities	DNA
Persons without disabilities	DNA

DNA = Data have not been analyzed. DNC = Data are not collected. DSU = Data are statistically unreliable.
*Data are for IHS service areas.

NOTE: THE TABLE ABOVE MAY HAVE CONTINUED FROM THE PREVIOUS PAGE.

A full dentition is defined as having 28 natural teeth, exclusive of third molars and teeth removed for orthodontic treatment or as a result of trauma. Most persons can keep their teeth for life with optimal personal, professional, and population-based preventive practices. Early tooth loss has been shown to be a predictor of eventual edentulism.[40] As teeth are lost, a person's ability to chew and speak decreases. A loss of or a withdrawal from social functioning can occur. Tooth loss can result from infection, unintentional injury, and head and neck cancer treatment. In addition, certain orthodontic and prosthetic services sometimes require the removal of teeth.

Despite an overall trend toward a reduction in tooth loss in the U.S. population,[1] older data indicate 25 percent of American Indians or Alaska Natives aged 35 to 44 years have fewer than 20 natural teeth;[4] among all persons aged 55 years and older, nearly 75 percent have fewer than 20 natural teeth. Females tend to have more teeth extracted than males of the same age group. African Americans are more likely than whites to have teeth extracted.[6] The percentage of whites who have never had a permanent tooth extracted is more than three times as great as for African Americans. Among all predisposing and enabling variables, low educational level often has been found to have the strongest and most consistent association with tooth loss.[41]

21-4. Reduce the proportion of older adults who have had all their natural teeth extracted.

Target: 20 percent.

Baseline: 26 percent of adults aged 65 to 74 years had lost all their natural teeth in 1997.

Target setting method: Better than the best.

Data sources: National Health Interview Survey (NHIS), CDC, NCHS; Oral Health Survey of Native Americans, 1999, IHS.

Adults Aged 65 to 74 Years, 1997 (unless noted)	Lost All Natural Teeth
	Percent
TOTAL	26
Race and ethnicity	
American Indian or Alaska Native	30* (1999)
Asian or Pacific Islander	DSU
Asian	DSU
Native Hawaiian and other Pacific Islander	DSU
Black or African American	30
White	25
Hispanic or Latino	24
Not Hispanic or Latino	26
Black or African American	30
White	26
Gender	
Female	27
Male	24
Education level	
Less than high school	39
High school graduate	26
At least some college	13
Disability status	
Persons with disabilities	34
Persons without disabilities	22

DNA = Data have not been analyzed. DNC = Data are not collected. DSU = Data are statistically unreliable.
*Data are for IHS service areas.

Despite a steady decline in the rate of complete tooth loss over the past several decades, 26 percent of persons aged 65 to 74 years had lost all of their natural teeth. The rate of complete tooth loss among African Americans is 30 percent whereas that for Hispanics is 24 percent. Among all persons aged 65 years and older, 30 percent had lost all of their natural teeth.[35] Low-income adults aged 65 years and older experience a higher rate of edentulism (48 percent in 1993).[32] Also, State-specific variations range from 13 to 47 percent in the self-reported prevalence of complete tooth loss.[42]

Among elderly persons, loss of all natural teeth can contribute to psychological, social, and physical impairment.[2] Even when missing teeth are replaced with well-constructed dentures, there may be limitations in speech, chewing ability, taste perception, and quality of life. Most tooth loss is the result of dental caries and periodontal disease. The level of edentulism reflects not only the cases of caries and periodontal disease but also the availability and use of appropriate professional services and community preventive services. Tooth loss can be prevented through education, early diagnosis, and regular dental care. Children and adults (and the health care professionals who serve them) must recognize the signs and symptoms of oral and systemic diseases and know the oral and general health care practices necessary to prevent them.

21-5. Reduce periodontal disease.

Target and baseline:

Objective	Reduction in Periodontal Disease in Adults Aged 35 to 44 Years	1988–94 Baseline	2010 Target
		Percent	
21-5a.	Gingivitis	48	41
21-5b.	Destructive periodontal disease	22	14

Target setting method: Better than the best.

Data sources: National Health and Nutrition Examination Survey (NHANES), CDC, NCHS; Oral Health Survey of Native Americans, 1999, IHS.

NOTE: THE TABLE BELOW MAY CONTINUE TO THE FOLLOWING PAGE.

Adults Aged 35 to 44 Years, 1988–94 (unless noted)	21-5a. Gingivitis	21-5b. Destructive Periodontal Disease
	Percent	
TOTAL	48	22
Race and ethnicity		
American Indian or Alaska Native	98* (1999)	54* (1999)
Asian or Pacific Islander	DSU	DSU
Asian	DNC	DNC
Native Hawaiian and other Pacific Islander	DNC	DNC
Black or African American	51	33
White	47	20

Healthy People 2010: Objectives for Improving Health

Adults Aged 35 to 44 Years, 1988–94 (unless noted)	21-5a. Gingivitis	21-5b. Destructive Periodontal Disease
	Percent	
Hispanic or Latino	DSU	DSU
Mexican American	64	24
Not Hispanic or Latino	DNA	DNA
Black or African American	51	33
White	45	20
Gender		
Female	45	15
Male	52	29
Education level		
Less than high school	60	35
High school graduate	52	28
At least some college	42	15
Disability status		
Persons with disabilities	DNA	DNA
Persons without disabilities	DNA	DNA

DNA = Data have not been analyzed. DNC = Data are not collected. DSU = Data are statistically unreliable.
*Data are for IHS service areas.
NOTE: THE TABLE ABOVE MAY HAVE CONTINUED FROM THE PREVIOUS PAGE.

Gingivitis is characterized by localized inflammation, swelling, and bleeding gum tissues without a loss of connective tissue or bone support. Gingivitis usually is reversible with proper daily oral hygiene and serves as a crude measure of a person's self-care practices.[43] Removal of dental plaque from the teeth on a daily basis is extremely important to prevent gingivitis, which can progress to destructive periodontal disease. Most plaque removal can be achieved by conscientious tooth brushing. The use of dental floss helps to remove dental plaque from tooth surfaces that touch one another.

Most young adults have some gingivitis. Cases of gingivitis are high among Hispanics, American Indians, Alaska Natives, and adults with low incomes.[4] Cases of gingivitis likely will remain a substantial problem and may increase as tooth loss from dental caries declines or as a result of the use of some systemic medications. Although not all cases of gingivitis progress to periodontal disease, all periodontal disease starts as gingivitis.[44] The major method available to prevent destructive periodontitis, therefore, is to prevent the precursor condition of gingivitis.

Periodontal disease is manifested by the loss of the connective tissue and bone that support the teeth.[45] It places a person at risk of eventual tooth loss unless appropriate treatment occurs.[45] The presence of one or more sites with 4 mm or propriate treatment occurs.[45] The presence of one or more sites with 4 mm or greater loss of tooth attachment to surrounding periodontal tissues has been used to measure the cases of destructive periodontal disease.[45] This measure has allowed the monitoring of changes in periodontal disease over time and distinguishes the status of select populations from one another. Other measurements under development may serve as indicators of periodontal disease in the future. Among adults, destructive periodontal disease may be associated with an increased risk of some systemic disease and is a leading cause of bleeding, pain, infection, tooth mobility, and tooth loss.[21, 22, 23, 24, 25, 26]

Tobacco use, especially cigarette smoking, is a significant risk factor for periodontal disease,[27] accounting for up to half of all cases of periodontitis.[46] Home-care oral hygiene practices, such as daily tooth brushing and flossing, reduce bacterial plaque on teeth and gingiva and help maintain periodontal health. The number of cases of periodontal disease in persons with poor oral hygiene is more than 20 times that for persons who have good oral care practices.[27] Recent research has suggested that bacteria associated with periodontal disease are associated with an increased risk of heart disease and stroke, premature births in some females, and respiratory infection in susceptible individuals.[21, 22, 23, 24, 26]

The cases and severity of destructive periodontal disease are measured by loss of tissue attachment to the tooth and gingival pocket depth. These measures increase with age and vary by socioeconomic status. The number of cases of periodontal disease is higher than the national average among American Indians and Alaska Natives, adults with less than a high school education, and migrant workers.[4] Unless preventive measures are taken, the problem of destructive periodontal disease will grow as the aging U.S. population retains more teeth later in life. More effective intervention across the entire adult age spectrum will be essential.

21-6. Increase the proportion of oral and pharyngeal cancers detected at the earliest stage.

Target: 50 percent.

Baseline: 35 percent of oral and pharyngeal cancers (stage I, localized) were detected in 1990–95.

Target setting method: Better than the best.

Data source: Surveillance, Epidemiology, and End Results (SEER), NIH, NCI.

Persons With Oral and Pharyngeal Cancers, 1990–95	Detected at Earliest Stage
	Percent
TOTAL	35
Race and ethnicity	
American Indian or Alaska Native	20
Asian or Pacific Islander	DNA
Asian	DNA
Native Hawaiian and other Pacific Islander	DNA
Black or African American	21
White	38
Hispanic or Latino	36
Not Hispanic or Latino	34
Black or African American	DNA
White	DNA
Gender	
Female	39
Male	34
Education level	
Less than high school	DNA
High school graduate	DNA
At least some college	DNA
Disability status	
Persons with disabilities	DNA
Persons without disabilities	DNA

DNA = Data have not been analyzed. DNC = Data are not collected. DSU = Data are statistically unreliable.

For many years, the proportion of oral and pharyngeal cancer lesions diagnosed at stage I has remained low at about 35 percent.[16] Increasing the proportion of lesions detected at the earliest stage of diagnosis improves the 5-year survival rate and is one strategy to reduce illness and deaths.

For example, the 5-year survival rate for early stage cancer is 81 percent but is only 22 percent among persons diagnosed with advanced stage cancer. Further, only 19 percent of African Americans with oral and pharyngeal cancers are diagnosed at the local stage (with 34 percent 5-year survival), compared to 38 percent of whites (with 56 percent 5-year survival).[16]

A higher proportion of oral and pharyngeal cancer lesions diagnosed at stage I and a lower number of deaths from oral and pharyngeal cancers would indicate that strategies to increase appropriate detection with comprehensive oral and pharyngeal cancer examinations and referral have been successful. Other outcome measures indicating success include a reduction in new cases of oral and pharyngeal cancers, reduced death rates, and an increase in 5-year survival rates.

21-7. Increase the proportion of adults who, in the past 12 months, report having had an examination to detect oral and pharyngeal cancers.

Target: 20 percent.

Baseline: 13 percent of adults aged 40 years and older reported having had an oral and pharyngeal cancer examination in 1998 (age adjusted to the year 2000 standard population).

Target setting method: Better than the best.

Data source: National Health Interview Survey (NHIS), CDC, NCHS.

NOTE: THE TABLE BELOW MAY CONTINUE TO THE FOLLOWING PAGE.

Adults Aged 40 Years and Older, 1998	Oral and Pharyngeal Cancer Examination in Past 12 Months
	Percent
TOTAL	13
Race and ethnicity	
American Indian or Alaska Native	DSU
Asian or Pacific Islander	12
Asian	12
Native Hawaiian and other Pacific Islander	DSU
Black or African American	7
White	14
Hispanic or Latino	6
Not Hispanic or Latino	14
Black or African American	7
White	15
Gender	
Female	14
Male	13

Adults Aged 40 Years and Older, 1998	Oral and Pharyngeal Cancer Examination in Past 12 Months
	Percent
Education level	
Less than high school	5
High school graduate	10
At least some college	19

DNA = Data have not been analyzed. DNC = Data are not collected. DSU = Data are statistically unreliable.
Note: Data age adjusted to the year 2000 standard population.
NOTE: THE TABLE ABOVE MAY HAVE CONTINUED FROM THE PREVIOUS PAGE.

Oral cancer detection is accomplished by a thorough extra-oral examination of the head and neck and an intra-oral examination including the tongue and the entire oral and pharyngeal mucosal tissues, lips, and intra- and extra-oral palpation of the lymph nodes. Although the sensitivity and specificity of the oral cancer examination have not been established in clinical studies, evidence clearly supports a better prognosis with early detection and treatment of oral cancer.[37] If suspicious tissues are detected during examination, definitive diagnostic tests are needed, such as biopsies, to make a firm diagnosis.

The occurrence of oral and pharyngeal cancers varies by race and ethnicity. For example, blacks and whites have 12.5 and 10.0 new cases per 100,000 per year, respectively; Hispanics and American Indians and Alaska Natives have only 6.5 and 8.8 new cases per year, respectively.[3]

Regular oral cancer examinations afford an opportunity for practitioners to discuss with patients primary prevention of these lesions—that is, avoiding known risk factors, such as the use of tobacco products and alcohol. The risk of oral cancer is increased 6 to 28 times in current smokers. Alcohol consumption is an independent risk factor and, when combined with the use of tobacco products, accounts for 90 percent of all oral cancers.[47] Individuals also should be advised to avoid other potential carcinogens, such as exposure to sunlight (risk factor for lip cancer) without protection (use of lip sunscreen and hats recommended). (See Focus Area 3. Cancer.)

Because more adults seek care from physicians than from dentists, medical personnel must be educated on the importance of routinely doing oral cancer detection examinations of patients at high risk, and they also must be trained in the proper procedures for these examinations.[48]

21-8. Increase the proportion of children who have received dental sealants on their molar teeth.

Target and baseline:

Objective	Increase in Children Receiving Dental Sealants on Their Molar Teeth	1988–94 Baseline	2010 Target
		Percent	
21-8a.	Children aged 8 years	23	50
21-8b.	Adolescents aged 14 years	15	50

Target setting method: Better than the best.

Data sources: National Health and Nutrition Examination Survey (NHANES), CDC, NCHS; Oral Health Survey of Native Americans, 1999, IHS; Hawai'i Children's Oral Health Assessment, 1999, State of Hawaii Department of Health.

NOTE: THE TABLE BELOW MAY CONTINUE TO THE FOLLOWING PAGE.

Children, Selected Ages, 1988–94 (unless noted)	Dental Sealants on Molars	
	21-8a. Aged 8 Years	**21-8b. Aged 14 Years**
	Percent	
TOTAL	23	15
Race and ethnicity		
American Indian or Alaska Native	55* (1999)	42* (1999)
Asian or Pacific Islander	DSU	DSU
Asian	DNC	DNC
Native Hawaiian and other Pacific Islander	20† (1999)	DNC
Black or African American	11	5
White	26	19
Hispanic or Latino	DSU	DSU
Mexican American	10	7
Not Hispanic or Latino	25	DNA
Black or African American	11	5
White	29	18
Gender		
Female	24	14
Male	22	16

Children, Selected Ages, 1988–94 (unless noted)	Dental Sealants on Molars	
	21-8a. Aged 8 Years	21-8b. Aged 14 Years
	Percent	
Education level (head of household)		
Less than high school	17	4
High school graduate	12	6
At least some college	35	28
Disability status		
Persons with disabilities	DNC	DNC
Persons without disabilities	DNC	DNC
Select populations		
3rd grade students	26	NA

DNA = Data have not been analyzed. DNC = Data are not collected. DSU = Data are statistically unreliable. NA = Not applicable.

*Data are for IHS service areas.

†Data are for Hawaii.

NOTE: THE TABLE ABOVE MAY HAVE CONTINUED FROM THE PREVIOUS PAGE.

Since the early 1970s, childhood dental caries in smooth tooth surfaces (those without pits and fissures) has declined markedly because of widespread exposure to fluorides. By 1986–87, approximately 90 percent of the decay in children's teeth occurred in tooth surfaces with pits and fissures, and almost two-thirds were found in the chewing surfaces alone.[31]

Pit-and-fissure sealants—plastic coatings applied to susceptible tooth surfaces—have been approved for use for many years and have been recommended by professional health associations and public health agencies. First permanent molars erupt into the mouth at about age 6 years. Placing sealants on these teeth shortly after their eruption protects them from the development of caries in areas of the teeth where food and bacteria are retained. If sealants were applied routinely to susceptible tooth surfaces in conjunction with the appropriate use of fluoride, most tooth decay in children could be prevented.[49]

Second permanent molars erupt into the mouth at about age 12 to 13 years. Pit-and-fissure surfaces of these teeth are as susceptible to dental caries as the first permanent molars of younger children. Therefore, young teens need to receive dental sealants shortly after the eruption of their second permanent molars.

21-9. Increase the proportion of the U.S. population served by community water systems with optimally fluoridated water.

Target: 75 percent.

Baseline: 62 percent of the U.S. population was served by community water systems with optimally fluoridated water in 1992.

Target setting method: 21 percent improvement.

Data source: CDC Fluoridation Census, CDC, NCCDPHP.

> Data for population groups currently are not collected.

Community water fluoridation is the procedure of adjusting the natural fluoride concentration of a community's water supply to a level that is best for the prevention of dental decay. In the United States, community water fluoridation has been the basis for the primary prevention of dental decay for nearly 55 years and has been recognized as 1 of 10 great achievements in public health of the 20th century.[50] It is an ideal public health method because it is effective, eminently safe, inexpensive, requires no cooperative effort or direct action, and does not depend on access or availability of professional services. It is equitable because the entire population benefits regardless of financial resources.[33]

Water fluoridation reduces or eliminates disparities in preventing dental caries among different socioeconomic, racial, and ethnic groups. Fluoridation helps to lower the cost of dental care and dental insurance and helps residents retain their teeth throughout life. Of the Nation's 50 largest cities, only 7 do not benefit from community water fluoridation.[33] The consumption of fluoridated water provides both systemic fluoride exposure to developing teeth and frequent topical exposure to erupted teeth, promoting remineralization of early caries among persons of all ages.

Operators of municipal water plants need to maintain targeted concentrations of fluoride in water in fluoridated communities. Ongoing education for water plant personnel must continue with appropriate surveillance by State and local health officials.

21-10. Increase the proportion of children and adults who use the oral health care system each year.

Target: 56 percent.

Baseline: 44 percent of persons aged 2 years and older in 1996 visited a dentist during the previous year.

Target setting method: Better than the best.

Data source: Medical Expenditure Panel Survey (MEPS), AHRQ.

Persons Aged 2 Years and Older, 1996	Dental Visit in Previous Year
	Percent
TOTAL	44
Race and ethnicity	
American Indian or Alaska Native	34
Asian or Pacific Islander	42
Asian	DSU
Native Hawaiian and other Pacific Islander	DSU
Black or African American	27
White	47
Hispanic or Latino	30
Not Hispanic or Latino	DNC
Black or African American	27
White	50
Gender	
Female	47
Male	41
Education level (aged 25 years and older)	
Less than high school	24
High school graduate	40
At least some college	55
Disability status	
Persons with disabilities	40
Persons without disabilities	45
Select populations	
Children aged 2 to 17 years	48
Children at first school experience (aged 5 years)	48
3rd grade students	DNC
Children, adolescents, and young adults aged 2 to 19 years; <200 percent of poverty level	20
Adults aged 18 years and older	43
Adults aged 65 years and older	41

Persons Aged 2 Years and Older, 1996	Dental Visit in Previous Year
	Percent
Dentate adults aged 18 years and older	DNC
Edentate adults aged 18 years and older	DNC
Adults aged 18 years and older with disabilities	DNC

DNA = Data have not been analyzed. DNC = Data are not collected. DSU = Data are statistically unreliable.

NOTE: THE TABLE ABOVE MAY HAVE CONTINUED FROM THE PREVIOUS PAGE.

Although appropriate home oral health care and population-based prevention are essential, professional care also is necessary to maintain optimal oral and craniofacial health. Oral health care is an important, but often neglected, component of total health care. Regular dental visits provide an opportunity for the early diagnosis, prevention, and treatment of oral and craniofacial diseases and conditions for persons of all ages, as well as for the assessment of self-care practices. Experts recommend that children as young as age 1 year be examined for evidence of developing ECC.[11] Further, parents should be advised to avoid feeding practices that may lead to ECC, and parents should be counseled about the appropriate use of fluoride and other preventive measures. Necessary tooth restorative care must be provided to avoid pain, abscesses, and the need for tooth extractions. Sealants should be placed shortly after the permanent molars erupt.

Adults who do not receive regular professional care can develop oral diseases that eventually require complex restorative treatment and may lead to tooth loss, systemic health problems, and even death in rare cases. As gums recede in adults, the root surfaces of teeth become susceptible to dental caries. As the U.S. population ages, root caries may become a significant dental problem for adults and, particularly, for seniors; one in every five persons will be aged 65 years or older by the year 2010. Adults susceptible to root caries should visit their dentists regularly for evaluation and treatment, if necessary.

Persons who have lost all their natural teeth are less likely to seek periodic dental care than those with teeth,[6] which, in turn, decreases the likelihood of early detection of oral cancer in those without teeth. Edentulism occurs most frequently among older adults who also have the greatest risk of developing oral cancer.

Persons with no natural teeth who lack regular dental care may develop soft tissue lesions from medications, systemic conditions, and exposure to tobacco, as well as from prosthetic appliances that are not fully functional or are not maintained properly. As they grow older, persons with and without teeth are at increased risk of oral and pharyngeal cancers, as well as autoimmune disorders and other chronic disabling conditions that have oral manifestations. People without teeth may be unaware that they are still at risk for oral diseases. Consequently, they may have long intervals between professional examinations. Coordination of care between physicians and dentists is essential for optimal general health and oral health.

21-11. Increase the proportion of long-term care residents who use the oral health care system each year.

Target: 25 percent.

Baseline: 19 percent of all nursing home residents received dental services in 1997.

Target setting method: 32 percent improvement. (Better than the best will be used when data are available.)

Data source: National Nursing Home Survey, CDC, NCHS.

> **Data for population groups currently are not analyzed.**

To improve the oral health of the Nation's elderly persons and persons with disabilities who reside in long-term care facilities, every resident needs to have access to oral health assessment and treatment. Federal regulations require nursing facilities certified under Medicare or Medicaid or both to ensure that each resident attains and maintains the highest practicable physical, psychosocial, and mental well-being.

For many nursing home residents, substantial anecdotal evidence suggests that neither dental assessments nor subsequent treatments are being provided effectively. Nursing home staff members and State surveyors who assess long-term care facilities for certification should receive appropriate training to enable them to recognize residents' needs correctly and to ensure that necessary oral health services are available.

Residents of institutions face several barriers to obtaining needed dental services. Often, residents have multiple chronic diseases, take medications that affect their oral health, or have diseases or disabilities that make brushing and flossing their teeth difficult or impossible.[51] A decline in physical and oral health, use of one or more of the many medications that cause dry mouth (xerostomia), and inadequate access to dental care increase the risks of oral diseases such as yeast infections (candidiasis), caries on the crowns and roots of teeth, gingivitis, oral mucosal lesions, and periodontal disease.

21-12. Increase the proportion of low-income children and adolescents who received any preventive dental service during the past year.

Target: 57 percent.

Baseline: 20 percent of children and adolescents under age 19 years at or below 200 percent of the Federal poverty level received any preventive dental service in 1996.

Target setting method: Better than the best.

Data source: Medical Expenditure Panel Survey (MEPS), AHRQ.

Children Under Age 19 Years at or Below 200 Percent of the Federal Poverty Level, 1996	Preventive Dental Visit in Past 12 Months
	Percent
TOTAL	20
Race and ethnicity	
American Indian or Alaska Native	DSU
Asian or Pacific Islander	DSU
Asian	DNC
Native Hawaiian and other Pacific Islander	DNC
Black or African American	13
White	25
Hispanic or Latino	16
Not Hispanic or Latino	DNA
Black or African American	DNA
White	DNA
Gender	
Female	21
Male	19

DNA = Data have not been analyzed. DNC = Data are not collected. DSU = Data are statistically unreliable.

Public policymakers have long recognized the need for programs to facilitate access to dental services for children from low-income households. Coverage for pediatric dental services has been required under Medicaid for more than two decades and is allowed, although not required, under the new State Children's Health Insurance Program, also known as SCHIP.[52]

Despite the potential for improved oral health status, only about 20 percent of Medicaid children were reported to have received any preventive dental services in 1993.[39] Current research also indicates that children from low-income households have higher caries rates and more unmet dental treatment needs than their higher income counterparts.[12]

21-13. (Developmental) Increase the proportion of school-based health centers with an oral health component.

Potential data source: School Health Policies and Programs Study (SHPPS), CDC, NCCDPHP.

In some rural areas and urban neighborhoods, where health and social problems are concentrated and few residents have health insurance or the personal means to pay for private health care, most children do not receive timely preventive procedures.[39] The burden of untreated caries falls heaviest on children from low-income families.[12, 29] Moreover, disparities in oral health status and the use of dental services persist among certain ethnic and racial groups.[6]

Increasingly, schools are being viewed as an effective way to improve access to health and social support services for vulnerable populations. Parents give permission for health center staff members to oversee the provision of health education and preventive and treatment services. School-affiliated strategies mobilize existing community resources to create referral networks for students and provide services in the school when appropriate, based on community needs, resources, standards, and requirements.[53] Few school-based health centers include an oral health component. School-based oral health services could enable the targeting of preventive services such as fluoride mouth rinses or tablets and dental sealants to underserved, low-income children. Services also could include screening, referral, and case management to ensure the timely receipt of treatment services from community practitioners. School-based health centers should have oral health services and educational materials that are culturally and linguistically appropriate.

Multiple models for school-based health centers are in place. They typically are funded from a mix of sources, both public and private. School-based health centers have been increasing in numbers nationwide. The number of school-based health centers nationally was estimated to be 1,157 in 1997–98; the proportion with a dental component, however, is thought to be low.[54]

21-14. Increase the proportion of local health departments and community-based health centers, including community, migrant, and homeless health centers, that have an oral health component.

Target: 75 percent.

Baseline: 34 percent of local jurisdictions and health centers had oral health components in 1997.

Target setting method: 19 percent improvement.

Data source: HRSA, Bureau of Primary Health Care (BPHC).

Although dentists donate more services than do physicians to individuals who cannot afford care,[55] persons who cannot afford routine dental care and who are not covered either by public programs or by private dental insurance often do not receive basic dental services. Access to care for children and adults continues to be a problem for many, particularly for economically disadvantaged populations.[29]

To eliminate disparities in the provision of health care, more opportunities for preventive and restorative dental services must be provided in areas where need is demonstrated. Some local health departments promote community-based preventive services and provide dental services to children and to some adults; most local health departments lack a dental component.[56] Other sources of health care are community, migrant, or homeless health centers, which are located in approximately 700 areas where a need has been documented. By the late 1990s, nearly 60 percent of community-based health centers had a dental component.[57] These centers, which strive to ensure that health education programs and oral health staff members are culturally competent and linguistically appropriate, extend dental care to groups that traditionally have limited access to dental services.

The need is great among many populations in the United States. These centers serve primarily certain racial and ethnic populations, who are more likely than whites to live or work in medically and dentally underserved areas. Rural and low-income urban select population communities are more likely to have a shortage of health care providers. More health care providers from certain racial and ethnic groups are needed because they are more likely than white health care providers to treat Medicaid or uninsured patients.[52, 58, 59, 60, 61]

21-15. Increase the number of States and the District of Columbia that have a system for recording and referring infants and children with cleft lips, cleft palates, and other craniofacial anomalies to craniofacial anomaly rehabilitative teams.

Target: All States and the District of Columbia.

Baseline: 23 States and the District of Columbia had systems for recording and referring children with craniofacial anomalies in 1997.

Target setting method: Total coverage.

Data source: Survey of State Dental Directors, Illinois State Health Department.

States should have an effective mechanism in place for identifying, recording, and referring for treatment infants with cleft lips or cleft palates or both. Cleft lip and cleft palate are reported in about 1 of 1,000 live births, and isolated cleft palate is reported in about 0.5 of 1,000 live births, making these three conditions among the most common birth defects.[19, 20]

Physicians and nurses in hospital nurseries are usually the first to examine newborns and are responsible for noting any congenital anomalies and describing them on the neonatal medical records. Therefore, hospital personnel must understand the definitions of congenital defects and abnormalities of the lips and palate, properly examine newborns, and correctly record any malformations.

Proper diagnosis is important because newborns with cleft lip or cleft palate should be referred immediately to an interdisciplinary core craniofacial team to assess these infants and to counsel the parents prior to discharge. Sending infants home without comprehensive instructions for their parents or caregivers can seriously compromise the health of the infants. Therefore, children need to be enrolled in a system that provides for continuity of care.[62] Surgical repair of the lips often is performed soon after birth, repair of the palate usually should be performed before age 18 months.[63] Appropriate intervention will minimize the extent to which physical and psychosocial trauma adversely affect child development.

21-16. Increase the number of States and the District of Columbia that have an oral and craniofacial health surveillance system.

Target: All States and the District of Columbia.

Baseline: No States or the District of Columbia had oral and craniofacial health surveillance systems in 1999.

Target setting method: Total coverage.

Data source: Association of State and Territorial Dental Directors.

State and local dental programs have been hampered severely in carrying out their programmatic activities to improve health because of a lack of State-specific oral health data.[56] The existence of surveillance systems within States to assess oral health needs is essential for determining trends in oral diseases, implementing and evaluating interventions, and identifying where resources are required to improve oral health status. Surveillance systems are not just data collection systems, but involve at least (1) a timely communication of findings to responsible parties and to the public and (2) the use of data to initiate and evaluate public health measures to prevent and control diseases and conditions.[64] An oral health surveillance system for a State should contain, at a minimum, a core set of measures that describe the status of important oral health conditions to serve as benchmarks for assessing progress in achieving good oral health.

21-17. (Developmental) Increase the number of Tribal, State (including the District of Columbia), and local health agencies that serve jurisdictions of 250,000 or more persons that have in place an effective public dental health program directed by a dental professional with public health training.

Potential data sources: Association of State and Territorial Dental Directors; IHS.

The ability to improve the health and quality of life for communities and individuals relies on population-based preventive programs and the public and private capacity to provide needed care. The capability to provide services depends on an adequate infrastructure at the Tribal, State, and local health department level. This infrastructure is seriously compromised; for example, in 1999 only 29 States had full-time State dental directors, 14 States had part-time directors, and 8 States had no director. Dental professionals in leadership positions who have public health training are needed in Tribal, State, and local health departments to implement necessary oral health programs. A survey found that two-thirds of 243 local health departments serving nearly 80 million persons in the United States in 1995 reported having a dental program, of which 62 percent were directed by dentists and 22 percent by dental hygienists; the other 16 percent were directed by nondental personnel. The level of public health training of these persons was not assessed.[56]

Related Objectives From Other Focus Areas

1. **Access to Quality Health Services**
   - 1-1.   Persons with health insurance
   - 1-2.   Health insurance coverage for clinical preventive services
   - 1-3.   Counseling about health behaviors
   - 1-4.   Source of ongoing care
   - 1-7.   Core competencies in health provider training
   - 1-8.   Racial and ethnic representation in health professions
   - 1-15. Long-term care services
2. **Arthritis, Osteopororsis, and Chronic Back Conditions**
   - 2-2.   Activity limitations due to arthritis
   - 2-3.   Personal care limitations
   - 2-7.   Seeing a health care provider
   - 2-8.   Arthritis education
3. **Cancer**
   - 3-1.   Overall cancer deaths
   - 3-6.   Oropharyngeal cancer deaths
   - 3-9.   Sun exposure and skin cancer
   - 3-10. Provider counseling about cancer prevention
   - 3-14. Statewide cancer registries
   - 3-15. Cancer survival
5. **Diabetes**
   - 5-1.   Diabetes education
   - 5-2.   New cases of diabetes
   - 5-3.   Overall cases of diagnosed diabetes
   - 5-4.   Diagnosis of diabetes
   - 5-15. Annual dental examinations
6. **Disability and Secondary Conditions**
   - 6-13. Surveillance and health promotion programs
7. **Educational and Community-Based Programs**
   - 7-1.   High school completion
   - 7-2.   School health education
   - 7-3.   Health-risk behavior information for college and university students
   - 7-4.   School nurse-to-student ratio
   - 7-5.   Worksite health promotion programs
   - 7-6.   Participation in employer-sponsored health promotion activities
   - 7-7.   Patient and family education
   - 7-10. Community health promotion programs
   - 7-11. Culturally appropriate and linguistically competent community health promotion programs
   - 7-12. Older adult participation in community health promotion activities

8. **Environmental Health**
   8-5.   Safe drinking water
11. **Health Communication**
   11-1. Households with Internet access
   11-2. Health literacy
   11-3. Research and evaluation of communication programs
   11-4. Quality of Internet health information sources
   11-6. Satisfaction with health care providers' communication skills
12. **Heart Disease and Stroke**
   12-1. Coronary heart disease (CHD) deaths
14. **Immunization and Infectious Diseases**
   14-3. Hepatitis B in adults and high-risk groups
   14-9. Hepatitis C
   14-10. Identification of persons with chronic hepatitis C
   14-28. Hepatitis B vaccination among high-risk groups
15. **Injury and Violence Prevention**
   15-1. Nonfatal head injuries
   15-17. Nonfatal motor vehicle injuries
   15-19. Safety belts
   15-20. Child restraints
   15-21. Motorcycle helmet use
   15-23. Bicycle helmet use
   15-24. Bicycle helmet laws
   15-31. Injury protection in school sports
16. **Maternal, Infant, and Child Health**
   16-6. Prenatal care
   16-8. Very low birth weight infants born at level III hospitals
   16-10. Low birth weight and very low birth weight
   16-11. Preterm births
   16-16. Optimum folic acid levels
   16-19. Breastfeeding
   16-23. Service systems for children with special health care needs
17. **Medical Product Safety**
   17-3. Provider review of medications taken by patients
   17-4. Receipt of useful information about prescriptions from pharmacies
   17-5. Receipt of oral counseling about medications from prescribers and
          dispensers
18. **Mental Health and Mental Disorders**
   18-5. Eating disorder relapses
19. **Nutrition and Overweight**
   19-1. Healthy weight in adults
   19-2. Obesity in adults
   19-3. Overweight or obesity in children and adolescents
   19-5. Fruit intake
   19-6. Vegetable intake
   19-11. Calcium intake
   19-15. Meals and snacks at school
   19-16. Worksite promotion of nutrition education and weight management

20. Occupational Safety and Health
    20-2. Work-related injuries
    20-3. Overexertion or repetitive motion
    20-10. Needlestick injuries

22. Physical Activity and Fitness
    22-4. Muscular strength and endurance
    22-5. Flexibility

23. Public Health Infrastructure
    23-1. Public health employee access to the Internet
    23-2. Public access to information and surveillance data
    23-3. Use of geocoding in health data systems
    23-4. Data for all population groups
    23-6. National tracking of Healthy People 2010 objectives
    23-7. Timely release of data on objectives
    23-8. Competencies for public health workers
    23-9. Training in essential public health services
    23-10. Continuing education and training by public health agencies
    23-11. Performance standards for essential public health services
    23-12. Health improvement plans
    23.13. Access to public health laboratory services
    23-14. Access to epidemiology services
    23-16. Data on public health expenditures
    23-17. Population-based prevention research

25. Sexually Transmitted Diseases
    25-5. Human papillomavirus infection

26. Substance Abuse
    26-12. Average annual alcohol consumption

27. Tobacco Use
    27-1. Adult tobacco use
    27-2. Adolescent tobacco use
    27-3. Initiation of tobacco use
    27-4. Age at first tobacco use
    27-5. Smoking cessation by adults
    27-7. Smoking cessation by adolescents
    27-8. Insurance coverage of cessation treatment
    27-11. Smoke-free and tobacco-free schools
    27-12. Worksite smoking policies
    27-14. Enforcement of illegal tobacco sales to minors laws
    27-15. Retail license suspension for sales to minors
    27-18. Tobacco control programs
    27-19. Preemptive tobacco control laws
    27-20. Tobacco product regulation
    27-21. Tobacco tax

Terminology

(A listing of abbreviations and acronyms used in this publication appears in Appendix H.)

Candidiasis (oral): Yeast or fungal infection that occurs in the oral cavity or pharynx or both.

Cleft lip or palate: A congenital opening or fissure occurring in the lip or palate.

Congenital anomaly: An unusual condition existing at, and usually before, birth.

Craniofacial: Pertaining to the head and face.

Dental caries (dental decay or cavities): An infectious disease that results in demineralization and ultimately cavitation of the tooth surface if not controlled or remineralized. Dental cavities may be either treated (filled) or untreated (unfilled).

Caries experience: The sum of filled and unfilled cavities, along with any missing teeth resulting from decay.

> **Early childhood caries (ECC):** Dental decay of the primary teeth of infants and young children (aged 1 to 5 years) often characterized by rapid destruction.

> **Root caries:** Dental decay that occurs on the root portion of a tooth. (In younger persons, root surfaces are usually covered by gum [gingival] tissue.)

Dentate: A condition characterized by having one or more natural teeth.

Edentulism/edentulous: A condition characterized by not having any natural teeth.

Endocarditis: Inflammation of the lining of the heart.

Fluoride: A compound of the element fluorine. Fluorine, the 13th most abundant element in nature, is used in a variety of ways to reduce dental decay.

Gingivitis: An inflammatory condition of the gum tissue, which can appear reddened and swollen and frequently bleeds easily.

Oral cavity: Mouth.

Oral health literacy: Based on the definition of health literacy,[65] the degree to which individuals have the capacity to obtain, process, and understand basic oral and craniofacial health information and services needed to make appropriate health decisions.

Periodontal disease: A cluster of diseases caused by bacterial infections and resulting in inflammatory responses and chronic destruction of the soft tissues and bone that support the teeth. Periodontal disease is a broad term encompassing several diseases of the gums and tissues supporting the teeth.

Pharynx: Throat.

Sealants: Plastic coatings applied to the surfaces of teeth with developmental pits and grooves (primarily chewing surfaces) to protect the tooth surfaces from collecting food, debris, and bacteria that promote the development of dental decay.

Soft tissue lesion: An abnormality of the soft tissues of the oral cavity or pharynx.

Squamous cell carcinoma: A type of cancer that occurs in tissues that line major organs.

Xerostomia: A condition in which the mouth is dry because of a lack of saliva.

References

[1] U.S. Department of Health and Human Services (HHS). *Oral Health in America: A Report of the Surgeon General*. Rockville, MD: HHS, National Institutes of Health, National Institute of Dental and Craniofacial Research, 2000.

[2] Reisine, S., and Locker, D. Social, psychological, and economic impacts of oral conditions and treatments. In: Cohen, L.K., and Gift, H.C., (eds.). *Disease Prevention and Oral Health Promotion: Socio-Dental Sciences in Action*. Copenhagen: Munksgaard and la Fédération Dentaire Internationale, 1995, 33-71.

[3] Landis, S.H.; Murray, T.; Bolden, S.; et al. Cancer statistics, 1999. *CA—A Cancer Journal for Clinicians* 49:8-31, 1999.

[4] White, B.A.; Weintraub, J.A.; Caplan, D.J.; et al. Toward improving the oral health of Americans: An overview of oral health status, resources, and care delivery. *Public Health Reports* 108:657-872, 1993.

[5] Riley, III, J.W.; Gilbert, G.H.; and Heft, M.W. Orofacial pain symptom prevalence: Selected sex differences in the elderly. *Pain* 76:97-104, 1998.

[6] National Center for Health Statistics (NCHS). *National Health and Nutrition Examination Survey III, 1988–1994*. Hyattsville, MD: Centers for Disease Control and Prevention (CDC), unpublished data.

[7] Ismail, A.I., and Sohn, W.A. A systematic review of clinical diagnostic criteria of early childhood caries. *Journal of Public Health Dentistry* 59(3):171-191, 1999.

[8] Milnes, A.R. Description and epidemiology of nursing caries. *Journal of Public Health Dentistry* 56:38-50, 1996.

[9] Horowitz, H.S. Research issues in early childhood caries. *Community Dentistry and Oral Epidemiology* 26(Suppl. 1):67-81, 1998.

[10] Reisine, S., and Douglass, J.M. Psychosocial and behavioral issues in early childhood caries. *Community Dentistry and Oral Epidemiology 26*:(Suppl. 1):32-34, 1998.

[11] American Academy of Pediatric Dentistry. *Handbook of Pediatric Dentistry*. Chicago, IL: the Academy, 1999.

[12] Vargas, C.M.; Crall, J.J.; and Schneider, D.A. Sociodemographic distribution of pediatric dental caries: NHANES III, 1988–1994. *Journal of the American Dental Association* 129:1229-1238, 1998.

[13] Kaste, L.S.; Selwitz, R.H.; Oldakowski, R.J.; et al. Coronal caries in the primary and permanent dentition of children and adolescents 1-17 years of age: United States, 1988–1991. *Journal of Dental Research* 75:631-641, 1996.

[14] National Institute of Dental Research. *Oral Health of United States. Adults: The National Survey of Oral Health in U.S. Employed Adults and Seniors: 1985–1986*. NIH Pub. No. 87-2868. Bethesda, MD: National Institutes of Health (NIH), 1986.

[15] Greenlee, R.T.; Murray, T.; Bolden, S.; et al. Cancer statistics, 2000. *CA—Cancer Journal for Clinicians* 50:7-33, 2000.

[16] NIH. *SEER Cancer Statistics Review 1973–1996*. Bethesda, MD, 1999 National Cancer Institute, NIH. <http://www.seer.ims.nci.nih.gov/Publications/CSR1973_1996> June 15, 1999.

[17] CDC, NCHS. National Health Interview Survey, 1998, unpublished data.

[18] Horowitz, A.M., and Nourjah, P.A. Patterns of screening for oral cancer among U.S. adults. *Journal of Public Health Dentistry* 56:331-335, 1996.

[19] Slavkin, H.C. Meeting the challenges of craniofacial-oral-dental birth defects. *Journal of the American Dental Association* 127:126-137, 1998.

[20] Tolarova, M., and Cervenka, J. Classification and birth prevalence of orofacial clefts. *American Journal of Medical Genetics* 75:126-137, 1998.

[21] Dasanayake, A.P. Poor periodontal health of the pregnant woman as a risk factor for low birth weight. *Annals of Periodontology* 3:206-211, 1998.

[22] Offenbacher, S.; Katz, V.; Fertik, G.; et al. Periodontal infection as a possible risk factor for preterm low birth weight. *Annals of Periodontology* 67(Suppl. 10):1103-1113, 1995.

[23] Davenport, E.S.; Williams, C.E.; Sterne, J.A.; et al. The East London study of maternal chronic periodontal disease and preterm low birth weight infants: Study design and prevalence data. *Annals of Periodontology* 3:213-221, 1998.

[24] Beck, J.D.; Offenbacher, S.; Williams, R.; et al. Periodontitis: A risk factor for coronary heart disease? *Annals of Periodontology* 3:127-141, 1998.

[25] Genco, R.J. Periodontal disease and risk for myocardial infarction and cardiovascular disease. *Cardiovascular Reviews and Reports* 19:34-40, 1998.

[26] Slavkin, H.C. Does the mouth put the heart at risk? *Journal of the American Dental Association* 130:109-113, 1999.

[27] Genco, R.J. Current view of risk factors for periodontal diseases. *Journal of Periodontology* 67(Suppl.):1041-1049, 1996.

[28] Dajani, A.S.; Taubert, K.A.; Wilson, W.; et al. Prevention of bacterial endocarditis: Recommendations by the American Heart Association. *Journal of the American Dental Association* 128:1142-1151, 1997.

[29] U.S. General Accounting Office (GAO). *Report of Congressional Requestors. Oral Health in Low-Income Populations.* GAO/HEHS-00-72. Washington, DC: GAO, 2000.

[30] American Dental Association (ADA). *Survey on Pre-Doctoral Dental Education Institutions, 1996–1997: Volume I, Academic Programs Enrollment and Graduates.* Chicago, IL: the Association, May 1997.

[31] Burt, B.A. Trends in caries prevalence in North American children. *International Dental Journal* 44(4 Suppl. 1):403-413, 1994.

[32] NCHS. *Healthy People 2000 Review, 1998–99.* Hyattsville, MD: Public Health Service, 1998.

[33] Hinman, A.R.; Sterritt, G.R.; and Reeves, T.R. The U.S. experience with fluoridation. *Community Dental Health* 13(Suppl. 2):5-9, 1996.

[34] CDC, NCHS. National Health Interview Survey, 1995; data tabulated by the Office of Analysis, Epidemiology, and Health Promotion, NCHS, CDC, 1999.

[35] CDC. National Health Interview Survey 1997. Unpublished data. Hyattsville, MD: CDC.

[36] Agency for Healthcare Research and Quality (AHRQ). Medical Expenditure Panel Survey (MEPS), unpublished data, 1996.

[37] Horowitz, A.M.; Goodman, H.S.; Yellowitz, J.A.; et al. The need for health promotion in oral cancer prevention and early detection. *Journal of Public Health Dentistry* 56:319-330, 1996.

[38] ADA, CDC, and NIH. *Proceedings: National Strategic Planning Conference for the Prevention and Control of Oral and Pharyngeal Cancer.* Atlanta, GA: CDC, 1997.

[39] U.S. Department of Health and Human Services, Office of Inspector General. *Children's Dental Services Under Medicaid: Access and Utilization.* Pub. No. OEI-09-93-00240. Washington, DC: the Agency, 1996. <http://www.dhhs.gov/progorg/oei/reports/a10.pdf>November 23, 1999.

[40] Eklund, S.A., and Burt, B.A. Risk factors for total tooth loss in the United States: Longitudinal analysis of national data. *Journal of Public Dentistry* 54:5-14, 1994.

[41] Burt, B.A., and Eklund, S.A. *Dentistry, Dental Practice, and the Community.* 5th ed. Philadelphia, PA: W.B. Saunders Co., 1999, 205-206.

[42] CDC. Total tooth loss among persons aged $\geq$ 65 years—selected States, 1995-97. *Morbidity and Mortality Weekly Report* 48:206-210, 1999.

[43] Consensus report on periodontal diseases: Epidemiology and diagnosis. *Annals of Periodontology* 1:216-222, 1996.

[44] Burt, B.A., and Eklund, S.A. *Dentistry, Dental Practice, and the Community.* 5th ed. Philadelphia, PA: W.B. Saunders Co., 1999, 237-238.

[45] Burt, B.A., and Eklund, S.A. *Dentistry, Dental Practice, and the Community.* 5th ed. Philadelphia, PA: W.B. Saunders Co., 1999, 237-258.

[46] Tomar, S.L., and Asma, S. Smoking-attributable periodontitis in the United States: Findings from NHANES III. *Journal of Periodontology* 71:743-751, 2000.

[47] Silverman, S. *Oral Cancer.* 4th ed. Hamilton, Ontario, Canada: American Cancer Society, B.C. Decker, Inc., 1998.

[48] Goodman, H.S.; Yellowitz, J.A.; and Horowitz, A.M. Oral cancer prevention: The role of family practitioners. *Archives of Family Medicine* 4:628-636, 1995.

[49] Proceedings. NIH Consensus Development Conference: Dental Sealants in the Prevention of Tooth Decay. *Journal of Dental Education* 48(2) (Suppl.), 1984.

[50] CDC. Fluoridation of drinking water to prevent dental caries. *Morbidity and Mortality Weekly Report* 48(41):933-940, 1999.

[51] Dey, A.N. Characteristics of elderly nursing home residents: Data from the 1995 nursing home surveys. *Advance Data* 289, July 2, 1997.

[52] Isman, R., and Isman, B. *Oral Health America White Paper: Access to Oral Health Services in the United States—1997 and Beyond.* Chicago, IL: Oral Health America, December 1997.

[53] Institute of Medicine, Committee on Comprehensive School Health Programs, Division of Health Sciences Policy. Allensworth, D.; Lawson, E.; Nicholson, L.; et al.; eds. *Schools and Health.* Washington, DC: National Academic Press, 1997.

[54] School of Public Health and Health Services, George Washington University. *Making the Grade: National Survey of State School-Based Health Centers Initiatives School Year 1997–98.* Washington, DC: University. <http://www.gwu.edu/~mtg/sbhc/98summ.html>January 29, 1999.

[55] Manski, R.J.; Moeller, J.F.; and Maas, W.R. Health expenditures: A comparison between dental expenditures and office-based medical expenditures, 1987. *Journal of the American Dental Association* 5:659-666, 1999.

[56] Lockwood, S.A. Characterization of dental programs administered by U.S. city/county health departments, 1995. Presented before the annual session of the American Association for Public Health Dentistry in Washington, DC, October 15, 1997.

[57] Community and Migrant Health Centers Dental Program. Q&A, Bases of Primary Health Care. Washington, DC: HHS, March 1998.

[58] Brown, L.J., and Lazar, V. Minority dentists: Why do we need them? In: *Closing the Gap.* U.S. Government Printing Office No: 1999-721-913/94337. Washington, DC: Office of Minority Health, 1999.

[59] Montoya, R.; Hayes-Bautista, D.; Gonzales, L.; et al. Minority dental school graduates: Do they serve minority communities? *American Journal of Public Health* 68(10):1017-1019, 1978.

[60] Spasik, S., and Holt, K., eds. Building Partnerships to Improve Children's Access to Medicaid Oral Health Services: National Conference Proceedings. Arlington, VA: National Center for Education in Maternal and Child Health, 1999.

[61] HHS, Health Resources and Services Administration. *Health Care Rx: Access for All. The President's Initiative on Race.* Rockville, MD: HHS, 1998.

[62] Tindund, R.S., and Holmefjord, A. Functional results with team care of cleft lip and palate patients in Bergen, Norway. *Folia Phoniatrica et Logopedica* 49:168-176, 1997.

[63] American Cleft Palate-Craniofacial Association. Parameters for the evaluation and treatment of patients with cleft lip/palate or other craniofacial anomalies. *Cleft Palate-Craniofacial Journal* 30(Suppl. 1):58, 1993.

[64] Teutsch, S.M., and Churchill, R.E., eds. *Principles and Practice of Public Health Surveillance.* New York, NY: Oxford University Press, 1994.

[65] HHS, NIH, National Library of Medicine (NLM). Selden, C.R.; Zorn, M.; Ratzan, S.; et al.; eds. *Health Literacy, January 1990 Through October 1999.* NLM Pub. No. CBM2000-1, February 2000, vi.

22

Physical Activity and Fitness

Co-Lead Agencies: Centers for Disease Control and Prevention
President's Council on Physical Fitness and Sports

Contents

Goal

Improve health, fitness, and quality of life through daily physical activity.

Overview

The 1990s brought a historic new perspective to exercise, fitness, and physical activity by shifting the focus from intensive vigorous exercise to a broader range of health-enhancing physical activities. Research has demonstrated that virtually all individuals will benefit from regular physical activity.[1] A Surgeon General's report on physical activity and health concluded that moderate physical activity can reduce substantially the risk of developing or dying from heart disease, diabetes, colon cancer, and high blood pressure.[1] Physical activity also may protect against lower back pain and some forms of cancer (for example, breast cancer), but the evidence is not yet conclusive.[2, 3]

Issues and Trends

On average, physically active people outlive those who are inactive.[4, 5, 6, 7, 8] Regular physical activity also helps to maintain the functional independence of older adults and enhances the quality of life for people of all ages.[9, 10, 11]

The role of physical activity in preventing coronary heart disease (CHD) is of particular importance, given that CHD is the leading cause of death and disability in the United States. Physically inactive people are almost twice as likely to develop CHD as persons who engage in regular physical activity. The risk posed by physical inactivity is almost as high as several well-known CHD risk factors, such as cigarette smoking, high blood pressure, and high blood cholesterol. Physical inactivity, though, is more prevalent than any one of these other risk factors. People with other risk factors for CHD, such as obesity and high blood pressure, may particularly benefit from physical activity.

Regular physical activity is especially important for people who have joint or bone problems and has been shown to improve muscle function, cardiovascular function, and physical performance.[12] However, people with arthritis (20 percent of the adult population) are less active than those without arthritis.[13] People with osteoporosis, a chronic condition affecting more than 25 million people in the United States, may respond positively to regular physical activity, particularly weight-bearing activities, such as walking,[14] and especially when combined with appropriate drug therapy and calcium intake. Increased bone mineral density has been positively associated with aerobic fitness, body composition, and muscular strength.[15]

Although vigorous physical activity is recommended for improved cardiorespiratory fitness, increasing evidence suggests that moderate physical activity also can have significant health benefits, including a decreased risk of CHD. For people who are inactive, even small increases in physical activity are associated with measurable health benefits. In addition, moderate physical activity is more readily adopted and maintained than vigorous physical activity.[16] As research continues to illustrate the links between physical activity and selected health outcomes, people will be able to choose physical activity patterns optimally suited to individual preferences, health risks, and physiologic benefits.

For individuals who do not engage in any physical activity during their leisure time, taking the first step toward developing a pattern of regular physical activity is important. Unfortunately, few individuals engage in regular physical activity despite its documented benefits. Only about 23 percent of adults in the United States report regular, vigorous physical activity that involves large muscle groups in dynamic movement for 20 minutes or longer 3 or more days per week. Only 15 percent of adults report physical activity for 5 or more days per week for 30 minutes or longer, and another 40 percent do not participate in any regular physical activity.

Public education efforts need to address the specific barriers that inhibit the adoption and maintenance of physical activity by different population groups. Older adults, for example, need information about safe walking routes. Persons with foot problems need to learn about proper foot care and footwear in order to reach appropriate activity levels. People with CHD and other chronic conditions must understand the importance of regular physical activity to maintain physical function. Each person should recognize that starting out slowly with an activity that is enjoyable and gradually increasing the frequency and duration of the activity are central to the adoption and maintenance of physical activity behavior. Along with the public education efforts, public programs in a variety of settings (recreation centers, worksites, health care settings, and schools) need to be developed, evaluated, and shared as potential models. The availability of group activities in the community is important for many.

Disparities

Disparities in levels of physical activity exist among population groups. The proportion of the population reporting no leisure-time physical activity is higher among women than men, higher among African Americans and Hispanics than whites, higher among older adults than younger adults, and higher among the less affluent than the more affluent. Participation in all types of physical activity declines strikingly as age or grade in school increases. In general, persons with lower levels of education and income are least active in their leisure time. Adults in North Central and Western States tend to be more active than those in the Northeastern and Southern States. People with disabilities and certain health conditions are less likely to engage in moderate or vigorous physical activity than are people without disabilities. Health promotion efforts need to identify barriers to physical

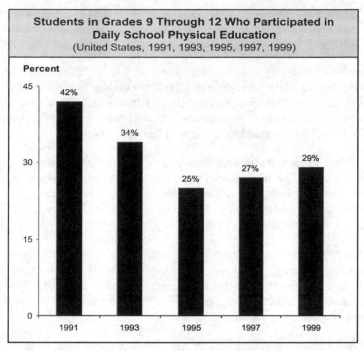

Students in Grades 9 Through 12 Who Participated in Daily School Physical Education
(United States, 1991, 1993, 1995, 1997, 1999)

Percent

- 1991: 42%
- 1993: 34%
- 1995: 25%
- 1997: 27%
- 1999: 29%

Source: CDC, NCHS. Youth Risk Behavior Surveillance System (YRBSS), 1991, 1993, 1995, 1997, 1999.

activity faced by particular population groups and develop interventions that address these barriers. [1]

Data demonstrate that major decreases in vigorous physical activity occur during grades 9 through 12. This decrease is more profound for girls than for boys, whether the measure is engaging in vigorous physical activity in general or in team sports. The President's Council on Physical Fitness and Sports concluded that because of the physical health and emotional benefits of physical activity, it should have an increasingly important role in the lives of girls.[17] Adolescents' interest and participation in physical activity differ by gender.[17] Therefore, strategies to increase the amount of physical activity for boys and girls must address these differences and must begin before the disparities in levels of physical activity manifest themselves. Compared to boys, girls are less likely to participate in team sports but more likely to participate in aerobics or dance. Often girls and boys perceive different benefits from physical activity, with boys viewing such activity as competition and girls as weight management. These factors must be considered in developing programs to address the needs of girls. Because boys are more likely than girls to have higher self-esteem and greater physical strength, programs addressing the needs of girls should provide instruction and experiences that increase their confidence and their opportunities to participate in activities, as well as social environments that support involvement in a range of physical activities.[17]

Opportunities

The Healthy People 2010 objectives offer opportunities to ensure that physical activity and fitness become part of regular healthy behavioral patterns. Encouraging any type or amount of physical activity in leisure time can provide important health benefits, compared to a sedentary lifestyle.

Activities that promote strength and flexibility are important because they may protect against disability, enhance functional independence, and encourage regular physical activity participation. These benefits are particularly important for older people—a good quality of life means being functionally independent and being able to perform the activities of daily living.

Young people are at particular risk for becoming sedentary as they grow older. Therefore, encouraging moderate and vigorous physical activity among youth is important. Because children spend most of their time in school, the type and amount of physical activity encouraged in schools are important components of a fitness program and a healthy lifestyle.

The major barriers most people face when trying to increase physical activity are time, access to convenient facilities, and safe environments in which to be active. Counseling by primary care providers about the need to participate in physical activity also is an important way to change behavior. In addition, facilities need to be accessible to people with disabilities.

Interim Progress Toward Year 2000 Objectives

Of the 13 physical activity and fitness objectives, 1 has been met—increasing worksite fitness programs. Four objectives show solid gains, indicating that the message about increased physical activity is reaching some segments of the population. The message that a sedentary lifestyle plays a role in both overweight and weight loss needs to be addressed better, as does the role primary care providers can play in counseling individuals to increase their daily activities. Both the quantity and quality of school physical education have slipped. Data to evaluate access and availability of community fitness facilities are not available.

Note: Unless otherwise noted, data are from the Centers for Disease Control and Prevention, National Center for Health Statistics, *Healthy People 2000 Review, 1998–99*.

Physical Activity and Fitness

Goal: Improve health, fitness, and quality of life through daily physical activity.

Number Objective Short Title

Physical Activity in Adults

22-1   No leisure-time physical activity

22-2   Moderate physical activity

22-3   Vigorous physical activity

Muscular Strength/Endurance and Flexibility

22-4   Muscular strength and endurance

22-5   Flexibility

Physical Activity in Children and Adolescents

22-6   Moderate physical activity in adolescents

22-7   Vigorous physical activity in adolescents

22-8   Physical education requirement in schools

22-9   Daily physical education in schools

22-10   Physical activity in physical education class

22-11   Television viewing

Access

22-12   School physical activity facilities

22-13   Worksite physical activity and fitness

22-14   Community walking

22-15   Community bicycling

Physical Activity in Adults

22-1. Reduce the proportion of adults who engage in no leisure-time physical activity.

Target: 20 percent.

Baseline: 40 percent of adults aged 18 years and older engaged in no leisure-time physical activity in 1997 (age adjusted to the year 2000 standard population).

Target setting method: Better than the best.

Data source: National Health Interview Survey (NHIS), CDC, NCHS.

NOTE: THE TABLE BELOW MAY CONTINUE TO THE FOLLOWING PAGE.

Adults Aged 18 Years and Older, 1997	No Leisure-Time Physical Activity
	Percent
TOTAL	40
Race and ethnicity	
American Indian or Alaska Native	46
Asian or Pacific Islander	42
Asian	42
Native Hawaiian and other Pacific Islander	41
Black or African American	52
White	38
Hispanic or Latino	54
Not Hispanic or Latino	38
Black or African American	52
White	36
Gender	
Female	43
Male	36
Education level (aged 25 years and older)	
Less than 9th grade	73
Grades 9 through 11	59
High school graduate	46
Some college or AA degree	35
College graduate or above	24

Adults Aged 18 Years and Older, 1997	No Leisure-Time Physical Activity
	Percent
Geographic location	
Urban	39
Rural	43
Disability status	
Persons with disabilities	56
Persons without disabilities	36
Select populations	
Age groups	
18 to 24 years	31
25 to 44 years	34
45 to 64 years	42
65 to 74 years	51
75 years and older	65
Persons with arthritis symptoms	43
Persons without arthritis symptoms	38

DNA = Data have not been analyzed. DNC = Data are not collected. DSU = Data are statistically unreliable.
Note: Age adjusted to the year 2000 standard population.

NOTE: THE TABLE ABOVE MAY HAVE CONTINUED FROM THE PREVIOUS PAGE.

22-2. Increase the proportion of adults who engage regularly, preferably daily, in moderate physical activity for at least 30 minutes per day.

Target: 30 percent.

Baseline: 15 percent of adults aged 18 years and older engaged in moderate physical activity for at least 30 minutes 5 or more days per week in 1997 (age adjusted to the year 2000 standard population).

Target setting method: Better than the best.

Data source: National Health Interview Survey (NHIS), CDC, NCHS.

Adults Aged 18 Years and Older, 1997	22-2. 30 Minutes of Activity 5 or More Days per Week	20 Minutes of Activity 3 or More Days per Week*
	Percent	
TOTAL	15	31
Race and ethnicity		
American Indian or Alaska Native	13	25
Asian or Pacific Islander	15	30
Asian	15	30
Native Hawaiian and other Pacific Islander	11	31
Black or African American	10	23
White	15	32
Hispanic or Latino	11	23
Not Hispanic or Latino	15	32
Black or African American	10	22
White	16	33
Gender		
Female	13	30
Male	16	31
Education level (aged 25 years and older)		
Less than 9th grade	7	13
Grades 9 through 11	11	21
High school graduate	14	28
Some college or AA degree	17	34
College graduate or above	17	38
Geographic location		
Urban	15	31
Rural	15	30
Disability status		
Persons with disabilities	12	23
Persons without disabilities	16	33
Select populations		
Age groups		
18 to 24 years	17	36
25 to 44 years	15	31

Adults Aged 18 Years and Older, 1997	22-2. 30 Minutes of Activity 5 or More Days per Week	20 Minutes of Activity 3 or More Days per Week*
	Percent	
45 to 64 years	14	30
65 to 74 years	16	31
75 years and older	12	23
Persons with arthritis symptoms	15	29
Persons without arthritis symptoms	15	32

DNA = Data have not been analyzed. DNC = Data are not collected. DSU = Data are statistically unreliable.
Note: Age adjusted to the year 2000 standard population.
*Data for 20 minutes of activity 3 or more days per week are displayed to further characterize the issue.

NOTE: THE TABLE ABOVE MAY HAVE CONTINUED FROM THE PREVIOUS PAGE.

22-3. **Increase the proportion of adults who engage in vigorous physical activity that promotes the development and maintenance of cardiorespiratory fitness 3 or more days per week for 20 or more minutes per occasion.**

Target: 30 percent.

Baseline: 23 percent of adults aged 18 years and older engaged in vigorous physical activity 3 or more days per week for 20 or more minutes per occasion in 1997 (age adjusted to the year 2000 standard population).

Target setting method: Better than the best.

Data source: National Health Interview Survey (NHIS), CDC, NCHS.

NOTE: THE TABLE BELOW MAY CONTINUE TO THE FOLLOWING PAGE.

Adults Aged 18 Years and Older, 1997	Vigorous Physical Activity
	Percent
TOTAL	23
Race and ethnicity	
American Indian or Alaska Native	19
Asian or Pacific Islander	17
Asian	16
Native Hawaiian and other Pacific Islander	24
Black or African American	17
White	24

Adults Aged 18 Years and Older, 1997	Vigorous Physical Activity
	Percent
Hispanic or Latino	16
Not Hispanic or Latino	24
Black or African American	17
White	25
Gender	
Female	20
Male	26
Education level (aged 25 years and older)	
Less than 9th grade	6
Grades 9 through 11	12
High school graduate	18
Some college or AA degree	24
College graduate and above	32
Geographic location	
Urban	24
Rural	21
Disability status	
Persons with disabilities	13
Persons without disabilities	25
Select populations	
Age groups	
18 to 24 years	32
25 to 44 years	27
45 to 64 years	21
65 to 74 years	13
75 years and older	6
Persons with arthritis symptoms	21
Persons without arthritis symptoms	24

DNA = Data have not been analyzed. DNC = Data are not collected. DSU = Data are statistically unreliable.
Note: Age adjusted to the year 2000 standard population.

NOTE: THE TABLE ABOVE MAY HAVE CONTINUED FROM THE PREVIOUS PAGE.

The adoption and maintenance of regular physical activity represent an important component of any health regime and provide multiple opportunities to improve and maintain health. Because the highest risk of death and disability is found among those who do no regular physical activity, engaging in any amount of physical activity is preferable to none. Physical activity should be encouraged as part of a daily routine. While moderate physical activity for at least 30 minutes a day is preferable, intermittent physical activity also increases caloric expenditure and may be important for those who cannot fit 30 minutes of sustained activity into their daily schedules. For even greater health benefits, vigorous physical activity is necessary. For most persons, the greatest opportunity for physical activity is associated with leisure time, because few occupations today provide sufficient vigorous or moderate physical activity to produce health benefits.

Engaging in moderate physical activity for at least 30 minutes per day will help ensure that sufficient calories are used to provide health benefits. A minimum level of intensity (for example, a brisk walk for 30 minutes per day) would, for most persons, result in an energy expenditure of about 600 to 1,100 calories per week.[18] If calorie intake remains constant, this expenditure translates into a weight loss of roughly one-sixth to one-third pound per week. Increases in daily activity to ensure a weekly expenditure of 1,000 calories would have significant individual and public health benefit for CHD prevention and deaths from all causes, especially for persons who are sedentary. Furthermore, this level of activity is feasible for most people even though the relative intensity of any activity will vary by age. Starting out slowly and gradually increasing the frequency and duration of physical activity is the key to successful behavior change. In the case of walking, the message becomes, "If you are not used to daily walking, then walk slowly and take short, frequent walks, gradually increasing distance and speed."

Muscular Strength/Endurance and Flexibility

22-4. Increase the proportion of adults who perform physical activities that enhance and maintain muscular strength and endurance.

Target: 30 percent.

Baseline: 18 percent of adults aged 18 years and older performed physical activities that enhance and maintain strength and endurance 2 or more days per week in 1998 (age adjusted to the year 2000 standard population).

Target setting method: Better than the best.

Data source: National Health Interview Survey (NHIS), CDC, NCHS.

NOTE: THE TABLE BELOW MAY CONTINUE TO THE FOLLOWING PAGE.

Adults Aged 18 Years and Older, 1998 (unless noted)	Strengthening and Endurance Exercises
	Percent
TOTAL	18
Race and ethnicity	
American Indian or Alaska Native	18
Asian or Pacific Islander	17
Asian	17
Native Hawaiian and other Pacific Islander	19
Black or African American	16
White	18
Hispanic or Latino	13
Not Hispanic or Latino	18
Black or African American	15
White	19
Gender	
Female	14
Male	21
Education level (aged 25 years and older)	
Less than 9th grade	4
Grades 9 through 11	8
High school graduate	11
Some college or AA degree	19
College graduate and above	26
Geographic location	
Urban	19
Rural	15
Disability status	
Persons with disabilities	14 (1997)
Persons without disabilities	20 (1997)
Select populations	
Age groups	
18 to 24 years (not age adjusted)	28
25 to 44 years (not age adjusted)	21
45 to 64 years (not age adjusted)	14

Adults Aged 18 Years and Older, 1998 (unless noted)	Strengthening and Endurance Exercises
	Percent
65 to 74 years (not age adjusted)	10
75 years and older (not age adjusted)	7
Persons with arthritis symptoms	18
Persons without arthritis symptoms	18

DNA = Data have not been analyzed. DNC = Data are not collected. DSU = Data are statistically unreliable.
Note: Age adjusted to the year 2000 standard population.

NOTE: THE TABLE ABOVE MAY HAVE CONTINUED FROM THE PREVIOUS PAGE.

22-5. Increase the proportion of adults who perform physical activities that enhance and maintain flexibility.

Target: 43 percent.

Baseline: 30 percent of adults aged 18 years and older did stretching exercises in the past 2 weeks in 1998 (age adjusted to the year 2000 standard population).

Target setting method: Better than the best.

Data source: National Health Interview Survey (NHIS), CDC, NCHS.

NOTE: THE TABLE BELOW MAY CONTINUE TO THE FOLLOWING PAGE.

Adults Aged 18 Years and Older, 1998 (unless noted)	Stretching Exercises
	Percent
TOTAL	30
Race and ethnicity	
American Indian or Alaska Native	26
Asian or Pacific Islander	34
Asian	34
Native Hawaiian and other Pacific Islander	42
Black or African American	26
White	30
Hispanic or Latino	22
Not Hispanic or Latino	31
Black or African American	27
White	31

Adults Aged 18 Years and Older, 1998 (unless noted)	Stretching Exercises
	Percent
Gender	
Female	30
Male	30
Family income level	
Below poverty	21
Near poverty	24
Middle/high income	34
Education level (aged 25 years and older)	
Less than high school	16
High school graduate	23
At least some college	36
Geographic location	
Urban	32
Rural	25
Disability status	
Persons with activity limitations	29 (1995)
Persons without activity limitations	31 (1995)
Select populations	
Age groups	
18 to 24 years	36
25 to 44 years	32
45 to 64 years	28
65 to 74 years	24
75 years and older	22
Persons with arthritis symptoms	DNA
Persons without arthritis symptoms	DNA

DNA = Data have not been analyzed. DNC = Data are not collected. DSU = Data are statistically unreliable.
Note: Age adjusted to the year 2000 standard population.

NOTE: THE TABLE ABOVE MAY HAVE CONTINUED FROM THE PREVIOUS PAGE.

All adults could benefit from physical activities designed to ensure functional independence throughout life. The specific physical fitness components that provide continued physical function as persons age include muscular strength/endurance and flexibility. Examples of these activities include weight training, resistance activities (using elastic bands or dumbbells), and stretching exercises (such as static stretching, yoga, or T'ai Chi Chuan).

Effective treatment of many chronic diseases and disorders has resulted in more years of life, but many of these extra years are spent with disabling conditions that prevent independent living and reduce the quality of life. Strengthening activities, while important for all age groups, are particularly important for older adults. Muscle strength declines with age, and there is a demonstrated relationship between muscle strength and physical function.[19] Age-related loss of strength may be lessened by strengthening exercises, enabling an individual to maintain a threshold level of strength necessary to perform basic weight-bearing activities, such as walking.[20, 21] Strength training also has been shown to preserve bone density in postmenopausal women.[9]

Physical activities that improve muscular strength/endurance and flexibility also improve the ability to perform tasks of daily living and may improve balance, thus preventing falls.[1] Activities of daily living have been identified as a scale to measure dependencies in basic self-care and other functions important for independent living and to avoid institutionalization. The performance of routine daily activities is particularly important to maintaining functional independence and social integration in older adults.[11]

Although flexibility may appear to be a minor component of physical fitness, the consequence of rigid joints affects all aspects of life, including walking, stooping, sitting, avoiding falls, and driving a vehicle. Lack of joint flexibility may adversely affect quality of life and will lead to eventual disability.[22] Activities such as static stretching or T'ai Chi Chuan routines, which consist of slow, graceful movements with low impact, have great promise for maintaining flexibility and can be appropriate for adults of any age.[23] Increasing public awareness of all these potential benefits of muscle strengthening and flexibility activities—and developing and making quality programs available and accessible—may encourage the pursuit of activities that promote muscular strength/endurance and flexibility.

Physical Activity in Children and Adolescents

22-6. Increase the proportion of adolescents who engage in moderate physical activity for at least 30 minutes on 5 or more of the previous 7 days.

Target: 35 percent.

Baseline: 27 percent of students in grades 9 through 12 engaged in moderate physical activity for at least 30 minutes on 5 or more of the previous 7 days in 1999.

Target setting method: Better than the best.

Data source: Youth Risk Behavior Surveillance System (YRBSS), CDC, NCCDPHP.

Students in Grades 9 Through 12, 1999 (unless noted)	Moderate Physical Activity		
	22-6. Both Genders	Females*	Males*
	Percent		
TOTAL	27	24	29
Race and ethnicity			
American Indian or Alaska Native	DSU	DSU	DSU
Asian or Pacific Islander	DSU	DSU	DSU
Asian	DSU	DSU	DSU
Native Hawaiian and other Pacific Islander	DSU	DSU	DSU
Black or African American	17	17	24
White	27	27	31
Hispanic or Latino	21	17	26
Not Hispanic or Latino	27	25	30
Black or African American	21	18	24
White	29	26	32
Parents' education level			
Less than high school	25 (1997)	25 (1997)	24 (1997)
High school graduate	21 (1997)	20 (1997)	21 (1997)
At least some college	20 (1997)	19 (1997)	20 (1997)
Select populations			
Grade levels			
9th grade	28	26	31
10th grade	26	25	27
11th grade	25	21	29
12th grade	27	24	29

DNA = Data have not been analyzed. DNC = Data are not collected. DSU = Data are statistically unreliable.
*Data for females and males are displayed to further characterize the issue.

22-7. Increase the proportion of adolescents who engage in vigorous physical activity that promotes cardiorespiratory fitness 3 or more days per week for 20 or more minutes per occasion.

Target: 85 percent.

Baseline: 65 percent of students in grades 9 through 12 engaged in vigorous physical activity 3 or more days per week for 20 or more minutes per occasion in 1999.

Target setting method: Better than the best.

Data source: Youth Risk Behavior Surveillance System (YRBSS), CDC, NCCDPHP.

NOTE: THE TABLE BELOW MAY CONTINUE TO THE FOLLOWING PAGE.

Students in Grades 9 Through 12, 1999 (unless noted)	Vigorous Physical Activity		
	22-7. Both Genders	Females*	Males*
	Percent		
TOTAL	65	57	72
Race and ethnicity			
American Indian or Alaska Native	DSU	DSU	DSU
Asian or Pacific Islander	DSU	DSU	DSU
Asian	DSU	DSU	DSU
Native Hawaiian and other Pacific Islander	DSU	DSU	DSU
Black or African American	56	49	64
White	68	60	75
Hispanic or Latino	61	50	72
Not Hispanic or Latino	65	58	73
Black or African American	56	47	65
White	67	60	75
Parents' education level			
Less than high school	50 (1997)	43 (1997)	60 (1997)
High school graduate	54 (1997)	45 (1997)	62 (1997)
At least some college	68 (1997)	57 (1997)	75 (1997)

Students in Grades 9 Through 12, 1999 (unless noted)	Vigorous Physical Activity		
	22-7. Both Genders	Females*	Males*
	Percent		
Select populations			
Grade levels			
9th grade	73	68	77
10th grade	65	56	73
11th grade	58	49	67
12th grade	61	52	71

DNA = Data have not been analyzed. DNC = Data are not collected. DSU = Data are statistically unreliable.
*Data for females and males are displayed to further characterize the issue.

NOTE: THE TABLE ABOVE MAY HAVE CONTINUED FROM THE PREVIOUS PAGE.

22-8. Increase the proportion of the Nation's public and private schools that require daily physical education for all students.

Target and baseline:

Objective	Increase in Schools Requiring Daily Physical Activity for All Students	1994 Baseline	2010 Target
		Percent	
22-8a.	Middle and junior high schools	17	25
22-8b.	Senior high schools	2	5

Target setting method: 47 percent improvement for middle and junior high schools; 150 percent improvement for senior high schools.

Data source: School Health Policies and Programs Study (SHPPS), CDC, NCCDPHP.

22-9. Increase the proportion of adolescents who participate in daily school physical education.

Target: 50 percent.

Baseline: 29 percent of students in grades 9 through 12 participated in daily school physical education in 1999.

Target setting method: Better than the best.

Data source: Youth Risk Behavior Surveillance System (YRBSS), CDC, NCCDPHP.

Students in Grades 9 Through 12, 1999 (unless noted)	Daily School Physical Education		
	22-9. Both Genders	Females*	Males*
	Percent		
TOTAL	29	26	32
Race and ethnicity			
American Indian or Alaska Native	DSU	DSU	DSU
Asian or Pacific Islander	DSU	DSU	DSU
Asian	DSU	DSU	DSU
Native Hawaiian and other Pacific Islander	DSU	DSU	DSU
Black or African American	28	25	33
White	28	26	31
Hispanic or Latino	40	36	45
Not Hispanic or Latino	28	25	30
Black or African American	29	26	33
White	28	26	31
Parents' education level			
Less than high school	29 (1997)	28 (1997)	30 (1997)
High school graduate	24 (1997)	22 (1997)	27 (1997)
At least some college	28 (1997)	25 (1997)	30 (1997)
Select populations			
Grade levels			
9th grade	42	40	44
10th grade	30	28	33
11th grade	20	17	24
12th grade	20	17	24

DNA = Data have not been analyzed. DNC = Data are not collected. DSU = Data are statistically unreliable.
*Data for females and males are displayed to further characterize the issue.

22-10. Increase the proportion of adolescents who spend at least 50 percent of school physical education class time being physically active.

Target: 50 percent.

Baseline: 38 percent of students in grades 9 through 12 were physically active in physical education class more than 20 minutes 3 to 5 days per week in 1999.

Target setting method: Better than the best.

Data source: Youth Risk Behavior Surveillance System (YRBSS), CDC, NCCDPHP.

Students in Grades 9 Through 12, 1999 (unless noted)	Physically Active in Physical Education Classes		
	22-10. Both Genders	Females*	Males*
	Percent		
TOTAL	38	32	45
Race and ethnicity			
American Indian or Alaska Native	DSU	DSU	DSU
Asian or Pacific Islander	DSU	DSU	DSU
Asian	DSU	DSU	DSU
Native Hawaiian and other Pacific Islander	DSU	DSU	DSU
Black or African American	32	24	41
White	40	33	46
Hispanic or Latino	41	35	47
Not Hispanic or Latino	38	31	45
Black or African American	32	25	37
White	40	33	45
Parents' education level			
Less than high school	28 (1997)	25 (1997)	32 (1997)
High school graduate	29 (1997)	24 (1997)	35 (1997)
At least some college	33 (1997)	27 (1997)	37 (1997)
Select populations			
Grade levels			
9th grade	55	48	62
10th grade	41	35	47
11th grade	29	24	35
12th grade	24	16	32

DNA = Data have not been analyzed. DNC = Data are not collected. DSU = Data are statistically unreliable.
*Data for females and males are displayed to further characterize the issue.

22-11. Increase the proportion of adolescents who view television 2 or fewer hours on a school day.

Target: 75 percent.

Baseline: 57 percent of students in grades 9 through 12 viewed television 2 or fewer hours per school day in 1999.

Target setting method: Better than the best.

Data source: Youth Risk Behavior Surveillance System (YRBSS), CDC, NCCDPHP.

NOTE: THE TABLE BELOW MAY CONTINUE TO THE FOLLOWING PAGE.

Students in Grades 9 through 12, 1999	Television 2 or Fewer Hours per School Day
	Percent
TOTAL	57
Race and ethnicity	
American Indian or Alaska Native	DSU
Asian or Pacific Islander	DSU
Asian	DSU
Native Hawaiian and other Pacific Islander	DSU
Black or African American	28
White	66
Hispanic or Latino	48
Not Hispanic or Latino	DNA
Black or African American	26
White	66
Gender	
Female	59
Male	56
Parents' education level	
Less than high school	DNC
High school graduate	DNC
At least some college	DNC

Students in Grades 9 through 12, 1999	Television 2 or Fewer Hours per School Day
	Percent
Select populations	
Grade levels	
9th grade	49
10th grade	54
11th grade	62
12th grade	67

DNA = Data have not been analyzed. DNC = Data are not collected. DSU = Data are statistically unreliable.
NOTE: THE TABLE ABOVE MAY HAVE CONTINUED FROM THE PREVIOUS PAGE.

The health benefits of moderate and vigorous physical activity are not limited to adults. Physical activity among children and adolescents is important because of the related health benefits (cardiorespiratory function, blood pressure control, and weight management) and because a physically active lifestyle adopted early in life may continue into adulthood. Even among children aged 3 to 4 years, those who were less active tended to remain less active after age 3 years than most of their peers.[24] These findings highlight the need for parents, educators, and health care providers to become positive role models and to be involved actively in the promotion of physical activity and fitness in children and adolescents.

Many children are less physically active than recommended, and physical activity declines during adolescence.[25, 26] One study found that one-quarter of U.S. children spend 4 hours or more watching television daily.[27] Schools are an efficient vehicle for providing physical activity and fitness instruction because they reach most children and adolescents. Participation in school physical education ensures a minimum amount of physical activity and provides a forum to teach physical activity strategies and activities that can be continued into adulthood. Findings suggest that the quantity and, in particular, the quality of school physical education programs have a significant positive effect on the health-related fitness of children and adolescents by increasing their participation in moderate to vigorous activities.[28, 29]

Studies have shown that spending 50 percent of physical education class time on physical activity is an ambitious but feasible target. Being active for at least half of physical education class time on at least half of the school days would provide a substantial portion of the physical activity time recommended for adolescents.[30] To achieve the benefits of school-based physical education equitably for all children, daily adaptive physical education programs should be available for children with special needs. School physical education requirements also are recommended for students in preschool and postsecondary programs.[31]

Physical education is the primary source of physical activity and fitness instruction. Health education and other courses, however, can highlight the importance of physical activity as a component of a healthy lifestyle. A well-designed health education curriculum can help students develop the knowledge, attitudes, behavioral skills, and confidence needed to adopt and maintain physically active lifestyles.[31] To maximize classroom time, instruction on physical activity also can be integrated into the lesson plans of other school subjects, such as mathematics, biology, and language arts. Programs that have included classroom instruction in physical activity have been effective in enhancing students' physical activity-related knowledge,[32] attitudes,[33] behavior,[34] and physical fitness.[35] (See Focus Area 7. Educational and Community-Based Programs.)

Access

22-12. (Developmental) Increase the proportion of the Nation's public and private schools that provide access to their physical activity spaces and facilities for all persons outside of normal school hours (that is, before and after the school day, on weekends, and during summer and other vacations).

Potential data source: School Health Policies and Programs Study (SHPPS), CDC, NCCDPHP.

22-13. Increase the proportion of worksites offering employer-sponsored physical activity and fitness programs.

Target: 75 percent.

Baseline: 46 percent of worksites with 50 or more employees offered physical activity and/or fitness programs at the worksite or through their health plans in 1998–1999.

Worksite Size	Worksite or Health Plan	Health Plan	Worksite
		Percent	
Total (50 or more employees)	46	22	36
50 to 99 employees	38	21	24
100 to 249 employees	42	20	31
250 to 749 employees	56	25	44
750 or more employees	68	27	61
Less than 50 employees		Developmental	

Target setting method: Better than the best.

Data source: National Worksite Health Promotion Survey, Association for Worksite Health Promotion (AWHP).

Participation in regular physical activity depends, in part, on the availability and proximity of community facilities and on environments conducive to physical activity. Studies of adult participation in physical activity have found that use generally decreases as facility distance from a person's residence increases.[36] People are unlikely to use community resources located more than a few miles away by car or more than a few minutes away by biking or walking.

One of the major barriers to youth participation in sports is lack of enough sports facilities.[37] Increased access to community physical activity facilities would, therefore, help increase youth physical activity. The availability of school facilities for physical activity programs also may be beneficial for crime and violence prevention and other social programs,[37] because most juvenile crime is committed between 3 and 8 p.m.

Schools need to work with community coalitions and community-based physical activity programs to take maximum advantage of school facilities for the benefit of children and adolescents and the community as a whole. The needs of all community members, including senior citizens and people with disabilities, need to be considered.

Worksite physical activity and fitness programs provide a mechanism for reaching large numbers of adults and have at least short-term effectiveness in increasing the physical activity and fitness of program participants.[38] Such programs should be provided in a culturally and linguistically competent manner. Evidence that worksite programs are cost-effective is growing. Such programs may even reduce employer costs for insurance premiums, disability benefits, and medical expenses.[39] Additional benefits for employers include increased productivity, reduced absenteeism, reduced employee turnover, improved morale, enhanced company image, and enhanced recruitment. Including family members and retirees in worksite programs can further increase benefits to employers and the community.[39]

As purchasers of group health and life insurance plans, employers can design employee benefit packages that include coverage for fitness club membership fees and community-based fitness classes. Employers also can offer reduced insurance premiums and rebates for employees who participate regularly in worksite fitness programs or who can document participation in regular physical activity.

22-14. Increase the proportion of trips made by walking.

Target and baseline:

Objective	Increase in Trips Made by Walking	Length of Trip	1995 Baseline*	2010 Target
			Percent	
22-14a.	Adults aged 18 years and older	Trips of 1 mile or less	17	25
22-14b.	Children and adolescents aged 5 to15 years	Trips to school of 1 mile or less	31	50

*Age adjusted to the year 2000 standard population.

Target setting method: 47 percent improvement for 22-14a and 68 percent improvement for 22-14b. (Better than the best will be used when data are available.)

Data source: Nationwide Personal Transportation Survey (NPTS), DOT.

NOTE: THE TABLE BELOW MAY CONTINUE TO THE FOLLOWING PAGE.

Adults Aged 18 Years and Older, 1995	22-14a. Trips of 1 Mile or Less Made by Walking
	Percent
TOTAL	17
Race and ethnicity	
American Indian or Alaska Native	DNC
Asian or Pacific Islander	DNC
Asian	DNC
Native Hawaiian and other Pacific Islander	DNC
Black or African American	DNC
White	DNC
Hispanic or Latino	DNC
Not Hispanic or Latino	DNC
Black or African American	DNC
White	DNC
Gender	
Female	17
Male	16

Adults Aged 18 Years and Older, 1995	22-14a. Trips of 1 Mile or Less Made by Walking
	Percent
Education level	
Less than high school	20
High school graduate	14
At least some college	18
Geographic location	
Urban	18
Rural	9
Select populations	
Age groups	
18 to 24 years	22
25 to 44 years	17
45 to 64 years	14
65 to 74 years	16
75 years and older	19

DNA = Data have not been analyzed. DNC = Data are not collected. DSU = Data are statistically unreliable.
Note: Age adjusted to the year 2000 standard population.

NOTE: THE TABLE ABOVE MAY HAVE CONTINUED FROM THE PREVIOUS PAGE.

NOTE: THE TABLE BELOW MAY CONTINUE TO THE FOLLOWING PAGE.

Children and Adolescents Aged 5 to 15 Years, 1995	22-14b. Trips to School of 1 Mile or Less Made by Walking
	Percent
TOTAL	31
Race and ethnicity	
American Indian or Alaska Native	DNC
Asian or Pacific Islander	DNC
Asian	DNC
Native Hawaiian and other Pacific Islander	DNC
Black or African American	DNC
White	DNC

Children and Adolescents Aged 5 to 15 Years, 1995	22-14b. Trips to School of 1 Mile or Less Made by Walking
	Percent
Hispanic or Latino	DNC
Not Hispanic or Latino	DNC
Black or African American	DNC
White	DNC
Gender	
Female	27
Male	35
Parents' education level	
Less than high school	DNC
High school graduate	DNC
At least some college	DNC
Geographic location	
Urban	32
Rural	27
Select populations	
Age groups	
5 to 9 years	27
10 to 15 years	35

DNA = Data have not been analyzed. DNC = Data are not collected. DSU = Data are statistically unreliable.
Note: Age adjusted to the year 2000 standard population.

NOTE: THE TABLE ABOVE MAY HAVE CONTINUED FROM THE PREVIOUS PAGE.

Walking is a very popular form of physical activity in the United States; however, people need the opportunity to walk safely. Over 75 percent of all trips less than 1 mile were made by automobile in 1995.[40] In addition, the number of walking trips as a percentage of all trips taken (of any distance) has declined over the years. Walking trips made by adults dropped from 9.3 percent in 1977 to 7.2 percent in 1990 and again to 5.4 percent in 1995. Walking has declined even more sharply for children.[40] These declines have negative implications for the health of adults and children.

22-15. Increase the proportion of trips made by bicycling.

Target and baseline:

Objective	Increase in Trips Made by Bicycling	Activity	1995 Baseline*	2010 Target
			Percent	
22-15a.	Adults aged 18 years and older	Trips of 5 miles or less	0.6	2.0
22-15b.	Children and adolescents aged 5 to15 years	Trips to school of 2 miles or less	2.4	5.0

*Age adjusted to the year 2000 standard population.

Target setting method: 233 percent improvement for 22-15a and 108 percent improvement for 22-15b. (Better than the best will be used when data are available.)

Data source: Nationwide Personal Transportation Survey (NPTS), DOT.

NOTE: THE TABLE BELOW MAY CONTINUE TO THE FOLLOWING PAGE.

Adults Aged 18 Years and Older, 1995	22-15a. Trips of 5 Miles or Less Made by Bicycling
	Percent
TOTAL	0.6
Race and ethnicity	
American Indian or Alaska Native	DNC
Asian or Pacific Islander	DNC
Asian	DNC
Native Hawaiian and other Pacific Islander	DNC
Black or African American	DNC
White	DNC
Hispanic or Latino	DNC
Not Hispanic or Latino	DNC
Black or African American	DNC
White	DNC
Gender	
Female	0.3
Male	0.9

Healthy People 2010: Objectives for Improving Health

Adults Aged 18 Years and Older, 1995	22-15a. Trips of 5 Miles or Less Made by Bicycling
	Percent
Education level	
Less than high school	0.6
High school graduate	0.5
At least some college	0.6
Geographic location	
Urban	0.6
Rural	0.3
Age groups	
18 to 24 years	1.4
25 to 44 years	0.6
45 to 64 years	0.3
65 to 74 years	0.3
75 years and older	0.1

DNA = Data have not been analyzed. DNC = Data are not collected. DSU = Data are statistically unreliable.
Note: Age adjusted to the year 2000 standard population.

NOTE: THE TABLE ABOVE MAY HAVE CONTINUED FROM THE PREVIOUS PAGE.

NOTE: THE TABLE BELOW MAY CONTINUE TO THE FOLLOWING PAGE.

Children and Adolescents Aged 5 to 15 Years, 1995	22-15b. Trips to School of 2 Miles or Less Made by Bicycling
	Percent
TOTAL	2.4
Race and ethnicity	
American Indian or Alaska Native	DNC
Asian or Pacific Islander	DNC
Asian	DNC
Native Hawaiian and other Pacific Islander	DNC
Black or African American	DNC
White	DNC

Children and Adolescents Aged 5 to 15 Years, 1995	22-15b. Trips to School of 2 Miles or Less Made by Bicycling
	Percent
Hispanic or Latino	DNC
Not Hispanic or Latino	DNC
Black or African American	DNC
White	DNC
Gender	
Female	1.7
Male	3.2
Parents' education level	
Less than high school	DNC
High school graduate	DNC
At least some college	DNC
Geographic location	
Urban	2.6
Rural	1.1
Select populations	
Age groups	
5 to 9 years	1.6
10 to 15 years	3.0

DNA = Data have not been analyzed. DNC = Data are not collected. DSU = Data are statistically unreliable.
Note: Age adjusted to the year 2000 standard population.
NOTE: THE TABLE ABOVE MAY HAVE CONTINUED FROM THE PREVIOUS PAGE.

Bicycling is another form of transportation that may be used by both children and adults for distances that may not be feasible, practical, or efficient to cover by walking. If the environment does not provide safe opportunities for physical activities such as walking and bicycling, adults and children likely will spend more time engaging in sedentary activities indoors. (See Focus Area 8. Environmental Health.) Sedentary activities such as watching television, playing video games, and using personal computers have contributed to increases in the cases of overweight individuals.[27]

1. **Access to Quality Health Services**
   - 1-2. Health insurance coverage for clinical preventive services
   - 1-3. Counseling about health behaviors
2. **Arthritis, Osteoporosis, and Chronic Back Conditions**
   - 2-2. Activity limitations due to arthritis
   - 2-3. Personal care limitations
   - 2-8. Arthritis education
   - 2-9. Cases of osteoporosis
   - 2-11. Activity limitations due to chronic back conditions
3. **Cancer**
   - 3-5. Colorectal cancer deaths
   - 3-7. Prostate cancer deaths
   - 3-9. Sun exposure and skin cancer
   - 3-10. Provider counseling about cancer prevention
4. **Chronic Kidney Disease**
   - 4-8. Medical therapy for persons with diabetes and proteinuria
5. **Diabetes**
   - 5-1. Diabetes education
   - 5-2. New cases of diabetes
   - 5-3. Overall cases of diagnosed diabetes
   - 5-4. Diagnosis of diabetes
   - 5-5. Diabetes deaths
   - 5-6. Diabetes-related deaths
   - 5-7. Cardiovascular disease deaths in persons with diabetes
6. **Disability and Secondary Conditions**
   - 6-2. Feelings and depression among children with disabilities
   - 6-3. Feelings and depression interfering with activities among adults with disabilities
   - 6-4. Social participation among adults with disabilities
   - 6-9. Inclusion of children and youth with disabilities in regular education programs
   - 6-10. Accessibility of health and wellness programs
   - 6-12. Environmental barriers affecting participation in activities
   - 6-13. Surveillance and health promotion programs
7. **Educational and Community-Based Programs**
   - 7-2. School health education
   - 7-3. Health-risk behavior information for college and university students
   - 7-5. Worksite health promotion programs
   - 7-6. Participation in employer-sponsored health promotion activities
   - 7-7. Patient and family education
   - 7-9. Health care organization sponsorship of community health promotion activities
   - 7-10. Community health promotion programs
   - 7-11. Culturally appropriate and linguistically competent community health promotion programs
   - 7-12. Older adult participation in community health promotion activities

8. **Environmental Health**
   8-1. Harmful air pollutants
   8-2. Alternative modes of transportation
   8-9. Beach closings
   8-20. School policies to protect against environmental hazards

9. **Family Planning**
   9-11. Pregnancy prevention education

11. **Health Communication**
    11-1. Households with Internet access
    11-4. Quality of Internet health information sources

12. **Heart Disease and Stroke**
    12-1. Coronary heart disease (CHD) deaths
    12-7. Stroke deaths
    12-9. High blood pressure
    12-10. High blood pressure control
    12-11. Action to help control blood pressure
    12-13. Mean total blood cholesterol levels
    12-14. High blood cholesterol levels
    12-16. LDL-cholesterol level in CHD patients

15. **Injury and Violence Prevention**
    15-1. Nonfatal head injuries
    15-2. Nonfatal spinal cord injuries
    15-13. Deaths from unintentional injuries
    15-14. Nonfatal unintentional injuries
    15-16. Pedestrian deaths
    15-18. Nonfatal pedestrian injuries
    15-21. Motorcycle helmet use
    15-23. Bicycle helmet use
    15-24. Bicycle helmet laws
    15-27. Deaths from falls
    15-28. Hip fractures
    15-29. Drownings
    15-31. Injury protection in school sports

16. **Maternal, Infant, and Child Health**
    16-3. Adolescent and young adult deaths
    16-12. Weight gain during pregnancy

17. **Medical Product Safety**
    17-2. Linked, automated information systems
    17-3. Provider review of medications taken by patients
    17-5. Receipt of oral counseling about medications from prescribers and dispensers

18. **Mental Health and Mental Disorders**
    18-5. Eating disorder relapses
    18-7. Treatment for children with mental health problems
    18-9. Treatment for adults with mental disorders

19. **Nutrition and Overweight**
    19-1. Healthy weight in adults
    19-2. Obesity in adults

19-3. Overweight or obesity in children and adolescents

19-16. Worksite promotion of nutrition education and weight management

20. Occupational Safety and Health

20-1. Work-related injury deaths

20-2. Work-related injuries

20-3. Overextension or repetitive motion

20-9. Worksite stress reduction programs

23. Public Health Infrastructure

23-2. Public access to information and surveillance data

23-5. Data for Leading Health Indicators, Health Status Indicators, and Priority Data Needs at Tribal, State, and local levels

23-17. Population-based prevention research

24. Respiratory Diseases

24-1. Deaths from asthma

24-2. Hospitalizations for asthma

24-3. Hospital emergency department visits for asthma

24-4. Activity limitations

24-5. School or work days lost

24-6. Patient education

24-7. Appropriate asthma care

25. Sexually Transmitted Diseases

25-11. Responsible adolescent sexual behavior

25-12. Responsible sexual behavior messages on television

26. Substance Abuse

26-9. Substance-free youth

26-14. Steroid use among adolescents

26-17. Perception of risk associated with substance abuse

26-23. Community partnerships and coalitions

27. Tobacco Use

27-1. Adult tobacco use

27-2. Adolescent tobacco use

27-3. Initiation of tobacco use

27-4. Age at first tobacco use

27-5. Smoking cessation by adults

27-7. Smoking cessation by adolescents

28. Vision and Hearing

28-9. Protective eyewear

Terminology

(A listing of abbreviations and acronyms used in this publication appears in Appendix H.)

Aerobic: Conditions or processes that occur in the presence of, or requiring, oxygen.[41]

Energy expenditure: The energy cost to the body of physical activity, usually measured in kilocalories.[41]

Functional independence: The ability to perform successfully and safely activities related to a daily routine with sufficient energy, strength/endurance, flexibility, and coordination.

Physical activity: Bodily movement that is produced by the contraction of skeletal muscle and that substantially increases energy expenditure.[1]

> **Moderate physical activity:** Activities that use large muscle groups and are at least equivalent to brisk walking. In addition to walking, activities may include swimming, cycling, dancing, gardening and yardwork, and various domestic and occupational activities.

> **Vigorous physical activity:** Rhythmic, repetitive physical activities that use large muscle groups at 70 percent or more of maximum heart rate for age. An exercise heart rate of 70 percent of maximum heart rate for age is about 60 percent of maximal cardiorespiratory capacity and is sufficient for cardiorespiratory conditioning. Maximum heart rate equals roughly 220 beats per minute minus age. Examples of vigorous physical activities include jogging/running, lap swimming, cycling, aerobic dancing, skating, rowing, jumping rope, cross-country skiing, hiking/backpacking, racquet sports, and competitive group sports (for example, soccer and basketball).

Physical fitness: A set of attributes that persons have or achieve that relates to the ability to perform physical activity.[1] Performance-related components of fitness include agility, balance, coordination, power, and speed.[42] Health-related components of physical fitness include body composition, cardiorespiratory function, flexibility, and muscular strength/endurance.[41]

> **Agility:** Ability to start, stop, and move the body quickly and in different directions.

> **Balance:** Ability to maintain a certain posture or to move without falling.

> **Body composition:** The relative amount of body weight that is fat and nonfat.

> **Cardiorespiratory function:** A health-related component of physical fitness that relates to the ability of the circulatory and respiratory systems to supply oxygen during physical activity.

> **Coordination:** Ability to do a task integrating movements of the body and different parts of the body.

> **Exercise (exercise training):** Planned, structured, and repetitive bodily movement done to improve or maintain one or more components of physical fitness.

> **Flexibility:** Ability to move a joint through the full range of motion without discomfort or pain.

> **Muscular endurance:** Ability of the muscle to perform repetitive contractions over a prolonged period of time.

> **Muscular strength:** Ability of the muscle to generate the maximum amount of force.

> **Power:** Ability to exert muscular strength quickly.

> **Speed:** Ability to move the whole body quickly.

Sedentary: Denotes a person who is relatively inactive and has a lifestyle characterized by a lot of sitting.[41]

References

[1] U.S. Department of Health and Human Services. *Physical Activity and Health: A Report of the Surgeon General*. Atlanta, GA: Centers for Disease Control and Prevention (CDC), National Center for Chronic Disease Prevention and Health Promotion, 1996.

[2] Frost, H.; Moffett, J.A.K.; Moser, J.S.; et al. Randomized controlled trial for evaluation of fitness programme for patients with chronic low back pain. *British Medical Journal* 310:151-154, 1995.

[3] McTiernan, A.; Stanford, J.L.; Weiss, N.S.; et al. Occurrence of breast cancer in relation to recreational exercise in women age 50-64 years. *Epidemiology* 7(6):598-604, 1996.

[4] Kujala, U.M.; Kaprio, J.; Sarna, S.; et al. Relationship of leisure-time physical activity and mortality: The Finnish twin cohort. *Journal of the American Medical Association* 279(6):440-444, 1998.

[5] Paffenbarger, R.S.; Hyde, R.T.; Wing, A.L.; et al. The association of changes in physical-activity level and other lifestyle characteristics with mortality among men. *New England Journal of Medicine* 328(8):538-545, 1993.

[6] Sherman, S.E.; D'Agostino, R.B.; Cobb, J.L.; et al. Physical activity and mortality in women in the Framingham Heart Study. *American Heart Journal* 128(5):879-884, 1994.

[7] Kaplan, G.A.; Strawbridge, W.J.; Cohen, R.D.; et al. Natural history of leisure-time physical activity and its correlates: Associations with mortality from all causes and cardiovascular disease over 28 years. *American Journal of Epidemiology* 144(8):793-797, 1996.

[8] Kushi, L.H.; Fee, R.M.; Folsom, A.R.; et al. Physical activity and mortality in postmenopausal women. *Journal of the American Medical Association* 277:1287-1292, 1997.

[9] Nelson, M.E.; Fiatarone, M.A.; Morganti, C.M.; et al. Effects of high-intensity strength training on multiple risk factors for osteoporotic fractures: A randomized controlled trial. *Journal of the American Medical Association* 272(24):1909-1914, 1994.

[10] LaCroix, A.Z.; Guralnik, J.M.; Berkman, L.F.; et al. Maintaining mobility in late life. II. Smoking, alcohol consumption, physical activity, and body mass index. *American Journal of Epidemiology* 137(8):858-869, 1993.

[11] Buchner, D.M. Preserving mobility in older adults. *Western Journal of Medicine* 167(4):258-264, 1997.

[12] Stenstrom, C.H. Home exercise in rheumatoid arthritis functional class II: Goal setting versus pain attention. *Journal of Rheumatology* 21(4):627-634, 1994.

[13] CDC. Prevalence of leisure-time physical activity among persons with arthritis and other rheumatic conditions—United States, 1990–91. *Morbidity and Mortality Weekly Report* 46(18):389-393, 1997.

[14] National Institutes of Health. Optimal calcium intake. In: *NIH Consensus Statement* 12(4):1-31, 1994.

[15] Snow-Harter, C.; Shaw, J.M.; and Matkin, C.C. Physical activity and risk of osteoporosis. In: Marcus, R.; Feldman, D.; and Kelsey, J., eds. *Osteoporosis.* San Diego, CA: Academic Press, 1996, 511-528.

[16] Pate, R.R.; Pratt, M.; Blair, S.N.; et al. Physical activity and public health: A recommendation from the Centers for Disease Control and Prevention and the American College of Sports Medicine. *Journal of the American Medical Association* 273(5):402-407, 1995.

[17] President's Council on Physical Fitness and Sports. *Physical Activity & Sport in the Lives of Girls.* Washington, DC: The President's Council on Physical Fitness and Sports, 1997.

[18] Stofan, J.R.; DiPietro, L.; Davis, D.; et al. Physical activity patterns associated with cardiorespiratory fitness and reduced mortality: The Aerobics Center Longitudinal Study. *American Journal of Public Health* 88(12):1807-1813, 1998.

[19] Brown, M.; Sinacore, D.R.; and Host, H.H. The relationship of strength to function in the older adult. *Journal of Gerontology* 50A:55-59, 1995.

[20] Tseng, B.S.; Marsh, D.R.; Hamilton, M.T.; et al. Strength and aerobic training attenuate muscle wasting and improve resistance to the development of disability with aging. *Journal of Gerontology* 50A:113-119, 1995.

[21] Evans, W.J. Effects of exercise on body composition and functional capacity of the elderly. *Journal of Gerontology* 50A:147-150, 1995.

[22] Cunningham, D.A.; Paterson, D.H.; Hinmann, J.E.; et al. P.A. Determinants of independence in the elderly. *Canadian Journal of Applied Physiology* 18(3):243-254, 1993.

[23] Lan, C.; Lai, J.S.; Chen, S.Y; et al. 12-month Tai Chi training in the elderly: Its effect on health fitness. *Medicine and Science in Sports and Exercise* 30(3):345-351, 1997.

[24] Pate, R.R.; Baranowski, T.; Dowda, M.; et al. Tracking of physical activity in young children. *Medicine and Science in Sports and Exercise* 28(1):92-96, 1996.

[25] Pate, R.R.; Long, B.J.; and Heath, G. Descriptive epidemiology of physical activity in adolescents. *Pediatric Exercise Science* 6:434-447, 1994.

[26] CDC. Youth risk behavior surveillance—United States, 1997. *Morbidity and Mortality Weekly Report* 47(55-3):1-89, 1998.

[27] Anderson, R.E.; Crespo, C.J.; Bartlett, S.J.; et al. Relationship of physical activity and television watching with body weight and level of fatness among children: Results from the Third National Health and Nutrition Examination Survey. *Journal of the American Medical Association* 279:938-942, 1998.

[28] McKenzie, T.L.; Nader, P.R.; Strikmiller, P.K.; et al. School physical education: Effect of the child and adolescent trial for cardiovascular health. *Preventive Medicine* 25(4):423-431, 1996.

[29] Sallis, J.F.; McKenzie, T.L.; Alcaraz, J.E.; et al. The effects of a 2-year physical education program (SPARK) on physical activity and fitness in elementary school students. *American Journal of Public Health* 87(8):1328-1334, 1997.

[30] Sallis, J.F., and Patrick, K. Physical activity guidelines for adolescents: Consensus statement. *Pediatric Exercise Science* 6:302-314, 1994.

[31] CDC. Guidelines for school and community programs to promote lifelong physical activity among young people. *Morbidity and Mortality Weekly Report* 46(RR-6):1-36, 1997.

[32] Killen, J.D.; Telch, M.J.; Robinson, T.N.; et al. Cardiovascular disease risk reduction for tenth graders: A multiple-factor school-based approach. *Journal of the American Medical Association* 260(12):1728-1733, 1988.

[33] Prokhorov, A.V.; Perry, C.L.; Kelder, S.H.; et al. Lifestyle values of adolescents: Results from Minnesota Heart Health Youth Program. *Adolescence* 28(111):637-647, 1993.

[34] Kelder, S.H.; Perry, C.L.; and Klepp, K.I. Community-wide youth exercise promotion: Long-term outcomes of the Minnesota Heart Health Program and the Class of 1989 study. *Journal of School Health* 63(5):218-223, 1993.

[35] Arbeit, M.L.; Johnson, C.C.; and Mott, D.S. The Heart Smart Cardiovascular School Health Promotion: Behavior correlates of risk factor change. *Preventive Medicine* 21(1):18-32, 1992.

[36] Sallis, J.F.; Hovell, M.F.; Hofstetter, C.R.; et al. Distance between homes and exercise facilities related to frequency of exercise among San Diego residents. *Public Health Reports* 105(2):179-185, 1990.

[37] Carnegie Council on Adolescent Development. *A Matter of Time: Risk and Opportunity in the Out-of-School Hours. Recommendations for Strengthening Community Programs for Youth.* New York, NY: Carnegie Corporation of New York, 1994.

[38] Cole, G.; Leonard, B.; Hammond, S.; et al. Using "stages of behavioral change" constructs to measure the short-term effects of a worksite-based intervention to increase moderate physical activity. *Psychological Reports* 82(2):615-618, 1998.

[39] Shephard, R.J. Employee health and fitness—state of the art. *Preventive Medicine* 12(5):644-653, 1983.

[40] U.S. Department of Transportation (DOT). *National Bicycling and Walking Study: Transportation Choices for a Changing America.* Pub. FH10A PD 94-023. Washington, DC: DOT, Federal Highway Administration, 1994.

[41] Kent, M. *The Oxford Dictionary of Sport's Science and Medicine.* Oxford, England: Oxford University Press, 1994.

[42] Howley, E.T., and Franks, B.O. *Health Fitness Instructors Handbook.* 3rd ed. Champaign, IL: Human Kinetics, 1997.

23

Public Health Infrastructure

Co-Lead Agencies: Centers for Disease Control and Prevention
Health Resources and Services Administration

Contents

Ensure that Federal, Tribal, State, and local health agencies have the infrastructure to provide essential public health services effectively.

Overview

The mission of public health is to fulfill "society's interest in assuring conditions in which persons can be healthy."[1] Public health engages both private and public organizations and individuals in accomplishing this mission. Responsibilities encompass preventing epidemics and the spread of disease, protecting against environmental hazards, preventing injuries, encouraging healthy behavior, helping communities to recover from disasters, and ensuring the quality and accessibility of health services.

Issues and Trends

The Nation's public health infrastructure is the resources needed to deliver the essential public health services to every community—people who work in the field of public health, information and communication systems used to collect and disseminate accurate data, and public health organizations at the State and local levels in the front lines of public health. The public health infrastructure is a complex web of practices and organizations that has been characterized as in "disarray."[1, 2]

Public health encompasses three core functions: *assessment* of information on the health of the community, comprehensive public health *policy development*, and *assurance* that public health services are provided to the community.[1] These functions have been defined further and expanded into 10 essential public health services.[2] (See chart on page 4 for full list from the *Public Health in America* statement.[3]) The totality of the public health infrastructure includes all governmental and nongovernmental entities that provide any of these services. Environmental health, occupational health and safety, mental health, and substance abuse are integral parts of public health. Service providers, such as managed care organizations, hospitals, nonprofit corporations, schools, faith organizations, and businesses, also are an integral part of the public health infrastructure in many communities.

Various reports and evaluations have described the continuing deterioration of the national public health system: health departments are closing, technology and information systems are outmoded, emerging and drug-resistant diseases threaten to overwhelm resources, and serious training inadequacies weaken the capacity of the public health workforce to address new threats and adapt to changes in the

Essential Public Health Services
1. Monitor health status to identify community health problems.
2. Diagnose and investigate health problems and health hazards in the community.
3. Inform, educate, and empower people about health issues.
4. Mobilize community partnerships to identify and solve health problems.
5. Develop policies and plans that support individual and community health efforts.
6. Enforce laws and regulations that protect health and assure safety.
7. Link people to needed personal health services and assure the provision of health care when otherwise unavailable.
8. Assure a competent public health and personal health care workforce.
9. Evaluate effectiveness, accessibility, and quality of personal and population-based health services.
10. Research for new insights and innovative solutions to health problems.

Source: Public Health Functions Steering Committee. *Public Health in America*, Fall 1994. http://www.health.gov/phfunctions/public.htm (January 1, 2000).

health care market.[1, 4] Conversely, interest in public health has led to the development of public health improvement plans in several States, including Illinois and Washington. In addition, private foundations have funded major national programs to improve health. For example, Turning Point: Collaborating for a New Century of Public Health Initiatives, supported by the Robert Wood Johnson Foundation and the W.K. Kellogg Foundation, helps develop more effective public health infrastructure by providing technical assistance to health departments at State and local levels.

All public health services depend on the presence of basic infrastructure. Every categorical public health program—childhood immunizations, infectious disease monitoring, cancer and asthma prevention, drinking water quality, injury prevention, and many others—requires health professionals who are competent in cross-cutting and technical skills, public health agencies with the capacity to assess and respond to community health needs, and up-to-date information systems. Federal public health agencies rely on the presence of infrastructure systems at the local and State levels to support the implementation of their programs.

In public health, a strong infrastructure provides the capacity to prepare for and respond to both acute and chronic threats to the Nation's health, whether they are bioterrorism attacks, emerging infections, disparities in health status, or increases in chronic disease and injury rates. Such an infrastructure serves as the foundation for planning, delivering, and evaluating public health. The public health infrastructure comprises the workforce, data and information systems, and public health organizations. Research also is a key activity of public health infrastructure in identifying opportunities to improve health, strengthen information systems and organizations, and make more effective and efficient use of resources.

Health data and surveillance systems provide information on illness, disability, and death from acute and chronic conditions; injuries; personal, environmental, and occupational risk factors; preventive and treatment services; and costs. To be most useful, public health data must be accessible, accurate, timely, and clearly stated and must adhere to strict confidentiality standards. The system must be linked with other data systems and must be linked with and integrated at the Federal, Tribal, State, and local levels. The systematic collection, analysis, interpretation, dissemination, and use of health data drive efforts to determine the health status of a population, plan prevention programs, and evaluate program effectiveness. Healthy People activities during the 1980s and 1990s have demonstrated the central role of data, focused attention on what is important to measure, and stimulated the development of new data systems.

Although Federal agencies take the lead in collecting national public health data, these agencies are only some of the many necessary partners that collect, analyze, and use public health data. Surveillance often involves active cooperation among Federal, Tribal, State, and local agencies. For example, the Vital Statistics Cooperative Program obtains information on births, deaths, marriages, and divorces from all 50 States, the District of Columbia, Puerto Rico, the U.S. Virgin Islands, and Guam. Programs in each area collect vital information from many sources in local communities, including funeral directors, medical examiners, coroners, hospitals, religious authorities, and justices of the peace. Other data collection systems, based on sample surveys rather than reports, depend on the participation of thousands of private citizens nationwide. And still other systems rely on the administrative records of public and private health care organizations.

If data are not available or are missing, problems can arise, especially for State and local health agencies. In particular, health problems may not be identified in high-risk populations, or the public intervention may not be timely enough. Information enables public health to direct preventive services and health promotion activities toward select populations.

The public health workforce must have up-to-date knowledge, skills, and abilities to deliver services effectively and carry out the core functions of assessment, policy development, and assurance of services. The importance of organizations in making a system effective often is overlooked. Yet, Tribal, State, and local public health agencies, in partnership with other community organizations, are essential to an effective public health system.

Because a national data system will not be available in the first half of the decade for tracking progress, one subject of interest concerning the public health infrastructure is not covered in this focus area's objectives. This topic represents a research and data collection agenda for the coming decade: increasing the proportion of Federal, Tribal, State, and local public and private employers that voluntarily adopt the Standard Occupational Classification (SOC) system to categorize public health personnel.

Disparities

A major goal of Healthy People 2010 is to eliminate health disparities. These disparities exist at all State and local levels but are not well delineated because of differences in public health systems. A better trained public health workforce, improved data and information systems, and more effective public health organizations will strengthen the public health infrastructure at all levels and help identify where disparities exist. Then targeted interventions and programs to eliminate the disparities can be developed.

Disparities among public health organizations and between the public and private health sectors are also of concern. For example, a diverse, highly skilled workforce must be recruited and trained to meet the challenges of the 21st century. Salary structures and disparities in staffing across jurisdictions, as well as between workers in the public and private sectors, will affect the ability of public health agencies to recruit and retain a high-quality workforce.

Opportunities

Several developments suggest opportunities to improve public health capacity nationwide.

The 1997 report *The Public Health Workforce: An Agenda for the 21st Century* recognized the need for a system to assure a stronger public health workforce.[5] The report identified five areas to be strengthened: national leadership, State and local leadership, workforce composition, curriculum development, and distance learning. Data systems are needed to track the extent to which the workforce has the knowledge, skills, and abilities to carry out its functions. With wide input from the public health community, the SOC system was updated in 1997 and 1998 to include an array of public health professions.[6] SOC will continue to be used in a number of national population- and employer-based surveys by the Bureau of Labor Statistics (U.S. Department of Labor), the Bureau of the Census (U.S. Department of Commerce), and the Bureau of Health Professions (U.S. Department of Health and Human Services). A standard classification may be useful in determining minimum levels of competency for each classification.

Healthy People 2000 did not have a specific focus area for public health infra-structure. Two objectives, however, did address broad infrastructure areas. One stated, "Increase to at least 90 percent the proportion of persons who are served by a local health department that is effectively carrying out the core functions of pub-lic health." Although selected studies have provided a snapshot of local health department effectiveness in carrying out the core functions,[7,8] systematic monitor-ing of this objective over time has not been done. However, efforts to define, achieve, and measure this objective have contributed to a more complete descrip-tion of infrastructure as well as a more detailed and expanded infrastructure goal.

The second objective stated, "Increase to at least 50 percent the proportion of counties that have established culturally and linguistically appropriate community health promotion programs for racial and ethnic minority populations." In 1996–97, baseline data for this objective were obtained for local health departments serving certain racial and ethnic groups comprising 10 percent or more of the population. Programs or interventions were most likely to be adapted in the areas of maternal and infant health (47 percent), nutrition (44 percent), and family plan-ning (42 percent). Adaptations were least likely to have been made for such groups in the areas of occupational safety and health (13 percent), mental health and mental disorders (18 percent), and food and drug safety and health (18 percent).

Healthy People 2000 had a specific priority area on data and surveillance. Several objectives from Healthy People 2000 have been modified and are included in Healthy People 2010 as Public Health Infrastructure objectives dealing with data and information systems.

Of the seven surveillance and data system objectives, progress has been made on six. A set of health status indicators appropriate to Federal, State, and local levels was developed, and all States monitor at least some indicators. National data sources to measure progress toward each of the Healthy People 2000 objectives were identified or created for 97 percent of objectives. Although difficult to quan-tify, progress toward filling data gaps is continuing, most recently through the *Healthy People 2000 Midcourse Review and 1995 Revisions,* when considerable attention was given to population groups at highest risk for premature death, dis-ease, or disability. The number of States that periodically publish data on Healthy People 2000 objectives has increased substantially. Systems for the transfer of data have expanded considerably in all States, with the expansion of the Internet playing a major role. Achieving the timely release of data appears to have moved away from the target; however, the measurement of progress for this objective is affected by the frequency of data collection.

Note: Unless otherwise noted, data are from the Centers for Disease Control and Prevention, National Center for Health Statistics, *Healthy People 2000 Review*, 1998–99.

Public Health Infrastructure

Goal: Ensure that Federal, Tribal, State, and local health agencies have the infrastructure to provide essential public health services effectively.

Number Objective Short Title

Data and Information Systems

23-1   Public health employee access to the Internet

23-2   Public access to information and surveillance data

23-3   Use of geocoding in health data systems

23-4   Data for all population groups

23-5   Data for Leading Health Indicators, Health Status Indicators, and Priority Data Needs at Tribal, State, and local levels

23-6   National tracking of Healthy People 2010 objectives

23-7   Timely release of data on objectives

Workforce

23-8   Competencies for public health workers

23-9   Training in essential public health services

23-10   Continuing education and training by public health agencies

Public Health Organizations

23-11   Performance standards for essential public health services

23-12   Health improvement plans

23-13   Access to public health laboratory services

23-14   Access to epidemiology services

23-15   Model statutes related to essential public health services

Resources

23-16   Data on public health expenditures

Prevention Research

23-17   Population-based prevention research

Healthy People 2010: Objectives for Improving Health

23-1. **(Developmental) Increase the proportion of Tribal, State, and local public health agencies that provide Internet and e-mail access for at least 75 percent of their employees and that teach employees to use the Internet and other electronic information systems to apply data and information to public health practice.**

Potential data sources: National Association of County and City Health Officials (NACCHO); Association of State and Territorial Health Officials (ASTHO); National Public Health Performance Standards Program, CDC, PHPPO; IHS.

Unpublished data from a 1999 survey of the National Association of County and City Health Officials showed 49 percent of local health department directors had continuous, high-speed access to the Internet at work. Further, 83 percent of local health departments had staff members who can search for and access public information on the Internet. The Bioterrorism Initiative, which began in 1999, is expected to generate information on Internet and e-mail capacity at State and local levels for responding to terrorist events; this information could be used in monitoring this objective.

All workers within a State or local public health agency need access to the Internet or other electronic information systems appropriate to their job functions. Access requires hardware (for example, computers, modems, CD-ROM drives), software that can browse the Internet and can be used to analyze health information databases, and training on the effective use of the Internet and database systems. Adequate capacity in public health informatics—the systematic application of information and computer science and technology to public health practice, research, and learning—is key to this objective. Public health agencies need to provide appropriate training on data sources and how to transform the data retrieved from these systems into information that can be used to develop public health policy.

23-2. **(Developmental) Increase the proportion of Federal, Tribal, State, and local health agencies that have made information available to the public in the past year on the Leading Health Indicators, Health Status Indicators, and Priority Data Needs.**

Potential data sources: CDC, NCHS; National Association of County and City Health Officials (NACCHO); Association of State and Territorial Health Officials

(ASTHO); National Public Health Performance Standards Program, CDC, PHPPO; IHS.

Leading Health Indicators are defined elsewhere in *Healthy People 2010*. (See Understanding and Improving Health.) Health Status Indicators and Priority Data Needs are those generated from objective 22.1 in Healthy People 2000[9, 10] This objective seeks to ensure that data collected at the national, Tribal, State, and local levels are electronically aggregated and available to and accessible by individuals and organizations. The objective includes publicly accessible communication through media (for example, print, television, and radio) or online systems, such as the Internet. In addition to data on Leading Health Indicators, Health Status Indicators, and Priority Data Needs, many other kinds of public health data need to be accessible to the public. These data include health outcomes; utilization statistics, such as the Health Plan Employer Data and Information Set (HEDIS) or similar measures from managed care organizations; infrastructure data; health risk data; and community report cards that provide a snapshot of a community's health. Efforts should be made to include other sources of data not widely used for public health assessment (for example, sources of socioeconomic, expenditure, and quality of life data).

23-3. Increase the proportion of all major national, State, and local health data systems that use geocoding to promote nationwide use of geographic information systems (GIS) at all levels.

Target: 90 percent.

Baseline: 45 percent of major national, State, and local health data systems geocoded records to street address or latitude and longitude in 2000.

Target setting method: 100 percent improvement.

Data source: CDC, NCHS.

Public health rests on information. The information technology revolution, including online systems, the Internet, and other electronic information systems, continues to expand both the volume and the accessibility of information. Increased use of geocoding in health data systems will provide the basis for more cost-effective disease surveillance and intervention. At the same time, challenges arise in synthesizing and disseminating the huge amount of available information as well as ensuring that the data are scientifically accurate and have appropriate safeguards for confidentiality.

The capacity to achieve national goals is related to the ability to target strategies to geographic areas.[11] Extension of geocoding capacities throughout health data systems will facilitate this ability. A GIS is a powerful tool combining geography, data, and computer mapping. With GIS, digital maps and databases are stored with linked georeferenced identifiers to facilitate rapid computer manipulation, analysis, and spatial display of information. Geocoding (street address matching or assignment of latitude and longitude) will be the basis for data linkage and analysis in the 21st century. The versatility of GIS supports the exploration of spatial relationships, patterns, and trends that otherwise would go unnoticed.[12] In 1999, 10 of 22 major health data systems, defined as data systems responsible for tracking five or more Healthy People 2010 objectives, geocoded data. However, public access to data below the county level is prohibited or severely restricted because of confidentiality and privacy issues. A major challenge in the coming decade will be to increase public access to GIS information without compromising confidentiality.[13] (See Tracking Healthy People 2010 for a discussion of these major health data systems.)

23-4. Increase the proportion of population-based Healthy People 2010 objectives for which national data are available for all population groups identified for the objective.

Target: 100 percent.

Baseline: 11 percent of the population-based objectives had national data for all select population groups in 2000.

Target setting method: Total coverage.

Data source: CDC, NCHS.

The capacity of the public health system to measure the health of all individuals requires special attention to groups that may not be identifiable in statewide or national databases. Lack of data for these groups can be the result of relatively small numbers of cases for rare events, small population groups, or other special circumstances. Better data-gathering systems are needed to track health objectives for such populations as racial and ethnic groups, persons with disabilities, specific Tribes, homeless persons, institutionalized persons (for example, in nursing homes and prisons), low-income persons, and students in special education.

National data indicate that some racial and ethnic groups often face higher rates of illness, disability, death, or other risk factors than the general population. Other groups, such as persons with low incomes, limited education, or disabilities, also have relatively poor health. Females and males also experience the burden of poor health in different ways. One of the overarching goals of Healthy People 2010 is to eliminate these health disparities. To assess progress toward this goal, data on population groups must be available.

23-5. (Developmental) Increase the proportion of Leading Health Indicators, Health Status Indicators, and Priority Data Needs for which data—especially for select populations— are available at the Tribal, State, and local levels.

Potential data sources: CDC, NCHS; IHS.

In 1997, 37 of 47 States and the District of Columbia had their own Healthy People 2000 plans.[14] The average number of objectives in the State plans was 113 but ranged from 20 to 308.[14] On average, baseline data were available for 76 percent of the States' objectives by 1997, although more than half of the data were 3 or more years old.[14]

Because of the lack of comparability between States, a set of Leading Health Indicators has been developed from the Healthy People 2010 objectives. (See Understanding and Improving Health.) These indicators can be monitored at the national, State, and local levels. They can be used in conjunction with States' objectives to evaluate the progress of Healthy People 2010 in communities.

Health Status Indicators and Priority Data Needs are those generated from objective 22.1 in Healthy People 2000.[9, 10] Select populations are those identified for each indicator that make up at least 10 percent of the population for the Tribal, State, or local area. State and local data are essential for the managers and providers who must assess health status and services and plan, carry out, and evaluate health programs. However, data were not available for all objectives at all State and local levels to evaluate the majority of Healthy People 2000 objectives. Therefore, a consensus process identified a small set of indicators that would be understandable, acceptable, outcome oriented, and measurable with available data and would imply specific interventions that compel action.[9] This process resulted in the set of Health Status Indicators. National data for these indicators are published regularly in the *Healthy People 2000 Review 1998–99.*[15]

An additional set of measures was considered that had important public health significance but could not be included because of insufficient data at the State and local levels. This set, known as Priority Data Needs, has been used to measure these additional indicators.[10] (State data are available for both the Health Status Indicators and Priority Data Needs at http://www.cdc.gov/nchswww/datawh/datawh.htm.)

An important function of these different sets of health indicators is to monitor progress toward the second goal of Healthy People 2010: to eliminate health disparities among population groups. Data for these indicators need to be available at the national, Tribal, State, and local levels. The objective's intent is to ensure the availability of sufficient and accurate data to evaluate these indicator sets at all geographic levels and for all select population groups.

23-6. Increase the proportion of Healthy People 2010 objectives that are tracked regularly at the national level.

Target: 100 percent.

Baseline: 82 percent of measurable objectives, including their subobjectives, were tracked at least every 3 years in 2000.

Target setting method: Total coverage for measurable objectives, including their subobjectives.

Data source: CDC, NCHS.

Frequent, regular feedback is needed to tailor strategies to achieve national objectives during a decade. Past efforts have been hampered by infrequent tracking of objectives. For adequate tracking of the objectives during the next decade, at least three data points (baseline, midpoint, final) are desirable to assess progress. Hence, objectives need to be measured at least every 3 years. In 2000, 66 percent of the measurable objectives, including their subobjectives, were tracked annually.

Healthy People 2010 contains more than 150 developmental objectives that lacked baseline data at initial publication but that were expected to have data points by 2004 to facilitate setting 2010 targets in the mid-decade review. Developmental objectives that do not have a baseline by the midcourse review will be dropped. Healthy People will succeed and lead to action only to the extent that regularly collected data can be used to track its objectives.

23-7. Increase the proportion of Healthy People 2010 objectives for which national data are released within 1 year of the end of data collection.

Target: 100 percent.

Baseline: 36 percent of the objectives, including their subobjectives, measured by major data systems were tracked with data released within 1 year of the end of data collection in 2000.

Target setting method: Total coverage (as measured by major data systems).

Data source: CDC, NCHS.

The utility of data depends on both the periodicity of data collection (see objective 23-6) and the timeliness of data release. In past years, a number of electronic data collection systems have been put in place in national, Tribal, State, and local data collection agencies (for example, electronic birth and death certificates, computer-assisted personal interview questionnaires, and computer-assisted telephone interview questionnaires). Some of these innovations, such as vital statistics data from electronic birth and death certificates, already are showing results in the more timely release of data. For others, the benefits of faster turnaround are still a few years away. The purpose of this objective is to ensure that health information is available to policymakers and the public shortly after data collection.

23-8. **(Developmental) Increase the proportion of Federal, Tribal, State, and local agencies that incorporate specific competencies in the essential public health services into personnel systems.**

Potential data sources: National Association of County and City Health Officials (NACCHO); Association of State and Territorial Health Officials (ASTHO); HRSA; IHS.

In addition to a basic knowledge of public health, all public health workers should have specific competencies in their areas of specialty, interest, and responsibility. Competent leaders, policy developers, planners, epidemiologists, funders, evaluators, laboratory staff, and others are necessary for a strong public health infrastructure. The workforce needs to know how to use information technology effectively for networking, communication, and access to information. A skilled workforce must be culturally and linguistically competent to understand the needs of and deliver services to select populations and to have sensitivity to diverse populations. Finally, technical competency in such areas as biostatistics, environmental and occupational health, the social and behavioral aspects of health and disease, and the practice of prevention in clinical medicine should be developed in the workforce.

Although the disciplines in a particular agency will vary according to the resources, policies, needs, and populations served, individual public health employees must have certain competencies or levels of expertise. Their combined areas of expertise enable the organization to provide essential public health services. Failure to include references to these competencies in the formal personnel system makes achieving standards difficult. Position descriptions or performance evaluations are likely sources of data for this objective.

National licensing and certification programs that measure competency already exist for nurses, physicians, dietitians, health educators, laboratory technicians, sanitarians, environmental health specialists, and many allied health professionals. Coordination with these national programs will be important to ensure that new certification efforts cover essential public health service concerns. At least one State, New Jersey, has licensing requirements for all local health officers.

23-9. **(Developmental) Increase the proportion of schools for public health workers that integrate into their curricula specific content to develop competency in the essential public health services.**

Potential data sources: Association of Schools of Public Health; American Association of Medical Colleges; HRSA's Bureau of Health Professions; American Association of Colleges of Nursing.

Healthy People 2010: Objectives for Improving Health

23-10. (Developmental) Increase the proportion of Federal, Tribal, State, and local public health agencies that provide continuing education to develop competency in essential public health services for their employees.

Potential data sources: National Association of County and City Health Officials (NACCHO); Association of State and Territorial Health Officials (ASTHO); IHS.

The above two objectives address training for both the current and future public health workforce. Tomorrow's public health workforce is being educated today by schools of public health, programs in public health accredited by the Council on Education for Public Health, and other graduate programs. These emerging leaders must be grounded in the areas of expertise needed to deliver essential public health services. This objective may be accomplished either by developing specific courses or by incorporating essential public health services into existing offerings, depending on the school or program.

There is an ongoing need to train and educate people who are currently employed in public health as new areas, problems, threats, and potential disasters emerge. For example, the threat of bioterrorism or the increased impact of any natural and technological disaster will require different training and areas of expertise so that public health workers can detect problems early, communicate rapidly, and respond effectively. A system for enabling career-long learning opportunities is desirable.

Although several disciplines have continuing education requirements as part of the licensing or certification process, this objective extends to all workers. Federal, Tribal, State, and local public health agencies do not necessarily have to provide the education, but they need to ensure its availability to employees. Employees in organizations that are not formally part of the public health system but that deliver health services also should have continuing education. Once an effective source of data is developed for this objective, a percentage of employees should be targeted annually for continuing education.

Public Health Organizations

23-11. (Developmental) Increase the proportion of State and local public health agencies that meet national performance standards for essential public health services.

Potential data source: National Public Health Performance Standards Program, CDC, PHPPO.

Experts in quality improvement have long asserted that "what gets measured gets done."[16] The measurement of performance is not new, nor is the concept foreign to most health departments. What is not being done, however, is comprehensive, systematic performance evaluation. Without standard performance indicators and systematic comparisons, public health lacks useful benchmarks for improvement.

National performance standards could be used to improve quality, increase accountability for dollars invested, and create credibility with internal and external constituents. National organizations, such as the Joint Commission on Accreditation of Healthcare Organizations and the National Commission on Quality Assurance, that work with performance measures in health care have models that can be followed.

A number of States have or are developing State-specific performance standards for local public health agencies. The Centers for Disease Control and Prevention (CDC), in conjunction with national, State, and local public health organizations, is developing national performance standards for State and local health departments.[17] These national standards, expected to be operational in 2000, are based on the essential public health services.

23-12. Increase the proportion of Tribes, States, and the District of Columbia that have a health improvement plan and increase the proportion of local jurisdictions that have a health improvement plan linked with their State plan.

Target and baseline:

Objective	Jurisdiction	1997 Baseline (unless noted)	2010 Target
			Percent
23-12a.	Tribes	Developmental	
23-12b.	States and the District of Columbia	78	100
23-12c.	Local jurisdictions	32 (1992–93)	80

Target setting method: Total coverage for Tribes, States, and the District of Columbia; 150 percent improvement for local jurisdictions.

Data sources: National Profile of Local Health Departments, National Association of County and City Health Officials (NACCHO); Association of State and Territorial Health Officials (ASTHO); IHS.

Planning is central to improving public health in any State or community. A health improvement plan (HIP) is a long-term, systematic effort to address health problems on the basis of the results of a community needs assessment. This plan is used by health and other governmental education and human service agencies, in collaboration with community partners, to set priorities and coordinate and target resources.

A HIP is critical for developing policies and defining actions to target efforts that promote health. It should define the vision for the health of the community inclusively and should be done in a timely way. Many States and localities have their own HIPs that may not be related to one another. Public health needs often exceed resources, and sufficient resources are never available. The health of a State or local community can be improved by setting priorities so available resources are used more efficiently.

Health improvement plans are, or should be, the link between Healthy People 2010 and the unique health needs of each State and local area. Plans should include all community interests and should tie health goals to other State goal-setting or benchmarking processes. Plans also will identify collaboration among partners to facilitate implementation and evaluation. State and local health departments have a leadership role in this process.

23-13. (Developmental) Increase the proportion of Tribal, State, and local health agencies that provide or assure comprehensive laboratory services to support essential public health services.

Potential data sources: CDC; Association of Public Health Laboratories; Association of State and Territorial Health Officials (ASTHO); National Association of County and City Health Officials (NACCHO).

Public health laboratories, in conjunction with clinical, environmental, and agricultural laboratories, constitute a national laboratory network that fulfills a critical role in assessing and assuring the health of populations and the environment. This role includes such activities and services as laboratory quality assessment and improvement, outbreak investigation, emergency preparedness and response, laboratory-based surveillance, population screening, and technology transfer. The national laboratory network also operates for the benefit of public health by helping to assure safe water, food, and air and by supporting programs such as newborn screening and lead-poisoning prevention.

23-14. (Developmental) Increase the proportion of Tribal, State, and local public health agencies that provide or assure comprehensive epidemiology services to support essential public health services.

Potential data sources: Council of State and Territorial Epidemiologists; IHS.

All communities need access to comprehensive epidemiology services so they can quickly detect, investigate, and respond to diseases in order to prevent unnecessary transmission. Epidemiologists carry out several essential public health services, including monitoring health status, diagnosing and investigating health problems and health hazards, and conducting evaluation and research.

23-15. (Developmental) Increase the proportion of Federal, Tribal, State, and local jurisdictions that review and evaluate the extent to which their statutes, ordinances, and bylaws assure the delivery of essential public health services.

Potential data sources: National Conference of State Legislators; Association of State and Territorial Health Officials (ASTHO); National Association of County and City Health Officials (NACCHO); IHS.

The statutes, ordinances, and charters that create the agency and set forth its powers and duties form the legal basis for any public health agency. General language in such a document usually states the agency's responsibility to preserve, promote, and protect the health of the persons in its jurisdiction. In addition, the agency usually is authorized to enforce multiple statutes that require it to control diseases (or classes of diseases), limit certain kinds of businesses (for example, restaurants and health facilities), and monitor the treatment of waste materials (for example, sewage and garbage). These authorities may be centralized in one agency or distributed across several. A review of State public health statutes shows significant variation from the accepted framework of the essential public health services.[18] Little correlation exists between the essential public health services identified in the mid-1990s and current statutes, as might be expected due to their antiquity.

Many laws, rules, regulations, and ordinances pertaining to public health are outmoded. Federal, Tribal, State, and local jurisdictions need to review their public health laws and consider a different conceptual approach for regulating public health. Rather than have a legal structure based on the provision of services for categorical health problems, communities might be better served and protected by a set of laws, statutes, and ordinances based on essential public health services. Without diminishing the role of each jurisdiction in tailoring a statute (ordinance, charter, or regulation) to local conditions and priorities, the Nation's public health infrastructure would be strengthened if jurisdictions had a model law and could use it regularly for improvements. Such a model should be developed and should contain examples of complete statutory language for key principles and provisions (such as establishment of agency powers, authority of the agency director, surveillance for conditions of public health importance, due process in enforcement actions to protect the public's health) and examples for drafting any other portion of the law.

23-16. (Developmental) Increase the proportion of Federal, Tribal, State, and local public health agencies that gather accurate data on public health expenditures, categorized by essential public health service.

Potential data sources: National Association of County and City Health Officials (NACCHO); Association of State and Territorial Health Officials (ASTHO); HHS, Operating Divisions; IHS.

Financial resources fuel the public health infrastructure. Understanding the Nation's investment in public health and the origin and destination of these financial resources is critical. To allocate resources appropriately and to ensure efficient performance, expenditures must be documented and explained. Documenting finances will allow communities to identify gaps in expenditures that they can help fill in partnership with public health agencies. State and local leaders need to know where gaps exist and how funding is changing in order to ensure that public health agencies can protect the Nation's health.

The Public Health Expenditures Project estimated and aggregated expenditures by Federal agencies and State health departments on the essential public health services.[19] The purpose was to understand the capacity to collect such data, apart from specific programmatic expenditures. Considerable difficulty was encountered during the project because expenditure information is not usually collected using this framework. Reporting requirements are different for different program areas and for different funding streams.

The Public Health Foundation (PHF) led a study of eight States that estimated expenditures by essential public health service.[19] A joint study by the National Association of County and City Health Officials, National Association of Local Boards of Health, and PHF reported the feasibility of collecting expenditure data by essential public health service at the local level.[20] These studies showed that reliable estimates of expenditures based on essential public health services can be produced, but that measuring investment in essential services must be integrated into existing data collection strategies and emerging initiatives.

A national perspective on the expenditure of financial resources related to essential public health services will help in allocating resources on a functional rather than a programmatic basis and in identifying where additional resources may be needed to assure a strong infrastructure at the Federal, Tribal, State, and local levels.

23-17. (Developmental) Increase the proportion of Federal, Tribal, State, and local public health agencies that conduct or collaborate on population-based prevention research.

Potential data sources: Association of Schools of Public Health; National Association of County and City Health Officials (NACCHO); Association of State and Territorial Health Officials (ASTHO); CDC Sentinel Network.

Research is the Nation's investment in the future. Public health research is both funded and conducted by Federal, State, and local public health agencies, academic institutions, private industry, and philanthropic institutions. Opportunities and incentives should be provided to attract new researchers and to encourage collaboration among Federal agencies, States, local communities, and academic institutions. These efforts should result in a research agenda for the Nation's public health infrastructure. The Federal Government has a strong commitment to health research, as evidenced by the billions of dollars allocated to the National Institutes of Health, the Centers for Disease Control and Prevention, the Agency for Healthcare Research and Quality, the Health Resources and Services Administration, and other U.S. Public Health Service agencies. State governments, private foundations, and private industry also are strong supporters of research. Most resources have been directed toward biomedical research, with more focus on individual diseases or risk factors than on population-based prevention.

Researchers and research organizations now recognize the value of including diverse populations and communities in their studies. Population-based prevention and clinical research must continue to include specific population groups, such as females, racial and ethnic groups, and persons who are either not served or are underserved. Research should be responsive to National, State, and local public health priorities and needs.

Strengthening the capacity to conduct population-based research is essential for improving the practice of public health. Research is defined by the *Code of Federal Regulations* as "a systematic investigation, including research development, testing, and evaluation, designed to develop or contribute to generalizable knowledge."[21] The primary goal of population-based public health research is to collect information that will form the basis for public health action.[22] Thus, the areas included in population-based public health research are public health surveillance, program evaluation, emergency response, and evidence-based guideline development and dissemination.

National, State, and local agencies and organizations conducting research require the collaboration and cooperation of the population being studied. Formal collaboration (such as a memorandum of agreement) between schools of public health and State or local health departments for the conduct of a specific project could be a measure for this objective.

Related Objectives From Other Focus Areas

1. **Access to Quality Health Services**
   - 1-7. Core competencies in health provider training
   - 1-8. Racial and ethnic representation in health professions
6. **Disability and Secondary Conditions**
   - 6-1. Standard definition of people with disabilities in data sets
   - 6-13. Surveillance and health promotion programs
7. **Educational and Community-Based Programs**
   - 7-10. Community health promotion programs
   - 7-11. Culturally appropriate and linguistically competent community health promotion programs
8. **Environmental Health**
   - 8-26. Information systems used for environmental health
11. **Health Communication**
   - 11-1. Households with Internet access
   - 11-3. Research and evaluation of communication programs
   - 11-4. Quality of Internet health information sources
   - 11-5. Centers of excellence
17. **Medical Product Safety**
   - 17-2. Linked, automated information systems
21. **Oral Health**
   - 21-16. Oral and craniofacial State-based surveillance system

Terminology

(A listing of abbreviations and acronyms used in this publication appears in Appendix H.)

Distance learning: A system and a process that connects learners with distributed learning resources characterized by (1) separation of place or time between instructor and learner, among learners, or between learners and learning resource and (2) interaction between the learner and the instructor, among learners, or between learners and learning resources conducted through one or more media. Use of electronic media is not required.

Epidemiology: Branch of medical science dealing with the distribution and determinants of health-related events in specified populations and the application of this study to the control of health problems.

Essential public health services: The services identified in *Public Health in America* (defined below): monitoring health status; diagnosing and investigating health problems; informing, educating, and empowering people; mobilizing community partnerships; developing policies and plans; enforcing laws and regulations; linking people to needed services; assuring a competent workforce; conducting evaluations; and conducting research.

Federal, State, or local public health agency: A government or nongovernment entity authorized to provide one or more essential public health services. Included are health, mental health, substance abuse, environmental health, occupational health, educational, and public health agencies.

Geocoding: The process of address matching and assignment of a street address to a corresponding latitude and longitude.

Geographic information system (GIS): Combines modern computer and supercomputing digital technology with data management systems to provide tools for the capture, storage, manipulation, analysis, and visualization of spatial data. Spatial data contain information, usually in the form of a geographic coordinate system, that gives the data location relative to the earth's surface. These spatial attributes enable previously disparate data sets to be integrated into a digital mapping environment.

Graduate program in public health: Any academic postbachelor's degree program that specifically trains public health workers. Included, for example, are programs in schools of public health, nursing, environmental health, medicine and dentistry, and veterinary medicine.

Health improvement plan (HIP): A plan made up of action steps to guide providers of essential public health services in addressing problems and gaps that have been identified in a needs assessment. A local plan should be linked to its State plan. Both plans should mobilize a variety of organizations to reduce health problems and improve the community's capacity to respond to public health needs. All providers of public health services—such as health departments, hospitals, schools, managed care providers under Medicaid, environmental health agencies, and medical and nursing organizations—should be included in a HIP. Health departments should play an especially active role in developing and implementing plans.

Health Status Indicators: Eighteen measures of health status defined in 1991 that represent a broad overview of a community's health and that can be used by various levels of government. Health Status Indicators include infant mortality, death rates for selected diseases, incidence rates of selected infectious diseases, measures regarding pregnancy and birth, childhood poverty, and air quality.

Leading Health Indicators: A set of 10 key determinants that influence health and can serve as a barometer for evaluating the health of the Nation. Leading Health Indicators include individual behaviors, the social and physical environment, and community health programs and address areas that most influence the health of individuals, communities, and the Nation. (See Understanding and Improving Health.)

Major health data systems: Data systems that provide tracking data for five or more national Healthy People 2010 objectives, including the Vital Statistics Cooperative Program, National Health Interview Survey, National Health and Nutrition Examination Survey, National Hospital Discharge Survey, and Behavioral Risk Factor Surveillance System.

Needs assessment: A formal process—which is the first step in a community health improvement process—of identifying problems and assessing the community's capacity to address health and social service needs. Examples include Assessment Protocol for Excellence in Public Health, Planned Approach to Community Health, Healthy Cities, and Model Standards.

Population-based prevention research: Research to identify effective public health prevention practices for particular populations.

Priority Data Needs: Sixteen measures of health status and risk behaviors of public health significance that were not included in the 1991 list of Health Status Indicators because of insufficient data at all levels of government. Subsequent to 1991, data sources have been developed for most of the Priority Data Needs. Priority Data Needs include indicators of selected chronic diseases, access to medical care, environmental exposures, and behavioral risks.

Public health and environmental health laboratory services: Laboratory services that include health and environmental assessment, surveillance, quality assurance, training, and consultation. These services also include a core set of tests in pathology, hematology, chemistry, microbiology, and environmental science.

Public Health in America: Statement that defines the public health vision and mission and describes the essential public health services. It was adopted in 1994 by the Public Health Functions Steering Committee, which included representatives of the U.S. Public Health Service agencies, American Public Health Association, Association of Schools of Public Health, Association of State and Territorial Health Officials, Environmental Council of the States, National Association of County and City Health Officials, National Association of State Alcohol and Drug Abuse Directors, National Association of State Mental Health Program Directors, and Public Health Foundation.

Public health informatics: The systematic application of information and computer science and technology to public health practice, research, and learning.

Public health infrastructure: The resources needed to deliver the essential public health services to every community—people who work in the field of public health, information and communication systems used to collect and disseminate accurate data, and public health organizations at the State and local levels in the front lines of public health.

Public health workers: Individuals who are responsible for providing the essential public health services whether or not they work in an official health agency. At the State level, many workers have public health responsibilities even though they may work for nonpublic health agencies, such as environmental, agricultural, and education departments. This definition does not include those workers who occasionally contribute to the public health effort while fulfilling other responsibilities. Public health workers also are defined in the SOC system used by the Bureau of Labor Statistics, Bureau of the Census, and Bureau of Health Professions. This system has been updated and expanded to include additional categories of public health workers.

References

[1] Institute of Medicine, Committee for the Study of the Future of Public Health. *The Future of Public Health*. Washington, DC: National Academy Press, 1988.

[2] Harrell, J.A., and Baker, E.L. The essential services of public health. *Leadership in Public Health* 3(3):27-31, 1994.

[3] Public Health Functions Steering Committee. *Public Health in America*. Fall 1994. <http://www.health.gov/phfuncions/public.htm>January 1, 2000.

[4] Baker, E.L.; Melton, R.J.; Stange, P.V.; et al. Health reform and the health of the public: Forging community health partnerships. *Journal of the American Medical Association* 272(16):1276-1282, 1994.

[5] Public Health Service (PHS). *The Public Health Workforce: An Agenda for the 21st Century*. Washington, DC: U.S. Department of Health and Human Services (HHS), 1997.

[6] Office of Management and Budget. 1998 Standard Occupational Classification. *Federal Register* 64(101):53136-53163, September 30, 1999.

[7] Richards, T.B.; Rogers, J.J.; Christenson, G.M.; et al. Evaluating local public health performance at a community level on a statewide basis. *Journal of Public Health Management and Practice* 1(4):70-83, 1995.

[8] Turnock, B.J.; Handler, A.; Hall, W.; et al. Local health department effectiveness in addressing the core functions of public health. *Public Health Reports* 109:478-484, 1994.

[9] Freedman, M.A. Health status indicators for the year 2000. *Statistical Notes*. No 1. Hyattsville, MD: National Center for Health Statistics (NCHS), 1991.

[10] Kim, I., and Kepple, K. Priority data needs: Sources for national, state, and local-level data and data collection systems. *Statistical Notes.* No. 15. Hyattsville, MD: NCHS, 1997.

[11] Yasnoff, W.A., and Sondik, E.J. Geographic information systems (GIS) in public health practice in the new millennium. *Journal of Public Health Management Practice* 5(4):ix, 1999.

[12] Croner, C.M.; Sperling, J.; and Broome, F.R. Geographic information systems (GIS): New perspectives in understanding human health and environmental relationships. *Statistics in Medicine* 15:1961-1977, 1996.

[13] Richards, T.B.; Croner, C.M.; Rushton, G.; et al. Geographic information systems and public health: Mapping the future. *Public Health Reports* 114:359-360, 1999.

[14] Public Health Foundation (PHF). *Measuring Health Objectives and Indicators: 1997 State and Local Capacity Survey.* Washington, DC: PHF, 1998.

[15] NCHS. *Healthy People 2000 Review, 1998–99.* Hyattsville, MD: PHS, 1999.

[16] Center for Accountability and Performance. *Performance Measurement: Concepts and Techniques.* 2nd ed. Washington, DC: American Society for Public Administration, 1998.

[17] Halverson, P.K.; Nicola, R.M.; and Baker, E.L. Performance measurement and accreditation of public health organizations: A call to action. *Journal of Public Health Management and Practice* 4(4):5-7, 1998.

[18] Gebbie, K. State public health laws: An expression of constituency expectations. *Journal of Public Health Management and Practice* 6(2):46-54, 2000.

[19] Elbert, K.W.; Barry, M.; Bialek, R.; and Garufi, M. *Measuring Expenditures for Essential Public Health Services.* Washington, DC: PHF, 1996.

[20] Barry, M.; Centra, L.; Pratt, E.; et al. *Where Do the Dollars Go? Measuring Local Public Health Expenditures.* Washington, DC: National Association of County and City Health Officials, National Association of Local Boards of Health, and PHF, 1998.

[21] HHS, National Institutes of Health, Office for Protection from Research Risks. *Protection of Human Subjects.* Revised June 18, 1991. <http://www.nih.gov/grants/oprr/humansubjects/45cfr46.htm> November 23, 1999.

[22] Snider, D.E., and Stroup, D.F. Defining research when it comes to public health. *Public Health Reports* 112:29-32, 1997.

24

Respiratory Diseases

Co-Lead Agencies: Centers for Disease Control and Prevention
National Institutes of Health

Contents

Goal

Promote respiratory health through better prevention, detection, treatment, and education efforts.

Overview

Asthma, chronic obstructive pulmonary disease (COPD), and obstructive sleep apnea (OSA) are a significant public health burden to the United States.[1] Specific methods of detection, intervention, and treatment exist that may reduce this burden. Several behaviors and diseases that affect the respiratory system, such as tuberculosis, lung cancer, acquired immunodeficiency syndrome (AIDS), pneumonia, occupational lung disease, and smoking, are covered in other chapters. (See Focus Area 3. Cancer, Focus Area 13. HIV, Focus Area 14. Immunization and Infectious Diseases, Focus Area 20. Occupational Safety and Health, Focus Area 25. Sexually Transmitted Diseases, and Focus Area 27. Tobacco Use.) Certain other important respiratory diseases, such as respiratory distress syndromes, sarcoidosis, and chronic sinusitis, which are difficult to define, detect, prevent, or treat, are not discussed in this chapter. Their omission, however, is not a reflection on the magnitude of the health problems associated with them.

Asthma and COPD are among the 10 leading chronic conditions causing restricted activity. After chronic sinusitis, asthma is the most common cause of chronic illness in children.[2] Methods are available to treat these respiratory diseases and promote respiratory health.

Asthma

Issues and Trends

Asthma is a serious and growing health problem. An estimated 14.9 million persons in the United States have asthma.[3] The number of people with asthma increased by 102 percent between 1979–80 and 1993–94.[4]

Asthma is responsible for about 500,000 hospitalizations,[3] 5,000 deaths,[3] and 134 million days[4] of restricted activity a year. Yet most of the problems caused by asthma could be averted if persons with asthma and their health care providers managed the disease according to established guidelines. Effective management of asthma comprises four major components: controlling exposure to factors that trigger asthma episodes, adequately managing asthma with medicine, monitoring the disease by using objective measures of lung function, and educating asthma patients to become partners in their own care.[2,5] Such prevention efforts are essential to interrupt the progression from disease to functional limitation and disability and to improve the quality of life for persons with asthma.

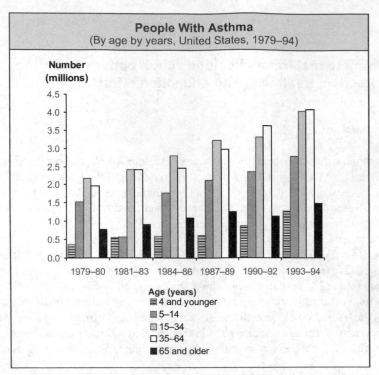

People With Asthma
(By age by years, United States, 1979–94)

Number (millions)

Age (years)
- 4 and younger
- 5–14
- 15–34
- 35–64
- 65 and older

Source: CDC, NCHS. Surveillance for Asthma—United States, 1960–1995. *Morbidity and Mortality Weekly Report* 47(SS-1);1-28, 1998.

In 1996, asthma was the 10th most common principal diagnosis in emergency department (ED) visits.[3] Among diseases commonly seen in outpatient departments, asthma was the ninth most frequent diagnosis in 1996.[6] In 1995, some 9 million physician office visits were made for asthma.[6] From 1990 to 1992, persons with asthma spent an estimated 64 million days in bed because of asthma, ranking asthma as the fourth highest chronic health condition.[4] The proportion of people with asthma who are limited in activity increased slightly from 19.4 percent in 1986–88 to 19.6 percent in 1994–96.[7]

Direct medical expenditures for asthma amounted to $3.64 billion in 1990, and indirect economic losses accounted for an additional $2.6 billion.[8] Of direct medical care costs, approximately 57 percent was spent on hospitalizations ($1.6 billion), outpatient hospital visits ($190 million), and ED visits ($295 million). Physician-related services accounted for 14 percent of the total expenditures, including $347 million for outpatient services. Prescription medications represented 30 percent of direct medical costs. Such facts highlight the significant cost of hospital care for asthma, compared to the more frequently used and less costly outpatient and pharmaceutical services.

Indirect costs—nonmedical economic losses such as days missed from work or school, caregiver costs, travel and waiting time, early retirement due to disability, and premature death—account for slightly less than 50 percent of the total costs of asthma. Data suggest that the uneven distribution of costs of asthma relates to nonscheduled acute or emergency care, indicating poor asthma management and suboptimal outcomes.[9, 10]

Environmental and occupational factors contribute to illness and disability from asthma. Decreases in lung function and a worsening of asthma have been associated with exposure to allergens, indoor pollutants (for example, tobacco smoke), and ambient air pollutants (for example, ozone, sulfur dioxide, nitrogen dioxide, acid aerosols, and particulate matter).[11, 12] Approximately 25 percent of children in the United States live in areas that exceed the Federal Government's standard for ozone.[13] Occupational factors cause or trigger asthma episodes in 5 to 30 percent of adults with the disease.[14] Environmental factors are associated with upper respiratory infections that contribute to illness and disability in children and adults.[15] (See Focus Area 8. Environmental Health.)

Disparities

Within the U.S. population, the health, economic, and social burdens of asthma vary. Disproportionate rates of death, hospitalization, ED use, and disability from asthma occur in certain age, gender, racial, and ethnic groups.

While the number of adults with asthma is greater than the number of children with asthma, the asthma rate is rising more rapidly in preschool-aged children than in any other group.[1] In 1995, the rate of self-reported asthma among children and adolescents under age 18 years was 7.5 percent, compared to 5.7 percent among the general population. The rates were higher in boys under age 18 years than in girls in the same age group. The rates of self-reported asthma were higher for women (6.7 percent) than men (5.2 percent) and higher for African Americans (6.7 percent) than whites (5.6 percent).[1] Among adults, women of all races have higher rates of illness and death from asthma than men.[16]

Death from asthma is two to six times more likely to occur among African Americans and Hispanics than among whites.[1] Although the number of deaths annually from asthma is low compared to other chronic diseases, the death rate for children aged 5 to 14 years and young adults aged 15 to 34 years doubled from 1979–80 to 1993–95 (from 1.5 to 3.7 deaths per million children aged 5 to 14 years and 2.8 to 6.3 deaths per million persons aged 15 to 34 years).[1] In 1993–95, death rates are slightly higher overall in women than in men.[1]

Rates of hospitalization for asthma demonstrate similar variations. Rates for African Americans are almost triple those for whites. Rates are higher among women than among men.[1] Asthma hospitalization rates have increased dramatically among children under age 5 years. From 1980 to 1993, the rate increased from 36 to 65 children hospitalized per 10,000 children under age 1 year. Some of this increase may be related to changes in diagnostic practices and changes in coding and reimbursement, but a large portion represents a true increase in illness and disability.

In the inner city, patients frequently use EDs for asthma care. In 1993 and 1994, African Americans were four times more likely than whites to visit an ED because of asthma.[1] Asthma patients in general and high-risk inner-city patients—in particular, those with a history of severe asthma who were hospitalized or visited the ED for asthma within the previous 2 years—need to be able to recognize the signs and symptoms of uncontrolled asthma and know how to respond appropriately.

The economic burden of asthma disproportionately affects patients with severe disease. Socioeconomic status, particularly poverty, appears to be an important contributing factor to asthma illness, disability, and death. In the United States, the rate of asthma cases for nonwhites is only slightly higher than for whites, yet the death, hospitalization, and ED-visit rates for nonwhites are more than twice those for whites.[1] Although reasons for these differences are unclear, they likely result from multiple factors: high levels of exposure to environmental tobacco smoke, pollutants, and environmental allergens (for example, house dust mites, cockroach particles, cat and dog dander, and possibly rodent dander and mold); a lack of access to quality medical care; and a lack of financial resources and social support to manage the disease effectively on a long-term basis.[17] Research into the role of socioeconomic factors is needed to identify additional prevention opportunities.

Opportunities

Scientific research has led to greater asthma control than was available in the early 1980s.[5] Effective management of asthma includes four components: avoiding or controlling the factors that may make asthma worse (for example, environmental and occupational allergens and irritants), taking appropriate medications tailored to the severity of the disease, objective monitoring of the disease by the patient and the health care professional, and actively involving the patient in managing the disease.[5] Effective asthma management reduces the need for hospitalizations and urgent care visits (in either an ED or physician's office) and enables patients to enjoy normal activities.[18, 19]

Advances in human genetics related to asthma are expected to provide better information about the contribution of genetic variation to the development of disease when people are exposed to certain environmental factors and variation in individual response to therapy. The use of this genetic information will improve targeted disease prevention and health management strategies for respiratory diseases.

Patient education is one of four components of effective asthma management.[5] Patients who are taught asthma self-management skills are able to manage and control their disease better than patients who do not receive education.[5] Patients need to learn to work with health care providers to optimize asthma care. Thus, both patients and health care providers need to be trained and educated on effective asthma management. Health outcomes for asthma—illness, disability, quality of life, and death—are related directly to the actions of health care professionals and patients. The National Asthma Education and Prevention Program (NAEPP) provides guidelines for diagnosis and management that should be incorporated into the curricula of health professional schools.[5, 20] Currently, there are no national data systems for tracking the training of health care providers in asthma management. Therefore, the issue is not covered in this focus area's objectives. It represents an important research and data collection agenda for the coming decade. In addition, research to identify the primary causes of development of asthma is a high priority. Such research can provide a scientific basis for efforts to prevent the development of asthma.

To control asthma effectively, asthma patients, particularly those on daily medication, need an asthma action plan developed under their physician's guidance. The plan spells out when and how to take medicines correctly, as well as what to do when asthma worsens. The treatment of persistent asthma emphasizes daily long-term therapy aimed at the underlying inflammation and preventing symptoms, rather than relying solely on treating symptoms with short-acting inhaled medication, such as a beta agonist medication. Use of more than one canister of the short-acting inhaled beta agonist medication per month is an indication of uncontrolled asthma and the need to start or increase long-term preventive therapy. Patients also need to work with health care providers during followup visits, particularly after being hospitalized, to make sure they understand and are able to follow the long-term management plan.

Working with local community groups to mobilize community resources for a comprehensive, culturally and linguistically competent approach to controlling asthma among high-risk populations is a priority. From a community-based perspective, States need to track occupational and environmental factors that cause or trigger asthma episodes. Such surveillance efforts should include collecting State-based data on the proportion of the population with asthma and monitoring occupational and environmental exposures and their impact on illness and disability related to asthma. Efforts directed to improving the environmental management of asthma also include reducing exposure to allergens and irritants, such as environmental tobacco smoke, and outdoor air pollution from ozone, sulfur dioxide, and particulate diesel matter. (See Focus Area 8. Environmental Health.)

Professional organizations, lay volunteer groups, Federal agencies, and the private sector have worked together and with NAEPP to implement a spectrum of asthma programs at national and local community levels. For example, numerous publications, media campaigns, and conferences target various audiences. Intensified efforts are planned to reach primary care providers, patients, and school personnel.[16, 20] A high-level work group convened by the U.S. Department of Health and Human Services in 1997 assessed the most urgent needs for tackling the growing problem of asthma. The work group's departmentwide strategic plan, Action Against Asthma, identified opportunities and presented a coordinated approach for improving asthma prevention and management.[16]

Issues and Trends

COPD includes chronic bronchitis and emphysema—both of which are character-ized by irreversible airflow obstruction and often exist together. Similar to asthma, COPD may be accompanied by an airway hyperresponsiveness. Most patients with COPD have a history of cigarette smoking. COPD worsens over time with continued exposure to a causative agent—usually tobacco smoke or sometimes a substance in the workplace or environment.

COPD occurs most often in older people. As much as 10 percent of the population aged 65 years and older is estimated to have COPD.[2] COPD has a major impact on health care, illness, disability, and death in the older population, and the magnitude of the problem is growing. Since 1980, the prevalence and age-adjusted death rate for COPD increased more than 30 percent.[2, 21, 22] Most of the increase occurred in people over age 65 years. Taking into account the expected aging of the U.S. population over the next 10 to 30 years as well as the improved management of other smoking-related diseases, any decline in the proportion of persons with COPD is unlikely without substantial changes in risk factors, mainly reductions in cigarette smoking. This is important for both men and women, given the modest decline in cigarette smoking rates from 1990 to 1995.[22]

Between 80 and 90 percent of COPD is attributable to cigarette smoking. How-ever, not all smokers develop COPD, and not all patients with COPD are smokers or have smoked in the past.[23, 24] Individual susceptibility to the adverse health effects of cigarette smoke on the lung appears to vary within the general popula-tion. Some 10 to 15 percent of smokers show a rate of decline in lung function that will result in COPD with severe disability. Smoking cessation is the only treatment that slows the decline. Susceptible smokers who stop smoking do not regain lost lung function,[25] but the rate of loss will return to what is normal for a nonsmoker.

How cigarette smoking causes COPD is an active area of research. The develop-ment of COPD—in particular, emphysema—is thought to be due to a chemical imbalance in the lungs caused by cigarette smoke.[26] In some individuals, emphy-sema occurs because of a genetic deficiency. Emphysema due to genetic defi-ciency, called familial emphysema, occurs even in nonsmokers, but smoking hastens its occurrence. Familial emphysema probably accounts for less than 5 percent of all cases of COPD.[27]

Smoking and occupational exposures together cause respiratory diseases and lung cancer.[28, 29] Miners, firefighters, metal workers, grain handlers, cotton workers, paper mill workers, agricultural workers, construction workers who handle ce-ment, and others employed in occupations associated with prolonged exposure to dusts, fumes, or gases develop significant airflow obstruction, coughing, phlegm, dyspnea, wheezing, and reduced lung function.[27, 29, 30]

Population studies have shown that chronic exposure to air pollution has an independent adverse effect on lung function.[31, 32] A multiyear study of the respiratory effects of long-term exposure to environmental tobacco smoke and air pollution reported that both long-term ozone and childhood exposure to maternal tobacco smoke were associated with diminished lung function in college students.[33] Viral infections also may contribute to susceptibility to COPD, and they are considered to play a role in the onset of airflow obstruction.

The direct costs of health care services and indirect costs through loss of productivity related to COPD amounted to $26 billion in 1998.[26] About 14 million persons in the United States have COPD—about 12.5 million have chronic bronchitis and 1.9 million have emphysema.[27] Emphysema has not increased, but since 1980, cases of chronic bronchitis increased 75 percent.[27]

Because national data systems will not be available in the first half of the decade for tracking progress, two subjects of interest concerning respiratory diseases are not addressed in this focus area's objectives. The first topic addresses increasing the proportion of primary care providers who are trained to provide culturally competent health services to racial and ethnic groups seeking care for chronic obstructive pulmonary disease. The second involves increasing the proportion of primary care providers who are trained to use appropriate lung function tests to recognize the early signs of chronic obstructive pulmonary disease before the disease becomes serious and disabling.

Disparities

Reliable statistics are not as available for COPD total cases, illness, disability, or death in African Americans, Hispanics, and other ethnic groups as for whites.[34, 35] From 1982 to 1984, the proportion of adults with COPD was 6.2 percent among whites and 3.2 percent among African Americans. In 1982, the age-adjusted COPD death rate for whites was 16.6 deaths per 1,000 population and 12.8 deaths per 1,000 for African Americans. Among the Hispanic groups studied, Puerto Ricans demonstrated a higher proportion of chronic bronchitis (2.9 percent) than Mexican Americans (1.7 percent) or Cuban Americans (1.7 percent).[34, 35]

In 1995, the proportion of the population with COPD was 5 percent in men aged 45 to 64 years and 11 percent in men aged 65 years and older. The proportion was 10 percent in women aged 45 to 64 years and 9 percent in women aged 65 to 74 years.

Death from COPD is more common in men than in women, and the death rate increases steeply with age.[27, 36] Men and women have similar COPD death rates before age 55 years, but the rate for men rises thereafter. At age 70 years, the rate for men is more than double that for women, and at age 85 years and older, the COPD death rate for men is 3.5 times that for women.[37] The proportion was 8 percent for whites aged 45 to 64 years and 10 percent for whites aged 65 years and older. The proportion of African Americans with COPD was 6 percent for those aged 45 to 64 years and 8 percent for those aged 65 years and older.[2] COPD death rates were lower in the Hispanic groups than in non-Hispanic whites; however, these rates have been increasing for Hispanics.[33]

Women might be more susceptible than men to developing COPD when exposed to risk factors such as tobacco smoke.[38] The beneficial effects of stopping smoking on the rate of lung function decline may be greater for women than men.[39]

Opportunities

Primary care physicians are in a key position to provide optimal care to patients with COPD and to provide counseling during clinical or health center visits to patients who smoke. Effective tests are available to screen patients for COPD, and primary care physicians need to be trained in the latest methods to detect and treat the disease.

Obstructive Sleep Apnea

Issues and Trends

Some 18 million persons in the United States were estimated to have OSA in 1993.[40] OSA affects all races, ages, and socioeconomic and ethnic groups.[41] Because OSA causes serious disturbances in normal sleep patterns, patients experience excessive daytime sleepiness and impaired performance. Common consequences of OSA range from personality changes and sexual dysfunction to falling asleep at work or while driving.[40, 41]

OSA symptoms include many repeated involuntary breathing pauses during sleep. The breathing pauses often are accompanied by choking sensations that may wake the patient. Other symptoms include intermittent snoring, awakening from sleep (poor sleep), early morning headaches, and excessive daytime sleepiness.

OSA can increase the seriousness of other lung diseases that decrease airflow, such as asthma and COPD. Cardiovascular deaths alone due to OSA have been estimated at 38,000 a year.[40] Individuals with OSA often do not recognize reductions in alertness, diminished productivity, and discord in interpersonal relationships as part of the syndrome. Persons affected by OSA, for example, are seven times more likely to be involved in multiple vehicular crashes.[42] In children, OSA can disrupt sleep. OSA also may cause daytime behavioral problems that affect workplace performance and affect their learning ability in school.

Infants with siblings or parents who have OSA inherit an increased risk of sudden infant death syndrome (SIDS).[43] This tragic sleep-related breathing disorder takes the lives of more infants than all other causes combined.

Disparities

OSA is prevalent particularly in men over age 50 years and in postmenopausal women, when hormonal changes appear to increase risk. The risk of OSA also is increased in certain racial and ethnic groups. Among young African Americans, the likelihood of experiencing OSA symptoms is twice that of young whites.[44] Nearly 50 percent of OSA patients have high blood pressure.[45, 46, 47]

Opportunities

A major factor in the pervasiveness of OSA's effects on health and society has been the failure to educate people—and especially health care practitioners—about the disorder. A wide range of behavioral, mechanical, and surgical treatments can be used to manage OSA symptoms. Providing persons at risk with culturally and linguistically appropriate information about OSA could enable them to prevent or lessen the effects of OSA. Improved awareness of OSA symptoms represents a major public health challenge.

Primary care providers are an important barometer of OSA awareness because they are a first stop for patients who are seeking appropriate diagnosis and treatment. However, only 79 cases of sleep disorder were diagnosed in a sample of 10 million patient records from 1989 and 1990.[40] In 1990 about a third of the medical schools in the United States offered no training in sleep medicine, and another third provided less than 2 hours on average for all sleep topics.[48] Data systems to track the training of health care providers in OSA over the decade are not currently available, and therefore the issue is not addressed in this focus area's objectives. However, it represents an important research and data collection agenda. In the absence of strong educational models for physicians, the risk remains high that OSA will be misdiagnosed and mismanaged.

The National Commission on Sleep Disorders Research[40] was established by the U.S. Congress in 1988 to assess the societal and economic impact of sleep disorders and the resources available to promote the prevention, diagnosis, and treatment of such disorders. In a 1994 report to Congress, the Commission concluded that even though the science of sleep disorders is not fully developed, such disorders can be prevented. The commission recommends that research on the natural history of sleep disorders be made an urgent national concern. Epidemiologic studies must be conducted to evaluate risk factors that lead to sleep disorders and to determine which sleep disorders lead to other serious health problems.

Interim Progress Toward Year 2000 Objectives

For the three objectives specific to asthma in Healthy People 2000, available data indicate movement away from the targets as the rate of hospitalizations and activity limitation increase and movement toward the target for increasing the proportion of persons with asthma who receive patient education. There were no objectives in Healthy People 2000 for COPD and OSA.

Note: Unless otherwise noted, data are from the Centers for Disease Control and Prevention, National Center for Health Statistics, Healthy People 2000 Review, 1998–99.

Respiratory Diseases

Goal: Promote respiratory health through better prevention, detection, treatment, and education efforts.

Number	Objective Short Title
Asthma	
24-1	Deaths from asthma
24-2	Hospitalizations for asthma
24-3	Hospital emergency department visits for asthma
24-4	Activity limitations
24-5	School or work days lost
24-6	Patient education
24-7	Appropriate asthma care
24-8	Surveillance systems
Chronic Obstructive Pulmonary Disease (COPD)	
24-9	Activity limitations due to chronic lung and breathing problems
24-10	Deaths from COPD
Obstructive Sleep Apnea (OSA)	
24-11	Medical evaluation and followup
24-12	Vehicular crashes related to excessive sleepiness

Select Age Groups, 1998	Asthma Deaths				
	24-1a. Children Under Age 5 Years	24-1b. Children Aged 5 to 14 Years	24-1c. Adolescents and Adults Aged 15 to 34 Years	24-1d. Adults Aged 35 to 64 Years	24-1e. Adults Aged 65 Years and Older
	Rate per Million				
Hispanic or Latino	DSU	DSU	3.7	16.4	84.5
Not Hispanic or Latino	2.1	3.5	6.9	17.8	86.2
Black or African American	8.3	10.3	21.9	54.0	133.5
White	DSU	2.0	3.9	12.8	80.6
Gender					
Female	1.4	2.7	4.3	22.3	99.1
Male	2.8	4.0	5.7	13.0	68.1
Education (aged 25 to 64 years)					
Less than high school	NA	NA	10.0*	31.0	NA
High school graduate	NA	NA	11.4*	22.9	NA
At least some college	NA	NA	3.9*	9.3	NA

DNA = Data have not been analyzed. DNC = Data are not collected. DSU = Data are statistically unreliable. NA = Not applicable.

*Data are for persons aged 25 to 34 years.

NOTE: THE TABLE ABOVE MAY HAVE CONTINUED FROM THE PREVIOUS PAGE.

24-2. Reduce hospitalizations for asthma.

Target and baseline:

Objective	Age Group	1998 Baseline	2010 Target
		Rate per 10,000	
24-2a.	Children under age 5 years	45.6	25
24-2b.	Children and adults aged 5 to 64 years*	12.5	7.7
24-2c.	Adults aged 65 years and older*	17.7	11

*Age adjusted to the year 2000 standard population.

Target setting method: Better than the best.

Data source: National Hospital Discharge Survey (NHDS), CDC, NCHS.

Asthma

24-1. Reduce asthma deaths.

Target and baseline:

Objective	Age Group	1998 Baseline	2010 Target
		Rate per Million	
24-1a.	Children under age 5 years	2.1	1.0
24-1b.	Children aged 5 to 14 years	3.3	1.0
24-1c.	Adolescents and adults aged 15 to 34 years	5.0	2.0
24-1d.	Adults aged 35 to 64 years	17.8	9.0
24-1e.	Adults aged 65 years and older	86.3	60.0

Target setting method: Better than the best.

Data source: National Vital Statistics System (NVSS), CDC, NCHS.

NOTE: THE TABLE BELOW MAY CONTINUE TO THE FOLLOWING PAGE.

	Asthma Deaths				
Select Age Groups, 1998	**24-1a. Children Under Age 5 Years**	**24-1b. Children Aged 5 to 14 Years**	**24-1c. Adolescents and Adults Aged 15 to 34 Years**	**24-1d. Adults Aged 35 to 64 Years**	**24-1e. Adults Aged 65 Years and Older**
	Rate per Million				
TOTAL	2.1	3.3	5.0	17.8	86.3
Race and ethnicity					
American Indian or Alaska Native	DSU	DSU	DSU	DSU	DSU
Asian or Pacific Islander	DSU	DSU	DSU	12.8	136.9
Asian	DNC	DNC	DNC	DNC	DNC
Native Hawaiian and other Pacific Islander	DNC	DNC	DNC	DNC	DNC
Black or African American	8.1	9.7	16.6	52.3	130.4
White	DSU	2.0	3.0	13.3	81.1

Select Age Groups, 1998	Asthma Hospitalizations		
	24-2a. Children Under Age 5 Years	24-2b. Children and Adults Aged 5 to 64 Years*	24-2c. Adults Aged 65 Years and Older*
	Rate per 10,000		
TOTAL	45.6	12.5	17.7
Race and ethnicity			
American Indian or Alaska Native	DSU	DSU	DSU
Asian or Pacific Islander	DSU	DSU	DSU
Asian	DNC	DNC	DNC
Native Hawaiian and other Pacific Islander	DNC	DNC	DNC
Black or African American	82.4	28.4	27.3
White	29.5	7.8	12.4
Hispanic or Latino	DSU	DSU	DSU
Not Hispanic or Latino	DSU	DSU	DSU
Black or African American	DSU	DSU	DSU
White	DSU	DSU	DSU
Gender			
Female	33.1	15.9	24.6
Male	57.6	9.0	8.5

DNA = Data have not been analyzed. DNC = Data are not collected. DSU = Data are statistically unreliable.
*Age adjusted to the year 2000 standard population.

24-3. Reduce hospital emergency department visits for asthma.

Target and baseline:

Objective	Age Group	1995–97 Baseline	2010 Target
		Rate per 10,000	
24-3a.	Children under age 5 years	150.0	80
24-3b.	Children and adults aged 5 to 64 years	71.1	50
24-3c.	Adults aged 65 years and older	29.5	15

Target setting method: Better than the best.

Data source: National Hospital Ambulatory Medical Care Survey (NHAMCS), CDC, NCHS.

NOTE: THE TABLE BELOW MAY CONTINUE TO THE FOLLOWING PAGE.

Select Age Groups, 1995–97	Hospital Emergency Department Visits for Asthma		
	24-3a. Children Under Age 5 Years	24-3b. Children and Adults Aged 5 to 64 Years	24-3c. Adults Aged 65 Years and Older
	Rate per 10,000		
TOTAL	150.0	71.1	29.5
Race and ethnicity			
American Indian or Alaska Native	DSU	DSU	DSU
Asian or Pacific Islander	DSU	DSU	DSU
Asian	DNC	DNC	DNC
Native Hawaiian and other Pacific Islander	DNC	DNC	DNC
Black or African American	407.2	191.7	90.8
White	101.7	53.4	23.1
Hispanic or Latino	DSU	DSU	DSU
Not Hispanic or Latino	DSU	DSU	DSU
Black or African American	DSU	DSU	DSU
White	DSU	DSU	DSU

Select Age Groups, 1995–97	Hospital Emergency Department Visits for Asthma		
	24-3a. Children Under Age 5 Years	24-3b. Children and Adults Aged 5 to 64 Years	24-3c. Adults Aged 65 Years and Older
	Rate per 10,000		
Gender			
Female	103.0	83.6	37.8
Male	195.5	57.9	17.9

DNA = Data have not been analyzed. DNC = Data are not collected. DSU = Data are statistically unreliable.
NOTE: THE TABLE ABOVE MAY HAVE CONTINUED FROM THE PREVIOUS PAGE.

24-4. Reduce activity limitations among persons with asthma.

Target: 10 percent.

Baseline: 20 percent of persons with asthma experienced activity limitations in activity in 1994–96 (age adjusted to the year 2000 standard population).

Target setting method: Better than the best.

Data source: National Health Interview Survey (NHIS), CDC, NCHS.

NOTE: THE TABLE BELOW MAY CONTINUE TO THE FOLLOWING PAGE.

Persons With Asthma, 1994–96	Experienced Activity Limitations
	Percent
TOTAL	20
Race and ethnicity	
American Indian or Alaska Native	DSU
Asian or Pacific Islander	DSU
Asian	DSU
Native Hawaiian and other Pacific Islander	DSU
Black or African American	26
White	18
Hispanic or Latino	22
Not Hispanic or Latino	19
Black or African American	26
White	18

Persons With Asthma, 1994–96	Experienced Activity Limitations
	Percent
Gender	
Female	21
Male	17
Family income level	
Poor	28
Near poor	20
Middle/high income	16

DNA = Data have not been analyzed. DNC = Data are not collected. DSU = Data are statistically unreliable.
Note: Age adjusted to the year 2000 standard population.

NOTE: THE TABLE ABOVE MAY HAVE CONTINUED FROM THE PREVIOUS PAGE.

24-5. (Developmental) Reduce the number of school or work days missed by persons with asthma due to asthma.

Potential data source: National Health Interview Survey (NHIS), CDC, NCHS.

24-6. Increase the proportion of persons with asthma who receive formal patient education, including information about community and self-help resources, as an essential part of the management of their condition.

Target: 30 percent.

Baseline: 8.4 percent of persons with asthma received formal patient education in 1998 (age adjusted to the year 2000 standard population).

Target setting method: Better than the best.

Data source: National Health Interview Survey (NHIS), CDC, NCHS.

NOTE: THE TABLE BELOW MAY CONTINUE TO THE FOLLOWING PAGE.

Persons With Asthma, 1998	Received Patient Education
	Percent
TOTAL	8.4
Race and ethnicity	
American Indian or Alaska Native	DSU
Asian or Pacific Islander	DSU
Asian	DSU
Native Hawaiian and other Pacific Islander	DSU

Persons With Asthma, 1998	Received Patient Education
	Percent
Black or African American	11.2
White	7.8
Hispanic or Latino	7.8
Not Hispanic or Latino	8.4
Black or African American	11.3
White	7.9
Gender	
Female	9.1
Male	7.1
Family income level	
Poor	7.2
Near poor	10.3
Middle/high income	8.4

DNA = Data have not been analyzed. DNC = Data are not collected. DSU = Data are statistically unreliable.
Note: Age adjusted to the year 2000 standard population.

NOTE: THE TABLE ABOVE MAY HAVE CONTINUED FROM THE PREVIOUS PAGE.

24-7. (Developmental) Increase the proportion of persons with asthma who receive appropriate asthma care according to the NAEPP Guidelines.

24-7a. Persons with asthma who receive written asthma management plans from their health care provider.

24-7b. Persons with asthma with prescribed inhalers who receive instruction on how to use them properly.

24-7c. Persons with asthma who receive education about recognizing early signs and symptoms of asthma episodes and how to respond appropriately, including instruction on peak flow monitoring for those who use daily therapy.

24-7d. Persons with asthma who receive medication regimens that prevent the need for more than one canister of short-acting inhaled beta agonists per month for relief of symptoms.

24-7e. Persons with asthma who receive followup medical care for long-term management of asthma after any hospitalization due to asthma.

24-7f. Persons with asthma who receive assistance with assessing and reducing exposure to environmental risk factors in their home, school, and work environments.

Potential data source: National Health Interview Survey (NHIS), CDC, NCHS.

24-8. **(Developmental) Establish in at least 25 States a surveillance system for tracking asthma death, illness, disability, impact of occupational and environmental factors on asthma, access to medical care, and asthma management.**

Potential data sources: Periodic surveys, Council of State and Territorial Epidemiologists and Public Health Foundation; Association of Schools of Public Health.

Chronic Obstructive Pulmonary Disease

24-9. **Reduce the proportion of adults whose activity is limited due to chronic lung and breathing problems.**

Target: 1.5 percent.

Baseline: 2.2 percent of adults aged 45 years and older experienced activity limitations due to chronic lung and breathing problems in 1997 (age adjusted to the year 2000 standard population).

Target setting method: Better than the best.

Data source: National Health Interview Survey (NHIS), CDC, NCHS.

NOTE: THE TABLE BELOW MAY CONTINUE TO THE FOLLOWING PAGE.

Adults Aged 45 Years and Older, 1997	Experienced Activity Limitations Due to Chronic Lung and Breathing Problems
	Percent
TOTAL	2.2
Race and ethnicity	
American Indian or Alaska Native	DSU
Asian or Pacific Islander	DSU
Asian	DSU
Native Hawaiian and other Pacific Islander	DSU
Black or African American	2.3
White	2.3

Adults Aged 45 Years and Older, 1997	Experienced Activity Limitations Due to Chronic Lung and Breathing Problems
	Percent
Hispanic or Latino	1.7
Not Hispanic or Latino	2.3
Black or African American	2.2
White	2.3
Gender	
Female	2.1
Aged 45 to 64 years	1.6
Aged 65 years and older	3.0
Male	2.5
Aged 45 to 64 years	1.6
Aged 65 years and older	4.1
Family income level	
Poor	5.2
Near poor	4.0
Middle/high income	1.8

DNA = Data have not been analyzed. DNC = Data are not collected. DSU = Data are statistically unreliable.
Note: Age adjusted to the year 2000 standard population.
NOTE: THE TABLE ABOVE MAY HAVE CONTINUED FROM THE PREVIOUS PAGE.

24-10. Reduce deaths from chronic obstructive pulmonary disease (COPD) among adults.

Target: 60 deaths per 100,000 adults.

Baseline: 119.4 deaths from COPD per 100,000 persons aged 45 years and older occurred in 1998 (age adjusted to the year 2000 standard population).

Target setting method: 50 percent improvement.

Data source: National Vital Statistics System (NVSS), CDC, NCHS.

Adults Aged 45 Years and Older, 1998	Chronic Obstructive Pulmonary Disease Deaths
	Rate per 100,000
TOTAL	119.4
Race and ethnicity	
American Indian or Alaska Native	79.6
Asian or Pacific Islander	48.6
Asian	DNC
Native Hawaiian and other Pacific Islander	DNC
Black or African American	85.3
White	124.3
Hispanic or Latino	52.5
Not Hispanic or Latino	122.8
Black or African American	87.2
White	127.9
Gender	
Female	98.8
Male	153.7
Education (aged 25 to 64 years)	
Less than high school	19.7
High school graduate	12.5
At least some college	4.4

DNA = Data have not been analyzed. DNC = Data are not collected. DSU = Data are statistically unreliable.
Note: Age adjusted to the year 2000 standard population.

Obstructive Sleep Apnea

24-11. (Developmental) Increase the proportion of persons with symptoms of obstructive sleep apnea whose condition is medically managed.

24-11a. Persons with excessive daytime sleepiness, loud snoring, and other signs associated with obstructive sleep apnea who seek medical evaluation.

24-11b. Persons with excessive daytime sleepiness, loud snoring, and other signs associated with obstructive sleep apnea who receive followup medical care for long-term management of their condition.

Potential data source: National Health Interview Survey (NHIS), CDC, NCHS.

24-12. (Developmental) Reduce the proportion of vehicular crashes caused by persons with excessive sleepiness.

Potential data source: National Health Interview Survey (NHIS), CDC, NCHS. Fatality Analysis Reporting System (FARS), U.S. Department of Transportation, National Highway Traffic Safety Administration.

Related Objectives From Other Focus Areas

1. **Access to Quality Health Services**
   1-10. Delay or difficulty in getting emergency care
7. **Educational and Community-Based Programs**
   7-8. Satisfaction with patient education
   7-11. Culturally appropriate and linguistically competent community health promotion programs
8. **Environmental Health**
   8-1. Harmful air pollutants
   8-2. Alternative modes of transportation
   8-3. Cleaner alternative fuels
   8-4. Airborne toxins
   8-14. Toxic pollutants
   8-16. Indoor allergens
   8-17. Office building air quality
   8-20. School policies to protect against environmental hazards
   8-23. Substandard housing
   8-26. Information systems used for environmental health
   8-27. Monitoring environmentally related diseases
   8-28. Local agencies using surveillance data for vector control
11. **Health Communication**
    11-6. Satisfaction with health care providers' communication skills
15. **Injury and Violence Prevention**
    15-15. Deaths from motor vehicle crashes
    15-17. Nonfatal motor vehicle injuries
20. **Occupational Safety and Health**
    20-1. Work-related injury deaths
    20-2. Work-related injuries
    20-4. Pneumoconiosis deaths
22. **Physical Activity and Fitness**
    22-6. Moderate physical activity in adolescents
    22-7. Vigorous physical activity in adolescents
23. **Public Health Infrastructure**
    23-2. Public access to information and surveillance data
    23-4. Data for all population groups
    23-6. National tracking of Healthy People 2010 objectives
    23-7. Timely release of data on objectives
    23-10. Continuing education and training by public health agencies

Terminology

(A listing of abbreviations and acronyms used in this publication appears in Appendix H.)

Ambulatory care: Medical care provided at hospital emergency and outpatient departments.

Asthma: A lung disease characterized by airway constriction, mucus secretion, and chronic inflammation, resulting in reduced airflow and wheezing, coughing, chest tightness, and difficulty breathing.

Chronic bronchitis: A lung disease characterized by the presence of chronic productive cough most days for 3 months in each of 2 successive years.

Chronic obstructive pulmonary disease (COPD): A lung disease characterized by airflow obstruction due to chronic bronchitis and emphysema, two diseases that often occur together. COPD is one of the most common respiratory conditions among adults worldwide and is the fourth leading cause of death in the United States.

Dyspnea: Shortness of breath.

Emphysema: Abnormal permanent enlargement of the airspaces in the lungs accompanied by coughing and difficulty breathing.

Epidemiologic studies: Studies of disease occurrence.

Obstructive sleep apnea (OSA): An illness characterized by snoring, partial or complete cessation of breathing during sleep, reductions in blood oxygen levels, severe sleep disruptions, and excessive daytime sleepiness. OSA is a chronic breathing problem with serious effects on individual health and productivity, including an inheritable risk of sudden infant deaths, behavior and learning disturbances, injury from accidents, and reduced quality of life.

Rate: The basic measure of disease occurrence that most clearly expresses the probability of risk of disease in a defined population over a specified period of time. A rate is defined as:

Number of events
Population at risk

References

[1] Mannino, D.M.; Homa, D.M.; Pertowski, C.A.; et al. Surveillance for asthma—United States, 1960–1995. *Morbidity and Mortality Weekly Report CDC Surveillance Summaries* 47(1):1-27, 1998.

[2] Benson, V., and Marano, M.A. Current estimates from the National Health Interview Survey, 1995. *Vital and Health Statistics* 10(199):1-428, 1998.

[3] National Heart, Lung, and Blood Institute (NHLBI). *Data Fact Sheet. Asthma Statistics.* Bethesda, MD: National Institutes of Health (NIH), Public Health Service (PHS), 1999.

[4] National Center for Health Statistics (NCHS). Current estimates from the National Health Interview Survey, 1990. *Vital and Health Statistics* 10(194), 1997.

[5] National Asthma Education and Prevention Program. *Expert Panel Report 2: Guidelines for the Diagnosis and Management of Asthma.* NIH Pub. No. 97-4051. Bethesda, MD: NIH, 1997.

[6] NCHS. Ambulatory care visits to physicians' offices, hospital outpatient departments, and emergency departments: United States, 1996. *Vital and Health Statistics* 13(134), 1998.

[7] NCHS. *Healthy People 2000 Review, 1998–99.* Hyattsville, MD: PHS, 1999.

[8] Weiss, K.B.; Gergen, P.J.; and Hodgson, T.A. An economic evaluation of asthma in the United States. *New England Journal of Medicine* 326:862-866, 1992.

[9] Sullivan, S.; Elixhauser, S.; Buist, A.S.; et al. National Asthma Education and Prevention Program working group report on the cost effectiveness of asthma care. *American Journal of Respiratory and Critical Care Medicine* 154(3, Part 2):584-595, 1996.

[10] Glaxco Canada. *The Costs of Asthma in Canada.* Princeton, NJ: Communications Media for Education, 1993.

[11] Koren, H.S. Environmental risk factors in atopic asthma. *International Archives of Allergy and Immunology* 113:65-68, 1997.

[12] Becklake, M.R., and Ernst, P. Environmental factors. *Lancet* 350(Suppl. 2):10-13, 1997.

[13] Office of Air Quality Planning and Standards, U.S. Environmental Protection Agency (EPA). *National Air Quality and Emissions Report, 1997.* CPA Pub. No. EPA 454/R-98-016. Research Triangle Park, NC: EPA, 1998.

[14] Schwartz, D.A., and Peterson, M.W. Occupational lung disease. *Advances in Internal Medicine* 42:269-312, 1997.

[15] Busse, W.W.; Gern, J.E.; and Dick, E.C. The role of respiratory viruses in asthma. *Ciba Foundation Symposium* 206:208-213, 1997.

[16] U.S. Department of Health and Human Services (HHS). *Action Against Asthma: A Strategic Plan for the Department of Health and Human Services.* Washington, DC: HHS, 2000.

[17] Wade, S.; Weil, C.; Holden, G.; et al. Psycho social characteristics of inner-city children with asthma: A description of the NCICAS psychosocial protocol. National Cooperative Inner-City Asthma Study. *Pediatric Pulmonology* 24:263-276, 1997.

[18] Evans, D.; Mellins, R.; Lobach, K.; et al. Improving care for minority children with asthma: Professional education in public health clinics. *Pediatrics* 99:157-164, 1997.

[19] Institute of Medicine. *Cleaning the Air: Asthma and Indoor Air Exposures.* Washington, DC: National Academy Press, 2000.

[20] NHLBI. *National Asthma Education and Prevention Program Summary Report.* Bethesda, MD: NIH, 1999.

[21] NCHS. *Health, United States, 1986.* Hyattsville, MD: NCHS, 1986.

[22] NCHS. *Health, United States, 1999 with Health and Aging Chartbook.* Hyattsville, MD: NCHS, 1999.

[23] Bone, R.C.; Dantzker, D.R.; and George, R.B. *Pulmonary and Critical Care Medicine.* St. Louis, MO: Mosby Year Book, 1993, Chapter G-1.

[24] Sherril, D.L.; Lebowitz, M.D.; and Burrows, B. Epidemiology of COPD. *Clinical Chest Medicine* 11:375-388, 1990.

[25] Fletcher, C., and Peto, R. The natural history of COPD. *British Medical Journal* 1:1645-1648, 1977.

[26] Fishman, A.P. *Pulmonary Diseases and Disorders.* 2nd ed. New York, NY: McGraw-Hill, Inc., 1998.

[27] NHLBI. *Morbidity and Mortality: 1998 Chartbook on Cardiovascular, Lung and Blood Diseases.* Bethesda, MD: NIH, 1998.

[28] Schwartz, D.A., and Peterson, M.W. Occupational lung disease. *Disease-A-Month* 44:41-84, 1998.

[29] Wynder, E.L., and Hoffmann, D. Tobacco and health: A societal challenge. *New England Journal of Medicine* 300:894-903, 1979.

[30] Bakke, S.; Baste, V.; Hanoa, R.; et al. Prevalence of obstructive lung disease in a general population: Relation to occupational title and exposure to some airborne agents. *Thorax* 46(12):863-870, 1991.

[31] Souza, M.B.; Saldiva, P.H.; Pope, III, C.A.; et al. Respiratory changes due to long-term exposure to urban levels of air pollution: A histopathologic study in humans. *Chest* 113:1312-1318, 1998.

[32] Dockery, D.W., and Brunekreef, B. Longitudinal studies of air pollution effects on lung function. *American Journal of Respiratory and Critical Care Medicine* 154(6, Part 2):S250-S256, 1996.

[33] Galizia, A., and Kinney, P.L. Long-term residence in areas of high ozone: Associations with respiratory health in a nationwide sample of nonsmoking young adults. *Environmental Health Perspectives* 107(8):675-679, 1999.

[34] Coultas, D.B.; Gong, Jr., H.; Grad, R.; et al. Respiratory diseases in minorities of the United States. *American Journal of Respiratory and Critical Care Medicine* 149:S93-S131, 1993.

[35] Gibson, K.F.; Aguayo, S.M.; Flowers, J.C.; et al. NHLBI special report. Respiratory diseases disproportionately affecting minorities. *Chest* 108:1380-1392, 1995.

[36] Higgins, M.W., and Keller, J.B. Trends in COPD morbidity and mortality in Tecumseh, Michigan. *Annual Review of Respiratory Diseases* 140:S42-S48, 1989.

[37] Feinlieb, M.; Rosenburg, H.M.; Collins, J.G.; et al. Trends in COPD morbidity and mortality in the United States. *American Journal of Respiratory Diseases* 140:S9-S18, 1989.

[38] Tashkin, D.P.; Altose, M.F.; Bleecker, E.R.; et al. The Lung Health Study: Airway responsiveness to inhaled methacholine in smokers with mild to moderate airflow limitation. *American Review of Respiratory Diseases* 145:301-310, 1992.

[39] Anthonisen, N.R.; Connell, J.E.; Kiley, J.P.; et al. Effects of smoking intervention and the use of an inhaled anticholinergic bronchodilator on the rate of decline of FEV1: The Lung Health Study. *Journal of the American Medical Association* 272:1497-1505, 1994.

[40] National Institute on Aging (NIA). *Wake Up America: A National Sleep Alert, Report of the National Commission on Sleep Disorders Research to the U.S. Congress and Department of Health and Human Services.* Bethesda, MD: NIA, 1994.

[41] Redline, S., and Strohl, K.P. Recognition and consequences of obstructive sleep apnea hypopnea syndrome. *Clinical Chest Medicine* 19:1-19, 1998.

[42] Young, T.; Blustein, J.; Finn, L.; et al. Sleep-disordered breathing and motor vehicle accidents in a population-based sample of employed adults. *Sleep* 20:608-613, 1997.

[43] Tischler, P.V.; Redline, S.; Ferrette, V.; et al. The association of sudden unexpected infant death with obstructive sleep apnea. *American Journal of Respiratory and Critical Care Medicine* 153:1857-1863, 1996.

[44] Redline, S. Epidemiology of sleep disordered breathing. *Seminars in Respiratory and Critical Care Medicine* 19(2):113-122.

[45] Fletcher, E.C.; DeBehunke, R.D.; Lovoi, M.S.; et al. Undiagnosed sleep apnea in patients with essential hypertension. *Annals of Internal Medicine* 103:190-195, 1995.

[46] Guilleminault, H.C.; Tilkian, A.; and Dement, W.C. The sleep apnea syndromes. *Annual Review of Medicine* 27:465-484, 1976.

[47] Carlson, J.T.; Hedner, J.A.; Ejnell, H.; et al. High prevalence of hypertension in sleep apnea patients independent of obesity. *American Journal of Respiratory and Critical Care Medicine* 150:72-77, 1994.

[48] Rosen, R.C.; Rosekind, M.; Rosevear, C.; et al. Physician education in sleep and sleep disorders: A national survey of U.S. medical schools. *Sleep* 16:249-254, 1993.

25

Sexually Transmitted Diseases

Lead Agency: Centers for Disease Control and Prevention

Contents

Promote responsible sexual behaviors, strengthen community capacity, and increase access to quality services to prevent sexually transmitted diseases (STDs) and their complications.

Overview

Sexually transmitted diseases (STDs) refer to the more than 25 infectious organisms transmitted primarily through sexual activity. STDs are among many related factors that affect the broad continuum of reproductive health agreed on in 1994 by 180 governments at the International Conference on Population and Development (ICPD). At ICPD, all governments were challenged to strengthen their STD programs.[1] STD prevention as an essential primary care strategy is integral to improving reproductive health.

Despite the burdens, costs, complications, and preventable nature of STDs, they remain a significant public health problem, largely unrecognized by the public, policymakers, and public health and health care professionals in the United States. STDs cause many harmful, often irreversible, and costly clinical complications, such as reproductive health problems, fetal and perinatal health problems, and cancer. In addition, studies of the worldwide human immunodeficiency virus (HIV) pandemic link other STDs to a causal chain of events in the sexual transmission of HIV infection.[2] (See Focus Area 13. HIV.)

Issues

A 1997 Institute of Medicine (IOM) report characterized STDs as "hidden epidemics of tremendous health and economic consequence in the United States" and stated, "STDs represent a growing threat to the Nation's health and that national action is urgently needed."[3] IOM's principal conclusion was that the United States needs to establish a much more effective national system for STD prevention, which takes into account the complex interaction between biological and social factors that sustain STD transmission in populations; focuses on preventing the disproportionate effect that STDs have on some population groups; applies proven, cost-effective behavioral and biomedical interventions; and recognizes that education, mass communication media, financing, and health care infrastructure policies must foster change in personal behaviors and in health care services.[3] (See Focus Area 23. Public Health Infrastructure.)

Biological factors. STDs are behavior-linked diseases that result from unprotected sex.[3] Several biological factors contribute to their rapid spread.

Asymptomatic nature of STDs. The majority of STDs either do not produce any symptoms or signs, or they produce symptoms so mild that they often are disregarded, resulting in a low index of suspicion by infected persons who should, but often do not, seek medical care. For example, as many as 85 percent of women and up to 50 percent of men with chlamydia have no symptoms.[4, 5, 6, 7] A person infected with HIV may be asymptomatic and may transmit the disease to another person. That person may, in turn, be infected for years but remain unaware until symptoms manifest themselves.

Lag time between infection and complications. Often, a long interval—sometimes years—occurs between acquiring a sexually transmitted infection and recognizing a clinically significant health problem. Examples are cervical cancer caused by human papillomavirus (HPV), liver cancer caused by hepatitis B virus infection,[8] and infertility and ectopic pregnancy resulting from unrecognized or undiagnosed chlamydia or gonorrhea.[9] The original infection often is asymptomatic, and, as a result, people frequently do not perceive a connection between the original sexually acquired infection and the resulting health problem.

Gender and age. Women are at higher risk than men for most STDs, and young women are more susceptible to certain STDs than are older women. The higher risk is partly because the cervix of adolescent females is covered with cells that are especially susceptible to STDs, such as chlamydia.[10]

Social and behavioral factors. The spread of STDs, especially in certain vulnerable population groups, is directly affected by social and behavioral factors. Social and cultural factors may cause serious obstacles to STD prevention by adversely influencing social norms regarding sex and sexuality.

Poverty and marginalization. STDs disproportionately affect disenfranchised persons and persons who are in social networks in which high-risk sexual behavior is common and either access to care or health-seeking behavior is compromised. Some disproportionately affected groups include sex workers (people who exchange sex for money, drugs, or other goods), adolescents, persons in detention, and migrant workers.[3] Without publicly supported STD services, many people in these categories would lack access to STD care.

Substance abuse, sex work, and STDs are closely connected, and substance abuse and sex work frequently are causes for arrest and detention. Studies show that comprehensive screening of incarcerated populations can be done successfully and safely within the criminal justice system.[11, 12, 13] Discussed below are several connected themes relevant to any discussion of poverty and marginalization issues.

Access to health care. Access to high-quality health care is essential for early detection, treatment, and behavior-change counseling for STDs. Often, groups with the highest rates of STDs are the same groups in which access to health services is most limited. This limitation relates to (1) lacking access to publicly supported

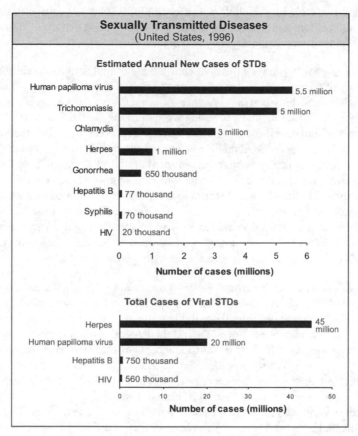

Sexually Transmitted Diseases
(United States, 1996)

Estimated Annual New Cases of STDs

Disease	Cases
Human papilloma virus	5.5 million
Trichomoniasis	5 million
Chlamydia	3 million
Herpes	1 million
Gonorrhea	650 thousand
Hepatitis B	77 thousand
Syphilis	70 thousand
HIV	20 thousand

Number of cases (millions)

Total Cases of Viral STDs

Disease	Cases
Herpes	45 million
Human papilloma virus	20 million
Hepatitis B	750 thousand
HIV	560 thousand

Number of cases (millions)

Source: American Social Health Association. *Sexually Transmitted Diseases in America: How Many Cases and at What Cost?* Menlo Park, CA: Kaiser Family Foundation, 1998.

STD clinics (present in only 50 percent of U.S. public health jurisdictions),[14] (2) having no health care coverage, (3) having coverage that imposes a copayment or deductible, or (4) having coverage that excludes the basic preventive health services that help avert STDs or their complications. (See Focus Area 1. Access to Quality Health Services.)

Substance abuse. Many studies document the association of substance abuse, especially the abuse of alcohol and drugs, with STDs.[15] At the population level, the introduction of new illicit substances into communities often can drastically alter sexual behavior in high-risk sexual networks, leading to the epidemic spread of STDs.[16] Behavioral factors that can increase STD transmission in a community include increases in the exchange of sex for drugs, increases in the number of anonymous sex partners, decreases in motivation to use barrier protection, and decreases in attempts to seek medical treatment. The nationwide syphilis epidemic of the late 1980s, for example, was fueled by increased crack cocaine use.[17] Other substances, including alcohol, may affect an individual's cognitive and negotiating skills before and during sex, lowering the likelihood that protection against STD transmission and pregnancy will be used.

Sexual coercion. Analysis of adolescent female sexual activity reveals the frequency of coercive behaviors and brings to light that not all young women enter sexual relationships as willing partners.[18] In fact, sexual coercion is a major problem for significant numbers of young women in the United States. In 1995, 16 percent of females whose first sexual intercourse took place when they were aged 15 years or under reported that it was not voluntary.[19] This aspect of adolescent sexual behavior demands increased national and local attention, both for social justice and for health reasons. Sexual violence against women contributes both directly and indirectly to STD transmission. Directly, women experiencing sexual violence are less able to protect themselves from STDs or pregnancy. Indirectly, research demonstrates that women with a history of involuntary sexual intercourse are more likely to have voluntary intercourse at earlier ages—a known risk factor for STDs—than women who are not sexually abused.[20]

Sexuality and secrecy. Perhaps the most important social factor contributing to the spread of STDs in the United States and the factor that most significantly separates the United States from those industrialized countries with low rates of STDs is the stigma associated with STDs and the general discomfort of people in the United States with discussing intimate aspects of life, especially those related to sex.[21] Sex and sexuality pervade many aspects of the Nation's culture, and people in the United States are fascinated with sexual matters. Paradoxically, while sexuality is considered a normal aspect of human functioning, people in the United States nevertheless are secretive and private about their sexual behavior. Talking openly and comfortably about sex and sexuality is difficult even in the most intimate relationships. One survey showed that, for married couples, about one-fourth of women and one-fifth of men had no knowledge of their partner's sexual history.[22] In its study, IOM stated, "The secrecy surrounding sexuality impedes sexuality education programs for adolescents, open discussion between parents and their children and between sex partners, balanced messages from mass media, education and counseling activities of health care professionals, and community activism regarding STDs."[23]

Changing sexual behaviors and sexual norms will be an important part of any long-term strategy to develop a more effective national system of STD prevention in the United States. A new sexual openness needs to become the norm to ensure that all sexual relationships are consensual, nonexploitive, and honest and to protect against disease and unintended pregnancy. This openness would allow (1) parents to talk frankly and comfortably with their children, and teachers and counselors with their students, about responsible behavior and avoiding risks (for example, abstaining from intercourse, delaying initiation of intercourse, reducing the number of sex partners, and increasing the use of effective barrier contraception), (2) sex partners to talk openly about safe behaviors, and (3) health care providers to talk comfortably and knowledgeably with patients about sexuality and sexual risk, to counsel them about risk avoidance, and to screen them regularly for STDs when indicated.[24] (See Focus Area 11. Health Communication.)

The entertainment industry, particularly television, has noticed interest in sexual themes. While people in the United States are bombarded by sexual messages and images, very little informed, high-quality STD prevention advice or discussion exists regarding contraception, sexuality, or the risks of early, unprotected sexual behavior. Popular television programs depict as many as 25 instances of sexual behaviors for every 1 instance of protected behavior or discussion about STDs or pregnancy prevention.[25] Media companies can play an important part in reshaping sexual behaviors and norms in the United States in the next decade.

Trends

STDs are common, costly, and preventable. Worldwide, an estimated 333 million cases of curable STDs occur annually.[26] In 1995, STDs were the most common reportable diseases in the United States.[27] They accounted for 87 percent of the top 10 infections most frequently reported to the Centers for Disease Control and Prevention (CDC) from State health departments. Of the top 10 infections, 5 were STDs (chlamydia, gonorrhea, AIDS, syphilis, and hepatitis B). Each year an estimated 15 million new STD infections occur in the United States, and nearly 4 million teenagers are infected with an STD.[28] The direct and indirect costs of the major STDs and their complications, including sexually transmitted HIV infection, are conservatively estimated at $17 billion annually.[3]

Despite recent progress toward controlling some STDs, when compared to other industrialized nations, the United States has failed to go far enough or fast enough in its national attempt to contain acute STDs and STD-related complications.[3] STD rates in this Nation exceed those in all other countries of the industrialized world (including the countries of western and northern Europe, Canada, Japan, and Australia). Through a sustained, collaborative, multifaceted approach, other countries have reduced significantly the burden of STDs on their citizens, an accomplishment the United States also should strive to achieve.

Disparities

All racial, cultural, economic, and religious groups are affected by STDs. People in all communities and sexual networks are at risk for STDs. Nevertheless, some population groups are disproportionately affected by STDs and their complications.

Gender disparities. Women suffer more frequent and more serious STD complications than men do. Among the most serious STD complications are pelvic inflammatory disease (PID), ectopic pregnancy, infertility, and chronic pelvic pain.[29] Women are biologically more susceptible to infection when exposed to a sexually transmitted agent. Often, STDs are transmitted more easily from a man to a woman.[30] Acute STDs (and even some complications) often are very mild or are completely asymptomatic in women. STDs are more difficult to diagnose in women due to the physiology and anatomy of the female reproductive tract. This combination of increased susceptibility and "silent" infection frequently can result in women being unaware of an STD, which results in delayed diagnosis and treatment.

STDs in pregnant women can cause serious health problems or death to the fetus or newborn.[31] Sexually transmitted organisms in the mother can cross the placenta to the fetus or newborn, resulting in congenital infection, or these organisms can reach the newborn during delivery, resulting in perinatal infections. Regardless of the route of infection, these organisms can permanently damage the brain, spinal cord, eyes, auditory nerves, or immune system. Even when the organisms do not reach the fetus or newborn directly, they can significantly complicate the pregnancy by causing spontaneous abortion, stillbirth, premature rupture of the membranes, or preterm delivery.[32] For example, women with bacterial vaginosis are 40 percent more likely to deliver a preterm, low birth weight infant than are mothers without this condition.[33, 34] (See Focus Area 16. Maternal, Infant, and Child Health.)

Age disparities. For a variety of behavioral, social, and biological reasons, STDs also disproportionately affect adolescents and young adults.[35] In 1997, females aged 15 to 19 years had the highest reported rates of both chlamydia and gonorrhea among women; males aged 20 to 24 years had the highest reported rates of both chlamydia and gonorrhea among men.[36] The herpes infection rate of white youth aged 12 to 19 years increased nearly fivefold from the period 1976–80 to the period 1988–94.[37] Indeed, because not all teenagers are sexually active, the actual rate of STDs in teens is probably higher than the observed rates suggest.[10] There are several contributing factors:

- Sexually active teenagers are at risk for STDs. In 1995, 50 percent of females aged 15 to 19 years interviewed for the National Survey of Family Growth (NSFG) indicated that they had had sexual intercourse.[19] In the same year, 54 percent of adolescent males in high school reported having had sexual intercourse, including 49 percent of white males, 62 percent of Hispanic males, and 81 percent of African American males.[38]

- Teenagers are increasingly likely to have more sex partners at earlier ages. Compounding this factor is the fact that these partners are active in sexual networks already highly infected with untreated STDs.[36] In 1971, 39 percent of sexually active adolescent females aged 15 to 19 years had more than one sex partner; in 1988 the percentage had increased to 62 percent.[39]

- Sexually active teenagers often are reluctant to obtain STD services, or they may face serious obstacles when trying to obtain them. In addition, health care providers often are uncomfortable discussing sexuality and risk reduction with their patients, thus missing opportunities to counsel and screen young people for STDs.[3]

Racial and ethnic disparities. Certain racial and ethnic groups (mainly African American and Hispanic populations) have high rates of STDs, compared with rates for whites. Race and ethnicity in the United States are risk markers that correlate with other fundamental determinants of health status, such as poverty, limited or no access to quality health care, fewer attempts to get medical treatment, illicit drug use, and living in communities with a high number of cases of STDs. National surveillance data may overrepresent STDs in racial and ethnic groups that are more likely to receive STD services from public-sector STD clinics where timely and complete illness reporting is generally the rule. However, studies using random sampling techniques document higher rates of STDs in marginalized populations, particularly African Americans as compared with whites.[37] Surveillance data from 1997 show:[36]

■ Although chlamydia is a widely distributed STD in population groups, it occurs more frequently in certain racial and ethnic groups.

■ African Americans (non-Hispanic blacks) accounted for about 77 percent of the total number of reported cases of gonorrhea—31 times the rate in whites (non-Hispanic whites). African American rates were on average about 24 times higher than those of white adolescents aged 15 to 19 years; the rate for African Americans aged 20 to 24 years was almost 28 times greater than that in whites. Gonorrhea rates in Hispanic persons were nearly three times the rate in whites.

■ The most recent syphilis epidemic occurred largely in heterosexual minority populations. Since 1990, rates of primary and secondary (P&S) syphilis have declined in all racial and ethnic groups except American Indians or Alaska Natives. However, rates for African Americans and Hispanics continue to be higher than those for whites. In 1997, African Americans accounted for about 82 percent of all reported cases of P&S syphilis.

■ In 1997, the rate of congenital syphilis was 113.5 per 100,000 live births in African Americans and 34.6 per 100,000 live births in Hispanics, compared with 3.3 per 100,000 live births in whites.

Finally, young heterosexual women, especially minority women, are increasingly acquiring HIV infection and developing AIDS. In 1998, 41 percent of reported AIDS cases in persons aged 13 to 24 years occurred in young women, and more than four of every five AIDS cases reported in women occurred in certain racial and ethnic groups (mostly African American or Hispanic).[40] The U.S. spread of HIV infection through heterosexual transmission closely parallels other STD epidemics.[2]

Compelling worldwide evidence indicates that the presence of other STDs increases the likelihood of both transmitting and acquiring HIV infection.[2] Prospective epidemiologic studies from four continents, including North America, have repeatedly demonstrated that when other STDs are present, HIV transmission is at least two to five times higher than when other STDs are not present. Biological studies demonstrate that when other STDs are present, an individual's susceptibility to HIV infection is increased, and the likelihood of a dually infected person (having HIV infection and another STD) infecting other people with HIV is increased. Conversely, effective STD treatment can slow the spread of HIV at the individual and community levels.

Opportunities

Prevention opportunities arise from an understanding of STD transmission dynamics. The rate of STD infection in a population is determined by the interaction of three principal factors:[41, 42]

- The rate at which uninfected individuals have sex with infected persons (rate of sex partner exchange or exposure).

- The probability that a susceptible exposed person actually will acquire the infection (transmission).

- The time period during which an infected person remains infectious and able to spread disease to others (duration).

Effective STD prevention requires effective population-level and individual-level interventions that can alter the natural course of these factors. IOM advised in its report, "Use of available information and interventions could have a rapid and dramatic impact on the incidence and prevalence of STDs in the United States. Many effective and efficient behavioral and biomedical interventions are available."[3]

Behavioral interventions can be brought to bear on exposure, transmission, and duration factors. They help persons abstain from sexual intercourse, delay initiation of intercourse, reduce the number of sex partners, and increase the use of effective physical barriers, such as condoms, or emerging chemical barriers, such as microbicides. Further attention must be given to helping parents become better at imparting STD information. Currently, a small percentage of adolescents receive STD prevention information from parents.[43] Schools are the main source of STD information for most teenagers,[43] indicating that school-based interventions can play a significant role in informing young people about STD exposure and transmission issues and in motivating them to modify their behaviors.[43] (See Focus Area 7. Educational and Community-Based Programs.) Both school-based health information and school-based health service programs are potentially beneficial to young persons.[44]

Mass media campaigns have been effective in bringing about significant changes in awareness, attitude, knowledge, and behaviors for other health problems, such as smoking.[45] National communication efforts are needed to help overcome widespread misinformation and lack of awareness about STDs.

Biomedical interventions can affect aspects of transmission and duration factors. Vaccines minimize the probability of infection, disease, or both, after exposure (transmission). While vaccines for some STDs are in various stages of development, the only effective and widely available STD vaccine is for hepatitis B.[46, 47] Unfortunately, hepatitis B vaccine coverage remains minimal, especially in high-risk groups, mainly due to a lack of awareness on the part of health care providers, limited opportunities to reach high-risk youth in traditional health care settings, and limited financial support for wide-scale implementation of this effective intervention. (See Focus Area 14. Immunization and Infectious Diseases.)

Correct and consistent condom use decreases STD transmission.[48] While condom use has been on the rise in the United States over the past few decades,[49] women who use the most effective forms of contraception (sterilization and hormonal contraception) are less likely to use condoms for STD prevention.[50, 51, 52] IOM stated in its report, "Because no single method of preventing STDs or pregnancy confers the maximum level of protection against both conditions, use of dual protection—that is, a condom and another effective contraceptive for pregnancy—is especially important. Not clear, however, is how well the public understands the need for dual protection against STDs and pregnancy."[3] Dual methods could prevent unwanted pregnancy and STDs.[53] Yet most sexually active young people do not employ this strategy.[54] (See Focus Area 9. Family Planning.)

Identifying and treating partners of persons with curable STDs to break the chain of transmission in a sexual network always have been integral to organized control programs.[55] Early antimicrobial prophylaxis of the exposed partner reduces the likelihood of transmission and thwarts infection. With partner treatment, the initially infected person benefits from a reduced risk of reinfection from an untreated partner, and the partner avoids acute infection and its potential complications. Future sex partners are protected by treating partners; thus, this treatment strategy also benefits the community.

Active partner notification and partner treatment generally have been the responsibility of personnel in public STD clinics. New approaches for getting more partners treated are being assessed both in traditional and nontraditional STD treatment settings. One approach actively involves initially infected patients in the process of referring their partners for evaluation and treatment.[56] Another approach uses new techniques to assess sexual networks in outbreak situations in order to identify infected patients and their partners more quickly.[57] Because most STD care in the United States is delivered in the private sector, private health care providers, managed-care organizations, and health departments need to work together to overcome barriers to rapid and effective treatment of the nonplan sex partners of health plan members.

Screening and treatment of STDs affect both transmission and duration factors. For curable STDs, screening and treatment can be cost-effective, or even cost-saving, in altering the period during which infected persons can infect others. Screening for STDs clearly meets the criteria for an effective preventive intervention.[58] For STDs that frequently are asymptomatic, screening and treatment benefit those who are likely to suffer severe complications (especially women) if infections are not detected and treated early.[59] For example, in a randomized controlled trial conducted in a large managed-care organization, chlamydia screening reduced by 56 percent new cases of subsequent pelvic inflammatory disease in a screened group.[60] Selective screening for chlamydia in the Pacific Northwest reduced the burden of disease in the screened population by 60 percent in 5 years.[61]

When combined with a new generation of sensitive and rapid diagnostic tests, some of which can be performed on a urine specimen, STD screening of specific high-risk populations in nontraditional settings appears to be a promising control strategy that expands access to underserved groups.[62] The success of screening programs will depend on the availability of funds, the willingness of communities and institutions to support them, and the availability of well-trained health care providers and of well-equipped and accessible laboratories.

Interim Progress Toward Year 2000 Objectives

Significant progress was made during the 1990s toward reducing the burden of the common bacterial STDs in the United States, such as gonorrhea, syphilis, and congenital syphilis—diseases for which national control programs have existed for the longest period. Encouraging data are emerging from a new and expanding chlamydia prevention program, suggesting that chlamydia screening is reducing disease burden and preventing complications. Nevertheless, STD complications, such as PID, continue to take a heavy toll on women's health and increase health care costs.

Because so many people are already infected, and millions more are infected annually, viral STDs continue to present challenges for prevention and control. One of the most serious health problems associated with STDs is sexually acquired HIV infection that is facilitated by the presence of an inflammatory or ulcerative STD in one or both sex partners. In 1998, females accounted for 23 percent of all AIDS cases in the United States, with African American and Hispanic females incurring a disproportionate share (similar to other STDs) of heterosexually transmitted HIV infection.[40] A nationally representative study showed that genital herpes infection is very common in the United States.[37] Nationwide, 45 million persons aged 12 years and older, or 1 out of 5 of the total adolescent and adult population, are infected with herpes simplex virus type 2. As many as 20 million persons in the United States already are infected with strains of the human papillomavirus, and an estimated 5.5 million new infections occur annually.[28]

Of the 17 STD-related Healthy People 2000 objectives, 10 either met or moved toward their targets. The Nation is making strides in efforts to reduce the occurrence of STDs, educate people about condom use, increase clinic services for HIV and other sexually transmitted diseases, and encourage abstinence from sexual intercourse among adolescents. Routine counseling by clinicians to prevent STDs has slipped away from its target. Two objectives have held steady: adolescents engaging in sexual intercourse and annual first-time consultations about genital herpes and warts. Another four could not be assessed.

Note: Unless otherwise noted, data are from the Centers for Disease Control and Prevention, National Center for Health Statistics, *Healthy People 2000 Review, 1998–99.*

Sexually Transmitted Diseases

Goal: Promote responsible sexual behaviors, strengthen community capacity, and increase access to quality services to prevent sexually transmitted diseases (STDs) and their complications.

Number   Objective Short Title

Bacterial STD Illness and Disability

25-1   Chlamydia

25-2   Gonorrhea

25-3   Primary and secondary syphilis

Viral STD Illness and Disability

25-4   Genital herpes

25-5   Human papillomavirus infection

STD Complications Affecting Females

25-6   Pelvic inflammatory disease (PID)

25-7   Fertility problems

25-8   Heterosexually transmitted HIV infection in women

STD Complications Affecting the Fetus and Newborn

25-9   Congenital syphilis

25-10   Neonatal STDs

Personal Behaviors

25-11   Responsible adolescent sexual behavior

25-12   Responsible sexual behavior messages on television

Community Protection Infrastructure

25-13   Hepatitis B vaccine services in STD clinics

25-14   Screening in youth detention facilities and jails

25-15   Contracts to treat nonplan partners of STD patients

Personal Health Services

25-16   Annual screening for genital chlamydia

25-17   Screening of pregnant women

25-18   Compliance with recognized STD treatment standards

25-19   Provider referral services for sex partners

Bacterial STD Illness and Disability

25-1. Reduce the proportion of adolescents and young adults with *Chlamydia trachomatis* infections.

Target and baseline:

Objective	Reduction in *Chlamydia trachomatis* infections	1997 Baseline	2010 Target
		Percent	
25-1a.	Females aged 15 to 24 years attending family planning clinics	5.0	3.0
25-1b.	Females aged 15 to 24 years attending STD clinics	12.2	3.0
25-1c.	Males aged 15 to 24 years attending STD clinics	15.7	3.0

Target setting method: Better than the best.

Data source: STD Surveillance System, CDC, NCHSTP.

NOTE: THE TABLE BELOW MAY CONTINUE TO THE FOLLOWING PAGE.

Persons Aged 15 to 24 Years Attending Clinics, 1997	Infected With Chlamydia		
	25-1a. Females (Family Planning Clinics)	25-1b. Females (STD Clinics)	25-1c. Males (STD Clinics)
	Percent		
TOTAL	5.0	12.2	15.7
Race and ethnicity			
American Indian or Alaska Native	6.3	13.1	12.6
Asian or Pacific Islander	4.7	12.0	16.6
Asian	DNC	DNC	DNC
Native Hawaiian and other Pacific Islander	DNC	DNC	DNC
Black or African American	DNC	DNC	DNC
White	DNC	DNC	DNC

Persons Aged 15 to 24 Years Attending Clinics, 1997	Infected With Chlamydia		
	25-1a. Females (Family Planning Clinics)	25-1b. Females (STD Clinics)	25-1c. Males (STD Clinics)
	Percent		
Hispanic or Latino	5.2	14.0	18.5
Not Hispanic or Latino	DNC	DNC	DNC
Black or African American	11.1	15.2	18.1
White	3.1	9.2	11.5
Family income level			
Poor	DNC	DNC	DNC
Near poor	DNC	DNC	DNC
Middle/high income	DNC	DNC	DNC

DNA = Data have not been analyzed. DNC = Data are not collected. DSU = Data are statistically unreliable.

NOTE: THE TABLE ABOVE MAY HAVE CONTINUED FROM THE PREVIOUS PAGE.

25-2. Reduce gonorrhea.

Target: 19 new cases per 100,000 population.

Baseline: 123 new cases of gonorrhea per 100,000 population occurred in 1997.

Target setting method: Better than the best.

Data source: STD Surveillance System, CDC, NCHSTP.

NOTE: THE TABLE BELOW MAY CONTINUE TO THE FOLLOWING PAGE.

Total Population, 1997	New Gonorrhea Cases		
	25-2. Both Genders	Females*	Males*
	Rate per 100,000		
TOTAL	123	119	125
Race and ethnicity			
American Indian or Alaska Native	100	131	67
Asian or Pacific Islander	20	21	18
Asian	DNC	DNC	DNC
Native Hawaiian and other Pacific Islander	DNC	DNC	DNC
Black or African American	DNC	DNC	DNC
White	DNC	DNC	DNC

Total Population, 1997	New Gonorrhea Cases		
	25-2. Both Genders	Females*	Males*
	Rate per 100,000		
Hispanic or Latino	69	72	67
Not Hispanic or Latino	DNC	DNC	DNC
Black or African American	808	714	912
White	26	32	20
Family income level			
Poor	DNC	DNC	DNC
Near poor	DNC	DNC	DNC
Middle/high income	DNC	DNC	DNC
Age			
15 to 24 years	512	617	414
25 to 34 years	198	161	235
35 to 44 years	71	40	101

DNA = Data have not been analyzed. DNC = Data are not collected. DSU = Data are statistically unreliable.
*Data for females and males are displayed to further characterize the issue.
NOTE: THE TABLE ABOVE MAY HAVE CONTINUED FROM THE PREVIOUS PAGE.

25-3. Eliminate sustained domestic transmission of primary and secondary syphilis.

Target: 0.2 cases per 100,000 population.

Baseline: 3.2 cases of primary and secondary syphilis per 100,000 population occurred in 1997.

Target setting method: Better than the best and consistent with the National Plan to Eliminate Syphilis from the United States, CDC, 1999.

Data source: STD Surveillance System, CDC, NCHSTP.

Total Population, 1997	Primary and Secondary Syphilis Cases		
	25-3. Both Genders	Females*	Males*
	Rate per 100,000		
TOTAL	3.2	2.9	3.6
Race and ethnicity			
American Indian or Alaska Native	2.0	1.8	2.3
Asian or Pacific Islander	0.3	0.4	0.3
Asian	DNC	DNC	DNC
Native Hawaiian and other Pacific Islander	DNC	DNC	DNC
Black or African American	DNC	DNC	DNC
White	DNC	DNC	DNC
Hispanic or Latino	1.6	1.0	2.1
Not Hispanic or Latino	DNC	DNC	DNC
Black or African American	22.0	19.3	25.0
White	0.5	0.5	0.6
Family income level			
Poor	DNC	DNC	DNC
Near poor	DNC	DNC	DNC
Middle/high income	DNC	DNC	DNC
Sexual orientation	DNC	DNC	DNC

DNA = Data have not been analyzed. DNC = Data are not collected. DSU = Data are statistically unreliable.
*Data for females and males are displayed to further characterize the issue.

The United States has a unique opportunity to eliminate syphilis within its borders. Syphilis is easy to detect and cure, given adequate access to and use of care. Nationally, it is at the lowest rate ever recorded and is confined to a very limited number of geographic areas. The last epidemic peaked in 1990, with the highest syphilis rate in 40 years. By 1997, the number of cases had declined by 84 percent.[62] In addition, where syphilis does persist in the United States, it disproportionately affects African Americans living in poverty. Although the black:white ratio for reported syphilis has decreased since the early 1990s, the 1997 primary and secondary syphilis rate for non-Hispanic blacks was still 44 times greater than that for non-Hispanic whites.[62] In 1997, of the 1,034 reported congenital syphilis cases with known race or ethnicity of the mother, non-Hispanic blacks and Hispanics accounted for 88 percent of these reported cases, while accounting for only

23 percent of the female population and 33 percent of all births.[62] The persistence of high rates of syphilis in the United States is a sentinel event identifying communities in which there is a fundamental failure of basic public health capacity to control infectious diseases and ensure reproductive health.

Elimination of syphilis would have far-reaching public health implications because it would remove two devastating consequences of the disease—increased likelihood of HIV transmission and compromised ability to have healthy babies due to spontaneous abortions, stillbirths, and multisystem disorders caused by congenital syphilis acquired from mothers with syphilis. Eliminating syphilis in the United States would be a landmark achievement because it would remove these direct health burdens and would significantly decrease one of this Nation's most glaring racial disparities in health.

While many other endemic diseases, such as polio, measles, and smallpox, have been eliminated through widespread use of vaccines, the strategies for syphilis elimination differ from these efforts largely because there currently is no vaccine. Five strategies are critical for eliminating syphilis from the United States. Two strategies—strengthened community involvement and partnerships and rapid outbreak response—will be new in many parts of the United States. The three remaining strategies—enhanced surveillance, expanded clinical and laboratory services, and enhanced health promotion—have been used for syphilis control and will be intensified and expanded for syphilis elimination.

Viral STD Illness and Disability

25-4. Reduce the proportion of adults with genital herpes infection.

Target: 14 percent.

Baseline: 17 percent of adults aged 20 to 29 years had genital herpes infection in 1988–94 (as measured by herpes simplex virus type 2 [HSV-2] antibody).

Target setting method: Better than the best.

Data source: National Health and Nutrition Examination Survey (NHANES), CDC, NCHS.

NOTE: THE TABLE BELOW MAY CONTINUE TO THE FOLLOWING PAGE.

Adults Aged 20 to 29 Years, 1988–94	Infected With Genital Herpes
	Percent
TOTAL	17
Race and ethnicity	
American Indian or Alaska Native	DSU
Asian or Pacific Islander	DSU

Adults Aged 20 to 29 Years, 1988–94	Infected With Genital Herpes
	Percent
Asian	DNC
Native Hawaiian and other Pacific Islander	DNC
Black or African American	34
White	15
Hispanic or Latino	DSU
Mexican American	15
Not Hispanic or Latino	DNA
Black or African American	33
White	15
Gender	
Female (all ages)	26
Male (all ages)	18
Family income level	
Poor	28
Near poor	14
Middle/high income	15
Age	
12 to 19 years*	6
20 to 29 years	17
30 to 39 years*	28
40 to 49 years*	27

DNA = Data have not been analyzed. DNC = Data are not collected. DSU = Data are statistically unreliable.
*Data for persons aged 12 to 19 years, 30 to 39 years, and 40 to 49 years are displayed to further characterize the issue.

NOTE: THE TABLE ABOVE MAY HAVE CONTINUED FROM THE PREVIOUS PAGE.

25-5. (Developmental) Reduce the proportion of persons with human papillomavirus (HPV) infection.

Potential data source: National Health and Nutrition Examination Survey (NHANES), CDC, NCHS.

Reducing the number of new HPV cases can help to minimize the overall number of cases of high-risk subtypes associated with cervical cancer in females aged 15 to 44 years. Over the past 15 years, molecular, biochemical, and epidemiologic data have firmly established the central role of several types of HPV (types 16, 18, 31, and 45) in the pathogenesis of cervical cancer.[63]

25-6. Reduce the proportion of females who have ever required treatment for pelvic inflammatory disease (PID).

Target: 5 percent.

Baseline: 8 percent of females aged 15 to 44 years required treatment for PID in 1995.

Target setting method: Better than the best.

Data source: National Survey of Family Growth (NSFG), CDC, NCHS.

Females Aged 15 to 44 Years, 1995	Treated for PID
	Percent
TOTAL	8
Race and ethnicity	
American Indian or Alaska Native	DSU
Asian or Pacific Islander	DSU
Asian	DNC
Native Hawaiian and other Pacific Islander	DNC
Black or African American	11
White	7
Hispanic or Latino	8
Not Hispanic or Latino	8
Black or African American	11
White	7
Family income level (aged 22 to 44 years)	
Poor	12
Near poor	11
Middle/high income	8
Education level (aged 22 to 44 years)	
Less than high school	14
High school graduate	9
At least some college	7

DNA = Data have not been analyzed. DNC = Data are not collected. DSU = Data are statistically unreliable.

PID is among the most serious threats to female reproductive capability. PID is caused most frequently by chlamydial infections and gonorrhea that ascend past the cervix into the upper reproductive tract.[64] More than 1 million women have an episode of PID annually.[65, 66] PID often results in scarring and either complete or partial blockage of the fallopian tubes. As a result, as many as one-quarter of women with acute PID experience serious long-term sequelae, most often an ectopic pregnancy or tubal factor infertility. Women who have had PID are 6 to 10 times more likely to have an ectopic pregnancy compared with women who have not had PID.[9] In 1992, approximately 9 percent of all pregnancy-related deaths were caused by ectopic pregnancy.[67]

25-7. Reduce the proportion of childless females with fertility problems who have had a sexually transmitted disease or who have required treatment for pelvic inflammatory disease (PID).

Target: 15 percent.

Baseline: 27 percent of childless females aged 15 to 44 years with fertility problems had a history of STDs or PID treatment in 1995.

Target setting method: 44 percent improvement.

Data source: National Survey of Family Growth (NSFG), CDC, NCHS.

NOTE: THE TABLE BELOW MAY CONTINUE TO THE FOLLOWING PAGE.

Childless Females Aged 15 to 44 Years With Fertility Problems, 1995	STD History or PID Treatment
	Percent
TOTAL	27
Race and ethnicity	
American Indian or Alaska Native	DSU
Asian or Pacific Islander	DSU
Asian	DNC
Native Hawaiian and other Pacific Islander	DNC
Black or African American	33
White	27
Hispanic or Latino	27
Not Hispanic or Latino	27
Black or African American	32
White	27
Education level (aged 22 to 44 years)	
Less than high school	30
High school graduate	27
At least some college	28

Childless Females Aged 15 to 44 Years With Fertility Problems, 1995	STD History or PID Treatment
	Percent
Age	
15 to 24 years	23
25 to 34 years	26
35 to 44 years	31

DNA = Data have not been analyzed. DNC = Data are not collected. DSU = Data are statistically unreliable.

NOTE: THE TABLE ABOVE MAY HAVE CONTINUED FROM THE PREVIOUS PAGE.

In 1995, there were approximately 24.2 million women aged 15 to 44 years who had not given birth to a child and had not had a sterilizing operation. Most of them (21.2 million) were presumed to be able to have a child. Perhaps these women were not aware of fertility problems (see Terminology) because they had not yet tested their fertility potential. This presumption is supported by the fact that most of these 21.2 million childless women were using contraception in 1995. While some fraction of them may remain voluntarily childless and never choose to test their fertility, most are likely to pursue childbearing at some point in the future. Approximately 2.3 million of these "untested" women in 1995 had a history of STDs or PID treatment, increasing the likelihood that some of them will experience a fertility problem in the future. If the social stigma associated with STDs resulted in any underreporting of STDs in this self-report survey, the 2.3 million women at risk for future fertility problems may be a low estimate.

At the time of the NSFG in 1995, nearly 3 million of the 24.2 million childless women had a fertility problem. A subset of this group, approximately 800,000 women, had a history of STDs or PID treatment. This subset comprised 27 percent of the women with known fertility problems, which may be a low estimate of the contribution made by previous STDs or PID to the fertility problems among childless women. Because bacterial STDs and PID may be asymptomatic when present and because diagnosing tubal factor infertility caused by PID is both difficult and expensive, many women with fertility problems may not be aware of having had an STD or PID in the past. Evidence has shown that reducing the burden of bacterial STDs in reproductive age women can dramatically reduce the amount of PID[60] and through this mechanism could reduce fertility problems.

25-8. (Developmental) Reduce HIV infections in adolescent and young adult females aged 13 to 24 years that are associated with heterosexual contact.

Potential data source: HIV/AIDS Surveillance System, CDC, NCHSTP.

25-9.   Reduce congenital syphilis.

Target: 1 new case per 100,000 live births.

Baseline: 27 new cases of congenital syphilis per 100,000 live births were reported in 1997.

Target setting method: Better than the best and consistent with the National Plan to Eliminate Syphilis from the United States, CDC, 1998.

Data sources: STD Surveillance System, CDC, NCHSTP; National Vital Statistics System (NVSS), CDC, NCHS.

Live Births, 1997	New Congenital Syphilis Cases
	Rate per 100,000
TOTAL	27
Mother's race and ethnicity	
American Indian or Alaska Native	11
Asian or Pacific Islander	8
Asian	DNC
Native Hawaiian and other Pacific Islander	DNC
Black or African American	DNC
White	DNC
Hispanic or Latino	34
Not Hispanic or Latino	DNC
Black or African American	123
White	4
Family income level	
Poor	DNC
Near poor	DNC
Middle/high income	DNC

DNA = Data have not been analyzed. DNC = Data are not collected. DSU = Data are statistically unreliable.

25-10. (Developmental) Reduce neonatal consequences from maternal sexually transmitted diseases, including chlamydial pneumonia, gonococcal and chlamydial *ophthalmia neonatorum*, laryngeal papillomatosis (from human papillomavirus infection), neonatal herpes, and preterm birth and low birth weight associated with bacterial vaginosis.

Potential data source: STD Surveillance System, CDC, NCHSTP.

Personal Behaviors

25-11. Increase the proportion of adolescents who abstain from sexual intercourse or use condoms if currently sexually active.

Target: 95 percent.

Baseline: 85 percent of adolescents in grades 9 through 12 abstained from sexual intercourse or used condoms in 1999 (50 percent had never had intercourse; 14 percent had intercourse but not in the past 3 months; and 21 percent currently were sexually active and used a condom at last intercourse).

Target setting method: 12 percent improvement.

Data source: Youth Risk Behavior Surveillance System (YRBSS), CDC, NCCDPHP.

NOTE: THE TABLE BELOW MAY CONTINUE TO THE FOLLOWING PAGE.

Students in Grades 9 Through 12, 1999	25-11. Abstained From Sexual Intercourse or Used Condom [Column a = b + c + d]	NOT Currently Sexually Active		Currently Sexually Active	
		Never Had Intercourse* [Column b]	No Intercourse in Past 3 Months* [Column c]	Used Condom at Last Intercourse * [Column d]	Did NOT Use Condom at Last Intercourse [Column e]
	Percent				
TOTAL	85	50	14	21	15
Race and ethnicity					
American Indian or Alaska Native	DSU	DSU	DSU	DSU	DSU
Asian or Pacific Islander	DSU	DSU	DSU	DSU	DSU

Students in Grades 9 Through 12, 1999	25-11. Abstained From Sexual Intercourse or Used Condom [Column a = b + c + d]	NOT Currently Sexually Active		Currently Sexually Active	
		Never Had Intercourse* [Column b]	No Intercourse in Past 3 Months* [Column c]	Used Condom at Last Intercourse* [Column d]	Did NOT Use Condom at Last Intercourse [Column e]
		Percent			
Asian	DNC	DNC	DNC	DNC	DNC
Native Hawaiian and other Pacific Islander	DNC	DNC	DNC	DNC	DNC
Black or African American	83	30	17	36	17
White	86	55	13	18	14
Hispanic or Latino	84	46	18	20	16
Not Hispanic or Latino	85	51	13	21	15
Black or African American	84	29	18	37	16
White	85	55	12	18	15
Gender					
Female	81	52	11	18	18
Male	87	48	16	23	13
Grade					
9th	90	61	12	17	10
10th	87	53	14	20	13
11th	84	47	15	22	16
12th	73	35	14	24	27
Sexual orientation	DNC	DNC	DNC	DNC	DNC
Select populations					
Number of sex partners (past 3 months)					
None	100	79	21	NA	NA
1	57	NA	NA	57	43

Healthy People 2010: Objectives for Improving Health

Students in Grades 9 Through 12, 1999	25-11. Ab-stained From Sexual Inter-course or Used Condom [Column a = b + c + d]	NOT Currently Sexually Active		Currently Sexually Active	
		Never Had Inter-course* [Column b]	No Inter-course in Past 3 Months* [Column c]	Used Con-dom at Last Inter-course* [Col-umn d]	Did NOT Use Condom at Last Inter-course [Column e]
	Percent				
2 to 3	62	NA	NA	62	38
4 or more	60	NA	NA	60	40

DNA = Data have not been analyzed. DNC = Data are not collected. DSU = Data are statistically unreliable. NA = Not applicable.

*Data for never had intercourse, had intercourse but not in the past 3 months, and currently sexually active and used a condom at last intercourse are displayed to further characterize the issue.

NOTE: THE TABLE ABOVE MAY HAVE CONTINUED FROM THE PREVIOUS PAGE.

Promoting responsible adolescent sexual behavior targets three protective behaviors that reduce the risk of STDs (including HIV infection) and unintended pregnancy. These behaviors are especially relevant to young people who, as a group, experience a disproportionate share of STDs and unintended pregnancies when they engage in sexual intercourse.[36, 37] The protective behaviors of interest are completely abstaining from sexual intercourse during adolescence (primary abstinence), reverting to abstinence for long periods of time after having had intercourse in the past (secondary abstinence), and at least using condoms (a single method that offers protection against both pregnancy and some STDs) consistently and correctly if regular intercourse is occurring. In 1999, 85 percent of high school youth demonstrated at least one of these behaviors. In contrast, the remaining 15 percent were sexually active and did not use a condom at last intercourse, placing them at high risk for STDs and unwanted pregnancy. Increasing and maintaining the proportion of youth who exhibit the above protective behaviors reduce the risks of HIV infection, other STDs, and unintended pregnancies for adolescents because the proportion of youth who are currently sexually active and do not use condoms will be reduced.

Various societal institutions (such as parents and families, schools, health care providers, postsecondary institutions, religious organizations, media, employers, community agencies that serve youth, celebrities, and government agencies) can positively influence the health and behaviors of the Nation's youth. Collaboration among these institutions can (1) help adolescents abstain from sexual intercourse, (2) help them overcome pressure to become sexually active prematurely, and (3) ensure accessible, confidential community counseling and clinical services for young people who are or have been sexually active.

Abstaining from sexual intercourse offers maximum protection to adolescents who are generally poorly prepared to deal with the physical and psychological consequences of HIV infection, other STDs, and pregnancy. Overall, 50 percent of high school youth fell into this category (see objective 25-11 population data table). Abstaining from sexual intercourse while in high school varied by race and ethnicity, for example, from 55 percent among white youth to 29 percent among African American youth. Abstaining from intercourse decreased as young people progressed through high school, from 61 percent among 9th graders to 35 percent among 12th graders. These data point out that while 61 percent of 9th graders had never had sexual intercourse, at least 39 percent had intercourse during or before 9th grade. Among the 39 percent, 12 percent had not had intercourse in the past 3 months, 17 percent were currently sexually active and used a condom at last intercourse, and the remaining 10 percent were sexually active and did not use a condom at last intercourse. These data suggest a need for counseling, support, education, and services for many young people even before high school begins.

Young people who have had sexual intercourse in the past but are not currently sexually active need special attention and services. Overall, 14 percent of high school youth fall into this category. Slightly more males (16 percent) than females (11 percent) fit into this category. More African American (18 percent) and Hispanic (18 percent) youth fit into this category than do white (12 percent) youth. Even if pregnancy were avoided in the past, the same may not be true for STDs. Some youth may have acquired viral or bacterial STDs that have not been recognized or treated. Previously sexually active adolescents need to be educated about this possibility, and medical evaluation and counseling are strongly suggested both to identify treatable conditions and to reinforce abstinence messages.

Young people who are currently sexually active also require special attention and services. This requirement applies both to the 21 percent of high school youth who were sexually active and used a condom at last intercourse and the remaining 15 percent of youth who were currently sexually active and did not use a condom at last intercourse. These data illustrate wide variation in current sexual activity by race/ethnicity. For African American high school youth, 53 percent were sexually active (37 percent were sexually active and used a condom at last intercourse, and 16 percent were sexually active but did not use a condom at last intercourse). For Hispanic youth, 36 percent were sexually active (20 percent were sexually active and used a condom, and 16 percent were sexually active and did not use a condom). Among white youth, 33 percent were sexually active (18 percent used a condom at last intercourse, and 15 percent did not use a condom). Also, fewer sex partners among currently sexually active youth does not equate with a much higher degree of condom use. Regardless of the number of sex partners in a given interval, approximately one of every two sexually active adolescents did not use a condom at last intercourse. For example, for adolescents who had four or more sex partners in the past 3 months, 40 percent of them would be considered to be at very high risk for STDs (including HIV infection) and possibly pregnancy by not using condoms consistently. Even for youth with one sex partner in the past 3 months, 43 percent did not use condoms consistently. In addition to reinforcing abstinence messages, adult counselors of currently sexually active adolescents must be aware that there is ongoing, very high risk of HIV infection, other STDs, and pregnancy. Responsible and influential adults should help young males and females gain easy access to high quality, confidential, comprehensive reproductive health care in their communities that can help them reduce HIV infection, STD, and pregnancy risk. This is especially true for adolescent females, who bear all the physical consequences of unintended pregnancy and bear disproportionate short- and long-term complications from STDs.

25-12. (Developmental) Increase the number of positive messages related to responsible sexual behavior during weekday and nightly prime-time television programming.

Potential data source: CDC, NCHSTP.

Television messages hold the potential to promote responsible sexual behaviors, such as abstinence, delaying sexual intercourse, or using effective methods to prevent STDs and pregnancy, such as use of condoms and hormonal contraception.

Community Protection Infrastructure

25-13. Increase the proportion of Tribal, State, and local sexually transmitted disease programs that routinely offer hepatitis B vaccines to all STD clients.

Target: 90 percent.

Baseline: 5 percent of State and local STD programs offered hepatitis B vaccines to clients in accordance with CDC guidelines in 1998.[46, 68] Tribal STD program data are developmental.

Target setting method: 85 percentage point improvement.

Data sources: Survey of STD Programs, National Coalition of STD Directors (NCSD); IHS.

Routine vaccination of infants is expected to produce a highly immune population to eliminate hepatitis B virus transmission in the United States. However, high rates of acute hepatitis B continue to occur in young adult risk groups, particularly persons with a history of another sexually transmitted disease and persons with multiple sex partners. Approximately 50 percent of new infections occur in persons with a sexual risk factor for transmission, and most of these persons have had a missed opportunity to be vaccinated. For example, 42 percent of acute hepatitis B cases reported in the CDC Sentinel Counties Study of Viral Hepatitis in 1996 had been treated for a sexually transmitted disease in the past.

25-14. **(Developmental) Increase the proportion of youth detention facilities and adult city or county jails that screen for common bacterial sexually transmitted diseases within 24 hours of admission and treat STDs (when necessary) before persons are released.**

Potential data sources: Annual Survey of Correctional Facilities, CDC, NCHSTP and National Institute of Justice; U.S. Department of Justice, Bureau of Justice Statistics.

25-15. **(Developmental) Increase the proportion of all local health departments that have contracts with managed care providers for the treatment of nonplan partners of patients with bacterial sexually transmitted diseases (gonorrhea, syphilis, and chlamydia).**

Potential data source: Survey of STD Programs, National Coalition of STD Directors (NCSD).

Personal Health Services

25-16. **(Developmental) Increase the proportion of sexually active females aged 25 years and under who are screened annually for genital chlamydia infections.**

Potential data sources: Family Planning Annual Report, OPA; STD Surveillance System, CDC, NCHSTP.

Routine screening for asymptomatic infection with *Chlamydia trachomatis* during pelvic examination is recommended for all sexually active female adolescents and for other women at high risk for chlamydial infection. While evidence is insufficient to make a recommendation concerning routine screening of sexually active males, in situations where asymptomatic chlamydial infection is high in males, screening using urine-based tests may be recommended to prevent spread of the infection.[58] Reported chlamydial infection rates in males are highest among those aged 20 to 24 years.

25-17. **(Developmental) Increase the proportion of pregnant females screened for sexually transmitted diseases (including HIV infection and bacterial vaginosis) during prenatal health care visits, according to recognized standards.**

Potential data source: STD Surveillance System, CDC, NCHSTP.

While evidence is insufficient to make a recommendation concerning routine screening of pregnant females for STDs, the benefits of early intervention in HIV-asymptomatic pregnant women, for example, are known. Similar benefits have been demonstrated in detecting and treating asymptomatic chlamydia infection in pregnancy.[58]

25-18. Increase the proportion of primary care providers who treat patients with sexually transmitted diseases and who manage cases according to recognized standards.

Target: 90 percent.

Baseline: 70 percent of primary care providers treated patients with STDs according to CDC STD Treatment Guidelines in 1988.

Target setting method: Retain 2000 target.

Data sources: National Disease and Therapeutic Index, IMS America; National Ambulatory Medical Care Survey (NAMCS), CDC, NCHS.

25-19. (Developmental) Increase the proportion of all sexually transmitted disease clinic patients who are being treated for bacterial STDs (chlamydia, gonorrhea, and syphilis) and who are offered provider referral services for their sex partners.

Potential data source: STD Surveillance System, CDC, NCHSTP.

Related Objectives From Other Focus Areas

1. **Access to Quality Health Services**
   - 1-3. Counseling about health behaviors
   - 1-7. Core competencies in health provider training
3. **Cancer**
   - 3-4. Cervical cancer deaths
   - 3-11. Pap tests
7. **Educational and Community-Based Programs**
   - 7-2. School health education
9. **Family Planning**
   - 9-8. Abstinence before age 15 years
   - 9-9. Abstinence among adolescents aged 15 to 17 years
   - 9-10. Pregnancy prevention and sexually transmitted disease (STD) protection
   - 9-11. Pregnancy prevention education
   - 9-12. Problems in becoming pregnant and maintaining a pregnancy
13. **HIV**
   - 13-5. New HIV cases
   - 13-6. Condom use
   - 13-9. HIV/AIDS, STD, and TB education in State prisons
   - 13-12. Screening for STDs and immunization for hepatitis B

14. **Immunization and Infectious Diseases**
    14-3. Hepatitis B in adults and high-risk groups
    14-28. Hepatitis B vaccination among high-risk groups
15. **Injury and Violence Prevention**
    15-35. Rape or attempted rape
    15-36. Sexual assault other than rape
16. **Maternal, Infant, and Child Health**
    16-1. Fetal and infant deaths
    16-6. Prenatal care
    16-10. Low birth weight and very low birth weight
    16-11. Preterm births

Terminology

(A listing of abbreviations and acronyms used in this publication appears in Appendix H.)

Bacterial and protozoal STDs: Refer to curable sexually transmitted infections caused by *Chlamydia trachomatis* (chlamydia), *Neisseria gonorrhoeae* (gonorrhea), *Treponema pallidum* (syphilis), *Haemophilus ducreyi* (chancroid), *Trichomonas vaginalis* (trichomoniasis), *bacterial vaginosis*, and other organisms.

Congenital syphilis: A condition in a fetus or newborn caused by infection with the syphilis bacteria from an untreated mother. Infected newborns show a wide spectrum of clinical signs, and only severe cases are clinically apparent at birth. Severe illness or death can result after birth if the newborn is not treated.

Fertility problems: Refer to the standard medical definitions of infertility (have not used contraception and have not become pregnant for 12 months or more) or impaired fecundity (women reporting no sterilizing operation and classified as finding it difficult or impossible to get pregnant or carry a baby to term).

Provider referral: Formerly called contact tracing, the process whereby health department personnel directly and confidentially notify the sex partners of infected individuals about their exposure to a sexually transmitted disease for the purposes of education, counseling, and referral to health care services.

STD complications: Refer to serious health problems that occur following an acute bacterial or viral STD. Among the most serious of these complications:

Cancer: Includes cervical cancer and its precursors (due to some strains of human papillomavirus) and liver cancer that can result after chronic infection with hepatitis B virus.

Infection of a fetus or newborn: Includes conditions such as congenital syphilis, neonatal herpes, HIV infection, eye infections, and pneumonia.

Pelvic inflammatory disease (PID): Can cause permanent damage to the female reproductive tract and lead to ectopic pregnancy, infertility, or chronic pelvic pain.

Preterm birth: Can result from maternal infection.

Sexually transmitted HIV infection: Can be facilitated by the presence of an inflammatory or ulcerative STD in one or both sex partners.

Syphilis elimination: Refers to the elimination of sustained domestic transmission of syphilis. Term means that there is no continuing transmission of the disease within a community or jurisdiction and absence of transmission within a jurisdiction except within 90 days of report of an imported case.

Viral STDs: Refer to the sexually transmitted viral infections—HIV infection, genital herpes, and HPV infection. Initial infections with these organisms may be asymptomatic or may cause only mild symptoms. Hepatitis B virus and hepatitis C virus can be transmitted through sexual activity.

References

[1] United Nations. *Report of the International Conference on Population and Development Cairo, Egypt, September 5-13, 1994.* New York, NY: United Nations, 1995.

[2] St. Louis, M.E.; Wasserheit, J.N.; and Gayle, H.D. (Editorial) Janus considers the HIV pandemic-harnessing recent advances to enhance AIDS prevention. *American Journal of Public Health* 87:10-12, 1997.

[3] Institute of Medicine (IOM). Eng, T.R., and Butler, W.T., eds. *The Hidden Epidemic: Confronting Sexually Transmitted Diseases.* Washington, DC: National Academy Press, 1997.

[4] Fish, A.; Fairweather, D.; Oriel, J.; et al. *Chlamydia trachomatis* infection in a gynecology clinic population: Identification of high-risk groups and the value of contact tracing. *European Journal of Obstetrics, Gynecology and Reproductive Biology* 31:67-74, 1989.

[5] Handsfield, H.; Jasman, L.; Roberts, P.; et al. Criteria for selective screening for *Chlamydia trachomatis* infection in women attending family planning clinics. *Journal of the American Medical Association* 255:1730-1734, 1986.

[6] Judson, F. Gonorrhea. *Medical Clinics of North America* 74:1353-1367, 1990.

[7] Stamm, W., and Holmes, K. *Chlamydia trachomatis* infections in the adult. In: Holmes, K.; Mardh, P.A.; Sparling, P.; et al.; eds. *Sexually Transmitted Diseases.* 2nd ed. New York, NY: McGraw-Hill, Inc., 1990, 181-193.

[8] Beasley, R.P.; Hwang, L.Y.; Lin, C.C.; et al. Hepatocellular carcinoma and hepatitis B virus. A prospective study of 22,707 men in Taiwan. *Lancet* 2(8256):1129-1133, 1981.

[9] Marchbanks, P.; Annegers, J.; Coulam, C.; et al. Risk factors for ectopic pregnancy: A population-based study. *Journal of the American Medical Association* 259:1823-1827, 1988.

[10] Cates, W. Epidemiology and control of sexually transmitted diseases in adolescents. In: Schydlower, M., and Shafer, M., eds. *AIDS and Other Sexually Transmitted Diseases.* Philadelphia, PA: Hanly & Belfus, Inc., 1990, 409-427.

[11] Blank, S.; McDonnell, D.; Rubin, et al. New approaches to syphilis control: Finding opportunities for syphilis treatment and congenital syphilis prevention in a women's correctional setting. *Sexually Transmitted Diseases* 24(4):218-228, 1997.

[12] Cohen, D.; Scribner, R.; Clark, J.; et al. The potential role of custody facilities in controlling sexually transmitted diseases. *American Journal of Public Health* 82:552-556, 1992.

[13] Oh, M.; Cloud, G.; Wallace, L.; et al. Sexual behavior and sexually transmitted diseases among male adolescents in detention. *Sexually Transmitted Diseases* 21:127-132, 1994.

[14] Landry, D., and Forrest, J. Public health departments providing STD services. *Family Planning Perspectives* 28:261-266, 1996.

[15] Beltrami, J.; Wright-DeAguero, L.; Fullilove, M.; et al. *Substance Abuse and the Spread of Sexually Transmitted Diseases.* Commissioned paper for the IOM Committee on Prevention and Control of STDs, 1997.

[16] Marx, R.; Aral, S.; Rolfs, R.; et al. Crack, sex, and STDs. *Sexually Transmitted Diseases* 18:92-101, 1991.

[17] Gunn, R.; Montes, J.; Toomey, K.; et al. Syphilis in San Diego County 1983–1992: Crack cocaine, prostitution, and the limitations of partner notification. *Sexually Transmitted Diseases* 22:60-66, 1995.

[18] Abma, J.; Driscoll, A.; and Moore, K. Young women's degree of control over first intercourse: An exploratory analysis. *Family Planning Perspectives* 30(1):12-18, 1998.

[19] Abma, J.; Chandra, A.; Mosher, W.; et al. Fertility, family planning, and women's health: New data from the 1995 National Survey of Family Growth. *Vital and Health Statistics* 23(19), 1997.

[20] Miller, B.; Monson, B.; and Norton, M. The effects of forced sexual intercourse on white female adolescents. *Child Abuse and Neglect* 19:1289-1301, 1995.

[21] Brandt, A. *No Magic Bullet: A Social History of Venereal Disease in the United States Since 1880.* New York, NY: Oxford University Press, Inc., 1985.

[22] EDK Associates. *The ABCs of STDs.* New York, NY: EDK Associates, 1995.

[23] IOM. *Summary—The Hidden Epidemic: Confronting Sexually Transmitted Diseases.* Washington, DC: National Academy Press, 1997.

[24] Lawrence, L. How OB-GYNs are failing women. *Glamour* 10:292, 1997.

[25] Lowry, D., and Schindler, J. Prime time TV portrayals of sex, "Safe sex and AIDS: A longitudinal analysis." *Journalism Quarterly* 70:628-637, 1993.

[26] Tsui, A.; Wasserheit, J.; and Haaga, J. *Reproductive Health in Developing Countries: Expanding Dimensions, Building Solutions.* Washington, DC: National Academy Press, 1997.

[27] Centers for Disease Control and Prevention (CDC). Ten leading national notifiable infectious diseases—United States, 1995. *Morbidity and Mortality Weekly Report* 45:883-884, 1996.

[28] American Social Health Association. *Sexually Transmitted Diseases in America: How Many Cases and at What Cost?* Menlo Park, CA: Kaiser Family Foundation, 1998.

[29] Chandra, A., and Stephen, E. Impaired fecundity in the United States: 1982–1995. *Family Planning Perspectives* 30(1):34-42, 1998.

[30] Holmes, K.; Johnson, D.; and Trostle, H. An estimate of the risk of men acquiring gonorrhea by sexual contact with infected females. *American Journal of Epidemiology* 91:170-174, 1970.

[31] Brunham, R.; Holmes, K.; and Embree, J. Sexually transmitted diseases in pregnancy. In: Holmes, K.; Mardh, P.; Sparling, P.; et al.; eds. *Sexually Transmitted Diseases.* 2nd ed. New York, NY: McGraw-Hill, Inc., 1990, 771-801.

[32] Goldenberg, R.L.; Andrews, W.W.; Yuan, A.C.; et al. Sexually transmitted diseases and adverse outcomes of pregnancy. *Clinics in Perinatology* 24(1):23-41, 1997.

[33] Hillier, S.; Nugent, R.; Eschenbach, D.; et al. Association between bacterial vaginosis and preterm delivery of a low-birth-weight infant. *New England Journal of Medicine* 333:1737-1742, 1995.

[34] Meis, P.J.; Goldenberg, R.L.; Mercer, G.; et al. The preterm prediction study: Significance of vaginal infections. *American Journal of Obstetrics and Gynecology* 173(4):1231-1235, 1995.

[35] Alan Guttmacher Institute. *Sex and America's Teenagers*. New York, NY: the Institute, 1994.

[36] CDC, Division of STD Prevention. *Sexually Transmitted Disease Surveillance, 1997*. U.S. Department of Health and Human Services (HHS), Public Health Service (PHS). Atlanta, GA: CDC, September 1998.

[37] Fleming, D.T.; McQuillan, G.M.; Johnson, R.E.; et al. Herpes Simplex Virus Type 2 in the United States, 1976 to 1994. *New England Journal of Medicine* 337:1105-1111, 1997.

[38] Warren, C.; Santelli, J.; Everett, S.; et al. Sexual behavior among U.S. high school students, 1990–1995. *Family Planning Perspectives* 30(4):170-172, 1998.

[39] Kost, I., and Forrest, J.D. American Women's sexual behavior and exposure to risk of sexually transmitted diseases. *Family Planning Perspectives* 24:244-254, 1992.

[40] CDC. *HIV/AIDS Surveillance Report, 1998* 10(No. 2), 1998.

[41] Anderson, R. The transmission dynamics of sexually transmitted diseases: The behavior component. In: Wasserheit, H.; Aral, S.; Holmes, K.; et al.; eds. *Research Issues in Human Behavior and Sexually Transmitted Diseases in the AIDS Era*. Washington, DC: American Society for Microbiology, 1991, 38-60.

[42] May, R., and Anderson, R. Transmission dynamics of HIV infection. *Nature* 326:137-142, 1987.

[43] American Social Health Association. Teenagers know more than adults about STDs, but knowledge among both groups is low. *STD News* 3:1, 5, 1996.

[44] Kirby, D. Sexuality and HIV education programs in schools. In: Garrison, J.; Smith, M.; and Besharov, D.; eds. *Sexuality and American Social Policy: A Seminar Series. Sex Education in the Schools*. Menlo Park, CA: Henry J. Kaiser Family Foundation, 1994, 1-41.

[45] Flay, B. Mass media and smoking cessation: A critical review. *American Journal of Public Health* 77:153-160, 1987.

[46] CDC. Hepatitis B virus: A comprehensive strategy for eliminating transmission in the United States through universal childhood vaccination: Recommendations of the Immunization Practices Advisory Committee (ACIP). *Morbidity and Mortality Weekly Report* 40(RR-13):1-20, 1991.

[47] CDC. Under vaccination for hepatitis B among young men who have sex with men—San Francisco and Berkeley, California, 1992–1993. *Morbidity and Mortality Weekly Report* 45:215-217, 1996.

[48] Roper, W.L.; Peterson, H.B.; and Curran, J.W. Commentary: Condoms and HIV prevention—clarifying the message. *American Journal of Public Health* 83:501-503, 1993.

[49] Piccinino, L., and Mosher, W. Trends in contraceptive use in the United States: 1982–1995. *Family Planning Perspectives* 30(1):4-10, 46, 1998.

[50] Anderson, J.; Brackbill, R.; and Mosher, W. Condom use for disease prevention among unmarried U.S. women. *Family Planning Perspectives* 28:25-28, 39, 1996.

[51] CDC. HIV-risk behaviors of sterilized and nonsterilized women in drug-treatment programs—Philadelphia, 1989–1991. *Morbidity and Mortality Weekly Report* 41:149-152, 1992.

[52] CDC. Surgical sterilization among women and use of condoms—Baltimore, 1989–1990. *Morbidity and Mortality Weekly Report* 41:568-575, 1992.

[53] Cates, W., and Stone, K. Family planning, sexually transmitted diseases, and contraceptive choice: A literature update. *Family Planning Perspectives* 24:75-84, 1992.

[54] IOM. Brown, S., and Eisenberg, L., eds. *Best Intentions: Unintended Pregnancy and the Well-Being of Children and Families.* Washington, DC: National Academy Press, 1995.

[55] Rothenberg, R., and Potterat, J. Strategies for management of sex partners. In: Holmes, K.; Mardh, P.A.; Sparling, P.; et al.; eds. *Sexually Transmitted Diseases.* 2nd ed. New York, NY: McGraw-Hill, Inc., 1990, 1081-1086.

[56] CDC. Alternate case-finding methods in a crack-related syphilis epidemic—Philadelphia. *Morbidity and Mortality Weekly Report* 40:77-80, 1991.

[57] Engelgau, M.; Woernle, C.; Rolfs, R.; et al. Control of epidemic early syphilis: The results of an intervention campaign using social networks. *Sexually Transmitted Diseases* 22:203-209, 1995.

[58] U.S. Preventive Services Task Force. *Guide to Clinical Preventive Services.* 2nd ed. Washington, DC: HHS, 1996.

[59] Hillis, S.; Nakashima, A.; Amsterdam, L.; et al. The impact of a comprehensive chlamydia prevention program in Wisconsin. *Family Planning Perspectives* 27:108-111, 1995.

[60] Scholes, D.; Stergachis, A.; Heidrich, F.; et al. Prevention of pelvic inflammatory disease by screening for cervical chlamydial infection. *New England Journal of Medicine* 334:1362-1366, 1996.

[61] Britton, T.; DeLisle, S.; and Fine, D. STDs and family planning clinics: A regional program for chlamydia control that works. *American Journal of Gynecological Health* 6:80-87, 1992.

[62] Division of STD Prevention. *Sexually Transmitted Disease Surveillance 1997 Supplement—Chlamydia Prevalence Monitoring Project Annual Report.* Atlanta, GA: HHS, PHS,CDC, 1998.

[63] Kiviat, N.; Koutsky, L.; and Paavonen, J. Cervical neoplasia and other STD- related genital tract neoplasias. In: Holmes, K.; Mardh, P.; Sparling, P.; et al.; eds. *Sexually Transmitted Diseases.* 3rd ed. New York, NY: McGraw-Hill, 1999, 811-831.

[64] Jossens, M.O.; Schacter, J.; and Sweet, R.L. Risk factors associated with pelvic inflammatory disease of differing microbial etiologies. *Obstetrics and Gynecology* 83:989-997, 1984.

[65] Washington, A.E., and Katz, P. Cost and payment source for pelvic inflammatory disease. Trends and projections, 1983 through 2000. *Journal of the American Medical Association* 266:2565-2569, 1991.

[66] Rolfs, R.T.; Galaid, E.I.; and Zaidi, A.A. Pelvic inflammatory disease: Trends in hospitalizations and office visits, 1979 through 1988. *American Journal of Obstetrics and Gynecology* 166:983-990, 1992.

[67] NCHS. Advanced report of final mortality statistisics, 1992. *Monthly Vital Statistics Report* 43(Suppl. 6), 1994.

[68] CDC. 1998 guidelines for treatment of sexually transmitted diseases. *Morbidity and Mortality Weekly Report* 47(RR-1):1-118, 1998.

26
Substance Abuse

Co-Lead Agencies: National Institutes of Health
Substance Abuse and Mental Health Services
Administration

Contents

Goal

Reduce substance abuse to protect the health, safety, and quality of life for all, especially children.

Overview

Substance abuse and its related problems are among society's most pervasive health and social concerns. Each year, about 100,000 deaths in the United States are related to alcohol consumption.[1] Illicit drug abuse and related acquired immunodeficiency syndrome (AIDS) deaths account for at least another 12,000 deaths. In 1995, the economic cost of alcohol and drug abuse was $276 billion.[2] This represents more than $1,000 for every man, woman, and child in the United States to cover the costs of health care, motor vehicle crashes, crime, lost productivity, and other adverse outcomes of alcohol and drug abuse.

Issues and Trends

A substantial proportion of the population drinks alcohol. Forty-four percent of adults aged 18 years and older (more than 82 million persons) report having consumed 12 or more alcoholic drinks in the past year.[3] Among these current drinkers, 46 percent report having been intoxicated at least once in the past year—nearly 4 percent report having been intoxicated weekly. More than 55 percent of current drinkers report having consumed five or more drinks on a single day at least once in the past year—more than 12 percent did so at least once a week. Nearly 20 percent of current drinkers report having consumed an average of more than two drinks per day. Nearly 10 percent of current drinkers (about 8 million persons) meet diagnostic criteria for alcohol dependence. An additional 7 percent (more than 5.6 million persons) meet diagnostic criteria for alcohol abuse.[4]

Alcohol use and alcohol-related problems also are common among adolescents.[5] Age at onset of drinking strongly predicts development of alcohol dependence over the course of the lifespan. About 40 percent of those who start drinking at age 14 years or under develop alcohol dependence at some point in their lives; for those who start drinking at age 21 years or older, about 10 percent develop alcohol dependence at some point in their lives.[6] Persons with a family history of alcoholism have a higher prevalence of lifetime dependence than those without such a history.[7]

Excessive drinking has consequences for virtually every part of the body. The wide range of alcohol-induced disorders is due (among other factors) to differences in the amount, duration, and patterns of alcohol consumption, as well as differences in genetic vulnerability to particular alcohol-related consequences.[8]

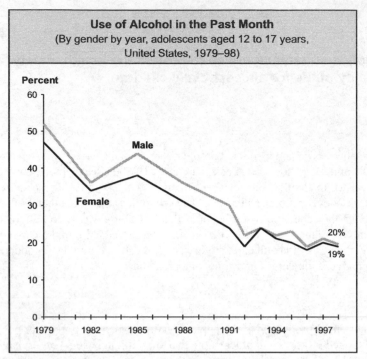

Use of Alcohol in the Past Month
(By gender by year, adolescents aged 12 to 17 years,
United States, 1979–98)

Percent

- Male
- Female

20%
19%

Source: SAMHSA, OAS. National Household Survey on Drug Abuse (NHSDA), preliminary data, June 1998.

Light-to-moderate drinking can have beneficial effects on the heart, particularly among those at greatest risk for heart attacks, such as men over age 45 years and women after menopause.[9] Moderate drinking generally refers to consuming one or two drinks per day. Moderate drinking, however, cannot be achieved by simply averaging the number of drinks. For example, consuming seven drinks on a single occasion will not have the same effects as consuming one drink each day of the week.

Long-term heavy drinking increases risk for high blood pressure, heart rhythm irregularities (arrhythmias), heart muscle disorders (cardiomyopathy), and stroke. Long-term heavy drinking also increases the risk of developing certain forms of cancer, especially of the esophagus, mouth, throat, and larynx.[10] Heavy alcohol use also increases risk for cirrhosis and other liver disorders[11] and worsens the outcome for patients with hepatitis C.[12] Drinking also may increase the risk for developing cancer of the colon and rectum.[10] Women's risk of developing breast cancer increases slightly if they drink two or more drinks per day.[13]

Alcohol use has been linked with a substantial proportion of injuries and deaths from motor vehicle crashes, falls, fires, and drownings.[11] It also is a factor in homicide, suicide, marital violence, and child abuse[14] and has been associated with high-risk sexual behavior.[11, 15, 16] Persons who drink even relatively small amounts of alcoholic beverages may contribute to alcohol-related death and injury in occupational incidents or if they drink before operating a vehicle.[11] In 1998, alcohol use was associated with 38 percent of all motor vehicle crash fatalities, a significantly lower percentage than in the 1980s.[17]

Although there has been a long-term drop in overall use, many people in the United States still use illicit drugs. In 1998, there were 13.6 million current users of any illicit drug in the total household population aged 12 years and older, representing 6.2 percent of the total population.[18] Marijuana is the most commonly used illicit drug, and 60 percent of users abuse marijuana only.[18] Among persons aged 12 years and older, 35.8 percent have used an illegal drug in their lifetime. Of these, more than 90 percent used marijuana or hashish, and approximately 30 percent tried cocaine.[18] Relatively rare in 1996, methamphetamine use began spreading in 1997.[18, 19]

Estimated rates of chronic drug use also are significant. Of the estimated 4.4 million chronic drug users in the United States in 1995, 3.6 million were chronic cocaine users (primarily crack cocaine), and 810,000 were chronic heroin users.[20]

Drug dependence is a chronic, relapsing disorder. Addicted persons frequently engage in self-destructive and criminal behavior. Research has confirmed that treatment can help end dependence on addictive drugs and reduce the consequences of addictive drug use on society. While no single approach for substance abuse and addiction treatment exists, comprehensive and carefully tailored treatment works.[21]

Drug use among adolescents aged 12 to 17 years doubled between 1992 and 1997, from 5.3 percent to 11.4 percent.[18] Youth marijuana use has been associated with a number of dangerous behaviors. Nearly 1 million youth aged 16 to 18 years (11 percent of the total) have reported driving in the past year at least once within 2 hours of using an illegal drug (most often marijuana).[22] Adolescents aged 12 to 17 years who smoke marijuana were more than twice as likely to cut class, steal, attack persons, and destroy property than those who did not smoke marijuana.[23] Drug and alcohol use by youth also is associated with other forms of unhealthy and unproductive behavior, including delinquency and high-risk sexual activity.

Illegal use of drugs, such as heroin, marijuana, cocaine, and methamphetamine, is associated with other serious consequences, including injury, illness, disability, and death as well as crime, domestic violence, and lost workplace productivity. Drug users and persons with whom they have sexual contact run high risks of contracting gonorrhea, syphilis, hepatitis, tuberculosis, and human immunodeficiency virus (HIV). The relationship between injection drug use and HIV/AIDS transmission is well known. Injection drug use also is associated with hepatitis B and C infections.[24] The use of cocaine, nitrates, and other substances can produce cardiac irregularities and heart failure, convulsions, and seizures. Cocaine use temporarily narrows blood vessels in the brain, contributing to the risk of strokes (bleeding within the brain) and cognitive and memory deficits.[25] Long-term consequences, such as chronic depression, sexual dysfunction, and psychosis, may result from drug use.

Substance abuse, including tobacco use and nicotine dependence, is associated with a variety of other serious health and social problems. An analysis of the epidemiologic evidence reveals that 72 conditions requiring hospitalization are wholly or partially attributable to substance abuse.[26]

Substance abuse contributes to cancers that, until recently, were thought to be unrelated. Advances in research techniques since the 1980s, including advanced brain imaging and the study of the effects of alcohol and drug abuse on individual cells, have helped to document the alteration of healthy systems by all forms of substance abuse, including marijuana use. Researchers have identified lasting brain and nervous system damage from drugs, including changes in nerve cell structure associated with alcohol and drug dependence. Other research has focused on the long-term effects of alcohol and drug abuse on the immune system as well as the effects of prenatal alcohol and drug exposure on the behavior and development of children.

Research confirms that a substantial number of frequent users of cocaine, heroin, and illicit drugs other than marijuana have co-occurring chronic mental health disorders. Some of these persons can be identified by their behavior problems at the time of their entry into elementary school.[27] Such youth tend to use substances at a young age and exhibit sensation-seeking (or "novelty-seeking") behaviors. These youth benefit from more intensive preventive interventions, including family therapy and parent training programs.[28, 29]

The stigma attached to substance abuse increases the severity of the problem. The hiding of substance abuse, for example, can prevent persons from seeking and continuing treatment and from having a productive attitude toward treatment. Compounding the problem is the gap between the number of available treatment slots and the number of persons seeking treatment for illicit drug use or problem alcohol use.

Disparities

Substance abuse affects all racial, cultural, and economic groups. Alcohol is the most commonly used substance, regardless of race or ethnicity, and there are far more persons who smoke cigarettes than persons who use illicit drugs. Usage rates for an array of substances reveal that for adolescents aged 12 to 17 years:

- Whites and Hispanics are more likely than African Americans to use alcohol.
- Whites are more likely than African Americans and Hispanics to use tobacco.

■ Whites and Hispanics are more likely than African Americans to use illicit drugs.

Additional findings include the following:

Substance Use in the Past Year, 1998						
	White, Not Hispanic		Hispanic		African American, Not Hispanic	
Substance	All Ages	Aged 12 to 17 Years	All Ages	Aged 12 to 17 Years	All Ages	Aged 12 to 17 Years
	Percent					
Alcohol	67.8	35.1	58.5	29.4	50.4	22.3
Cigarette	30.8	26.9	29.6	20.4	31.2	16.2
Any illicit drug	10.4	16.9	10.5	17.4	13.0	14.0
Marijuana	8.4	14.6	8.2	14.4	10.6	12.1
Cocaine	1.7	1.9	2.3	2.5	1.9	DSU
Inhalants	1.0	3.4	0.9	2.8	0.3	1.0
Heroin	0.1	DSU	0.1	DSU	0.2	DSU

DSU = Data are statistically unreliable.
Source: National Household Survey on Drug Abuse: Population Estimates 1998, SAMHSA.

Older adolescents and adults with co-occurring substance abuse and mental health disorders need explicit and appropriate treatment for their disorders. Those who suffer from co-occurring disorders, however, frequently are turned away from treatment designed for one or the other problem but not for both. (See Focus Area 18. Mental Health and Mental Disorders.)

The population aged 65 years and older faces risks for alcohol-related problems, although this group consumes comparatively low amounts of alcoholic beverages.[30] Adverse alcohol-drug interaction can put older people in the hospital, since many take multiple medications. In addition, many cases of memory deficits and dementia now are understood to result from alcoholism.[31]

Opportunities

The direct application of prevention and treatment research knowledge is particularly important in solving substance abuse problems. Developing adaptations of research-proven programs for diverse racial and ethnic populations, field testing them with high-quality process and outcome evaluations, and providing them where they are most needed are critical. Interventions appropriate to the population to be served, including interventions to address gaps in substance abuse treatment capacity, must be identified and implemented by Federal, Tribal, regional, State, and community-based providers in a variety of settings.

Scientific research has identified many opportunities to prevent alcohol-related problems. For example, studies indicate that school-based programs focused on altering perceived peer-group norms about alcohol use[32, 33] and developing skills in resisting peer pressures to drink[34, 35, 36] reduce alcohol use among participating students. Communitywide programs involving school curricula, peer leadership, parental involvement and education, and community task forces also have reduced alcohol use among adolescents.[37]

Raising the minimum legal drinking age to 21 years was accompanied by reduced alcohol consumption, traffic crashes, and related fatalities among young persons under age 21 years.[38] Reductions in alcohol-related traffic crashes are associated with many policy and program measures[39]—among them, administrative revocation of licenses for drinking and driving[40] and lower legal blood alcohol limits for youth[41] and adults.[42] Community programs involving multiple city departments and private citizens have reduced driving after drinking and traffic deaths and injuries.[43] In addition, a combination of community mobilization, media advocacy, and enhanced law enforcement has been shown to reduce alcohol-related traffic crashes and sales of alcohol to minors.[44]

Higher prices or taxes for alcoholic beverages are associated with lower alcohol consumption and lower levels of a wide variety of adverse outcomes—including the probability of frequent beer consumption by young persons,[45] the probability of adults drinking five or more drinks on a single occasion,[46] death rates from cirrhosis[47] and motor vehicle crashes,[48, 49] frequency of drinking and driving,[50] and some categories of violent crime.[51] One study suggests that, among adults, the effect of alcoholic beverage prices on frequency of heavy drinking varies with knowledge of the health consequences of heavy drinking: better informed heavy drinkers are more responsive to price changes.[52]

In college settings, brief one-on-one motivational counseling has proved effective in reducing alcohol-related problems among high-risk drinkers.[53] Research on the effect of the density of alcohol outlets on violence is inconclusive.[54, 55]

Many opportunities to prevent drug-related problems have been identified. Core strategies for preventing drug abuse among youth include raising awareness, educating and training parents and others, strengthening families, providing alternative activities, building skills and confidence, mobilizing and empowering communities, and employing environmental approaches. Studies indicate that making youth and others aware of the health, social, and legal consequences associated with drug abuse has an impact on use. Parents also play a primary role in helping their children understand the dangers of substance abuse and in communicating their expectation that drug and alcohol use will not be tolerated. Research suggests that improving parent/child attachment and supervision and monitoring also protect youth from substance abuse. Alternative activities for youth teach social skills and provide an alternative to substance abuse. According to one study, programs that help young persons develop psychosocial and peer resistance skills are more successful than other programs in preventing drug abuse.[21] Findings suggest that having community partnerships in place for sustained periods of time produces significant results in decreasing alcohol and drug use in males. Literature shows that having "buy-in" from local participants greatly enhances the success of any endeavor. Studies also show that changing norms is extremely effective in reducing substance abuse and related problems.[21]

For substance abuse prevention to be effective, people need access to culturally, linguistically, and age-appropriate services; job training and employment; parenting training; general education; more behavioral research; and programs for women, dually diagnosed patients, and persons with learning disabilities. Particular attention must be given to young persons under age 18 years who have an addicted parent because these youth are at increased risk for substance abuse. Because alcoholism and drug abuse continue to affect lesbians, gay men, and transgendered persons at two to three times the rate of the general population,[56] programs that address the special risks and requirements of these population groups also are needed. Government, employers, the faith community, and other organizations in the private and nonprofit sectors must increase their level of cooperation and coordination to ensure that multiple service needs are met.

The prevention and treatment of substance abuse require that all abused substances be addressed—from tobacco and alcohol to marijuana and other illicit drugs. Tobacco prevention and treatment are equally important parts of a comprehensive substance abuse prevention program. (See Focus Area 27. Tobacco Use.)

Interim Progress Toward Year 2000 Objectives

Of the 20 substance abuse objectives in Healthy People 2000, 2 have met or surpassed their targets. More than 90 percent of worksites with 50 or more employees have adopted policies on alcohol and drugs (1995), exceeding the Healthy People 2000 target of 60 percent. One additional target has been met—monitoring access to treatment programs by underserved persons (1996).

Progress has been made toward other objectives. Alcohol-related motor vehicle crash deaths declined to 6.5 per 100,000 population (1996), attributed in part to passage of State laws mandating administrative license revocation (ALR), setting maximum blood alcohol concentration (BAC) levels of 0.08 percent for drivers aged 21 years and older, and establishing zero tolerance for alcohol in the blood of drivers under age 21 years. The cirrhosis death rate declined to 7.4 per 100,000 population (1995), although the rate for American Indians or Alaska Natives remains significantly higher than that of other groups. Average age of first use of harmful substances by adolescents aged 12 to 17 years has increased. In addition, past-month use of alcohol by adolescents aged 12 to 17 years has declined, as has steroid use by high school seniors.

Less progress has been made toward other targets. Past-month use of marijuana and cigarettes among adolescents aged 12 to 17 years has increased since 1994.

Among high school seniors, both perception of harm and perception of social disapproval of substance abuse have declined. For the total population, rates of drug-related deaths and drug-abuse-related emergency department (ED) visits have increased.

Note: Unless otherwise noted, data are from the Centers for Disease Control and Prevention, National Center for Health Statistics, *Healthy People 2000 Review, 1998–99.*

Substance Abuse

Goal: Reduce substance abuse to protect the health, safety, and quality of life for all, especially children.

Number Objective Short Title

Adverse Consequences of Substance Use and Abuse

26-1   Motor vehicle crash deaths and injuries

26-2   Cirrhosis deaths

26-3   Drug-induced deaths

26-4   Drug-related hospital emergency department visits

26-5   Alcohol-related hospital emergency department visits

26-6   Adolescents riding with a driver who has been drinking

26-7   Alcohol- and drug-related violence

26-8   Lost productivity

Substance Use and Abuse

26-9   Substance-free youth

26-10   Adolescent and adult use of illicit substances

26-11   Binge drinking

26-12   Average annual alcohol consumption

26-13   Low-risk drinking among adults

26-14   Steroid use among adolescents

26-15   Inhalant use among adolescents

Risk of Substance Use and Abuse

26-16   Peer disapproval of substance abuse

26-17   Perception of risk associated with substance abuse

Treatment for Substance Abuse

26-18   Treatment gap for illicit drugs

26-19   Treatment in correctional institutions

26-20   Treatment for injection drug use

26-21   Treatment gap for problem alcohol use

State and Local Efforts

Adverse Consequences of Substance Use and Abuse

26-1. Reduce deaths and injuries caused by alcohol- and drug-related motor vehicle crashes.

Target and baseline:

Objective	Reduction in Consequences of Motor Vehicle Crashes	1998 Baseline	2010 Target
		Per 100,000 Population	
26-1a.	Alcohol-related deaths	5.9	4
26-1b.	Alcohol-related injuries	113	65
26-1c.	Drug-related deaths	Developmental	
26-1d.	Drug-related injuries	Developmental	

Target setting method: Consistent with the U.S. Department of Transportation for 26-1a; 42 percent improvement for 26-1b.

Data sources: Fatality Analysis Reporting System (FARS), DOT, NHTSA; General Estimates System (GES), DOT.

NOTE: THE TABLE BELOW MAY CONTINUE TO THE FOLLOWING PAGE.

Total Population, 1998 (unless noted)	Alcohol-Related Motor Vehicle Crashes	
	26-1a. Deaths	26-1b. Injuries
	Rate per 100,000	
TOTAL	5.9	113
Race and ethnicity		
American Indian or Alaska Native	19.2 (1995)	DNC
Asian or Pacific Islander	2.4 (1995)	DNC
Asian	DNC	DNC
Native Hawaiian and other Pacific Islander	DNC	DNC
Black or African American	6.4 (1995)	DNC
White	6.0 (1995)	DNC

Total Population, 1998 (unless noted)	Alcohol-Related Motor Vehicle Crashes	
	26-1a. Deaths	26-1b. Injuries
	Rate per 100,000	
Hispanic or Latino	DNA	DNC
Not Hispanic or Latino	DNA	DNC
Black or African American	DNA	DNC
White	DNA	DNC
Gender		
Female	2.3	DNA
Male	9.2	DNA
Education level		
Less than high school	DNC	DNC
High school graduate	DNC	DNC
At least some college	DNC	DNC
Select populations		
Age group		
Persons aged 15 to 24 years	13.5	DNA

DNA = Data have not been analyzed. DNC = Data are not collected. DSU = Data are statistically unreliable.
NOTE: THE TABLE ABOVE MAY HAVE CONTINUED FROM THE PREVIOUS PAGE.

Progress has been achieved in reducing the rate of alcohol-related driving fatalities, which declined from 9.8 deaths per 100,000 population in 1987 to 5.9 deaths per 100,000 in 1998. However, fatal injuries caused by motor vehicle crashes in which either a driver or nonoccupant (that is, pedestrian or bicyclist) was under the influence of alcohol or drugs remain a serious problem in the United States.

Of particular concern is the fatality rate among Native Americans and persons aged 15 to 24 years. In 1994, the alcohol involvement rate in fatal traffic crashes for American Indian or Alaska Native men was four times higher (28 per 100,000 population) than for the general population. For persons aged 15 to 24 years, the rate was 11.7 per 100,000 population in 1997. Based on these rates, about 3 in every 10 persons in the United States will be involved in an alcohol-related crash sometime in their lives. The alcohol-related traffic fatality rate for youth, however, has decreased by more than 50 percent since 1982, from 22 deaths per 100,000 population to 10 deaths per 100,000 population in 1996.[57] The National Highway Traffic Safety Administration estimates that since 1975, over 18,220 lives have been saved by enforcement of minimum drinking age laws.[57]

The number of children who are victims of alcohol- and drug-related traffic crashes also is significant. In 1998, of traffic crashes in which 2,990 children under age 16 years were killed, nearly 21 percent were alcohol related.[58]

Crash-related injuries also are a serious problem. In 1998, crash-related injuries totaled 3,192,000, compared to 41,471 crash-related deaths.[58] A reduction in all injuries resulting from alcohol- and drug-related driving is needed. Such injuries significantly contribute to emergency department use and overall health care costs and cause personal tragedies for families.

Although alcohol and its relationship to motor vehicle crashes has been studied more extensively than other substances, tracking drug-related fatalities and injuries is needed. This extension will promote the understanding that driving while under the influence of drugs is a serious problem and will help reduce drug-related fatalities.

Reductions in motor vehicle crashes are the result, in part, of many policy and program measures—among them, raising the minimum legal drinking age to 21 years,[59] administrative revocation of licenses for drinking and driving,[60] lower legal blood alcohol limits for youth[41] and adults,[42] and higher prices through increased taxation of alcoholic beverages.[48, 49] Higher prices for alcoholic beverages also are associated with reduced frequency of drinking and driving.[50] In addition, community programs involving multiple city departments and private citizens have reduced both driving after drinking and traffic deaths and injuries.[43]

26-2. Reduce cirrhosis deaths.

Target: 3.0 deaths per 100,000 population.

Baseline: 9.5 cirrhosis deaths per 100,000 population occurred in 1998 (age adjusted to the year 2000 standard population).

Target setting method: Better than the best.

Data source: National Vital Statistics System (NVSS), CDC, NCHS.

NOTE: THE TABLE BELOW MAY CONTINUE TO THE FOLLOWING PAGE.

Total Population, 1998	Cirrhosis Deaths
	Rate per 100,000
TOTAL	9.5
Race and ethnicity	
American Indian or Alaska Native	25.9
Asian or Pacific Islander	3.5
Asian	DNC
Native Hawaiian and other Pacific Islander	DNC
Black or African American	9.9
White	9.4

Total Population, 1998	Cirrhosis Deaths
	Rate per 100,000
Hispanic or Latino	15.4
Not Hispanic or Latino	9.0
Black or African American	10.2
White	8.8
Gender	
Female	6.0
Male	13.4
Education level (aged 25 to 64 years)	
Less than high school	19.9
High school graduate	14.2
At least some college	5.7

DNA = Data have not been analyzed. DNC = Data are not collected. DSU = Data are statistically unreliable.
Note: Age adjusted to the year 2000 standard population.

NOTE: THE TABLE ABOVE MAY HAVE CONTINUED FROM THE PREVIOUS PAGE.

Sustained heavy alcohol consumption is the leading cause of cirrhosis, 1 of the 10 leading causes of death in the United States.[61, 62, 63, 64, 65] Cirrhosis occurs when healthy liver tissue is replaced with scarred tissue until the liver is unable to function effectively. Changes in alcohol consumption patterns over time are associated with changes in the death rate from cirrhosis. Improvements in disease management and in the availability of treatment for alcoholism, however, also may have contributed to a decline in cirrhosis deaths since 1973. In addition, higher State excise tax rates on distilled spirits are associated with lower death rates from cirrhosis.[47]

26-3. Reduce drug-induced deaths.

Target: 1.0 death per 100,000 population.

Baseline: 6.3 drug-induced deaths per 100,000 population occurred in 1998 (age adjusted to the year 2000 standard population).

Target setting method: Better than the best.

Data source: National Vital Statistics System (NVSS), CDC, NCHS.

Total Population, 1998	Drug-Induced Deaths
	Rate per 100,000
TOTAL	6.3
Race and ethnicity	
American Indian or Alaska Native	7.0
Asian or Pacific Islander	1.2
Asian	DNC
Native Hawaiian and other Pacific Islander	DNC
Black or African American	8.8
White	6.1
Hispanic or Latino	6.2
Not Hispanic or Latino	6.2
Black or African American	9.1
White	6.0
Gender	
Female	3.9
Male	8.6
Education level (aged 25 to 64 years)	
Less than high school	19.1
High school graduate	14.6
At least some college	5.3

DNA = Data have not been analyzed. DNC = Data are not collected. DSU = Data are statistically unreliable.
Note: Age adjusted to the year 2000 standard population.

Causes of drug-induced deaths include drug psychosis, drug dependence, suicide, and intentional and accidental poisoning that result from illicit drug use. Declining initiation, number of cases, and intensity of drug abuse should be reflected in fewer drug-induced deaths. However, the prevention of suicide, accidental poisoning, and fatal interaction among medications contributes to changes in the statistics measured in this objective.

26-4. Reduce drug-related hospital emergency department visits.

Target: 350,000 visits per year.

Baseline: 542,544 hospital emergency department visits were drug-related in 1998.

Target setting method: 35 percent improvement.

Data source: Drug Abuse Warning Network (DAWN), SAMHSA.

Data for population groups currently are not collected.

Drug-related hospital emergency department (ED) visits are another major indicator of the harmful effects of drugs. In hospital EDs, a "drug-related episode" is defined as one resulting from the nonmedical use of a drug. This includes the unprescribed use of prescription drugs, use of drugs contrary to approved labeling, and use of illicit drugs. Episodes are abstracted from medical records by hospital staff or hired clerks. To be counted as having a drug-related episode, the ED patient must be aged 6 years or older and meet four criteria: the patient was treated in the hospital's ED; the presenting problem was induced by or related to drug use; the case involved the nonmedical use of a legal drug or any use of an illegal drug; and the patient's reason for taking the substance(s) included dependence, suicide attempt or gesture, or psychic effects.

"Suicide attempt or gesture" and dependence were the most frequently cited motives for taking a substance that resulted in an ED episode, with each accounting for 35 percent of all episodes in 1998. In 1998, 55 percent of the drug-related ED episodes occurred among adolescents and adults aged 16 to 34 years and 44 percent among persons aged 35 years and older. Whites accounted for 54 percent of drug-related ED episodes. African Americans and Hispanics accounted for 25 percent and 11 percent, respectively.[66]

26-5. (Developmental) Reduce alcohol-related hospital emergency department visits.

Potential data source: National Hospital Ambulatory Medical Care Survey (NHAMCS), CDC, NCHS.

Alcohol consumption is associated with a wide range of events that can result in ED visits—among them, motor vehicle crashes, violence, and alcohol poisoning. In 1996, alcohol-related hospital ED visits (2.2 million) accounted for 2.4 percent of all ED visits.[67] Visits related to both alcohol and drugs accounted for an additional 0.4 percent. However, these figures, based on a national probability survey of hospital EDs, are probably underestimates because information on alcohol involvement often is missing from ED medical records.[67]

An analysis of 1995 data from the same survey found that alcohol-related visits are 1.6 times as likely as other ED visits to be injury related; in 20 percent of alcohol-related visits, the principal diagnosis is alcohol abuse or alcohol dependence.[68] Other studies, based on smaller samples and different measures of alcohol involvement, suggest a large proportion of young persons and trauma victims are intoxicated when they visit the ED.[69, 70, 71]

Screening for alcohol problems in the ED offers an opportunity for early intervention and appropriate referral of patients and may reduce subsequent illness, injury, and death.[72] Policy measures that reduce specific alcohol-related problems[11]—for example, motor vehicle crashes or violence—also may help reduce alcohol-related ED visits.

26-6. Reduce the proportion of adolescents who report that they rode, during the previous 30 days, with a driver who had been drinking alcohol.

Target: 30 percent.

Baseline: 33 percent of students in grades 9 through 12 reported riding during the previous 30 days with a driver who had been drinking alcohol in 1999.

Target setting method: Better than the best.

Data source: Youth Risk Behavior Surveillance System (YRBSS), CDC, NCCDPHP.

NOTE: THE TABLE BELOW MAY CONTINUE TO THE FOLLOWING PAGE.

Students in Grades 9 Through 12, 1999	Rode With Drinking Driver During Previous 30 Days
	Percent
TOTAL	33
Race and ethnicity	
American Indian or Alaska Native	DSU
Asian or Pacific Islander	DSU
Asian	DSU
Native Hawaiian and other Pacific Islander	DSU
Black or African American	34
White	33
Hispanic or Latino	40
Not Hispanic or Latino	32
Black or African American	34
White	32

Students in Grades 9 Through 12, 1999	Rode With Drinking Driver During Previous 30 Days
	Percent
Gender	
Female	32
Male	34
Family income level	
Poor	DNC
Near poor	DNC
Middle/high income	DNC

DNA = Data have not been analyzed. DNC = Data are not collected. DSU = Data are statistically unreliable.
NOTE: THE TABLE ABOVE MAY HAVE CONTINUED FROM THE PREVIOUS PAGE.

Health risk behaviors that contribute to the leading causes of illness, death, and social problems among youth and adults often are established during youth, extend into adulthood, and are interrelated. In the United States, 72 percent of all deaths among school-aged youth and young adults result from four causes: motor vehicle crashes, other unintentional injuries, homicide, and suicide. Many high school students practice behaviors that may increase their likelihood of death from these four causes. Hispanic students are more likely than African American or white students to ride with a driver who has been drinking.

Rates of adolescents riding with a driver who had been drinking alcohol across State surveys ranged from 19.7 percent to 48 percent (median: 34.1 percent). Across the local surveys, the rates ranged from 18.1 percent to 39.1 percent (median: 31.4 percent).[73] Reducing the number of adolescents who ride in a motor vehicle with another adolescent driver who has been drinking is an important step to decrease motor-vehicle related deaths and injuries.

26-7. (Developmental) Reduce intentional injuries resulting from alcohol- and illicit drug-related violence.

Potential data source: National Crime Victimization Survey (NCVS), U.S. Department of Justice, Bureau of Justice Statistics.

A review of the literature found that the percentage of homicide offenders who were drinking when they committed the offense ranged from 7 percent to 85 percent, with most studies finding the figure greater than 60 percent.[74] Drugs, and most commonly alcohol, also are a factor in a significant number of firearm-related deaths.[75] In 1996, juvenile and adult arrestees testing positive for drugs had been arrested frequently for violent offenses, such as robbery, assault, and weapons offenses. Two-thirds of victims who experienced violence by an intimate (a current or former spouse, boyfriend, or girlfriend) reported that alcohol had been involved. Among spousal victims, three out of four incidents involved an offender who was drinking. Thirty-one percent of strangers who were victimized believed that the offender was using alcohol.[76] Efforts are under way to establish targeted prevention and treatment programs aimed at reducing violence related to or caused by alcohol and drug use.[77, 78] Efforts are under way to develop surveillance systems aimed at reinforcing local community activities.[79]

26-8. (Developmental) Reduce the cost of lost productivity in the workplace due to alcohol and drug use.

Potential data source: Periodic estimates of economic costs of alcohol and drug use, NIH, NIAAA and NIDA.

The economic cost of alcohol and drug abuse in the United States was estimated at $276 billion for 1995,[2] with about $167 billion attributed to alcohol abuse and $110 billion to drug abuse. Productivity losses accounted for $119 billion of the costs of alcohol abuse and $77 billion of the costs of drug abuse.

The majority of alcohol-related productivity losses (62 percent) were attributed to alcohol-related illness. These costs, measured as impaired earnings among those with a history of alcohol dependence, may result from increased unemployment, poor job performance, and limited career advancement. The adverse effects of early alcohol use on educational attainment may underlie these effects. Productivity losses were greatest for males who started drinking before age 15 years.

For drug abuse, most (56 percent) of the estimated productivity losses were associated with crime, including lost earnings of victims (3 percent) and incarcerated perpetrators (26 percent) of drug-related crime and foregone legitimate earnings because of participation in the drug trade (28 percent). Studies from offender populations have found early onset of drinking and drug use and high dropout rates; these findings may reflect causal linkages.[2]

As indicators of the adverse consequences of alcohol and drug misuse, estimates of lost productivity have important limitations, including concerns about statistical and methodological issues and data quality and completeness. For example, productivity losses cannot be observed directly, implying some inherent imprecision in these estimates, so that changes in productivity losses may not be detected. Also, there is persistent uncertainty in quantifying the causal roles of alcohol and drugs in generating productivity losses. Finally, some likely effects on productivity are omitted from current estimates, mainly because suitable data are lacking. These measurement concerns notwithstanding, efforts to reduce or delay alcohol and drug use may lead to significant reductions in productivity losses over the long run.

26-9. Increase the age and proportion of adolescents who remain alcohol and drug free.

Target and baseline:

Objective	Increase in Average Age of First Use in Adolescents Aged 12 to 17 Years	1998 Baseline	2010 Target
		Average Age in Years	
26-9a.	Alcohol	13.1	16.1
26-9b.	Marijuana	13.7	17.4

Target setting method: Better than the best for alcohol use; consistent with Office of National Drug Control Policy for marijuana use.

Data source: National Household Survey on Drug Abuse (NHSDA), SAMHSA.

NOTE: THE TABLE BELOW MAY CONTINUE TO THE FOLLOWING PAGE.

Adolescents Aged 12 to 17 Years, 1998	26-9a. First Alcohol Use	26-9b. First Marijuana Use
	Average Age in Years	
TOTAL	13.1	13.7
Race and ethnicity		
American Indian or Alaska Native	13.0	12.8
Asian or Pacific Islander	13.3	13.7
Asian	DNC	DNC
Native Hawaiian and other Pacific Islander	DNC	DNC
Black or African American	13.1	13.8
White	13.1	13.7
Hispanic or Latino	13.2	13.5
Not Hispanic or Latino	13.1	13.8
Black or African American	13.1	13.8
White	13.1	13.8
Gender		
Female	13.2	13.7
Male	13.0	13.7

Adolescents Aged 12 to 17 Years, 1998	26-9a. First Alcohol Use	26-9b. First Marijuana Use
	Average Age in Years	
Family income level		
Poor	12.6	13.5
Near poor	12.6	13.3
Middle/high income	13.2	13.8
Sexual orientation	DNC	DNC

DNA = Data have not been analyzed. DNC = Data are not collected. DSU = Data are statistically unreliable.

NOTE: THE TABLE ABOVE MAY HAVE CONTINUED FROM THE PREVIOUS PAGE.

Target and baseline:

Objective	Increase in High School Seniors Never Using Substances	1998 Baseline	2010 Target
		Percent	
26-9c.	Alcoholic beverages	19	29
26-9d.	Illicit drugs	46	56

Target setting method: Better than the best.

Data source: Monitoring the Future Study, NIH, NIDA.

NOTE: THE TABLE BELOW MAY CONTINUE TO THE FOLLOWING PAGE.

High School Seniors, 1998	26-9c. Never Used Alcoholic Beverages	26-9d. Never Used Any Illicit Drugs
	Percent	
TOTAL	19	46
Race and ethnicity		
American Indian or Alaska Native	DSU	DSU
Asian or Pacific Islander	DNC	DNC
Asian	DSU	DSU
Native Hawaiian and other Pacific Islander	DNC	DNC
Black or African American	28	55
White	16	44

High School Seniors, 1998	26-9c. Never Used Alcoholic Beverages	26-9d. Never Used Any Illicit Drugs
	Percent	
Hispanic or Latino	18	43
Not Hispanic or Latino	DNC	DNC
Black or African American	DNC	DNC
White	DNC	DNC
Gender		
Female	19	50
Male	18	43
Family income level		
Poor	DNC	DNC
Near poor	DNC	DNC
Middle/high income	DNC	DNC
Sexual orientation	DNC	DNC

DNA = Data have not been analyzed. DNC = Data are not collected. DSU = Data are statistically unreliable.

NOTE: THE TABLE ABOVE MAY HAVE CONTINUED FROM THE PREVIOUS PAGE.

An important goal of U.S. policy for the prevention of substance abuse among youth is to increase the percentage of young persons who reach adulthood without using tobacco, illicit drugs, or alcohol. (See Focus Area 27. Tobacco Use.) Strengthening the ability of children and teenagers to reject all such substances is an important and critical element in prevention activities because the required skills and attitudes can carry over into adulthood, long after family constraints and other influences have lost their effectiveness.[80]

From 1985 until 1995, the percentage of high school seniors who reported they had never used tobacco, drugs, or alcohol increased dramatically.[81] This increase clearly demonstrated the value of the national investment in prevention because it followed many years of virtually no change in the percentage of high school seniors who reported they had never used any substance.

To achieve overall prevention goals, local activities are important. Some of the best prevention approaches involve comprehensive, multistrategy prevention interventions. Comprehensive community-based programs include interventions that influence individual behavior and attitudes through education, for example, and interventions that change environments through controls on the availability of substances. Comprehensive programs must be applied universally to the general population and in a more intensive fashion to selected and indicated groups and persons known to be at high risk for serious drug problems or to targeted groups of persons already exhibiting early signs of drug use. Meeting the need to sustain universal preventive interventions, selective preventive interventions, and indicated preventive interventions requires coordination among schools, State and local governments, businesses, the faith community, civic groups, and other elements of the community.

26-10. Reduce past-month use of illicit substances.

26-10a. Increase the proportion of adolescents not using alcohol or any illicit drugs during the past 30 days.

Target: 89 percent.

Baseline: 79 percent of adolescents aged 12 to 17 years reported no alcohol or illicit drug use in the past 30 days in 1998.

Target setting method: Better than the best.

Data source: National Household Survey on Drug Abuse (NHSDA), SAMHSA.

NOTE: THE TABLE BELOW MAY CONTINUE TO THE FOLLOWING PAGE.

Adolescents Aged 12 to 17 Years, 1998	26-10a. No Alcohol or Illicit Drug Use in Past 30 Days	No Alcohol Use in Past 30 Days*	No Illicit Drug Use in Past 30 Days*
	Percent		
TOTAL	79	81	90
Race and ethnicity			
American Indian or Alaska Native	72	76	87
Asian or Pacific Islander	87	89	94
Asian	DNC	DNC	DNC
Native Hawaiian and other Pacific Islander	DNC	DNC	DNC
Black or African American	82	87	90
White	77	79	90
Hispanic or Latino	79	81	90
Not Hispanic or Latino	79	81	90
Black or African American	82	87	90
White	77	79	90
Gender			
Female	79	81	91
Male	78	81	90

Adolescents Aged 12 to 17 Years, 1998	26-10a. No Alcohol or Illicit Drug Use in Past 30 Days	No Alcohol Use in Past 30 Days*	No Illicit Drug Use in Past 30 Days*
	Percent		
Family income level			
Poor	75	79	84
Near poor	80	84	89
Middle/high income	79	81	91
Sexual orientation	DNC	DNC	DNC

DNA = Data have not been analyzed. DNC = Data are not collected. DSU = Data are statistically unreliable.
*Data for no alcohol use and no illicit drug use are displayed to further characterize the issue.

NOTE: THE TABLE ABOVE MAY HAVE CONTINUED FROM THE PREVIOUS PAGE.

26-10b. Reduce the proportion of adolescents reporting use of marijuana during the past 30 days.

Target: 0.7 percent.

Baseline: 8.3 percent of adolescents aged 12 to 17 years reported marijuana use in the past 30 days in 1998.

Target setting method: Better than the best (consistent with the Office of National Drug Control Policy).

Data source: National Household Survey on Drug Abuse (NHSDA), SAMHSA.

NOTE: THE TABLE BELOW MAY CONTINUE TO THE FOLLOWING PAGE.

Adolescents Aged 12 to 17 Years, 1998	26-10b. Use of Marijuana in Past 30 Days
	Percent
TOTAL	8.3
Race and ethnicity	
American Indian or Alaska Native	8.9
Asian or Pacific Islander	4.3
Asian	DNC
Native Hawaiian and other Pacific Islander	DNC
Black or African American	8.4
White	8.5

Adolescents Aged 12 to 17 Years, 1998	26-10b. Use of Marijuana in Past 30 Days
	Percent
Hispanic or Latino	7.6
Not Hispanic or Latino	8.4
Black or African American	8.3
White	8.7
Gender	
Female	7.9
Male	8.6
Family income level	
Poor	14.7
Near poor	8.5
Middle/high income	7.8
Sexual orientation	DNC

DNA = Data have not been analyzed. DNC = Data are not collected. DSU = Data are statistically unreliable.

NOTE: THE TABLE ABOVE MAY HAVE CONTINUED FROM THE PREVIOUS PAGE.

26-10c. Reduce the proportion of adults using any illicit drug during the past 30 days.

Target: 2.0 percent.

Baseline: 5.8 percent of adults aged 18 years and older used any illicit drug during the past 30 days in 1998.

Target setting method: Better than the best (consistent with Office of National Drug Control Policy).

Data source: National Household Survey on Drug Abuse (NHSDA), SAMHSA.

NOTE: THE TABLE BELOW MAY CONTINUE TO THE FOLLOWING PAGE.

Adults Aged 18 Years and Older, 1998	26-10c. Illicit Drug Use in Past 30 Days
	Percent
TOTAL	5.8
Race and ethnicity	
American Indian or Alaska Native	8.4
Asian or Pacific Islander	2.5
Asian	DNC
Native Hawaiian and other Pacific Islander	DNC

Adults Aged 18 Years and Older, 1998	26-10c. Illicit Drug Use in Past 30 Days
	Percent
Black or African American	8.2
White	5.6
Hispanic or Latino	5.5
Not Hispanic or Latino	5.8
Black or African American	8.0
White	5.7
Gender	
Female	4.0
Male	7.8
Education level	
Less than high school	6.6
High school graduate	6.2
At least some college	5.3
Sexual orientation	DNC

DNA = Data have not been analyzed. DNC = Data are not collected. DSU = Data are statistically unreliable.
NOTE: THE TABLE ABOVE MAY HAVE CONTINUED FROM THE PREVIOUS PAGE.

Past-month use of any illicit drug and marijuana was about the same in 1997 as in 1996 and most of the 1990s for adults aged 18 years and older.[82] However, young adults aged 18 to 25 years continued to be the age group with the highest rates of use. In 1998, past-month use of drugs decreased among adolescents aged 12 to 17 years. However, the 1998 rates of past month use of any illicit drug (9.9 percent) and marijuana (8.3 percent) were significantly higher than the 1997 rates of use by this age group (11.4 percent and 9.4 percent, respectively). Furthermore, past-month use of illicit drugs by youths was significantly higher in 1997 than at any time during the 4 years between 1991 and 1994. Past-month use of alcohol was about the same in 1998 as in 1997.[82]

The first goal of the 1999 National Drug Control Strategy is to "educate and enable America's youth to reject illegal drugs as well as alcohol and tobacco."[83] In response to this goal, specific targets for the reduction of drug use among adolescents aged 12 to 17 years have been established under the Youth Substance Abuse Prevention Initiative (YSAPI). These targets, which have a baseline of 1996 and goals for the year 2002 (7 years), are as follows:

■ Reverse the upward trend and reduce past-month use of marijuana among adolescents aged 12 to 17 years by 20 percent (1996 baseline: 7.1 percent; target: 5.7 percent in 2002).

■ Reduce past-month use of any illicit drugs among adolescents aged 12 to 17 years by 20 percent (1996 baseline: 9.0 percent; target: 7.2 percent in 2002).

■ Reduce past-month use of alcohol among adolescents aged 12 to 17 years by 10 percent (1996 baseline: 18.8 percent; target: 16.9 percent in 2002).

These targets were used as the basis for identifying Healthy People 2010 objectives.

Adopting a multicomponent approach to youth substance abuse prevention may increase the long-term effectiveness of prevention efforts. This approach includes focusing on mobilizing and leveraging resources, raising public awareness, and countering pro-use messages. Several strategies may be effective, such as increasing the involvement of parents and parent groups at the local level, increasing the number of adult volunteers involved in drug prevention at the local level, changing normative attitudes among youth from "everyone's using drugs" to "everyone has better things to do than drugs," and increasing the proportion of youth participating in positive skill-building activities.

26-11. Reduce the proportion of persons engaging in binge drinking of alcoholic beverages.

Target and baseline:

Objective	Reduction in Students Engaging in Binge Drinking During Past 2 Weeks	1998 Baseline	2010 Target
		Percent	
26-11a.	High school seniors	32	11
26-11b.	College students	39	20

Target setting method: Better than the best for 26-11a; 49 percent improvement for 26-11b. (Better than the best will be used when data are available.)

Data source: Monitoring the Future Study, NIH, NIDA.

High School Seniors and College Students, 1998	Engaged in Binge Drinking During Past 2 Weeks	
	26-11a. High School Seniors	26-11b. College Students
	Percent	
TOTAL	32	39
Race and ethnicity		
American Indian or Alaska Native	DSU	DSU
Asian or Pacific Islander	DNC	DNC
Asian	DSU	DSU
Native Hawaiian and other Pacific Islander	DNC	DNC
Black or African American	12	DNA
White	36	DNA
Hispanic or Latino	28	DNA
Not Hispanic or Latino	DNC	DNC
Black or African American	DNC	DNC
White	DNC	DNC
Gender		
Female	24	31
Male	39	52
Family income level		
Poor	DNC	DNC
Near poor	DNC	DNC
Middle/high income	DNC	DNC
Sexual orientation	DNC	DNC

DNA = Data have not been analyzed. DNC = Data are not collected. DSU = Data are statistically unreliable.

Target and baseline:

Objective	Reduction in Adults and Adolescents Engaging in Binge Drinking During Past Month	1998 Baseline	2010 Target
		Percent	
26-11c.	Adults aged 18 years and older	16.6	6.0
26-11d.	Adolescents aged 12 to 17 years	7.7	2.0

Target setting method: Better than the best.

Data source: National Household Survey on Drug Abuse (NHSDA), SAMHSA.

Select Age Groups, 1998	Engaged in Binge Drinking During Past Month	
	26-11c. Adults Aged 18 Years and Older	26-11d. Adolescents Aged 12 to 17 Years
	Percent	
TOTAL	16.6	7.7
Race and ethnicity		
American Indian or Alaska Native	DSU	11.1
Asian or Pacific Islander	10.1	2.4
Asian	DNC	DNC
Native Hawaiian and other Pacific Islander	DNC	DNC
Black or African American	13.3	3.2
White	17.2	6.8
Hispanic or Latino	17.2	6.3
Not Hispanic or Latino	16.5	7.9
Black or African American	12.7	2.9
White	17.3	9.3
Gender		
Female	8.8	6.6
Male	25.0	8.7
Family income level		
Poor	20.2	8.7
Near poor	14.5	5.3
Middle/high income	16.7	8.0
Sexual orientation	DNC	DNC

DNA = Data have not been analyzed. DNC = Data are not collected. DSU = Data are statistically unreliable.

Binge drinking is a national problem, especially among males and young adults. Nearly 15 percent of persons aged 12 years or older reported binge drinking in the past 30 days, with young adults aged 18 to 25 years more likely (27 percent) than all other age groups to have engaged in binge drinking. In all age groups, more males than females engaged in binge drinking: among adults, the ratio was two or three to one. Rates of binge drinking varied little by educational attainment. People with some college, however, were more likely than those with less than a high school education to binge drink.

The perceived acceptance of problematic drug-using behavior among family, peers, and society influences an adolescent's decision to use or avoid alcohol, tobacco, and drugs. The perception that alcohol use is socially acceptable correlates with the fact that more than 80 percent of youth in the United States consume alcohol before their 21st birthday, whereas the lack of social acceptance of other drugs correlates with comparatively lower rates of use. Similarly, widespread societal expectations that young persons will engage in binge drinking may encourage this highly dangerous form of alcohol consumption.[5]

Passage of higher minimum purchase ages for alcoholic beverages during the mid-1980s reduced but did not eliminate underaged drinking.[59] Many States are examining the use of additional restrictions and penalties for alcoholic beverage retailers to ensure compliance with the minimum purchase age.

To address the problem of binge drinking and reduce access to alcohol by underaged persons, several additional policies and strategies may be effective, including:

- Tougher State restrictions and penalties for alcoholic beverage retailers to ensure compliance with the minimum purchase age.

- Restrictions on the sale of alcoholic beverages at recreational facilities and entertainment events where minors are present.

- Improved enforcement of State laws prohibiting distribution of alcoholic beverages to anyone under age 21 years and more severe penalties to discourage distribution to underaged persons.

- Implementation of server training and standards for responsible hospitality.[84, 85] (Management and server training educates waitresses, waiters, bartenders, and supervisory staff on ways to avoid serving alcohol to minors and intoxicated persons.) States could require periodic server training or use the regulatory authority of alcohol distribution licensing to mandate a minimal level of training for individual servers.

- Institution of a requirement that college students reporting to student health services following a binge drinking incident receive an alcohol screening that would identify the likelihood of a health risk. An alcohol screening would provide student health services with the information needed to assess the student's drinking and refer the student to an appropriate intervention.

- Restrictions on marketing to underaged populations, including limiting advertisements and promotions. Although alcohol advertising has been found to have little or no effect on overall consumption,[86, 87] this strategy may reduce the demand that results in illicit purchase or binge consumption.

- Higher prices for alcoholic beverages. Higher prices are associated with reductions in the probability of frequent beer consumption by young persons[45] and in the probability of adults drinking five or more drinks on a single occasion.[46]

Binge drinking among women of childbearing age (defined as 18 to 44 years) also is a problem because of the risk for prenatal alcohol exposures. Approximately half of the pregnancies in the United States are unintended,[88] and most women do not know they are pregnant until after the sixth week of gestation.[89] Such prenatal alcohol exposures can result in fetal alcohol syndrome and other alcohol-related neurodevelopmental disorders.[90]

26-12. Reduce average annual alcohol consumption.

Target: 2 gallons.

Baseline: 2.18 gallons of ethanol per person aged 14 years and older were consumed in 1997.

Target setting method: 9 percent improvement.

Data source: Alcohol Epidemiologic Data System (AEDS), NIH, NIAAA.

Annual estimates of per capita consumption for persons aged 14 years and older provide a valuable means for monitoring trends in U.S. alcohol consumption. These estimates are based on population figures as they relate to information on beverage sales, tax receipt data, or both. The data come primarily from States, with some data provided by beverage industry sources.

An overall downward trend in per-person ethanol consumption, after a peak in 1981 of 2.76 gallons, masks substantial differences in consumption trends for different types of alcoholic beverages. Per-person consumption of beer, wine, and distilled spirits declined during the 1990s. The sharpest decline occurred for distilled spirits, down by more than 40 percent since its peak in the 1970s. The downward trend in alcohol consumption can be attributed to a variety of factors, including changing lifestyles and heightened awareness of the health and safety risks of excessive alcohol consumption.

Consumption of alcohol can be influenced by laws and regulations, particularly minimum drinking age laws[91] and those that affect the prices of alcoholic beverages. A substantial and growing body of economic research has established that consumption of beer, wine, and distilled spirits declines in response to increases in the prices or taxes associated with these beverages.[11] Most studies have found that demand for beer is less responsive to price changes than are demands for wine and distilled spirits. In addition, evidence suggests important differences in the price responsiveness of light, moderate, and heavy drinkers. The heaviest-drinking 5 percent of drinkers (who report about four or more standard drinks per day and consume 36 percent of all alcohol)[46] and heavy drinkers who are ill-informed about health problems associated with heavy drinking[52] may not respond significantly to price changes. These findings suggest the importance of using a range of effective prevention and treatment interventions.

26-13. Reduce the proportion of adults who exceed guidelines for low-risk drinking.

Target and baseline:

Objective	Reduction in Adults Exceeding Guidelines for Low-Risk Drinking	1992 Baseline	2010 Target
		Percent	
26-13a.	Females	72	50
26-13b.	Males	74	50

Target setting method: Better than the best.

Data source: National Longitudinal Alcohol Epidemiologic Survey, NIH, NIAAA.

Current Drinkers Aged 21 Years and Older, 1992	26-13a. Females Exceeding Guideline	26-13b. Males Exceeding Guideline
	Percent	
TOTAL	72	74
Race and ethnicity		
American Indian or Alaska Native	85	97
Asian or Pacific Islander	64	53
Asian	DNC	DNC
Native Hawaiian and other Pacific Islander	DNC	DNC
Black or African American	65	75
White	72	74
Hispanic or Latino	72	80
Not Hispanic or Latino	72	74
Black or African American	65	74
White	72	74
Education level		
Less than high school	72	75
High school graduate	73	78
At least some college	71	72

DNA = Data have not been analyzed. DNC = Data are not collected. DSU = Data are statistically unreliable.

Males may be at risk for alcohol-related problems if they drink more than 14 drinks per week or more than 4 drinks per occasion.[92] Females may be at risk if they drink more than seven drinks per week or more than three drinks per occasion.[92] (A drink is defined as 0.54 ounces of ethanol—about the amount of alcohol in 12 ounces of regular beer, 5 ounces of wine, or 1.5 ounces of 80-proof distilled spirits.) Most persons who exceed these guidelines do so by drinking more than the specified maximum number of drinks per occasion at least once a year. Drinking more than the per-occasion maximum impairs mental performance and physical coordination, increasing the risk of injury.

Guidelines for males and females differ in part because females metabolize alcohol less efficiently than males (so they are at greater risk for some health problems than males who drink the same amount). Females also have less body water than males, so they become more intoxicated than males after drinking the same amount of alcohol.[93] Both males and females have less body water as they age. Older persons can lower their risk of alcohol problems by drinking no more than one drink a day.[94]

Some persons should not drink any alcohol.[92, 95] They include:

- Children and adolescents.
- Females who are pregnant or considering pregnancy.
- Persons who are alcohol dependent.
- Persons with health problems (for example, ulcers) that may be made worse by drinking alcohol.
- Persons who are taking prescription or over-the-counter drugs that interact with alcohol.
- Persons who plan to drive or engage in other activities requiring attention or skill.

26-14. Reduce steroid use among adolescents.

Target and baseline:

Objective	Reduction in Steroid Use Among Adolescents in Past Year	1998 Baseline	2010 Target
		Percent	
26-14a.	8th graders	1.2	0.4
26-14b.	10th graders	1.2	0.4
26-14c.	12th graders	1.7	0.4

Target setting method: Better than the best.

Data source: Monitoring the Future Study, NIH, NIDA.

Adolescents, 1998	Steroid Use in Past Year		
	26-14a. 8th Graders	26-14b. 10th Graders	26-14c. 12th Graders
	Percent		
TOTAL	1.2	1.2	1.7
Race and ethnicity			
American Indian or Alaska Native	DSU	DSU	DSU
Asian or Pacific Islander	DNC	DNC	DNC
Asian	DSU	DSU	DSU
Native Hawaiian and other Pacific Islander	DNC	DNC	DNC
Black or African American	0.7	0.5	0.9
White	1.1	1.3	1.5
Hispanic or Latino	1.4	1.2	2.4
Not Hispanic or Latino	DNC	DNC	DNC
Black or African American	DNC	DNC	DNC
White	DNC	DNC	DNC
Gender			
Female	0.7	0.6	0.3
Male	1.6	1.9	2.8
Family income level			
Poor	DNC	DNC	DNC
Near poor	DNC	DNC	DNC
Middle/high income	DNC	DNC	DNC

DNA = Data have not been analyzed. DNC = Data are not collected. DSU = Data are statistically unreliable.

The self-administration by athletes of so-called performance-enhancing substances has led to risky injection practices. These substances include steroids and over-the-counter stimulant drugs and herbs, with steroids the most common. Nonmedical use of steroids poses serious problems since such use is illegal and dangerous. Behavior and health problems associated with steroid use include suicides, homicides, liver damage, and heart attacks.[96]

Many substance abuse researchers believe that attempts to enhance athletic performance with steroids and other substances reduce the perceived negative consequences of substance abuse and increase the likelihood of using illicit drugs for other purposes. In addition, limited access to needles and other equipment results in a high rate of needle-sharing among adolescent teammates who inject performance-enhancing substances. While steroid use by male athletes has attracted the most attention, information suggests that adolescent females are increasing their use of steroids.[96]

26-15. Reduce the proportion of adolescents who use inhalants.

Target: 0.7 percent.

Baseline: 2.9 percent of adolescents aged 12 to 17 years used inhalants in the past year in 1998.

Target setting method: Better than the best.

Data source: National Household Survey on Drug Abuse (NHSDA), SAMHSA.

NOTE: THE TABLE BELOW MAY CONTINUE TO THE FOLLOWING PAGE.

Adolescents Aged 12 to 17 Years, 1998	Inhalant Use in Past Year
	Percent
TOTAL	2.9
Race	
American Indian or Alaska Native	DSU
Asian or Pacific Islander	DSU
Asian	DNC
Native Hawaiian and other Pacific Islander	DNC
Black or African American	DNA
White	DNA
Hispanic or Latino	2.8
Not Hispanic or Latino	DNA
Black or African American	1.0
White	3.4
Gender	
Female	3.0
Male	2.8
Family income level	
Poor	DNA
Near poor	DNA
Middle/high income	DNA
Regions	
Northeast	2.3
North central	3.0
South	2.6
West	3.8

Adolescents Aged 12 to 17 Years, 1998	Inhalant Use in Past Year
	Percent
Sexual orientation	DNC

DNA = Data have not been analyzed. DNC = Data are not collected. DSU = Data are statistically unreliable.

NOTE: THE TABLE ABOVE MAY HAVE CONTINUED FROM THE PREVIOUS PAGE.

Approximately 12.6 million, or 5.8 percent, of the civilian household population aged 12 years and older in 1998 reported lifetime inhalant use. About 2.0 million persons (0.9 percent) used inhalants in the past year, and 713,000 persons (0.4 percent) used them in the past month. Among adolescents aged 12 to 17 years between 1997 and 1998, there was a significant decrease in the lifetime rate of inhaling amyl nitrate (from 0.8 percent in 1997 to 0.3 percent in 1998), spray paint (from 2.2 percent in 1997 to 1.4 percent in 1998), nitrous oxide (2.3 percent in 1997 to 1.5 percent in 1998), and other aerosol sprays from 1.9 percent in 1997 to 1.1 percent in 1998. Among adolescents, there were no significant differences between males and females in the use of inhalants.[18]

Overall, important age, racial and ethnic, and regional differences were found in the number of cases of inhalant use in 1998. Although the rate of current use of inhalants was similar among young adults (aged 18 to 25 years) and adolescents (aged 12 to 17 years), young adults had higher lifetime rates of inhalant use than did adolescents. Over all age groups, whites and Hispanics were more likely than African Americans to report lifetime and past-year inhalant use, and in most age groups, rates of inhalant use were higher among whites than among Hispanics. Respondents living in metropolitan areas were more likely to have used inhalants at least once in their lifetime than were those in nonmetropolitan areas. Residents of the Western region were more likely than those in other regions to have used inhalants in the past year.[18]

Risk of Substance Use and Abuse

26-16. Increase the proportion of adolescents who disapprove of substance abuse.

Target and baseline:

Objective	Increase in Adolescents Who Disapprove of Having One or Two Alcoholic Drinks Nearly Every Day	1998 Baseline	2010 Target
		Percent	
26-16a.	8th graders	77	83
26-16b.	10th graders	75	83
26-16c.	12th graders	69	83

Increase in Adolescents Who Disapprove of Trying Marijuana or Hashish Once or Twice	1998 Baseline	2010 Target
	Percent	
8th graders	69	72
10th graders	56	72
12th graders	52	72

ag method: Better than the best.

: Monitoring the Future Study, NIH, NIDA.

NOTE: THE TABLE BELOW MAY CONTINUE TO THE FOLLOWING PAGE.

ts, 1998	Disapprove of Trying Marijuana or Hashish		
	26-16d. 8th Graders	26-16e. 10th Graders	26-16f. 12th Graders
	Percent		
AL	69	56	52
thnicity			
rican Indian or Alaska e	DSU	DSU	DSU
or Pacific Islander	DNC	DNC	DNC
sian	DSU	DSU	DSU
ative Hawaiian and other acific Islander	DNC	DNC	DNC
k or African American	71	61	59
e	69	53	48
anic or Latino	64	59	61
Hispanic or Latino	DNC	DNC	DNC
ack or African American	DNC	DNC	DNC
hite	DNC	DNC	DNC
ale	71	57	55
	68	55	47
ome level			
	DNC	DNC	DNC
poor	DNC	DNC	DNC
le/high income	DNC	DNC	DNC

Target setting method: Better than the be

Data source: Monitoring the Future Study,

Adolescents, 1998	
TOTAL	
Race and ethnicity	
American Indian or Alaska Native	
Asian or Pacific Islander	
Asian	
Native Hawaiian and other Pacific Islander	
Black or African American	
White	
Hispanic or Latino	
Not Hispanic or Latino	
Black or African American	
White	
Gender	
Female	
Male	
Family income level	
Poor	
Near poor	
Middle/high income	
Sexual orientation	

DNA = Data have not been analyzed. DNC = Data are not

Target and

Objective

26-16d.
26-16e.
26-16f.

Target sett

Data sourc

Adolesce	
TOT	
Race and	
Ame Nat	
Asia	
A	
N F	
Bla	
Wh	
His	
Not	
Gender	
Fer	
Ma	
Family in	
Poc	
Ne	
Mic	

Adolescents, 1998	Disapprove of Trying Marijuana or Hashish		
	26-16d. 8th Graders	26-16e. 10th Graders	26-16f. 12th Graders
	Percent		
Sexual orientation	DNC	DNC	DNC

DNA = Data have not been analyzed. DNC = Data are not collected. DSU = Data are statistically unreliable.

NOTE: THE TABLE ABOVE MAY HAVE CONTINUED FROM THE PREVIOUS PAGE.

Disapproval of substance abuse is inversely related to adolescents' reports of use. For example, multiyear tracking of the results of the Monitoring the Future Study indicates that marijuana use among youth declines as the percentage of youth expressing disapproval of the drug increases. Similarly, an increase in marijuana use among youth during the early 1990s coincided with an apparent decline in the percentage of parents and peers expressing strong disapproval.

26-17. Increase the proportion of adolescents who perceive great risk associated with substance abuse.

Target and baseline:

Objective	Increase in Adolescents Aged 12 to 17 Years Perceiving Great Risk Associated With Substance Abuse	1998 Baseline	2010 Target
		Percent	
26-17a.	Consuming five or more alcoholic drinks at a single occasion once or twice a week	47	80
26-17b.	Smoking marijuana once per month	31	80
26-17c.	Using cocaine once per month	54	80

Target setting method: Better than the best (consistent with Office of National Drug Control Policy).

Data source: National Household Survey on Drug Abuse (NHSDA), SAMHSA.

NOTE: THE TABLE BELOW MAY CONTINUE TO THE FOLLOWING PAGE.

Adolescents Aged 12 to 17 Years, 1998	Perceived Risk From		
	26-17a. Alcohol	26-17b. Marijuana	26-17c. Cocaine
	Percent		
TOTAL	47	31	54
Race and ethnicity			
American Indian or Alaska Native	47	26	64

Adolescents Aged 12 to 17 Years, 1998	Perceived Risk From		
	26-17a. Alcohol	26-17b. Marijuana	26-17c. Cocaine
	Percent		
Asian or Pacific Islander	43	26	42
Asian	DNC	DNC	DNC
Native Hawaiian and other Pacific Islander	DNC	DNC	DNC
Black or African American	57	34	61
White	45	31	54
Hispanic or Latino	51	35	54
Not Hispanic or Latino	46	30	54
Black or African American	58	34	62
White	44	29	54
Gender			
Female	50	31	54
Male	44	31	55
Family income level			
Poor	43	29	56
Near poor	53	39	60
Middle/high income	46	30	53
Sexual orientation	DNC	DNC	DNC

DNA = Data have not been analyzed. DNC = Data are not collected. DSU = Data are statistically unreliable.

NOTE: THE TABLE ABOVE MAY HAVE CONTINUED FROM THE PREVIOUS PAGE.

The perception of risk in using illegal drugs is an important factor in decreasing drug use. As perception of harmfulness decreases, use tends to increase.[18] Therefore, youth need to be informed of the many risks, such as HIV infection, associated with use of alcohol, tobacco, and illegal drugs. (See Focus Area 27. Tobacco Use.) People who use or abuse drugs or alcohol sometimes reported being so high or intoxicated that they forgot to use a condom.[18] Therefore, informing youth about the connection between substance use and abuse and other problem behaviors, such as unsafe sex, dating violence, and suicide, is important.

The percentage of adolescents aged 12 to 17 years who perceive great risk associated with substance abuse is on the decline.[18] The percentage perceiving great risk in using marijuana once a month decreased from 40 percent (1990) to 30.8 percent in 1998. The percentage of youth perceiving great risk in using cocaine once a month decreased from 63 percent in 1994 to 54.3 percent in 1998. Perception of risk in having five or more drinks once or twice a week decreased from 58 percent in 1992 to 47 percent in 1998.[18]

The attitude of influential adults about alcohol and drugs is another critical predictor of attitudes in youth. Many adults who have regular contact with youth communicate ambivalent messages about alcohol and drug use.[97] In addition, more than 11 million children and adolescents under age 18 years have at least one parent who is addicted to alcohol or drugs.[98] As a result, the messages about harm and risk that they receive are sometimes impacted by family dynamics and denial. Risk and harm messages targeted to youth must therefore take this into account.

Treatment for Substance Abuse

26-18. (Developmental) Reduce the treatment gap for illicit drugs in the general population.

Potential data source: National Household Survey on Drug Abuse (NHSDA), SAMHSA.

The treatment gap is the difference between the number of persons who need treatment for the use of illicit drugs and the number of persons who are receiving treatment in a given year. Despite the widely acknowledged problem of drug abuse in the United States, accepted estimates of the number of persons who need treatment and the number who receive treatment are not available.[99, 100] It is estimated that 5.3 million persons are most in need of treatment.[77] National efforts are under way to estimate better the size of the gap, to develop strategies to expand capacity, and to eliminate barriers to access for those in need. These strategies involve seeking changes in financial barriers created by funding constraints and inadequate health and disability insurance coverage[101] and improvements in gender-specific and culturally appropriate treatment methods.[102]

Strategies address the specific and unique needs of select populations, including adolescents,[103] females, and elderly persons.[104]

26-19. (Developmental) Increase the proportion of inmates receiving substance abuse treatment in correctional institutions.

Potential data source: Uniform Facilities Data Set Survey of Correctional Facilities, OAS, SAMHSA.

Much attention has been focused on the link between substance abuse and criminality, in part because of the large increase in the number of individuals incarcerated for drug-related offenses, such as possession, trafficking, and crimes of violence. In general, criminal offenders frequently have high occurrences of a substance abuse history, may or may not have previously received treatment, and without treatment have a greater likelihood of committing a criminal offense.[105, 106, 107]

26-20. Increase the number of admissions to substance abuse treatment for injection drug use.

Target: 200,000 admissions.

Baseline: 167,960 admissions for injection drug use were reported in 1997.

Target setting method: 19 percent improvement.

Data source: Treatment Episodes Data System, OAS, SAMHSA.

The 167,960 admissions to treatment for injection drug use indicates a large unmet need for treatment in this group, because estimates of injection drug users in the Nation are as high as 810,000.[83] Better data are needed on this group's need for treatment. Because of the consequences associated with HIV/AIDS, injection drug users are a high priority population group needing substance abuse treatment. HIV infection among females and infants in the United States can be traced primarily to contaminated drug "works" and to sexual relations with infected drug users. Pediatric AIDS is a particularly virulent problem among the children of persons involved in drug-related lifestyles. To address these problems, substance abuse treatment must be provided for injection drug users. Such treatment will be most effective against HIV if it includes information, counseling, and other assistance on how to prevent HIV and unintended pregnancy.

26-21. (Developmental) Reduce the treatment gap for alcohol problems.

Potential data source: National Household Survey on Drug Abuse, SAMHSA.

Although alcohol problems are diverse and vary along many dimensions, they can be described in part by their duration (acute, intermittent, chronic) and severity (mild, moderate, substantial, severe).[108] As with illicit drugs, availability of resources and access to clinically appropriate and effective treatment for alcohol problems are limited.[11, 108] The size of the gap is not well defined. Wide variability exists among jurisdictions in total treatment capacity and in how that capacity is distributed among settings and modalities.[11, 108]

Increasing the availability of treatment for alcohol problems is critical because of the pervasive impact these problems have on all aspects of society.[109, 110] Alcohol problems have an effect on such important components of human capital as level of school attainment, work experience, health status, and family structure. Strategies to be employed here are similar to those needed to improve access to appropriate primary, rehabilitative, and long-term care through addressing the many barriers that exist at multiple levels.[111] Key patient-level barriers include lack of knowledge or skepticism about the effectiveness of treatment and lack of money or insurance coverage to pay for treatment. System-level barriers include lack of trained personnel, stigma, lack of health and disability insurance coverage, and inadequate reimbursement for clinically necessary services through public funding mechanisms such as the Substance Abuse Prevention and Treatment Services Block Grant and Medicaid.[112, 113]

26-22. (Developmental) Increase the proportion of persons who are referred for followup care for alcohol problems, drug problems, or suicide attempts after diagnosis or treatment for one of these conditions in a hospital emergency department.

Potential data source: National Hospital Ambulatory Medical Care Survey (NHAMCS), CDC, NCHS.

Alcohol problems, drug problems, and suicide attempts frequently cause ED visits, but these conditions may be overlooked during the visit or inadequately addressed when plans for followup are made. Some ED patients are treated for physical manifestations of alcohol problems, drug problems, or suicide attempts and released without appropriate evaluation, treatment, or referral for underlying behavioral risk factors that may cause a repeat ED visit.[114] These risk factors include hazardous patterns of alcohol consumption, use of illicit drugs, and predisposition to suicidal thoughts or actions. The effectiveness of ED interventions for these risk factors is determined by how well the affected patients are evaluated and treated in the ED and by the extent of communication and coordination with other settings and organizations in the community.[115] EDs are strategically well positioned to ensure appropriate referrals for followup care, but underlying behavioral risk factors must be identified and appropriate followup services must be available.

26-23. (Developmental) Increase the number of communities using partnerships or coalition models to conduct comprehensive substance abuse prevention efforts.

Potential data source: Community Partnerships Data, SAMHSA.

A comprehensive program of interventions at the community level is crucial to effective substance abuse prevention.[116, 117] Such programs enable communities to address issues related to their environments, not just their at-risk populations. Improving the environment means changing local ordinances and policies, coordinating local prevention services, increasing resident participation, communicating with the local media on how they portray local communities, and addressing numerous other conditions. Because of the diversity of communities, no single partnership model is expected to be the sole model used. However, desirable procedures and practices, such as how a community should get mobilized, now are being promoted.[117]

A recent 48-community study demonstrates that community partnerships showing statistically significant reductions in substance abuse shared a number of common characteristics. These include a communitywide vision that reflects the consensus of diverse groups and citizens throughout the community; a strong core of community partners; an inclusive, broad membership of organizations from all parts of the community; an ability to avoid or resolve conflict; decentralized groups that implement a large number of locally tailored prevention programs that effectively target local causes of drug use and empower residents to take action and make decisions; low staff turnover; and extensive prevention activities and support for improvements in local prevention policies.[118]

26-24. Extend administrative license revocation laws, or programs of equal effectiveness, for persons who drive under the influence of intoxicants.

Target: All States and the District of Columbia.

Baseline: 41 States and the District of Columbia had administrative license revocation laws for persons who drive under the influence of intoxicants in 1998.

Target setting method: Total coverage.

Data source: DOT, NHTSA.

Administrative license revocation (ALR) has proven to be a successful deterrent to driving while under the influence of intoxicants. ALR laws provide for administrative action separate from the judicial process that follows when a person is arrested for driving under the influence of alcohol or drugs. Colorado, Illinois, Maine, New Mexico, North Carolina, and Utah observed significant reductions in alcohol-related fatal crashes following the implementation of ALR laws. A 1991 study examined the costs and benefits of the procedure and found that reinstatement fees assessed to offenders more than covered the expenses of the program and that States also benefited from the cost savings of fewer nighttime crashes. Another study found that ALR reduced fatal crashes an average of 9 percent during late-night hours when drivers are most likely to have been drinking alcohol. As a result of an ALR publicity campaign, the rate of fatal crashes during late-night hours was further reduced.[119]

26-25. Extend legal requirements for maximum blood alcohol concentration levels of 0.08 percent for motor vehicle drivers aged 21 years and older.

Target: All States and the District of Columbia.

Baseline: 16 States had legal requirements for maximum blood alcohol concentration levels of 0.08 percent for motor vehicle drivers aged 21 years and older in 1998.

Target setting method: Total coverage.

Data source: DOT, NHTSA.

More than 80 percent of the drivers involved in fatal crashes had blood alcohol concentration (BAC) levels exceeding 0.08 percent. An average man weighing 170 pounds must consume in 1 hour more than four drinks on an empty stomach to reach a 0.08 BAC level.[120] Most States that have enacted 0.08 BAC legislation experienced significant decreases in alcohol-related fatal crashes. For example, a 12 percent reduction in alcohol-related fatalities occurred in California in 1990, the year 0.08 legislation and an ALR law went into effect.[120]

As of August 1998, 50 States and the District of Columbia had established BAC cutoff levels of 0.00, 0.01, or 0.02 to define driving under the influence for individuals under age 21 years. A zero tolerance law makes driving with any measurable amount of alcohol in the blood illegal for persons under age 21 years. Because young drivers place such a high value on their driver's licenses, the threat of license revocation has proved to be an effective sanction for this age group.[120]

Related Objectives From Other Focus Areas

1. **Access to Quality Health Services**
   1-1. Persons with health insurance
   1-2. Health insurance coverage for clinical preventive services
   1-3. Counseling about health behaviors
   1-4. Source of ongoing care
   1-5. Usual primary care provider
   1-6. Difficulties or delays in obtaining needed health care
   1-7. Core competencies in health provider training
   1-8. Racial and ethnic representation in the health professions
   1-10. Delay or difficulty in getting emergency care
   1-11. Rapid prehospital emergency care
   1-12. Single toll-free number for poison control centers
   1-13. Trauma care systems
   1-14. Special needs of children

3. **Cancer**
   3-10. Provider counseling about cancer prevention

6. **Disability and Secondary Conditions**
   6-2. Feelings and depression among children with disabilities

7. **Educational and Community-Based Programs**
   7-1. High school completion
   7-2. School health education
   7-3. Health-risk behavior information for college and university students
   7-4. School nurse-to-student ratio
   7-5. Worksite health promotion programs
   7-6. Participation in employer-sponsored health promotion activities
   7-7. Patient and family education
   7-8. Satisfaction with patient education

7-9. Health care organization sponsorship of community health promotion activities

7-10. Community health promotion programs

7-11. Culturally appropriate and linguistically competent community health promotion programs

7-12. Older adult participation in community health promotion activities

9. Family Planning

9-8. Abstinence before age 15 years

9-9. Abstinence among adolescents aged 15 to 17 years

9-10. Pregnancy prevention and sexually transmitted disease (STD) protection

9-11. Pregnancy prevention education

9-12. Problems in becoming pregnant and maintaining a pregnancy

13. HIV

13-3. AIDS among persons who inject drugs

13-4. AIDS among men who have sex with men and who inject drugs

13-8. HIV counseling and education for persons in substance abuse treatment

13-12. Screening for STDs and immunization for hepatitis B

13-13. Treatment according to guidelines

14. Immunization and Infectious Diseases

14-28. Hepatitis B vaccination among high-risk groups

15. Injury and Violence Prevention

15-12. Emergency department visits

15-13. Deaths from unintentional injuries

15-14. Nonfatal unintentional injuries

15-15. Deaths from motor vehicle crashes

15-16. Pedestrian deaths

15-17. Nonfatal motor vehicle injuries

15-18. Nonfatal pedestrian injuries

15-29. Drownings

15-32. Homicides

15-37. Physical assaults

16. Maternal, Infant, and Child Health

16-17. Prenatal substance exposure

16-18. Fetal alcohol syndrome

17. Medical Product Safety

17-3. Provider review of medications taken by patients

18. Mental Health and Mental Disorders

18-6. Primary care screening and assessment

18-10. Treatment for co-occurring disorders

18-13. State plans addressing cultural competence

23. Public Health Infrastructure

23-2. Public access to information and surveillance data

23-3. Use of geocoding in health data systems

23-4. Data for all population groups

23-5. Data for Leading Health Indicators, Health Status Indicators, and Priority Data Needs at Tribal, State, and local levels

23-6. National tracking of Healthy People 2010 objectives

23-7. Timely release of data on objectives

23-8. Competencies for public health workers

23-9. Training in essential public health services

23-10. Continuing education and training by public health agencies

23-11. Performance standards for essential public health services

23-12. Health improvement plans

23-14. Access to epidemiology services

23-15. Model statutes related to essential public health services

23-16. Data on public health expenditures

23-17. Population-based prevention research

25. **Sexually Transmitted Diseases**

25-11. Responsible adolescent sexual behavior

25-12. Responsible sexual behavior messages on television

25-13. Hepatitis B vaccine services in STD clinics

25-14. Screening in youth detention facilities and jails

27. **Tobacco Use**

27-1. Adult tobacco use

27-2. Adolescent tobacco use

27-3. Initiation of tobacco use

27-4. Age at first tobacco use

27-5. Smoking cessation by adults

27-6. Smoking cessation during pregnancy

27-7. Smoking cessation by adolescents

27-8. Insurance coverage of cessation treatment

27-9. Exposure to tobacco smoke at home among children

27-10. Exposure to environmental tobacco smoke

27-11. Smoke-free and tobacco-free schools

27-12. Worksite smoking policies

27-13. Smoke-free indoor air laws

27-14. Enforcement of illegal tobacco sales to minors laws

27-15. Retail license suspension for sales to minors

27-16. Tobacco advertising and promotion targeting adolescents and young adults

27-17. Adolescent disapproval of smoking

27-18. Tobacco control programs

27-19. Preemptive tobacco control laws

27-20. Tobacco product regulation

27-21. Tobacco tax

Terminology

(A listing of abbreviations and acronyms used in this publication appears in Appendix H.)

Administrative license revocation (ALR): Legal procedure that allows an arresting officer to confiscate immediately the driver's license of a driver who is found with a blood alcohol concentration (BAC) at or above the legally set limit or who refuses to take a BAC test. The officer usually issues a temporary driving permit valid for a short time, often 15 to 20 days, then notifies the offender of his or her right to an administrative hearing to appeal the revocation. If there is no appeal or if revocation is upheld, the offender loses his or her driver's license for a set period (90 days in most States for a first offense and longer for subsequent offenses).

Alcohol abuse: A maladaptive pattern of alcohol use that leads to clinically significant impairment or distress, as manifested by one or more of the following occurring within a 12-month period: recurrent alcohol use resulting in a failure to fulfill major role obligations at work, school, or home; recurrent alcohol use in physically hazardous situations; recurrent alcohol-related legal problems; continued alcohol use despite having persistent or recurrent social or interpersonal problems caused or exacerbated by the effects of alcohol. In the literature on economic costs, alcohol abuse means any cost-generating aspect of alcohol consumption; this definition differs from the clinical use of the term, which involves specific diagnostic outcomes.

Alcohol dependence: A maladaptive pattern of alcohol use that leads to clinically significant impairment or distress, as manifested by three or more of the following occurring at any time in the same 12-month period: tolerance; withdrawal; often taking alcohol in larger amounts or over a longer period than was intended; persistent desire or unsuccessful efforts to cut down or control alcohol use; spending a great deal of time in activities necessary to obtain alcohol or recover from its effects; giving up or reducing important social, occupational, or recreational activities because of alcohol use; continued alcohol use despite knowledge of having a persistent or recurrent physical or psychological problem that is likely to have been caused or exacerbated by alcohol.

Alcohol-related crash: A motor vehicle crash in which either a driver or a nonmotorist (usually a pedestrian) had a measurable or estimated BAC of 0.01 grams per deciliter (g/dL) or above.

Binge drinking: The National Household Survey on Drug Abuse defines binge drinking as drinking five or more drinks on the same occasion on at least 1 day in the past 30 days. The Monitoring the Future Study defines binge drinking as drinking five or more drinks on the same occasion during the past 2 weeks.

Blood alcohol concentration (BAC): The amount of alcohol in the bloodstream measured as a percentage, by weight, of alcohol in the blood in grams per deciliter (g/dL). Legal intoxication has been defined by States to occur at ranges from as low as 0.05 g/dL to as high as 0.10 g/dL.

Chronic drug use: Use of any heroin or cocaine more than 10 days in the past month.

Co-occurring disorders: The simultaneous presence of two or more disorders, such as the coexistence of a mental health disorder and substance abuse problem.

Current drinkers: Persons who have consumed at least 12 drinks of any kind of alcohol in the past year.

Drug dependence: A pattern of drug use leading to clinically significant impairment or distress, as manifested by three or more of the following occurring at any time in the same 12-month period: tolerance; withdrawal; use in larger amounts or over a longer period of time than intended; persistent desire or unsuccessful efforts to cut down; spending a great deal of time in activities necessary to obtain drug(s); giving up or reducing important social, occupational, or recreational activities; continued use despite knowledge of having a persistent or recurrent physical or psychological problem.

Fatal crash: A police-reported crash involving a motor vehicle in transport on a traffic way in which at least one person dies within 30 days of the crash.

Hepatitis B and C: Viral infections of the liver spread through contact with infected blood products, injection use of drugs, and needle-sharing.

Indicated preventive interventions: Interventions targeted to reach high-risk individuals who are identified as having minimal but detectable signs or symptoms foreshadowing substance abuse or biological or familial markers indicating predisposition for substance abuse, even though they do not meet DSM-III-R diagnostic levels at the current time.

Inhalants: Fumes or gases from common household substances, such as glues, aerosols, butane, and solvents, that are inhaled to produce a high.

Injection drug use: The use of a needle and syringe to inject illicit drugs (for example, heroin, cocaine, steroids) into the vein, muscle, skin, or below the skin. Injection drug use places the user at great risk for transmitting or contracting a number of bloodborne infectious diseases, including HIV, hepatitis B, and hepatitis C.

Selective preventive interventions: Interventions targeted to individuals or a subgroup of the population whose risk of developing substance abuse is significantly higher than average. The risk may be imminent, or it may be a lifetime risk. The basis may be biological, psychological, or environmental.

Substance abuse: The problematic consumption or illicit use of alcoholic beverages, tobacco products, and drugs, including misuse of prescription drugs.

Universal preventive interventions: Interventions targeted to the public or a whole population group that has not been identified on the basis of individual risk. The intervention is desirable for everyone in that group. Universal interventions have advantages in terms of cost and overall effectiveness for large populations.

References

[1] McGinnis, J.M., and Foege, W.H. Actual causes of death in the United States. *Journal of the American Medical Association* 270:2207-2212, 1993.

[2] Harwood, H.; Fountain, D.; and Livermore, G. *The Economic Costs of Alcohol and Drug Abuse in the United States, 1992.* NIH Pub. No. 98-4327. Rockville, MD: National Institutes of Health (NIH), 1998.

[3] Dawson, D.A.; Grant, B.F.; Chou, S.P.; et al. Subgroup variation in U.S. drinking patterns: Results of the 1992 National Longitudinal Alcohol Epidemiologic Study. *Journal of Substance Abuse* 7:331-344, 1995.

[4] National Institute on Alcohol Abuse and Alcoholism (NIAAA). Unpublished analysis of 1992 data.

[5] O'Malley, P.M.; Johnston, L.D.; and Bachman, J.F. Alcohol use among adolescents. *Alcohol Health & Research World* 22(2):85-93, 1998.

[6] Grant, B.F., and Dawson, D.A. Age at onset of alcohol use and its association with DSM-IV alcohol abuse and dependence: Results from the National Longitudinal Alcohol Epidemiologic Survey. *Journal of Substance Abuse* 9:103-110, 1997.

[7] Grant, B.F. The impact of a family history of alcoholism on the relationship between age at onset of alcohol use and DSM-IV alcohol dependence. *Alcohol Health & Research World* 22(2):144-148, 1998.

[8] NIAAA. *Eighth Special Report to the U.S. Congress on Alcohol and Health.* Rockville, MD: NIH, 1994.

[9] Zakhari, S. Alcohol and the cardiovascular system: Molecular mechanisms for beneficial and harmful action. *Alcohol Health & Research World* 21(1):21-29, 1997.

[10] NIAAA. Alcohol and cancer. *Alcohol Alert.* No. 21. Rockville, MD: NIH, 1993.

[11] NIAAA. *Ninth Special Report to the U.S. Congress on Alcohol and Health From the Secretary of Health and Human Services.* NIH Pub. No. 97-4017. Rockville, MD: NIH, 1997.

[12] NIH, National Institute on Drug Abuse (NIDA). *Preventing Drug Use Among Children and Adolescents: A Research-Based Guide*. NIDA, NIH Pub. No. 97-4212. Rockville, MD: NIH, NIDA, 1997.

[13] Reichmann, M.E. Alcohol and breast cancer. *Alcohol Health & Research World* 18(3):182-184, 1994.

[14] Roizen, J. Issues in the epidemiology of alcohol and violence. In: Martin, S., ed. *Alcohol and Interpersonal Violence: Fostering Multidisciplinary Perspectives*. NIH Pub. No. 93-3496. Rockville, MD: NIH, 1993.

[15] Strunin, L., and Hingson, R. Alcohol, drugs, and adolescent sexual behavior. *International Journal of the Addictions* 27(2):129-146, 1992.

[16] Strunin, L., and Hingson, R. Alcohol use and risk for HIV infection. *Alcohol Health & Research World* 17(1):35-38, 1993.

[17] U.S. Department of Transportation (DOT), National Highway Traffic Safety Administration (NHTSA). *Traffic Safety Facts*. Washington, DC: NHTSA, 1998.

[18] U.S. Department of Health and Human Services (HHS), Substance Abuse and Mental Health Services Administration (SAMHSA). *1998 National Household Survey on Drug Abuse*. Rockville, MD: SAMHSA, 2000.

[19] Community Epidemiology Work Group. *Epidemiological Trends in Drug Abuse: Advance Report*. Rockville, MD: NIDA, 1998.

[20] Office of National Drug Control Policy (ONDCP). *What America's Users Spend on Illegal Drugs, 1995–1998*. Washington, DC: U.S. Government Printing Office (GPO), 1997.

[21] HHS. *The National Structured Evaluation of Alcohol and Other Drug Abuse Prevention*. Rockville, MD: HHS, 1994.

[22] HHS. *Driving After Drug or Alcohol Use: Findings from the 1996 National Household Survey on Drug Abuse*. Rockville, MD: SAMHSA, 1998.

[23] HHS, SAMHSA. *Analyses of Substance Abuse and Treatment Need Issues*. Rockville, MD: SAMHSA, 1997.

[24] Garfien, R.S.; Vlahov, D.; Galai, N.; et al. Viral infections in short-term injection drug users: The prevalence of the hepatitis C, hepatitis B, human immunodeficiency, and human T-lymphotropic virus. *American Journal of Public Health* 86:655-661, 1996.

[25] Kaufman, M.J.; Levin, J.M.; Ross, M.H.; et al. Cocaine-induced cerebral vasoconstriction detected in humans with magnetic resonance angiography. *Journal of the American Medical Association* 279:376-380, 1998.

[26] Merrill, J.; Fox, K.; and Chang, H. *The Cost of Substance Abuse to America's Health Care System: Report 1. Medicaid Costs*. New York, NY: Center on Addiction and Substance Abuse, 1993.

[27] Shedler, J., and Block, J. Adolescent drug use and psychological health: A longitudinal inquiry. *American Psychologist* 45(5):612-630, 1990.

[28] Dishion, T.J.; Andrews, D.W.; Kavanagh, K.; et al. Preventive interventions for high-risk youth: The Adolescent Transitions Program. In: Peters, R.D., and McMahon, R.J., eds. *Preventing Childhood Disorders, Substance Abuse and Delinquency*. Thousand Oaks, CA: Sage Publications, 1996, 184-214.

[29] Kumpfer, K.L. Prevention of alcohol and drug abuse: A critical review of risk factors and prevention strategies. In: Shaffer, D.; Philips, I.; and Enzer, N.; eds. *Prevention of Mental Disorders, Alcohol and Other Drug Use in Children and Adolescents.* Office for Substance Abuse Prevention (OSAP), Monograph 2. DHHS Pub. No. (ADM) 92-1646. Rockville, MD: OSAP, 1992, 309-371.

[30] Dufour, M., and Fuller, R.K. Alcohol in the elderly. *Annual Review of Medicine* 46:123-132, 1995.

[31] Parsons, O.A., and Nixon, S.J. Neurobehavioral sequelae of alcoholism. *Neurological Clinics* 11(1):205-218, 1993.

[32] Pentz, M.A.; Dwyer, J.H.; MacKinnon, D.P.; et al. A multi-community trial for primary prevention of adolescent drug abuse. *Journal of the American Medical Association* 261(22):3259-3266, 1989.

[33] MacKinnon, D.P.; Johnson, C.A.; Pentz, M.A.; et al. Mediating mechanisms in a school-based drug prevention program: First-year effects of the Midwestern Prevention Project. *Health Psychology* 10(3):164-172, 1991.

[34] Dielman, T.E.; Kloska, D.D.; Leech, S.L.; et al. Susceptibility to peer pressure as an explanatory variable for differential effectiveness of an alcohol misuse prevention program in elementary schools. *Journal of School Health* 62(6):233-237, 1992.

[35] Shope, J.T.; Copeland, L.A.; Maharg, R.; et al. Assessment of adolescent refusal skills in an alcohol misuse prevention study. *Health Education Quarterly* 20(3):373-390, 1993.

[36] Botvin, G.J.; Baker, E.; Dusenbury, L.; et al. Long-term follow up results of a randomized drug abuse prevention trial in a white middle-class population. *Journal of the American Medical Association* 273(14):1106-1112, 1995.

[37] Perry, C.L.; Williams, C.L.; Veblen-Mortenson, S.; et al. Project Northland: Outcomes of a community wide alcohol use prevention program during early adolescence. *American Journal of Public Health* 86(7):956-965, 1996.

[38] O'Malley, P.M., and Wagenaar, A.C. Effects of minimum drinking age laws on alcohol use, related behaviors and traffic crash involvement among American youth: 1976–1987. *Journal of Studies on Alcohol* 52(5):478-491, 1991.

[39] Hingson, R. Prevention of drinking and driving. *Alcohol Health & Research World* 20(4):219-226, 1996.

[40] Zador, P.L.; Lund, A.K.; Fields, M.; et al. *Fatal Crash Involvement and Laws Against Alcohol Impaired Driving.* Arlington, VA: Institute for Highway Safety, 1989.

[41] Hingson, R.; Heeren, T.; and Winter, M. Lower legal blood alcohol limits for young drivers. *Public Health Reports* 109(6):738-744, 1994.

[42] Hingson, R.; Heeren, T.; and Winter, M. Lowering state legal blood alcohol limits to 0.08 percent: The effect on fatal motor vehicle crashes. *American Journal of Public Health* 86(9):1297-1299, 1996.

[43] Hingson, R.; McGovern, T.; Howland, J.; et al. Reducing alcohol-impaired driving in Massachusetts: The Saving Lives Program. *American Journal of Public Health* 86(6):791-797, 1996.

[44] Holder, H.D.; Saltz, R.F.; Grube, J.W.; et al. Summing up: Lessons from a comprehensive community prevention trial. *Addiction* 92(Suppl. 2): S293-S301, 1997.

[45] Coate, D., and Grossman, M. Effects of alcoholic beverage prices and legal drinking ages on youth alcohol use. *Journal of Law and Economics* 31:145-171, 1988.

[46] Manning, W.G.; Blumberg, L.; and Moulton, L.H. The demand for alcohol: The differential response to price. *Journal of Health Economics* 14(2):123-148, 1995.

[47] Cook, P.J., and Tauchen, G. The effect of liquor taxes on heavy drinking. *Bell Journal of Economics* 13(2):379-390, 1982.

[48] Chalopuka, F.J.; Saffer, H.; and Grossman, M. Alcohol-control policies and motor-vehicle fatalities. *Journal of Legal Studies* 22:161-186, 1993.

[49] Ruhm, C.J. Alcohol policies and highway vehicle fatalities. *Journal of Health Economics* 15:435-454, 1996.

[50] Kenkel, D.S. Drinking, driving, and deterrence: The effectiveness and social costs of alternative policies. *Journal of Law and Economics* 36(2):877-933, 1993.

[51] Cook, P.J., and Moore, M.J. Economic perspectives on reducing alcohol-related violence. In: Martin, S.E., ed. *Alcohol and Interpersonal Violence: Fostering Multidisciplinary Perspectives.* NIH Pub. No. 93-3496. Rockville, MD: NIH, 1993.

[52] Kenkel, D.S. New estimates of the optimal tax on alcohol. *Economic Inquiry* 34:296-319, 1996.

[53] Marlatt, G.A.; Baer, J.S.; and Larimer, M. Preventing alcohol abuse in college students: A harm-reduction approach. In: Boyd, G.M.; Howard, J.; and Zucker, R.A.; eds. *Alcohol Problems among Adolescents: Current Directions in Prevention Research.* Hillsdale, NJ: Lawrence Erlbaum Associates, 1995.

[54] Scribner, R.A.; MacKinnon, D.P.; and Dwyer, J.H. Relative risk of assaultive violence and alcohol availability in Los Angeles County. *American Journal of Public Health* 85:335-340, 1995.

[55] Gorman, D.M.; Speer, P.W.; Labouvie, E.W.; et al. Risk of assaultive violence and alcohol availability in New Jersey. *American Journal of Public Health* 88:97-100, 1998.

[56] McKirnan, D.J., and Peterson, P.L. Alcohol and drug use among homosexual men and women: Epidemiology and population characteristics. *Addictive Behaviors* 14:545-553, 1989.

[57] NHTSA. *1996 Youth Fatal Crash and Alcohol Facts.* Washington, DC: DOT, 1997.

[58] NHTSA. *Traffic Safety Facts 1998.* Pub. No. DOT-HS808983. Washington, DC: NHTSA, 1999.

[59] O'Malley, P.M., and Wagenaar, A.C. Effects of minimum drinking age laws on alcohol use, related behaviors and traffic crash involvement among American youth: 1976–1987. *Journal of Studies on Alcohol* 52(5):478-491, 1991.

[60] Zador, P.L.; Lund, A.K.; Fields, M.; et al. Fatal crash involvement and laws against alcohol impaired driving. Arlington, VA: Institute for Highway Safety, 1989.

[61] Hasin, D.; Grant, B.; and Harford, T. Male and female differences in liver cirrhosis mortality in the United States, 1961–1985. *Journal of Studies on Alcohol* 51:123-129, 1990.

[62] Popham, R.; Schmidt, W.; and Israelstam, S. Heavy alcohol consumption and physical health problems: A review of epidemiologic evidence. In: Smart, R.G.; Cappell, H.D.;

Glaser, F.B.; et al.; eds. *Recent Advances in Alcohol and Drug Problems*. No. 8. New York, NY: Plenum Press, 1984, 149-182.

[63] Schmidt, W. Effects of alcohol consumption on health. *Journal of Public Health Policy* 1:25-40, 1980.

[64] U.S. Bureau of the Census. *Statistical Abstract of the United States: 1997*. 117th ed. Washington, DC: U.S. Department of Commerce, 1997.

[65] Saadatamand, F.; Stinson, F.S.; Grant, B.F.; et al. *Surveillance Report* No. 45: *Liver Cirrhosis Mortality in the United States—1970–1994*. Rockville, MD: NIAAA, Division of Biometry and Epidemiology, Alcohol Epidemiologic Data System, 1997.

[66] HHS, SAMHSA, Office of Applied Studies. *Year-End 1998 Emergency Department Data from the Drug Abuse Warning Network*. Rockville, MD: SAMHSA, 1999.

[67] McCaig, L.F., and Stussman, B.J. *National Hospital Ambulatory Medical Care Survey: 1996 Emergency Department Summary. Advance Data From Vital and Health Statistics*. No. 293. Hyattsville, MD: National Center for Health Statistics, 1997.

[68] Li, G.; Keyl, P.M.; Rothman, R.; et al. Epidemiology of alcohol-related emergency department visits. *Academic Emergency Medicine* 5(8):788-795, 1998.

[69] Barnett, N.P.; Spirito, A.; Colby, S.M.; et al. Detection of alcohol use in adolescent patients in the emergency department. *Academic Emergency Medicine* 5(6):607-612, 1998.

[70] Meropol, S.B.; Moscati, R.M.; Lillis, K.A.; et al. Alcohol-related injuries among adolescents in the emergency department. *Annals of Emergency Medicine* 26(2):221-223, 1995.

[71] Rivara, F.P.; Jurkovich, G.J.; Gurney, J.G.; et al. The magnitude of acute and chronic alcohol abuse in trauma patients. *Archives of Surgery* 128(8):907-912, 1993.

[72] D'Onofrio, G.; Bernstein, E.; Bernstein, J.; et al. Patients with alcohol problems in the emergency department. Part 1: Improving detection. Substance Abuse Task Force, Society for Academic Emergency Medicine. *Journal of the Academy of Emergency Medicine* 5(12):1200-1209, 1998.

[73] HHS, CDC. *Youth Risk Behavior Survey*. Atlanta, GA: CDC, 1999.

[74] Murdoch, D., and Ross, R.O. Alcohol and crimes of violence. *International Journal of the Addictions* 25(9):1065-1081, 1990.

[75] Pacific Center for Violence Prevention. *Preventing Youth Violence: Reducing Access to Firearms*. San Francisco, CA: the Center, 1994.

[76] U.S. Department of Justice (DOJ), Bureau of Justice Statistics (BJS). *National Crime Victimization Survey*. Washington, DC: BJS, 1997.

[77] ONDCP. *The National Drug Control Strategy, 1999: A Ten Year Plan*. Washington, DC: GPO, 1999.

[78] DOJ. *National Symposium on Alcohol Abuse and Crime: Recommendations to the Office of Justice Programs*. Washington, DC: Office of Justice Programs (OJP), 1998.

[79] Doherty, M.; Edberg, M.; Cohen, M.; et al. The violence data exchange team: Developing a local data collection network to monitor community violence. Presented at the Society for Applied Anthropology Annual Meeting in Seattle, WA, March 1997.

[80] Hansen, W. School-based substance abuse prevention: A review of the state of the art curriculum, 1980–1990. *Health Education Research* 7(3):403-430, 1992.

[81] Johnston, L.; O'Malley, P.; and Bachman, J. *National Survey Results on Drug Use From the Monitoring the Future Study, 1975–1995.* Vol. I: Secondary School Students. Rockville, MD: NIDA, 1996.

[82] HHS, SAMHSA. *National Household Survey on Drug Abuse: Population Estimates 1996.* Rockville, MD: SAMHSA, 1997.

[83] ONDCP. *The National Drug Control Strategy: 1999.* Washington, DC: GPO, 1999.

[84] Saltz, R. Research needs and opportunities in server intervention programs. *Health Education Quarterly* 16(3):429-438, 1989.

[85] Holder, H.D., and Wagenaar, A.C. Mandated server training and reduced alcohol-involved traffic crashes: A time series analysis of the Oregon experience. *Accident Analysis and Prevention* 26:89-97, 1994.

[86] Nelson, J.P., and Moran, J.R. Advertising and United States alcoholic beverage demand: System-wide estimates. *Applied Economics* 27(12):1225-1236, 1995.

[87] Saffer, H. Alcohol advertising and alcohol consumption: Econometric studies. In: Martin, S.E., and Mail, P., eds. *The Effects of the Mass Media on the Use and Abuse of Alcohol.* NIAAA Research Monograph No. 28. NIH Publication No. 95-3743. Bethesda, MD: NIH, 1995.

[88] Henshaw, S.K. Unintended pregnancy in the United States. *Family Planning Perspectives* 30:24-29, 1998.

[89] CDC. Unpublished data, February 1999.

[90] CDC. Alcohol consumption among pregnant and childbearing-aged women, United States, 1991 and 1995. *Morbidity and Mortality Weekly Report* 46:346-350, 1997.

[91] Wagenaar, A.C. Minimum drinking age and alcohol availability to youth: Issues and research needs. In: Hilton, M.E., and Bloss, G., eds. *Economics and the Prevention of Alcohol-Related Problems.* NIAAA Research Monograph No. 25. NIH Pub. No. 93-3513. Rockville, MD: NIH, NIAAA, 1993.

[92] NIAAA. *The Physicians' Guide to Helping Patients With Alcohol Problems.* NIH Pub. No. 95-3769. Rockville, MD: NIH, 1995.

[93] NIAAA. Alcohol and Women. *Alcohol Alert.* No. 10. Rockville, MD: NIH, 1990.

[94] Dufour, M.C.; Archer, L.; and Gordis, E. Alcohol and the elderly. Health promotion and disease prevention. *Clinics in Geriatric Medicine* 8:127-141, 1992.

[95] U.S. Department of Agriculture and HHS. *Nutrition and Your Health: Dietary Guidelines for Americans.* 4th ed. Washington, DC: GPO, 1995.

[96] Yesalis, C.E.; Barsukiewicz, C.K.; Epstein, A.N.; et al. Trends in anabolic-androgenic steroid use among adolescents. *Archives of Pediatrics and Adolescent Medicine* 151(12):1197-1206, 1997.

[97] Ellis, D.; Zucker, R.; and Fitzgerald, H. The role of family influences in development and risk. *Alcohol Health & Research World* 21(3):218-226, 1997.

[98] Eigen, L., and Rowden, D.A. A methodology and current estimate of the number of children of alcoholics in the U.S. *Children of Alcoholics, Selected Readings.* Rockville, MD: National Association of Children of Alcoholics, 1995.

[99] Woodward, A.; Einstein, J.; Gfroerer, J.; et al. The drug abuse treatment gap: Recent estimates. *Health Care Financing Review* 18(3):1-13, 1997.

[100] Simeone, R.S.; Rhodes, W.R.; and Hunt, D.E. A plan for estimating the number of hardcore drug users in the United States. *The International Journal of Addictions* 30:637-657, 1995.

[101] Buck, J.A., and Umland, B. Covering mental health and substance abuse services. *Health Affairs* 16:120-126, 1997.

[102] Weisner, C., and Schmidt, L. Alcohol and drug problems among diverse health and social service populations. *American Journal of Public Health* 83:824-829, 1993.

[103] Harrison, P.A.; Fulkerson, J.A.; and Beebe, T.J. DSM-IV substance use disorder criteria for adolescents: A critical examination based on a statewide school survey. *American Journal of Psychiatry* 155:486-492, 1998.

[104] HHS, SAMHSA, Center for Substance Abuse Treatment (CSAT). *Substance Abuse Among Older Adults.* Treatment Improvement Protocol 26. Rockville, MD: SAMHSA, 1998.

[105] CSAT. *Planning for Alcohol and Other Drug Treatment for Adults in the Criminal Justice System.* Treatment Improvement Protocol 17. Rockville, MD: SAMHSA, 1995.

[106] Mumola, C.J. *Substance Abuse and Treatment, State and Federal Prisoners, 1997.* Washington, DC: DOJ, OJP, BJS, 1999.

[107] Anglin, M.D., and Hser, Y. Criminal justice and the drug-abusing offender: Policy issues of coerced treatment. *Behavioral Sciences and the Law* 9:243-267, 1991.

[108] Institute of Medicine. *Broadening the Base of Treatment for Alcohol Problems.* Washington, DC: National Academy Press, 1990.

[109] Harwood, H.J., Fountain, D.; and Livermore, G. *Economic Costs of Alcohol Abuse and Alcoholism. Recent Developments in Alcoholism.* Vol. 14: The Consequences of Alcoholism. New York, NY: Plenum Press, 1998.

[110] Sindelar, J. Social costs of alcohol. *Journal of Drug Issues* 28:763-780, 1998.

[111] McCrady, B.S., and Lagenbucher, J.W. Alcohol treatment and health care system reform. *Archives of General Psychiatry* 53:737-746, 1996.

[112] NIAAA. *Improving the Delivery of Alcohol Treatment and Prevention Services: A National Plan for Alcohol Services Research.* Rockville, MD: NIH, 1997.

[113] Sing, M.; Hik, S; Smolkin, S.; et al. *The Costs and Effects of Parity for Mental Health and Substance Abuse Benefits.* Rockville, MD: SAMHSA, 1998.

[114] Medical Association Commission on Emergency Medical Services. Pediatric emergencies. (Excerpt from Guidelines for Categorization of Hospital Emergency Capabilities.) *Pediatrics* 85:879-887, 1990.

[115] U.S. Consumer Product Safety Commission (CPSC), Division of Hazard and Injury Data Systems. *Hospital-Based Pediatric Emergency Resource Survey.* Bethesda, MD: CPSC, 1997.

[116] Philips, J., and Springer, J.F. Implementation of community interventions: Lessons learned. *Secretary's Youth Substance Abuse Prevention Initiative: Resource Papers. Regional Technical Assistance Workshop Pre-Publication Documents.* Rockville, MD: Center for Substance Abuse Prevention (CSAP), 1997, 159-178.

[117] Yin, R.K.; Kaftarian, S.J.; Yu, P.; et al. Outcomes from CSAP's community partnership program: Findings from the National Cross-Site Evaluation. *Evaluation and Program Planning* 20:345-355, August 1997.

[118] Community Partnership Program Study, SAMHSA, CSAP, 1999.

[119] NHTSA. *License Revocation: State Legislative Fact Sheet.* Washington, DC: DOT, 1996.

[120] NHTSA. *0.08 BAC Illegal Per Se Level: State Legislative Fact Sheet.* Washington, DC: DOT, 1996.

27

Tobacco Use

Lead Agency: Centers for Disease Control and Prevention

Contents

Reduce illness, disability, and death related to tobacco use and exposure to secondhand smoke.

Overview

Scientific knowledge about the health effects of tobacco use has increased greatly since the first Surgeon General's report on tobacco was released in 1964.[1, 2] Cigarette smoking causes heart disease, several kinds of cancer (lung, larynx, esophagus, pharynx, mouth, and bladder), and chronic lung disease. Cigarette smoking also contributes to cancer of the pancreas, kidney, and cervix. Smoking during pregnancy causes spontaneous abortions, low birth weight, and sudden infant death syndrome.[3]

Other forms of tobacco are not safe alternatives to smoking cigarettes. Use of spit tobacco causes a number of serious oral health problems, including cancer of the mouth and gum, periodontitis, and tooth loss.[1, 4] Cigar use causes cancer of the larynx, mouth, esophagus, and lung.[5] In recent years, reports have shown an increase in the popularity of bidis.[6] Bidis are small brown cigarettes, often flavored, consisting of tobacco hand-rolled in tendu or temburni leaf and secured with a string at one end. Research shows that bidis are a significant health hazard to users, increasing the risk of coronary heart disease and cancer of the mouth, pharynx and larynx, lung, esophagus, stomach, and liver.[7]

Issues and Trends

Tobacco use is responsible for more than 430,000 deaths per year among adults in the United States, representing more than 5 million years of potential life lost.[8] If current tobacco use patterns persist in the United States, an estimated 5 million persons under age 18 years will die prematurely from a smoking-related disease.[9] Direct medical costs related to smoking total at least $50 billion per year;[10] direct medical costs related to smoking during pregnancy are approximately $1.4 billion per year.[11]

Evidence is accumulating that shows maternal tobacco use is associated with mental retardation and birth defects such as oral clefts. Exposure to secondhand smoke also has serious health effects.[12, 13, 14] Researchers have identified more than 4,000 chemicals in tobacco smoke; of these, at least 43 cause cancer in humans and animals.[13] Each year, because of exposure to secondhand smoke, an estimated 3,000 nonsmokers die of lung cancer, and 150,000 to 300,000 infants and children under age 18 months experience lower respiratory tract infections.[13, 14] Asthma and other respiratory conditions often are triggered or worsened by tobacco smoke. (See Focus Area 8. Environmental Health; Focus Area 16. Maternal, Infant, and Child Health; and Focus Area 24. Respiratory Diseases.)

Studies also have found that secondhand smoke exposure causes heart disease among adults.[15, 16] Data reported from a study of the U.S. population aged 4 years and older indicated that among nontobacco users, 88 percent had detectable levels of serum cotinine, a biological marker for exposure to secondhand smoke.[17] Both home and workplace environments have contributed to the widespread exposure to secondhand smoke. Data from a 1996 study indicated that 22 percent of U.S. children and adolescents under age 18 years (approximately 15 million children and adolescents) were exposed to secondhand smoke in their homes.[18]

Smoking among adults declined steadily from the mid-1960s through the 1980s. However, smoking among adults appears to have leveled off in the 1990s. The rate of smoking among adults in 1997 was 25 percent.[19]

Tobacco use and addiction usually begin in adolescence. Furthermore, tobacco use may increase the probability that an adolescent will use other drugs. (See Focus Area 26. Substance Abuse.) Among adults in the United States who have ever smoked daily, 82 percent tried their first cigarette before age 18 years, and 53 percent became daily smokers before age 18 years.[20] Preventing tobacco use among youth has emerged as a major focus of tobacco control efforts.

Tobacco use among adolescents increased in the 1990s after decreasing in the 1970s and 1980s. Data from the 1999 Monitoring the Future Study indicated that past-month smoking among 8th, 10th, and 12th graders was 18, 26, and 35 percent, respectively. These rates represent increases of 20 to 33 percent since 1991.[21] Data from the Youth Risk Behavior Survey revealed that past-month smoking among 9th to 12th graders rose from 28 percent in 1991 to 36 percent in 1997.[22] Past-month spit tobacco use among 9th to 12th graders was 9 percent in 1997 (2 percent among females and 16 percent among males).[22] In 1997, past-month cigar use among 9th to 12th graders was 22 percent (11 percent of females and 31 percent of males).[22]

Youth are put at increased risk of initiating tobacco use by sociodemographic, environmental, and personal factors. Sociodemographic risk factors include coming from a family with low socioeconomic status. Environmental risk factors include accessibility and availability of tobacco products, cigarette advertising and promotion practices, the price of tobacco products, perceptions that tobacco use is normal, peers' and siblings' use and approval, and lack of parental involvement. Personal risk factors include low self-image and low self-esteem, the belief that tobacco use provides a benefit, and the lack of ability to refuse offers to use tobacco.[20]

Overwhelming evidence indicates that nicotine found in tobacco is addictive and that addiction occurs in most smokers during adolescence.[20, 23] Among students who were high school seniors during 1976–86, 44 percent of daily smokers

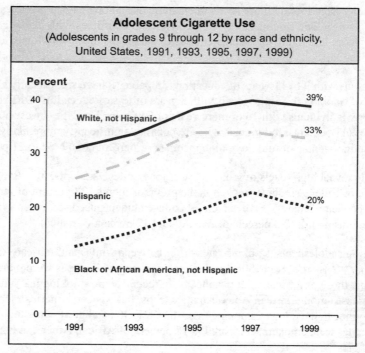

Adolescent Cigarette Use
(Adolescents in grades 9 through 12 by race and ethnicity,
United States, 1991, 1993, 1995, 1997, 1999)

Percent

- White, not Hispanic — 39%
- Hispanic — 33%
- Black or African American, not Hispanic — 20%

Source: CDC, NCCDPHP. Youth Risk Behavior Surveillance System (YRBSS), 1991, 1993, 1995, 1997, 1999.

believed that in 5 years they would not be smoking. Followup studies, however, indicated that 5 to 6 years later 73 percent of these persons remained daily smokers.[20] In 1995, 68 percent of current smokers wanted to quit smoking completely, and 46 percent of the current daily smokers had stopped smoking for at least 1 day during the preceding 12 months.[19] Less than 3 percent of current smokers stopped smoking permanently.[24]

Disparities

Men are more likely to smoke than women (26 percent compared to 22 percent).[19] Disparities in tobacco use exist among certain racial and ethnic populations. American Indians or Alaska Natives (35 percent) are more likely to smoke than other racial and ethnic groups, with considerable variations in percentages by Tribe.[25] Hispanics (18 percent) and Asians or Pacific Islanders (13 percent) are less likely to smoke than other groups. Regional and local data, however, reveal much higher smoking levels among specific population groups of Hispanics and Asians or Pacific Islanders.[25] Smoking levels among Vietnamese and Korean Asian Americans are higher than previously reported, according to a 1997 multilingual survey.[26]

Studies have found higher levels of cigarette use among gay men and lesbians than among heterosexuals.[27, 28, 29, 30] Gay men and lesbians with higher education levels are less likely to use cigarettes as frequently as those with lower levels of education.[28]

Persons with 9 to 11 years of education (38 percent) have significantly higher levels of smoking than individuals with 8 years or less of education or 12 years or more. Individuals with 16 or more years of education have the lowest smoking rates (11 percent). Individuals who are poor are significantly more likely to smoke than individuals of middle or high income (34 percent compared to 21 percent).[19]

Data reveal high levels of tobacco use among college students. In 1995, 29 percent of college students smoked in the previous month (28 percent of females and 30 percent of males). Five percent of college students used spit tobacco in the previous month (0.3 percent of females and 12 percent of males).[31]

Among adolescents, smoking rates differ between whites and African Americans.[21, 22] By the late 1980s, smoking rates among white teens were more than triple those of African American teens. In recent years, smoking has started to increase among African American male teens, but African American female teens continue to have lower smoking rates. In 1997, 40 percent of white high school females were smokers, compared to 17 percent of African American high school females.[22]

Spit tobacco use among adolescents also differs significantly by students' gender, race, and ethnicity. In 1997, 15.8 percent of male high school students currently used spit tobacco, compared to only 1.5 percent of female high school students. Current spit tobacco use was 12.2 percent for non-Hispanic whites, 2.2 percent for non-Hispanic African Americans, and 5.1 percent for Hispanics.[22]

Opportunities

Efforts to reduce tobacco use in the United States have shifted from focusing primarily on smoking cessation for individuals to more population-based interventions. Such interventions emphasize prevention of initiation, reduction of exposure to environmental tobacco smoke, and policy changes in health care systems to promote smoking cessation.[20, 32, 33, 34, 35, 36, 37] Federal, State, and local government agencies and numerous health organizations have joined together to develop and implement population-based approaches.

Community research studies and evidence from California, Florida, Massachusetts, and Oregon have shown that comprehensive programs can be effective in reducing average cigarette consumption per person. Both California and Massachusetts increased cigarette excise taxes and designated a portion of the revenues for comprehensive tobacco control programs. Data from these States indicate that (1) increasing excise taxes on cigarettes is one of the most cost-effective short-term strategies to reduce tobacco consumption among adults and to prevent initiation among youth and (2) the ability to sustain lower consumption increases when the tax increase is combined with an antismoking campaign.[38] In addition, recent data from Florida indicate that past-month smoking decreased significantly among public middle school students (19 percent to 15 percent) and high school students (27 percent to 25 percent) from 1998 to 1999 following implementation of a comprehensive program to prevent and reduce tobacco use among youth in that State.[39]

As education programs for school-aged youth are developed and proven effective in preventing initiation and in cessation, these programs should be included in quality health education curricula at the grade level. Education should aim to prevent initiation among youth, provide knowledge about effective cessation methods, and increase understanding of the health effects of tobacco use. (See Focus Area 7. Educational and Community-Based Programs.)

The goals of comprehensive tobacco prevention and reduction efforts include preventing people from starting to use tobacco, helping people quit using tobacco, reducing exposure to secondhand smoke, and identifying and eliminating disparities in tobacco use among population groups. To address these goals, community programs, media interventions, policy and regulatory activities, and surveillance and evaluation programs are being implemented. Specifically, the following elements are used to build capacity to implement and support tobacco use prevention and control interventions: a focus on change in social norms and environments that support tobacco use, policy and regulatory strategies, community participation, establishment of public and private partnerships, strategic use of media, development of local programs, coordination of statewide and local activities, linkage of school-based activities to community activities, and use of data collection and evaluation techniques to monitor program impact.

The importance of these various strategic elements has been demonstrated in a number of States, such as Arizona, California, Florida, Massachusetts, and Oregon.[40] In these and other States, tobacco control programs are supported through funding from the Federal Government, private foundations, State tobacco taxes, State lawsuit settlements, and other sources. These programs address issues such as reducing exposure to secondhand smoke, restricting minors' access to tobacco, treating nicotine addiction, limiting the impact of tobacco advertising, increasing the price of tobacco products, and directly regulating the product (for example, requiring product ingredient reporting). Tobacco control programs and materials should be culturally and linguistically appropriate.

Of the 26 tobacco-related objectives, 3 have been met: reducing the rate of lung cancer deaths, reducing the rate of oral cancer deaths, and increasing the number of States that have tobacco control plans.

Sixteen additional objectives are showing progress. These include reducing cigarette smoking among adults, which declined in the early part of the 1990s and then leveled off, and reducing children's exposure to secondhand smoke, which also declined. Some objectives, though showing progress, are far from their targets. For example, although 13 States have laws limiting smoking in public places and worksites, few ban smoking or limit it to separately ventilated areas in private workplaces or restaurants. As of December 31, 1998, only one State had met the objective for private worksites, and three had met it for restaurants. All 50 States and the District of Columbia have laws prohibiting the sale of tobacco to minors. However, the objective on enforcement of minors' access laws to achieve illegal buy rates of no more than 20 percent is far from being met: in fiscal year 1998, only 12 States had met this target. Although Healthy People 2000 data indicate that smoking among adolescents is declining somewhat, other surveys indicate that smoking among youth increased through 1997 and remained unchanged or declined somewhat in 1998 and 1999. Two additional objectives that include the use of and perception of harm from using drugs, alcohol, and cigarettes by high school seniors show mixed progress; for cigarettes there is slight progress.

Three objectives (perception of social disapproval of cigarette smoking among adolescents, States with preemptive clean indoor air laws, and smoking cessation during pregnancy) are moving away from the targets.

Data beyond baseline were not available for two objectives (tobacco product advertising and promotion to youth, and health plans offering treatment for nicotine addiction).

Note: Unless otherwise noted, data are from the Centers for Disease Control and Prevention, National Center for Health Statistics, *Healthy People 2000 Review, 1998–99*.

Tobacco Use

Goal: Reduce illness, disability, and death related to tobacco use and exposure to secondhand smoke.

Number Objective Short Title

Tobacco Use in Population Groups

27-1   Adult tobacco use

27-2   Adolescent tobacco use

27-3   Initiation of tobacco use

27-4   Age at first tobacco use

Cessation and Treatment

27-5   Smoking cessation by adults

27-6   Smoking cessation during pregnancy

27-7   Smoking cessation by adolescents

27-8   Insurance coverage of cessation treatment

Exposure to Secondhand Smoke

27-9   Exposure to tobacco smoke at home among children

27-10   Exposure to environmental tobacco smoke

27-11   Smoke-free and tobacco-free schools

27-12   Worksite smoking policies

27-13   Smoke-free indoor air laws

Social and Environmental Changes

27-14   Enforcement of illegal tobacco sales to minors laws

27-15   Retail license suspension for sales to minors

27-16   Tobacco advertising and promotion targeting adolescents and young adults

27-17   Adolescent disapproval of smoking

27-18   Tobacco control programs

27-19   Preemptive tobacco control laws

27-20   Tobacco product regulation

27-21   Tobacco tax

Tobacco Use in Population Groups

27-1. Reduce tobacco use by adults.

Target and baseline:

Objective	Reduction in Tobacco Use by Adults Aged 18 Years and Older	1998 Baseline*	2010 Target
		Percent	
27-1a.	Cigarette smoking	24	12
27-1b.	Spit tobacco	2.6	0.4
27-1c.	Cigars	2.5	1.2
27-1d.	Other products	Developmental	

*Age adjusted to the year 2000 standard population.

Target setting method: Better than the best.

Data source: National Health Interview Survey (NHIS), CDC, NCHS.

NOTE: THE TABLE BELOW MAY CONTINUE TO THE FOLLOWING PAGE.

Adults Aged 18 Years and Older, 1998 (unless noted)	27-1a. Cigarette Smoking	27-1b. Spit Tobacco	27-1c. Cigars
	Percent		
TOTAL	24	2.6	2.5
Race and ethnicity			
American Indian or Alaska Native	35	DSU	DSU
Asian or Pacific Islander	13	DSU	DSU
Asian	13	DSU	DSU
Native Hawaiian and other Pacific Islander	17	DSU	DSU
Black or African American	25	1.1	1.9
White	25	2.9	2.6
Hispanic or Latino	19	0.5	1.3
Not Hispanic or Latino	25	2.8	2.6
Black or African American	25	1.1	1.9
White	25	3.2	2.8

Adults Aged 18 Years and Older, 1998 (unless noted)	27-1a. Cigarette Smoking	27-1b. Spit Tobacco	27-1c. Cigars
	Percent		
Gender			
Female	22	0.3	0.2
Male	26	4.9	4.9
Family income level			
Poor	34	3.0	2.2
Near poor	31	3.0	2.7
Middle/high income	21	2.6	2.6
Education level (aged 25 years and older)			
Less than high school	34	4.1	2.4
Less than 9 years	27	3.8	2.5
9 to 11 years	38	3.9	2.3
High school graduate	29	2.6	2.4
At least some college	17	1.7	2.7
13 to 15 years	24	2.2	2.7
16 years or more	11	1.2	2.6
Disability status			
Persons with disabilities	33 (1997)	DNA	DNA
Persons without disabilities	23 (1997)	DNA	DNA
Sexual orientation	DNC	DNC	DNC
Select populations			
Age groups (not age adjusted)			
18 to 24 years	28 (1997)	3.5 (1997)	2.2 (1997)
25 to 44 years	27 (1997)	3.2 (1997)	2.8 (1997)
45 to 64 years	25 (1997)	1.7 (1997)	3.0 (1997)
65 years and older	11 (1997)	1.8 (1997)	0.9 (1997)

DNA = Data have not been analyzed. DNC = Data are not collected. DSU = Data are statistically unreliable.
Note: Age adjusted to the year 2000 standard population.

NOTE: THE TABLE ABOVE MAY HAVE CONTINUED FROM THE PREVIOUS PAGE.

27-2. Reduce tobacco use by adolescents.

Target and baseline:

Objective	Reduction in Tobacco Use by Students in Grades 9 Through 12	1999 Baseline	2010 Target
		Percent	
27-2a.	Tobacco products (past month)	40	21
27-2b.	Cigarettes (past month)	35	16
27-2c.	Spit tobacco (past month)	8	1
27-2d.	Cigars (past month)	18	8

Target setting method: Better than the best.

Data source: Youth Risk Behavior Surveillance System (YRBSS), CDC, NCCDPHP.

NOTE: THE TABLE BELOW MAY CONTINUE TO THE FOLLOWING PAGE.

Students in Grades 9 Through 12, 1999 (unless noted)	Current Tobacco Use (used cigarettes, spit tobacco, or cigars on 1 or more of the 30 days preceding the survey)		
	27-2a. Both Genders	Females*	Males*
	Percent		
TOTAL	40	37	44
Race and ethnicity			
American Indian or Alaska Native	DSU	DSU	DSU
Asian or Pacific Islander	DSU	DSU	DSU
Asian	DSU	DSU	DSU
Native Hawaiian and other Pacific Islander	DSU	DSU	DSU
Black or African American	34	23	28
White	33	41	49
Hispanic or Latino	35	33	38
Not Hispanic or Latino	41	37	44
Black or African American	25	22	29
White	45	40	49

Students in Grades 9 Through 12, 1999 (unless noted)	Current Tobacco Use (used cigarettes, spit tobacco, or cigars on 1 or more of the 30 days preceding the survey)		
	27-2a. Both Genders	Females*	Males*
	Percent		
Parents' education level			
Less than high school	41 (1997)	36 (1997)	48 (1997)
High school graduate	46 (1997)	41 (1997)	51 (1997)
At least some college	43 (1997)	35 (1997)	48 (1997)
Sexual orientation	DNC	DNC	DNC
Select populations			
Grade			
9th grade	32	30	33
10th grade	40	38	42
11th grade	42	37	47
12th grade	50	43	57

DNA = Data have not been analyzed. DNC = Data are not collected. DSU = Data are statistically unreliable.
*Data for females and males are displayed to further characterize the issue.

NOTE: THE TABLE ABOVE MAY HAVE CONTINUED FROM THE PREVIOUS PAGE.

NOTE: THE TABLE BELOW MAY CONTINUE TO THE FOLLOWING PAGE.

Students in Grades 9 Through 12, 1999 (unless noted)	Current Cigarette Smoking (smoked cigarettes on 1 or more of the 30 days preceding the survey)		
	27-2b. Both Genders	Females*	Males*
	Percent		
TOTAL	35	35	35
Race and ethnicity			
American Indian or Alaska Native	DSU	DSU	DSU
Asian or Pacific Islander	DSU	DSU	DSU
Asian	DSU	DSU	DSU
Native Hawaiian and other Pacific Islander	DSU	DSU	DSU
Black or African American	20	19	22
White	39	40	38

Students in Grades 9 Through 12, 1999 (unless noted)	Current Cigarette Smoking (smoked cigarettes on 1 or more of the 30 days preceding the survey)		
	27-2b. Both Genders	Females*	Males*
	Percent		
Hispanic or Latino	33	32	34
Not Hispanic or Latino	35	35	35
Black or African American	20	18	22
White	39	39	38
Parents' education level			
Less than high school	39 (1997)	37 (1997)	43 (1997)
High school graduate	40 (1997)	39 (1997)	41 (1997)
At least some college	35 (1997)	33 (1997)	37 (1997)
Sexual orientation	DNC	DNC	DNC
Selection populations			
Grade			
9th grade	28	29	26
10th grade	35	36	34
11th grade	36	36	36
12th grade	43	41	46

DNA = Data have not been analyzed. DNC = Data are not collected. DSU = Data are statistically unreliable.
*Data for females and males are displayed to further characterize the issue.

NOTE: THE TABLE ABOVE MAY HAVE CONTINUED FROM THE PREVIOUS PAGE.

NOTE: THE TABLE BELOW MAY CONTINUE TO THE FOLLOWING PAGE.

Students in Grades 9 Through 12, 1999 (unless noted)	Current Spit Tobacco Use (used spit tobacco on 1 or more of the 30 days preceding the survey)		
	27-2c. Both Genders	Females*	Males*
	Percent		
TOTAL	8	1	14
Race and ethnicity			
American Indian or Alaska Native	DSU	DSU	DSU
Asian or Pacific Islander	DSU	DSU	DSU
Asian	DSU	DSU	DSU
Native Hawaiian and other Pacific Islander	DSU	DSU	DSU

Students in Grades 9 Through 12, 1999 (unless noted)	Current Spit Tobacco Use (used spit tobacco on 1 or more of the 30 days preceding the survey)		
	27-2c. Both Genders	Females*	Males*
	Percent		
Black or African American	1	1	2
White	10	2	18
Hispanic or Latino	4	2	6
Not Hispanic or Latino	8	1	15
Black or African American	1	0	3
White	10	2	19
Parents' education level			
Less than high school	8 (1997)	1 (1997)	18 (1997)
High school graduate	9 (1997)	1 (1997)	17 (1997)
At least some college	10 (1997)	2 (1997)	16 (1997)
Sexual orientation	DNC	DNC	DNC
Select populations			
Grade			
9th grade	7	2	12
10th grade	7	1	13
11th grade	8	2	15
12th grade	9	1	17

DNA = Data have not been analyzed. DNC = Data are not collected. DSU = Data are statistically unreliable.
*Data for females and males are displayed to further characterize the issue.

NOTE: THE TABLE ABOVE MAY HAVE CONTINUED FROM THE PREVIOUS PAGE.

NOTE: THE TABLE BELOW MAY CONTINUE TO THE FOLLOWING PAGE.

Students in Grades 9 Through 12, 1999 (unless noted)	Current Cigar Use (smoked cigars on 1 or more of the 30 days preceding the survey)		
	27-2d. Both Genders	Females*	Males*
	Percent		
TOTAL	18	10	25
Race and ethnicity			
American Indian or Alaska Native	DSU	DSU	DSU

Students in Grades 9 Through 12, 1999 (unless noted)	Current Cigar Use (smoked cigars on 1 or more of the 30 days preceding the survey)		
	27-2d. Both Genders	Females*	Males*
	Percent		
Asian or Pacific Islander	DSU	DSU	DSU
Asian	DSU	DSU	DSU
Native Hawaiian and other Pacific Islander	DSU	DSU	DSU
Black or African American	14	13	16
White	19	9	29
Hispanic or Latino	17	12	22
Not Hispanic or Latino	18	10	26
Black or African American	14	12	16
White	19	9	28
Parents' education level			
Less than high school	19 (1997)	11 (1997)	29 (1997)
High school graduate	21 (1997)	11 (1997)	32 (1997)
At least some college	23 (1997)	11 (1997)	32 (1997)
Sexual orientation	DNC	DNC	DNC
Select populations			
Grade			
9th grade	14	9	18
10th grade	18	11	25
11th grade	18	9	27
12th grade	22	11	34

DNA = Data have not been analyzed. DNC = Data are not collected. DSU = Data are statistically unreliable.
*Data for females and males are displayed to further characterize the issue.

NOTE: THE TABLE ABOVE MAY HAVE CONTINUED FROM THE PREVIOUS PAGE.

Effective prevention approaches for reducing tobacco use among adolescents include school-based prevention programs as an integral part of communitywide strategies that address the overall social context of tobacco use.[20, 32] School-based tobacco prevention programs identify the social influences that promote tobacco use among youth and teach skills to resist these influences. Such programs have demonstrated consistent and significant reductions or delays in adolescent smoking.[20, 41] The effects dissipate over time if they are not followed by additional educational interventions or linkages to community programs. Studies have shown that the effectiveness of school-based tobacco prevention programs appears to be strengthened by (1) booster sessions or further application of the programs and (2) communitywide programs involving parents, school policies, mass media, youth access, and community organizations.[42, 43, 44, 45, 46, 47] A multicomponent approach to school-based tobacco use prevention[48] also may increase the long-term effectiveness of prevention efforts. (See Focus Area 7. Educational and Community-Based Programs.)

27-3. (Developmental) Reduce the initiation of tobacco use among children and adolescents.

Potential data source: National Household Survey on Drug Abuse (NHSDA), SAMHSA.

27-4. Increase the average age of first use of tobacco products by adolescents and young adults.

Target and baseline:

Objective	Increase in Average Age of First Tobacco Use	1997 Baseline	2010 Target
		Average Age of First Cigarette Use, in Years	
27-4a.	Adolescents aged 12 to 17 years	12	14
27-4b.	Young adults aged 18 to 25 years	15	17

Target setting method: Better than the best.

Data source: National Household Survey on Drug Abuse (NHSDA), SAMHSA.

NOTE: THE TABLE BELOW MAY CONTINUE TO THE FOLLOWING PAGE.

Adolescents and Young Adults, 1997	First Cigarette Use	
	27-4a. Aged 12 to 17 Years	27-4b. Aged 18 to 25 Years
	Average Age in Years	
TOTAL*	12	15
Race and ethnicity		
American Indian or Alaska Native	12	14
Asian or Pacific Islander	13	15
Black or African American	13	16
White	12	15
Hispanic or Latino	13	15

Adolescents and Young Adults, 1997	First Cigarette Use	
	27-4a. Aged 12 to 17 Years	27-4b. Aged 18 to 25 Years
	Average Age in Years	
Not Hispanic or Latino*	12	15
Black or African American	12	15
White	13	16
Gender		
Female	13	15
Male	12	15
Family income level		
Poor	DNA	DNA
Near poor	DNA	DNA
Middle/high income	DNA	DNA
Sexual orientation	DNC	DNC

DNA = Data have not been analyzed. DNC = Data are not collected. DSU = Data are statistically unreliable.
*Total for not Hispanic or Latino excludes all race categories other than black and white.
NOTE: THE TABLE ABOVE MAY HAVE CONTINUED FROM THE PREVIOUS PAGE.

Because tobacco use is linked with numerous adverse health outcomes, reducing tobacco use will reduce illness, disability, and death across a spectrum of conditions, including heart disease, cancer, and chronic lung disease. (See Related Objectives From Other Focus Areas section.)

Assessing the number of cases of tobacco use among both adults and adolescents is a critical element of public health surveillance. Indeed, in 1996 the Council of State and Territorial Epidemiologists added adult cigarette smoking as a notifiable condition, the first time that a behavior rather than a disease was designated a notifiable condition.[49]

Because the majority of initiation of tobacco use occurs in adolescence,[20] direct measures of tobacco use in adolescence are important health indicators. Measures of use in adulthood provide an assessment of use that has extended beyond experimentation and initiation. Evidence indicates substitution of tobacco products among both adults and youth, so measuring the use of multiple products (cigarettes, spit tobacco, and cigars at a minimum) is important.

27-5. Increase smoking cessation attempts by adult smokers.

Target: 75 percent.

Baseline: 41 percent of adult smokers aged 18 years and older stopped smoking for 1 day or longer because they were trying to quit in 1998 (age adjusted to the year 2000 standard population).

Target setting method: Better than the best.

Data source: National Health Interview Survey (NHIS), CDC, NCHS.

NOTE: THE TABLE BELOW MAY CONTINUE TO THE FOLLOWING PAGE.

Adults Aged 18 Years and Older, 1998 (unless noted)	Stopped Smoking 1 Day or Longer Because They Were Trying To Quit
	Percent
TOTAL	41
Race and ethnicity	
American Indian or Alaska Native	42
Asian or Pacific Islander	44
Asian	38
Native Hawaiian and other Pacific Islander	DSU
Black or African American	45
White	40
Hispanic or Latino	38
Not Hispanic or Latino	41
Black or African American	45
White	40
Gender	
Female	42
Male	39
Family income level	
Poor	40
Near poor	42
Middle/high income	43
Education level (aged 25 years and older)	
Less than high school	38
Under 9 years	36

Adults Aged 18 Years and Older, 1998 (unless noted)	Stopped Smoking 1 Day or Longer Because They Were Trying To Quit
	Percent
9 to 11 years	39
High school graduate	36
At least some college	42
13 to 15 years	42
16 years or more	43
Disability status	
Persons with disabilities	44 (1997)
Persons without disabilities	42 (1997)
Sexual orientation	DNC
Select populations	
Age groups (not age adjusted)	
18 to 24 years	52
25 to 44 years	42
45 to 64 years	37
65 years and older	35

DNA = Data have not been analyzed. DNC = Data are not collected. DSU = Data are statistically unreliable.
Note: Age adjusted to the year 2000 standard population.
NOTE: THE TABLE ABOVE MAY HAVE CONTINUED FROM THE PREVIOUS PAGE.

27-6. Increase smoking cessation during pregnancy.

Target: 30 percent.

Baseline: 14 percent of females aged 18 to 49 years stopped smoking during the first trimester of their pregnancy in 1998.

Target setting method: Better than the best.

Data source: National Health Interview Survey (NHIS), CDC, NCHS.

NOTE: THE TABLE BELOW MAY CONTINUE TO THE FOLLOWING PAGE.

Pregnant Females Aged 18 to 49 Years, 1998 (unless noted)	Stopped Smoking
	Percent
TOTAL	14
Race and ethnicity	
American Indian or Alaska Native	DSU
Asian or Pacific Islander	DSU

Pregnant Females Aged 18 to 49 Years, 1998 (unless noted)	Stopped Smoking
	Percent
Asian	DSU
Native Hawaiian and other Pacific Islander	DSU
Black or African American	DSU
White	14
Hispanic or Latino	DSU
Not Hispanic or Latino	14
Black or African American	DSU
White	14
Family income level	
Poor	DSU
Near poor	12
Middle/high income	22
Education level	
Less than 12 years	DSU
Less than 9 years	DSU
9 to 11 years	DSU
High school graduate	14
13 years or more	12
13 to 15 years	10
16 years or more	DSU
Disability status	
Persons with activity limitations	DSU (1991)
Persons without activity limitations	12 (1991)

DNA = Data have not been analyzed. DNC = Data are not collected. DSU = Data are statistically unreliable.

NOTE: THE TABLE ABOVE MAY HAVE CONTINUED FROM THE PREVIOUS PAGE.

27-7. Increase tobacco use cessation attempts by adolescent smokers.

Target: 84 percent.

Baseline: 76 percent of ever-daily smokers in grades 9 through 12 had tried to quit smoking in 1999.

Target setting method: Better than the best.

Data source: Youth Risk Behavior Surveillance System (YRBSS), CDC, NCCDPHP.

Students in Grades 9 Through 12 Who Were Ever Daily Smokers (Ever Smoked Every Day for 30 Days), 1999 (unless noted)	Tried To Quit		
	27-7. Both Genders	Females*	Males*
	Percent		
TOTAL	76	81	71
Race and ethnicity			
American Indian or Alaska Native	DSU	DSU	DSU
Asian or Pacific Islander	DSU	DSU	DSU
Asian	DNC	DNC	DNC
Native Hawaiian and other Pacific Islander	DNC	DNC	DNC
Black or African American	81	82	80
White	76	80	72
Hispanic or Latino	72	75	69
Not Hispanic or Latino	76	81	72
Black or African American	80	80	79
White	76	79	73
Parents' education level			
Less than high school	69 (1997)	81 (1997)	57 (1997)
High school graduate	79 (1997)	82 (1997)	76 (1997)
At least some college	72 (1997)	76 (1997)	69 (1997)
Sexual orientation	DNC	DNC	DNC
Select populations			
Grade			
9th grade	72	74	69
10th grade	81	84	78
11th grade	74	79	67
12th grade	78	85	73

DNA = Data have not been analyzed. DNC = Data are not collected. DSU = Data are statistically unreliable.
*Data for females and males are displayed to further characterize the issue.

27-8. Increase insurance coverage of evidence-based treatment for nicotine dependency.

Target and baseline:

Objective	Increase in Insurance Coverage of Evidence-Based Treatment for Nicotine Dependency	1998 Baseline (unless noted)	2010 Target
		Percent	
27-8a.	Managed care organizations	75 (1997–98)	100
		Number	
27-8b.	Medicaid programs in States and the District of Columbia	24	51
27-8c.	All insurance	Developmental	

Target setting method: Total coverage of FDA-approved pharmacotherapies and behavioral therapies.

Data sources: Addressing Tobacco in Managed Care Survey, Robert Wood Johnson Foundation; (Medicaid data) Health Policy Tracking Service, National Conference of State Legislators.

Nearly 70 percent of current smokers want to quit smoking, and approximately 45 percent have quit smoking for at least 1 day because they were trying to quit.[19] However, only about 2.5 percent of current smokers stop smoking permanently each year.[24] Smoking cessation has major and immediate health benefits for men and women of all ages. For example, people who quit smoking before age 50 years have half the risk of dying in the next 15 years compared with people who continue to smoke.[2]

In 1996, the Agency for Health Care Policy and Research (AHCPR, now the Agency for Healthcare Research and Quality) sponsored an expert panel that produced an evidence-based guideline that evaluated smoking cessation interventions available at the time and concluded that the efficacy of intervention increases with intensity.[50] The results clearly showed that a variety of smoking cessation interventions are effective: (1) simple advice to quit by a clinician (30 percent increase in cessation), (2) individual and group counseling (doubles cessation rates), (3) telephone hotlines and helplines (40 percent increase in cessation), and (4) nicotine replacement therapy (up to double the cessation rates). This guideline will be updated in 2000.

AHCPR's guideline recommended that smoking cessation treatments (both pharmacotherapy and counseling) be provided as paid services and that providers be reimbursed for delivering effective smoking cessation interventions. AHCPR concluded that effective reduction of tobacco use will require health care systems to make institutional changes resulting in systematic identification of, and intervention with, all tobacco users at every visit.[50]

Almost 44 percent of high school seniors who smoke report that they would like to stop smoking. About 30 percent of high school seniors who smoke report that they have tried to stop smoking but failed to do so.[51] Although many teen smokers want to quit or have tried to quit smoking, almost no proven interventions exist for tobacco use cessation among teenagers. Research is under way to assess effective cessation methods for young persons, but expanded research efforts are needed.

Data reported from a study of managed care organizations indicated that 75 percent of plans either partially or fully covered one or more smoking cessation interventions. Full coverage was provided most often for self-help materials and smoking cessation classes, whereas more costly interventions, such as pharmaceutical treatments for nicotine addiction, were less frequently covered in full.[52] According to other data, Medicaid coverage of smoking cessation services, including counseling and nicotine replacement therapies, varied by State.[53] (See Focus Area 1. Access to Quality Health Services.)

Exposure to Secondhand Smoke

27-9. Reduce the proportion of children who are regularly exposed to tobacco smoke at home.

Target: 10 percent.

Baseline: 27 percent of children aged 6 years and under lived in a household where someone smoked inside the house at least 4 days per week in 1994.

Target setting method: Better than the best.

Data source: National Health Interview Survey (NHIS), CDC, NCHS.

NOTE: THE TABLE BELOW MAY CONTINUE TO THE FOLLOWING PAGE.

Children Aged 6 Years and Under, 1994	Lived in Household Where Someone Smoked Inside the House at Least 4 Days a Week
	Percent
TOTAL	27
Race and ethnicity	
American Indian or Alaska Native	DSU
Asian or Pacific Islander	23
Asian	DSU
Native Hawaiian and other Pacific Islander	DSU
Black or African American	28
White	27

Children Aged 6 Years and Under, 1994	Lived in Household Where Someone Smoked Inside the House at Least 4 Days a Week
	Percent
Hispanic or Latino	20
Not Hispanic or Latino	29
Black or African American	28
White	29
Gender	
Female	28
Male	27
Family income	
Poor	38
Near poor	33
Middle/high income	19

DNA = Data have not been analyzed. DNC = Data are not collected. DSU = Data are statistically unreliable.

NOTE: THE TABLE ABOVE MAY HAVE CONTINUED FROM THE PREVIOUS PAGE.

27-10. Reduce the proportion of nonsmokers exposed to environmental tobacco smoke.

Target: 45 percent.

Baseline: 65 percent of nonsmokers aged 4 years and older had a serum cotinine level above 0.10 ng/mL in 1988–94 (age adjusted to the year 2000 standard population).

Target setting method: Better than the best.

Data source: National Health and Nutrition Examination Survey (NHANES), CDC, NCHS.

Nonsmokers Aged 4 Years and Older, 1988–94	Serum Cotinine Levels >0.10 ng/mL
	Percent
TOTAL	65
Race and ethnicity	
American Indian or Alaska Native	DSU
Asian or Pacific Islander	DSU
Asian	DNC
Native Hawaiian and other Pacific Islander	DNC
Black or African American	81
White	63
Hispanic or Latino	DSU
Mexican American	53
Not Hispanic or Latino	66
Black or African American	81
White	63
Gender	
Female	61
Male	69
Education level (aged 25 years and older)	
Less than high school	71
High school graduate	67
At least some college	55
Sexual orientation	DNC
Select populations	
Age groups (not age adjusted)	
4 to 11 years	68
12 to 19 years	69
20 to 44 years	67
45 to 64 years	65
65 years and older	51

DNA = Data have not been analyzed. DNC = Data are not collected. DSU = Data are statistically unreliable.
Note: Age adjusted to the year 2000 standard population.

27-11. Increase smoke-free and tobacco-free environments in schools, including all school facilities, property, vehicles, and school events.

Target: 100 percent.

Baseline: 37 percent of middle, junior high, and senior high schools were smoke-free and tobacco-free in 1994.

Target setting method: Retain year 2000 target.

Data source: School Health Policies and Programs Study (SHPPS), CDC, NCCDPHP.

27-12. Increase the proportion of worksites with formal smoking policies that prohibit smoking or limit it to separately ventilated areas.

Target: 100 percent.

Baseline: 79 percent of worksites with 50 or more employees had formal smoking policies that prohibited or limited smoking to separately ventilated areas in 1998–99.

Target setting method: Retain year 2000 target.

Data source: National Worksite Health Promotion Survey, Association for Worksite Health Promotion (AWHP).

27-13. Establish laws on smoke-free indoor air that prohibit smoking or limit it to separately ventilated areas in public places and worksites.

Target and baseline:

Objective	Jurisdictions With Laws on Smoke-Free Air	1998 Baseline	2010 Target
		Number	
	States and the District of Columbia		
27-13a.	Private workplaces	1	51
27-13b.	Public workplaces	13	51
27-13c.	Restaurants	3	51
27-13d.	Public transportation	16	51
27-13e.	Day care centers	22	51
27-13f.	Retail stores	4	51
27-13g.	**Tribes**	Developmental	
27-13h.	**Territories**	Developmental	

Target setting method: Retain year 2000 target.

Data source: State Tobacco Activities Tracking and Evaluation System (STATE System), CDC, NCCDPHP, OSH.

In 1996, only 37 percent of adult nontobacco users were aware enough of their exposure to report having been exposed to secondhand smoke either at home or at work.[17] Both home and workplace environments contributed significantly to widespread exposure to secondhand smoke in the United States.[17] An alarming level of secondhand smoke exposure at home was reported. Exposure ranged from 12 percent of children aged 17 years and under in Utah to 34 percent of children in Kentucky.[18]

A 1992–93 National Cancer Institute survey found that significant numbers of workers, especially those in blue-collar and service occupations, reported smoke-free workplace policy rates considerably lower than the overall rate of 46 percent.[54] Least likely to have a smoke-free policy were food service workers— waiters, waitresses, cooks, bartenders, and counter help. Of these 5.5 million workers, 22 percent were teenagers. In a 1993 study, food service workers were estimated to have a 50 percent increased risk of dying from lung cancer compared to the general population, with the higher risk attributed in part to their workplace exposure to secondhand smoke.[55]

Policy, educational, and clinical interventions can reduce secondhand smoke exposure among the population. Policy approaches include the voluntary adoption of worksite restrictions, enactment of clean indoor air laws, and enforcement of restrictions. Public education campaigns and local community efforts to limit smoking in public places in California and Massachusetts have been associated with reported reductions in the exposure of both adults and children to secondhand smoke.[33, 34]

A study published in 1996 concluded that a portion of children's respiratory diseases and their associated illness may be prevented by decreasing or eliminating their exposure to secondhand smoke.[56]

Another study concluded that secondhand smoke exposure worsens asthma and each year leads to 500,000 visits to physicians by children.[57] The American Academy of Pediatrics has recommended that pediatricians inform parents about the health hazards of secondhand smoke and provide guidance on smoking cessation.[58] (See Focus Area 8. Environmental Health and Focus Area 24. Respiratory Diseases.)

27-14. Reduce the illegal sales rate to minors through enforcement of laws prohibiting the sale of tobacco products to minors.

Target and baseline:

Objective	Jurisdictions With a 5 Percent or Less Illegal Sales Rate to Minors	1998 Baseline	2010 Target
		Number	
27-14a.	States and the District of Columbia	0	51
27-14b.	Territories	0	All

Target setting method: Based on published literature and expert opinion.

Data source: State Synar Enforcement Reporting, SAMHSA, CSAP.

27-15. Increase the number of States and the District of Columbia that suspend or revoke State retail licenses for violations of laws prohibiting the sale of tobacco to minors.

Target: All States and the District of Columbia.

Baseline: 34 States with some form of retail licensure could suspend or revoke the license for violation of minors' access laws in 1998.

Target setting method: Total coverage.

Data source: State Tobacco Activities Tracking and Evaluation System (STATE System), CDC, NCCDPHP, OSH.

Restricting minors' access to tobacco products is one core element in a comprehensive approach to tobacco use prevention. In 1997, of the 30 percent of students who purchased their cigarettes from a gas station or store in the month preceding a survey, 67 percent of them were not asked for proof of age.[59] Earlier data indicated that only about half of smokers aged 12 to 17 years were ever asked to show proof of age when they tried to purchase cigarettes.[60] Data revealed that self-service tobacco displays make it easier for minors to purchase or steal tobacco products. In a 1995 survey, stores with self-service displays were 61 percent more likely to sell tobacco to minors than stores without self-service displays.[61]

Although all States prohibit the sale of tobacco products to minors, enforcement of laws has been limited until recent years. States and localities have undertaken a number of measures to reduce minors' access, including policy establishment, retail licensure, enforcement activities, compliance checks, retailer education, and youth involvement. State restrictions on tobacco vending machines vary, with the most stringent restrictions banning vending machines except in areas inaccessible to minors. Not all States have retail licensure systems. Among those that do, not all will suspend or revoke licenses for violation of State minors' access laws. Federal policy initiatives require the active participation of State and local communities to ensure effective implementation.[35, 62] In addition to efforts to address the purchase of tobacco products by minors, tobacco control initiatives also must target social sources of tobacco for young people, including friends, siblings, and parents.

27-16. (Developmental) Eliminate tobacco advertising and promotions that influence adolescents and young adults.

Potential data source: American Legacy Foundation and National Association of Attorneys General.

27-17. Increase adolescents' disapproval of smoking.

Target and baseline:

Objective	Increase in Adolescents' Disapproval of Smoking	1998 Baseline	2010 Target
		Percent	
27-17a.	8th grade	80	95
27-17b.	10th grade	75	95
27-17c.	12th grade	69	95

Target setting method: Retain year 2000 target.

Data source: Monitoring the Future Study (MTF), NIH, NIDA.

NOTE: THE TABLE BELOW MAY CONTINUE TO THE FOLLOWING PAGE.

Adolescents, 1998	Disapproval of Smoking One or More Packs of Cigarettes Daily		
	27-17a. 8th Graders	27-17b. 10th Graders	27-17c. 12th Graders
	Percent		
TOTAL	80	75	69
Race and ethnicity			
American Indian or Alaska Native	DSU	DSU	DSU
Asian or Pacific Islander	DNC	DNC	DNC
Asian	DSU	DSU	DSU
Native Hawaiian and other Pacific Islander	DNC	DNC	DNC
Black or African American	DNC	DNC	DNC
White	DNC	DNC	DNC

Adolescents, 1998	Disapproval of Smoking One or More Packs of Cigarettes Daily		
	27-17a. 8th Graders	27-17b. 10th Graders	27-17c. 12th Graders
	Percent		
Hispanic or Latino	76	81	76
Not Hispanic or Latino	DNC	DNC	DNC
Black or African American	82	83	82
White	81	72	64
Gender			
Female	83	79	73
Male	77	72	64
Parents' education level			
Less than high school	DNC	DNC	DNC
High school graduate	DNC	DNC	DNC
At least some college	DNC	DNC	DNC
Sexual orientation	DNC	DNC	DNC

DNA = Data have not been analyzed. DNC = Data are not collected. DSU = Data are statistically unreliable.
NOTE: THE TABLE ABOVE MAY HAVE CONTINUED FROM THE PREVIOUS PAGE.

Attitudes of adolescents regarding the acceptability of tobacco use provide an indication of their susceptibility to tobacco use.[20] The 1994 Surgeon General's report on tobacco concluded that the following are all risk factors for tobacco use among adolescents: adolescents' perceptions that tobacco use is the norm, peers' and siblings' approval of tobacco use, and the belief that tobacco use provides benefits. The report further concluded that for spit tobacco use, insufficient knowledge among youth of the health effects also is a factor.[20]

27-18. (Developmental) Increase the number of Tribes, Territories, and States and the District of Columbia with comprehensive, evidence-based tobacco control programs.

Potential data sources: State Tobacco Activities Tracking and Evaluation System (STATE System), CDC, NCCDPHP, OSH; IHS.

Evidence indicates that comprehensive tobacco control programs are effective. Investments in such programs to date, however, have been seriously limited. Data from California and Massachusetts indicate that the ability to sustain reductions in per capita consumption due to excise tax increases is greater when the tax increase is combined with a comprehensive tobacco control program. Per capita cigarette consumption in California and Massachusetts, two States with such programs, has declined two to three times faster than in the rest of the Nation. In addition, the rapid rise in youth smoking rates experienced nationwide was slowed in both California and Massachusetts as a result of the combined effects of a tax increase and a strong tobacco control program.[38] Other analyses suggest that comprehensive programs, including media campaigns, have reduced the rate of increase in youth smoking in States with programs funded by excise taxes (such as Massachusetts), compared with the rest of the Nation.[63]

In the Minnesota Heart Health Program, smoking rates were reduced by approximately 40 percent in the intervention community with a combined school-based curriculum, community-based activities, and mass media interventions.[46] Furthermore, a preliminary report on the effectiveness of the American Stop Smoking Intervention Study (ASSIST) indicated that in 1993–94, per capita cigarette consumption was 7 percent less in the 17 ASSIST States than in the remaining States (excluding California).[64]

Limiting the appeal of tobacco products to young people involves both restricting tobacco advertising and promotions and countering the ability of pro-tobacco messages to reach large segments of the population quickly and efficiently. Because of their appeal, the mass media can serve as a powerful tool for tobacco control. Television and radio stations, magazines, and other media can deliver information and educational messages directly to targeted audiences, build public support for tobacco control programs and policies, reinforce social norms supporting the nonuse of tobacco, and counteract the pro-use messages and images of tobacco marketing and public relations campaigns.

An essential element in programs for reducing tobacco's appeal to youth is to change the current social environment that reinforces the acceptability of tobacco use.[20, 32, 40] This change requires strategies to counter the billions of dollars worth of tobacco advertising and promotion that bombard young people with false and misleading messages and images about tobacco.[20, 32] An integral part of the Arizona, California, and Massachusetts tobacco control programs has been paid counteradvertising campaigns to deglamorize and denormalize tobacco use, especially among young people, with unequivocal messages about the negative effects of tobacco use on health, performance, and appearance.[33, 34, 36, 37] Preliminary results indicate that the media programs have reached youth, adults, and multicultural populations in those States and have achieved their program objectives.

27-19. Eliminate laws that preempt stronger tobacco control laws.

Target: Zero States.

Baseline: 30 States had preemptive tobacco control laws in the areas of clean indoor air, minors' access laws, or marketing in 1998.

Target setting method: Retain year 2000 target.

Data source: State Tobacco Activities Tracking and Evaluation System (STATE System), CDC, NCCDPHP, OSH.

Preemptive State laws limit the ability of State and local programs to address major areas of tobacco control, in particular smoke-free indoor air and minors' access policies. A preemptive State tobacco control law prevents local jurisdictions from enacting restrictions that are more restrictive than or vary from State law. The tobacco industry attempts to promote such laws as health promotion efforts that ensure a uniform set of restrictions for all communities. Such laws, however, usually afford less protection and prevent local governments from adopting more restrictive provisions in the future.[65] Preemptive laws have led, for example, to weaker public health standards, loss of community education involved in the passage of local ordinances, more difficulty with enforcement at the local level, and lower compliance with the laws.[66, 67] Several national organizations have expressed opposition to the enactment of preemptive laws, including the American Public Health Association, the Institute of Medicine, and a working group of State attorneys general.

27-20. (Developmental) Reduce the toxicity of tobacco products by establishing a regulatory structure to monitor toxicity.

Potential data source: FDA.

Over the past several years, new technology and the increasing availability of alternative forms of nicotine delivery have prompted discussion of a "harm reduction" approach to tobacco control. Part of this discussion has focused on making tobacco products safer, while acknowledging that there is no such thing as a "safe cigarette." Approaches proposed and debated include the reduction of tar and nicotine levels in tobacco products, the reduction of tobacco-specific nitrosamines, and the reduction of specific additives in tobacco products.

Issues raised by products or technologies that purport to reduce risk require the establishment of an appropriate scientific and regulatory framework within the Federal Government. Much work needs to be done before scientific and regulatory agencies are in a position to evaluate the issues raised by these technologies and to inform the public about risks.

A framework also is needed to ensure that the ongoing activities of Federal agencies, such as the collection of information about tobacco product ingredients and the establishment of protocols for measuring tar and nicotine yields, better serve public health needs. For example, an inadequate method for testing tar and nicotine yields has led to inaccurate information about the tar and nicotine smokers actually receive and a misperception among smokers about the safety of so-called low-tar cigarettes.[68] In addition, information provided by tobacco companies about additives in tobacco products is protected from release to the public.[69]

27-21. Increase the average Federal and State tax on tobacco products.

Target and baseline:

Objective	Increase in Combined Federal and Average State Tax	1998 Baseline	2010 Target
27-21a.	Cigarettes	$0.63*	$2
27-21b.	Spit tobacco	Developmental[†]	

*24 cent Federal tax; 38.9 cent average State tax in 1998.

[†]2.7 cent Federal tax in 1999; 7 States and the District of Columbia did not tax smokeless tobacco products in 1999.

Target setting method: Expert opinion; comparison to international tax rates.

Data source: The Tax Burden on Tobacco, The Tobacco Institute.

As with almost all consumer products, the demand for cigarettes decreases as price increases. An increase in the excise tax on tobacco products would reduce rates of use of both cigarettes and spit tobacco among adults and youth. Economists agree that a 10 percent increase in the price of cigarettes will reduce overall smoking among adults by approximately 4 percent.[63, 70] Data suggest that the prevention effect on youth would be at least as large if not larger.[63, 70]

Likewise, increasing the tax on smokeless tobacco products would reduce demand. Economists have found that a 10 percent increase in the price of spit tobacco products will decrease male youth demand by 5.9 percent.[71]

A 1989 report predicted that for every 10 percent increase in the price of cigarettes, there would be a 7.6 to 12 percent decrease in teen smoking participation rates (that is, whether teens smoke at all).[72] The report concluded that among teens, smoking participation responds more strongly to price than does the amount of daily cigarette consumption. Studies conducted since the release of this report reinforce and support these conclusions.[63, 70, 71] Data also indicate that earmarking funds from an excise tax increase for tobacco prevention and control programs increases both public support for the proposed tax and the public health impact of the price increase.[38, 73]

Related Objectives From Other Focus Areas

1. Access to Quality Health Services
    1-2. Health insurance coverage for clinical preventive services
    1-3. Counseling about health behaviors

3. Cancer
    3-1. Overall cancer deaths
    3-2. Lung cancer deaths

Terminology

(A listing of abbreviations and acronyms used in this publication appears in Appendix H.)

Consumption: The amount of tobacco products consumed or used by the population. Consumption usually is measured in units, such as the number of cigarettes smoked or pounds of spit tobacco used over a given period of time.

Counteradvertising: The placement of pro-health advertisements on TV, on radio, in print, on billboards, on movie trailers, on the Internet, and in other media.

Illegal buy rate: Rate of illegal sales to minors in compliance checks to assess adherence to minors' tobacco access laws.

Nicotine dependency: Highly controlled or compulsive use, use despite harmful effects, withdrawal upon cessation of use, and recurrent drug craving.

Notifiable condition: A disease or risk factor that is reported to the Centers for Disease Control and Prevention by the States and the District of Columbia.

Pharmacotherapy: Medical treatment using pharmaceuticals or drugs.

Preemptive laws: Legislation prohibiting any local jurisdiction from enacting restrictions more stringent than State law or restrictions that may vary from State law.

Secondhand smoke: A mixture of the smoke exhaled by smokers and the smoke that comes from the burning end of the tobacco product.

Serum cotinine: A biological marker for tobacco use and exposure to environmental tobacco smoke measured in the blood. Cotinine is a breakdown product of nicotine.

Spit tobacco: Chewing tobacco, snuff, or smokeless tobacco.

References

[1] U.S. Department of Health and Human Services (HHS). *Reducing the Health Consequences of Smoking: 25 Years of Progress. A Report of the Surgeon General.* HHS Pub. No. (CDC) 89-8411. Atlanta, GA: HHS, Public Health Service (PHS), Centers for Disease Control (CDC), National Center for Chronic Disease Prevention and Health Promotion (NCCDPHP), Office on Smoking and Health (OSH), 1989.

[2] HHS. *The Health Benefits of Smoking Cessation. A Report of the Surgeon General.* HHS Pub. No. (CDC) 90-8416. Atlanta, GA: HHS, PHS, CDC, NCCDPHP, OSH, 1990.

[3] DiFranza, J.R., and Lew, R.A. Effect of maternal cigarette smoking on pregnancy complications and sudden infant death syndrome. *Journal of Family Practice* 40(4):385-394, 1995.

[4] HHS. *The Health Consequences of Using Smokeless Tobacco. A Report of the Advisory Committee to the Surgeon General.* NIH Pub. No. 86-2874. Bethesda, MD: HHS, PHS, CDC, Center for Health Promotion and Education (CHPE), OSH, 1986.

[5] HHS. *The Health Consequences of Smoking: Cancer. A Report of the Surgeon General.* Rockville, MD: HHS, PHS, CDC, CHPE, OSH, 1982.

[6] CDC. Bidi use among urban youth—Massachusetts, March-April 1999. *Morbidity and Mortality Weekly Report* 48(36):796-799, 1999.

[7] Gupta, P.C.; Hammer, III, J.E.; Murti, P.R.; eds. *Control of Tobacco-Related Cancers and Other Diseases; Proceedings of an International Symposium.* Bombay, India: Tata Institute of Fundamental Research, Oxford University Press, 1992.

[8] CDC. Cigarette smoking-attributable mortality and years of potential life lost—United States, 1984. *Morbidity and Mortality Weekly Report* 46(20):444-451, 1997.

[9] CDC. Projected smoking-related deaths among youth—United States. *Morbidity and Mortality Weekly Report* 45:971-974, 1996.

[10] CDC. Medical-care expenditures attributable to cigarette smoking—United States, 1993. *Morbidity and Mortality Weekly Report* 43(26):469-472, 1994.

[11] CDC. Medical-care expenditures attributable to cigarette smoking during pregnancy—United States, 1995. *Morbidity and Mortality Weekly Report* 46:1048-1050, 1997.

[12] HHS. *The Health Consequences of Involuntary Smoking. A Report of the Surgeon General.* Rockville, MD: HHS, PHS, CDC, CHPE, OSH, 1986.

[13] U.S. Environmental Protection Agency (EPA). *Respiratory Health Effects of Passive Smoking: Lung Cancer and Other Disorders.* EPA Pub. No. EPA/600/6-90/006F. Washington, DC: EPA, 1992.

[14] California Environmental Protection Agency. *Health Effects of Exposure to Environmental Tobacco Smoke.* Final Report. Sacramento, CA: the Agency, Office of Environmental Health Hazard Assessment, 1997.

[15] Glantz, S.A., and Parmely, W.W. Passive smoking and heart disease: Mechanism and risk. *Journal of the American Medical Association* 273:1047-1053, 1995.

[16] Howard, G.; Wagenknech, L.E.; Burke, G.E.; et al. Cigarette smoking and progression of atherosclerosis. *Journal of the American Medical Association* 279(2):119-124, 1998.

[17] Pirkle, J.L.; Flegal, K.M.; Bernet, J.T.; et al. Exposure of the U.S. population to environmental tobacco smoke. *Journal of the American Medical Association* 275:1233-1240, 1996.

[18] CDC. State-specific prevalence of cigarette smoking among adults, and children's and adolescents' exposure to environmental tobacco smoke—United States. *Morbidity and Mortality Weekly Report* 46:1038-1043, 1997.

[19] CDC, NCHS. National Health Interview Survey. Unpublished data, 1998.

[20] HHS. *Preventing Tobacco Use Among Young People: A Report of the Surgeon General.* Atlanta, GA: HHS, PHS, CDC, NCCDPHP, OSH, 1994.

[21] HHS. Drug use among teenagers leveling off. *HHS News,* December 17, 1999.

[22] CDC. Tobacco use among high school students—United States, 1997. *Morbidity and Mortality Weekly Report* 47:229-233, 1998.

[23] HHS. *The Health Consequences of Smoking: Nicotine Addiction. A Report of the Surgeon General.* Washington, DC: U.S. Government Printing Office, 1988.

[24] CDC. Smoking cessation during previous year among adults—United States, 1990 and 1991. *Morbidity and Mortality Weekly Report* 42:504-507, 1993.

[25] HHS. *Tobacco Use Among U.S. Racial/Ethnic Minority Groups—African Americans, American Indians, and Alaska Natives, Asian Americans and Pacific Islanders, and Hispanics: A Report of the Surgeon General.* Atlanta, GA: HHS, PHS, CDC, NCCDPHP, OSH, 1998.

[26] National Asian Women's Health Organization. *Smoking Among Asian Americans: A National Tobacco Survey.* San Francisco, CA: the Organization, 1998.

[27] Goebel, K. Lesbians and gays face tobacco targeting. *Tobacco Control* 3:65-67, 1994.

[28] Skinner, W.F. The prevalence and demographic predictors of illicit and licit drug use among lesbians and gay men. *American Journal of Public Health* 84(8):1307-1310, 1994.

[29] Penkower, L.; Dew, M.A.; Kingsley, L.; et al. Behavioral, health and psychosocial factors and risk for HIV infection among sexually active homosexual men: The Multicenter AIDS Cohort Study. *American Journal of Public Health* 81(2):194-196, 1991.

[30] Arday, D.A.; Edlin, B.R.; Giovino, G.A.; et al. Smoking, HIV infection, and gay men in the United States. *Tobacco Control* 2:156-158, 1993.

[31] CDC. Youth Risk Behavior Surveillance: National College Health Risk Behavior Survey—United States, 1995. *Morbidity and Mortality Weekly Report* 46(SS-6):1-56, 1997.

[32] HHS. *Strategies to Control Tobacco Use in the United States: A Blueprint for Public Health Action in the 1990s.* Smoking and Tobacco Control Monograph 1. NIH Pub. No. 92-3316. Bethesda, MD: HHS, PHS, National Institutes of Health (NIH), National Cancer Institute (NCI), 1991.

[33] Pierce, J.P.; Evans, N.; Farkas, A.J.; et al. *Tobacco Use in California: An Evaluation of the Tobacco Control Program, 1989-93.* La Jolla, CA: University of California, San Diego, 1994.

[34] Abt Associates, Inc., for the Massachusetts Department of Public Health. *Independent Evaluation of the Massachusetts Tobacco Control Program.* 2nd Annual Report. Cambridge, MA: Abt Associates, Inc., 1996.

[35] Gostin, L.O.; Arno, P.S.; and Brandt, A.M. FDA regulation of tobacco advertising and youth smoking. Historical, social, and constitutional perspectives. *Journal of the American Medical Association* 277:410-418, 1997.

[36] Tobacco Education Oversight Committee. *Toward a Tobacco-Free California: Exploring a New Frontier.* Report to the California Legislature. February 1993, 69.

[37] Arizona Tobacco Use Prevention Plan <http://www.hs.state.az.us/aztepp>May 12, 1999.

[38] CDC. Cigarette smoking before and after an excise tax increase and an antismoking campaign. *Morbidity and Mortality Weekly Report* 45:966-970, 1996.

[39] CDC. Tobacco use among middle and high school students—Florida, 1998 and 1999. *Morbidity and Mortality Weekly Report* 48:248-253, 1999.

[40] Pechacek, T.F.; Asthma, S.; and Eriksen, M.P. Tobacco: Global burden and community solutions. In: Yusuf, S.; Cairns, J.A.; Camm, A.J.; et al.; eds. *Evidence Based Cardiology.* London, England: BMJ Books, 1998, 165-178.

[41] Glynn, T. Essential elements of school-based smoking prevention programs. *Journal of School Health* 59(5):181-188, 1989.

[42] Botvin, G.J.; Renick, N.L.; and Baker, E. The effects of scheduling format and booster sessions on a broad-spectrum psychosocial smoking prevention. *Journal of Behavioral Medicine* 6(4):359-379, 1983.

[43] Perry, C.L.; Klepp, K.I.; and Sillers, C. Community-wide strategies for cardiovascular health: The Minnesota Heart Health Program youth program. *Health Education Research* 4(1):87-101, 1989.

[44] Pentz, M.A.; Dwyer, J.H.; MacKinnon, D.P.; et al. A multicommunity trial for primary prevention of adolescent drug abuse. Effects on drug use prevalence. *Journal of the American Medical Association* 261(2):3259-3266, 1989.

[45] Vartianen, E.; Fallonen, U.; McAlister, A.L.; et al. Eight-year follow-up results of an adolescent smoking prevention program: The North Karelia Youth Project. *American Journal of Public Health* 80(1):78-79, 1990.

[46] Perry, C.L.; Kelder, S.H.; Murray, D.M.; et al. Community-wide smoking prevention: Long-term outcomes of the Minnesota Heart Health Program and the Class of 1989 Study. *American Journal of Public Health* 82(9):1210-1216, 1992.

[47] Botvin, G.J.; Baker, E.; Dusenbury, L.; et al. Long-term follow-up results of a randomized drug abuse prevention trial in a white middle-class population. *Journal of the American Medical Association* 273(14):1106-1112, 1995.

[48] CDC. Guidelines for school health programs to prevent tobacco use and addiction. *Morbidity and Mortality Weekly Report* 43:1-18, 1994.

[49] CDC. Addition of prevalence of cigarette smoking as a nationally notifiable condition—June 1996. *Morbidity and Mortality Weekly Report* 45:537, 1996.

[50] HHS. *Smoking Cessation: Clinical Practice Guideline.* No. 18. HHS Pub. No. (AHCPR) 96-0692. Washington, DC: HHS, PHS, Agency for Health Care Policy and Research, 1996.

[51] Monitoring the Future Project 1997. *Public Use Data Tapes, 1992–95.* 1992–95 combined data. Ann Arbor, MI: University of Michigan, Institute for Social Research.

[52] McPhillips-Tangrum, C. Results from the first annual survey on addressing tobacco in managed care. *Tobacco Control* 7:S11-S13, 1998.

[53] Zebrek, A. *Medicaid and Indigent Care: Smoking Cessation.* Washington, DC: Health Policy Tracking Service, 1998.

[54] Gerlach, K.; Shopland, D.R.; Hartman, A.M.; et al. Workplace smoking policies in the United States: Results from a national survey of more than 100,000 workers. *Tobacco Control* 6:199-206, 1997.

[55] Siegel, M. Involuntary smoking in the restaurant workplace. *Journal of the American Medical Association* 270:490-493, 1993.

[56] Mannino, D.M.; Siegel, M.; Husten, C.; et al. Environmental tobacco smoke exposure and health effects in children: Results from the 1991 National Health Interview Survey. *Tobacco Control* 5:13-18, 1996.

[57] DiFranza, J.R., and Lew, R.A. Morbidity and mortality in children associated with the use of tobacco products by other people. *Pediatrics* 97:560-568, 1996.

[58] American Academy of Pediatrics, Committee on Environmental Health. Environmental tobacco smoke: A hazard to children. *Pediatrics* 99:639-642, 1997.

[59] Kann, L.; Kinchen, S.A.; William, B.I.; et al. Youth risk behavior surveillance—United States, 1997. *Morbidity and Mortality Weekly Report* 47(SS-3):1-89, 1998.

[60] CDC. Accessibility of tobacco products to youths aged 12-17—United States, 1989–1993. *Morbidity and Mortality Weekly Report* 45:125-130, 1996.

[61] Widley, M.B.; Woodruff, S.I.; Pamplone, S.Z.; et al. Self-service sale of tobacco: How it contributes to youth access. *Tobacco Control* 4:355-361, 1995.

[62] Substance Abuse and Mental Health Services Administration. Tobacco Regulation for Substance Abuse Prevention and Treatment Block Grants. Final Rule. *Federal Register* (16)13:1492-1500, 1996.

[63] Chaloupka, F., and Grossman, M. *National Bureau of Economic Research Working Paper.* No. 5740. Cambridge, MA: National Bureau of Economic Research, 1996.

[64] Manley, M.; Pierce, J.P.; Gilpin, E.A.; et al. Impact of the American Stop Smoking Intervention Study on cigarette consumption. *Tobacco Control* 6:S12-S16, 1997.

[65] Conlisk, E.; Siegel, M.; Lengerich, E.; et al. The status of local smoking regulations in North Carolina following a state preemption bill. *Journal of the American Medical Association* 273:805-807, 1995.

[66] Jordan, J.; Pertschuk M.; and Carol, J. *Preemption in Tobacco Control: History, Current Issues, and Future Concerns.* No. 97-0424. Berkeley, CA: Americans for Nonsmokers' Rights/Western Consortium for Public Health, 1994.

[67] Fishman, J.A.; Allison, H.; Knowles, S.B.; et al. State laws on tobacco control—United States. *Morbidity and Mortality Weekly Report* 48(SS-3):21-62, 1998.

[68] HHS. *The FTC Cigarette Test Method for Determining Tar, Nicotine, and Carbon Monoxide Yields of U.S. Cigarettes: A Report of the NCI Expert Committee.* NIH Pub. No. 96-4028. Bethesda, MD: HHS, PHS, NIH, NCI, 1996.

[69] Public Law 99-252, Section 4. The Comprehensive Smokeless Tobacco and Health Education Act of 1986.

[70] U.S. Department of Treasury (DOT). *The Economic Costs of Smoking in the United States and the Benefits of Comprehensive Tobacco Legislation.* Department of Treasury Working Paper Series. Washington, DC: DOT, 1998.

[71] Chaloupka, F.J.; Tauras, J.A.; and Grossman, M. Public policy and youth smokeless tobacco use. *Southern Economic Journal* 64(2):503-516, 1997.

[72] General Accounting Office. *Teen Smoking: Higher Excise Tax Should Significantly Reduce the Number of Smokers. A Report to the Honorable Michael A. Andrews, House of Representatives.* GAO/HRD 89-119. Rockville, MD: GAO, 1989.

[73] CDC. Tobacco tax initiative—Oregon, 1996. *Morbidity and Mortality Weekly Report* 46:246-248, 1997.

28

Vision and Hearing

Lead Agency: National Institutes of Health

Contents

Goal

Improve the visual and hearing health of the Nation through prevention, early detection, treatment, and rehabilitation.

Overview

Among the five senses, people depend on vision and hearing to provide the primary cues for conducting the basic activities of daily life. At the most basic level, vision and hearing permit people to navigate and to stay oriented within their environment. These senses provide the portals for language, whether spoken, signed, or read. They are critical to most work and recreation and allow people to interact more fully. For these reasons, vision and hearing are defining elements of the quality of life. Either, or both, of these senses may be diminished or lost because of heredity, aging, injury, or disease. Such loss may occur gradually, over the course of a lifetime, or traumatically in an instant. Conditions of vision or hearing loss that are linked with chronic and disabling diseases pose additional challenges for patients and their families. From the public health perspective, the prevention of either the initial impairment or additional impairment from these environmentally orienting and socially connecting senses requires significant resources. Prevention of vision or hearing loss or their resulting disabling conditions through the development of improved disease prevention, detection, or treatment methods or more effective rehabilitative strategies must remain a priority.

Vision

Issues and Trends

Vision is an essential part of everyday life, depended on constantly by people at all ages. Vision affects development, learning, communicating, working, health, and quality of life. In the United States, an estimated 80 million people have potentially blinding eye diseases, 3 million have low vision, 1.1 million people are legally blind, and 200,000 are more severely visually impaired.[1]

In 1981, the economic impact of visual disorders and disabilities was approximately $14.1 billion per year.[2] By 1995, this figure was estimated to have risen to more than $38.4 billion—$22.3 billion in direct costs and another $16.1 billion in indirect costs each year.[3]

Estimates of the number of people in the United States with visual impairment vary with its definition. Legal blindness represents an artificial distinction and has little value for rehabilitation but is a significant policy issue, determining eligibility for certain disability benefits from the Federal Government. Because of their reliance on narrow definitions of visual impairment, many estimates of the number of people with low vision are understated. When low vision is more broadly defined as visual problems that hamper the performance and enjoyment of everyday activities, almost 14 million persons are estimated to have low vision. Visual impairment is 1 of the 10 most frequent causes of disability in the United States.[4] In children, visual impairment is associated with developmental delays and the need for special educational, vocational, and social services, often into adulthood. In adults, visual impairment may result in loss of personal independence, decreased quality of life, and difficulty in maintaining employment. Impairment may lead to the need for disability payment, vocational and social services, and nursing home or assisted living placement.

The leading causes of visual impairment are diabetic retinopathy, cataract, glaucoma, and age-related macular degeneration (AMD). People with diabetes are at risk of developing diabetic retinopathy, a major cause of blindness. Because early diagnosis and timely treatment have been shown to prevent vision loss in more than 90 percent of patients, health care practice guidelines recommend an annual dilated eye examination for all people with diabetes.[5, 6] Studies indicate, however, that many people with diabetes do not get an annual dilated eye examination. An estimated 50 percent of patients are diagnosed too late for treatment to be effective. People with diabetes also are more likely to have cataracts and glaucoma.

Glaucoma is a major public health problem in this country. The disease causes progressive optic nerve damage that, if left untreated, leads to blindness. An estimated 3 million people in the United States have the disease;[7] of these, as many as 120,000 are blind as a result.[8] Furthermore, glaucoma is the number one cause of blindness in African Americans. Treatments to slow the progression of the disease are available. However, at least half of the people who have glaucoma are not receiving treatment because they are unaware of their condition. Blindness from glaucoma is believed to impose significant costs annually on the Federal Government in Social Security benefits, lost tax revenues, and health care expenditures.

While important strides have been made in the prevention and treatment of eye disease, there is no cure for many causes of vision loss, particularly AMD. In addition to being a leading cause of blindness in the United States, AMD is a leading cause of low vision. People with low vision often cannot perform daily routine activities, such as reading the newspaper, preparing meals, or recognizing faces of friends. The inability to see well affects functional capabilities and social interactions and can lead to a loss of independence.

Myopia, or nearsightedness, is a common condition in which images of distant objects are focused in front of, instead of on, the retina. Myopia occurs in approximately 25 percent of the U.S. population.[9] In children, myopia is found in 2 percent of those entering first grade and 15 percent of those entering high school.[10]

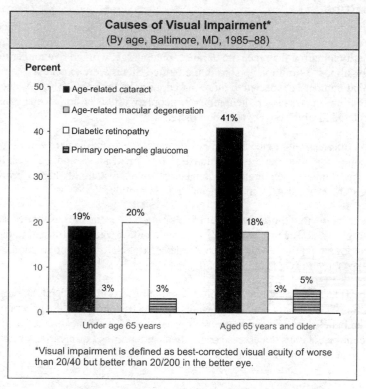

Causes of Visual Impairment*
(By age, Baltimore, MD, 1985–88)

Percent

- ■ Age-related cataract
- ▨ Age-related macular degeneration
- ☐ Diabetic retinopathy
- ▤ Primary open-angle glaucoma

Under age 65 years: 19%, 3%, 20%, 3%

Aged 65 years and older: 41%, 18%, 3%, 5%

*Visual impairment is defined as best-corrected visual acuity of worse than 20/40 but better than 20/200 in the better eye.

Source: Rahmani, B.; Tielsch, J.; Katz, J.; et al. The cause-specific prevalence of visual impairments in an urban population: The Baltimore Eye Survey. *Ophthalmology* 103(11):1721–1725, November 1996.

Many infants and young children are at high risk for vision problems because of hereditary, prenatal, or perinatal factors. These individuals need to be identified and tested early and annually to make sure their eyes and visual system are functioning normally. Research in the 1980s and 1990s found that amblyopia, a leading cause of visual impairment in children, results from visual problems in very early life.[11] These problems can be prevented or reversed with early detection and appropriate intervention.

While nothing medically can be done for patients with low vision, their quality of life can be greatly improved. Many low vision services and devices are available to help patients maintain their independence. Generally, devices fall into two categories: visual and adaptive. Visual devices use lenses or combinations of lenses to provide magnification. They include such aids as magnifying spectacles, hand-held magnifiers, stand magnifiers, computer monitors with large type, and closed-circuit televisions. Adaptive devices include large-print reading materials (books, newspapers), check writing guides, and high-contrast watch dials. Also in this latter category are auditory aids, such as talking computers.

Disparities

More than two-thirds of visually impaired adults are over age 65 years. Although no gender differences exist in the number of older adults with vision problems, more women are visually impaired than men are because, on average, women live longer than men do. By 1999, almost 34 million persons in the United States were expected to be over age 65 years; that number is expected to more than double by the year 2030.[12] As the population of older adults grows larger, the number of people with visual impairment and other aging-related disabilities is expected to increase.

African Americans are twice as likely to be visually impaired as are whites of comparable socioeconomic status.[1] Studies conducted in the United States and the West Indies have shown that primary open-angle glaucoma exists in a substantially higher proportion of Caribbean blacks and African Americans than in whites.[7, 13, 14]

Hispanics have three times the risk of developing type 2 diabetes as whites, and they also have a higher risk of complications.[15] Available data suggest that visual impairment may be an important public health problem in the Mexican-Hispanic population.[16] There also is a higher rate of myopia in Asian children.[17]

Many barriers still need to be overcome in reducing vision disorders. Among the major prevention strategies are educating health care professionals and the general population about the benefits of prevention, improving access to quality health care across socioeconomic classes to decrease disparities, and gaining cooperation of families in the screening and treatment of infants and children.

Opportunities

Blindness and visual impairment from most eye diseases and disorders can be reduced with early detection and treatment. Most eye diseases, however, lack symptoms until vision is lost. Vision that is lost cannot be restored. Therefore, early intervention through regular vision exams needs to be emphasized. Health education programs directed at groups at higher risk for eye diseases and disorders are essential in preventing blindness and visual impairments. The incorporation of vision into health education programs can be beneficial to participants and to agencies seeking to provide quality care to their clients.

The prevention of blindness and visual impairment and the promotion of eye health often result in improved health status and reduced risk factors for illness, disability, and death from diseases and injuries across all age groups. Translation of scientific advances can help people who are blind and visually impaired maintain their quality of life and independence.

Issues and Trends

An estimated 28 million people in the United States are deaf or hard of hearing.[18] Some 1,465,000 individuals aged 3 years or older are deaf in both ears.[19] Deafness or hearing impairment may be caused by genetic factors, noise or trauma, sensitivity to certain drugs or medications, and viral or bacterial infections.

Language is the set of rules that allow for the sharing of thoughts, ideas, and emotions. Speaking is one way that language can be expressed. Language also is expressed in writing or through sign language by some groups of individuals. In some cases, language can be expressed in additional ways by people who have neurological disorders. The most intensive period for development of language, either spoken or signed, is during the first 3 years of life. This is the period when the brain is developing and maturing. The skills associated with effective acquisition of language, either speech or sign, depend on exposure to, and manipulation of, these communication tools. Early identification of deafness or hearing loss is a critical factor in preventing or ameliorating language delay or disorder in children who are deaf or hard of hearing, allowing appropriate intervention or rehabilitation to begin while the developing brain is ready. Early identification and intervention have lifelong implications for the child's understanding and use of language.

The standard estimate of congenital hearing loss (1 in 1,000 live births) appears to underestimate actual congenital hearing loss as reported in data from States with universal newborn screening programs. Estimates based on emerging data place the number at 2 to 3 per 1,000 live births.[20] These data do not include children who are born with normal hearing but have late-onset or progressive hearing loss. Hearing loss often is sufficient to prevent the spontaneous development of spoken language.[21, 22, 23, 24] More than 50 percent of childhood hearing impairments are believed to be of genetic origin.[25] Earliest possible identification of infant hearing loss has been endorsed widely as critical for the developing child. Minimal hearing loss also is an important factor in school success and psychosocial development.[26]

Estimates for the average age of diagnosis of hearing loss in infants and children range from 14 months[27] to around 3 years.[28] This delay of diagnosis is significant in terms of time lost for rehabilitation and time lost during unique opportunities provided by brain development in the infant and young child for language acquisition, spoken or signed. Nearly 15 percent of children have a low-frequency or high-frequency hearing loss.[29] Strategies for intervention or rehabilitation depend on the kind of hearing loss, age of onset, services available, and family preferences. Strategies include hearing aids, augmentative and assistive devices, oral-auditory instruction, sign language instruction, interpreter services, cued speech, cochlear implant, or combinations of these devices and strategies.

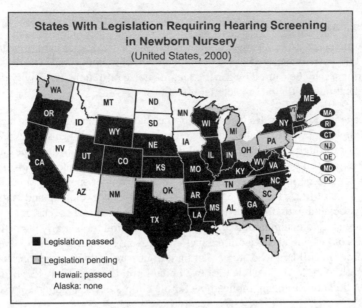

**States With Legislation Requiring Hearing Screening
in Newborn Nursery**
(United States, 2000)

■ Legislation passed
□ Legislation pending
Hawaii: passed
Alaska: none

Source: American Speech-Language-Hearing Association.
<http://www.asha.org/infant_hearing/overview.htm> May 19, 2000.

More than 300 inherited syndromes involve hearing impairment.[30, 31] Hereditary hearing loss can be either syndromic (accompanied by other characteristics, such as visual impairment) or nonsyndromic (where hearing loss is the only identifiable characteristic). Not all hereditary hearing loss is present at birth. Some hereditary hearing loss may be progressive or may appear later in childhood or adulthood as late-onset hearing impairment or deafness. One cause of late-onset hearing loss is otosclerosis. Otosclerosis, an abnormal growth of bone in the middle ear, results in gradual loss of hearing and affects 1 out of 100 adults in the U.S. population. Another form of hearing loss is Meniere's disease,[32] which causes bilateral, often fluctuating, hearing loss in 20 to 40 percent of cases, usually in conjunction with balance disorder and tinnitus.

Otitis media, or middle ear infection, accounts for 24.5 million visits to doctors' offices[33] and is the most frequent reason cited for taking children to the emergency department.[34] Health care costs for otitis media in the United States have been reported to be $3 billion to $5 billion per year.[35] Otitis media often occurs in repeated bouts, causing periods of hearing loss that can affect children during the critical time for language and speech acquisition and hamper children in a variety of learning environments.

Approximately 10 million persons in the United States have permanent, irreversible hearing loss from noise or trauma.[36] Additionally, 30 million people are estimated to be exposed to injurious levels of noise each day. Noise-induced hearing loss (NIHL) is the most common occupational disease and the second most self-reported occupational illness or injury.[37] In industry-specific studies, 44 percent of carpenters and 48 percent of

Healthy People 2010: Objectives for Improving Health

plumbers reported they had a perceived hearing loss.[38] Ninety percent of coal miners are estimated to have a hearing impairment by age 52 years,[39] and 70 percent of male metal and nonmetal miners will experience a hearing impairment by age 60 years.[40] (See Focus Area 20. Occupational Safety and Health.)

Data indicate that people are losing hearing earlier in life and that men are more frequently affected in the 35- to 60-year-old age group.[41] Noise-induced hearing loss can be the result of a traumatic, sudden level of impulse noise, such as an explosion, that can leave an individual immediately and permanently deafened; the result of continuing exposure to high levels of sound in the workplace or in recreational settings; the consequence of years of exposure causing subtle, progressive damage; or exacerbated due to individual vulnerability to noise. Noise-induced hearing loss is related to noise level, proximity to the harmful sound, time of exposure, and individual susceptibility. Many of these causes can be controlled by prevention. Prevention of noise-induced hearing loss is necessary for people both on and off the job.

Disparities

The work environment of the 21st century will require intense use of communication and information skills and technologies. The individual who has a communication disability, disorder, or difference will be at a disadvantage.

Data show that students with disabilities, including hearing impairment and deafness, are disproportionately disadvantaged.[42] The average reading level for deaf persons aged 18 years is estimated at the fourth grade.[43] Early intervention for language acquisition, spoken or signed, can improve later ability to use language. Hearing impairments also are a major barrier to health care access and information.[44, 45] (See Focus Area 6. Disability and Secondary Conditions.)

Older people also are a major concern in terms of hearing health disparity. Presbycusis, the loss of hearing associated with aging, affects about 30 percent of adults who are aged 65 years and older.[46] About half of the population over age 75 years has a significant hearing loss.[47] As the population ages and lives longer, these numbers are increasing. Only about one-fourth of those who could benefit from a hearing aid actually use one.[48] More than 8 percent of the population aged 70 years and older report both hearing and vision impairment.[49] With the exception of increased hearing loss in men, there are no currently available data on these disparities.

Opportunities

Two activities have yielded opportunity for early identification and intervention for infants who are born deaf or with hearing impairments. As of 1999, 20 States had laws requiring hearing screening in the newborn nursery. Early identification allows for language acquisition, either spoken or signed, during the critical time period when the child is developing communication skills. Research in the field of molecular genetics has identified genes that contribute to hereditary hearing impairment. The potential exists for early identification and intervention for hearing impairment. Identifying individuals who may experience late-onset or progressive hearing loss provides time to make the appropriate treatment or rehabilitation options available.

Public education can promote hearing health and behavior to reduce noise-induced hearing loss, which is a fully preventable condition. An education effort, WISE EARS!,[50] has been launched by a coalition of government agencies headed by the National Institute on Deafness and Other Communication Disorders at the National Institutes of Health and the National Institute on Occupational Safety and Health at the Centers for Disease Control and Prevention. They have joined with State agencies; some 70 public interest, advocacy, and patient organizations; businesses; industries; and unions as well as health professional organizations in a national effort to educate the public about ear defense. The education effort focuses both on the public, with special emphasis on children, and on the workforce and has important World Wide Web-based components.

A further opportunity exists with noise-induced hearing loss prevention. Tinnitus, a ringing, buzzing, or roaring in the ears, is a symptom that accompanies many forms of hearing loss and can be debilitating. Data indicate that tinnitus affects almost 15 percent of adults aged 45 years and older.[51] Because tinnitus often is associated with preventable noise-induced hearing loss, hearing protection is key to reducing one important cause of tinnitus.

Assistive technologies are providing additional strategies for individuals with disabilities. For individuals who are deaf or hard of hearing, improved technologies will facilitate their ability to have an equal opportunity in the workplace and in society. (See Focus Area 6. Disability and Secondary Conditions.)

Early identification for improved intervention strategies, prevention of noise-induced hearing loss through health education, and the development of innovations in assistive technology could improve significantly the hearing health of the Nation.

Interim Progress Toward Year 2000 Objectives

Three Healthy People 2000 objectives addressed vision and hearing. Two of these objectives, to reduce the number of cases of significant hearing impairment and to reduce the number of cases of significant visual impairment, have shown progress toward the targets. One objective, early detection of significant hearing impairment, shows no change from baseline.

Note: Unless otherwise noted, data are from the Centers for Disease Control and Prevention, National Center for Health Statistics, *Healthy People 2000 Review, 1998–99.*

Vision and Hearing

Goal: Improve the visual and hearing health of the Nation through prevention, early detection, treatment, and rehabilitation.

Number	Objective Short Title
Vision	
28-1	Dilated eye examinations
28-2	Vision screening for children
28-3	Impairment due to refractive errors
28-4	Impairment in children and adolescents
28-5	Impairment due to diabetic retinopathy
28-6	Impairment due to glaucoma
28-7	Impairment due to cataract
28-8	Occupational eye injury
28-9	Protective eyewear
28-10	Vision rehabilitation services and devices
Hearing	
28-11	Newborn hearing screening, evaluation, and intervention
28-12	Otitis media
28-13	Rehabilitation for hearing impairment
28-14	Hearing examination
28-15	Evaluation and treatment referrals
28-16	Hearing protection
28-17	Noise-induced hearing loss in children
28-18	Noise-induced hearing loss in adults

Vision

28-1. (Developmental) Increase the proportion of persons who have a dilated eye examination at appropriate intervals.

Potential data source: National Health Interview Survey (NHIS), CDC, NCHS.

Many eye diseases and disorders have no symptoms or early warning signs. Dilated eye examinations should be performed at appropriate intervals to detect changes in the retina or optic nerve or both. Eye care professionals can view the back of the eye for subtle changes and, if necessary, initiate treatment at the right time.

28-2. (Developmental) Increase the proportion of preschool children aged 5 years and under who receive vision screening.

Potential data source: National Health Interview Survey (NHIS), CDC, NCHS.

Many vision problems begin well before children reach school. Every effort must be made to ensure that, before they reach age 5 years, children receive a screening examination from their health care provider. Early recognition of disease results in more effective treatment that can be sight-saving or even life-saving.

28-3. (Developmental) Reduce uncorrected visual impairment due to refractive errors.

Potential data source: National Health and Nutrition Examination Survey (NHANES), CDC, NCHS.

28-4. Reduce blindness and visual impairment in children and adolescents aged 17 years and under.

Target: 20 per 1,000 children and adolescents aged 17 years and under.

Baseline: 25 per 1,000 children and adolescents aged 17 years and under were blind or visually impaired in 1997.

Target setting method: Better than the best.

Data source: National Health Interview Survey (NHIS), CDC, NCHS.

Children and Adolescents Aged 17 Years and Under, 1997	Blindness and Visual Impairment
	Rate per 1,000
TOTAL	25
Race and ethnicity	
American Indian or Alaska Native	DSU
Asian or Pacific Islander	DSU
Asian	DSU
Native Hawaiian or other Pacific Islander	DSU
Black or African American	27
White	24
Hispanic or Latino	23
Not Hispanic or Latino	25
Black or African American	27
White	25
Gender	
Female	24
Male	26
Family income level	
Poor	39
Near poor	30
Middle/high income	20
Disability status	
Persons with disabilities	92
Persons without disabilities	19

DNA = Data have not been analyzed. DNC = Data are not collected. DSU = Data are statistically unreliable.

28-5. (Developmental) Reduce visual impairment due to diabetic retinopathy.

Potential data source: National Health Interview Survey (NHIS), CDC, NCHS.

28-6. (Developmental) Reduce visual impairment due to glaucoma.

Potential data source: National Health Interview Survey (NHIS), CDC, NCHS.

28-7. (Developmental) Reduce visual impairment due to cataract.

Potential data source: National Health Interview Survey (NHIS), CDC, NCHS.

28-8. (Developmental) Reduce occupational eye injury.

Potential data sources: Annual Survey of Occupational Injuries and Illnesses (ASOII), U.S. Department of Labor, Bureau of Labor Statistics; National Electronic Injury Surveillance System (NEISS), CPSC, and NIOSH.

28-9. (Developmental) Increase the use of appropriate personal protective eyewear in recreational activities and hazardous situations around the home.

Potential data source: National Health Interview Survey (NHIS), CDC, NCHS.

Almost all eye injuries can be prevented. Many sports and recreation activities, including baseball, basketball, tennis, racquetball, and hockey, carry some risk of eye injury. Some injuries may go unnoticed because only one eye is involved. Activities at home, such as cooking and yard work, also may present eye injury risk.

28-10. (Developmental) Increase vision rehabilitation.

28-10a. Increase the use of rehabilitation services by persons with visual impairments.

28-10b. Increase the use of visual and adaptive devices by persons with visual impairments.

Potential data source: National Health Interview Survey (NHIS), CDC, NCHS.

Hearing

28-11. (Developmental) Increase the proportion of newborns who are screened for hearing loss by age 1 month, have audiologic evaluation by age 3 months, and are enrolled in appropriate intervention services by age 6 months.

Potential data sources: State-based Early Hearing Detection and Intervention (EHDI) Program Network, CDC and/or specific State data.

28-12. Reduce otitis media in children and adolescents.

Target: 294 visits per 1,000 children and adolescents under age 18 years.

Baseline: 344.7 visits per 1,000 children and adolescents under age 18 years were for otitis media in 1997.

Target setting method: Better than the best.

Data sources: National Ambulatory Medical Care Survey (NAMCS), CDC, NCHS; National Hospital Ambulatory Medical Care Survey (NHAMCS), CDC, NCHS.

Children and Adolescents Under Age 18 Years, 1997	Visits for Otitis Media
	Rate per 1,000
TOTAL	344.7
Race and ethnicity	
American Indian or Alaska Native	DSU
Asian or Pacific Islander	DSU
Asian	DNC
Native Hawaiian or other Pacific Islander	DNC
Black or African American	294.9
White	369.1
Hispanic or Latino	DSU
Not Hispanic or Latino	DSU
Gender	
Female	321.8
Male	366.5
Age	
Under 3 years	1,160.4
3 to 5 years	456.6
6 to 17 years	113.8
Family income level	
Poor	DNC
Near poor	DNC
Middle/high income	DNC
Disability status	
Persons with activity limitations	DNC
Persons without activity limitations	DNC

DNA = Data have not been analyzed. DNC = Data are not collected. DSU = Data are statistically unreliable.

28-13. (Developmental) Increase access by persons who have hearing impairments to hearing rehabilitation services and adaptive devices, including hearing aids, cochlear implants, or tactile or other assistive or augmentative devices.

Potential data sources: National Health Interview Survey (NHIS), CDC, NCHS; National Health and Nutrition Examination Survey (NHANES), CDC, NCHS.

28-14. (Developmental) Increase the proportion of persons who have had a hearing examination on schedule.

Potential data sources: National Health Interview Survey (NHIS), CDC, NCHS; National Health and Nutrition Examination Survey (NHANES), CDC, NCHS.

Audiologic screening serves both primary and secondary prevention purposes, resulting in prevention and amelioration of the effects of hearing loss using developmentally appropriate assessment and treatment. Differing milestones and screening strategies are needed for pediatric populations depending upon their status for impairment screening, disorder screening, or disability screening and their age from birth through 18 years. In the adult population, both impairment and disability screening should occur every decade after age 18 years until age 50 years with more frequent monitoring after age 50 years.[52]

28-15. (Developmental) Increase the number of persons who are referred by their primary care physician for hearing evaluation and treatment.

Potential data sources: National Ambulatory Medical Care Survey (NAMCS), CDC, NCHS; National Health Interview Survey (NHIS), CDC, NCHS.

28-16. (Developmental) Increase the use of appropriate ear protection devices, equipment, and practices.

Potential data source: National Health Interview Survey (NHIS), CDC, NCHS.

Noise-induced hearing loss (NIHL) can be caused by one-time exposure to an impulse noise, such as gunfire or an explosion, or by repeated exposure to sounds at various levels over an extended period of time from sources such as combustion engines, electric motors, or woodworking equipment. The effects of NIHL may be immediate hearing loss that is permanent—resulting from an impulse sound that severely damages the structures of the inner ear—and may be accompanied by tinnitus. Tinnitus is a ringing, buzzing, or roaring in the ears or head. Hearing loss and tinnitus may be experienced in one or both ears. Tinnitus may continue constantly or intermittently throughout a lifetime. The damage that occurs slowly over years of continuous exposure to loud noise is accompanied by various changes in the structure of the hair cells. It also results in hearing loss and tinnitus. Both forms of hearing loss can be prevented. For the worker, hearing conservation involves engineering controls, noise monitoring and measuring, employee notification, audiometric testing and evaluation, health education, and followup that includes hearing protection and fitting and/or audiologic/otologic evaluation.[53, 54] For the public, knowledge of potentially dangerous noise, fitting and use of hearing protection, careful product selection, and audiologic/otologic evaluation are all significant factors in prevention of NIHL.

28-17. (Developmental) Reduce noise-induced hearing loss in children and adolescents aged 17 years and under.

Potential data source: National Health and Nutrition Examination Survey (NHANES), CDC, NCHS.

28-18. (Developmental) Reduce adult hearing loss in the noise-exposed public.

Potential data sources: National Health Interview Survey (NHIS), CDC, NCHS; National Health and Nutrition Examination Survey (NHANES), CDC, NCHS.

Related Objectives From Other Focus Areas

5. **Diabetes**
    5-13. Annual dilated eye examinations
6. **Disability and Secondary Conditions**
    6-11. Assistive devices and technology
20. **Occupational Safety and Health**
    20-11. Work-related, noise-induced hearing loss

Terminology

(A listing of abbreviations and acronyms used in this publication appears in Appendix H.)

Age-related macular degeneration (AMD): Deterioration of the macula that results in a loss of sharp central vision.

Amblyopia: Developmental abnormality of the central nervous system that causes impaired vision in one or both eyes.

Assistive devices: Technical tools and devices used to aid individuals who have communication disorders in performing actions, tasks, and activities. Examples of assistive devices include alphabet boards, text telephones (TT/TTY/TDD), and text-to-speech conversion software. (See Focus Area 6. Disability and Secondary Conditions.)

Audiologic evaluation: Tests and procedures that measure the ability to hear. Identifies type and degree of hearing loss. Included are tests of conduction, speech perception and speech discrimination, and case history; can include a central test battery. Evaluation can include recommendations about appropriate assistive devices.

Augmentive devices: Tools that help individuals with limited or absent speech to communicate, such as communication boards, pictographs (symbols that look like the things they represent), and ideographs (symbols representing ideas).

Cataract: Cloudiness of the lens that may prevent a clear image from forming on the retina.

Cochlear implant: Medical device that bypasses damaged structures in the inner ear and directly stimulates the auditory nerve, allowing some deaf individuals to hear and to maintain or develop speech and language.

Cued speech: Method of communication that combines speech reading with a system of handshapes placed near the mouth to help deaf or hard-of-hearing individuals differentiate words that look similar on the lips (for example, "bunch" versus "punch") or understand words when the lips do not move (for example, "kick").

Diabetic retinopathy: Complication of diabetes that damages the retina.

Dilate: Process by which the pupil is temporarily enlarged with special eyedrops, allowing the eyecare specialist to view the fundus better.

Ear infection: See *Otitis media*.

Fundus: Interior posterior lining of the eye that includes the retina, optic nerve, and macula.

Hearing aid: Electronic device that brings amplified sound to the ear. A hearing aid usually consists of a microphone, amplifier, and receiver.

Hereditary hearing loss: Hearing loss passed down through generations of a family—that is, with a genetic basis.

Legal blindness: Determines eligibility for benefits from the Federal Government; however, it has little or no value for rehabilitation purposes.

Low vision (limited vision): A visual impairment, not correctable by standard eyeglasses or contact lenses, medication, or surgery, that interferes with an individual's ability to perform activities of daily living.

Meniere's disease: Inner ear disorder that can affect both hearing and balance and can cause episodes of vertigo, hearing loss, tinnitus, and the sensation of fullness in the ear.

Myopia: Nearsightedness, or the ability to see close objects more clearly than distant objects. Myopia may be compensated for with glasses or contact lenses.

Noise-induced hearing loss: Hearing loss that is caused by either a one-time exposure to very loud sound(s) or by repeated exposure to sounds at various loudness levels over an extended period of time. Hearing loss may be temporary or permanent.

Nonsyndromic hereditary hearing loss: Hearing loss or deafness that is inherited and is not associated with other inherited features.

Open angle glaucoma: Disease characterized by increased intraocular pressure that damages the optic nerve.

Optic nerve: Bundle of over 1 million nerve fibers that carry visual messages from the retina to the brain.

Oral-auditory instruction: Techniques used with persons who have hearing loss to improve their ability to speak—for example, speechreading, communication management, language and auditory skill development, and counseling.

Otitis media: Commonly called ear infection; an inflammation of the middle ear caused by viral or bacterial infection.

Otosclerosis: An abnormal growth of bone in the middle ear that results in gradual loss of hearing and affects 1 out of 100 adults in the U.S. population.

Presbycusis: Loss of hearing that gradually occurs because of inner or middle ear changes in some individuals as they grow older.

Rehabilitation: As used in this focus area, addresses the needs in daily living skills that are directly related to vision or hearing loss.

Retina: Light-sensitive layer of tissue that lines the back of the eyeball. The retina sends visual impulses through the optic nerve to the brain.

Sign language: Hand movements, gestures, and facial expressions that convey grammatical structure and meaning.

Syndromic hereditary hearing loss: Hearing loss or deafness that is inherited or passed down through generations of a family along with other features.

Tactile devices: Mechanical instruments that make use of touch to help individuals to communicate who have certain disabilities, such as deafness and blindness.

Tinnitus: Sensation of a ringing, roaring, or buzzing sound in the ears or head. Tinnitus is often associated with various forms of hearing impairment.

Visual aid: Optical and nonoptical devices that help people with low vision make use of their remaining sight.

Visual field: Entire area that can be seen when the eye is looking forward, including peripheral vision.

References

[1] Teilsch, J.M.; Sommer, A.; Will, K..; et al. Blindness and visual impairment in an American urban population. The Baltimore Eye Survey. *Archives of Ophthalmology* 108:286-290, 1990.

[2] Hu, T. *Economic Costs of Visual Disorders and Disabilities, Special Report to the National Eye Institute (NEI), National Institutes of Health (NIH), United States.* 1981.

[3] Ellwein, L. Personal communication. Bethesda, MD: NIH, NEI, 1998.

[4] Verbrugge, L.M., and Patrick, D.L. Seven chronic conditions: Their impact on U.S. adults' activity levels and use of medical services. *American Journal of Public Health* 85:173-182, 1995.

[5] Ferris, I. The Early Treatment Diabetic Retinopathy Study Research Group. How Effective are Treatments for Diabetic Retinopathy? *Journal of the American Medical Association* 269(10):1290-1291, 1993.

[6] American Diabetes Association. Clinical practice recommendations 1999. *Diabetes Care* 22(Suppl. 1):S70-S73.

[7] Rahmani, B.; Tielsch, J.; Katz, J.; et al. The cause-specific prevalence of visual impairment in an urban population, the Baltimore Eye Survey. *Ophthalmology* 103(11):1721-1726, 1996.

[8] Kahn, H.A., and Moorhead, H.B. *Statistics on Blindness in the Model Reporting Area, 1969–70.* Pub. No. (NIH) 73-427. Washington, DC: U.S. Department of Health, Education, and Welfare, Public Health Service, 1973, 120-143.

[9] Sperduto, R.D.; Siegel, D.; Roberts, J.; et al. Prevalence of myopia in the United States. *Archives of Ophthalmology* 101(3):405–407, 1983.

[10] Zadnik, K. The Glenn A. Fry Award lecture 1995. Myopia development in childhood. *Optometry and Vision Science* 74(8):603-608, 1997.

[11] Levi, D.M., and Carkeet, A.C. Amblyopia: A consequence of abnormal visual development. In Simons, K., ed. *Early Visual Development—Normal and Abnormal.* New York: Oxford University Press, 1993, 391-408.

[12] U.S. Bureau of the Census. Population Projections. http://www.census.gov/population/ www/projections/projections/popproj.html>November 24, 1999.

[13] Klein, B.E.K.; Klein, R.; Sponsel, W.; et al. Prevalence of glaucoma, the Beaver Dam Eye Study Group. *Ophthalmology* 99(10):1499-1504, 1992.

[14] Leske, M.C.; Connell, A.M.; Wu, S.Y.; et al. Distribution of intraocular pressure, the Barbados Eye Study Group. *Archives of Ophthalmology* 1158:1051-1057, 1997.

[15] National Institute of Diabetes and Digestive and Kidney Diseases. *Diabetes in America.* 2nd ed. Washington, DC: U.S. Department of Health and Human Services (HHS), NIH, 1995.

[16] Novella, A.C.; Wise, P.H.; and Kleinman, D.V. Hispanic Health. Time for data, time for action. *Journal of the American Medical Association* 265(2):253-255, 1991.

[17] Voo, I.; Lee, D.; and Oelrich, F. Prevalences of ocular conditions among Hispanic, white, Asian and Black immigrant students examined by the UCLA Mobile Eye Clinic. *Journal of the American Optometric Association* 69(4):255-261, 1998.

[18] National Institute on Deafness and Other Communication Disorders (NIDCD). *National Strategic Research Plan: Hearing and Hearing Impairment.* Bethesda, MD: HHS, NIH, 1996.

[19] Collins, J.G. Prevalence of selected chronic conditions: United States 1990–1992. National Center for Health Statistics. *Vital and Health Statistics* 10(194):1-89, 1997.

[20] Reports of prevalence from State programs. [Texas, 3.14 per 1,000] Albright, K., and O'Neal, J. The Newborn With Hearing Loss: Detection in the Nursery. *Pediatrics* (102):142-146, 1998; [Hawaii, 1.4 per 1,000] Mason, J.A., and Herrmann, K.R. Universal Infant Hearing Screening By Automated Auditory Brainstem Response Measurement. *Pediatrics* (101):221-228, 1998; [New Jersey, 2.9 per 1,000] Barsky-Firsker, L., and Sun, S. Universal Newborn Hearing Screenings: A Three-Year Experience. *Pediatrics* 99(6):E4, 1997; [Colorado, 2.56 per 1,000] NCHAM *Sound Ideas* (2):3, 1998.

[21] Yoshinaga-Itano, C., and Apuzzo, M.L. Identification of hearing loss after 18 months is not early enough. *American Annals of the Deaf* 143(5):380-387, 1998.

[22] Joint Committee on Infant Hearing Screening. 1994 Position Statement. *American Speech-Language-Hearing Association* 36(12):38-41, 1994.

[23] Yoshinaga-Itano, C.; Sedy, A.; Coulter, D.; et al. Language of early and later-identified children with hearing loss. *Pediatrics* 102(5):1161-1171, 1998.

[24] NIDCD. Recommendations of the NIDCD Working Group on Early Identification Hearing Impairment on Acceptable Protocols for Use in State-Wide Universal Newborn Hearing Screening Programs, 1997. <www.nih.gov/nidcd/news/97/recomnd.htm>June 27, 2000.

[25] Morton, N.E. Genetic epidemiology of hearing impairment. *Annals of the New York Academy of Science* 630:16-31, 1991.

[26] Bess, F.H.; Dodd-Murphy, J.; and Parker, R.A. Children with minimal sensorineural hearing loss: Prevalence, educational performance and functional status. *Ear and Hearing* (19)5:339-354, 1998.

[27] American Academy of Pediatrics. Newborn and infant hearing loss: detection and intervention. *Pediatrics* 103(2):527-530, 1999.

[28] NIDCD. Recommendations of the NIDCD Working Group on Early Identification of Hearing Impairment on Acceptable Protocols for Use in State-Wide Universal Newborn Hearing Screening Programs (1997). <http://www.nih.gov/recomnd.htm>.

[29] Niskar, A.S.; Kieszak, S.M.; Holmes, A.; et al. Prevalence of hearing loss among children 6 to 19 years of age—the Third National Health and Nutrition Examination Survey. *Journal of the American Medical Association* 279(14):1071-1075, 1998.

[30] Gorlin, R.J.; Toriello, H.V.; and Cohen, M.M. *Hereditary Hearing Loss and Its Syndromes.* New York, NY: Oxford University Press, 1995.

[31] Van Camp, G., and Smith, R.J.H. Hereditary Hearing Loss Homepage <http://dnalab0www.uia.ac.be/dnalab/hhh> and Morton, N.E. Genetic epidemiology of hearing impairment. *Annals of New York Academy of Science* 630:16-31, 1991.

[32] NIDCD. *Because You Asked About Meniere's Disease.* Washington, DC: HHS, 1-7.

[33] Schappert, S.M. Office visits for otitis media: United States, 1975–90. *Advance Data* 13(137):17, 1992.

[34] Freid, V.M.; Makuc, D.M.; and Rooks, R.N. Ambulatory health care visits by children: Principal diagnosis and place of visit. *Vital and Health Statistics* 13(137):17, 1-23, 1998.

[35] Alsarraf, R.; Jung, C.J.; Perkins, J.; et al. Otitis media health status evaluation: A pilot study for the investigation of cost-effective outcomes of recurrent acute otitis media treatment. *Annals of Otology, Rhinology and Laryngology* 107(2):120-128, 1998.

[36] NIDCD. *Fact Sheet on Noise-Induced Hearing Loss.* Washington, DC: HHS, 1998.

[37] National Institute for Occupational Safety and Health (NIOSH). *Fact Sheet: Work-Related Hearing Loss.* Washington, DC: HHS, 1999.

[38] Lusk, S.L.; Kerr, M.J.; and Kauffman, S.A. Use of hearing protection and perceptions of noise exposure and hearing loss among construction workers. *American Industrial Hygiene Association Journal* 59:566-570, 1998.

[39] Franks, J.R. *Analysis of Audiograms for a Large Cohort of Noise-Exposed Miners.* Cincinnati, OH: HHS, Centers for Disease Control and Prevention, NIOSH, Division of Biomedical and Behavioral Science, 1996.

[40] Mine Safety and Health Administration. Health Standards for Occupational Noise Exposure in Coal, Metal, and Nonmetal Mines: Proposed Rule. *Federal Register* 61:243:66347-66397, December 17, 1996.

[41] Wallhagen, M.I.; Strawbridge, W.J.; Cohen, R.D.; et al. An Increasing prevalence of hearing impairment and associated risk factors over three decades of the Alameda County Study. *American Journal of Public Health* 87(3):440-442, 1997.

[42] HHS, NIDCD. *Economic and Social Realities of Communication Difference and Disorder.* Bethesda, MD: NIH, 1998.

[43] Kelly, L.P. Using silent motion pictures to teach complex syntax to adult deaf readers. *Journal of Deaf Studies and Deaf Education* 3(3):217-230, 1998.

[44] Steinburg, A.G. Issues in providing mental health services to hearing-impaired persons. *Hospital & Community Psychiatry* 42(4):380-389, 1991.

[45] Steinburg, A.G.; Sullivan, V.J.; and Montoya, L.A. Lipreading the stirrups: An investigation of deaf women's perspectives of their health, health care, and providers. Paper presented at National Health Service Corps 25th Anniversary Meeting in Washington, DC, in 1998.

[46] Gates, G.A.; Cooper, Jr., J.C.; Kannel, W.B.; et al. Hearing in the elderly: The Framingham Cohort, 1983–1985. Part I. Basic audiometric test results. *Ear and Hearing* 11(4):247-256, 1990.

[47] Cruickshanks, K.J.; Wiley, T.L.; Tweed, T.S.; et al. Prevalence of hearing loss in older adults in Beaver Dam, Wisconsin: The Epidemiology of Hearing Loss Study. *American Journal of Epidemiology* 148(9):879-886, 1998.

[48] Popelka, M.M.; Cruickshanks, K.J.; Wiley, T.L.; et al. Low prevalence of hearing aid use among older adults with hearing loss: The Epidemiology of Hearing Loss Study. *Journal of the American Geriatrics Society* 46(9):1075-1078, 1998.

[49] Klein, R.; Cruickshanks, K.F.; Klein, B.E.K.; et al. Is age-related maculopathy related to hearing loss? *Archives of Ophthalmology* 116(3):360-365, 1998.

[50] NIDCD. WISE EARS! (For full listing of coalition members:)<http://www.nih.gov/nidcd/health/wise>December 15, 1999.

[51] Ries, P.W. Prevalence and characteristics of persons with hearing trouble, United States, 1990–91. *Vital and Health Statistics* 10(188), 1994.

[52] American Speech-Language-Hearing Association. *Guidelines for Audiologic Screening.* Rockville, MD: the Association, 1997.

[53] Lusk, S.L.; Kerr, J.J.; Ronis, R.L.; et al. Applying the Health Promotion Model to development of a worksite intervention. *American Journal of Health Promotion* 13(4):219-227, 1999.

[54] Lusk, S.L.; Hogan, M.M.; and Ronis, D.L. Test of the Health Promotion Model as a causal model of construction workers' use of hearing protection. *Research in Nursing & Health* 20(3):183-194, 1997.

1995

Healthy People Consortium expanded to include all State mental health, substance abuse, and environmental agencies to encourage their participation in the development of the objectives and their use of the objectives at State and local levels.

September 12-13, 1996

CDC/NCHS convenes APHA, ASTHO, and NACCHO with States in the CDC Assessment Initiative to examine the data successes and challenges with Healthy People 2000. States participating include Iowa, Kansas, Ohio, Oregon, Minnesota, Missouri, and South Carolina.

October 1996 to February 1997

Healthy People Consortium member focus groups review Healthy People 2000 evaluating what has been useful and should be preserved and what should be recast.

November 15, 1996

Healthy People Consortium Meeting in New York, New York, *Building the Prevention Agenda for 2010: Lessons Learned.* Keynote speaker Dr. Ilona Kickbusch, Director of the Division of Health Promotion, Education, and Communication of the World Health Organization, delivers keynote address.

1997 and ongoing:

Agencies of the U.S. Department of Health and Human Services begin to lead Healthy People Work Groups to develop draft objectives for public review and comment.

April 21, 1997

Secretary's Council on National Health Promotion and Disease Prevention holds a public meeting on the Healthy People 2010 objectives. The Council reviews lessons learned from Healthy People 2000, addresses the need to improve data collection, and discusses the proposed framework for Healthy People 2010, which incorporates two overarching goals: increase years of healthy life and eliminate health disparities.

May 14, 1997

Measuring Performance Lessons Learned and Challenges Ahead, a Federal interagency conference, is held to examine issues in performance measurement under the Government Performance and Results Act (GPRA) focused on the linkage between Healthy People and annual GPRA measures.

July 1997

Release of *Stakeholder's Report*, announcing the results of the Consortium focus group process, on www.health.gov/healthypeople.

July 1997

Partnership for Prevention, a Healthy People Consortium member, with support from the Robert Wood Johnson Foundation, establishes the Healthy People Business Advisory Council to increase the involvement of the business community in Healthy People 2010 development.

September 15, 1997, to December 15, 1997

Developing Objectives for Healthy People 2010 is released in printed and electronic form on the Internet for a 90-day public comment period on the goals, objectives, and framework of Healthy People.

November 7, 1997

Healthy People Consortium Meeting in Indianapolis, Indiana, Reducing Health Disparities: How Far Have We Come? Keynote speakers representing minority population groups address disparities in health.

December 17, 1997

Nearly 800 comments are received on the Healthy People 2010 framework and are available to the public on the Internet at www.health.gov/healthypeople.

February 19-20, 1998

Symposium on National Strategies for Renewing Health for All at the Pan American Health Organization engages 24 countries from the Western Hemisphere in using health targets. Healthy People represents the United States contribution to "World Health for All" strategy.

March 6, 1998

U.S. Department of Health and Human Services Working Group on Sentinel Objectives releases the *Leading Health Indicators for Healthy People 2010* report, which describes the potential uses for and provides examples of possible approaches to sentinel objectives.

April 30, 1998

Annual Secretary's Council public meeting takes place. The Council endorses the goal of eliminating health disparities and affirms that one target should be set for all population groups. The Council discusses the proposed draft objectives for 2010 and approves the development of leading health indicators, a set of selected objectives chosen to capture the state of the Nation's health.

April to October 1998

Getting Started for 2010, a series of five audio conferences, features national and State successes and challenges in using health objectives. All 50 States participate.

August 1998

Institute of Medicine (IOM) releases its *Preliminary Report on the Leading Health Indicators*.

September 15, 1998, to December 15, 1998

Healthy People 2010: Draft for Public Comment, containing the draft of 531 objectives proposed in 26 focus areas, is released for public comment. Comments accepted via the Internet, by mail, and at regional meetings.

September 17-18, 1998

CDC/NCHS holds a workshop on measuring years of healthy life, resulting in a report called *Identifying Summary Measures for Healthy People 2010.*

October 5-6, 1998

Two hundred and sixty-eight people attend the Regional Healthy People Meeting in Philadelphia, Pennsylvania, to provide input on developing Healthy People 2010 objectives.

October 21-22, 1998

Two hundred and thirty-six people attend the Regional Healthy People Meeting in New Orleans, Louisiana, to provide input on developing Healthy People 2010 objectives.

November 5-6, 1998

Four hundred and fifty-six people attend the Regional Healthy People Meeting in Chicago, Illinois, to provide input on developing Healthy People 2010 objectives.

November 13, 1998

Four hundred and sixty-nine people attend the Public Hearing and Healthy People Consortium Meeting, Building the Next Generation of Healthy People, in Washington, D.C., with speakers Dr. Julius Richmond and Dr. David Satcher.

December 2-3, 1998

Three hundred and nineteen people attend the Regional Healthy People Meeting in Seattle, Washington, to provide input on developing Healthy People 2010 objectives.

December 9-10, 1998

Three hundred and fifty-four people attend the Regional Healthy People Meeting in Sacramento, California, to provide input on developing Healthy People 2010 objectives.

December 17, 1998

More than 11,000 public comments on the draft Healthy People 2010 objectives are received from people in every State, the District of Columbia, and Puerto Rico. Comments can be viewed at www.health.gov/healthypeople.

January 1999

IOM produces the report *Leading Health Indicators for Healthy People 2010: Second Interim Report.* The report summarizes the efforts of the IOM Committee on Leading Health Indicators for Healthy People 2010 to develop sample sets of leading health indicators.

January 25, 1999

The Partnerships for Health in the New Millennium Conference Planning Committee, comprising representatives from the Healthy People Consortium, Partnerships for Networked Consumer Health Information Steering Committee, academia, State and local government, and private organizations, identifies plenary speakers, develops the program, and sets criteria for sessions for the conference.

April 1999

IOM produces the report *Leading Health Indicators for Healthy People 2010: Final Report*, detailing IOM's development of three sets of leading health indicators.

April 23, 1999

Annual Secretary's Council public meeting takes place. The Council reviews the IOM's report on leading health indicators and endorses the general form of the emerging set of Leading Health Indicators, discusses and helps refine the proposed draft objectives for 2010, and approves plans for launching Healthy People 2010 in January 2000.

June 1999 and ongoing

State and local Healthy People 2010 plans are developed.

June 1999

Focus groups on Leading Health Indicators are conducted.

September 1999

Healthy People 2010 Toolkit: A Field Guide to Health Planning is released as a resource for State and local planning. The Toolkit includes national and State examples of engaging partners, setting objectives, and sustaining the initiatives. *Healthy People 2010 Toolkit* is available on the Internet at www.health.gov/healthypeople/state/toolkit.

January 25, 2000

Assistant Secretary for Health and Surgeon General David Satcher releases *Healthy People 2010* (Conference Edition) at the Partnerships for Health in the New Millennium conference in Washington, D.C.

Healthy People 2010 is the product of a national effort that has involved individuals, organizations, and agencies from across the United States. Work on the report began in 1996 with a meeting of the Healthy People 2000 Consortium and the convening of focus groups. A public comment period in 1997 and testimony from six public hearings in 1998 provided valuable public input. The development of the objectives was guided by the Secretary's Council on National Health Promotion and Disease Prevention Objectives for 2010, chaired by Donna E. Shalala with David Satcher as Vice Chair, and by the Healthy People Steering Committee, currently chaired by Nicole Lurie. The 28 focus areas were developed by work groups coordinated by lead agency scientists from the Federal Government.

Preparation of the report was sponsored by the U.S. Department of Health and Human Services, through a project coordinated by the Office of Disease Prevention and Health Promotion under the leadership of Claude Earl Fox, Susanne A. Stoiber, Linda D. Meyers, and Randolph F. Wykoff.

Principal staff responsibility for the project belonged to Deborah R. Maiese and Mary Jo Deering. Mark S. Smolinski had primary responsibility for the introductory section. Carter R. Blakey and Janice T. Radak provided critical editorial support. Other current and former staff members from the Office of Disease Prevention and Health Promotion who helped in the coordination and development of Healthy People 2010 included DelShaun Adams, Paul Ambrose, David Baker, Gloria Barnes, Cynthia Baur, Phyllis Carroll, Christine Cichetti, Ellis Davis, Tom Eng, Kenneth Fisher, Yolande Gary, Kristine Gebbie, Toni M. Goodwin, Kate-Louise Gottfried, Miryam Granthon, Matthew Guidry, Raymond Han, Jim Harrell, Leslie Hsu, Sally Jones, Woodie Kessel, Lindsay Kim, Paul Kim, Ann Marie Lee, Joan Lyon, Rika Maeshiro, Kathryn McMurry, Robin Moore, Phyllis Morgan, Cindy Nordlie, Emmeline Ochiai, Jerome Paulson, Dalton Paxman, Irene Randell, Natiqua Riley, Kiven Robinson, Gloria Robledo, Janet Samorodin, Sandy Saunders, Stephanie Smith, India Stroman, Tom Vischi, and Kelly Woodward. Preventive Medicine Residents and medical students providing research assistance included Madhavi Battineni, Joy L. Bottoms, Wayne Brandes, Dominic Cheung Chow, Penny Shelton-Hoffman, Robin McFee, J. Patrick Moulds, Alex Nettles, Elpidoforos Soteriades, Peter Thornquist, Edward Van Oeveren, Stephanie Weller, and Amanda Williams. J. Michael McGinnis and Robert Valdez were consultants to the 2010 development.

Linda Bailey and Mark S. Smolinski coordinated the development of the Leading Health Indicators. This effort was guided by an interagency work group and the Healthy People Steering Committee which included Lois Albarelli, David R. Arday, David Atkins, Delton Atkinson, Olivia Carter-Pokras, Lynn Cates, Melissa H. Clarke, Marsha G. Davenport, Tuei Doong, Margaret Gilliam, Chuck Gollmar, William R. Harlan, Jim Harrell, Suzanne G. Haynes, Wanda K. Jones, Diane

Justice, Nicole Lurie, Evelyn Kappeler, Richard J. Klein, Mary Ann MacKenzie, John Monahon, J. Henry Montes, Paul W. Nannis, Eileen Parish, Kate Rickard, Carol Roddy, Theresa Rogers, Dorita Sewell, Mary Beth Skupien, Philip B. Smith, Christine G. Spain, Matthew Stagner, Irma Tetzloff, Betsy L. Thompson, Martina Vogel-Taylor, and Diane K. Wagener. The National Academy of Sciences, Institute of Medicine, Committee on Leading Health Indicators for Healthy People 2010 included Susan Allan, Roger Bulger, Carole A. Chrvala, Donna D. Duncan, Neal Halfon, Barbara S. Hulka, Thomas J. Kean, Kelly Norsingle, Scott C. Ratzan, Stephen C. Schoenbaum, Mark Smith, Shoshanna Sofaer, Kathleen Stratton, and Robert B. Wallace.

The Division of Health Promotion Statistics of the National Center for Health Statitics, Centers for Disease Control and Prevention, provided statistical advice and developed data for the Healthy People objectives. Diane K. Wagener served as Acting Division Director, and staff members included Jeanette Guyton-Krishnan, Elizabeth Jackson, Richard J. Klein, Cheryl Rose, Colleen Ryan, J. Fred Seitz, Thomas Socey, Kathleen Turczyn, Jennie Wald, and Jean Williams.

Social & Health Services, Ltd., the National Health Information Center and ODPHP contractor, developed the Healthy People Web site and handled the production of the *Healthy People 2010* document under the leadership of Lewis Eigen and Ramona Arnett. Nancy Klein managed the editing and production of the document. Other contributing staff members from SHS included Mark Akbayrak, Anwar Aziz, Tamara Bailey, Keith Barbour, Stacey Berry, Amy Bielski, Tiffanie Bilbrey, Tobie Bilbrey, Barbara Blue, Doreen Bonnett, Christine Botsford, Sharon Boyd, Qiana Bowie, Nicole Carson, Edward Cavanagh, Alyson Chmielewski, Jody Cole, David Cummings, Rosemarie Dempsey, Carolyn Diaz, Vivian Doidge, Bryan Elrod, Bradley Eng-Kohn, Bryce Gaylor, Jaime Geyer, Jennifer Geyer, Char Glendening, Ayanna Grant, Adriane Griffen, Deborah Hill, Alfred R. Imhoff, Denise Jones, Susan Kanaan, William Keating, John Klein, Linda Lee, Lilian Lopez, George Mitchell, Mary Moien, Eric Moore, Melanie Morrow, William Niles, Michael Peck, Kevin Pierson, Elaine Rahbar, Ann Redmon, Anne Restino, Carli Richard, Jeff Rife, Sheldon Robinson, Charles Scott, Tanya Singer, Adil Sisman, Sedat Sisman, Ugur Sisman, Steve Sonner, Craig Steinburg, Henry Stryker, Mary Sy, Emily Tinkler, Lisa R. Van Wagner, Van Wall, Arlene Weitzman, Dennis Williams, Todd Witiak, Ralph Yang, and Mike Zhang.

IQ Solutions handled the production of *Healthy People 2010: Understanding and Improving Health*. IQ staff members included Ted Buxton, E.J. King-Carter, Michael Huddleston, Jim Libbey, Josue Martinez, Craig Packer, Meredith Pond, and Karen Stroud.

While it is not possible to recognize everyone who made contributions to Healthy People 2010, their efforts were invaluable to the development of the final product.

Appendix C. The Secretary's Council on National Health Promotion and Disease Prevention Objectives for 2010

Approved on September 5, 1996, and announced in the *Federal Register* on October 21, 1996, the Secretary's Council on National Health Promotion and Disease Prevention Objectives for 2010 was established to oversee the development and implementation of Healthy People 2010. The Secretary of Health and Human Services (HHS) chairs this Council, with the Assistant Secretary for Health and Surgeon General sitting as vice chair. Members include all former Assistant Secretaries for Health and all current heads of HHS operating divisions. The Council meets yearly to guide the implementation policies of Healthy People 2010.

Members

(as of August 1, 2000)

Chair

Donna E. Shalala, Ph.D.
Secretary of Health and Human Services

Vice Chair

David Satcher, M.D., Ph.D.
Assistant Secretary for Health and Surgeon General

Former Assistant Secretaries for Health

Edward N. Brandt, Jr., M.D., Ph.D.
Merlin K. DuVal, M.D.
Charles C. Edwards, M.D.
Philip R. Lee, M.D.
James O. Mason, M.D., Dr.P.H.
Julius B. Richmond, M.D.
Robert E. Windom, M.D.

HHS Operating Division Heads

Administration for Children and Families	Olivia Golden, Ph.D.
Administration on Aging	Jeanette C. Takamura, Ph.D.
Agency for Healthcare Research and Quality	John M. Eisenberg, M.D.
Centers for Disease Control and Prevention	Jeffrey P. Koplan, M.D., M.P.H.
Food and Drug Administration	Jane E. Henney, M.D.
Health Care Financing Administration	Nancy-Ann Min DeParle
Health Resources and Services Administration	Claude Earl Fox, M.D., M.P.H.
Indian Health Service	Michael Trujillo, M.D., M.P.H.
National Institutes of Health	Ruth Kirschstein, M.D. (Acting)
Substance Abuse and Mental Health Services Administration	Nelba Chavez, Ph.D.

Chair

Nicole Lurie, M.D., M.S.P.H.
Principal Deputy Assistant Secretary for Health
Office of Public Health and Science
U.S. Department of Health and Human Services
Humphrey Building, Room 716G
200 Independence Avenue, S.W.
Washington, DC 20201
(202) 690-7694/Fax (202) 690-6960

Vice Chair

Randolph W. Wykoff, M.D., M.P.H., T.M.
Deputy Assistant Secretary for Health
Office of Disease Prevention and Health
Promotion
U.S. Department of Health and Human Services
Humphrey Building, Room 738G
200 Independence Avenue, S.W.
Washington, DC 20201
(202) 401-6295/Fax (202) 690-7054
E-mail: rwykoff@osophs.dhhs.gov

Administration on Aging

Diane Justice, M.P.A.
Deputy Assistant Secretary for Aging
Humphrey Building, Room 309F
200 Independence Avenue, S.W.
Washington, DC 20201
(202) 401-4634/Fax (202) 401-7741
E-mail: djustice@aoa.gov

Lois Albarelli
Program Specialist
Division of Program Management and
Analysis
Office of State and Community Programs
Administration on Aging
Cohen Building, Room 4745
330 Independence Avenue, S.W.
Washington, DC 20201
(202) 619-2621/Fax (202) 260-1012
E-mail: lalbarelli@ban-gate.aoa.dhhs.gov

Administration for Children and Families

Mary Ann MacKenzie
Senior Strategic Planner
Office of Planning, Research, and Evaluation
Administration for Children and Families
Aerospace Building, 7th Floor West
370 L'Enfant Promenade, S.W.
Washington, DC 20447
(202) 401-5272/Fax (202) 205-3598
E-mail: ml@acf.dhhs.gov

Agency for Healthcare Research and Quality

David Atkins, M.D., M.P.H.
Medical Officer
Center for Practice and Technology
Assessment
Agency for Healthcare Research and Quality
6010 Executive Boulevard, Suite 300
Rockville, MD 20852
(301) 594-4016/Fax (301) 594-4027
E-mail: datkins@ahrq.gov

Kate Rickard
Program Analyst
Center for Practice and Technology
Assessment
Agency for Healthcare Research and Quality
6010 Executive Boulevard, Suite 300
Rockville, MD 20852
(301) 594-2431/Fax (301) 594-4027
E-mail: krickard@ahrq.gov

Centers for Disease Control and Prevention

Veronica P. Alvarez, M.P.A.
Program Analyst
Office of Program Planning and Evaluation
Centers for Disease Control and Prevention
Building 16, Room 5145, MS D23
1600 Clifton Road, N.E.
Atlanta, GA 30333
(404) 639-7136/Fax (404) 639-7181
E-mail: vba3@cdc.gov

Chuck Gollmar
Deputy Director
Office of Program Planning and Evaluation
Centers for Disease Control and Prevention
Building 16, Room 5145, MS D23
1600 Clifton Road, N.E.
Atlanta, GA 30333
(404) 639-7070/Fax (404) 639-7171
E-mail: cwg2@cdc.gov

Food and Drug Administration

Marlene E. Haffner, M.D., M.P.H., RADM
Director
Office of Orphan Products Development
Food and Drug Administration
Parklawn Building, Room 8-73, HF-35
5600 Fishers Lane
Rockville, MD 20857
(301) 827-3666/Fax (301) 443-4915
E-mail: mhaffner@oc.fda.gov

Health Care Financing Administration

David R. Arday, M.D., M.P.H.
Medical Epidemiologist
Office of Clinical Standards and Quality,
S3-02-01
Health Care Financing Administration
7500 Security Boulevard
Baltimore, MD 21244-1850
(410) 786-3528/Fax (410) 786-4005
E-mail: darday@hcfa.gov

Marsha Davenport, M.D., M.P.H.
Chief Medical Officer
Office of Strategic Planning, C3-20-11
Health Care Financing Administration
7500 Security Boulevard
Baltimore, MD 21244-1850
(410) 786-6693/Fax (410) 786-6511
E-mail: davenport@hcfa.gov

Health Resources and Services Administration

Paul Nannis, M.S.W.
Director
Office of Planning, Evaluation, and
Legislation
Health Resources and Services
Administration
Parklawn Building, Room 14-33
5600 Fishers Lane
Rockville, MD 20857
(301) 443-2460/Fax (301) 443-9270
E-mail: pnannis@hrsa.gov

Melissa Clarke, M.P.A.
Senior Health Policy and Program Analyst
Healthy People 2000/2010 Coordinator
Office of Planning, Evaluation, and
Legislation
Health Resources and Services
Administration
Parklawn Building, Room 14-33
5600 Fishers Lane
Rockville, MD 20857
 (301) 443-5277/Fax (301) 443-9270
E-mail: mclarke@hrsa.gov

Indian Health Service

Phil Smith, M.D., M.P.H.
Clinical Consultant
Division of Clinical and Preventive Services
Indian Health Service
Parklawn Building, Room 6A-55
5600 Fishers Lane
Rockville, MD 20857
(301) 443-3024/Fax (301) 594-6213
E-mail: psmith@hqe.ihs.gov

National Institutes of Health

William R. Harlan, M.D.
Associate Director for Disease Prevention
Building 31, Room 1B03
31 Center Drive, MSC 2082
National Institutes of Health
Bethesda, MD 20892-2082
(301) 496-1508/Fax (301) 480-7660
E-mail: wh27v@nih.gov

Martina Vogel-Taylor, MT (ASCP)
Senior Program Analyst
Building 31, Room 1B03
31 Center Drive, MSC 2082
National Institutes of Health
Bethesda, MD 20892-2082
(301) 496-6614/Fax (301) 480-9654
E-mail: martinav@nih.gov

Office of the Assistant Secretary for Planning and Evaluation

Eileen Salinsky
Director, Division of Public Health Policy
Office of Health Policy
Office of the Assistant Secretary for Planning
and Evaluation
U.S. Department of Health and Human Services
Humphrey Building, Room 431E
200 Independence Avenue, S.W.
Washington, DC 20201
(202) 690-6051/Fax (202) 401-7321
E-mail: esalinsk@osaspe.dhhs.gov

Office of Minority Health

Tuei Doong, M.P.H.
Deputy Director for Minority Health
Office of Minority Health
Rockwall II Building, Suite 1000
5515 Security Lane
Rockville, MD 20857
(301) 443-5084/Fax (301) 594-0767 or
(301) 443-8280
E-mail: tdoong@osophs.dhhs.gov

Office of Population Affairs

Evelyn Kappeler
Public Health Analyst
Office of Population Affairs
Suite 200 West
4350 East West Highway
Bethesda, MD 20814
(301) 594-7608/Fax (301) 594-5980
E-mail: ekappeler@osophs.dhhs.gov

Office on Women's Health

Wanda K. Jones, Dr.P.H.
Deputy Assistant Secretary for Health
(Women's Health)
Office on Women's Health
Humphrey Building, Room 712E
200 Independence Avenue, S.W.
Washington, DC 20201
(202) 690-7650/Fax (202) 401-4005
E-mail: wjones@osophs.dhhs.gov

President's Council on Physical Fitness and Sports

Christine Spain, M.A.
Director
Research, Planning, and Special Projects
President's Council on Physical Fitness and
Sports
Humphrey Building, Room 731H
200 Independence Avenue, S.W.
Washington, DC 20201
(202) 690-5148/Fax (202) 690-5211
E-mail: cspain@osophs.dhhs.gov

Substance Abuse and Mental Health Services Administration

Margaret Gilliam
Public Health Analyst
Office of Policy and Program Coordination
Substance Abuse and Mental Health Services
Administration
Parklawn Building, Room 12C-26
5600 Fishers Lane
Rockville, MD 20857
(301) 443-6067/Fax (301) 594-6159
E-mail: mgilliam@samhsa.gov

Dorita Sewell, Ph.D.
Healthy People Coordinator
Office of Policy and Program Coordination
Substance Abuse and Mental Health Services
Administration
Parklawn Building, Room 12C-26
5600 Fishers Lane
Rockville, MD 20857
(301) 443-6067/Fax (301) 594-6159
E-mail: dsewell@samhsa.gov

Office of Disease Prevention and Health Promotion Staff

Randolph W. Wykoff, M.D., M.P.H., T.M.
(202) 401-6295
E-mail: rwykoff@osophs.dhhs.gov

Ellis Davis (202) 260-2873
E-mail: edavis@osophs.dhhs.gov

Matthew Guidry, Ph.D. (202) 401-7780
E-mail: mguidry@osophs.dhhs.gov

Miryam Granthon (202) 690-6245
E-mail: mgranthon@osophs.dhhs.gov

Phyllis Morgan (202)205-8385
E-mail: pmorgan@osophs.dhhs.gov

Emmeline Ochiai (202) 260-9281
E-mail: eochiai@osophs.dhhs.gov

Office of Disease Prevention and Health
Promotion
Humphrey Building, Room 738G
200 Independence Ave., S.W.
Washington, D.C. 20201
(202) 401-6295/Fax (202) 205-9478

Centers for Disease Control/National Center for Health Statistics Statistical Advisors

Richard Klein, M.P.H.
Chief
Data Monitoring and Analysis Branch
Division of Health Promotion Statistics
National Center for Health Statistics
Centers for Disease Control and Prevention
6525 Belcrest Road, Room 770
Hyattsville, MD 20782
(301) 458-4013/Fax (301) 458-4036
E-mail: rjk6@cdc.gov

Diane K. Wagener, Ph.D.
Acting Director
Division of Health Promotion Statistics
National Center for Health Statistics
Centers for Disease Control and Prevention
6525 Belcrest Road, Room 770
Hyattsville, MD 20782
(301) 458-4013/Fax (301) 458-4036
E-mail: dkw1@cdc.gov

1. Access to Quality Health Services

David Atkins, M.D., M.P.H.
Medical Officer
Center for Practice and Technology Assessment
Agency for Healthcare Research and Quality
6010 Executive Boulevard, Suite 300
Rockville, MD 20852
(301) 594-4016/Fax (301) 594-4027
E-mail: datkins@ahrq.gov

Melissa Clarke, M.P.A.
Senior Health Policy and Program Analyst
Healthy People 2000/2010 Coordinator
Office of Planning, Evaluation, and Legislation
Health Resources and Services Administration
Parklawn Building, Room 14-33
5600 Fishers Lane
Rockville, MD 20857
(301) 443-5277/Fax (301) 443-9270
E-mail: mclarke@hrsa.gov

Paul Nannis, M.S.W.
Director
Office of Planning, Evaluation, and Legislation
Health Resources and Services Administration
Parklawn Building, Room 14-33
5600 Fishers Lane
Rockville, MD 20857
(301) 443-2460/Fax (301) 443-9270
E-mail: pnannis@hrsa.gov

Kathryn Rickard, M.P.A.
Program Analyst
Center for Practice and Technology Assessment
Agency for Healthcare Research and Quality
6010 Executive Boulevard, Suite 300
Rockville, MD 20852
(301) 594-2431/Fax (301) 594-4027
E-mail: krickard@ahrq.gov

2. Arthritis, Osteoporosis, and Chronic Back Conditions

Charles G. Helmick, M.D.
Medical Epidemiologist
Health Care and Aging Studies Branch
Division of Adult and Community Health
National Center for Chronic Disease Prevention and Health Promotion
Centers for Disease Control and Prevention
4770 Buford Highway, N.E., MS K45
Atlanta, GA 30341
(770) 488-5456/Fax (770) 488-5964
E-mail: cgh1@cdc.gov

Reva Lawrence, M.P.H.
Epidemiologist/Data Systems Program Officer
National Institute of Arthritis and Musculoskeletal and Skin Diseases
National Institutes of Health
45 Center Drive, MS 6500
Bethesda, MD 20892
(301) 594-5014/Fax (301) 402-2406
E-mail: rl27b@nih.gov

Paul Scherr, Ph.D., D.Sc.
Supervisory Epidemiologist
National Center for Chronic Disease Prevention and Health Promotion
Centers for Disease Control and Prevention
4770 Buford Highway, N.E., MS K45
Atlanta, GA 30341
(770) 488-5454/Fax (770) 488-5964
E-mail: pas0@cdc.gov

3. Cancer

Barry Portnoy, Ph.D.
Cancer Planning and Program Officer
National Cancer Institute
National Institutes of Health
Building 31, Room 10A49
31 Center Drive, MSC 2580
Bethesda, MD 20892-2580
(301) 496-9569/Fax (301) 496-9931
E-mail: bp22z@nih.gov

Karen Richard, M.P.A.
Public Health Advisor
National Center for Chronic Disease
Prevention and Health Promotion
Division of Cancer Prevention and Control
Centers for Disease Control and Prevention
4770 Buford Highway, N.E., MS K64
Atlanta, GA 30341
(770) 488-4737/Fax (770) 488-4760
E-mail: kmr4@cdc.gov

4. Chronic Kidney Disease

Lawrence Agodoa, M.D.
Program Director
Division of Kidney Urologic and
Hematologic Diseases
National Institute of Diabetes and Digestive
and Kidney Diseases
National Institutes of Health
Building 45, Room 6AS-13B
45 Center Drive
Bethesda, MD 20892-6600
(301) 594-7717/Fax (301) 480-3510
E-mail: la21j@nih.gov

5. Diabetes

Benjamin Burton, Ph.D.
Emeritus Scientist
National Institute of Diabetes and Digestive
and Kidney Diseases
National Institutes of Health
Building 45, Room 6AN38J
45 Center Drive
Bethesda, MD 20892
(301) 594-8867/Fax (301) 480-4237
E-mail: burtonb@extra.niddk.nih.gov

Bill Foster, M.D.
Senior Staff Physician
National Institute of Diabetes and Digestive
and Kidney Diseases
National Institutes of Health
Building 31, Room 9A21
45 Center Drive
Bethesda, MD 20892
(301) 435-2991/Fax (301) 496-2830
E-mail: fosterb@hq.niddk.nih.gov

Frank M. Vinicor, M.D.
Director
Division of Diabetes Translation
National Center for Chronic Disease
Prevention and Health Promotion
Centers for Disease Control and Prevention
4770 Buford Highway, N.E., MS K10
Atlanta, GA 30341-3724
(770) 488-5000/Fax (770) 488-5966
E-mail: fxv1@cdc.gov

6. Disability and Secondary Conditions

Chris Kochtitzky, M.S.P.
Policy Analyst
National Center for Environmental Health
Centers for Disease Control and Prevention
4770 Buford Highway, N.E., MS F29
Atlanta, GA 30341-3724
(770) 488-7114/Fax (770) 488-7024
E-mail: csk3@cdc.gov

Don Lollar, Ed.D.
Director
Office on Disability and Health
National Center for Environmental Health
Centers for Disease Control and Prevention
4770 Buford Highway, N.E., MS F35
Atlanta, GA 30341-3724
(770) 488-7094/Fax (770) 488-7075
E-mail: DCL5@cdc.gov

Katherine Seelman, Ph.D.
Director
National Institute on Disability and
Rehabilitation Research
U.S. Department of Education
Switzer Building, Room 3060
330 C Street, S.W.
Washington, DC 20202
(202) 205-8134/Fax (202) 205-8997
E-mail: kate_seelman@ed.gov

Lisa Sinclair, M.P.H.
Health Policy Analyst
Office on Disability and Health
National Center for Environmental Health
Centers for Disease Control and Prevention
4770 Buford Highway, N.E., MS F35
Atlanta, GA 30341-3724
(770) 488-7667
E-mail: lvs4@cdc.gov

As of August 1, 2000

7. Educational and Community-Based Programs

Melissa Clarke, M.P.A.
Senior Health Policy and Program Analyst
Healthy People 2000/2010 Coordinator
Office of Planning, Evaluation and
Legislation
Health Resources and Services
Administration
Parklawn Building, Room 14-33
5600 Fishers Lane
Rockville, MD 20857
(301) 443-5277/Fax (301) 443-9270
E-mail: mclarke@hrsa.gov

Catherine A. Hutsell, M.P.H.
Health Education Specialist
Community Health and Program Services
Branch
Division of Adult and Community Health
National Center for Chronic Disease
Prevention and Health Promotion
Centers for Disease Control and Prevention
4770 Buford Highway, N.E., MS K30
Atlanta, GA 30341-3717
(770) 488-5438/Fax (770) 488-5974
E-mail: czh2@cdc.gov

Brick Lancaster, M.A., CHES
Associate Director for Health Education
Practice and Policy
Division of Adult and Community Health
National Center for Chronic Disease
Prevention and Health Promotion
Centers for Disease Control and Prevention
4770 Buford Highway, N.E., MS K45
Atlanta, GA 30341-3724
(770) 488-5269/Fax (770) 488-5964
E-mail: bxl0@cdc.gov

Paul Nannis, M.S.W.
Director
Office of Planning, Evaluation, and
Legislation
Health Resources and Services
Administration
Parklawn Building, Room 14-33
5600 Fishers Lane
Rockville, MD 20857
(301) 443-2460/Fax (301) 443-9270
E-mail: pnannis@hrsa.gov

David McQueen, Sc.D.
Associate Director for Global Health
Promotion
National Center for Chronic Disease
Prevention and Health Promotion
Centers for Disease Control and Prevention
4770 Buford Highway, N.E., MS K45
Atlanta, GA 30341-3724
(770) 488-5414/Fax (770) 488-5971
E-mail: dvm0@cdc.gov

8. Environmental Health

David Evans
Senior Program Analyst
Office of Policy and External Affairs
Agency for Toxic Substances and Disease
Registry
1600 Clifton Road, N.E., MS E60
Atlanta, GA 30333
(404) 639-0506/Fax (404) 639-0522
E-mail: eevans@cdc.gov

David Homa, Ph.D., M.P.H.
Epidemiologist
Air Pollution and Respiratory Health Branch
Division of Environmental Hazards and
Health Effects
National Center for Environmental Health
Centers for Disease Control and Prevention
1600 Clifton Road, N.E., MS E17
Atlanta, GA 30333
(404) 639-2544/Fax (404) 639-2560
E-mail: dgh3@cdc.gov

William Jirles, M.P.H.
Program Analyst
Office of Policy, Planning, and Evaluation
National Institute of Environmental Health
Sciences
National Institutes of Health
Building 101, Room B222
111 Alexander Drive, MS B2-08
Research Triangle Park, NC 27709
(919) 541-2637/Fax (919) 541-4737
E-mail: jirles@niehs.nih.gov

Chris Kochtitzky, M.S.P.
Policy Analyst
Office of Planning, Evaluation, and
Legislation
National Center for Environmental Health
Centers for Disease Control and Prevention
4770 Buford Highway, N.E., MS F29
Atlanta, GA 30341-3724
(770) 488-7114/Fax (770) 488-7024
E-mail: csk3@cdc.gov

Mark McClanahan, Ph.D.
Health Studies Branch
Division of Environmental Hazards and
Health Effects
National Center for Environmental Health
Centers for Disease Control and Prevention
1600 Clifton Road, N.E., MS E23
Atlanta, GA 30333
(404) 639-2562/Fax (404) 639-2565
E-mail: mam4@cdc.gov

Sheila Newton, Ph.D.
Director
Office of Policy, Planning, and Evaluation
National Institute of Environmental Health
Sciences
National Institutes of Health
Building 101, Room B250
111 Alexander Drive, MS B2-08
Research Triangle Park, NC 27709
(919) 541-3484/Fax (919) 541-4737
E-mail: newton1@niehs.nih.gov

John Schelp, M.P.A.
Office of Policy, Planning, and Evaluation
National Institute of Environmental Health
Sciences
National Institutes of Health
Building 101, Room B218
111 Alexander Drive, MS B2-08
Research Triangle Park, NC 27709
(919) 541-5723/Fax (919) 541-2260
E-mail: schelp@niehs.nih.gov

9. Family Planning

Evelyn Kappeler
Senior Policy Analyst
Office of Population Affairs
Office of Public Health and Science
Suite 200 West
4350 East West Highway
Bethesda, MD 20814
(301) 594-7608/Fax (301) 594-5980
E-mail: ekappeler@osophs.dhhs.gov

10. Food Safety

Elisa L. Elliot, Ph.D.
Microbiologist
Center for Food Safety and Applied
Nutrition
Food and Drug Administration
200 C Street, S.W., HFS-615
Washington, DC 20204
(202) 205-4018/Fax (202) 260-0136
E-mail: Elisa.Elliot@cfsan.fda.gov

Ruth Etzel, M.D., Ph.D.
Director
Division of Epidemiology and Risk
Assessment
Food Safety and Inspection Service
U.S. Department of Agriculture
Franklin Court Building, Room 3718
1400 Independence Avenue, S.W.
Washington, DC 20250
(202) 501-7373/Fax (202) 501-6982
E-mail: ruth.etzel@usda.gov

11. Health Communication

Cynthia Baur, Ph.D.
Policy Advisor, Interactive Health
Communication
Office of Disease Prevention and Health
Promotion
Office of Public Health and Science
200 Independence Avenue, S.W., Room
738G
Washington, DC 20201
(202) 205-2311/Fax (202) 205-0463
E-mail: cbaur@osophs.dhhs.gov

Mary Jo Deering, Ph.D.
Director
Health Communication and Telehealth Staff
Office of Disease Prevention and Health
Promotion
Office of Public Health and Science
200 Independence Avenue, S.W., Room
738G
Washington, DC 20201
(202) 260-2652/Fax (202) 205-0463
E-mail: mdeering@osophs.dhhs.gov

12. Heart Disease and Stroke

Robinson Fulwood, Ph.D., M.S.P.H.
Senior Manager for Public Health Program
Development
Office of Prevention, Education, and
Control
National Heart, Lung, and Blood Institute
National Institutes of Health
Building 31, Room 4A03
31 Center Drive MSC 2480
Bethesda, MD 20892-2480
(301) 496-0554/Fax (301) 480-4907
E-mail: fulwoodr@nih.gov

Kurt Greenlund, Ph.D.
National Center for Chronic Disease
Prevention and Health Promotion
Centers for Disease Control and Prevention
4770 Buford Highway, N.E., MS K47
Atlanta, GA 30341-3717
(770) 488-2572/Fax (770) 488-8151
E-mail: keg9@cdc.gov

Claude Lenfant, M.D.
Director
National Heart, Lung, and Blood Institute
National Institutes of Health
31 Center Drive MSC 2486
Bethesda, MD 20892-2486
(301) 496-5166/Fax (301) 480-4907

George Mensah, M.D.
Chief, Cardiovascular Health
National Center for Chronic Disease
Prevention and Health Promotion
Centers for Disease Control and Prevention
4770 Buford Highway, N.E., MS K47
Atlanta, GA 30341-3717
(770) 488-8009/Fax (770) 488-8151
E-mail: ghm8@cdc.gov

Zhi-Jie Zheng, M.D., Ph.D.
Senior Epidemiologist
National Center for Chronic Disease
Prevention and Health Promotion
Centers for Disease Control and Prevention
4770 Buford Highway, N.E., MS K47
Atlanta, GA 30341-3717
(770) 488-8058/Fax (770) 488-8151
E-mail: zzheng@cdc.gov

13. HIV

Shelley Gordon
Public Health Analyst
Office of Policy and Program Development
HIV/AIDS Bureau
Health Resources and Services
Administration
Parklawn Building, Room 7-20
5600 Fishers Lane
Rockville, MD 20857
(301) 443-9684/Fax (301) 443-3323
E-mail: sgordon@hrsa.gov

Emily DeCoster, M.P.H.
Office of Policy and Program Development
HIV/AIDS Bureau
Health Resources and Services
Administration
Parklawn Building, Room 7-20
5600 Fishers Lane
Rockville, MD 20857
(301) 443-1381/Fax (301) 443-3323
E-mail: edecoster@hrsa.gov

Gena Hill, M.P.H.
Program Analyst
Office of Planning, Policy, and Coordination
National Center for HIV, STD, and TB
Prevention
Centers for Disease Control and Prevention
1600 Clifton Road, N.E., MS E07
Atlanta, GA 30333
(404) 639-8008/Fax (404) 639-8600
E-mail: gfh5@cdc.gov

Eva Margolies-Seiler
Associate Director for Planning, Policy, and
Coordination
National Center for HIV, STD, and TB
Prevention
Centers for Disease Control and Prevention
1600 Clifton Road, N.E., MS E07
Atlanta, GA 30333
(404) 639-8008/Fax (404) 639-8600
E-mail: eam1@cdc.gov

14. Immunization and Infectious Diseases

Jennifer Brooks, M.P.H.
Program Analyst
Office of Policy, Planning, and Legislation
National Center for Infectious Diseases
Centers for Disease Control and Prevention
1600 Clifton Road, N.E., MS C12
Atlanta, GA 30333
(404) 639-4915/Fax (404) 639-2715
E-mail: jlc9@cdc.gov

James Hughes, M.D.
Director
National Center for Infectious Diseases
Centers for Disease Control and Prevention
1600 Clifton Road, N.E., MS C12
Atlanta, GA 30333
(404) 639-3401/Fax (404) 639-3039
E-mail: jmh2@cdc.gov

Martin Landry
Associate Director
Planning, Evaluation, and Legislation
National Immunization Program
Centers for Disease Control and Prevention
1600 Clifton Road, N.E., MS E05
Atlanta, GA 30333
(404) 639-8200/Fax (404) 639-8626
E-mail: mgl0@cdc.gov

Walter Orenstein, M.D.
Director
National Immunization Program
Centers for Disease Control and Prevention
1600 Clifton Road, N.E., MS E05
Atlanta, GA 30333
(404) 639-8200/Fax (404) 639-8626
E-mail: wao1@cdc.gov

Rosemary Ramsey
Associate Director
Policy, Planning, and Legislation
National Center for Infectious Diseases
Centers for Disease Control and Prevention
1600 Clifton Road, N.E., MS C12
Atlanta, GA 30333
(404) 639-3484/Fax (404) 639-2715
E-mail: rbr2@cdc.gov

Nicole Smith, M.P.H., M.P.P.
Program Analyst
Office of Planning, Evaluation, and
Legislation
National Immunization Program
Centers for Disease Control and Prevention
1600 Clifton Road, N.E., MS E05
Atlanta, GA 30333
(404) 639-8711/Fax (404) 639-8626
E-mail: nbs8@cdc.gov

15. Injury and Violence Prevention

LaTanya Butler
Deputy Director
Division of Unintentional Injury
National Center for Injury Prevention and
Control
Centers for Disease Control and Prevention
4770 Buford Highway, N.E., MS K63
Atlanta, GA 30341-3724
(770) 488-4652/Fax (770) 488-1317
E-mail: lab1@cdc.gov

Alex Crosby, M.D., M.P.H.
Medical Epidemiologist
Division of Violence Prevention
National Center for Injury Prevention and
Control
Centers for Disease Control and Prevention
4770 Buford Highway, N.E., MS K60
Atlanta, GA 30341
(770) 488-4272/Fax (770) 488-4349
E-mail: aec1@cdc.gov

Tim W. Groza, M.P.A.
Public Health Advisor
National Center for Injury Prevention and Control
Centers for Disease Control and Prevention
4770 Buford Highway, N.E., MS K63
Atlanta, GA 30341-3724
(770) 488-4676/Fax (770) 488-1317
E-mail: twg1@cdc.gov

Martha Highsmith
Program Analyst
Division of Violence Prevention
National Center for Injury Prevention and Control
Centers for Disease Control and Prevention
4770 Buford Highway, N.E., MS K60
Atlanta, GA 30341-3724
(770) 488-4276/Fax (770) 488-4349
E-mail: mah3@cdc.gov

Laura Yerdon Martin
Assistant Director for Policy and Planning (Acting)
Division of Violence Prevention
National Center for Injury Prevention and Control
Centers for Disease Control and Prevention
4770 Buford Highway, N.E., MS K60
Atlanta, GA 30341-3724
(770) 488-4074/Fax (404) 488-4349
E-mail: lym1@cdc.gov

16. Maternal, Infant, and Child Health

Myra Tucker, M.P.H., RN
Maternal, Infant, and Child Health
Epidemiology Team Leader
Pregnancy and Infant Health Branch
Division of Reproductive Health
National Center for Chronic Disease
Prevention and Health Promotion
Centers for Disease Control and Prevention
4770 Buford Highway, N.E., MS K23
Atlanta, GA 30341
(770) 488-5187/Fax (770) 488-5628
E-mail: mjt2@cdc.gov

Charlotte Dickinson, Ph.D.
Planning and Communications Officer
National Center for Environmental Health
Centers for Disease Control and Prevention
4770 Buford Highway, N.E., MS F34
Atlanta, GA 30341-3724
(770) 488-7155/Fax (770) 488-7156
E-mail: cmd1@cdc.gov

Stella Yu, Sc.D., M.P.H.
Statistician
Maternal and Child Health Bureau
Health Resources and Services Administration
Parklawn Building, Room 18A-55
5600 Fishers Lane
Rockville, MD 20857
(301) 443-0695/Fax (301) 443-4842
E-mail: syu@hrsa.gov

17. Medical Product Safety

Linda Brophy, R.N., M.N., M.P.H.
Special Assistant
Office of Post-Marketing Drug Risk Assessment
Center for Drug Evaluation and Research
Food and Drug Administration
Parklawn Building, MS HFD 400
5600 Fishers Lane
Rockville, MD 20857
(301) 827-3193/Fax (301) 443-9664
E-mail: brophyl@cder.fda.gov

18. Mental Health and Mental Disorders

Michele Edwards, M.S., A.C.S.W.
Healthy People Coordinator
Center for Mental Health Services
Substance Abuse and Mental Health
Services Administration
Parklawn Building, Room 17C-06
5600 Fishers Lane
Rockville, MD 20857
(301) 443-7790 x8/Fax (301) 443-7912
E-mail: medwards@samhsa.gov

Doreen S. Koretz, Ph.D.
Associate Director for Prevention
Chief, Developmental Psychopathology and
Prevention Research Branch
National Institute of Mental Health
National Institutes of Health
Neuroscience Center Building, Room 6196
6001 Executive Boulevard
Bethesda, MD 20892-9617
(301) 443-5944/Fax (301) 480-4415
E-mail: dkoretz@nih.gov

19. Nutrition and Overweight

Nancy T. Crane, M.S., M.P.H., R.D.
Nutritionist
Division of Nutrition Science and Policy
Office of Nutritional Products, Labeling,
and Dietary Supplements (HFS-830)
Center for Food Safety and Applied
Nutrition
Food and Drug Administration
200 C Street, S.W.
Washington, DC 20204
(202) 205-5615/Fax (202) 205-5532
E-mail: ncrane@cfsan.fda.gov

Van S. Hubbard, M.D., Ph.D.
Director, NIH Division of Nutrition
Research Coordination, and
Chief, Nutritional Sciences Branch
National Institute of Diabetes and Digestive
and Kidney Diseases
National Institutes of Health
Rockledge 1, Suite 8048
6705 Rockledge Drive MSC 7973
Bethesda, MD 20892-7973
(301) 594-8822/Fax (301) 480-3768
E-mail: vh16h@nih.gov or
van_hubbard@nih.gov

Christine J. Lewis, Ph.D., R.D.
Director
Office of Nutritional Products, Labeling,
and Dietary Supplements (HFS-800)
Center for Food Safety and Applied
Nutrition
Food and Drug Administration
200 C Street, S.W.
Washington, DC 20204
(202) 205-4561/Fax (202) 205-5295
E-mail: clewis1@cfsan.fda.gov

Pamela E. Starke-Reed, Ph.D.
Deputy Director
NIH Division of Nutrition Research
Coordination
National Institute of Diabetes and Digestive
and Kidney Diseases
National Institutes of Health
Rockledge 1, Suite 8048
6705 Rockledge Drive, MSC 7973
Bethesda, MD 20892-7973
(301) 594-8805/Fax (301) 480-3768
E-mail: ps39p@nih.gov

20. Occupational Safety and Health

Lore Jackson Lee
Program Analyst
Office of Policy and Legislation
National Institute for Occupational Safety
and Health
Centers for Disease Control and Prevention
200 Independence Avenue, S.W., Room 715H
Washington, DC 20201
(202) 205-8898/Fax (202) 260-4464
E-mail: laj2@cdc.gov

21. Oral Health

Alice M. Horowitz, Ph.D.
Senior Scientist
National Institute of Dental and Craniofacial
Research
National Institutes of Health
Building 45, Room 3AN-44B
45 Center Drive, MSC 6401
Bethesda, MD 20892-6401
(301) 594-5391/Fax (301) 480-8254
E-mail: alice.horowitz@nih.gov

Candace M. Jones, M.P.H.
Health Resources and Services
Administration
Parklawn Building, Room 6A-30
5600 Fishers Lane
Rockville, MD 20857
(301) 443-1106/Fax (301) 594-6610
E-mail: jonesc@hqe.ihs.gov

As of August 1, 2000

Stuart A. Lockwood, D.M.D., M.P.H.
Dental Officer
Surveillance Investigation Research Branch
Division of Oral Health
National Center for Chronic Disease
Prevention and Health Promotion
Centers for Disease Control and Prevention
4770 Buford Highway, N.E., MS F10
Atlanta, GA 30341
(770) 488-6067/Fax (770) 488-6080
E-mail: sal4@cdc.gov

22. Physical Activity and Fitness

Carol Macera, Ph.D.
Senior Epidemiologist
Division of Nutrition and Physical Activity
National Center for Chronic Disease
Prevention and Health Promotion
Centers for Disease Control and Prevention
4770 Buford Highway, N.E., MS K46
Atlanta, GA 30341-3724
(770) 488-5018/Fax (770) 488-5473
E-mail: cam4@cdc.gov

Christine Spain
Director
Research, Planning, and Special Projects
President's Council on Physical Fitness and
Sports
Office of Public Health and Science
200 Independence Avenue, S.W., Room 731
Washington, DC 20201
(202) 690-5148/Fax (202) 690-5211
E-mail: cspain@osophs.dhhs.gov

23. Public Health Infrastructure

Carol Roddy, J.D.
Senior Advisor to the Administrator
Center for Public Health Practice
Health Resources and Services
Administration
Parklawn Building, Room 14-15
5600 Fishers Lane
Rockville, MD 20857
(301) 443-4034/Fax (301) 443-0192
E-mail: croddy@hrsa.gov

Diane Rodill, Ph.D.
Center for Public Health Practice
Health Resources and Services
Administration
Parklawn Building, Room 14-15
5600 Fishers Lane
Rockville, MD 20857
(301) 443-0062/Fax (301) 443-0192
E-mail: drodill@hrsa.gov

Pomeroy Sinnock, Ph.D.
Division of Public Health
Public Health Practice Program Office
Centers for Disease Control and Prevention
4770 Buford Highway, N.E., MS K39
Atlanta, GA 30341-3724
(770) 488-2469/Fax (770) 488-2489
E-mail: pxs1@cdc.gov

24. Respiratory Diseases

Robinson Fulwood, Ph.D., M.S.P.H.
Senior Manager for Public Health Program
Development
Office of Prevention, Education, and
Control
National Heart, Lung, and Blood Institute
National Institutes of Health
Building 31, Room 4A03
31 Center Drive MSC 2480
Bethesda, MD 20892-2480
(301) 496-0554/Fax (301) 480-4907
E-mail: fulwoodr@nih.gov

William Jirles, M.P.H.
Office of Policy, Planning, and Evaluation
National Institute of Environmental Health
Sciences
National Institutes of Health
Building 101, Room B222
111 Alexander Drive, MS B2-08
Research Triangle Park, NC 27709
(919) 541-2637/Fax (919) 541-4737
E-mail: jirles@niehs.nih.gov

Carol Johnson, M.P.H.
Air Pollution and Respiratory Health Branch
Division of Environmental Hazards and
Health Effects
National Center for Environmental Health
Centers for Disease Control and Prevention
1600 Clifton Road, N.E., MS E17
Atlanta, GA 30333
(404) 639-2556/Fax (404) 639-2560
E-mail: cxj3@cdc.gov

Marshall Plaut, M.D.
Chief
Allergic Mechanisms Section
Division of Allergy, Immunology, and
Transplantation
National Institute of Allergy and Infectious
Diseases
National Institutes of Health
6700-B Rockledge Drive, Room 5146
Bethesda, MD 20892-7640
(301) 496-8973/Fax (301) 402-2571
E-mail: mp27s@nih.gov

Stephen Redd, M.D.
Chief
Air Pollution and Respiratory Health Branch
Division of Environmental Hazards and
Health Effects
National Center for Environmental Health
Centers for Disease Control and Prevention
1600 Clifton Road, N.E., MS E17
Atlanta, GA 30341
(404) 639-2549/Fax (404) 639-2560
E-mail: scr1@cdc.gov

Daniel Rotrosen, M.D.
Director
Division of Allergy, Immunology, and
Transplantation
National Institute of Allergy and Infectious
Diseases
National Institutes of Health
6700-B Rockledge Drive, Room 5142
Bethesda, MD 20892-7640
(301) 496-1886/Fax (301) 402-2571
E-mail: drl7@nih.gov

25. Sexually Transmitted Diseases

Dana M. Shelton
Assistant Director for Policy, Planning, and
External Relations
Division of STD Prevention
National Center for HIV, STD, and TB
Prevention
Centers for Disease Control and Prevention
1600 Clifton Road, N.E., MS E02
Atlanta, GA 30333
(404) 639-8260/Fax (404) 639-8608
E-mail: dzs8@cdc.gov

26. Substance Abuse

Wendy Davis
Special Assistant to the Director
Office of Policy and Planning
Center for Substance Abuse Prevention
Substance Abuse and Mental Health
Services Administration
Rockwall II Building, Room 950
5600 Fishers Lane
Rockville, MD 20857
(301) 443-9913/Fax (301) 443-6394
E-mail: wdavis@samhsa.gov

Susan Farrell, Ph.D.
Acting Deputy Director
Division of Biometry and Epidemiology
National Institute on Alcohol Abuse and
Alcoholism
National Institutes of Health
Willco Building, Room 514
6000 Executive Boulevard
Bethesda, MD 20892-7005
(301) 443-1274/Fax (301) 443-7043
E-mail: sf128t@nih.gov

James D. Colliver, Ph.D.
Epidemiology Research Branch, DESPR
National Institute on Drug Abuse
National Institutes of Health
Suite 5153 MSC 9589
6001 Executive Boulevard
Bethesda, MD 20892-9589
(301) 402-1846/Fax (301) 443-2636
E-mail: jcollive@mail.nih.gov

Ann Mahony, M.P.H.
Senior Program Management Officer
Office of Policy, Coordination, and Planning
Center for Substance Abuse Treatment
Substance Abuse and Mental Health
Services Administration
Rockwall II Building, Room 619
5600 Fishers Lane
Rockville, MD 20857
(301) 443-7924/Fax (301) 480-6077
E-mail: amahony@samhsa.gov

27. Tobacco Use

Karil Bialostosky, M.S.
Senior Health Policy Analyst
Office on Smoking and Health
Centers for Disease Control and Prevention
200 Independence Ave, S.W., Room 317-B
Washington, DC 20201
(202) 205-9231/Fax (202) 205-8313
E-mail: kfb3@cdc.gov

28. Vision and Hearing

Marin P. Allen, Ph.D.
Chief
Office of Health Communication and Public
Liaison
National Institute on Deafness and Other
Communication Disorders
National Institutes of Health
Building 31, Room 3C35
31 Center Drive, MSC 2320
Bethesda, MD 20892-2320
(301) 496-7243 or 402-0252/Fax
(301) 402-0018
E-mail: ma51v@nih.gov

Judith Cooper, Ph.D.
Chief, Scientific Programs Branch
National Institute on Deafness and Other
Communication Disorders
National Institutes of Health
EPS400C, MSC 7180
6120 Executive Boulevard
Bethesda, MD 20892-7180
(301) 496-5061/Fax (301) 402-6251
E-mail: judith_cooper@nih.gov

Michael Davis
Associate Director for Science Policy and
Legislation
National Eye Institute
National Institutes of Health
Building 31, Room 6A23
31 Center Drive, MSC 2510
Bethesda, MD 20892-2510
(301) 496-4308/Fax (301) 402-3799
E-mail: mpd@nei.nih.gov

Rosemary Janiszewski, M.S., CHES.
Deputy Director
Scientific Programs Branch
Office of Communication, Health
Education, and Public Liaison
National Eye Institute
National Institutes of Health
Building 31, Room 6A32
31 Center Drive, MSC 2510
Bethesda, MD 20892-2510
(301) 496-5248/Fax (301) 402-1065
E-mail: rjaniszewski@nei.nih.gov

Adolescent Health

Trina Anglin, M.D., Ph.D.
Chief, Office of Adolescent Health
Maternal and Child Health Bureau
Health Resources and Services
Administration
Parklawn Building, Room 18A-39
5600 Fishers Lane
Rockville, MD 20857
(301) 443-4291/Fax (301) 443-1296
E-mail: tanglin@hrsa.gov

Casey Hannan, M.P.H.
Health Education Specialist
Division of Adolescent and School Health
National Center for Chronic Disease
Prevention and Health Promotion
Centers for Disease Control and Prevention
4770 Buford Highway, N.E., MS K29
Atlanta, GA 30341-3724
(770) 488-3190/Fax (770) 488-3110
E-mail: clh8@cdc.gov

Lloyd J. Kolbe, Ph.D.
Director, Division of Adolescent and School
Health
National Center for Chronic Disease
Prevention and Health Promotion
Centers for Disease Control and Prevention
4770 Buford Highway, N.E., MS K29
Atlanta, GA 30341-3724
(770) 488-3254/Fax (770) 488-3110
E-mail: ljk3@cdc.gov

Health of Racial/Ethnic Minority Populations

Georgia Buggs
Special Assistant to the Director
Office of Minority Health
5515 Security Lane, Room 1000
Rockville, MD 20852
(301) 443-5084/Fax (301) 594-0767
E-mail: gbuggs@osophs.dhhs.gov

Olivia Carter-Pokras
Director, Division of Policy and Data
Office of Minority Health
5515 Security Lane, Room 1000
Rockville, MD 20852
(301) 443-9923/Fax (301) 443-8280
E-mail: ocarter@osophs.dhhs.gov

Tuei Doong
Deputy Director
Office of Minority Health
5515 Security Lane, Room 1000
Rockville, MD 20852
(301) 443-5084/Fax (301) 594-0767
E-mail: tdoong@osophs.dhhs.gov

Betty Lee Hawks
Special Assistant to the Director
Office of Minority Health
5515 Security Lane, Room 1000
Rockville, MD 20852
(301) 443-5084/Fax (301) 594-0767
E-mail: bhawks@osophs.dhhs.gov

Women's Health

Theresa Brown
Staff Assistant
DHHS Office on Women's Health
200 Independence Avenue, S.W., Room
728F
Washington, DC 20201
(202) 690-7650/Fax (202) 260-6537
E-mail: tbrown@osophs.dhhs.gov

Miryam Granthon
Healthy People Consortium Coordinator
Office of Disease Prevention and Health
Promotion
200 Independence Avenue, S.W., Room
738G
Washington, DC 20201
(202) 690-6245/Fax (202) 205-9478
E-mail: mgranthon@osophs.dhhs.gov

Suzanne Haynes, Ph.D.
Assistant Director for Science
DHHS Office on Women's Health
200 Independence Avenue, S.W., Room
728F
Washington, DC 20201
(202) 690-7650/Fax (202) 260-6537
E-mail: shaynes@osophs.dhhs.gov

1. Access to Quality Health Services

Barbara Altman, Agency for Healthcare Research and Quality, Rockville, MD

Sania Amr, Health Care Financing Administration, Baltimore, MD

Jean Athey, Health Resources and Services Administration, Rockville, MD

David Atkins, Agency for Healthcare Research and Quality, Rockville, MD

Jessica Banthin, Agency for Healthcare Research and Quality, Rockville, MD

Sharon Barrett, Health Resources and Services Administration, Rockville, MD

Arlene Bierman, Agency for Healthcare Research and Quality, Rockville, MD

Dana Bradshaw, U.S. Air Force, Washington, DC

Georgia Buggs, Office of Minority Health, Rockville, MD

Ronald Carlson, Health Resources and Services Administration, Rockville, MD

Dorothy Carter, U.S. Air Force, Washington, DC

Joseph Chin, Health Care Financing Administration, Baltimore, MD

Evelyn Christian, Health Resources and Services Administration, Rockville, MD

Melissa Clarke, Health Resources and Services Administration, Rockville, MD

Carol Crecy, Administration on Aging, Washington, DC

Wendy Davis, Substance Abuse and Mental Health Services Administration, Rockville, MD

Laura Diaz-Baker, Health Resources and Services Administration, Rockville, MD

Joan Edmondson, Centers for Disease Control and Prevention, Atlanta, GA

Russell Eggert, U.S. Air Force, Washington, DC

Anne Elixhauser, Agency for Healthcare Research and Quality, Rockville, MD

Carol Galaty, Health Resources and Services Administration, Rockville, MD

Kate Gottfried, Office of Disease Prevention and Health Promotion, Washington, DC

Betty Hambleton, Health Resources and Services Administration, Rockville, MD

Mary Hand, National Institutes of Health, Bethesda, MD

Christian Hanson, Centers for Disease Control and Prevention, Atlanta, GA

William Harlan, National Institutes of Health, Bethesda, MD

Jeff Harris, Centers for Disease Control and Prevention, Atlanta, GA

June Horner, Health Resources and Services Administration, Rockville, MD

Miguel Kamat, Office of Minority Health, Rockville, MD

Mireille Kanda, Administration for Children and Families, Washington, DC

Evelyn Kappeler, Office of Population Affairs, Washington, DC

Lynn Kazemekas, Agency for Healthcare Research and Quality, Rockville, MD

Woodie Kessel, Office of Disease Prevention and Health Promotion, Washington, DC

Richard Klein, Centers for Disease Control and Prevention, Hyattsville, MD

Bonnie Lefkowitz, Health Resources and Services Administration, Rockville, MD

Doug Lloyd, Health Resources and Services Administration, Rockville, MD

Rika Maeshiro, Office of Disease Prevention and Health Promotion, Washington, DC

Ann Mahony, Substance Abuse and Mental Health Services Administration, Rockville, MD

Deborah Maiese, Office of Disease Prevention and Health Promotion, Washington, DC

Saralyn Mark, Office on Women's Health, Washington, DC

Merle McPherson, Health Resources and Services Administration, Washington, DC

Jean Moody-Williams, EMSC National Resource Center, Rockville, MD

Paul Nannis, Health Resources and Services Administration, Rockville, MD

Patrick O'Brien, Indian Health Service, Tulsa, OK

Karen Pane, Health Resources and Services Administration, Rockville, MD

Eileen Parish, Food and Drug Administration, Rockville, MD

Daniel Pollock, Centers for Disease Control and Prevention, Atlanta, GA

Kathryn Rickard, Agency for Healthcare Research and Quality, Rockville, MD

Gail Ritchie, Substance Abuse and Mental Health Services Administration, Rockville, MD

Bill Robinson, Health Resources and Services Administration, Rockville, MD

Theresa Rogers, Centers for Disease Control and Prevention, Atlanta, GA

Sheera Rosenfeld, Health Resources and Services Administration, Rockville, MD

Colleen Ryan, Centers for Disease Control and Prevention, Hyattsville, MD

Kenneth Schachter, Centers for Disease Control and Prevention, Atlanta, GA

Ray Seltzer, Agency for Healthcare Research and Quality, Rockville, MD

Dorita Sewell, Substance Abuse and Mental Health Services Administration, Rockville, MD

Mary Beth Skupien, Indian Health Service, Rockville, MD

Mark Smolinski, Office of Public Health and Science, Washington, DC

David Snyder, Health Resources and Services Administration, Rockville, MD

Lynn Soban, Office of Disease Prevention and Health Promotion, Washington, DC

Daniel Stryer, Agency for Healthcare Research and Quality, Rockville, MD

Robert Sullivan, Department of Veterans Affairs, Durham, NC

Irma Tetzloff, Administration on Aging, Washington, DC

Betsy Thompson, Centers for Disease Control and Prevention, Atlanta, GA

Craig Vanderwagen, Indian Health Service, Rockville, MD

Joan Van Nostrand, Health Resources and Services Administration, Rockville, MD

Lyman Van Nostrand, Health Resources and Services Administration, Rockville, MD

Martina Vogel-Taylor, National Institutes of Health, Bethesda, MD

Robin Weinick, Agency for Healthcare Research and Quality, Rockville, MD

Valerie Welsh, Office of Minority Health, Rockville, MD

Gerald Zelinger, Health Care Financing Administration, Baltimore, MD

2. Arthritis, Osteoporosis, and Chronic Back Conditions

Gunner Andersson, Rush-Presbyterian-St. Luke's Medical Center, Chicago, IL

Barbara Bowman, Centers for Disease Control and Prevention, Atlanta, GA

Teresa Brady, Centers for Disease Control and Prevention, Atlanta, GA

Leigh Callahan, University of North Carolina School of Medicine, Chapel Hill, NC

Tim Carey, University of North Carolina, Chapel Hill, NC

Doyt Conn, Emory University School of Medicine, Atlanta, GA

David Felson, Boston University School of Medicine, Boston, MA

Larry Fine, Centers for Disease Control and Prevention, Cincinnati, OH

Jamila Fonseka, Centers for Disease Control and Prevention, Atlanta, GA

Deborah Galuska, Centers for Disease Control and Prevention, Atlanta, GA

Charles Helmick, Centers for Disease Control and Prevention, Atlanta, GA

Rosemarie Hirsch, Centers for Disease Control and Prevention, Hyattsville, MD

Marc Hochberg, University of Maryland School of Medicine, Baltimore, MD

Reva Lawrence, National Institutes of Health, Bethesda, MD

Matthew Liang, Brigham and Women's Hospital, Boston, MA

Anne Looker, Centers for Disease Control and Prevention, Hyattsville, MD

Kate Lorig, Stanford University School of Medicine, Palo Alto, CA

Robert Meenan, Boston University School of Public Health, Boston, MA

Susan Nesci, Arthritis Foundation, Rocky Hill, CT

Diane Orenstein, Centers for Disease Control and Prevention, Atlanta, GA

Laurie Piacitelli, Centers for Disease Control and Prevention, Cincinnati, OH

Paul Scherr, Centers for Disease Control and Prevention, Atlanta, GA

Judy Stevens, Centers for Disease Control and Prevention, Atlanta, GA

Annette Swezey, Arthritis and Back Pain Center, Santa Monica, CA

Robert L. Swezey, Arthritis and Back Pain Center, Santa Monica, CA

Kathleen Turczyn, Centers for Disease Control and Prevention, Hyattsville, MD

Diane Wagener, Centers for Disease Control and Prevention, Hyattsville, MD

Edward Yelin, University of California Arthritis Research Group, San Francisco, CA

Ping Zhang, Centers for Disease Control and Prevention, Atlanta, GA

3. Cancer

Nelvis Castro, National Institutes of Health, Bethesda, MD

Ralph Coates, Centers for Disease Control and Prevention, Atlanta, GA

Brenda Edwards, National Institutes of Health, Bethesda, MD

William Harlan, National Institutes of Health, Bethesda, MD

Betty Hawks, Office of Minority Health, Rockville, MD

Elizabeth Jackson, Centers for Disease Control and Prevention, Hyattsville, MD

Richard Klein, Centers for Disease Control and Prevention, Hyattsville, MD

Nancy Lins, American Cancer Society, Atlanta, GA

Deborah Maiese, Office of Disease Prevention and Health Promotion, Washington, DC

Barry Portnoy, National Institutes of Health, Bethesda, MD

Marion Primas, Office on Women's Health, Bethesda, MD

Barbara Reilley, Centers for Disease Control and Prevention, Atlanta, GA

Karen Richard, Centers for Disease Control and Prevention, Atlanta, GA

Ray Seltzer, Agency for Healthcare Research and Quality, Rockville, MD

Gloria Stables, National Institutes of Health, Bethesda, MD

Judith Swan, National Institutes of Health, Bethesda, MD

Nancy Wartow, Administration on Aging, Washington, DC

4. Chronic Kidney Disease

D.W. Chen, Health Resources and Services Administration, Rockville, MD

Paul Eggers, Health Care Financing Administration, Baltimore, MD

Andrew Narva, Indian Health Service, Albuquerque, NM

Colleen Ryan, Centers for Disease Control and Prevention, Hyattsville, MD

Jerry Tokars, Centers for Disease Control and Prevention, Atlanta, GA

5. Diabetes

Kelly Acton, Indian Health Service, Albuquerque, NM

Lois Albarelli, Administration on Aging, Washington, DC

Terence Albright, American Podiatric Medical Association, Chicago, IL

Kate Alich, Massachusetts Department of Public Health, Boston, MA

Lawrence Blonde, Ochsner Clinic, New Orleans, LA

Benjamin Burton, National Institutes of Health, Bethesda, MD

Mary Clark, The Links, Inc., Sterling, VA

Lorelei de Cora, American Indian Talking Circles, Winnebago, NE

Jane Delgado, National Coalition of Hispanic Health and Human Services Organizations, Washington, DC

Michael Duenas, American Optometric Association, Chattahoochee, FL

Richard Eastman, National Institutes of Health, Bethesda, MD

John Eisenberg, Agency for Healthcare Research and Quality, Rockville, MD

Rick Ferris, National Institutes of Health, Bethesda, MD

Barbara Fleming, Health Care Financing Administration, Baltimore, MD

Willis Foster, National Institutes of Health, Bethesda, MD

Wilfred Fujimoto, University of Washington, Seattle, WA

Glenn Gastwirth, American Podiatric Medical Association, Bethesda, MD

Robert Goldstein, Juvenile Diabetes Foundation, Inc., New York, NY

Linda Jackson, National Caucus and Center on Black Aged, Inc., Washington, DC

Joan Jacobs, Office of Minority Health, Rockville, MD

Stephen Jiang, Association of Asian/Pacific Community Health, Oakland, CA

Paula Jorisch, Administration on Developmental Disabilities, Washington, DC

Richard Kahn, American Diabetes Association, Alexandria, VA

Richard Klein, Centers for Disease Control and Prevention, Hyattsville, MD

Claresa Levetan, Medlantic Clinical Research Center, Washington, DC

Saralyn Mark, Office on Women's Health, Washington, DC

Kathy Mulcahy, American Association of Diabetes Educators, Chicago, IL

Henry Pacheco, National Council of La Raza, Washington, DC

Leonard Pogach, Veterans Health Administration, East Orange, NJ

David Robinson, National Institutes of Health, Bethesda, MD

William Robinson, Health Resources and Services Administration, Rockville, MD

Yvette Roubideaux, University of Arizona, Tucson, AZ

Colleen Ryan, Centers for Disease Control and Prevention, Hyattsville, MD

Darian Schaubert, North Dakota Department of Health, Bismarck, ND

Earl W. Schurman, Department of Health and Mental Hygiene, Baltimore, MD

Stephen Spann, American Academy of Family Physicians, Houston, TX

Chris Tobin, Atlanta, GA

Lorraine Valdez, Indian Health Service, Albuquerque, NM

6. Disability and Secondary Conditions

Michelle Adler, Social Security Administration, Baltimore, MD

Lynda Anderson, University of Minnesota, Minneapolis, MN

David Auxter, Research Institute for Independent Living, KS

Allan Bergman, United Cerebral Palsy, Washington, DC

Dyanne Bostain, Regent University, Virginia Beach, VA

David Braddock, University of Illinois, Chicago, IL

David Brown, National Council on Disability, Washington, DC

Roberta Carlin, Spina Bifida Association of America, Washington, DC

Andrea Censky, Paralyzed Veterans of America, Washington, DC

Evey Chernow, American Speech-Language-Hearing Association, Rockville, MD

Kate Ciacco-Palatianos, Indian Health Service, Rockville, MD

Melissa Clarke, Health Resources and Services Administration, Rockville, MD

Marie Clements, UNIM Life Insurance Company

Diane Coleman, National Council on Disability, Washington, DC

Fred Cowell, Paralyzed Veterans of America, Washington, DC

Marsha Davenport, Health Care Financing Administration, Rockville, MD

Speed Davis, Disability Advocate Specialist, Arlington, VA

Gay Girolami, Pathways Awareness Foundation, Chicago, IL

Murray Goldstein, United Cerebral Palsy, Washington, DC

David Gray, Washington University, St. Louis, MO

Bob Griss, Center on Disability and Health, Washington, DC

David Hamel, Rhode Island Department of Health, Providence, RI

Bryna Helfer, Traumatic Brain Injury Technical Assistance Center, Alexandria, VA

Richard Hemp, University of Illinois at Chicago, Chicago, IL

Elaine Holland, American Academy of Pediatrics, Washington, DC

Anne-Marie Hughey, National Council on Independent Living, Washington, DC

Elizabeth Jackson, Centers for Disease Control and Prevention, Hyattsville, MD

Corrine Kirchner, American Foundation for the Blind, New York, NY

Fred Krause, Brain Injury Association of America, Alexandria, VA

Charles Lakin, University of Minnesota, Minneapolis, MN

Carol Locust, National Council on Disability, Washington, DC

Michael Marge, American Association on Health and Disability, Fayetteville, NY

Kathy Martinez, World Institute on Disability, Oakland, CA

Suzanne McDermott, University of South Carolina, Columbia, SC

Kathy McGinley, Association for Retarded Citizens, Washington, DC

Jack McNeil, U.S. Department of Commerce, Washington, DC

Dot Nary, National Council on Independent Living, Washington, DC

Els Nieuwenhuijenson, University of Michigan, Ann Arbor, MI

Kathryn O'Connell, Rehabilitation Counselor, Syracuse, NY

Diane Paul-Brown, American Speech-Language-Hearing Association, Rockville, MD

Louis Quatrano, National Institutes of Health, Bethesda, MD

Jim Rimmer, University of Illinois, Chicago, IL

Sunny Roller, University of Michigan, Ann Arbor, MI

Marcia Roth, North Carolina Department of Health and Human Services, Raleigh, NC

Shirley Ryan, National Council on Disability, Washington, DC

Julie Sargent, Kansas Department of Health, Topeka, KS

Donna Scandlin, University of North Carolina, Chapel Hill, NC

Tom Seekins, University of Montana, Missoula, MT

Raymond Seltzer, Agency for Healthcare Research and Quality, Rockville, MD

Dorita Sewell, Substance Abuse and Mental Health Services Administration, Rockville, MD

James Steen, Administration on Aging, Washington, DC

Frances Stevens, New York State Department of Health, Albany, NY

Marie Strahan, Social Security Administration, Baltimore, MD

Alexa Stuifgergen, University of Texas, Austin, TX

Paul Tupper, Massachusetts Department of Health, Boston, MA

Don Wagner, University of Cincinnati, Cincinnati, OH

Lesa Walker, Texas Department of Health, Austin TX

Sylvia Walker, Howard University, Washington, DC

Reginald Wells, Administration for Children and Families, Washington, DC

Sandy Welner, Gynecological Care for Women with Disabilities, Silver Spring, MD

Glen White, University of Kansas, Lawrence, KS

Gale Whiteneck, Craig Hospital, Englewood, CO

7. Educational and Community-Based Programs

Mike Adams, Centers for Disease Control and Prevention, Atlanta, GA

Lois Albarelli, Administration on Aging, Washington, DC

Lynda Anderson, Centers for Disease Control and Prevention, Atlanta, GA

Elaine Auld, Society for Public Health Education, Washington, DC

Carol Brown, National Association of City and County Health Officials, Washington, DC

Ellen Capwell, Ohio Department of Health, Columbus, OH

Larry Chapman, Summex Corporation, Seattle, WA

Melissa Clarke, Health Resources and Services Administration, Rockville, MD

Ashley Coffield, Partnership for Prevention, Washington, DC

Kevin Costigan, Administration for Children and Families, Washington, DC

Nancy Couey-Pegg, Centers for Disease Control and Prevention, Atlanta, GA

Carolyn Crump, University of North Carolina, Chapel Hill, NC

Stephen Fawcett, University of Kansas, Lawrence, KS

Jennifer Fiedelholtz, Health Resources and Services Administration, Rockville, MD

Mary Frase, U.S. Department of Education, Washington, DC

Robinson Fulwood, National Institutes of Health, Bethesda, MD

Carol Galaty, Health Resources and Services Administration, Rockville, MD

Barbara Giloth, University of Illinois, Chicago, IL

Adrienne Goode, Substance Abuse and Mental Health Services Administration, Rockville, MD

Jim Grizzell, California Polytechnic Institute, Pomona, CA

Jeanette Guyton-Krishnan, Centers for Disease Control and Prevention, Hyattsville, MD

Casey Hannan, Centers for Disease Control and Prevention, Atlanta, GA

Suzanne Haynes, Office on Women's Health, Washington, DC

Amy Holmes-Chavez, Centers for Disease Control and Prevention, Atlanta, GA

Marita Hopmann, Administration for Children and Families, Washington, DC

Elizabeth Howze, Centers for Disease Control and Prevention, Atlanta, GA

Ellen Jones, Mississippi Department of Health, Jackson, MS

Laura Kann, Centers for Disease Control and Prevention, Atlanta, GA

Richard Klein, Centers for Disease Control and Prevention, Hyattsville, MD

Lloyd Kolbe, Centers for Disease Control and Prevention, Atlanta, GA

Marshall Kreuter, Centers for Disease Control and Prevention, Atlanta, GA

Brick Lancaster, Centers for Disease Control and Prevention, Atlanta, GA

Mae Lee, Centers for Disease Control and Prevention, Atlanta, GA

Joe Leutsinger, Union Pacific Railroads, Omaha, NE

Laura Lippman, U.S. Department of Education, Washington, DC

Douglas Lloyd, Health Resources and Services Administration, Rockville, MD

Rose Marie Matulionis, Association of State and Territorial Directors of Health Promotion and Public Health Education, Washington, DC

Marilyn McMillen, U.S. Department of Education, Washington, DC

Paul Nannis, Health Resources and Services Administration, Rockville, MD

Donna Nichols, Texas Department of Health, Austin, TX

Michael O'Donnell, American Journal of Health Promotion, Keego Harbor, MI

Guadalupe Pacheco, Office of Minority Health, Rockville, MD

Kathleen Palmes, Continental Health Promotion, Blacksburg, VA

Stephanie Pronk, William Mercer, Inc., Minneapolis, MN

Robin Rager, Texas Women's University, Denton, TX

Rebecca Reeve, University of Virginia, Charlottesville, VA

Elena Rios, Office on Women's Health, Washington, DC

Angel Roca, Centers for Disease Control and Prevention, Atlanta, GA

Colleen Ryan, Centers for Disease Control and Prevention, Hyattsville, MD

Randy Schwartz, Maine Department of Human Services, Augusta, ME

Dorita Sewell, Substance Abuse and Mental Health Services Administration, Rockville, MD

Kathleen Shannon, Health Resources and Services Administration, Bethesda, MD

Dana Silverman, Centers for Disease Control and Prevention, Atlanta, GA

Rob Simmons, Christiana Care Health Services, Wilmington, DE

Ray Sinclair, Centers for Disease Control and Prevention, Cincinnati, OH

Marc Tomlinson, National Association of City and County Health Officials, Washington, DC

Mary Turner, American Association of Retired Persons, Washington, DC

Lyman Van Nostrand, Health Resources and Services Administration, Rockville, MD

Mary Wachacha, Indian Health Service, Rockville, MD

Margaret Washnitzer, Administration for Children and Families, Washington, DC

Nancy B. Watkins, Centers for Disease Control and Prevention, Atlanta, GA

Valerie Welsh, Office of Minority Health, Rockville, MD

Mark Wilson, University of Georgia, Athens, GA

Susan Wooley, American School Health Association, Kent, OH

Joseph Zogby, Health Resources and Services Administration, Rockville, MD

8. Environmental Health

Christa Alonso, Centers for Disease Control and Prevention, Atlanta, GA

Henry Anderson, Council of State and Territorial Epidemiologists, Milwaukee, WI

Tim Baker, Centers for Disease Control and Prevention, Atlanta, GA

Ron Banks, Department of Health and Human Services, San Francisco, CA

Pat Bohan, Centers for Disease Control and Prevention, Atlanta, GA

Sherry Brady, Centers for Disease Control and Prevention, Atlanta, GA

Sonia Buist, University of Oregon Health Sciences Center, Portland, OR

Arden Calvert, U.S. Environmental Protection Agency, Washington, DC

Brad Campbell, Council on Environmental Quality, Washington, DC

Craig Carlson, American Association of Health Plans, Washington, DC

Olivia Carter-Pokras, Office of Minority Health, Washington, DC

Bruce Chelikowsky, Indian Health Service, Rockville, MD

Melissa Clarke, Health Resources and Services Administration, Rockville, MD

Tom Doremus, Public Health Foundation, Washington, DC

Dick Durrett, Indian Health Service, Rockville, MD

Emilio Esteban, Centers for Disease Control and Prevention, Atlanta, GA

David Evans, Centers for Disease Control and Prevention, Atlanta, GA

Robinson Fulwood, National Institutes of Health, Bethesda, MD

Ginger Gist, National Environmental Health Association, Washington, DC

Mike Hadrick, U.S. Environmental Protection Agency, Washington, DC

Burl Haigwood, Clean Fuels Foundation, Washington, DC

Barbara Hatcher, American Public Health Association, Washington, DC

Suzanne Haynes, Office on Women's Health, Washington, DC

Sharon Heber, Florida Department of Health, Tallahassee, FL

David Homa, Centers for Disease Control and Prevention, Atlanta, GA

Polly Hoppin, Office of Deputy Assistant Secretary for Science Policy, Washington, DC

Fen Hunt, U.S. Department of Agriculture, Washington, DC

David Jacobs, U.S. Department of Housing and Urban Development, Washington, DC

William Jirles, National Institutes of Health, Research Triangle Park, NC

Eric Juzenas, American Public Health Association, Washington, DC

Rick Karlin, American Water Works Association, Denver, CO

Rita Kelliher, Association of Schools of Public Health, Washington, DC

Tom Kennedy, Association of State and Territorial Solid Waste Management Officials, Washington, DC

Chris Kochtitzky, Centers for Disease Control and Prevention, Atlanta, GA

Vanessa Leiby, Association of State Drinking Water Administrators, Washington, DC

Deborah Maiese, Office of Disease Prevention and Health Promotion, Washington, DC

David Manino, Centers for Disease Control and Prevention, Atlanta, GA

Floyd Maveaux, Howard University, Washington, DC

Mark McClanahan, Centers for Disease Control and Prevention, Atlanta, GA

Leyla McCurdy, American Lung Association, Washington, DC

Kathleen Meade, National Recycling Coalition, Washington, DC

Pam Meyer, Centers for Disease Control and Prevention, Atlanta, GA

Melinda Moore, Centers for Disease Control and Prevention, Atlanta, GA

Sheila Newton, National Institutes of Health, Research Triangle Park, NC

Tim O'Leary, Association of State and Territorial Health Officials, Washington, DC

Horst Otterstetter, Pan American Health Organization, Washington, DC

Gib Parrish, Centers for Disease Control and Prevention, Atlanta, GA

Don Patterson, Centers for Disease Control and Prevention, Atlanta, GA

Dalton Paxman, Office of Disease Prevention and Health Promotion, Washington, DC

Carol Pertowski, Centers for Disease Control and Prevention, Atlanta, GA

Rossanne Philen, Centers for Disease Control and Prevention, Atlanta, GA

Marshall Plaut, National Institutes of Health, Bethesda, MD

Stephen Redd, Centers for Disease Control and Prevention, Atlanta, GA

Beth Resnick, National Association of County and City Health Officials, Washington, DC

Robbie Roberts, Environmental Council of the States, Washington, DC

Theresa Rogers, Centers for Disease Control and Prevention, Atlanta, GA

Don Ryan, Alliance to End Childhood Lead Poisoning, Washington, DC

Mike Sage, Centers for Disease Control and Prevention, Atlanta, GA

Richard Saul, Administration for Children and Families, Washington, DC

Roberta Savage, Association of State and Interstate Water Pollution Control Authorities, Washington, DC

John Schelp, National Institutes of Health, Research Triangle Park, NC

Fred Seitz, Centers for Disease Control and Prevention, Hyattsville, MD

Bruce Sidwell, U.S. Environmental Protection Agency, Washington, DC

Rose Ann Soloway, American Association of Poison Control Centers, Washington, DC

Richard Walling, Office of International and Refugee Health, Rockville, MD

Ron White, American Lung Association, Washington, DC

Bill Wilkinson, Bicycle Federation of America, Washington, DC

Drusilla Yorke, U.S. Environmental Protection Agency, Washington, DC

9. Family Planning

Joyce Abma, Centers for Disease Control and Prevention, Hyattsville, MD

Christine Bachrach, National Institutes of Health, Bethesda, MD

Georgia Buggs, Office of Minority Health, Rockville, MD

Cynthia Daliard, The Alan Guttmacher Institute, Washington, DC

Rachel Gold, The Alan Guttmacher Institute, Washington, DC

Kate Gottfried, Office of Disease Prevention and Health Promotion, Washington, DC

Joel Greenspan, Centers for Disease Control and Prevention, Atlanta, GA

Matthew Guidry, Office of Disease Prevention and Health Promotion, Washington, DC

Jeanette Guyton-Krishnan, Centers for Disease Control and Prevention, Hyattsville, MD

Leslie Hardy, Office of the Assistant Secretary for Planning and Evaluation, Washington, DC

Brad Hendrick, Office of Population Affairs, Bethesda, MD

Evelyn Kappeler, Office of Population Affairs, Bethesda, MD

Mariana Kastrinakis, Office of Population Affairs, Bethesda, MD

Lisa Koonin, Centers for Disease Control and Prevention, Atlanta, GA

Thomas Kring, Office of Population Affairs, Bethesda, MD

Mary Kay Larson, Centers for Disease Control and Prevention, Atlanta, GA

Laura Duberstein Lindberg, Urban Institute, Washington, DC

William Mosher, Centers for Disease Control and Prevention, Hyattsville, MD

Susan Moskosky, Office of Population Affairs, Bethesda, MD

Susan Newcomer, National Institutes of Health, Bethesda, MD

Linda Peterson, Centers for Disease Control and Prevention, Hyattsville, MD

John Santelli, Centers for Disease Control and Prevention, Atlanta, GA

Fred Seitz, Centers for Disease Control and Prevention, Hyattsville, MD

Mary Shiffer, Administration for Child and Families, Washington, DC

Susheela Singh, The Alan Guttmacher Institute, New York, NY

Wendy Turnbull, The Alan Guttmacher Institute, Washington, DC

Stephanie Ventura, Centers for Disease Control and Prevention, Hyattsville, MD

Susan Woods, Office on Women's Health, Washington, DC

10. Food Safety

Lise Borel, B ELASTIC Inc., West Chester, PA

Melissa Chun, U.S. Environmental Protection Agency, Washington, DC

Melissa Clarke, Health Resources and Services Administration, Rockville, MD

Elisa Elliot, Food and Drug Administration, Washington, DC

Ruth Etzel, U.S. Department of Agriculture, Washington, DC

Sandy Facinoli, U.S. Department of Agriculture, Washington, DC

Sara Fein, Food and Drug Administration, Washington, DC

Ann Furlong, Food Allergy Network, Fairfax, VA

Bing Garthright, Food and Drug Administration, Washington, DC

Brenda Halbrook, U.S. Department of Agriculture, Washington, DC

Marcia Headrick, Food and Drug Administration, Rockville, MD

George J. Jackson, Food and Drug Administration, Washington, DC

Rick Kirchoff, National Association of State Departments of Agriculture, Washington, DC

Chris Kochtitzky, Centers for Disease Control and Prevention, Atlanta, GA

Sandra Lancaster, Conference for Food Protection, Little Rock, AR

Priscilla Levine, U.S. Department of Agriculture, Washington, DC

Glenda Lewis, Food and Drug Administration, Washington, DC

Kathryn McMurry, Office of Disease Prevention and Health Promotion, Washington, DC

Holly McPeak, U.S. Department of Agriculture, Washington, DC

Tim O'Leary, Association of State and Territorial Health Officials, Washington, DC

Eileen Parish, Food and Drug Administration, Washington, DC

Clifford Purdy, Food and Drug Administration, Atlanta, GA

Beth Resnick, National Association of County and City Health Officials, Washington, DC

Sheila Richburg, Joint Institute for Food Safety and Applied Nutrition, College Park, MD

Bruce Sidwell, U.S. Environmental Protection Agency, Washington, DC

Dennis Thayer, National Restaurant Association, Washington, DC

Kathleen Turczyn, Centers for Disease Control and Prevention, Hyattsville, MD

Tom Van Gilder, Centers for Disease Control and Prevention, Atlanta, GA

Tom Wilcox, Food and Drug Administration, Washington, DC

Betsy Woodward, Association of Food and Drug Officials, Tallahassee, FL

Juanita Yates, Food and Drug Administration, Washington, DC

11. Health Communication

Elaine Auld, Society for Public Health Education, Washington, DC

Michael Barnes, Brigham Young University, Salt Lake City, UT

Allan Braslow, Agency for Healthcare Research and Quality, Rockville, MD

Cynthia Baur, Office of Disease Prevention and Health Promotion, Washington, DC

Jose T. Carneiro, Office of Minority Health Resource Center, Silver Spring, MD

Blake Crawford, Office of Minority Health, Rockville, MD

Mary Jo Deering, Office of Disease Prevention and Health Promotion, Washington, DC

Connie Dresser, National Institutes of Health, Bethesda, MD

Tom Eng, Institute for Interactive Health Communication, Washington, DC

Vicki Freimuth, Centers for Disease Control and Prevention, Atlanta, GA

Sarah Gegenheimer, Office of the Assistant Secretary for Public Affairs, Washington, DC

Leslie Hsu, Office of Disease Prevention and Health Promotion, Washington, DC

Elizabeth Jackson, Centers for Disease Control and Prevention, Hyattsville, MD

Linda Johnston, Health Resources and Services Administration, Rockville, MD

Cynthia Jorgensen, Centers for Disease Control and Prevention, Atlanta, GA

Sandy Kappert, Health Care Financing Administration, Baltimore, MD

Fred Kroger, Centers for Disease Control and Prevention, Atlanta, GA

Naomi Kulakòw, Food and Drug Administration, Washington, DC

Mary Agnes Laureno, Health Care Financing Administration, Baltimore, MD

R. Craig Lefebvre, Prospect Associates, Silver Spring, MD

James Lindenberger, Best Start Social Marketing, Tampa, FL

Donna Lloyd-Kolkin, Society for Public Health Education, New Hope, PA

Rose Marie Matulionis, Association of State and Territorial Directors of Health Promotion and Public Health Education, Washington, DC

Andrew Maxfield, Centers for Disease Control and Prevention, Washington, DC

Charlotte Mehuron, Health Resources and Services Administration, Rockville, MD

Scott Ratzan, Academy for Educational Development, Washington, DC

Gale Riddles, Indian Health Service, Rockville, MD

Valerie Scardino, Office on Women's Health, Washington, DC

Stephanie Smith, Office of Disease Prevention and Health Promotion, Washington, DC

Sue Stableford, Maine AHEC Health Literacy Center, University of New England, Biddeford, ME

Tim Tinker, Agency for Toxic Substances and Disease Registry, Atlanta, GA

Jean Wooldridge, Fred Hutchinson Cancer Center, Seattle, WA

12. Heart Disease and Stroke

Georgia Buggs, Office of Minority Health, Rockville, MD

James Cleeman, National Institutes of Health, Bethesda, MD

Karen Donato, National Institutes of Health, Bethesda, MD

Robinson Fulwood, National Institutes of Health, Bethesda, MD

Mary Hand, National Institutes of Health, Bethesda, MD

Suzanne Haynes, Office on Women's Health, Washington, DC

Elizabeth Jackson, Centers for Disease Control and Prevention, Hyattsville, MD

Richard Klein, Centers for Disease Control and Prevention, Hyattsville, MD

Deborah Maiese, Office of Disease Prevention and Health Promotion, Washington, DC

Gregory Morosco, National Institutes of Health, Bethesda, MD

Nancy Poole, National Institutes of Health, Bethesda, MD

Edward Roccella, National Institutes of Health, Bethesda, MD

Frederick Rohde, National Institutes of Health, Bethesda, MD

Dana Silverman, Centers for Disease Control and Prevention, Atlanta, GA

Patricia Turner, National Institutes of Health, Bethesda, MD

Martina Vogel-Taylor, National Institutes of Health, Bethesda, MD

13. HIV

Marty Bond, Substance Abuse and Mental Health Services Administration, Rockville, MD

David Brownell, Centers for Disease Control and Prevention, Atlanta, GA

Georgia Buggs, Office of Minority Health, Rockville, MD

Christine Cagle, Centers for Disease Control and Prevention, Atlanta, GA

Pat Campiglia, Administration for Children and Families, Washington, DC

Emily DeCoster, Health Resources and Services Administration, Rockville, MD

Gary Edgar, Centers for Disease Control and Prevention, Atlanta, GA

Paul Gaist, National Institutes of Health, Bethesda, MD

Shelley Gordon, Health Resources and Services Administration, Rockville, MD

Dawn Gnesda, Centers for Disease Control and Prevention, Atlanta, GA

Randy Graydon, Health Care Financing Administration, Baltimore, MD

Leslie Hardy, Office of the Assistant Secretary for Planning and Evaluation, Washington, DC

Glen Harelson, Office of HIV/AIDS Policy, Washington, DC

Gena Hill, Centers for Disease Control and Prevention, Atlanta, GA

Evelyn Kappeler, Office of Populations Affairs, Bethesda, MD

Richard Klein, Centers for Disease Control and Prevention, Hyattsville, MD

Deborah Maiese, Office of Disease Prevention and Health Promotion, Washington, DC

Gerry McQuillan, Centers for Disease Control and Prevention, Hyattsville, MD

John Miles, Centers for Disease Control and Prevention, Atlanta, GA

Fran Page, Office on Women's Health, Washington, DC

Donald Pohl, Food and Drug Administration, Rockville, MD

Rebecca Rosenberg, Office on Women's Health, Washington, DC

Alex Ross, Health Resources and Services Administration, Rockville, MD

Colleen Ryan, Centers for Disease Control and Prevention, Hyattsville, MD

John Seggerson, Centers for Disease Control and Prevention, Atlanta, GA

Eva M. Seiler, Centers for Disease Control and Prevention, Atlanta, GA

Dorita Sewell, Substance Abuse and Mental Health Services Administration, Rockville, MD

Laura Shelby, Indian Health Service, Albuquerque, NM

Mark Smolinski, Office of Disease Prevention and Health Promotion, Washington, DC

Jack Spencer, Centers for Disease Control and Prevention, Atlanta, GA

Carmen Villar, Centers for Disease Control and Prevention, Atlanta, GA

Phyllis Zucker, Agency for Healthcare Research and Quality, Rockville, MD

14. Immunization and Infectious Diseases

Jon Abramson, American Academy of Pediatrics, Winston-Salem, NC

Lois Albarelli, Administration on Aging, Washington, DC

Angela Bauer, Centers for Disease Control and Prevention, Atlanta, GA

Jennifer Brooks, Centers for Disease Control and Prevention, Atlanta, GA

Jim Buehler, Centers for Disease Control and Prevention, Atlanta, GA

Virginia Burggraf, American Nurses Association, Washington, DC

Gail Cassell, American Society for Microbiology, Indianapolis, IN

Jim Cheek, Indian Health Service, Albuquerque, NM

Anthony Chen, Asian Pacific Task Force on Hepatitis B Immunization, Seattle, WA

Melissa Clarke, Health Resources and Services Administration, Rockville, MD

José Cordero, Centers for Disease Control and Prevention, Atlanta, GA

George Counts, National Institutes of Health, Bethesda, MD

Fran DuMelle, American Lung Association, Washington, DC

Catherine Ehlen, American Association of Health Plans, Washington, DC

Judy English, Association for Professionals in Infection Control and Epidemiology, Inc, Falls Church, VA

Walter Faggett, National Medical Association, Washington, DC

Pierce Gardner, American College of Physicians, Stony Brook, NY

Helene Gayle, Centers for Disease Control and Prevention, Atlanta, GA

Bruce Gellin, Infectious Diseases Society of America, Nashville, TN

Mary Gilchrist, American Society for Microbiology, Iowa City, IA

Rita Goodman, Health Resources and Services Administration, Bethesda, MD

Claire Hannan, Association of State and Territorial Health Officials, Washington, DC

Gena Hill, Centers for Disease Control and Prevention, Atlanta, GA

Alan Hinman, Task Force for Child Survival and Development, Decatur, GA

Linda Horsch, Health Care Financing Administration, Dallas, TX

James Hughes, Centers for Disease Control and Prevention, Atlanta, GA

John Iskauder, Council of State and Territorial Epidemiologists, Columbia, SC

Michael Johnson, Health Resources and Services Administration, Rockville, MD

David Kelly, Health Resources and Services Administration, Rockville, MD

Joel Kuritsky, Centers for Disease Control and Prevention, Atlanta, GA

Martin Landry, Centers for Disease Control and Prevention, Atlanta, GA

Roland Levandowski, Food and Drug Administration, Rockville, MD

John Livengood, Centers for Disease Control and Prevention, Atlanta, GA

Steve MacDonald, Council of State and Territorial Epidemiologists, Olympia, WA

Mark Magenheim, Centers for Disease Control and Prevention, Sarasota, FL

Louis Mahoney, Health Resources and Services Administration, Rockville, MD

Alison Mawle, Centers for Disease Control and Prevention, Atlanta, GA

Joanne Mitten, Association of State and Territorial Directors of Health Promotion and Health Education, Boise, ID

John Modlin, CDC Advisory Committee on Immunization Practices, Lebanon, NH

Amy Nevel, U.S. Department of Health and Human Services, Washington, DC

Charles Nolan, CDC Advisory Committee for TB Elimination, Seattle, WA

Patricia Nolan, Association of State and Territorial Health Officials, Providence, RI

Walter Orenstein, Centers for Disease Control and Prevention, Atlanta, GA

Stephen Ostroff, Centers for Disease Control and Prevention, Atlanta, GA

Walter Page, National Tuberculosis Controllers Association, Atlanta, GA

Georges Peter, National Vaccine Advisory Committee, Providence, RI

Gregory Poland, National Coalition for Adult Immunization, Rochester, MN

Carol Pozsik, National TB Controllers Association, Columbia, SC

Michele Puryear, Health Resources and Services Administration, Rockville, MD

Rosemary Ramsey, Centers for Disease Control and Prevention, Atlanta, GA

Margaret Rennels, American Academy of Pediatrics, Baltimore, MD

Theresa Rogers, Centers for Disease Control and Prevention Atlanta, GA

Colleen Ryan, Centers for Disease Control and Prevention, Hyattsville, MD

John Seggerson, Centers for Disease Control and Prevention, Atlanta, GA

Eva Seiler, Centers for Disease Control and Prevention, Atlanta, GA

Steve Sepe, Centers for Disease Control and Prevention, Atlanta, GA

Dorita Sewell, Substance Abuse and Mental Health Services Administration, Rockville, MD

Diane Simpson, Centers for Disease Control and Prevention, Atlanta, GA

Nicole Smith, Centers for Disease Control and Prevention, Atlanta, GA

Mark Smolinski, Office of Disease Prevention and Health Promotion, Washington, DC

Cassandra Sparrow, The Congress of National Black Churches, Washington, DC

Samuel Stanley, American Society of Tropical Medicine and Hygiene, St. Louis, MO

Mary Thorngren, Coalition of Spanish Speaking Mental Health Organizations, Washington, DC

James Tierney, Interamerican College of Physicians and Surgeons, New York, NY

Tom Tonniges, American Academy of Pediatrics, Elk Grove Village, IL

Bill Watson, All Kids Count, Atlanta, GA

Peggy Webster, National Foundation for Infectious Diseases, Bethesda, MD

Burton Wilcke, Association of Public Health Laboratories, Burlington, VT

Walter Williams, Centers for Disease Control and Prevention, Atlanta, GA

Robert Wright, Centers for Disease Control and Prevention, Hyattsville, MD

Quentin Young, American Public Health Association, Washington, DC

Richard Zimmerman, American Academy of Family Physicians, Pittsburgh, PA

15. Injury and Violence Prevention

Lee Annest, Centers for Disease Control and Prevention, Atlanta GA

Meri-K Appy, National Fire Protection Association, Quincy, MA

Bernard Auchter, U.S. Department of Justice, Washington, DC

Sharon Barrett, Health Resources and Services Administration, Bethesda, MD

Lisa Cohen Barrios, Centers for Disease Control and Prevention, Atlanta, GA

Alan Berman, American Association of Suicidology, Washington, DC

Stephanie Bryn, Health Resources and Services Administration, Rockville, MD

Gail Burns-Smith, Connecticut Sexual Assault Crisis Services, Inc., East Hartford, CT

LaTanya Butler, Centers for Disease Control and Prevention, Atlanta, GA

Robert Carson, Office of Minority Health, Rockville, MD

Alex Crosby, Centers for Disease Control and Prevention, Atlanta, GA

Mary Ann Danello, Consumer Product Safety Commission, Bethesda, MD

Lemyra DeBruyn, Centers for Disease Control and Prevention, Atlanta, GA

Carol Delany, Health Resources and Services Administration, Rockville, MD

Chhanda Dutta, National Institute on Aging, Bethesda, MD

Lois Fingerhut, Centers for Disease Control and Prevention, Hyattsville, MD

Cathy Gotschall, National Highway Traffic Safety Administration, Washington, DC

Tim Groza, Centers for Disease Control and Prevention, Atlanta, GA

Matthew Guidry, Office of Disease Prevention and Health Promotion, Washington, DC

Lyne Heneson, Administration on Children, Youth, and Families, Washington, DC

Martha Highsmith, Centers for Disease Control and Prevention, Atlanta, GA

Patti Horgas, Psychiatric and Addiction Treatment Center, Manassas, VA

Sandra Howard, Office of the Assistant Secretary for Planning and Evaluation, Washington, DC

Sarah Ingersoll, U.S. Department of Justice, Washington, DC

Lynn Jenkins, Centers for Disease Control and Prevention, Washington, DC

Ann Mahony, Substance Abuse and Mental Health Services Administration, Rockville, MD

Laura Yerdon Martin, Centers for Disease Control and Prevention, Atlanta, GA

Angela Mickalide, National SAFE KIDS Campaign, Washington, DC

Tom Minnich, Federal Emergency Management Agency, Emmitsburg, MD

Eve Moscicki, National Institutes of Health, Rockville, MD

Catherine Nolan, Head Start, Washington, DC

Emmeline Ochiai, Office of Disease Prevention and Health Promotion, Washington, DC

Mary Overpeck, National Institutes of Health, Rockville, MD

Francess Page, Office on Women's Health, Washington, DC

Jane Pearson, National Institutes of Health, Bethesda, MD

Craig Perkins, U.S. Department of Justice, Washington, DC

Ken Powell, Centers for Disease Control and Prevention, Atlanta, GA

Michael Rand, U.S. Department of Justice, Washington, DC

Bill Riley, Administration for Children and Families, Washington, DC

Theresa Rogers, Centers for Disease Control and Prevention, Atlanta, GA

Ann Rosewater, U.S. Department of Health and Human Services, Washington, DC

Fred Seitz, Centers for Disease Control and Prevention, Hyattsville, MD

Dorita Sewell, Substance Abuse and Mental Health Services Administration, Rockville, MD

Jerry Silverman, U.S. Department of Health and Human Services, Washington, DC

Richard Smith, Indian Health Service, Rockville, MD

Barbara Smothers, National Institute on Alcohol Abuse and Alcoholism, Bethesda MD

Rose Ann Soloway, American Association of Poison Control Centers, Washington, DC

Kathleen Somers, Centers for Disease Control and Prevention, Atlanta, GA

Carl Spurlock, Kentucky Injury Prevention Center, Lexington, KY

Judith Lee Stone, Advocates for Highway and Auto Safety, Washington, DC

Carol Thornhill, Administration on Aging, Washington, DC

Bill Tremblay, Brain Injury Association, Alexandria, VA

Louise Vis, National SAFE KIDS Campaign, Washington, DC

Valerie Welsh, Office of Minority Health, Rockville, MD

Jerry Weyrauch, Suicide Prevention Advocacy Network-USA, Marietta, GA

Stacey Williams-Diggs, Office of Minority Health, Rockville, MD

Sarah Yerkes, National Fire Protection Association, Washington, DC

16. Maternal, Infant, and Child Health

Myron Adams, Jr., Centers for Disease Control and Prevention, Atlanta, GA

Sue Ann Anderson, Food and Drug Administration, Washington, DC

Trude Bennett, University of North Carolina, Chapel Hill, NC

Candice Bowman, Agency for Healthcare Research and Quality, Rockville, MD

Coleen Boyle, Centers for Disease Control and Prevention, Atlanta, GA

Geogia Buggs, Office of Minority Health, Rockville, MD

Charlotte Catz, National Institutes of Health, Rockville, MD

Melissa Clarke, Health Resources and Services Administration, Rockville, MD

Isabelle Danel, Centers for Disease Control and Prevention, Atlanta, GA

Ellis Davis, Office of Disease Prevention and Health Promotion, Washington, DC

Charlotte Dickinson, Centers for Disease Control and Prevention, Atlanta, GA

David Erickson, Centers for Disease Control and Prevention, Atlanta, GA

Ricarda Goins-Mills, Office of Minority Health, Rockville, MD

Patricia Hufford, Health Care Financing Administration, Baltimore, MD

Solomon Iyasu, Centers for Disease Control and Prevention, Atlanta, GA

Elizabeth Jackson, Centers for Disease Control and Prevention, Hyattsville, MD

Evelyn Kappeler, Office of Population Affairs, Bethesda, MD

Woodie Kessel, Office of Disease Prevention and Health Promotion, Washington, DC

John Kiely, Centers for Disease Control and Prevention, Hyattsville, MD

Milton Kotelchuck, University of North Carolina, Chapel Hill, NC

Richard Klein, Centers for Disease Control and Prevention, Hyattsville, MD

Cara Kruletwitch, National Institutes of Health, Bethesda, MD

Brenda Lisi, Health Resources and Services Administration, Rockville, MD

Joyce Martin, Centers for Disease Control and Prevention, Hyattsville, MD

Amy Nevel, Office of the Assistant Secretary for Planning and Evaluation, Washington, DC

Joann Petrini, March of Dimes Foundation, White Plains, NY

Jonelle Rowe, Office on Women's Health, Washington, DC

Russ Scarato, Health Resources and Services Administration, Rockville, MD

Renee Schwalberg, Maternal and Child Health Information Resource Center, Washington, DC

Dorita Sewell, Substance Abuse and Mental Health Services Administration, Rockville, MD

Philip Smith, Indian Health Service, Rockville, MD

Vince Smeriglio, National Institutes of Health, Rockville, MD

Stella Yu, Health Resources and Services Administration, Rockville, MD

17. Medical Product Safety

William R. Archer, Texas Department of Health, Austin, TX

Linda Hiddemen Barondess, Geriatric Society, New York, NY

Mark Blumenthal, American Botanical Council, Austin, TX

Mark D. Boesen, American Association of Colleges of Pharmacy, Alexandria, VA

Debra Bowen, Food and Drug Administration, Rockville, MD

Robert Britain, National Electrical Manufacturers Association, Rosslyn, VA

W. Ray Bullman, National Council on Patient Information and Education, Washington, DC

Craig Carlson, American Association of Health Plans, Washington, DC

Geoffrey Cheung, National Institutes of Health, Bethesda, MD

Mike Cohen, Institute for Safe Medication Practices, Huntington Valley, PA

MaryPat Couig, Food and Drug Administration, Rockville, MD

Diane Cousins, U.S. Pharmacopeia, Rockville, MD

Joseph Cranston, American Medical Association, Washington, DC

Cynthia Culmo, Texas Department of Health, Austin, TX

Rick Davey, American Red Cross, Washington, DC

Jane Delgado, National Coalition of Hispanic Health and Human Services Organizations, Washington, DC

Gary Dennis, National Medical Association, Washington, DC

Jarilyn Dupont, Food and Drug Administration, Rockville, MD

Christine Everett, Food and Drug Administration, Rockville, MD

Harmon Eyer, American Cancer Society, Atlanta, GA

Merle Fossen, Academy of Managed Care Pharmacy, Alexandria, VA

John A. Gans, American Pharmacy Association, Washington, DC

Susan Gardner, Food and Drug Administration, Rockville, MD

Margaret Garikas, American Medical Association, Washington, DC

Linda Golodner, National Consumer League, Washington, DC

Kay Gregory, American Association of Blood Banks, Bethesda, MD

Tessie Guillermo, Asian and Pacific Islander American Health Forum, San Francisco, CA

Jeanette Guyton-Krishnan, Centers for Disease Control and Prevention, Hyattsville, MD

Deborah Henderson, Food and Drug Administration, Rockville, MD

Betty Hiner, Food and Drug Administration, Rockville, MD

Melissa Hines, National Black Nurses Association, Washington, DC

Edna Kane-Williams, American Association of Retired Persons, Washington, DC

Toby Litovitz, American Association of Poison Control Centers, Washington, DC

Henri R. Manasse, Jr., American Society of Health System Pharmacists, Bethesda, MD

Iris Masucci, Food and Drug Administration, Rockville, MD

John May, National Association of Boards of Pharmacy, Gaithersburg, MD

Gilberto Moreno, Association for Advancement of Mexican-Americans,

Fred G. Paavola, Health Resources and Services Administration, Washington, DC

Rossanne Philen, Centers for Disease Control and Prevention, Atlanta, GA

Jerry Phillips, Food and Drug Administration, Rockville, MD

Susie Razzano, Food and Drug Administration, Rockville, MD

Mary Rouleau, Consumer Federation of America, Washington, DC

N. Lee Rucker, National Council on Patient Information and Education, Washington, DC

Joe M. Sanders, Jr., American Academy of Pediatrics, Elk Grove Village, IL

Ellen Tabak, Food and Drug Administration, Rockville, MD

Marlene Tandy, Health Industry Manufacturers Association, Washington, DC

Hugh Tilson, Glaxo Wellcome, Research Triangle Park, NC

Kathleen Turcyzn, Centers for Disease Control and Prevention, Rockville, MD

Janet Whitley, Food and Drug Administration, Rockville, MD

18. Mental Health and Mental Disorders

Crystal Blyler, Substance Abuse and Mental Health Services Administration, Rockville, MD

Robert Carson, Office of Minority Health, Rockville, MD

Marie Danforth, Substance Abuse and Mental Health Services Administration, Rockville, MD

Paolo Del Vecchio, Substance Abuse and Mental Health Services Administration, Rockville, MD

Robert DeMartino, Substance Abuse and Mental Health Services Administration, Rockville, MD

Michele Edwards, Substance Abuse and Mental Health Services Administration, Rockville, MD

Theodora Fine, Substance Abuse and Mental Health Services Administration, Rockville, MD

Peggy Gilliam, Substance Abuse and Mental Health Services Administration, Rockville, MD

Ingrid Goldstrom, Substance Abuse and Mental Health Services Administration, Rockville, MD

Marilyn Henderson, Substance Abuse and Mental Health Services Administration, Rockville, MD

Kevin Hennessy, U.S. Department of Health and Human Services, Washington, DC

Cille Kennedy, National Institutes of Health, Bethesda, MD

Doreen Koretz, National Institutes of Health, Bethesda, MD

Ronald Manderscheid, Substance Abuse and Mental Health Services Administration, Rockville, MD

Dave Moriarty, Centers for Disease Control and Prevention, Atlanta, GA

Eve Moscicki, National Institutes of Health, Rockville, MD

William Narrow, National Institutes of Health, Bethesda, MD

Jane Pearson, National Institutes of Health, Bethesda, MD

Juan Ramos, National Institutes of Health, Bethesda, MD

Cheryl Reese, National Institutes of Health, Bethesda, MD

Gail Ritchie, Substance Abuse and Mental Health Services Administration, Rockville, MD

Fred Seitz, Centers for Disease Control and Prevention, Hyattsville, MD

Dorita Sewell, Substance Abuse and Mental Health Services Administration, Rockville, MD

Paul Sirovatka, National Institutes of Health, Bethesda, MD

Shelagh Smith, Substance Abuse and Mental Health Services Administration, Rockville, MD

Diane Sondheimer, Substance Abuse and Mental Health Services Administration, Rockville, MD

Benedetto Vitiello, National Institutes of Health, Bethesda, MD

Mary Westcott, Substance Abuse and Mental Health Services Administration, Rockville, MD

19. Nutrition and Overweight

Cynthia Amis, Office of Minority Health, Rockville, MD

Rajen Anand, U.S. Department of Agriculture, Washington, DC

Marietta Anthony, Food and Drug Administration, Rockville, MD

Karil Bialostosky, Centers for Disease Control and Prevention, Hyattsville, MD

Barbara Bowman, Centers for Disease Control and Prevention Atlanta, GA

Ronette Briefel, Centers for Disease Control and Prevention, Hyattsville, MD

Dorothy Caldwell, U.S. Department of Agriculture, Alexandria, VA

Linda Cleveland, U.S. Department of Agriculture, Beltsville, MD

Carolyn Clifford, National Institutes of Health, Rockville, MD

Paul M. Coates, National Institutes of Health, Bethesda, MD (former work group co-chair through January 2000)

Mary Cogswell, Centers for Disease Control and Prevention, Atlanta, GA

Nancy Crane, Food and Drug Administration, Washington, DC

Ellis Davis, Office of Disease Prevention and Health Promotion, Washington, DC

Tuei Doong, Office of Minority Health, Rockville, MD

Nancy Ernst, National Institutes of Health, Bethesda, MD

Christine Everett, Food and Drug Administration, Rockville, MD

Elizabeth Frazao, U.S. Department of Agriculture, Washington, DC

Gilman Grave, National Institutes of Health, Bethesda, MD

William Harlan, National Institutes of Health, Bethesda, MD

Jay Hirchman, U.S. Department of Agriculture, Alexandria, VA

Van Hubbard, National Institutes of Health, Bethesda, MD

Yvonne Jackson, Administration on Aging, Washington, DC

Barbara Keir, Texas Department of Health, Austin, TX

Laura Kettel-Kahn, Centers for Disease Control and Prevention, Atlanta, GA

Sooja Kim, National Institutes of Health, Bethesda, MD

Carol Kramer-LeBlanc, U.S. Department of Agriculture, Washington, DC

Susan Krebs-Smith, National Institutes of Health, Bethesda, MD

Sarah Kuester, Centers for Disease Control and Prevention, Atlanta, GA

Naomi Kulakow, Food and Drug Administration, Washington, DC

William Lands, National Institutes of Health, Rockville, MD

Christine Lewis, Food and Drug Administration, Washington, DC

Deborah Maiese, Office of Disease Prevention and Health Promotion, Washington, DC

Bernadette Marriott, National Institutes of Health, Bethesda, MD

Joan McGowan, National Institutes of Health, Bethesda, MD

Kathryn McMurry, Office of Disease Prevention and Health Promotion, Washington, DC

Robert Mehnert, National Institutes of Health, Bethesda, MD

Linda Meyers, Office of Disease Prevention and Health Promotion, Washington, DC

Alanna Moshfegh, U.S. Department of Agriculture, Beltsville, MD

Jean Pennington, National Institutes of Health, Bethesda, MD

Ann Prendergast, Health Resources and Services Administration, Rockville, MD

Susan Schappert, Centers for Disease Control and Prevention, Hyattsville, MD

Jules Selden, National Institutes of Health, Rockville, MD

Bettylou Sherry, Centers for Disease Control and Prevention, Atlanta, GA

Rochelle Small, National Institutes of Health, Rockville, MD

Gloria Stables, National Institutes of Health, Bethesda, MD

Pamela Starke-Reed, National Institutes of Health, Bethesda, MD

Karen Strauss, Indian Health Service, Rockville, MD

Susanne Strickland, National Institutes of Health, Bethesda, MD

Linda Thomas, National Institutes of Health, Bethesda, MD

Richard Troiano, National Institutes of Health, Bethesda, MD

Kathleen Turczyn, Centers for Disease Control and Prevention, Hyattsville, MD

Howell Wechsler, Centers for Disease Control and Prevention, Atlanta, GA

Violet Woo, Office of Minority Health, Rockville, MD

Susan Yanovski, National Institutes of Health, Bethesda, MD

20. Occupational Safety and Health

Lani Boldt, Centers for Disease Control and Prevention, Spokane, WA

John Breslin, Centers for Disease Control and Prevention, Pittsburgh, PA

Robert Castellan, Centers for Disease Control and Prevention, Morgantown, WV

Lawrence Fine, Centers for Disease Control and Prevention, Cincinnati, OH

John Franks, Centers for Disease Control and Prevention, Cincinnati, OH

Joanna Friedrich, U.S. Department of Labor, Washington, DC

James Grosch, Centers for Disease Control and Prevention, Cincinnati, OH

DeLon Hull, Centers for Disease Control and Prevention, Cincinnati, OH

Lore Jackson Lee, Centers for Disease Control and Prevention, Washington, DC

Lynn Jenkins, Centers for Disease Control and Prevention, Morgantown, WV

James Jones, Centers for Disease Control and Prevention, Cincinnati, OH

Boris Lushniak, Centers for Disease Control and Prevention, Cincinnati, OH

Edward Petsonk, Centers for Disease Control and Prevention, Morgantown, WV

Robert Roscoe, Centers for Disease Control and Prevention, Cincinnati, OH

Fred Seitz, Centers for Disease Control and Prevention, Hyattsville, MD

John Sestito, Centers for Disease Control and Prevention, Cincinnati, OH

Kenneth Weber, Centers for Disease Control and Prevention, Morgantown, WV

21. Oral Health

Myron Allukian, Jr., Boston Department of Health, Boston, MA

Jay Anderson, Health Resources and Services Administration, Bethesda, MD

Eric Bothwell, Indian Health Service, Rockville, MD

Brian Burt, University of Michigan, Ann Arbor, MI

Stephen Corbin, Oral Health America, Rockville, MD

James Crall, American Academy of Pediatric Dentistry, Farmington, CT

Ann Drum, Health Resources and Services Administration, Rockville, MD

Thomas Drury, National Institutes of Health, Bethesda, MD

Scott Dubowsky, Academy of General Dentistry, Bayonne, NJ

Caswell Evans, National Institutes of Health, Bethesda, MD

Harold Goodman, Association of State and Territorial Dental Directors, Baltimore, MD

Kevin Hardwick, National Institutes of Health, Bethesda, MD

Lawrence Hill, Association of Community Dental Programs, Cincinnati, OH

Cynthia Hodge, National Dental Association, Nashville, TN

Herschel Horowitz, Dental Public Health Consultant, Bethesda, MD

Robert Isman, American Public Health Association, Sacramento, CA

Elizabeth Jackson, Centers for Disease Control and Prevention, Hyattsville, MD

Marjorie Jeffcoat, American Association of Dental Research, Birmingham, AL

Rebecca King, North Carolina Department of Health and Human Services, Raleigh, NC

Dushanka Kleinman, National Institutes of Health, Bethesda, MD

Jay Kumar, New York State Department of Health, Albany, NY

G.M. Nana Lopez, Hispanic Dental Association, Austin, TX

William R. Maas, Centers for Disease Control and Prevention, Atlanta, GA

Mark Macek, Centers for Disease Control and Prevention, Hyattsville, MD

Dolores M. Malvitz, Centers for Disease Control and Prevention, Atlanta, GA

Kathleen Mangskau, American Dental Hygienists' Association, Bismarck, ND

Don Marianos, U.S. Public Health Service, retired, Pinetop, AZ

Lawrence Meskin, University of Colorado Health Science Center, Denver, CO

David Moss, U.S. Army, Great Lakes, IL

Linda Niessan, Baylor College of Dentistry, Dallas, TX

John P. Rossetti, Health Resources and Services Administration, Rockville, MD

R. Gary Rozier, University of North Carolina, Chapel Hill, NC

Lois Salzman, National Institutes of Health, Bethesda, MD (deceased)

Don Schneider, Health Care Financing Administration, Baltimore, MD

Sandra L. Shire, Food and Drug Administration, Rockville, MD

Mark Siegal, Ohio Department of Health, Columbus, OH

Harold C. Slavkin, National Institutes of Health, Bethesda, MD

Paul E. Stubbs, American Dental Association, Georgetown, TX

Scott Tomar, Centers for Disease Control and Prevention, Atlanta, GA

Clemencia M. Vargas, Centers for Disease Control and Prevention, Hyattsville, MD

Jane Weintraub, University of California, San Francisco, CA

Robert Weyant, University of Pittsburgh, Pittsburgh, PA

B. Alex White, American Association of Public Health Dentistry, Portland, OR

22. Physical Activity and Fitness

Melissa Clarke, Health Resources and Services Administration, Rockville, MD

Paul Coates, National Institutes of Health, Bethesda, MD

William Dietz, Centers for Disease Control and Prevention, Atlanta, GA

Henry Doan, Administration on Children, Youth, and Families, Washington, DC

Karen Donato, National Institutes of Health, Bethesda, MD

Tuei Doong, Office of Minority Health, Rockville, MD

Gilman Grave, National Institutes of Health, Bethesda, MD

Matthew Guidry, Office of Disease Prevention and Health Promotion, Washington, DC

William Harlan, National Institutes of Health, Bethesda, MD

Van Hubbard, National Institutes of Health, Bethesda, MD

Naomi Kulakow, Food and Drug Administration, Washington, DC

Donald Lollar, Centers for Disease Control and Prevention, Atlanta, GA

Richard Lymn, National Institutes of Health, Bethesda, MD

Carol Macera, Centers for Disease Control and Prevention, Atlanta, GA

Mary Ann Mackenzie, Administration for Children and Families, Washington, DC

Saralyn Mark, Office on Women's Health, Washington, DC

Charlotte Schoenborn, Centers for Disease Control and Prevention, Hyattsville, MD

Dorita Sewell, Substance Abuse and Mental Health Services Administration, Rockville, MD

Denise Sofka, Health Resources and Services Administration, Rockville, MD

Christine Spain, President's Council on Physical Activity and Fitness, Washington, DC

Moya Thompson, Administration on Aging, Washington, DC

Kathleen Turczyn, Centers for Disease Control and Prevention, Hyattsville, MD

Martina Vogel-Taylor, National Institutes of Health, Bethesda, MD

Howell Wechsler, Centers for Disease Control and Prevention, Atlanta, GA

Evelyn Yee, Administration on Aging, Washington, DC

23. Public Health Infrastructure

David Arday, Health Care Financing Administration, Baltimore, MD

Elaine Auld, Society of Public Health Education, Washington, DC

Edward Baker, Centers for Disease Control and Prevention, Atlanta, GA

Ned Baker, National Association of Local Boards of Health, Bowling Green, OH

Doris Barnette, Health Resources and Services Administration, Rockville, MD

Mike Barry, Public Health Foundation, Washington, DC

Scott Becker, Association of State and Territorial Public Health Laboratory Directors, Washington, DC

Georges Benjamin, Maryland Department of Health and Hygiene, Baltimore, MD

Bobbie Berkowitz, Robert Wood Johnson Foundation, Seattle, WA

Patricia Berry, Vermont Department of Health, Burlington, VT

Ronald Bialek, Public Health Foundation, Washington, DC

Neal Brandes, Robert Wood Johnson Foundation, Princeton, NJ

Carol Brown, National Association of County and City Health Officials, Washington, DC

Michelle Browne, Health Care Financing Administration, Baltimore, MD

Jackie Bryan, Association of State and Territorial Health Officials, Washington, DC

Debra Burns, Minnesota Department of Health, St. Paul, MN

LaTanya Butler, Centers for Disease Control and Prevention, Atlanta, GA

Marjorie Cahn, National Institutes of Health, Bethesda, MD

D.W. Chen, Health Resources and Services Administration, Rockville, MD

Melissa Clarke, Health Resources and Services Administration, Rockville, MD

Ashley Coffield, Partnership for Prevention, Washington, DC

Liza Corso, National Association of County and City Health Officials, Washington, DC

Mary Jo Deering, Office of Disease Prevention and Health Promotion, Washington, DC

Doug Drabkowski, Association of State and Territorial Public Health Laboratory Directors, Washington, DC

Ron Elble, Zanesville, OH

Pauline Feldman, Health Care Financing Administration, Baltimore, MD

Florence Fiori, Health Resources and Services Administration, Rockville, MD

Michael Fishman, Health Resources and Services Administration, Rockville, MD

Alison Foster, Association of Schools of Public Health, Washington, DC

Michael Fraser, National Association of County and City Health Officials, Washington, DC

Keith Frazier, Tyler County Health Department, Tyler, TX

Kristine Gebbie, Columbia University, New York, NY

Michael Gemmell, Association of Schools of Public Health, Washington, DC

Charles Godue, World Health Organization, Washington, DC

Lawrence Gostin, Georgetown/Johns Hopkins University, Washington, DC

Tim Groza, Centers for Disease Control and Prevention, Atlanta, GA

Paul Halverson, Centers for Disease Control and Prevention, Atlanta, GA

William Harlan, National Institutes of Health, Bethesda, MD

Brad Hendrick, Office of Population Affairs, Bethesda, MD

Dave Heppel, Health Resources and Services Administration, Rockville, MD

Martha Highsmith, Centers for Disease Control and Prevention, Atlanta, GA

Helen Howerton, Administration for Children and Families, Washington, DC

Deane Johnson, Centers for Disease Control and Prevention, Atlanta, GA

Tamara Lewis Johnson, Health Resources and Services Administration, Bethesda, MD

Laura Kahn, Centers for Disease Control and Prevention, Atlanta, GA

Wendy Katz, Association of Schools of Public Health, Washington, DC

Richard Klein, Centers for Disease Control and Prevention, Hyattsville, MD

Brick Lancaster, Centers for Disease Control and Prevention, Atlanta, GA

Monica Larrieu, World Health Organization, Washington, DC

Jeffrey Lake, Virginia Department of Health, Richmond, VA

Roz Lasker, New York Academy of Medicine, New York, NY

Barry Levy, American Public Health Association, Sherborn, MA

Louis Lex, Iowa Department of Public Health, Des Moines, IA

Joshua Lipsman, Alexandria Health Department, Alexandria, VA

Douglas Lloyd, Health Resources and Services Administration, Rockville, MD

Steven Macdonald, Washington State Department of Health, Olympia, WA

Deborah Maiese, Office of Disease Prevention and Health Promotion, Washington, DC

Rose Marie Martinez, Mathematica Policy Research, Inc., Washington, DC

Michael McGinnis, National Academy of Sciences, Washington, DC

Dick Melton, Utah Department of Health, Salt Lake City, UT

Jeff Mero, Washington Health Foundation, Seattle, WA

Michael Millman, Health Resources and Services Administration, Rockville, MD

Thomas Milne, National Association of County and City Health Officials, Washington, DC

Roscoe Moore, Jr., Office of International and Refugee Health, Rockville, MD

Anthony Moulton, Centers for Disease Control and Prevention, Atlanta, GA

Paul Nannis, Health Resources and Services Administration, Rockville, MD

Jane Nelson, Rollins School of Public Health at Emory University, Atlanta, GA

Ray Nicola, Centers for Disease Control and Prevention, Atlanta, GA

Samuel Nixon, Congress of National Black Churches, Washington, DC

Mark O'Brien, Association of Schools of Public Health, Washington, DC

Mary Jo O'Brien, Lewin Group, Fairfax, VA

Anne O'Connor, Centers for Disease Control and Prevention, Atlanta, GA

Barry Portnoy, National Institutes of Health, Bethesda, MD

Edwin Pratt, Jr., National Association of the Local Boards of Health, Marion, MA

Dixie Ray, Indiana University, Indianapolis, IN

Patricia Reynolds, Agency for Healthcare Research and Quality, Rockville, MD

Jud Richland, American College of Preventive Medicine, Washington, DC

Sara Riedel, Association of Schools of Public Health, Washington, DC

Gail Ritchie, Substance Abuse and Mental Health Services Administration, Rockville, MD

Carol Roddy, Health Resources and Services Administration, Rockville, MD

Theresa Rogers, Centers for Disease Control and Prevention, Atlanta, GA

Colleen Ryan, Centers for Disease Control and Prevention, Hyattsville, MD

John Saccenti, National Association of Local Boards of Health, Kendall Park, NJ

Eileen Salinsky, Lewin Group, Fairfax, VA

Margaret Schmelzer, Wisconsin Department of Health, Madison, WI

Fred Seitz, Centers for Disease Control and Prevention, Hyattsville, MD

Dorita Sewell, Substance Abuse and Mental Health Services Administration, Rockville, MD

Pomeroy Sinnock, Centers for Disease Control and Prevention, Atlanta, GA

MaryBeth Skupein, Sault Ste. Marie Health and Human Services, Sault Ste. Marie, MI

Hugh Sloan, U.S. Public Health Service, Denver, CO

Mark Smolinski, Office of Disease Prevention and Health Promotion, Washington, DC

Laverne Snow, Utah Department of Health, Salt Lake City, UT

Cassandra Sparrow, Congress of National Black Churches, Washington, DC

Kathleen Turczyn, Centers for Disease Control and Prevention, Hyattsville, MD

Bernard Turnock, University of Illinois, Chicago, IL

Joan Valas, National Association of Local Boards of Health, Park Ridge, NJ

Martina Vogel-Taylor, National Institutes of Health, Bethesda, MD

Beth Vumbaco, Meridian Health and Human Services, Meridian, CT

Diane Wagener, Centers for Disease Control and Prevention, Hyattsville, MD

Nancy Warren, State and Territorial Public Health Laboratory Directors, Washington, DC

Valerie Welsh, Office of Minority Health, Rockville, MD

24. Respiratory Diseases

Robinson Fulwood, National Institutes of Health, Bethesda, MD

William Jirles, National Institutes of Health, Bethesda, MD

Carol Johnson, Centers for Disease Control and Prevention, Atlanta, GA

Christopher Kochtitzky, Centers for Disease Control and Prevention, Atlanta, GA

Sheila Newton, National Institutes of Health, Research Triangle Park, NC

Dalton Paxman, Office of Disease Prevention and Health Promotion, Washington, DC

Marshall Plaut, National Institutes of Health, Bethesda, MD

Stephen Redd, Centers for Disease Control and Prevention, Atlanta, GA

Susan Rogus, National Institutes of Health, Bethesda, MD

Daniel Rotrosen, National Institutes of Health, Bethesda, MD

Fred Seitz, Centers for Disease Control and Prevention, Hyattsville, MD

Virginia Taggart, National Institutes of Health, Bethesda, MD

Michael Twery, National Institutes of Health, Bethesda, MD

Martina Vogel-Taylor, National Institutes of Health, Bethesda, MD

Gail Weinmann, National Institutes of Health, Bethesda, MD

25. Sexually Transmitted Diseases

Linda Alexander, American Social Health Association, Research Triangle Park, NC

Margaret Anderson, Society for the Advancement of Women's Health Research, Washington, DC

Georgia Buggs, Office of Minority Health, Washington, DC

Carol Cassell, Centers for Disease Control and Prevention, Atlanta, GA

Anjani Chandra, Centers for Disease Control and Prevention, Hyattsville, MD

James Cheek, Indian Health Service, Albuquerque, NM

Marty Goldberg, National Coalition of STD Directors, Philadelphia, PA

Rita Goodman, Health Resources and Services Administration, Rockville, MD

Joel Greenspan, Centers for Disease Control and Prevention, Atlanta, GA

Leslie Hardy, Office of the Assistant Secretary for Planning and Evaluation, Washington, DC

Brad Hendrick, Office of Population Affairs, Bethesda, MD

Evelyn Kappeler, Office of Population Affairs, Bethesda, MD

Richard Klein, Centers for Disease Control and Prevention, Hyattsville, MD

Eva Margolies-Seiler, Centers for Disease Control and Prevention, Atlanta, GA

Bill Mosher, Centers for Disease Control and Prevention, Hyattsville, MD

Frank Beadle de Palomo, Academy for Educational Development, Washington, DC

Molly Parece, Centers for Disease Control and Prevention, Atlanta, GA

Linda Piccinino, Centers for Disease Control and Prevention, Hyattsville, MD

Leah Robin, Centers for Disease Control and Prevention, Atlanta, GA

Audrey Rogers, National Institutes of Health, Rockville, MD

Colleen Ryan, Centers for Disease Control and Prevention, Hyattsville, MD

Laura Shelby, Indian Health Service, Albuquerque, NM

Jack Spencer, Centers for Disease Control and Prevention, Atlanta, GA

Karen Turner, Administration on Children, Youth, and Families, Washington, DC

Carmen Villar, Centers for Disease Control and Prevention, Atlanta, GA

Susan F. Wood, Office on Women's Health, Washington, DC

Beverly Wright, Centers for Disease Control and Prevention, Rockville, MD

26. Substance Abuse

Rebecca Ashery, Substance Abuse and Mental Health Services Administration, Rockville, MD

David Atkins, Agency for Healthcare Research and Quality, Rockville, MD

Gail Beaumont, U.S. Department of Education, Washington, DC

Janice Berger, Health Resources and Services Administration, Rockville, MD

Robert Carson, Office of Minority Health, Rockville, MD

Javier Cordova, Office of National Drug Control Policy, Washington, DC

Linda Crosset, Centers for Disease Control and Prevention, Atlanta, GA

Darie Davis, Office of National Drug Control Policy, Washington, DC

Herman Diesenhaus, Substance Abuse and Mental Health Services Administration, Rockville, MD

Jane Dion, U.S. Department of Transportation, Washington, DC

Adrienne Goode, Substance Abuse and Mental Health Services Administration, Rockville, MD

Miryam Granthon, Office of Disease Prevention and Health Promotion, Washington, DC

Jack Gustafson, National Association of State Alcohol and Drug Abuse Directors, Washington, DC

Jan Howard, National Institutes of Health, Rockville, MD

Elizabeth Jackson, Centers for Disease Control and Prevention, Hyattsville, MD

Sehwan Kim, Database ER, Inc., Tampa, FL

Herbert Kleber, Columbia University, New York, NY

Richard Klein, Centers for Disease Control and Prevention, Hyattsville, MD

Craig Love, Brown University, Providence, RI

Nataki MacMurray, Office of National Drug Control Policy, Washington, DC

Winnie Mitchell, Substance Abuse and Mental Health Services Administration, Rockville, MD

Juana Mora, Glendale, CA

Doris Moseley, Health Resources and Services Administration, Rockville, MD

Pam McDonnell Perry, Substance Abuse and Mental Health Services Administration, Rockville, MD

Gloria Rodriguez, Avance, Inc., San Antonio, TX

Beatrice Rouse, Substance Abuse and Mental Health Services Administration, Rockville, MD

Mel Segal, Substance Abuse and Mental Health Services Administration, Rockville, MD

Dorita Sewell, Substance Abuse and Mental Health Services Administration, Rockville, MD

Jeffrey Thompson, Weyerhauser Company, Federal Way, VA

Tom Vischi, Office of Disease Prevention and Health Promotion, Washington, DC

Alex Wagenaar, University of Minnesota, Minneapolis, MN

Flavia Walden, Fort Washington, MD

Gina Woods, U.S. Department of Justice, Washington, DC

27. Tobacco Use

Myron Allukian, Boston Public Health Commission, Boston, MA

Victoria Almquist, National Association of Children's Hospitals and Related Institutions, Alexandria, VA

David Altman, Bowman Gray School of Medicine, Winston-Salem, NC

Alejandro Arias, Substance Abuse and Mental Health Services Administration, Rockville, MD

Linda Bailey, Centers for Disease Control and Prevention, Washington, DC

Cathy Backinger, National Institutes of Health, Bethesda, MD

Brenda Bell Caffee, African American Tobacco Education Network, Sacramento, CA

Harriett Bennett, Agency for Healthcare Research and Quality, Rockville, MD

Alvina Bey-Bennett, National Medical Association, Washington, DC

Michele Bloch, American Medical Women's Association, Rockville, MD

David Bourne, Arkansas Department of Health, Little Rock, AR

Phillip Brown, National Association of County and City Health Officials, Washington, DC

Anne Cahill, American Association of Health Plans, Washington, DC

Diane Canova, American Heart Association, Washington, DC

Julia Carol, Americans for Non-Smokers' Rights, Berkeley, CA

Frank Chaloupka, University of Illinois, Chicago, IL

Moon Chen, Ohio State University, Columbus, OH

Portia Choi, Maternal and Child Health Program, Bakersfield, CA

Melissa Clarke, Health Resources and Services Administration, Rockville, MD

Nathaniel Cobb, Indian Health Service, Albuquerque, NM

Ashley Coffield, Partnerships for Prevention, Washington, DC

Kathleen Conlan, Laborers' Health and Safety Fund of North America, Washington, DC

Linda Crossett, Centers for Disease Control and Prevention, Atlanta, GA

Michael Cummings, Roswell Park Cancer Institute, Buffalo, NY

Ronald Davis, Henry Ford Health System, Detroit, MI

Richard Daynard, Northeastern University School of Law, Boston, MA

Jack Dillenberg, Oral Health America, Phoenix, AZ

Virginia Ernster, University of California, San Francisco, CA

Marie Falon, National Association of Local Boards of Health, Bowling Green, OH

Michael Fiore, University of Wisconsin Medical School, Madison, WI

Stanton Glantz, University of California, San Francisco, CA

Donna Grande, American Medical Association/Robert Wood Johnson Foundation, Chicago, IL

Miryam Granthon, Office of Disease Prevention and Health Promotion, Washington, DC

Ellen Gritz, Anderson Cancer Center, Houston, TX

Charles Gruder, University of California, Oakland, CA

Jim Guillory, University of Health Sciences, Kansas City, MO

Roger Hartman, Tricare Management Activity, Falls Church, VA

Kathleen Harty, American Medical Association, Chicago, IL

Betty Hawks, Office of Minority Health, Rockville, MD

Jack Henningfield, Pinney Associates, Bethesda, MD

Felicia Hodge, Center for American Indian Research and Education, Berkeley, CA

Amanda Holm, National Association of County and City Health Officials, Washington, DC

Amy Holmes-Chavez, Centers for Disease Control and Prevention, Atlanta, GA

Alice Horowitz, National Institutes of Health, Bethesda, MD

Thomas Houston, American Medical Association, Chicago, IL

Kara Jacobson, USQA Center for Health Care Research, Atlanta, GA

Mona Lisa James, Kalamazoo County Human Services Department, Nazareth, MI

Jane Jasek, American Dental Association, Chicago, IL

Pamela Johnson, Administration for Children and Families, Washington, DC

Denyse Jones, TriCities Tobacco Reduction Coalition, Detroit, MI

Rhys Jones, American Association of Public Health Dentistry, Cedar Rapids, IA

Eric Juzenas, American Public Health Association, Washington, DC

Nancy Kaufman, Robert Wood Johnson Foundation, Princeton, NJ

Lore Jackson Lee, Centers for Disease Control and Prevention, Washington, DC

Rod Lew, Association of Asia-Pacific Community Health Organizations, Oakland, CA

Kerri Lopes, Indian Health Clinic, Portland, OR

Deborah Maiese, Office of Disease Prevention and Health Promotion, Washington, DC

Marc Manley, National Institutes of Health, Rockville, MD

Gerardo Marin, University of San Francisco, San Francisco, CA

Tim McAfee, Group Health Cooperative of Puget Sound, Seattle, WA

Carol McPhillips, Prudential Center for Health Care Research, Atlanta, GA

Robert Mecklenburg, National Institutes of Health, Potomac, MD

Robin Mermelstein, University of Illinois, Chicago, IL

Robert Merritt, Centers for Disease Control and Prevention, Atlanta, GA

Jane Moore, Association of State and Territorial Health Officers, Washington, DC

Jane Moore, Oregon Health Division, Portland, OR

Mildred Morse, Morse Enterprises, Inc., Silver Spring, MD

Ernestine Murray, Agency for Healthcare Research and Quality, Rockville, MD

Jerald Newberry, National Education Association, Washington, DC

Jeannette Noltenius, Latino Council on Alcohol and Tobacco, Washington, DC

William Novelli, National Center for Tobacco-Free Kids, Washington, DC

Tracy Orleans, Robert Wood Johnson Foundation, Princeton, NJ

Lynn Pahland, Department of Defense, Falls Church, VA

Karen Pane, Health Resources and Services Administration, Rockville, MD

James Pirkle, Centers for Disease Control and Prevention, Atlanta, GA

Susan Polan, Partnership for Prevention, Washington, DC

Amelie Ramirez, Baylor College of Medicine, Houston, TX

Charles Robbins, State University of New York, Stony Brook, NY

Theresa Rogers, Centers for Disease Control and Prevention, Atlanta, GA

Rosemary Rosso, Federal Trade Commission, Washington, DC

Richard Rothenberg, Emory University School of Medicine, Atlanta, GA

Gary Rudman, Teenage Research Unlimited, Northbrook, IL

Janet Samorodin, Office of Disease Prevention and Health Promotion, Washington, DC

Randy Schwartz, Bureau of Health, Augusta, ME

Liling Sherry, Northwest Portland Area Indian Health Board, Portland, OR

Danielle Skripak, American Association of Health Plans, Washington, DC

John Slade, St. Peter's Medical Center, New Brunswick, NJ

Mary Smith, U.S. Environmental Protection Agency, Washington, DC

Judy Sopenski, Stop Teenage Addiction to Tobacco, Springfield, MA

Adria Thomas, National School Boards Association, Alexandria, VA

Ron Todd, American Cancer Society, Atlanta, GA

Elizabeth Toledo, National Organization for Women, Washington, DC

Kathleen Turczyn, Centers for Disease Control and Prevention, Hyattsville, MD

Lucretia Vigil, National Coalition of Hispanic Health and Human Services Organizations, Washington, DC

David Votaw, Centers for Disease Control and Prevention, Cincinnati, OH

Sheri Watson-Hyde, American Heart Association, Washington, DC

Ronald White, American Lung Association, Washington, DC

Kerrie Wilson, National Government Relations Office, Washington, DC

Lee Wilson, Substance Abuse and Mental Health Services Administration, Rockville, MD

Carol Wright, Great Lakes Inter-Tribal Council, Lac du Flambeau, WI

Mitchell Zeller, Food and Drug Administration, Rockville, MD

28. Vision and Hearing

Kate Achelpohl, Vision Council of America, Arlington, VA

Lois Albarelli, Administration on Aging, Washington, DC

Ed Bettinardi, Low Vision Council, Littleton, CO

Norma K. Bowyer, American Optometric Association, Morgantown, WV

Tricia Shelby Brown, American Association of Retired Persons, Washington, DC

John Cahill, New York State Health Department, Albany, NY

Evelyn Cherow, American Speech-Language-Hearing Association, Rockville, MD

Amy Donahue, National Institutes of Health, Bethesda, MD

Sharon Fujikawa, American Academy of Audiology and University of California, Irvine, Medical Center, Orange, CA

Jeanette Guyton-Krishnan, Centers for Disease Control and Prevention, Hyattsville, MD

Maureen Hannley, American Academy of Otolaryngology—Head and Neck Surgery, Alexandria, VA

Howard Hoffman, National Institutes of Health, Bethesda, MD

Lisa Holden-Pitt, U.S. Department of Education, Washington, DC

Paul Holland, Indian Health Service, East Glacier Park, MT

James Iciek, National Academy of Opticianry, Landover, MD

Larry L. Jackson, Centers for Disease Control and Prevention, Morgantown, WV

Carrie Kovar, American Academy of Ophthalmology, Washington, DC

Andrew G. Lee, University of Iowa Hospital and Clinics, Iowa City, IA

Max Lum, Centers for Disease Control and Prevention, Washington, DC

John P. Madison, National Technical Institute for the Deaf, Rochester, NY

Deborah Maiese, Office of Disease Prevention and Health Promotion, Washington, DC

Janice Marshall, Contact Lens Manufacturing Association, Bethesda, MD

John Massare, Contact lens Institute of Ophthalmologists, Metarie, LA

Nancy Nadler, League for the Hard of Hearing, New York, NY

Kathryn S. Porter, Centers for Disease Control and Prevention, Hyattsville, MD

Jinan B. Saaddine, Centers for Disease Control and Prevention, Atlanta, GA

Ed Schilling, Contact Lens Institute, Landover, MD

John Shoemaker, Prevent Blindness America, Schaumburg, IL

Donna Sorkin, Alexander Graham Bell Association for the Deaf and Hard of Hearing, Washington, DC

Robert Sperduto, National Institutes of Health, Bethesda, MD

Cynthia Stuen, Lighthouse International, New York, NY

Jo Svochak, Contact Lens Manufacturers Association, Euless, TX

Althea Turk, The Links, Atlanta, GA

Carlos Ugarte, National Institutes of Health, Bethesda, MD

Martina Vogel-Taylor, National Institutes of Health, Bethesda, MD

John Whitener, American Optometric Association, Alexandria, VA

Bill Wilson, Vision Council of America, Arlington, VA

Adolescent Health

Trina Anglin, Health Resources and Services Administration, Rockville, MD

Robert Blum, University of Minnesota, Minneapolis, MN

Claire Brindis, National Adolescent Health Information Center, San Francisco, CA

Brett Brown, Child Trends, Inc., Washington, DC

Georgia Buggs, Office of Minority Health, Rockville, MD

Steve Conley, Virginia Department of Health, Richmond, VA

Denise Dougherty, Agency for Healthcare Research and Quality, Rockville, MD

Juanita Evans, Health Resources and Services Administration, Rockville, MD

Missy Fleming, American Medical Association, Chicago, Il

Peggy Gilliam, Substance Abuse and Mental Health Services Administration, Rockville, MD

Miryam Granthon, Office of Disease Prevention and Health Promotion, Washington, DC

Casey Hannan, Centers for Disease Control and Prevention, Atlanta, GA

Catherine Hess, Association of Maternal and Child Health Programs, Washington, DC

David Kaplan, American Academy of Pediatrics, Denver, CO

Michele Kipke, Institute of Medicine/National Research Council, Washington, DC

Lloyd Kolbe, Centers for Disease Control and Prevention, Atlanta, GA

William Modzeleski, U.S. Department of Education, Washington, DC

Susan Newcomer, National Institutes of Health, Bethesda, MD

Jonelle Rowe, Office on Women's Health, Washington, DC

Ann Segal, Office of the Assistant Secretary for Planning and Evaluation, Washington, DC

Fred Seitz, Centers for Disease Control and Prevention, Hyattsville, MD

Dana Silverman, Centers for Disease Control and Prevention, Atlanta, GA

Gail Slap, Society for Adolescent Medicine, Philadelphia, PA

Shepherd Smith, Institute for Youth Development, Herndon, VA

Barbara Starfield, Johns Hopkins University, Baltimore, MD

Women's Health

Marietta Anthony, Food and Drug Administration, Washington, DC

M. Carolyn Aoyama, Health Resources and Services Administration, Bethesda, MD

Magda Barini-Garcia, Health Resources and Services Administration, Bethesda, MD

Sharon E. Barrett, Health Resources and Services Administration, Bethesda, MD

Michael Brown, Centers for Disease Control and Prevention, Atlanta, GA

Theresa Brown, Office on Women's Health, Washington, DC

Tina Chung, Office of International Health, Rockville, MD

Dottie M. Crockett, Health Resources and Services Administration, Bethesda, MD

Marsha G. Davenport, Health Care Financing Administration, Baltimore, MD

Roselyn Payne Epps, National Institutes of Health, Bethesda, MD

Leonard G. Epstein, Health Resources and Services Administration, Bethesda, MD

Christine M. Everett, Food and Drug Administration, Rockville, MD

Linda Franklin, Agency for Healthcare Research and Quality, Rockville, MD

Kimberly Geissman, Centers for Disease Control and Prevention, Atlanta, GA

Miryam Granthon, Office of Disease Prevention and Health Promotion, Washington, DC

Yvonne T. Green, Centers for Disease Control and Prevention, Atlanta, GA

Marcy L. Gross, Agency for Healthcare Research and Quality, Rockville, MD

Betty B. Hambleton, Health Resources and Services Administration, Rockville, MD

Leslie M. Hardy, Office of the Assistant Secretary for Planning and Evaluation, Washington, DC

Betty Lee Hawks, Office of Minority Health, Rockville, MD

Suzanne Haynes, Office on Women's Health, Washington, DC

Helen V. Howerton, Administration on Children and Families, Washington, DC

Carrie P. Hunter, National Institutes of Health, Bethesda, MD

Elizabeth Jackson, Centers for Disease Control and Prevention, Hyattsville, MD

Tamara Lewis Johnson, Health Resources and Services Administration, Bethesda, MD

Helen M. Kavanagh, Health Resources and Services Administration, Bethesda, MD

Louis Kiger, Indian Health Service, Rockville, MD

Reva C. Lawrence, National Institutes of Health, Bethesda, MD

Richard W. Lymn, National Institutes of Health, Bethesda, MD

Saralyn Mark, Office on Women's Health, Washington, DC

Pamela McDonald-Perry, Substance Abuse and Mental Health Services Administration, Rockville, MD

Joan A. McGowan, National Institutes of Health, Bethesda, MD

Susan Moskosky, Office of Population Affairs, Bethesda, MD

Frances E. Page, Office on Women's Health, Washington, DC

Deborah L. Parham, Health Resources and Services Administration, Bethesda, MD

Estella Parrott, National Institutes of Health, Bethesda, MD

Wendy Perry, Agency for Healthcare Research and Quality, Rockville, MD

Kimberley Peters, Centers for Disease Control and Prevention, Hyattsville, MD

Vivian W. Pinn, National Institutes of Health, Bethesda, MD

Barry Portnoy, National Institutes of Health, Bethesda, MD

Marion Elizabeth Primas, Health Resources and Services Administration, Bethesda, MD

Louis Quatrano, National Institutes of Health, Bethesda, MD

Elena Rios, Office on Women's Health, Washington, DC

Laurie Robinson, Office on Women's Health, Boston, MA

Jonelle C. Rowe, Office on Women's Health, Washington, DC

Margaret I. Scarlett, Office of HIV/AIDS Policy, Washington, DC

Ulonda Shamwell, Substance Abuse and Mental Health Services Administration, Rockville, MD

Kathleen M. Shannon, Health Resources and Services Administration, Bethesda, MD

Audrey Sheppard, Food and Drug Administration, Rockville, MD

Christine G. Spain, President's Council on Physical Fitness and Sports, Washington, DC

Dora Warren, Centers for Disease Control and Prevention, Atlanta, GA

Nancy J. Wartow, Administration on Aging, Washington, DC

Susan F. Wood, Office on Women's Health, Washington, DC

Deborah Von Zinkernagel, Office of HIV/AIDS Policy, Washington, DC

Academy of General Dentistry

Aerobics and Fitness Association of America

Alcohol and Drug Problems Association

Alexander Graham Bell Association for the Deaf and Hard of Hearing

Alliance for Aging Research

Alliance for Health

African-American Calworks Coalition

Amateur Athletic Union

American Academy of Audiology

American Academy of Child and Adolescent Psychiatry

American Academy of Family Physicians

American Academy of Nursing

American Academy of Nurse Practitioners

American Academy of Ophthalmology

American Academy of Optometry

American Academy of Orthopaedic Surgeons

American Academy of Otolaryngology–Head and Neck Surgery

American Academy of Pain Management

American Academy of Pediatric Dentistry

American Academy of Pediatrics

American Academy of Physical Medicine and Rehabilitation

American Academy of Physician Assistants

American Alliance for Health, Physical Education, and Dance

American Art Therapy Association

American Association for Clinical Chemistry

American Association for Dental Research

American Association for Health Education

American Association for Marriage and Family Therapy

American Association for Respiratory Care

American Association for the Advancement of Science

American Association for World Health

American Association of Certified Orthopedists

American Association of Colleges of Nursing

American Association of Colleges of Osteopathic Medicine

American Association of Colleges of Pharmacy

American Association of Colleges for Teacher Education

American Association of Dental Schools

American Association of Family and Consumer Services

American Association of Health Plans

American Association of Homes for the Aging

American Association of Occupational Health Nurses

American Association of Pathologists' Assistants

American Association of Public Health Dentistry

American Association of Public Health Physicians

American Association of Retired Persons

American Association of School Administrators

American Association of Suicidiology

American Association of University Affiliated Programs for Persons with Developmental Disabilities

American Association on Health and Disability

American Association on Mental Retardation

American Cancer Society

American College Health Association

American College of Acupuncture

American College of Cardiology

American College of Clinical Pharmacy

American College of Emergency Physicians

American College of Gastroenterology

American College of Health Care Administrators

American College of Health Care Executives

American College of Nurse-Midwives

American College of Nutrition

American College of Obstetricians and Gynecologists

American College of Occupational and Environmental Medicine

American College of Physicians

American College of Preventive Medicine

American College of Radiology

American College of Sports and Medicine

American Correctional Health Services Association

American Council on Alcoholism

American Council on Exercise

American Counseling Association

American Dental Association

American Dental Hygienists' Association

American Diabetes Association

American Dietetic Association

American Disability Prevention and Wellness Association

American Federation of Teachers

American Geriatrics Society

American Health Lawyers Association

American Health Quality Association

American Heart Association

American Highway Users Alliance

American Hospital Association

American Indian Health Care Association

American Institute for Preventive Medicine

American Kinesiotherapy, Inc.

American Liver Association

American Lung Association

American Meat Institute

American Medical Association

American Medical Rehabilitation Providers Association

American Medical Student Association

American Music Therapy Association

American Nurses Association

American Obesity Association

American Occupational Therapy Association

American Optometric Association

American Orthopaedic Society for Sports Medicine

American Osteopathic Academy of Sports Medicine

American Osteopathic Association

American Osteopathic Healthcare Association

American Pharmaceutical Association

American Physical Therapy Association

American Podiatric Medical Association

American Psychological Association

American Psychiatric Association

American Psychiatric Nurses Association

American Public Health Association

American Red Cross

American Rehabilitation Counseling Association

American Running and Fitness Association

American School Food Service Association

American School Health Association

American Social Health Association

American Society for Clinical Nutrition

American Society for Gastrointestinal Endoscopy

American Society for Microbiology

American Society for Nutritional Sciences

American Society for Parental and Enteral Nutrition

American Society for Pharmacology and Experimental Therapeutics

American Society of Addiction Medicine

American Society of Consultant Pharmacists

American Society of Health System Pharmacists

American Society of Human Genetics

American Speech-Language-Hearing Association

American Spinal Injury Foundation

American Statistical Association

American Thoracic Society

American Trauma Society

American Veterinary Medical Association

Aquatic Exercise Association

Arthritis Foundation

Asian and Pacific Islander American Health Forum

Asociacion Nacional Pro Personas Mayores

Association for Applied Psychophysiology and Biofeedback

Association for Education and Rehabilitation

Association for Hospital Medical Education

Association for Professionals in Infection Control and Epidemiology

Association for the Advancement of Automotive Medicine

Association for the Care of Children's Health

Association for Vital Records and Health Promotion

Association for Worksite Health Promotion

Association of Academic Health Centers

Association of American Indian Physicians

Association of American Medical Colleges

Association of Asian Pacific Community Health Organizations

Association of Clinical Scientists

Association of Community Health Nursing Educators

Association of Food and Drug Officials

Association of Maternal and Child Health Programs

Association of Occupational and Environmental Clinics

Association of Pediatric Oncology Nurses

Association of Public Health Laboratories

Association of Rehabilitation Nurses

Association of Schools and Colleges of Optometry

Association of Schools of Allied Health Professions

Association of Schools of Public Health

Association of State and Territorial Chronic Disease Program Directors

Association of State and Territorial Dental Directors

Association of State and Territorial Directors of Health Promotion and Public Health Education

Association of State and Territorial Directors of Nursing

Association of State and Territorial Health Officials

Association of State and Territorial Public Health Laboratory Directors

Association of State and Territorial Public Health Nutrition Directors

Association of State and Territorial Public Health Social Workers

Association of Teachers of Preventive Medicine

Association of Technical Personnel in Ophthalmology

Association of Women's Health, Obstetric, and Neonatal Nurses

Asthma and Allergy Foundation of America

Blue Cross and Blue Shield Association

Boy Scouts of America

Brain Injury Association

Camp Fire Boys and Girls

Campaign for Tobacco-Free Kids

Cardiovascular Credentialing International

Catholic Health Association of the United States

Center for Science in the Public Interest

Center to Prevent Handgun Violence

Coalition for Consumer Health and Safety

Coalition for Healthier Cities and Communities

College of American Pathologists

Consortium of Social Science Associations

Consumer Federation of America

Contact Lens Manufacturers Association

Council for Responsible Nutrition

Council of Citizens with Low Vision International

Council of Medical Specialty Societies

Council of Regional Networks for Genetic Services

Council of State and Territorial Epidemiologists

Council of the Great City Schools

Emergency Nurses Association

Employee Assistance Professional Association

Environmental Council of the States

Eye Bank Association of America

Farm Safety 4 Just Kids

Federation of American Societies for Experimental Biology

Federation of Behavioral, Psychological, and Cognitive Sciences

Food Marketing Institute

Future Homemakers of America

Gay and Lesbian Medical Association

General Federation of Women's Clubs

Gerontological Society of America

Girl Scouts of the United States of America

Global Health Council

Grocery Manufacturers of America

Health Industry Manufacturers Association

Health Insurance Association of America

Health Ministers Association

Health Science Communications Association

Healthier People Network

Healthy Mothers, Healthy Babies

HIV Prevention Education Project

Hope Worldwide

Institute of Food Technologists

International Association for Dental Research

International Health, Racquet, and Sports Association

International Hearing Society

International Lactation Consultant Association

International Life Sciences Institute

International Patient Education Council

La Leche League International

Lamaze International

League for the Hard of Hearing

Learning Disabilities Association of America

Lighthouse International

Lions Club International

Living with Lupus

Low Vision Council

Macular Degeneration Partnership

March of Dimes Birth Defects Foundation

Maternity Center Association

Medical Library Association

Men's Health Network

Midwives Alliance of North America

Migrant Clinicians Network

Mothers Against Drunk Driving

NARAL—Reproductive Freedom and Choice

National Academy of Opticianry

National AIDS Fund

National Alliance for the Mentally Ill

National Alliance of Black School Educators

National Alliance of Nurse Practitioners

National Alliance of Senior Citizens

National Asian Pacific American Families Against Substance Abuse

National Asian Women's Health Organization

National Association for Family and Community Education

National Association for Healthcare Quality

National Association for Home Care

National Association for Human Development

National Association for Parents of Children with Visual Impairments

National Association for Public Employee Wellness

National Association for Public Health

National Association for Public Health Statistics and Information Systems

National Association for Public Worksite Health Promotion

National Association for Sport and Physical Education

National Association for the Visually Handicapped

National Association of Biology Teachers

National Association of Childbearing Centers

National Association of Children's Hospitals and Related Institutions

National Association of Community Health Centers

National Association of Counties

National Association of County and City Health Officials

National Association of Elementary School Principals

National Association of Governor's Councils on Physical Fitness and Sports

National Association of Local Boards of Health

National Association of Music Therapy

National Association of Neonatal Nurses

National Association of Neighborhoods

National Association of Optometrists and Opticians

National Association of Pediatric Nurse Associates and Practitioners

National Association of Physical Activity and Health Promotion

National Association of Rehabilitation Facilities

National Association of Retail Druggists

National Association of School Nurses

National Association of School Psychologists

National Association of Secondary School Principals

National Association of Social Workers

National Association of State Alcohol and Drug Abuse Directors

National Association of State Mental Health Program Directors

National Association of State Network Program Coordinators

National Association of State School Nurse Consultants

National Association of Vision Professionals

National Athletic Trainers' Association

National Black Nurses Association

National Black Women's Health Project

National Board of Medical Examiners

National Center for Health Education

National Civic League

National Coalition Against Sexual Assault

National Commission Against Drunk Driving

National Committee to Prevent Child Abuse

National Community Pharmacists Association

National Conference of State Legislatures

National Consumers League

National Council for Adoption

National Council for the Education of Health Professionals in Health Promotion

National Council of La Raza

National Council on Alcoholism and Drug Dependence

National Council on Community Hospitals

National Council on Health Laboratory Services

National Council on Patient Information and Education

National Council on Safe-Help and Public Health

National Council on the Aging

National Dairy Council

National Education Association

National Environmental Health Association

National Family Planning and Reproductive Health Association

National Federation for Specialty Nursing Organizations

National Federation of State High School Associations

National Food Processors Association

National 4-H Council

National Head Injury Foundation

National Health Council

National Health Lawyers Association

National Healthy Mothers, Healthy Babies Coalition

National Hispanic Council on Aging

National Hispanic Medical Association

National Hispanic Nurses Association

National Inhalant Prevention Coalition

National Institute for Fitness and Sports

National Institute on Managed Care

National Kidney Foundation

National League for Nursing

National League of Cities

National Lesbian and Gay Health Association

National Medical Association

National Mental Health Association

National Middle School Association

National Minority AIDS Council

National Minority Health Association

National Nurses Society on Addictions

National Optometric Association

National Organization for Women

National Organization of Mothers of Twins Club

National Organization on Adolescent Pregnancy, Parenting, and Prevention

National Osteoporosis Foundation

National Pediculosis Association

National Peer Helpers Association

National Pest Control Association

National PTA

National Recreation and Park Association

National SAFE KIDS Campaign

National Safety Council

National School Boards Association

National Society of Allied Health

National Strength and Conditioning Association

National Stroke Association

National Wellness Institute

National Women's Health Network

Network of Employers for Traffic Safety

North American Association for the Study of Obesity

Nursing Network on Violence Against Women

Oncology Nursing Society

Opticians Association of America

Oral Health America

Pan American Health Organization

Partnership for Prevention

People's Medical Society

Pharmaceutical Researchers and Manufacturers of America

Physicians for a Violence-Free Society

Planned Parenthood Federation of America

Poison Prevention Week Council

Population Association of America

Prevent Blindness America

Prevention of Blindness Society of the Metropolitan Area

Produce for Better Health Foundation

Produce Marketing Association

Public Health Institute

Road Runners Club of America

Salt Institute

Salvation Army

Sexuality Information and Education Council of United States

Shape Up America!

Society for Academic Emergency Medicine

Society for Adolescent Medicine

Society for Healthcare Epidemiology of America

Society for Healthcare Strategy and Market Development

Society for Nutrition Education

Society for Public Health Education

Society for the Advancement of Women's Health Research

Society of Behavioral Medicine

Society of General Internal Medicine

Society of Prospective Medicine

Society of State Directors of Health, Physical Education, and Recreation

Spina Bifida Association of America

State Family Planning Administrators

Stop Teenage Addiction to Tobacco

Student Athletic Trainers' Association

Sugar Association

Take Off Pounds Sensibly (TOPS) Club

The Arc, a National Organization on Mental Retardation

The Federation of Behavioral, Psychological, and Cognitive Sciences

The National Alliance for Hispanic Health

Unitarian Universalist, Seventh Principle Project

United Methodist Association of Health and Welfare Ministries

United States Eye Injury Registry

United Way of America

U.S. Chamber of Commerce

U.S. Conference of Mayors

Visiting Nurse Association of America

Voluntary Hospital Association of America

Washington Business Group on Health

Western Consortium for Public Health

Wellness Councils of America

Women's Sports Foundation

Wound, Ostomy, and Continence Nurses Society

YMCA of the USA

YWCA of the USA

AAMC	Association of American Medical Colleges
AAP	American Academy of Pediatrics
AAPCC	American Association of Poison Control Centers
ABCs	Active Bacterial Core Surveillance
ABLES	Adult Blood Lead Epidemiology and Surveillance
ACE	angiotensin-converting enzyme
ACF	Administration on Children and Families
ACIP	Advisory Committee on Immunization Practices
ACS	American Cancer Society
ADA	American Diabetes Association
ADA	American Dietetic Association
ADA	Americans with Disabilities Act
ADE	adverse drug experience
ADHD	attention deficit/hyperactivity disorder
ADLs	activities of daily living
ADPKD	autosomal dominant polycystic kidney disease
ADR	adverse drug reaction
AF	atrial fibrillation
AFDC	Aid to Families with Dependent Children
AGI	Alan Guttmacher Institute
AHA	American Heart Association
AHCPR	(See AHRQ)
AHEC	Area Health Education Center
AHRQ	Agency for Healthcare Research and Quality, formerly Agency for Health Care Policy and Research (AHCPR)
AHS	American Housing Survey
AIDS	acquired immunodeficiency syndrome
AIRS	Aerometric Information Retrieval System
ALA	American Lung Association
ALR	administrative license revocation
AMA	American Medical Association
AMD	age-related macular degeneration
AMI	acute myocardial infarction
AoA	Administration on Aging
AODM	adult-onset diabetes mellitus
aP	acellular pertussis
APEX/PH	Assessment Protocol for Excellence in Public Health

APHIS	Animal and Plant Health Inspection Service
APNCU	Adequacy of Prenatal Care Utilization Index
ARS	Agricultural Research Service
ASD	adult spectrum of disease
ASHP	American Society for Health-Systems Pharmacists
ASOII	Annual Survey of Occupational Injuries and Illnesses
ASPE	Assistant Secretary for Planning and Evaluation
ASPH	Association of Schools of Public Health
ASSIST	American Stop Smoking Intervention Study
ASTDHPPHE	Association of State and Territorial Directors of Health Promotion and Public Health Education
ASTHO	Association of State and Territorial Health Officials
ATPM	Association of Teachers of Preventive Medicine
ATSDR	Agency for Toxic Substances and Disease Registry
AV	arteriovenous
AWHP	Association for Worksite Health Promotion
AZT	zidovudine (formerly azidothymidine)
BAC	blood alcohol concentration
BEST	Biomonitoring of Environmental Status and Trends
BHPr	Bureau of Health Professions
BJS	Bureau of Justice Statistics
BLL	blood lead level
BLS	Bureau of Labor Statistics
BMD	bone mineral density
BMI	body mass index
BOC	U.S. Bureau of the Census
BPHC	Bureau of Primary Health Care
BRFS	Behavioral Risk Factor Survey
BRFSS	Behavioral Risk Factor Surveillance System
BUN	blood urea nitrogen
CAD	coronary artery disease
CAHPS	Consumer Assessment of Health Plans Survey
CD	conduct disorder
CDC	Centers for Disease Control and Prevention
CFOI	Census of Fatal Occupational Injuries
CFR	Child Fatality Review Process
CFRT	Child Fatality Review Team
CFSAN	Center for Food Safety and Applied Nutrition

CHIP	Child Health Insurance Program
CHD	coronary heart disease
CMHS	Center for Mental Health Services
CNS	central nervous system
COPD	chronic obstructive pulmonary disease
CPR	cardiopulmonary resuscitation
CPS	clinical preventive services
CPSC	Consumer Product Safety Commission
CPT	current procedural terminology
CRC	colorectal cancer
CSAP	Center for Substance Abuse Prevention
CSAT	Center for Substance Abuse Treatment
CSFII	Continuing Survey of Food Intakes by Individuals
CSREES	Cooperative State Research, Education, and Extension Service
CSTE	Council of State and Territorial Epidemiologists
CVD	cardiovascular disease
CVM	Center for Veterinary Medicine
DALYs	disability-adjusted life years
DANS	Data Analysis System
DASH	Division of Adolescent and School Health
DAWN	Drug Abuse Warning Network
DM	diabetes mellitus
DNA	data not analyzed
DNC	data not collected
DOC	U.S. Department of Commerce
DoD	U.S. Department of Defense
DOE	U.S. Department of Energy
DOJ	U.S. Department of Justice
DOL	U.S. Department of Labor
DOQI	dialysis outcomes quality initiative
DOT	U.S. Department of Transportation
DQIP	Diabetes Quality Improvement Project
DRE	digital rectal examination
DSU	data statistically unreliable
DTaP	diphtheria-tetanus-pertussis vaccine
DTBE	Division of Tuberculosis Elimination
DVD	digital video disk

DWI	driving while intoxicated
EAP	employee assistance program
ECA	Environmental Catchment Area
ECC	early childhood caries
ECG	electrocardiogram
ECP	emergency contraceptive pills
ED	emergency department
ED	U.S. Department of Education
EDF	Environmental Defense Fund
EIA	Energy Information Administration
EME	established market economies
EMS	emergency medical services
EMT	emergency medical technician
EMTALA	Emergency Medical Treatment and Active Labor Act
EPA	Environmental Protection Agency
EPACT	Energy Policy Act of of 1992
EPC	Evidence-based Practice Center
EPCRA	Emergency Planning and Community Right-To-Know Act
EPO	Epidemiology Program Office
ER	emergency room
ERS	Economic Research Service
ESRD	end-stage renal disease
ETS	environmental tobacco smoke
FARS	Fatality Analysis Reporting System
FAS	fetal alcohol syndrome
FBI	Federal Bureau of Investigation
FDA	Food and Drug Administration
FEMA	Federal Emergency Management Agency
FHA	Federal Highway Administration
FOBT	fecal occult blood test
FPL	Federal poverty level
FSIS	Food Safety and Inspection Service
FSS	Food Safety Survey
GAO	General Accounting Office
GBD	global burden of disease
GBS	group B streptococcal; group B *Streptococcus*
GDM	gestational diabetes mellitus
GED	General Education Development

GES	General Estimates System
GFR	glomerular filtration rate
GHG	greenhouse gas
GIS	geographic information system
GISP	Gonococcal Isolate Surveillance Project
GMPs	good manufacturing practices
GPRA	Government Performance and Results Act
HAART	highly active antiretroviral therapy
HACCP	Hazard Analysis Critical Control Point
HALYs	health-adjusted life years
HAV	hepatitis A virus
HBIG	hepatitis B immune globulin
HBsAg	hepatitis B surface antigen
HBV	hepatitis B virus
HCBS	Home and Community-Based Services
HCFA	Health Care Financing Administration
HCUP	Health Care Cost and Utilization Project
HCV	hepatitis C virus
HDL	high-density lipoprotein
HEDIS	Health Plan Employer Data and Information Set
HEI	Healthy Eating Index
HepB	hepatitis B
HERS	Heart and Estrogen/Progestin Replacement Study
HHS	U.S. Department of Health and Human Services
Hib	Hæmophilus influenzæ type B
Hi-Ethics	Health Internet Ethics
HIP	health improvement plan
HIV	human immunodeficiency virus
HMO	health maintenance organization
HPSA	health professional shortage area
HPV	human papillomavirus
HRQOL	health-related quality of life
HRSA	Health Resources and Services Administration
HSV-2	herpes simplex virus type 2
HUD	U.S. Department of Housing and Urban Development
IAQ	indoor air quality
ICA	International Communication Association
ICAN	Inter-Agency Council on Child Abuse and Neglect

ICARIS	Injury Control and Risk Survey
ICD	International Classification of Diseases
ICIDH-2	International Classification of Impairments, Disabilities, and Handicaps; International Classification of Functioning and Disability
ICPD	International Conference on Population and Development
ICU	intensive care unit
IDDM	insulin-dependent diabetes mellitus
IDUs	injection drug users
IgA	immunoglobulin A
IHS	Indian Health Service
IM	infant mortality
IOM	Institute of Medicine
IPV	inactivated poliovirus vaccine
IPV	intimate partner violence
IRIS	Integrated Risk Information System
IRMO	Information Resources Management Office
IT	information technology
IUD	intrauterine device
IUGR	intrauterine growth retardation
JCAHO	Joint Commission for the Accreditation of Healthcare Organizations
JODM	juvenile-onset diabetes mellitus
LBP	low back pain
LBW	low birth weight
LDL	low-density lipoprotein
LPN	licensed practical nurse
LTC	long-term care
MAC	*Mycobacterium avium* complex
MADDSP	Metropolitan Atlanta Developmental Disabilities Surveillance Program
MCHB	Maternal and Child Health Bureau
MCL	maximum contaminant level
MCO	managed care organization
MDS	minimum data set
MEPS	Medical Expenditure Panel Survey
MMR	measles, mumps, and rubella vaccine
MMWR	Morbidity and Mortality Weekly Report
MSA	metropolitan statistical area

MSM	men who have sex with men
MUA/P	Medically Underserved Area/Population
NA	not applicable
NAAQS	National Ambient Air Quality Standards
NACCHO	National Association of County and City Health Officials
NACO	National Association of Counties
NAEPP	National Asthma Education and Prevention Program
NAMCS	National Ambulatory Medical Care Survey
NaSH	National Surveillance System for Hospital Health Care Workers
NBDPN	National Birth Defects Prevention Network
NBS	newborn screening
NCA	National Communication Association
NCANDS	National Child Abuse and Neglect Data System
NCCAN	National Center for Child Abuse and Neglect
NCCDPHP	National Center for Chronic Disease Prevention and Health Promotion
NCC MERP	National Coordinating Council for Medication Error Reporting and Prevention
NCEH	National Center for Environmental Health
NCEP	National Cholesterol Education Program
NCES	National Center for Educational Statistics
NCHSR	National Center for Health Services Research
NCHS	National Center for Health Statistics
NCHSTP	National Center for HIV, STD, and TB Prevention
NCI	National Cancer Institute
NCID	National Center for Infectious Diseases
NCIPC	National Center for Injury Prevention and Control
NCPA	National Community Pharmacy Association
NCPIE	National Council on Patient Information and Education
NCPS	National Center for Prevention Services
NCQA	National Committee for Quality Assurance
NCRSR	National Congenital Rubella Syndrome Registry
NCSD	National Coalition of STD Directors
NCSDR	National Commission on Sleep Disorders Research
NCUTLO	National Committee on Uniform Traffic Laws and Ordinances
NCVHS	National Committee on Vital and Health Statistics
NCVS	National Crime Victimization Survey
NEISS	National Electronic Injury Surveillance System

NETSS	National Electronic Telecommunications System for Surveillance
NFIRS	National Fire Incidence Reporting System
NHAMCS	National Hospital Ambulatory Medical Care Survey
NHANES	National Health and Nutrition Examination Survey
NHBPEP	National High Blood Pressure Education Program
NHDS	National Hospital Discharge Survey
NHII	national health information infrastructure
NHIS	National Health Interview Survey
NHLBI	National Heart, Lung, and Blood Institute
NHSDA	National Household Survey on Drug Abuse
NHTSA	National Highway Traffic Safety Administration
NIAAA	National Institute on Alcohol Abuse and Alcoholism
NICHD	National Institute of Child Health and Human Development
NIDA	National Institute on Drug Abuse
NIDCR	National Institute of Dental and Craniofacial Research, formerly National Institute of Dental Research (NIDR)
NIDDK	National Institute of Diabetes and Digestive and Kidney Diseases
NIDDM	non-insulin-dependent diabetes mellitus
NIDR	(See NIDCR)
NIDRR	National Institute on Disability and Rehabilitation Research
NIEHS	National Institute of Environmental Health Sciences
NIH	National Institutes of Health
NIHL	noise-induced hearing loss
NIJ	National Institute of Justice
NIMH	National Institute of Mental Health
NIOSH	National Institute for Occupational Safety and Health
NIP	National Immunization Program
NIS	National Immunization Survey
NLM	National Library of Medicine
NME	new molecular entity
NNDSS	National Notifiable Disease Surveillance System
NNHS	National Nursing Home Survey
NNISS	National Nosocomial Infections Surveillance System
NOES	National Occupational Exposure Survey
NOPUS	National Occupant Protection Use Survey
NORA	National Occupational Research Agenda
NPCR	National Program of Cancer Registries

NPL	National Priorities List
NPSF	National Patient Safety Foundation
NPTS	National Personal Transportation Survey
NRDC	Natural Resources Defense Council
NRT	nicotine replacement therapy
NSAIDs	nonsteroidal antiinflammatory drugs
NSAM	National Survey of Adolescent Males
NSBA	National School Boards Association
NSEPs	needle and syringe exchange programs
NSFG	National Survey of Family Growth
NSSPM	National Surveillance System for Pneumoconiosis Mortality
NTDs	neural tube defects
NTOF	National Traumatic Occupational Fatalities Surveillance System
NTOMS	National Treatment Outcomes Monitoring System
NVAP	National Vaccine Advisory Committee
NVSS	National Vital Statistics System
NWHPS	1999 National Worksite Health Promotion Survey
OAR	Office of Air and Radiation
OAS	Office of the Assistant Secretary
OASD	Office of the Assistant Secretary of Defense
OASH	Office of the Assistant Secretary for Health
OCAN	Office of Child Abuse and Neglect
OCD	occupational contact dermatitis
ODH	Office on Disability and Health
ODPHP	Office of Disease Prevention and Health Promotion
OMB	Office of Management and Budget
ONDCP	Office of National Drug Control Policy
OPA	Office of Population Affairs
OPEL	Office of Planning, Evaluation, and Legislation
OPHS	Office of Public Health and Science
OPPTS	Office of Pollution, Prevention, and Toxic Substances
OPV	oral polio vaccine
ORA	Office of Research and Analysis
OSA	obstructive sleep apnea
OSDs	occupational skin diseases or disorders
OSERS	Office of Special Education and Rehabilitative Services
OSH	Office of the Secretary of Health

OSHA	Occupational Safety and Health Administration
OSWER	Office of Solid Waste Enforcement and Remediation
OTC	over the counter
PAHO	Pan American Health Organization
PATCH	Planned Approach to Community Health
PATH	Projects for Assistance in Transition from Homelessness
PCBs	polychlorinated biphenyls
PCC	Poison Control Center
PCP	*Pneumocystis carinii* pneumonia
PCPFS	President's Council on Physical Fitness and Sports
PEP	postexposure prophylaxis
PHF	Public Health Foundation
PHS	Public Health Service
PID	pelvic inflammatory disease
PIR	poverty-income ratio
PKU	phenylketonuria
POS	point-of-service
PPO	preferred provider organization
P&S	primary and secondary
PSA	prostate-specific antigen
PWD	people with disabilities
PWSS	Potable Water Surveillance System
QALYs	quality-adjusted life years
QuIC	Quality Interagency Coordination
QOL	quality of life
RBC	red blood cell
RCRA	Resource Conservation and Recovery Act
RN	registered nurse
ROPs	rollover protection systems
RRT	renal replacement therapy
RTECS®	Registry of Toxic Effects of Chemical Substances
SAMHSA	Substance Abuse and Mental Health Services Administration
SAPT	Substance Abuse Prevention and Treatment
SCHIP	State Children's Health Intervention Program
SDWA	Safe Drinking Water Act
SDWIS	Safe Drinking Water Information System
SEDs	serious emotional disturbances
SEER	Surveillance, Epidemiology, and End Results

SES	socioeconomic status
SHPPS	School Health Policies and Programs Study
SIDS	sudden infant death syndrome
SIPP	Survey of Income and Program Participation
SMI	serious mental illness
SOC	Standard Occupational Classification
SPF	sun protective factor
STD	sexually transmitted disease
SUD	substance use disorder
TB	tuberculosis
TESS	Toxic Exposure Surveillance System
TRI	Toxics Release Inventory
TRUS	transrectal ultrasonography
TSDF	treatment, storage, and disposal facilities
TST	tuberculin skin testing
UA	urban area
UMTA	Urban Mass Transit Authority
USDA	U.S. Department of Agriculture
USGS	U.S. Geological Survey
USP	U.S. Pharmacopeia
USPSTF	U.S. Preventive Services Task Force
USRDS	U.S. Renal Data System
UST	underground storage tank
UV	ultraviolet light
VA	U.S. Department of Veterans Affairs
VAERS	Vaccine Adverse Event Reporting System
VAPP	vaccine-associated paralytic polio
VLBW	very low birth weight
VMT	vehicle miles traveled
VPDs	vaccine-preventable diseases
VSD	Vaccine Safety Datalink
WHO	World Health Organization
WIC	Women, Infants, and Children
wP	whole cell pertussis
YHL	years of healthy life
YPLL	years of potential life lost

YRBS	Youth Risk Behavior Survey
YRBSS	Youth Risk Behavior Surveillance System
YSAPI	Youth Substance Abuse Prevention Initiative

Index

Editor's Note:

With the exception of the section on Understanding and Improving Health and the Reader's Guide, the page numbers are hyphenated, with the number preceding the hyphen referring to the chapter and the number following the hyphen referring to the page; hence, 5-12 means chapter 5, page 12. Each Focus Area has an alphabetized list of Terminology at the end of the chapter. A list of abbreviations and acronyms may be found in Appendix H.

Because the elimination of health disparities among different segments of the population is one of Healthy People 2010's overarching goals, select population groups are discussed extensively throughout this document. The index, however, does not provide specific page numbers for each population group.

For references to racial, ethnic, and other population groups, readers are directed to Understanding and Improving Health, pages 12 through 16; the Reader's Guide, pages RG-1 through RG-10; the disparities section of each Focus Area's Overview; and the population data tables that appear with more than 200 objectives. The electronic versions of Healthy People 2010—available at http://www.health.gov/healthypeople/ or on CD-ROM—may be searched in a variety of ways, including by more than 100 keywords.

A

Ability days, 2-3

Abstinence as part of young adult education, 9-26—9-28, 25-25—25-29

Abuse prevention. *See* Violence prevention.

Access to health care, Leading Health Indicator. *See* Understanding and Improving Health, pp. 44-45.

Access to quality health services—Focus Area 1. *See also* Health insurance.

access to, 1-20—1-24

clinical preventive services, 1-4—1-5, 1-13—1-14

components of system, 1-3

disparities, 1-7—1-9

emergency services, 1-5—1-6, 1-30—1-31, 1-33—1-34

long-term care services, 1-6, 1-34—1-36

medical homes for special health care needs, 16-49—16-50

patient and family health education, 7-21—7-22

patient health education and promotion, 7-6

primary care, 1-5, 5-7—5-8

rehabilitative services, 1-6, 1-34—1-36, 28-16

service systems for special health care needs, 16-50—16-51

STDs and, 25-4—25-5

Acellular pertussis vaccine, 14-4, 14-12

Acquired immunodeficiency syndrome. *See* AIDS; HIV.

Activity. *See* Physical activity.

Activity limitations. *See also* Disabilities.

arthritis and, 2-11—2-14

chronic back conditions and, 2-20—2-21

Acute myocardial infarctions (AMI), 12-10

Addictive disorders, mental disorders and, 18-6—18-7, 18-20

Administrative license revocation (ALR), 26-9, 26-46

Adolescent health. *See also* Teenagers.

alcohol use, 26-3

binge drinking, 26-29—26-33

calcium recommended daily intakes, 19-34

chlamydia, 25-15—25-16, 25-30

contraception use, 9-23—9-26, 13-18

death rates, 16-21—16-23

dental caries in, 21-11—21-16

disabilities, 6-10—6-11, 6-20

drownings, 15-40—15-42

drug use, 26-5

emotional disturbances and, 18-6

externalizing disorders, 18-7

health instruction in schools, 7-4—7-5, 7-14

HIV, 13-16

homicides, 15-43—15-44

inhalants use, 26-37—26-38

marijuana use, 26-26—26-27

mental health and, 18-3, 18-16—18-17

motor vehicle crashes, 15-25—15-26, 26-13—26-14

noise-induced hearing loss, 28-17

otitis media, 28-14—28-15

overweight or obesity in, 19-4, 19-13—19-16

perceived risk of substance abuse, 26-41—26-43

physical activity and, 22-17—22-25

physical fighting among, 15-51—15-52

preventing alcohol and drug use, 26-22—26-29

proportion engaging in sexual intercourse, 9-20—9-22

quality of school meals and snacks, 19-40

riding with a driver drinking alcohol, 26-19—26-20

safety belt use, 15-29—15-30

sale of tobacco products to, 27-29

sexual behavior and STDs, 25-25—25-29

smoking and, 27-12—27-14, 27-15—27-18

smoking cessation attempts, 27-21—27-22

spit tobacco use, 27-6, 27-14—27-15

steroid use, 26-35—26-37

substance abuse

disapproval, 26-38—26-41

past-month use, 26-25—26-27

suicide, 18-12—18-14

tobacco use, 27-4—27-5, 27-12—27-18

tobacco use disapproval, 27-30—27-31

unintended pregnancy and, 9-5—9-6, 9-19—9-20

vaccine coverage levels, 14-39—14-40, 14-42—14-44

weapons carried on school property, 15-52—15-54

Adolescents. *See* Editor's Note, I-1.

Key to page numbering: 1-62, Understanding and Improving Health; RG-1—RG-10, Reader's Guide; 1-1—1-47, Focus Area 1. Access to Quality Health Services; 2-1—2-28, Focus Area 2. Arthritis, Osteoporosis, and Chronic Back Conditions; and so forth. Understanding and Improving Health, Reader's Guide, and Focus Areas 1-14 are in Volume I; Focus Areas 15-28 and the Appendices are in Volume II.

Adult-onset diabetes. *See* Diabetes.
Adverse events. *See also* Medication errors.
  elderly persons and adverse drug events,
    17-7
  integrated system for monitoring and
    reporting events, 17-12—17-13
  sources of risk, 17-3—17-5
  vaccines and, 14-49—14-50
Affective disorders, 18-4—18-5
Aflatoxins, 10-5
African Americans. *See* Editor's Note, I-1.
Age factors
  arthritis, 2-6
  chronic kidney disease and, 4-4
  diabetes and, 5-5
  disability rates, 6-4
  heart disease and, 12-4—12-5
  STDs and, 25-8—25-9
  stroke and, 12-4—12-5
  susceptibility of foodborne infections
    caused by *Campylobacter* species,
      10-6, 10-7
  vertebral fractures due to osteoporosis and,
    2-19—2-20
Age groups. *See* Editor's Note, I-1.
Age-related macular degeneration, 28-4
Agoraphobia, suicide and, 18-20
AIDS. *See also* HIV.
  ACTG-076, 13-25
  blood transfusions and, 13-7, 13-10,
    17-4—17-5
  costs of, 13-5
  education programs for students,
    7-14—7-16
  men who have sex with men and, 13-15
  occurrence of, 13-3, 13-5—13-7,
    13-13—13-14
  perinatal transmission, 13-7
  prevention education in prison systems,
    13-19
  STDs and, 25-9—25-10
  time interval between AIDS diagnosis and
    death, 13-24—13-25
  time interval between HIV diagnosis and
    AIDS diagnosis, 13-24
  zidovudine therapy, 13-7, 13-15
Air quality
  adverse health effects from toxic
    emissions, 8-17—8-18

chronic obstructive pulmonary disease and,
    24-9
  EPA standards, 8-15
  lung cancer and, 3-12
  motor vehicle emissions and, 8-5,
    8-16—8-17
  nonattainment areas, 8-5, 8-10, 8-15
  in office buildings, 8-24—8-25
  scope of problem, 8-5, 8-7
  smoking policies, 27-27—27-28
Alaska Natives. *See* Editor's Note, I-1.
Alcohol use. *See also* Substance abuse.
  abuse, 26-3
  administrative license revocation, 26-9,
    26-46
  adolescents riding with a drinking driver,
    26-19—26-20
  alcohol dependence, 26-3
  annual consumption, 26-33
  binge drinking, 26-29—26-33
  blood alcohol concentration, 26-9,
    26-46—26-27
  cirrhosis death rate, 26-15—26-16
  counseling services, 1-17
  disapproval by adolescents, 26-39
  drownings and, 15-41
  education programs for students,
    7-14—7-16
  fetal alcohol syndrome and, 16-5, 16-45
  fetal mortality and, 16-18
  followup care after emergency department
    treatment, 26-45
  hospital emergency department visits,
    26-18—26-19
  infant health and, 16-5, 16-43—16-45
  lost productivity in the workplace, 26-21
  low-risk drinking guidelines, 26-34—26-25
  mental disorders and, 18-6—18-7
  motor vehicle crash deaths and, 15-7,
    15-32
  occurrence of, 26-3—26-4
  oral cancer and, 21-25
  oropharyngeal cancer and, 3-17
  preventing adolescent use, 26-22—26-29
  risks of, 26-4
  treatment lag, 26-44—26-45
  violence and, 26-20—26-21

Allergens
  food allergies and, 10-5—10-6, 10-14
  indoor levels, 8-24
Alternative fuels, 8-16—8-17
Alzheimer's disease, 18-4, 18-8
Amblyopia, 28-5
American Indians or Alaska Natives. See
  Editor's Note, I-1.
Amputations, diabetes and, 5-3, 5-22—5-23
Anaphylaxis, food-induced, 10-5,
  10-14—10-15
Anemia
  among low-income females in third
    trimester of pregnancy, 19-37—19-38
  causes of, 19-38
Angioplasty, 12-11
Anhedonia, depression and, 18-19
Animal feeds. See Food safety.
Anorexia nervosa relapse rates,
  18-15—18-16
Antibiotic-resistant infections, 14-16—14-18
Antibiotics
  common cold and, 14-32—14-33
  ear infections and, 14-31—14-32
  intensive care unit use, 14-35
Antimicrobial resistance
  food safety and, 10-13
  infectious diseases and, 14-22—14-35
Antiretroviral therapy for HIV infection, 13-6,
  13-23
Anxiety disorders
  adults receiving treatment for,
    18-18—18-20
  occurrence of, 18-5
Apnea. See Obstructive sleep apnea.
Area Health Education Centers (AHECs),
  7-23
Arteriovenous fistulas, use for vascular
  access in hemodialysis, 4-14—4-15
Arthritis—Focus Area 2
  activity limitations, 2-11—2-14
  costs of, 2-4
  disparities, 2-6
  education interventions, 2-16
  employment rate and, 2-14—2-15
  Haemophilus influenzae type b and, 14-5
  joint symptoms, 2-11—2-14
  medical management of, 2-16
  mental health and, 2-14

  occurrence of, 2-3
  pain and, 2-11
  physical activity and, 22-3
  public health impact, 2-3—2-4
  racial disparities in rate of knee
    replacements, 2-15—2-16
  risk factors, 2-7
Asian Americans; Asians or Pacific
  Islanders. See Editor's Note, I-1.
Aspirin, diabetes and, 5-29—5-30
Assaults
  by current or former intimate partners,
    15-46—15-47
  occurrence of, 15-5, 15-51
  work-related, 20-14
Assisted living, 1-34
Assistive technology, disabilities and, 6-21
Asthma. See also Respiratory diseases;
  Environmental health.
  absence from school or work due to
    asthma, 24-18
  activity limitations and, 24-17—24-18
  appropriate care, 24-19—24-20
  beta antagonists, 24-7
  costs of, 8-9, 24-4—24-5
  death rates, 8-8—8-9, 8-11, 24-13—24-14
  disparities, 24-5—24-6
  environmental health and, 8-8
  hospital emergency department visits,
    24-16—24-17
  hospitalization rates, 8-11, 24-14—24-15
  hospitalization rates for pediatric cases,
    1-27—1-29
  indoor allergen levels and, 8-24
  management of, 24-3, 24-7
  occurrence of, 8-8, 24-3—24-4
  patient education, 24-18—24-19
  surveillance systems, 24-20
Atherosclerotic disease. See Cardiovascular
  disease.
Atrial fibrillation (AF), 12-5
Attempted rape, 15-47—15-48
Attention deficit/hyperactivity disorder
  (ADHD), 18-7
Automobiles. See Motor vehicles.
Azidothymidine (AZT). See Zidovuline
  therapy.

Key to page numbering: 1-62, Understanding and Improving Health; RG-1—RG-10, Reader's Guide;
1-1—1-47, Focus Area 1. Access to Quality Health Services; 2-1—2-28, Focus Area 2. Arthritis,
Osteoporosis, and Chronic Back Conditions; and so forth. Understanding and Improving Health,
Reader's Guide, and Focus Areas 1-14 are in Volume I; Focus Areas 15-28 and the Appendices are
in Volume II.

B

Back conditions. *See* Chronic back conditions.

Bacterial meningitis, 14-6, 14-15—14-16

Balloon angioplasty, 12-11

Barium enema, use in colorectal cancer diagnosis, 3-15

Beach closings, 8-20

Benzene, 8-17

Bicycling
head injuries and, 15-13
helmet use, 15-33—15-34
motor vehicle emissions and, 8-16
for physical activity, 22-30—22-32

Binge drinking, 26-29—26-33

Binge eating. *See* Bulimia nervosa.

Biological products. *See* Medical product safety.

Birth control. *See* Contraception.

Birth defects
fetal alcohol syndrome and, 16-45
fetal mortality and, 16-3, 16-15—16-16, 16-18—16-19

Blacks. *See* Editor's Note, I-1.

Blindness. *See also* Vision.
diabetes and, 5-3
occurrence of, 28-3
prevention of 28-6—28-7

Blood alcohol concentration (BAC), 26-9, 26-46—26-27

Blood lead levels (BLLs)
lead-based paints and, 8-21—8-22
work exposures, 20-14—20-15

Blood pressure. *See* High blood pressure.

Blood supply safety, 17-5, 17-16

Blood transfusions, AIDS and, 13-7, 13-10, 17-4—17-5

Blood-glucose monitoring, diabetes and, 5-30—5-31

Body mass index (BMI), 12-10, 19-5, 19-10, 19-14—19-15

Bone mineral density (BMD), osteoporosis and, 2-17—2-18

Bones, calcium intake and, 19-34

Breast cancer
death rates, 3-12—3-13
risk factors, 3-13
screening, 3-6

Breastfeeding
infant health and, 16-5—16-6, 16-46—16-48
iron deficiency prevention, 19-39

Bronchitis, 24-8—24-9

Brownfields, 8-23

Bulimia nervosa relapse rates, 18-15—18-16

C

Calcium
blood pressure and, 19-35
deficiencies, 19-3—19-4, 19-33—19-35
osteoporosis and, 19-34—19-35
recommended daily intakes, 19-34
salt consumption and, 19-32

Campylobacter species, foodborne illness due to, 10-6—10-8, 10-10—10-11

Cancer—Focus Area 3. *See also* specific cancers.
costs of, 3-3
death rates, 3-3—3-4, 3-10—3-19
dietary factors, 19-3, 19-29—19-30
disparities, 3-4—3-6
occurrence of, 3-3
overweight or obesity and, 19-5
physician counseling for prevention, 3-22
population-based State registries, 3-27
screening, 3-6—3-7, 3-22
sites of new cases, 3-4
survival rate, 3-28
tobacco use and, 27-3

Cardiopulmonary resuscitation (CPR), 12-17

Cardiovascular disease (CVD). *See* Heart disease.

Caregivers, people with disabilities and, 6-22

Cataracts, 28-14

CD4+ testing, 13-23

Cellulitis, *Haemophilus influenzae* type b and, 14-5

Centers for excellence, health communication and, 11-17

Cerebral palsy among infants, 16-38—16-39

Cerebrovascular disease. *See* Stroke.

Cervical cancer
death rates, 3-13—3-14
Medicare coverage of screenings, 1-15
screening, 3-6—3-7, 3-14

Cesarean births, 16-30—16-31

Key to page numbering: 1-62, Understanding and Improving Health; RG-1—RG-10, Reader's Guide; 1-1—1-47, Focus Area 1. Access to Quality Health Services; 2-1—2-28, Focus Area 2. Arthritis, Osteoporosis, and Chronic Back Conditions; and so forth. Understanding and Improving Health, Reader's Guide, and Focus Areas 1-14 are in Volume I; Focus Areas 15-28 and the Appendices are in Volume II.

Chemotherapy, oral health and, 21-5
Child health—Focus Area 16
asthma and, 8-8
bacterial meningitis and, 14-15—14-16
blindness or visual impairment,
28-12—28-13
calcium recommended daily intakes, 19-34
courses of antibiotics for ear infections,
14-31—14-32
death rates, 16-19—16-20
deaths resulting from injury, 15-4, 15-17
dental caries in, 21-3—21-4, 21-11—21-13
diabetes, 5-3
disabilities, 16-6
drownings, 15-41—15-42
education opportunities for children with
disabilities, 6-20
emergency pediatric care, 1-33—1-34
emotional disturbances and, 18-6
externalizing disorders, 18-7
food allergies, 10-5
growth retardation among low-income
children, 19-16—19-18
health instruction in schools, 7-4—7-5, 7-14
hepatitis B virus infections, 14-12—14-13
hospitalization rates for pediatric asthma,
1-27—1-29
iron deficiencies, 19-36—19-37
lead poisoning, 8-21—8-22
maltreatment of, 15-45—15-46
medical homes for special health care
needs, 16-49—16-50
mental disorders, 18-3, 18-7,
18-13—18-14, 18-16—18-17
noise-induced hearing loss, 28-17
otitis media in, 28-14—28-15
overweight or obesity in, 19-4,
19-13—19-16
population-based immunization registries,
14-41—14-42
quality of school meals and snacks, 19-40
regular dental visits for low-income
children, 21-31—21-32
sepsis from sickling hemoglobinopathies,
16-49
service systems for special health care
needs, 16-50—16-51
source of ongoing care, 1-20
special health care needs, 16-49—16-51

suffocation death rate, 15-20—15-21
toxoplasmosis rates, 10-12
vaccination programs, 14-5
vaccine coverage levels, 14-35—14-41
vision disorders and, 28-4—28-5
Child restraints, use of, 15-30
Childbirth classes, 16-28—16-29
Childhood injury prevention, counseling
services regarding, 1-17
Children. *See* Child health; Editor's
Note, I-1.
Chlamydia. *See* Sexually transmitted
diseases.
Cholesterol
heart disease and, 12-3, 12-7, 12-9, 12-29
high blood levels, 12-27—12-28
high-density lipoprotein, 12-10
low-density lipoprotein, 12-29
mean total blood levels, 12-25—12-26
screening, 12-8—12-9, 12-28—12-29
Chronic back conditions—Focus Area 2.
See also Disabilities.
activity limitation and, 2-20—2-21
disparities, 2-7
ergonomic interventions, 2-8
occurrence of, 2-6
prevention interventions, 2-8
risk factors, 2-21
work-related injuries, 20-12
Chronic kidney disease—Focus Area 4
angio-tensin-converting enzyme and, 4-7
cardiovascular disease complications,
4-11—4-12
costs of, 4-5
counseling necessary prior to renal
replacement therapy, 4-13—4-14
diabetes and, 4-4—4-7, 4-19—4-20
dialysis, 4-4—4-5, 4-14—4-15
disparities, 4-5—4-6
end-stage renal disease, 4-3—4-4,
4-10—4-14, 4-19—4-20
interventions, 4-7
occurrence of, 4-3—4-4
renal replacement therapy, 4-13—4-15
risk factors, 4-7
transplantation, 4-3—4-7
transplantation waiting list, 4-16—4-18
treated chronic kidney failure, 4-3—4-4,
4-10—4-14

---

*Key to page numbering: 1-62, Understanding and Improving Health; RG-1—RG-10, Reader's Guide;
1-1—1-47, Focus Area 1. Access to Quality Health Services; 2-1—2-28, Focus Area 2. Arthritis,
Osteoporosis, and Chronic Back Conditions; and so forth. Understanding and Improving Health,
Reader's Guide, and Focus Areas 1-14 are in Volume I; Focus Areas 15-28 and the Appendices are
in Volume II.*

Chronic obstructive pulmonary disease
(COPD)
   activity limitation, 24-20—24-21
   death rates, 24-21—24-22
   disparities, 24-9—24-10
   smoking and, 24-8
Chronic renal insufficiency, 4-3
Cigarette smoking. See Tobacco use.
Cigars. See Tobacco use.
Cirrhosis death rate, 26-15—26-16
Cleft lip and palate, 21-5, 21-34—21-35
Clinical preventive care, 1-4—1-5,
   1-13—1-14
Clinical preventive services (CPS). See
   Access to quality health services.
Clot-dissolving therapy. See thrombolytic
   agents.
Cocaine. See Drug use.
Cochlear implants, 28-16
Cognitive-behavioral treatment, anorexia
   nervosa and, 18-16
Colds, antibiotics and, 14-32—14-33
Colleges
   binge drinking among students,
      26-29—26-33
   health instruction for students, 7-14—7-16
Colonoscopy, use in colorectal cancer
   diagnosis, 3-15
Colorectal cancer (CRC)
   death rates, 3-14—3-15
   Medicare coverage of screenings, 1-15
   proportion of adults receiving screening
      examinations, 3-24—3-25
   risk factors, 3-15
   screening, 3-7
Communication disorders. See Disabilities.
Communications. See Health
   communication.
Community-based programs—
   Focus Area 7. See also Educational
      programs.
   culturally and linguistically appropriate
      health promotion programs,
      7-23—7-24
   disparities, 7-8
   environmental health, 8-7
   health centers with oral health component,
      21-33—21-34
   health promotion programs, 7-22—7-24

patient and family health education,
   7-21—7-22
people with disabilities and, 6-17—6-18
prevention programs, 11-4
Condoms
   HIV prevention and, 13-8,
      13-16—13-18
   STDs and, 25-11
   use among adolescents, 9-23—9-26,
      13-18, 25-25—25-29
Conduct problems, 18-7
Confidentiality in health communication, 11-8
Congenital heart defects, infant deaths due
   to, 16-15—16-16
Congenital rubella syndrome, 14-12, 16-39
Congenital syphilis. See Sexually transmitted
   diseases.
Congestive heart failure. See Heart disease.
Conjugate vaccines, 14-5—14-6
Contraception
   emergency contraceptive pills, 9-17—9-18
   health insurance coverage, 9-29—9-30
   male involvement, 9-18—9-19
   methods, 9-3—9-5
   misinformation concerning, 9-8
   oral contraceptives, 9-26
   rates of use, 9-14—9-17
   use among adolescents, 9-23—9-26
   young adult education, 9-26—9-28
Coping skills. See also Mental health.
   stress and, 18-9
Coronary artery bypass surgery, 12-11
Coronary heart disease (CHD). See Heart
   disease.
Coronary stenting, 12-11
Correctional institutions. See also Jail
   system; Juvenile justice system; Prison
   systems.
   substance abuse treatment, 26-43
Cotinine, serum, 27-25—27-26
Counseling services
   health behaviors, 1-15—1-18
   health insurance coverage, 1-15
   medication use and risks, 17-15
   nutrition, 19-42—19-44
Cryptosporidiosis, 8-6
Cubans; Cuban Americans. See Editor's
   Note, I-1.
Cyclospora cayetanensis, 10-11

Key to page numbering: 1-62, Understanding and Improving Health; RG-1—RG-10, Reader's Guide;
1-1—1-47, Focus Area 1. Access to Quality Health Services; 2-1—2-28, Focus Area 2. Arthritis,
Osteoporosis, and Chronic Back Conditions; and so forth. Understanding and Improving Health,
Reader's Guide, and Focus Areas 1-14 are in Volume I; Focus Areas 15-28 and the Appendices are
in Volume II.

D

Dairy products
  calcium and, 19-35
  trans-fatty acids and, 19-30
Data and information systems, 3-27,
  8-29—8-30, 17-12—17-14, 23-19
Day care facilities and vaccine coverage
  levels for children, 14-38
Deafness. *See also* Hearing.
Defibrillation, 12-11—12-12
Dementia. *See* Alzheimer's disease; Mental
  health.
Dental caries
  among children, 21-11—21-13
  early childhood caries, 21-3
  fluoride and, 21-4, 21-28
  sealants, 21-4, 21-26—21-27
  tooth extraction and, 21-17—21-18
  untreated, 21-4, 21-13—21-16
Dental examinations, diabetes and,
  5-28—5-29
Dental health. *See* Oral health.
Depression. *See also* Mental health.
  adults receiving treatment for,
    18-18—18-19
  among elderly, 18-8
  costs of, 18-19
  disabilities and, 6-10—6-12
  gender factors, 18-8
  occurrence of, 18-4—18-5
  postpartum, 16-26
Dermatitis, 20-15—20-16
Determinants of health, 18-20
Developing countries, environmental health
  and, 8-7—8-8
Developmental disabilities, among infants,
  16-38—16-39
Device errors, 17-6
Devices. *See* Medical product safety.
Diabetes—Focus Area 5
  amputations and, 5-3, 5-22—5-23
  aspirin consumption, 5-29—5-30
  cardiovascular disease and, 5-3,
    5-20—5-21
  chronic kidney disease and, 4-4—4-7,
    4-19—4-20
  complications, 5-3
  costs of, 5-4
  death rates, 5-17—5-20

dental examinations, 5-28—5-29
diabetic retinopathy, 28-13
diagnosis rates, 5-16—5-17
diet and nutrition counseling and education,
  19-42—19-44
dietary factors, 19-3
dilated eye examinations, 5-25—5-26
disparities, 5-8—5-9
education interventions, 5-12—5-13
foot examinations, 5-26—5-27
foot ulcers, 5-21
glycosylated hemoglobin screening,
  5-24—5-25
heart disease and, 12-8, 12-10
hospitalization rates, 1-27—1-29
macrovascular complications, 5-25
microalbumin screening, 5-23
microvascular complications, 5-25
overweight or obesity and, 19-5
pregnancy and, 5-21
self-blood-glucose-monitoring, 5-30—5-31
stroke and, 12-8, 12-10
transition points, 5-9
types of, 5-3, 5-13—5-16
vision disorders and, 28-4
Dialysis. *See also* Chronic kidney disease.
  arteriovenous fistula use for vascular
    access, 4-14—4-15
  health care coverage, 4-5
  limitations of, 4-4
Diarrhea, reduction in infants through
  breastfeeding, 16-47
Diet. *See* Nutrition. *See also* Obesity;
  Overweight.
Digital divide, 11-9
Digital rectal examinations (DRE), 3-18
Dilated eye examinations, diabetes and,
  5-25—5-26
Diphtheria vaccine, 14-4, 14-12
Disabilities—Focus Area 6. *See also*
  Editor's Note, I-1.
  Americans with Disabilities Act (ADA), 6-3,
    6-20—6-21
  assistive devices, 6-21
  caregivers, 6-22
  causes of, 2-4
  childhood disabilities, 16-6

Key to page numbering: 1-62, Understanding and Improving Health; RG-1—RG-10, Reader's Guide;
1-1—1-47, Focus Area 1. Access to Quality Health Services; 2-1—2-28, Focus Area 2. Arthritis,
Osteoporosis, and Chronic Back Conditions; and so forth. Understanding and Improving Health,
Reader's Guide, and Focus Areas 1-14 are in Volume I; Focus Areas 15-28 and the Appendices are
in Volume II.

*Key to page numbering: 1-62, Understanding and Improving Health; RG-1—RG-10, Reader's Guide;
1-1—1-47, Focus Area 1. Access to Quality Health Services; 2-1—2-28, Focus Area 2. Arthritis,
Osteoporosis, and Chronic Back Conditions; and so forth. Understanding and Improving Health,
Reader's Guide, and Focus Areas 1-14 are in Volume I; Focus Areas 15-28 and the Appendices are
in Volume II.*

family planning, 9-8
health instruction in schools, 7-4—7-5,
  7-14—7-16
health promotion programs for elderly
  persons, 7-25—7-26
high blood pressure control, 12-8
high school graduation rates, 7-12—7-13
nurse-to-student ratio in schools, 7-17
nutrition programs in schools, 19-6
patient and family education from health
  care organizations, 7-21—7-22
reproductive health issues for young adults,
  9-26—9-28
worksite nutrition or weight management
  programs, 19-41—19-42
worksite programs, 7-5, 7-18—7-21
Elderly persons. See Editor's Note, I-1.
adverse drug events, 17-7
Alzheimer's disease, 18-4
asthma
  deaths, 24-13—24-14
  emergency department visits,
    24-16—24-17
  hospitalization for, 24-14—24-15
calcium recommended daily intakes, 19-34
congestive heart failure hospitalization
  rates, 12-18—12-19
depression and, 18-8
health promotion activity, 7-25—7-26
heart disease and, 12-4—12-5
hip fracture, 15-39—15-40
leisure-time physical activity, 22-8—22-9
medication reviews, 17-14
mental disorders, 18-3—18-4, 18-8, 18-22
pneumococcal infections, 14-16—14-17
pneumonia or influenza, hospitalization for,
  1-27—1-29
stroke and, 12-4—12-5
tooth extraction, 21-18—21-20
vaccination, 14-45-14-49
vertebral fractures, hospitalization for, 2-18
Elevated serum creatinine, cardiovascular
  disease complications from, 4-12
Emergency contraceptive pills (ECP),
  9-17—9-18
Emergency departments (EDs), 1-5—1-6,
  1-30, 24-16—24-17
Emergency medical services (EMS). See
  Access to quality health services.

Emotional problems. See Mental health.
Emphysema, 24-8—24-9
Employer-sponsored programs
  health promotion programs, 7-18—7-21
  insurance plans, 1-15
  nutrition programs, 19-41—19-42
  weight management programs,
    19-41—19-42
Employment rates
  arthritis and, 2-14—2-15
  for people with disabilities, 6-18—6-19
End-stage renal disease (ESRD). See
  Chronic kidney disease.
Endurance, physical activity and,
  22-13—22-15, 22-17
Energy recovery, toxic pollutants from,
  8-23—8-24
Environmental health—Focus Area 8. See
  also Respiratory diseases.
air quality, 8-5, 8-9—8-10, 8-15—8-18
communities, 8-7
components of, 8-3
developing countries and, 8-7—8-8
disaster planning, 8-26
disease monitoring, 8-30
disparities, 8-10—8-11
education programs for students,
  7-14—7-16
energy recovery and, 8-23—8-24
global community, 8-7—8-10, 8-31—8-32
hazardous waste, 8-6, 8-21—8-22
homes, 8-21—8-22
indoor air quality, 8-24—8-26
information systems, 8-29
infrastructure, 8-28—8-32
lead-based paints and, 8-21—8-22,
  8-26—8-27
municipal solid waste, 8-24
pesticides and, 8-6—8-7, 8-28—8-29
substandard housing, 8-27
surveillance, 8-28—8-32
toxic substances, 8-6
urban sprawl and, 8-9
vector control programs, 8-30
water quality, 8-6, 8-18—8-20, 8-31—8-32
Environmental quality, Leading Health
  Indicator. See Understanding and
  Improving Health, pp. 40-41.

Environmental tobacco smoke (ETS), 27-24, 27-28

Epiglottitis, *Haemophilus influenzae* type b and, 14-5

Errors. *See also* Medical product safety, medication or device errors, 17-6

Escherichia coli O157:H7, foodborne illness due to, 10-8, 10-10—10-12

Estrogen replacement therapy, osteoporosis and, 2-9, 19-35

Ethanol-blended fuels, 8-17

Ethnic groups. *See* Editor's Note, I-1.

Ethnicity. *See* Editor's Note, I-1.

Exercise. *See also* Physical activity. counseling services regarding, 1-17

Externalizing disorders, 18-7

Eye examinations, diabetes and, 5-25—5-26

Eye injury. *See* Injuries and injury prevention.

F

Falls
  death rate, 15-37—15-38
  head and spinal cord injuries, 15-13
  hip fracture rates, 15-39—15-40

Families, access to health care, 1-22—1-24

Family planning—Focus Area 9. *See also* Pregnancy.
  abortions, 9-6, 9-20
  barriers to, 9-7
  consequences of unintended pregnancies, 9-5—9-6
  contraception use among adolescents, 9-23—9-26
  contraceptive use, 9-3—9-5, 9-14—9-17
  costs of, 9-7—9-8
  costs of unintended pregnancies, 9-6
  disparities, 9-6—9-7
  education for young adults on reproductive health issues, 9-26—9-28
  emergency contraception, 9-17—9-18
  health insurance coverage of contraceptive services and supplies, 9-29—9-30
  for homeless women, 9-7—9-8
  impaired fecundity, 9-28—9-29
  male involvement, 9-18—9-19
  for people with disabilities, 9-8
  proportion of adolescents engaging in sexual intercourse, 9-20—9-22

public education, 9-8
  spacing pregnancies, 9-12—9-14
  for substance abusers, 9-7
  unintended pregnancy rates, 9-3—9-4, 9-11—9-12, 9-16—9-17, 9-19—9-20

Fats, consumption of, 19-25—19-30

Fecal occult blood tests, 3-15

Females. *See* Editor's Note, I-1.

Fetal alcohol syndrome (FAS), 16-5, 16-45

Fetal mortality
  occurrence of, 16-4, 16-12—16-13
  risk factors, 16-18

Fighting. *See also* Violence prevention. among adolescents, 15-51—15-52

Firearms
  death rates, 15-14
  loaded and unlocked firearms in homes, 15-15
  nonfatal injuries, 15-15—15-16

Fires, residential, 15-6, 15-34—15-37

Fitness. *See* Physical activity.

Flexibility, physical activity and, 22-15—22-17

Fluoridated water. *See* Oral health.

Fluoride, dental caries and, 21-4, 21-28

Folic acid
  maternal levels of, 16-41—16-42
  neural tube defects and, 16-6, 19-4

Food insecurity. *See* Food security.

Food labels, nutrition information and, 19-7

Food security, 19-5, 19-44—19-46

Food safety—Focus Area 10
  allergen risk, 10-5—10-6, 10-14—10-15
  antimicrobial-resistant pathogens, 10-4, 10-13
  chemical contaminants, 10-4—10-5
  costs of foodborne illnesses, 10-3
  disparities, 10-6—10-7
  emerging pathogens, 10-4, 10-10—10-13
  environmental health and, 8-9
  foodborne death rates, 10-3
  foodborne illness rates, 10-3
  global food supply, 10-4—10-5
  naturally occurring toxins, 10-4—10-5
  parasites, 10-11—10-12
  pesticides and, 10-4—10-5, 10-16
  preparation practices and, 10-4

Key to page numbering: 1-62, Understanding and Improving Health; RG-1—RG-10, Reader's Guide; 1-1—1-47, Focus Area 1. Access to Quality Health Services; 2-1—2-28, Focus Area 2. Arthritis, Osteoporosis, and Chronic Back Conditions; and so forth. Understanding and Improving Health, Reader's Guide, and Focus Areas 1-14 are in Volume I; Focus Areas 15-28 and the Appendices are in Volume II.

retail employee training, 10-4,
10-15—10-16
storage practices and, 10-4
Foot examinations, diabetes and,
5-26—5-27
Foot ulcers, diabetes and, 5-21
Fractures
hip, 15-39—15-40
osteoporosis and, 2-7—2-8, 2-18—2-20
Fruit, consumption of, 3-6, 3-15, 12-7, 19-3,
19-6, 19-8, 19-18—19-19, 19-24—19-25

G
Galactosemia screening, 16-48
Gallbladder disease, overweight or obesity
and, 19-5
Gay men. *See* Editor's Note, I-1.
Gender. *See* Editor's Note, I-1.
Generalized anxiety disorder, adults
receiving treatment for, 18-18—18-20
Genetic counseling, developmental
disabilities and, 16-39
Genetic markers, diabetes and, 5-6
Genital herpes. *See* Sexually transmitted
diseases.
Geocoding, 23-10—23-11
Geographic information systems (GIS),
23-10—23-11
Geographic location. *See* Editor's Note, I-1.
Gestation length as cause of infant death,
16-3—16-4
Gestational diabetes, 5-21
Gingivitis, 21-21
Glaucoma, 28-4, 28-13
Global environmental health, 8-7—8-10,
8-31—8-32
Glycosylated hemoglobin, diabetes and,
5-24—5-25
Gonorrhea. *See* Sexually transmitted
diseases.
Grain products
consumption of, 19-22—19-25
folic acid fortification, 16-42
Group B *Streptococcus* (GBS)
bacterial meningitis and, 14-6
rate of new infections, 14-28—14-29
Growth retardation, low-income children and,
19-16—19-18

Gynecologic examinations, health insurance
coverage for, 1-15

H
Haemophilus influenzae type b (Hib)
bacterial meningitis and, 14-6
developmental disabilities and, 16-39
invasive diseases caused by, 14-5—14-6
vaccine, 14-4—14-6, 14-12
Hashish, disapproval of by adolescents,
26-40—26-41
Hazardous substances, 8-6
hazardous waste sites, 8-22—8-23
Head injuries
bicycle helmet use and, 15-33—15-34
hospitalization rate for, 15-11—15-12
Health behaviors, counseling services
regarding, 1-15—1-18
Health care services. See Access to quality
health services. *See also*
Community-based programs; Educational
programs; Managed care organizations.
Health care workers and needlestick injuries,
20-17—20-18
Health communication—Focus Area 11
attributes of effective communication, 11-4
audience-centered perspectives,
11-6—11-7
centers for excellence, 11-17
community-centered prevention, 11-4
digital divide, 11-9
disparities, 11-9—11-10
health literacy, 11-9, 11-15
interactive media and, 11-7—11-8,
11-13—11-17
Internet and, 11-7—11-8, 11-13—11-15
Leading Health Indicators, 11-5
mass media and, 11-7
multidimensional interventions, 11-6
national health information infrastructure,
11-10
privacy and confidentiality, 11-8
provider-patient communication, 11-8,
11-17—11-18
research and evaluation, 11-15—11-16,
11-17
targeting specific population segments,
11-6—11-7

*Key to page numbering: 1-62, Understanding and Improving Health; RG-1—RG-10, Reader's Guide;
1-1—1-47, Focus Area 1. Access to Quality Health Services; 2-1—2-28, Focus Area 2. Arthritis,
Osteoporosis, and Chronic Back Conditions; and so forth. Understanding and Improving Health,
Reader's Guide, and Focus Areas 1-14 are in Volume I; Focus Areas 15-28 and the Appendices are
in Volume II.*

Health departments, role in health education and promotion, 7-7
Health improvement plans, 23-16—23-17
Health insurance
  contraception coverage, 9-29—9-30
  coverage for nicotine dependency treatment, 27-23—27-24
  employer-sponsored plans, 1-15
  preventive services coverage, 1-15
  proportion of people with insurance, 1-6
Health literacy, 7-16, 11-9, 11-15, 21-5
Health maintenance organizations (HMO). See also Managed care organizations.
  coverage of contraceptive services and supplies, 9-30
  monitoring and reporting adverse events, 17-12—17-13
  preventive services, 1-9
Health professionals' training, 1-26, 23-14—23-15
Health status, 21-23
Health status indicators, 23-9—23-12
Health-related quality of life issues. See Quality-of-life issues.
Healthy cities, 7-3, 7-22
Healthy communities, 7-3, 7-22
Healthy People 2010 objectives
  defined, RG-2—RG-10
  short titles. See Understanding and Improving Health, pp. 53-62.
  target setting, RG-8
Hearing—Focus Area 28
  adaptive devices, 28-16
  deafness, 28-7
  disparities, 28-9
  examinations, 28-16
  otitis media and, 28-8, 28-14—28-15
  protection devices, equipment, and practices, 28-16—28-17
  referral for evaluation and treatment, 28-16
  rehabilitation services, 28-16
  screening newborns, 28-8, 28-14
Hearing aids, 28-16
Heart attacks. See Heart disease.
Heart defects, infant deaths due to, 16-15—16-16
Heart disease—Focus Area 12. See also High blood pressure; Cholesterol.
  age factors, 12-4—12-5

alcohol use, 26-4
artery-opening therapy, 12-17
atrial fibrillation, 12-5
cholesterol levels and, 12-3, 12-7, 12-9, 12-29
chronic kidney failure and, 4-11—4-12
congestive heart failure and, 12-18—12-19
death rates, 12-4, 12-6—12-17
diabetes and, 5-3, 5-20—5-21
diet and nutrition counseling and education, 19-42—19-44
dietary factors, 19-3, 19-29
disparities, 12-5—12-7
early treatment of, 12-11—12-12, 12-17
electric shock therapy, 12-17
heart attacks, 12-10—12-12, 12-17, 26-4
overweight or obesity and, 12-7, 19-5
physical activity and, 12-7, 22-3—22-4
recurrences, 12-12
saturated fatty acids and, 19-29
screening, 12-13
smoking and, 12-8, 27-4
treatment adherence difficulties, 12-12—12-13
Heavy metals, exposure to, 8-28—8-29
Height loss, vertebral fractures due to osteoporosis and, 2-20
Helicobacter pylori, 14-30
Hemodialysis. See Dialysis.
Hepatitis A virus (HAV)
  high-risk populations, 14-19
  rate of new cases, 14-18—14-19
  risk to international travelers, 14-27—14-28
  vaccine, 14-4—14-5
Hepatitis B virus (HBV)
  high-risk populations, 14-44—14-45
  HIV infection and, 13-21—13-22
  infections in children and infants, 14-12—14-13
  needlestick injuries, 20-17—20-18
  occurrence of, 14-13—14-15
  surface antigen screening, 17-4
  vaccines, 14-12, 25-29
Hepatitis C virus (HCV)
  chronically infected persons, 14-23—14-24
  needlestick injuries, 20-17—20-18
  rate of new cases, 14-22—14-23
High blood pressure
  calcium intake and, 19-35

Key to page numbering: 1-62, Understanding and Improving Health; RG-1—RG-10, Reader's Guide; 1-1—1-47, Focus Area 1. Access to Quality Health Services; 2-1—2-28, Focus Area 2. Arthritis, Osteoporosis, and Chronic Back Conditions; and so forth. Understanding and Improving Health, Reader's Guide, and Focus Areas 1-14 are in Volume I; Focus Areas 15-28 and the Appendices are in Volume II.

Page I-14   Healthy People 2010

chronic kidney disease and, 4-7
control of, 12-22—12-24
education campaign, 12-8
heart disease and, 12-12
occurrence of, 12-20—12-21
overweight or obesity and, 19-5
salt consumption and, 19-32
screening, 12-8, 12-24—12-25
stroke and, 12-4, 12-6, 12-7
High-density lipoprotein (HDL), 12-10
Hispanics or Latinos. *See* Editor's Note, I-1.
HIV (human immunodeficiency virus)—
  Focus Area 13
antiretroviral therapy, 13-6, 13-23
breastfeeding and, 16-5
condom use and, 13-8, 13-16—13-18
contraception use among adolescents and,
  9-25—9-26
counseling and testing in prison systems,
  13-19—13-20
death rates, 13-23—13-24
determinants of transmission, 13-7
disparities, 13-8—13-10
drug use and, 13-14—13-15
education programs for students,
  7-14—7-16
emergence of, 17-4
hepatitis B virus and, 13-21—13-22
interventions, 13-8
male involvement in prevention of, 9-18
needlestick injuries, 20-17—20-18
occurrence of, 13-6, 13-16
opportunities, 13-10
perinatal transmission, 13-7, 13-25
prevention education in prison systems,
  13-19
serostatus testing, 13-18
STDs and, 13-21—13-22, 25-9—25-10,
  25-23
substance abuse and, 9-7
time interval between HIV diagnosis and
  AIDS diagnosis, 13-24
treatment guidelines, 13-22—13-24
tuberculosis and, 13-20—13-21
young adult education, 9-26—9-28
zidovudine therapy, 13-7, 13-25
Home health care, 1-34
Homeless persons
family planning for, 9-7—9-8

mental disorders and, 18-14—18-15
Homes
blood lead levels and age of housing, 8-8
environmental health, 8-8
fires, 15-6, 15-34—15-35
indoor allergen levels, 8-24
lead-based paints, 8-21—8-22, 8-26—8-27
medical homes for special care needs,
  16-49—16-50
radon levels, 8-12, 8-25—8-26
smoke alarm use, 15-36—15-37
substandard housing, 8-27
Homicides
occurrence of, 15-4—15-6, 15-43—15-45
work-related, 20-5, 20-13—20-14
Hospice care, 1-34
Hospitalization rates
for ambulatory-care-sensitive conditions,
  1-27—1-29
for asthma, 24-14—24-15
for congestive heart failure, 12-18—12-19
for head injuries, nonfatal, 15-11—15-12
for peptic ulcer disease, 14-29—14-31
for spinal cord injuries, nonfatal,
  15-12—15-13
for vertebral fractures, 2-18
Hospitals
antibiotic use among intensive care unit
  patients, 14-35
emergency departments, 1-5—1-6,
  1-42—15-43, 24-16—24-17,
  26-18—26-19
infections acquired by intensive care unit
  patients, 14-34
level III, 16-29—16-30
patient and family health education,
  7-21—7-22
pediatric emergency care, 1-33—1-34
Housing. *See* Homes.
Human immunodeficiency virus. *See* HIV.
  See also AIDS.
Human papillomavirus (HPV)
cervical cancer and, 3-14
occurrence of infections, 25-20
Humped backs, vertebral fractures due to
osteoporosis and, 2-20
Hunger. *See* Food security.
Hyperlipidemia, diet and nutrition counseling
and education, 19-42—19-44

*Key to page numbering: 1-62, Understanding and Improving Health; RG-1—RG-10, Reader's Guide;
1-1—1-47, Focus Area 1. Access to Quality Health Services; 2-1—2-28, Focus Area 2. Arthritis,
Osteoporosis, and Chronic Back Conditions; and so forth. Understanding and Improving Health,
Reader's Guide, and Focus Areas 1-14 are in Volume I; Focus Areas 15-28 and the Appendices are
in Volume II.*

Index   Page I-15

Hypertension. *See* High blood pressure.
Hypothyroidism screening, 16-6, 16-48

*Key to page numbering: 1-62, Understanding and Improving Health; RG-1—RG-10, Reader's Guide;
1-1—1-47, Focus Area 1. Access to Quality Health Services; 2-1—2-28, Focus Area 2. Arthritis,
Osteoporosis, and Chronic Back Conditions; and so forth. Understanding and Improving Health,
Reader's Guide, and Focus Areas 1-14 are in Volume I; Focus Areas 15-28 and the Appendices are
in Volume II.*

falls, death rate, 15-37—15-38
firearms and, 15-14—15-16
fractures, 2-7—2-8, 2-18—2-20,
15-39—15-40
graduated driver licensing model laws,
15-32—15-33
head injuries, nonfatal, 15-11—15-12
hospital emergency department visits,
15-22—15-23
motor vehicle crash death rates, 15-3,
15-4, 15-25—15-26
motorcycle helmet use, 15-31
nonfatal motor vehicle crash injuries, 15-4
nonfatal pedestrian injuries on public roads,
15-28—15-29
pedestrian death rate, 15-26—15-27
poisonings, 15-17—15-20
programs for students, 7-14—7-16
protective gear for school-sponsored
physical activities, 15-43
residential fire death rate, 15-34—15-35
safety belt use, 15-29—15-30
spinal cord injuries, nonfatal, 15-12—15-13
suffocation, 15-20—15-21
surveillance systems, 15-21
trauma care systems, 1-32
unintentional injuries, 15-4—15-5, 15-24
unintentional injury death rate,
15-23—15-24
**Injury and Violence, Leading Health
Indicator.** See Understanding and
Improving Health, pp. 38-39.
Insulin-dependent diabetes. See Diabetes.
Insurance. See Health insurance.
Intensive care units (ICUs)
antibiotic use among patients, 14-35
hospital-acquired infections, 14-34
Intentional injuries. See Injuries and injury
prevention.
International travel, infectious diseases and,
14-27—14-28
Internet
access for public health employees, 23-9
access rates, 11-13—11-14
for health communication, 11-7—11-8,
11-13—11-17
Intrauterine growth retardation (IUGR), 16-5
Intravenous polio vaccine (IPV),
14-49—14-50

Iron deficiencies, 19-3—19-4, 19-36—19-39

J
Jail system. See also Correctional
institutions; Juvenile justice system;
Prison systems.
mental illness diversion programs, 18-20
STD screening, 25-30
Japanese Americans. See Editor's Note, I-1.
Joint symptoms, arthritis and, 2-11—2-14
Juvenile diabetes. See Diabetes.
Juvenile justice system. See also
Correctional institutions; Jail system;
Prison systems.
mental disorder screening, 18-17
STD screening, 25-30

K
Kidney disease. See Chronic kidney
disease.
Knee replacements and racial disparities,
2-15—2-16

L
Laboratories, in support of public health
services, 23-17
Latex allergies, 20-5
Latinos. See Editor's Note, I-1.
Lead
poisoning, 8-21—8-22
work exposures, 20-14—20-15
Lead-based paints, 8-21—8-22, 8-26—8-27
Leading Health Indicators
identified, See Understanding and
Improving Health, pp. 24-45.
public health infrastructure and, 23-9,
23-11—23-12
Lesbians. See Editor's Note, I-1.
Life satisfaction. See Quality-of-life issues.
Limitation in activity. See Activity limitations.
Listeria monocytogenes
bacterial meningitis and, 14-6
foodborne illness due to, 10-8,
10-10—10-11
Literacy, health communication and, 11-9,
11-15
Long-term care services, 1-6

*Key to page numbering: 1-62, Understanding and Improving Health; RG-1—RG-10, Reader's Guide;
1-1—1-47, Focus Area 1. Access to Quality Health Services; 2-1—2-28, Focus Area 2. Arthritis,
Osteoporosis, and Chronic Back Conditions; and so forth. Understanding and Improving Health,
Reader's Guide, and Focus Areas 1-14 are in Volume I; Focus Areas 15-28 and the Appendices are
in Volume II.*

Index   Page I-17

Low back pain (LBP). *See* Chronic back conditions.
Low birth weight (LBW)
  as cause of infant death, 16-3—16-4
  developmental disabilities and, 16-39
  occurrence of, 16-32—16-33
  long-term disabilities and, 16-5
  risk factors, 16-5
Low-density lipoprotein (LDL), 12-29
Lung cancer
  death rates, 3-11—3-12
  risk factors, 3-12
Lyme disease, rate of new cases, 14-21—14-22

M

Major depressive disorder, 18-19
Malaria, risk to international travelers, 14-27—14-28
Males. *See* Editor's Note, I-1.
Mammography
  barriers for people with disabilities and, 6-6—6-7
  breast cancer death reduction, 3-13
  health insurance coverage, 1-15
  Medicare coverage, 1-15
  proportion of women receiving mammograms, 3-26—3-27
Managed care organizations (MCOs). *See also* Health maintenance organizations.
  diabetes management and, 5-7
  patient and family health education, 7-21—7-22
  patient health education and promotion, 7-6
  STD treatment of nonplan patients, 25-30
Manic depressive illness, 18-4—18-5
Manufacturing process, toxic pollutants from, 8-23—8-24
Marijuana
  disapproval by adolescents, 26-40—26-41
  infant health and, 16-44—16-45
  use, 26-5, 26-26—26-27
Maternal health—Focus Area 16. *See also* Child health; Infant health.
  alcohol use and, 16-43—16-45
  cesarean birth, 16-30—16-31
  childbirth classes, 16-28—16-29
  death rate, 16-23—16-24
  disparities, 16-7—16-8

folic acid intake, 16-41—16-42
illicit drug use and, 16-43—16-45
illness and complications due to pregnancy, 16-24—16-26
intrauterine growth retardation and, 16-5
mortality causes, 16-6—16-7
prenatal care, 16-26—16-28
tobacco use and, 16-43—16-45
weight gain during pregnancy, 16-36
Measles
  occurrence of, 14-5, 14-8
  resurgence of, 14-4, 14-37
  vaccine, 14-4, 14-12
Measles, mumps, rubella vaccine (MMR), 14-4, 14-12
Medicaid
  family planning programs, 9-6—9-7
  vaccination programs for children, 14-5
Medical homes for special health care needs, 16-49—16-50
Medical product safety—Focus Area 17
  automated information systems, 17-13—17-14
  benefit-risk system, 17-3
  blood supply, 17-5, 17-16
  counseling on appropriate use and risks of medications, 17-15—17-16
  disparities, 17-7
  information technology and, 17-8
  integrated system for monitoring and reporting adverse events, 17-12—17-13
  known side effects of pharmaceuticals, 17-5—17-6
  management of risk, 17-5—17-7
  medication or device errors, 17-6
  medication reviews for elderly patients, 17-14
  prescription drug information, 17-14—17-15
  product defects, 17-5
  risk communication, 17-8—17-9
  sources of risk, 17-3—17-5
Medical schools
  preventive care training, 1-24—1-25
  proportion of degrees awarded to members of racial and ethnic groups, 1-25—1-26

Key to page numbering: 1-62, Understanding and Improving Health; RG-1—RG-10, Reader's Guide; 1-1—1-47, Focus Area 1. Access to Quality Health Services; 2-1—2-28, Focus Area 2. Arthritis, Osteoporosis, and Chronic Back Conditions; and so forth. Understanding and Improving Health, Reader's Guide, and Focus Areas 1-14 are in Volume I; Focus Areas 15-28 and the Appendices are in Volume II.

Medicare, 2-8, 6-18
  End-Stage Renal Disease Program, 4-6
  kidney disease costs, 4-5
  preventive services coverage, 1-15
Medications
  automated information systems,
    17-13—17-14
  counseling on appropriate use and risks,
    17-15—17-16
  errors, 17-4, 17-6, 17-13, 17-14
  informational materials, 17-14—17-15
  known side effects, 17-5—17-6
  medication reviews for elderly patients,
    17-14
  product defects, 17-5
Medicine. See Medications.
Melanoma, 3-7. See also Skin cancer.
  death rates, 3-18—3-19
  risk factors, 3-19
Men. See Editor's Note, I-1.
Meningitis
  bacterial, 14-6, 14-15—14-16
  developmental disabilities and, 16-39
  Haemophilus influenzae type b and,
    14-5—14-6
Meningococcal disease, rate of new cases,
  14-20
Menopause
  bone loss rate, 2-8
  counseling services, 1-16—1-18
Mental disorders. See Mental health.
Mental health—Focus Area 18
  addictive disorders and, 18-6—18-7, 18-20
  adults receiving treatment for,
    18-17—18-20
  affective disorders, 18-4—18-5
  among children, 18-7, 18-13—18-14,
    18-16—18-17
  among elderly persons, 18-3—18-4,
    18-8, 18-22
  anxiety disorders, 18-5, 18-18—18-20
  arthritis and, 2-4, 2-14
  burden of disability study, 18-3
  consumers' satisfaction with mental health
    services, 18-21
  costs of, 18-5—18-6
  crisis interventions for elderly persons,
    18-22

cultural competence of mental health plans,
    18-21
  defined, 18-3
  depression, 18-18—18-19
  disabilities and, 6-10—6-12
  disparities, 18-7—18-9
  eating disorders, 18-8, 18-15—18-16
  emotional disturbances, 18-6
  employment of persons with serious mental
    illness, 18-15
  externalizing disorders, 18-7
  homeless persons and, 18-14—18-15
  jail diversion programs, 18-20
  juvenile justice facility screening, 18-17
  occurrence of, 18-3—18-4
  percentage of people seeking treatment,
    18-5
  resilience and, 18-9
  schizophrenia, 18-4, 18-18—18-19
  screening and assessment, 18-16
  screening elderly persons, 18-22
  serious mental illness, 18-14—18-15,
    18-18—18-20
  state activities, 18-21—18-22
  stigma of, 18-9
  stress and, 18-9
  substance abuse and, 18-20
  suicide, 18-12—18-14
  treatment options, 18-5
  treatment services for elderly persons,
    18-22
Mental Health, Leading Health Indicator.
  See Understanding and Improving Health,
    pp. 36-37.
Mental illness
  defined, 18-3
  occurrence of, 18-4
Mental retardation
  among infants, 16-38—16-39
  fetal alcohol syndrome and, 16-45
Metals. See Heavy metals.
Methylene chloride, 8-17
Mexicans; Mexican Americans. See Editor's
  Note, I-1.
Microalbumin, diabetes and, 5-23
Microalbuminuria, chronic kidney disease
  risk from, 4-7
Milk, calcium and, 19-35
Monounsaturated fatty acids, 19-30

Key to page numbering: 1-62, Understanding and Improving Health; RG-1—RG-10, Reader's Guide;
1-1—1-47, Focus Area 1. Access to Quality Health Services; 2-1—2-28, Focus Area 2. Arthritis,
Osteoporosis, and Chronic Back Conditions; and so forth. Understanding and Improving Health,
Reader's Guide, and Focus Areas 1-14 are in Volume I; Focus Areas 15-28 and the Appendices are
in Volume II.

Mothers. *See* Editor's Note, I-1.
Motor vehicles
  adolescents riding with a driver drinking
    alcohol, 26-19—26-20
  alcohol use and, 26-46—26-47
  alcohol-related crashes, 15-32
  child restraint use, 15-30
  crashes due to excessive sleepiness
    caused by obstructive sleep apnea,
    24-23
  deaths due to crashes, 15-3, 15-4,
    15-25—15-26, 15-32
  emissions, 8-5, 8-16—8-17
  graduated driver licensing model laws,
    15-32—15-33
  nonfatal injuries due to crashes,
    15-27—15-28
  safety belt use, 15-29—15-30
  work-related deaths, 20-5
Motorcycles
  head injuries and, 15-13
  helmet use, 15-31
Mumps
  occurrence of, 14-5
  vaccine, 14-4, 14-12
Muscular strength, physical activity and,
  22-13—22-15, 22-17
Mycobacterium avium, 13-23
Mycobacterium tuberculosis, 13-27
Mycotoxins, 10-5
Myocardial infarctions. *See* Heart attacks.
Myopia, 28-4

N
National health information infrastructure,
  11-10
Native Americans. *See* American Indians or
  Alaska Natives; Editor's Note, I-1.
Native Hawaiians or other Pacific Islanders.
  See Editor's Note, I-1.
Nearsightedness, 28-4
Needle and syringe exchange programs,
  13-19
Needlesticks injuries, 20-17—20-18
Neisseria meningitidis
  bacterial meningitis and, 14-6
  meningococcal disease and, 14-20
Neonates
  mortality rate, 16-3, 16-13—16-15

STDs and, 25-25
Neural tube defects, 16-6, 16-40
Newborn screening programs, 16-48—16-49
Nicotine. *See also* Smoking; Tobacco use.
  dependency treatment, 27-23—27-24
Noise-induced hearing loss, 28-8,
  28-16—28-17
Nonattainment areas, 8-5, 8-10
Noninsulin-dependent diabetes. *See*
  Diabetes.
Nursing home care, 1-34
  pressure ulcer occurrence, 1-33—1-36
  regular dental visits for residents, 21-31
Nutrition—Focus Area 19. *See also*
  Obesity; Overweight.
  ABCs for health, 19-3
  anemia among low-income females in third
    trimester of pregnancy, 19-37—19-38
  away-from-home foods and, 19-7,
    19-30—19-32
  calcium deficiencies, 19-3—19-4,
    19-33—19-35
  caloric intake from fat, 12-14
  counseling services, 1-17, 19-43—19-44
  diabetes and, 5-4—5-5
  disease and, 19-3
  disparities, 19-5
  education programs for students,
    7-14—7-16
  fat consumption, 19-25—19-30
  folic acid intake, 19-4
  Food Guide Pyramid, 19-3, 19-6
  food insecurity and, 19-5, 19-44—19-46
  food label information, 19-7
  fruit consumption, 19-18—19-19,
    19-24—19-25
  grain product consumption, 19-22—19-25
  growth retardation among low-income
    children, 19-16—19-18
  heart disease and, 12-7
  iron deficiencies, 19-3—19-4,
    19-36—19-39
  proportion of adults at a healthy weight,
    19-10—19-11, 19-10—19-20
  quality of school meals and snacks, 19-40
  sodium consumption, 19-30—19-32
  stroke and, 12-7
  vegetable consumption, 19-20—19-22,
    19-24—19-25

Key to page numbering: 1-62, Understanding and Improving Health; RG-1—RG-10, Reader's Guide; 1-1—1-47, Focus Area 1. Access to Quality Health Services; 2-1—2-28, Focus Area 2. Arthritis, Osteoporosis, and Chronic Back Conditions; and so forth. Understanding and Improving Health, Reader's Guide, and Focus Areas 1-14 are in Volume I; Focus Areas 15-28 and the Appendices are in Volume II.

worksite nutrition or weight management programs, 19-41—19-42

O

Obesity. *See also* Nutrition; Overweight.
adults and, 19-11—19-13
body mass index (BMI), 19-5, 19-11, 19-15
causes of, 19-15
children and, 19-13—19-16
clinical practice guidelines, 12-10
costs of, 19-5
diabetes and, 5-4—5-5
disease risks, 19-5
heart disease and, 12-7
occurrence of, 12-14
proportion of adults at a healthy weight, 19-10—19-11
stroke and, 12-7
Obstructive sleep apnea (OSA)
disparities, 24-10—24-11
management of, 24-22
vehicular crashes due to excessive sleepiness caused by apnea, 24-23
Occupational contact dermatitis (OCD), 20-15
Occupational safety and health—Focus Area 20
assaults, 20-14
blood lead concentrations, 20-14—20-15
cost of work-related injuries, 20-3
deaths from work-related injuries, 20-6, 20-9—20-10
disparities, 20-6
eye injuries, 28-14
hearing protection, 28-16—28-17
homicides, 20-13—20-14
needlestick injuries, 20-17—20-18
overexertion injuries, 20-11—20-12
pneumoconiosis deaths, 20-12—20-13
repetitive motion injuries, 20-11—20-12
skin diseases or disorders, 20-15—20-16
stress reduction programs, 20-16—20-17
work-related injuries and illnesses, 20-3
work-related injuries resulting in medical treatment, lost time from work, or restricted work activity, 20-11
Older adults. *See* Elderly persons; Editor's Note, I-1.
Omega-3 polyunsaturated fatty acids, 19-29

Oppositional-defiant disorder, 18-7
Oral and pharyngeal cancers, 21-5, 21-22—21-25. *See also* Oropharyngeal cancer.
Oral health—Focus Area 21. *See also* Teeth.
chemotherapy and, 21-5
cleft lip and palate, 21-5, 21-34—21-35
community-based health centers with oral health component, 21-33—21-34
craniofacial health surveillance system, 21-35
dental caries, 21-3—21-4, 21-11—21-16
dental sealants, 21-4, 21-26—21-27
disparities, 21-7
long-term care residents, 21-31
oral and pharyngeal cancers, 21-5, 21-22—21-25
periodontal disease, 21-20—21-22
public dental health programs, 21-35—21-36
radiotherapy and, 21-5
regular dental visits and, 21-28—21-32
school-based health centers with oral health component, 21-32—21-33
surveillance system, 21-35
tooth extraction among elderly persons, 21-18—21-20
tooth extraction due to dental caries or periodontal disease, 21-17—21-18
water fluoridation and, 21-4, 21-28
Oral polio vaccine (OPV), 14-49
Organophosphate pesticides. *See* pesticides.
Oropharyngeal cancer. *See also* Oral and pharyngeal cancers.
death rate, 3-16—3-17
Osteoarthritis, 2-6—2-7
overweight or obesity and, 19-5
Osteopenia, 2-5
Osteoporosis—Focus Area 2
bone mineral density (BMD) and, 2-17—2-18
calcium intake and, 19-34—19-35
disparities, 2-7
estrogen replacement therapy and, 19-35
fractures and, 2-18—2-20
occurrence of, 2-18
people with disabilities and, 6-6

Key to page numbering: 1-62, Understanding and Improving Health; RG-1—RG-10, Reader's Guide; 1-1—1-47, Focus Area 1. Access to Quality Health Services; 2-1—2-28, Focus Area 2. Arthritis, Osteoporosis, and Chronic Back Conditions; and so forth. Understanding and Improving Health, Reader's Guide, and Focus Areas 1-14 are in Volume I; Focus Areas 15-28 and the Appendices are in Volume II.

Otitis media
  breastfeeding and, 16-47
  courses of antibiotics for, 14-31—14-32
  hearing disorders and, 28-8, 28-14—28-15
Overexertion injuries, 20-11—20-12
Over-the-counter drugs. *See* Medications.
Overweight—Focus Area 19. *See also*
  Nutrition; Obesity.
  among children and adolescents, 19-4,
    19-13—19-16
  assessment of, 12-10
  body mass index, 19-5
  breast cancer and, 3-13
  causes of, 19-15
  chronic back conditions and, 2-21
  clinical practice guidelines, 12-10
  coronary heart disease and, 12-7
  defined, 19-4
  diabetes and, 5-4—5-5
  disabilities and, 6-7
  disease risks, 19-5
  occurrence, 12-14
  proportion of adults at a healthy weight,
    19-10—19-11
  stroke and, 12-7
**Overweight and Obesity, Leading Health
Indicator.** *See* Understanding and
  Improving Health, pp. 28-29.
Ozone, 8-5

P

Pacific Islanders. *See* Editor's Note, I-1.
Pain, arthritis and, 2-11
Paints, lead-based, 8-21—8-22, 8-26—8-27
Panic disorder, suicide and, 18-20
Pap test
  cervical cancer death reduction, 3-14
  health insurance coverage, 1-15
  proportion of women receiving tests,
    3-23—3-24
Parasites. *See* Food safety.
Pathogens. *See* Food safety.
Pedalcycles. *See* Bicycling.
Pedestrians
  deaths on public roads, 15-26—15-27
  nonfatal injuries on public roads,
    15-28—15-29
Pelvic inflammatory disease (PID), 16-26,
  25-21—25-23

Pelvic pain, STDs and, 25-7
Penicillin-resistant infections, 14-16—14-18
Peptic ulcer disease, hospitalization rates
  for, 14-29—14-31
Perchloroethylene, 8-17
Performance-enhancing substances,
  26-35—26-37
Perinatal mortality, 16-12—16-13
Periodontal disease. *See also* Oral health.
  occurrence of, 21-20—21-22
  tobacco use and, 21-22
  tooth extraction and, 21-17—21-18
Periodontitis, diabetes and, 5-29
Personal care activities, arthritis and,
  2-12—2-14
Pertussis vaccine, 14-4, 14-12, 14-50
Pesticides
  environmental health and, 8-6—8-7, 8-23
  food safety and, 10-4—10-5, 10-16
  urine concentrations of metabolites,
    8-28—8-29
Pfiesteria piscicida, 8-6
Pharmacies
  automated information systems,
    17-13—17-14
  counseling on appropriate use and risks of
    medications, 17-15—17-16
Pharyngeal cancer. *See* Oral and
  pharyngeal cancers.
Phenylketonuria screening (PKU), 16-6,
  16-48
Physical activity—Focus Area 22
  access to school facilities outside of school
    hours, 22-25—22-26
  adolescents and, 22-17—22-25
  arthritis and, 22-3
  asthma and, 24-17—24-18
  bicycling, 22-30—22-32
  chronic obstructive pulmonary disease and,
    24-20—24-21
  coronary heart disease and, 22-3—22-4
  counseling services, 1-17
  diabetes and, 5-4—5-5
  disabilities and, 6-7
  disparities, 22-4—22-6
  education programs for students,
    7-14—7-16
  endurance and, 22-13—22-15, 22-17
  flexibility and, 22-15—22-17

*Key to page numbering: 1-62, Understanding and Improving Health; RG-1—RG-10, Reader's Guide;
1-1—1-47, Focus Area 1. Access to Quality Health Services; 2-1—2-28, Focus Area 2. Arthritis,
Osteoporosis, and Chronic Back Conditions; and so forth. Understanding and Improving Health,
Reader's Guide, and Focus Areas 1-14 are in Volume I; Focus Areas 15-28 and the Appendices are
in Volume II.*

heart disease and, 12-7
moderate physical activity, 22-9—22-11,
    22-17—22-18
muscular strength and, 22-13—22-15,
    22-17
no leisure-time physical activity, 22-8—22-9
percentage of population engaging in,
    12-14
physician counseling for cancer prevention,
    3-22
protective gear for school-sponsored
    activities, 15-43
school physical education programs, 22-5,
    22-20—22-22
stroke and, 12-7
television and, 22-23—22-25
vigorous physical activity, 22-11—22-13,
    22-19—22-20
walking, 22-27—22-29
weight status and, 19-16
worksite programs, 22-25—22-26
**Physical Activity, Leading Health
Indicator**. See Understanding and
    Improving Health, pp. 26-27.
Physical assaults, 15-51
Physical examinations and health insurance
    coverage, 1-15
Pneumococcal infections
    ear infections, 14-32
    penicillin-resistant infections, 14-16—14-18
    rate of new cases, 14-16—14-18
    vaccination rates, 14-5, 14-45—14-49
Pneumoconiosis, 20-12—20-13
Pneumocystis carinii (PCP), 13-23
Pneumonia
    Haemophilus influenzae type b and, 14-5
    hospitalization rates, 1-27—1-29
Poison control centers (PCCs), 1-31—1-32
Poisonings
    costs of, 15-20
    death rate, 15-18—15-20
    nonfatal poisonings, 15-17—15-18
Polio
    eradication, 14-37
    intravenous polio vaccine, 14-49—14-50
    oral polio vaccine, 14-49
    vaccine, 14-12
    vaccine-associated paralytic polio, 14-49
Polyunsaturated fatty acids, 19-30

Postmenopausal women and estrogen
    replacement therapy, 19-35
Postneonatal mortality, 16-14—16-15
Postpartum depression, 16-26
Poverty level. *See also* Editor's Note, I-1.
    health insurance coverage and, 1-9
    persons with source of ongoing care, 1-9
    STDs and, 25-4
Pregnancy. *See also* Contraception; Family
    planning.
    abortions, 9-6, 9-20, 16-44
    AIDS transmission, 13-7
    alcohol use, 16-5, 16-43—16-45
    anemia among low-income females in third
        trimester, 19-37—19-38
    childbirth classes, 16-28—16-29
    consequences of unintended pregnancies,
        9-5—9-6
    costs of unintended pregnancies, 9-6
    counseling services, 1-16—1-17
    ectopic, 16-6, 16-26, 25-7
    education programs for students,
        7-14—7-16
    folic acid levels, 16-41—16-42
    gestational diabetes, 5-21
    hepatitis B virus screening, 14-12—14-13
    HIV transmission, 13-4, 13-7, 13-25
    illicit drug use and, 16-43—16-45
    impaired fecundity, 9-28—9-29
    iron deficiencies, 19-38—19-39
    listeriosis risks, 10-11
    maternal illness and complications due to,
        16-24—16-26
    prenatal care, 16-26—16-28
    risk among adolescents, 9-22
    smoking cessation, 27-20—27-21
    smoking during, 16-5
    spacing pregnancies, 9-12—9-14
    STD screening, 25-30—25-31
    STDs and, 25-8
    tobacco use and, 16-43—16-45, 27-3
    toxoplasmosis risks, 10-12
    unintended pregnancy rates, 9-3—9-4,
        9-11—9-12, 9-16—9-17, 9-19—9-20
    weight gain, 16-36
Prescription drugs. *See* Medications.
Pressure ulcers, occurrence among nursing
    home residents, 1-33—1-36
Preterm births, 16-33—16-44, 16-34—16-36

---

*Key to page numbering: 1-62, Understanding and Improving Health; RG-1—RG-10, Reader's Guide;
1-1—1-47, Focus Area 1. Access to Quality Health Services; 2-1—2-28, Focus Area 2. Arthritis,
Osteoporosis, and Chronic Back Conditions; and so forth. Understanding and Improving Health,
Reader's Guide, and Focus Areas 1-14 are in Volume I; Focus Areas 15-28 and the Appendices are
in Volume II.*

Preterm infants, 16-5
Preventive care, barriers to, 1-4—1-5
Preventive services. *See* Access to quality
health services.
Primary care. *See* Access to quality health
Services.
Prison systems. *See also* Correctional
institutions; Jail system; Juvenile
justice system.
education in HIV/AIDS, STD, and TB
prevention, 13-19
HIV counseling and testing, 13-19—13-20
Privacy in health communication, 11-8
Product defects, 17-5. *See also* Medical
product safety.
Product safety. *See* Medical product safety.
Prostate cancer
death rates, 3-17—3-18
risk factors, 3-7
Prostate-specific antigen test (PSA), 3-18
Proteinuria
cardiovascular disease complications, 4-12
chronic kidney disease and, 4-20
Public dental health programs, 21-35—25-36
Public education. *See* Educational
programs.
Public health. *See* Public health
Infrastructure.
Public health infrastructure—Focus
Area 23.
continuing education for employees, 23-15
data availability, 23-11
disparities, 23-6
epidemiology services, 23-17
essential services, 23-4
evaluation of statutes, ordinances, and
bylaws, 23-18
expenditures, 23-19
functions of, 23-3
geographic information systems,
23-10—23-11
health improvement plans, 23-16—23-17
Health Status Indicators and, 23-9—23-10,
23-11—23-12
Internet access for employees, 23-9
laboratory services, 23-17
Leading Health Indicators and,
23-9—23-10, 23-11—23-12

national performance standards,
23-15—23-16
personnel competencies, 23-14
population-based prevention research,
23-20
Priority Data Needs and, 23-9—23-10,
23-11—23-12
release of data, 23-13
school curricula, 23-14
tracking objectives, 23-12—23-13
Puerto Ricans, *See* Editor's Note, I-1.
Purging. *See* Bulimia nervosa.

Q

Quality of health care. *See* Access to quality
health services.
Quality-of-life issues
arthritis and, 2-11
disabilities and, 6-16—16-17
Healthy People 2010 Goal 1. *See*
Understanding and Improving Health,
pp. 8-10.

R

Race. *See* Editor's Note, I-1.
Racial and ethnic groups. *See* Editor's Note,
I-1.
Radioactive wastes, 8-6
Radiotherapy, oral health and, 21-5
Radon in homes, 8-12, 8-25—8-26
Rape, 15-47—15-48
Rectal examinations. *See* Digital rectal
examinations.
Recycling of municipal solid waste, 8-24
Rehabilitation services
vision, 28-14
hearing, 28-16
Rehabilitative services, 1-6, 1-34—1-36
Renal replacement therapy, 4-13—4-15
Repetitive motion injuries, 20-11—20-12
Resilience, mental disorders and, 18-9
Respiratory diseases—Focus Area 24. *See
also* Asthma; Chronic obstructive
pulmonary disease (COPD);
Environmental health; Obstructive sleep
apnea (OSA)
asthma, 1-27—1-29, 8-8—8-9, 8-24
chronic obstructive pulmonary disease,
24-8—24-10, 24-20—24-22

*Key to page numbering: 1-62, Understanding and Improving Health; RG-1—RG-10, Reader's Guide;
1-1—1-47, Focus Area 1. Access to Quality Health Services; 2-1—2-28, Focus Area 2. Arthritis,
Osteoporosis, and Chronic Back Conditions; and so forth. Understanding and Improving Health,
Reader's Guide, and Focus Areas 1-14 are in Volume I; Focus Areas 15-28 and the Appendices are
in Volume II.*

environmental health and, 8-8—8-9

indoor allergen levels and, 8-24

obstructive sleep apnea, 24-10—24-11, 24-22—24-23

overweight or obesity and, 19-5

Respiratory distress syndrome, as cause of infant death, 16-3

Respiratory infections, breastfeeding and, 16-47

Responsible Sexual Behavior, Leading Health Indicator. *See* Understanding and Improving Health, pp.34-35.

Retail food industry, 10-4, 10-15—10-16

Rheumatic conditions, objectives of treatment, 2-11—2-16

Rheumatoid arthritis, 2-7

Rubella

occurrence of, 14-5

outbreaks, 14-12

vaccine, 14-4, 14-12

S

Safety belts, use of, 15-29—15-30

Salmonella serotype Enteritidis, foodborne illness due to, 10-8, 10-12

Salmonella species, foodborne illness due to, 10-8, 10-10—10-11, 10-13

Salt, consumption of, 19-32

Sanitation, water quality and, 8-31—8-32

Saturated fat, consumption of, 19-25—19-27, 19-29—19-30

Schizophrenia

adults receiving treatment for, 18-18—18-19

gender factors, 18-8

occurrence of, 18-4

Schools. *See also* Educational programs; Medical schools.

access to physical activity facilities outside of school hours, 22-25—22-26

environmental health of, 8-26

graduation rates, 7-12—7-13

health centers with oral health component, 21-32—21-34

health instruction for students, 7-4—7-5, 7-14—7-16

nurse-to-student ratio, 7-17

nutrition education, 19-6

physical education programs, 22-5, 22-20—22-22

protective gear for school-sponsored physical activities, 15-43

quality of school meals and snacks, 19-40

smoke- and tobacco-free, 27-27

vaccine coverage levels for children, 14-38

weapon carrying by adolescents on school property, 15-52—15-54

Screening tests, health insurance coverage of, 1-15

Secondary disease prevention, 1-4

diabetes and, 5-23

Secondhand smoke. *See* Environmental tobacco smoke.

Self-blood-glucose-monitoring, diabetes and, 5-30—5-31

Senior centers, health education and promotion by, 7-8

Sepsis from sickling hemoglobinopathies, 16-49

Serious emotional disturbances (SED), 18-3

Serious mental illness (SMI)

adults receiving treatment for, 18-18—18-19

employment and, 18-15

homeless persons and, 18-14—18-15

jail diversion programs, 18-20

Serum cotinine, 27-25—27-26

Serum creatinine, cardiovascular disease complications caused by elevation, 4-12

Sexual activity. *See also* Sexually transmitted diseases.

HIV and, 13-3—13-4

proportion of adolescents engaging in sexual intercourse, 9-20—9-22

television program messages, 25-29

Sexual assault, 15-48—15-50

Sexual orientation. *See* Editor's Note, I-1.

Sexually transmitted diseases—Focus Area 25

adolescent sexual behavior and, 25-25—25-29

behavioral factors, 25-4—25-7

biological factors, 25-3—25-4

cervical cancer and, 3-14

chlamydia, 16-26, 25-9, 25-15—25-16, 25-30

Key to page numbering: 1-62, Understanding and Improving Health; RG-1—RG-10, Reader's Guide; 1-1—1-47, Focus Area 1. Access to Quality Health Services; 2-1—2-28, Focus Area 2. Arthritis, Osteoporosis, and Chronic Back Conditions; and so forth. Understanding and Improving Health, Reader's Guide, and Focus Areas 1-14 are in Volume I; Focus Areas 15-28 and the Appendices are in Volume II.

Index   Page I-25

congenital syphilis, 25-24
contraception use among adolescents,
    9-25—9-26
counseling services, 1-17
disparities, 25-7—25-10
education programs for students,
    7-14—7-16
genital herpes, 25-19—25-20
gonorrhea, 16-26, 25-9, 25-16—25-17
hepatitis B vaccines, 25-29
HIV and, 13-8, 13-21—13-22, 25-9—25-10,
    25-23
human papillomavirus infection, 25-20
infertility and, 25-22—25-23
male involvement in prevention of, 9-18
management of, 25-31
neonatal consequences, 25-25
occurrence of, 25-5
pelvic inflammatory disease and, 16-26
prevention, 25-11
prevention education in prison systems,
    13-19
referral services for sex partners, 25-31
risk among adolescents, 9-22
screening during pregnancy, 25-30—25-31
screening in youth detention facilities and
    jails, 25-30
social factors, 25-4—25-7
spread of infection in a population, 25-10
syphilis, 25-9, 25-17—25-19, 25-24
television program messages concerning
    sexual behavior, 25-29
treatment of nonplan patients by managed
    care providers, 25-30
vaccines, 25-11, 25-29
young adult education, 9-26—9-28
Sickle cell disease
developmental disabilities and, 16-39
screening, 16-6, 16-48
sepsis, 16-49
Side effects
known side effects of pharmaceuticals,
    17-5—17-6
sources of risk from medical products,
    17-3—17-5
Sight impairments. See Disabilities.
Sigmoidoscopy, use in colorectal cancer
    screening, 3-15
Skin cancer. See also Melanoma.

occurrence of, 3-3
prevention, 3-7
protective measures, 3-19—3-21
Skin diseases or disorders, occupational,
    20-15—20-16
Sleep apnea, overweight or obesity and,
    19-5
Smoke alarms, 15-36—15-37
Smoking. See also Tobacco use.
adolescent cessation attempts,
    27-21—27-22
among adolescents, 27-4—27-5,
    27-12—27-14, 27-15—27-18
among adults, 27-10—27-11
cessation attempts, 27-19—27-20
cessation counseling services, 1-17
cessation during pregnancy, 27-20—27-21
chronic obstructive pulmonary disease and,
    24-8
environmental smoke exposure,
    27-24—27-28
health insurance coverage for cessation
    counseling, 1-15
heart disease and, 12-8, 12-10, 27-4
lung cancer and, 3-12
occurrence, 12-14
oropharyngeal cancer and, 3-17
Social activity participation, disabilities and,
    6-13—6-14
Social support, disabilities and, 6-14—6-15
Socioeconomic status (SES). See Editor's
    Note, I-1.
Sodium, consumption of, 19-30—19-32
Sources of ongoing care, 1-18—1-20
Special health care needs
medical homes for, 16-49—16-50
service systems for, 16-50—16-51
Spina bifida, 16-6, 16-40
Spinal cord injuries, hospitalization rate for,
    15-12—15-13
Spit tobacco. See also Tobacco use.
adolescent use, 27-6, 27-14—27-15
Steroids, use among adolescents,
    26-35—26-37
Streptococcus, Group B
bacterial meningitis and, 14-6
rate of new infections, 14-28—14-29
Streptococcus pneumoniae, bacterial
    meningitis and, 14-6

Key to page numbering: 1-62, Understanding and Improving Health; RG-1—RG-10, Reader's Guide;
1-1—1-47, Focus Area 1. Access to Quality Health Services; 2-1—2-28, Focus Area 2. Arthritis,
Osteoporosis, and Chronic Back Conditions; and so forth. Understanding and Improving Health,
Reader's Guide, and Focus Areas 1-14 are in Volume I; Focus Areas 15-28 and the Appendices are
in Volume II.

*Key to page numbering: 1-62, Understanding and Improving Health; RG-1—RG-10, Reader's Guide;
1-1—1-47, Focus Area 1. Access to Quality Health Services; 2-1—2-28, Focus Area 2. Arthritis,
Osteoporosis, and Chronic Back Conditions; and so forth. Understanding and Improving Health,
Reader's Guide, and Focus Areas 1-14 are in Volume I; Focus Areas 15-28 and the Appendices are
in Volume II.*

disparities, 27-5—27-6
education programs for students,
7-14—7-16
fetal mortality and, 16-18
infant health and, 16-5, 16-43—16-45
insurance coverage for nicotine
dependency treatment, 27-23—27-24
oral cancer and, 21-25
periodontal disease and, 21-22
physician counseling for cancer prevention,
3-22
pregnancy and, 27-3
sales to minors, 27-29
tax on tobacco products, 27-34
tobacco control laws, 27-32—27-33
toxicity monitoring and reduction, 27-33
Tobacco Use, Leading Health Indicator.
See Understanding and Improving Health,
pp. 30-31.
Toxic substances. See also Lead.
environmental health and, 8-6, 8-28—8-29
food safety and, 10-4—10-5
Toxoplasma gondii, 10-12
Trans-fatty acids, 19-29—19-30
Transfusions. See Blood transfusions.
Transplantation of kidneys, 4-3—4-7,
4-16—4-18
Trauma care systems, 1-32
Treated chronic kidney failure. See End-
stage renal disease.
Treatment, storage, and disposal facilities,
8-10
Tuberculosis (TB)
curative therapy, 14-25—14-26
detection of, 14-27
HIV testing and, 13-20—13-21
latent infections, 14-27
prevention education in prison systems,
13-19
rate of new cases, 14-24—14-25
Type 1 diabetes. See Diabetes.
Type 2 diabetes. See Diabetes.
Typhoid risk to international travelers,
14-27—14-28

U
Underground storage tanks (USTs), 8-23
Uninsured persons, 1-14
with source of ongoing care, 1-20

vaccination programs for children, 14-5
Unintended pregnancy. See Pregnancy.
Unintentional injuries. See Injuries and injury
prevention.
Universities and health instruction for
students, 7-14—7-16
Urban sprawl, 8-9
Urinary microalbumin, diabetes and, 5-23

V
Vaccine-associated paralytic polio (VAPP),
14-49
Vaccine-preventable diseases, 14-4—14-5,
14-7—14-8, 14-11—14-12, 14-37—14-40
Vaccines. See also Immunization.
conjugate vaccines, 14-5—14-6
coverage levels, 14-35—14-49
financing for, 14-5
function of, 14-3—14-4
hepatitis A virus, 14-4—14-5
measles and, 14-4
population-based registries, 14-41—14-42
safety, 14-49—14-50
vaccination rates, 14-5
Varicella vaccine, 14-4, 14-12
Vector control programs, 8-30
Vegetables, consumption of, 19-20—19-22,
19-24—19-25
Vertebral fractures, osteoporosis and,
2-18—2-20
Very low birth weight (VLBW), 16-3—16-5,
16-29—16-30, 16-32—16-33
Violence prevention—Focus Area 15. See
also Injuries and injury prevention.
alcohol-related violence, 26-20—26-21
disparities, 15-6—15-7
drug-related violence, 26-20—26-21
homicide rate, 15-43—15-45
maltreatment of children, 15-45—15-46
physical assault by current or former
intimate partners, 15-46—15-47
physical assault rate, 15-51
physical fighting among adolescents,
15-51—15-52
programs for students, 7-14—7-16
rape or attempted rape rates,
15-47—15-48
sexual assault, 15-48—15-50
STDs and, 25-6

Key to page numbering: 1-62, Understanding and Improving Health; RG-1—RG-10, Reader's Guide; 1-1—1-47, Focus Area 1. Access to Quality Health Services; 2-1—2-28, Focus Area 2. Arthritis, Osteoporosis, and Chronic Back Conditions; and so forth. Understanding and Improving Health, Reader's Guide, and Focus Areas 1-14 are in Volume I; Focus Areas 15-28 and the Appendices are in Volume II.

weapon carrying by adolescents on school
property, 15-52—15-54
Vision—Focus Area 28
adaptive devices, 28-5
cataracts, 28-14
causes of impairment, 28-5
childhood blindness or visual impairment,
28-12—28-13
costs of disorders, 28-3
diabetic retinopathy, 28-13
dilated eye examinations, 28-12
disparities, 28-6
glaucoma, 28-13
occupational eye injury, 28-14
protective eyewear, 28-14
refractive error correction, 28-12
screening for preschool children, 28-12
vision rehabilitation, 28-14
visual devices, 28-5
Vitamin D, 19-35

W
Walking
as alternative mode of transportation, 8-16
for physical activity, 22-27—22-29
Waste
environmental health and, 8-6
hazardous sites, 8-22—8-23
populations in census tracts surrounding
waste treatment, storage, and
disposal facilities, 8-10
recycling of municipal solid waste, 8-24
Water fluoridation, dental caries and, 21-4,
21-28
Water quality
beach closings, 8-20
community water system safety, 8-18
fish contamination, 8-20
global environmental hazards, 8-31—8-32
percentage of population served by private
wells, 8-18
in rivers, lakes, and estuaries, 8-19—8-20
scope of problem, 8-6
waterborne disease outbreaks, 8-18—8-19
Water supply management, 8-19
Weapons carried by adolescents on school
property, 15-52—15-54
Weight status. See also Obesity;
Overweight.

body mass index for healthy weight, 19-10,
19-15
excessive thinness risks, 19-15
physical activity and, 19-16
proportion of adults at a healthy weight,
19-10—19-11
Well-child care, health insurance coverage
for, 1-15
"Westernization," diabetes and, 5-4—5-5
Whites. See Editor's Note, I-1.
Women. See Editor's Note, I-1.
Work-related issues. See also Occupational
safety and health.
chronic back conditions, 2-21
health promotion programs, 7-5,
7-18—7-21
HIV infection, 13-10
lost productivity due to alcohol and drug
use, 26-21
lung cancer and, 3-12
nutrition programs, 19-41—19-42
smoking policies, 27-27
weight management programs,
19-41—19-42
worksite physical activity programs,
22-25—22-26
World Wide Web. See Internet.

Y
Years of potential life lost (YPLL), injuries
and, 15-4, 15-6
Young adults. See Editor's Note, I-1.
AIDS, new cases of, 13-9
binge drinking, 26-29—26-33
chlamydia screening, 25-30
death rates, 16-21—16-23
education of reproductive health issues,
9-26—9-28
graduated driver licensing model laws,
15-32—15-33
occurrence of death due to injuries, 15-4
Youth. See Editor's Note, I-1.

Z
Zidovudine therapy, 13-7, 13-25

---

*Key to page numbering: 1-62, Understanding and Improving Health; RG-1—RG-10, Reader's Guide;
1-1—1-47, Focus Area 1. Access to Quality Health Services; 2-1—2-28, Focus Area 2. Arthritis,
Osteoporosis, and Chronic Back Conditions; and so forth. Understanding and Improving Health,
Reader's Guide, and Focus Areas 1-14 are in Volume I; Focus Areas 15-28 and the Appendices are
in Volume II.*

Order Form

Name: _____

Address: _____

City, State, Zip: _____

Daytime phone: _____

Email: _____

☐ Personal check

☐ Credit Card ☐ VISA ☐ Mastercard ☐ American Express ☐ Discover
(check one)

Card Number: _____

Expiration: _____ Signature: _____

Title	ISBN	Price	Quantity	Subtotal
Healthy People 2010 **two volume set**	1-883205-75-1 1-883205-78-6	$75.00	_____	_____
U.S. Department of Health and Human Services				
Healthy People 2010-2nd Edition **paperback, one combined volume**	1-58808-110-9	$49.50	_____	_____
Clinician's Handbook of Preventive **Services, 2nd edition**	1-883205-32-8	$20.00	_____	_____
U.S. Public Health Service				
Guide to Clinical Preventive Services, **2nd & 3rd editions**	1-883205-13-1	$24.00	_____	_____
United States Preventive Services Task Force				

Subtotal _____

Shipping and Handling $7.50 per 2010 _____

hard cover set of two volumes _____

Other titles: S&H $4.00 each _____

Total _____

Please include 5.75% sales tax for orders from the District of Columbia.

Send your order to: Reiter's Scientific & Professional Books
2021 K Street, N.W.
Washington, D.C. 20006

Information: 800-591-2713   Fax: 202-296-9103   E-mail: books@reiters.com

Order Form

Name: _____

Address: _____

City, State, Zip: _____

Daytime phone: _____

Email: _____

☐ Personal check

☐ Credit Card   ☐ VISA ☐ Mastercard ☐ American Express ☐ Discover
   (check one)

Card Number: _____

Expiration: _____ Signature: _____

Title	ISBN	Price	Quantity	Subtotal

Healthy People 2010
   two volume set
U.S. Department of Health and
   Human Services
	1-883205-75-1
	1-883205-78-6
		$75.00	_____	_____

Healthy People 2010-2nd Edition **paperback, one combined volume**	1-58808-110-9	$49.50	_____	_____
Clinician's Handbook of Preventive **Services, 2nd edition** U.S. Public Health Service	1-883205-32-8	$20.00	_____	_____
Guide to Clinical Preventive Services, **2nd & 3rd editions** United States Preventive Services Task Force	1-883205-13-1	$24.00	_____	_____

Subtotal _____

Shipping and Handling $7.50 per 2010 _____

hard cover set of two volumes _____

Other titles: S&H $4.00 each _____

Total _____

Please include 5.75% sales tax for orders from the District of Columbia.

Send your order to: Reiter's Scientific & Professional Books
2021 K Street, N.W.
Washington, D.C. 20006

Information: 800-591-2713 Fax: 202-296-9103 E-mail: books@reiters.com